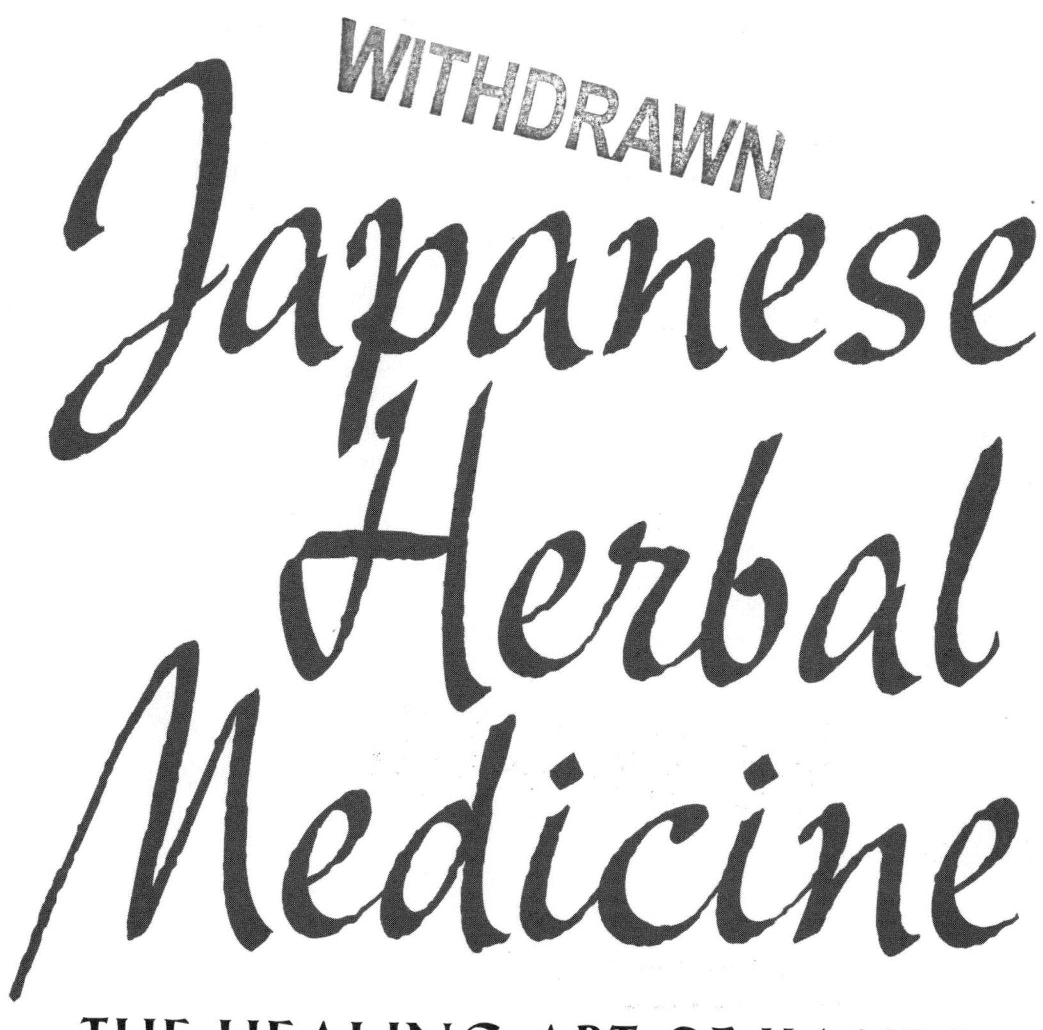

THE HEALING ART OF KAMPO

Robert Rister

AVERY PUBLISHING GROUP
Garden City Park • New York

The therapeutic procedures in this book are based on the training, personal experiences, and research of the author. Because each person and situation is unique, the author and publisher urge the reader to check with a qualified health professional before using any procedure where there is any question to appropriateness when there is any question regarding the presence or treatment of any abnormal health condition.

The publisher does not advocate the use of any particular diet or treatment, but believes the information presented in this book should be available to the public.

Because there is always some risk involved, the author and publisher are not responsible for any adverse effects or consequences resulting from the use of any of the suggestions, preparations, or procedures described in this book. Please do not use the book if you are unwilling to assume the risk. Feel free to consult with a physician or other qualified health professional. It is a sign of wisdom, not cowardice, to seek a second or third opinion.

Cover design: Doug Brooks and William Gonzalez
Typesetters: Gary A. Rosenberg & Liz Johnson
In-house editor: Lisa James

Avery Publishing Group, Inc.
120 Old Broadway
Garden City Park, New York 11040
1-800-548-5757
www.averypublishing.com

Cataloging-in-Publication Data

Rister, Robert.
Japanese herbal medicine : the healing art of kampo / by Robert Rister.
p. cm.
Includes bibliographical references and index.
ISBN 0-89529-836-8
1. Herbs—Therapeutic use—Japan. I. Title.
RM666.H33 R57 1999
615'.321'0952—dd21
98-53401
CIP

Printed in the United States of America

10 9 8 7 6 5 4 3 2 1

Contents

Acknowledgments, vii
Preface, ix
How to Use This Book, xi

Introduction, 1

PART ONE Understanding Kampo

Chapter 1 What Is Kampo?, 5
Chapter 2 Buying and Using Kampo Herbs, 13
Chapter 3 The Medicines of Kampo, 17
Chapter 4 The Formulas of Kampo, 109

PART TWO Disorders Treated With Kampo

Acne, 143
AIDS, 143
Alcoholism, 145
Allergies, Food, 146
Allergies, Respiratory, 147
Alzheimer's Disease, 149
Anemia, 150
Angina, 151
Anxiety, 152
Asthma, 154
Atherosclerosis, 157
Attention Deficit Disorder/Attention Deficit Hyperactivity Disorder (ADD/ADHD), 158

Bedwetting, Children's, 160
Bladder Cancer, 161
Bladder Infection (Cystitis), 163
Bleeding Gums, 164
Boils, 165
Bone Cancer, 166
Breast Cancer, 168
Bronchitis and Pneumonia, 171
Burns, 173

Cancer, 174
Cataracts, 175
Cervical Cancer, 176
Chemotherapy Side Effects, 178
Chronic Fatigue Syndrome, 181
Cirrhosis, Alcoholic, 183
Colds, 184
Colorectal Cancer, 186
Congestive Heart Failure, 189
Conjunctivitis, 191
Constipation, 192

Depression, 194
Diabetes, 196
Diabetic Retinopathy, 200
Diarrhea, 201

Ear Infections, 203
Eczema, 205
Endometrial Cancer, 207
Endometriosis, 208
Eye Disorders, 210
  Bags Beneath the Eyes, 210
  Bloodshot Eyes, 210
  Blurred Vision, 211
  Floaters, 211

Fibrocystic Breast Disease, 212
Fibroids (Uterine Myomas), 214

Gallstones, 216
Gastritis, 217
Glaucoma, 218

Hair Loss, 219
Hangover, 220
Headaches, 221
Hemorrhoids, 222
Hepatitis, 223
Herpes, 225
High Blood Pressure (Hypertension), 226
High Cholesterol, 229
HIV Infection, 231
Hodgkin's Disease, 233
Hyperthyroidism, 234
Hypothyroidism, 235

Impotence, 236
Incontinence, 237
Indigestion, 238
    Belching, 238
    Bloating and Flatulence, 239
    Heartburn, 239
    Hiccups, 240
Infertility, Female, 240
Infertility, Male, 241
Influenza, 242
Insomnia, 243
Irritable Bowel Syndrome, 244

Kidney Cancer (Renal Cell Carcinoma), 245
Kidney Disease, 247
Kidney Stones, 248

Leukemia, 249
Liver Cancer, 251
Lung Cancer, 253
Lupus, 254

Macular Degeneration, 256
Mastitis, 257
Measles, 258
Melanoma, 259
Memory Problems, 260
Ménière's Disease, 262
Menopause-Related Problems, 263
Menstrual Problems, 265
Migraine, 267
Multiple Sclerosis, 268
Mumps, 269

Nosebleed, 270

Obesity, 270
Osteoarthritis, 272
Ovarian Cancer, 273
Ovarian Cysts, 274

Pelvic Inflammatory Disease, 275
Peptic Ulcer, 276
Premenstrual Syndrome (PMS), 278
Prostate Cancer, 279
Prostate Enlargement, Benign, 280
Psoriasis, 281

Radiation Therapy Side Effects, 282
Rheumatoid Arthritis, 283

Seizure Disorders, 285
Sinusitis, 286
Skin Cancer (Basal Cell Carcinoma), 287
Stomach Cancer, 288
Strep Throat, 289
Stress, 290
Stroke, 291

Tinnitus (Ringing in the Ears), 292
Tuberculosis, 293

Yeast Infections, 294

Appendices

Appendix A Sources of Kampo Services and Products, 299
Appendix B Identifying Japanese Medicinal Herbs, 309
Appendix C Glossary, 326

References, 333
Index, 399

To my father,
whose life is evidence
of the power of faith and medicine
together to heal.

Acknowledgments

Kampo is an art traditionally passed from master to student. I am indebted to my teachers, Drs. Helmut Bacowsky and Michiko Okita. Through years of instruction, they taught me from their practice of traditional Japanese healing arts combined with modern clinical practice and scientific research. Although any shortcomings in this book are solely attributable to me, any strengths in this book are to be credited to Drs. Bacowsky and Okita.

The writing of this book would not have been possible without the help of many people. Tsumura and Company of Tokyo provided copies of Japanese technical journals I used in researching this book. Georg Treipl provided some of the European texts also consulted in writing this book. Linguist and teacher Tommi Urbanski edited an early version of this book and supported my attempts to communicate in her native language, Japanese. Dr. Helmut Wiedenfeld and Dr. Shannon Mar offered helpful information about the pharmacology of Japanese herbs. Laurie Radford and Dr. Albert Radford helped me with the botanical identification and nomenclature of the herbs. Dr. Jim Duke gave helpful advice concerning the planning of the book. Kampo physicians Drs. Gouen Wang, Qian Zhi Wu, and Gary Stier provided indispensable background information on Kampo as a healing art. I also acknowledge the constructive criticisms of Drs. Subhuti Dharmananda and Bill Egloff, and the help of Julie Joe, Daniel Steinhauser, Kramer Wetzel, Donald McLachlan, and Sanoma Ruffino.

The writing of this book also would not have been possible without the patient support of Avery Publishing Group. Editor Lisa James conquered the formidable task of fact-checking and cross-indexing every entry in this book. She also asked me hundreds of pertinent questions clarifying the text. Her suggestions formed the basis for writing many explanatory passages throughout this book.

I am especially grateful to publisher Rudy Shur, who initially approached me with the idea of writing this book. He then took on the task of teaching me to write in simple language without sacrificing adherence to strict principles of scientific documentation. When the project took longer than either of us expected, he extended the resources and support of Avery to the completion of this book.

Preface

This book is about one of the world's great systems of natural medicine. The Japanese system of herbalism, Kampo, is a unique healing tradition designed not only to treat disease but to return people to health. Kampo aims to go beyond defeating disease, to create a *greater* state of stamina and vigor than the person experienced before illness.

The curative art of Kampo combines herbs to relieve carefully defined patterns of symptoms, and then to recreate the healthful conditions of balance that existed in body, mind, and spirit before disease struck. Kampo herbs give the person the exact energy he or she needs to return to the fundamentally sound, vibrant, and robust state of health people were created to enjoy. Kampo is an ancient system, faithful to herbal formulas used for centuries throughout the Orient, but also a modern system, withstanding the scrutiny of cutting-edge scientific technique. Most importantly, Kampo is a person-oriented system. It is a Japanese adaptation and refinement of ancient Oriental healing practices designed to give the greatest benefit in the simplest form to the greatest number of people. Kampo can be used both in clinical practice and personal health maintenance, and can be used within the context of conventional Western medicine.

I first became aware of the healing art of Kampo on a trip not to Japan but to the Philippine island of Luzon in 1984. My schedule had not offered many sightseeing opportunities, so on one long weekend my hosts, Rogelio and Nora Bandala, and their daughter Naomi, took me to the remote Mountain Province to see the famed rice terraces of Banaue. Arriving just before nightfall, we had allowed ourselves barely enough time to take in the vista before retreating to a hostel. We made plans for the next day, but our schemes were not to be.

Even though it was the island's "dry" season, during the night unimaginable torrents of tropical rain and typhoon-force winds lashed Banaue. When we ventured out the next morning, all the roads out of town were inundated by mud. A quick call to Manila revealed that both my hosts and I would be in serious trouble with our respective employers if we didn't reach the capital city in three days. We decided to walk across the safest sections of the mudslides to try to hitch a ride to Manila. An Austrian tourist, Dr. Helmut Bacowsky, joined us. Dr. Bacowsky was a physician and medical school professor who had just launched a career researching Kampo.

In just a few kilometers we had kicked the mud off our boots and reached a jeepney, a decorated, open-air taxi. Nora and Naomi rode inside while Rogelio, Helmut, and I took turns clinging to the outside of a succession of jeepneys until we reached a bus terminal. From the terminal we rode a 1940s-vintage bus into Manila.

On that ride, Dr. Bacowsky and I began a ten-year conversation about Kampo. Through a decade of correspondence, calls, and visits, Helmut generated an infectious enthusiasm for natural medicine in general and Japanese herbalism in particular. For years, Dr. Bacowsky and his wife, Dr. Michiko Okita, sent me books in German (a language I didn't read in 1984) on herbalism and electromagnetic fields, original research articles in a number of languages about vitamins and natural supplements, and notes in Japanese (another language I didn't read in 1984) about Kampo. In reading these dozens of studies, I found many that were logically ill-founded, but many more that were based on the best scientific standards. As I slowly breached the language gap, my interest in Kampo grew, but I wasn't sufficiently interested in the field to make it my full-time vocation until 1994.

Two events made 1994 a watershed year for my interest in Kampo. Although I had been plagued by migraine headaches all of my adult life, that year migraines became for me not monthly but weekly events. With each migraine I temporarily lost the ability to speak. My normal vision was replaced by a falling curtain of kaleidoscopic colors and patterns. I did what my HMO told me to do and went to see their neurologist. Before my neurologist was able to schedule a full battery of tests, she prescribed a drug that required weekly blood tests to monitor its toxicity.

Prior to 1994, I was overweight, but I hadn't gained a pound in almost ten years. After I started the medication, even ten miles of daily biking and a rigorously vegetarian diet failed to keep my weight from ballooning by sixty pounds. Already balding, I found that almost all of my hair fell out. I developed drug-induced hepatitis. Having had no signs of diabetes in years of annual physicals, I developed severe hyperglycemia. I was hungry and thirsty twenty-four hours a day.

Even worse, I discovered that the medication I was given for migraines could have an especially undesirable side effect—increasing the frequency and severity of migraines. Weekly migraines became daily migraines. Migraines that lasted minutes became migraines that lasted hours.

Before the months of medical testing were complete, I had to quit my job, sell my assets, and give up my daily exercise routine. When all the tests were finally done, I went to see my neurologist. To my utter astonishment, the doctor told me she had uncovered no cause for my disease. Naturally, I asked her what basis she had then for continuing to prescribe the health-wrecking medication. She replied that I had no choice but to continue her prescription at an increased dosage, and added in an off-handed way, "We will confirm my diagnosis on your autopsy."

At this point I decided it was time I tried Kampo for myself. My first step was to find another neurologist who would supervise my withdrawal from the medications that were doing me harm. Then I needed to locate a Kampo practitioner to make another diagnosis and give me the herbs I hoped would remedy my situation.

The first office visit with my Kampo physician took about two hours. After probing my lifestyle and health history for indications of yin and yang, hot and cold, excess and deficiency, and superficial and interior complaints, the doctor went into his herb room. I could hear grinding and hacking, cutting and stirring. About fifteen minutes later I was presented with six bags of mixed herbs. The doctor gave me instructions on how to brew the herbs and sent me home.

For four years, I did not have another migraine nor any other form of headache. Nor did I experience any of the other symptoms that accompanied the attacks. However, my blood-sugar levels remained dangerously high, despite trying more than two dozen treatment regimens that included combinations of insulin with various prescription and herbal medicines. Finally, a prescription drug called Rezulin worked, but caused signs of serious liver damage. I needed the medicine to control the diabetes, and so turned again to Kampo for an answer. My Kampo practitioner found a formula that controlled Rezulin's side effects.

Since starting to use Kampo myself, I have devoted my professional energies to writing scientifically conscientious books about natural medicines. I have had a part in translating and editing an herbal reference guide for physicians and manufacturers of plant medicines, and I have written a book and articles about nutritional supplements. Kampo, however, is the form of natural medicine I use myself.

This book is based not only on the historical records of Japanese herbal medicine but also on over 1,000 contemporary scientific studies conducted in Japan, the United States, China, and Europe. Just as I required years of information to adopt Kampo for my personal use, the Japanese medical establishment required several decades of scientific testing to re-adopt Kampo for clinical use. Kampo involves not only ancient discoveries, but also recent discoveries. Conversely, even though Kampo formulas can be understood chemically, they also can be understood intuitively. Every Kampo formula has been proven effective in restoring health to hundreds of millions of people throughout Japan, China, and the rest of East Asia. Every Kampo formula has been used successfully for hundreds—and in most cases, thousands—of years. Furthermore, every Kampo formula has been subjected to at least preliminary scientific testing. Almost all of the individual Kampo herbs have also been subjected to rigorous testing.

In the first part of this book, I explain the Oriental system of medicine from which Kampo was born. I then discuss how to buy and use herbal medicines, and describe the Kampo herbs and formulas used in this book. In the second part, I recommend specific herbs and formulas for a number of disorders. I also provide information on how to find Kampo medicines and practitioners, and some scientific background on the herbs used.

Telling you what you need to know to enjoy the healing art of Kampo is why I have written this book. I want to thank you for choosing to read my work. I hope to make understanding this centuries-old healing system a little easier for you. And I hope that Kampo will be for you, as it has been for millions of others and myself, not just the treatment for disease but an avenue to better health than you have ever known before.

How to Use This Book

This book is a comprehensive guide for the layperson seeking to use Kampo, a Japanese healing system that relieves disease as it brings the whole person to a greater state of health. The subject of extensive scientific research, Kampo can be used in the context of disease treatment as understood by conventional Western medicine. At the same time, every herb and herbal formula Kampo uses is faithful to the writings of the ancient sages in Japan and China, and can be completely explained in terms of traditional Oriental medicine. Kampo can treat short- and long-term illnesses that threaten comfort, health, or life itself. This book has been designed to be an easy-to-use reference to Kampo's herbal remedies.

While not every remedy in this book will work for every person, every person can find a remedy within Kampo. Kampo's choice of remedy is matched to the complete pattern of one's physical, emotional, and even spiritual symptoms. The basic unit of treatment is not the herb, but the herbal formula. Herbs are combined into formulas to heal complex patterns of disease symptoms. These fixed combinations act as a single unit, creating a harmony of effects that corrects the entire range of symptoms. However, herbs can be used singly. When some symptoms are controlled by other means—including massage, meditation, nutrition, spiritual discipline, or Western medicine—individual herbs may be all that is needed to round out a treatment plan.

This book offers explanations that provide the most concise means of choosing among treatments. It will often be simple to match the symptoms of minor complaints and short-term illnesses to the applicable Kampo remedy, and one's own self-assessment of the condition can be verified with a doctor. But for serious illnesses and chronic conditions a health care professional should always be consulted.

This book is divided into two parts. In Part One, Chapter 1 discusses how the Japanese simplified and updated China's traditional medicine into the system now known as Kampo. This chapter discusses the concepts and principles found in Oriental medicine, and how Kampo is compatible with both the experimental rigor of scientific medicine and with the wealth of experience found in Oriental medicine. Chapter 2 provides information on buying and using medicinal herbs, including where they can be found and what forms are available. Chapter 3 describes the Japanese medicinal herbs used in this book. Each entry gives a description of the herb, how it is viewed in terms of both Kampo and conventional Western medicine, and notes on how the herb should be used, including tea-making directions where applicable. Chapter 4 is a guide to the Kampo formulas used in this book. Each entry explains both how the formula is used in traditional Kampo and how it is used to treat the health conditions Westerners are familiar with, along with the formula's ingredients and a brief summary of scientific research.

Part Two is an alphabetical listing of the health conditions that are treatable with Kampo. Each entry contains a brief discussion of the condition in mainstream medical terms, so the diagnosis made by one's physician can be matched with its corresponding Kampo diagnosis. The entry then describes how Kampo views the condition before giving the treatment options, including both individual herbs and formulas, that Kampo has to offer.

Almost all of the conditions listed in Part Two respond to treatment with single herbs. All of these conditions also respond to Kampo formulas. Whether one chooses to use Japanese medicinal herbs singly or in formulas, Part Two will state what to expect from Kampo treatment. In general, individual herbs are used when the condition is almost under control except for one or two prominent symptoms, and formulas are used if there is a chronic condition or multiple symptoms exist. Should there be any question regarding what therapies to use, consult both a medical doctor and a Kampo or TCM practitioner.

An important point to remember is that herbal remedies take longer to work than regular over-the-counter or prescription remedies. The herbs and formulas in Kampo are especially gentle. Bringing the whole body back into balance, especially in someone who is suffering a long-term imbalance, will not be an instant process. Herbs should be effective within three to four weeks, while formulas should show results within three to four months. Exceptions to these guidelines are given in Part Two where applicable.

This book also includes appendices giving sources of Kampo products and information on how to identify the herbs used, including a glossary for easy reference. In addition, technical references are given to document the information contained in this book.

This book is not a manual for self-diagnosis. Any attempt to diagnose or treat an illness requires the direction of a physician. If it is difficult to find a Kampo practitioner in any specific region, refer to Appendix A.

Introduction

We tend to think of medicine in terms of disease—diagnose the disorder, then prescribe the appropriate drug. But what if there were medicines designed not for diseases but for people?

There are. Kampo, a traditional Japanese system of herbalism, is a person-centered form of medicine that consists of several hundred formulas, each of which has been matched over hundreds of years to a precise set of symptoms. Symptoms in Kampo refer not to a particular disease but to the person's overall state of health, known as one's *sho*. Diagnosis in Kampo does not just describe part of the individual's experience of health captured as a disease, but instead characterizes the individual's entire physical, mental, social, and emotional condition. This is done through a system of observations that are stated in terms of opposites—heat and cold, for example.

For each *sho*, Kampo offers a precise herbal formula to bring the health of the whole individual back into balance. Many different medically defined diseases can result in the same set of symptoms, and the same medically defined disease can result in many different sets of symptoms. But in Kampo, matching herbal treatment to the one diagnostic *sho* describing the person almost always restores balance and health. In addition, many of the individual herbs that go into the formulas are also employed by themselves.

One of Kampo's greatest advantages is its power to heal gently, without causing serious side effects. Medications can cause toxic reactions, when dosage is miscalculated; allergic reactions, when the person is sensitive; damage to a developing fetus; and abnormal cell growth. Medications can also have paradoxical effects, worsening the conditions they are designed to treat. Long-term use of some prescription drugs can result in drug dependence and addiction.

The side effects of drugs are not only known to exist, they are considered acceptable. A standard pharmacy textbook asserts, "If a drug is claimed to have no side effects, then there is a strong suspicion that it also has no significant benefit." The standard definition of a safe drug is a drug for which serious side effects are unlikely and for which the risk-benefit ratio is acceptable. The standard way to deal with side effects is, of course, to offer additional medication. While only a small percentage of people will experience side effects, this is of little comfort to you if you happen to be one of those people.

Kampo employs combinations of minimally processed herbs. Unlike a standard medication that consists of one or occasionally two active chemical compounds plus carrier compounds and a buffer, Kampo formulas utilize combinations of whole herbs that contain dozens, and in many cases, hundreds, of active ingredients. The advantage of these formulas is that the many different active ingredients act on the body, and on each other, simultaneously. This serves both to make the primary ingredients more effective and to prevent the toxic reactions that lead to side effects. As a result, bodily imbalances are corrected without creating additional problems. Some individual herbs themselves can have side effects, but these, in general, pose less of a potential problem than their synthetic counterparts.

Kampo comes from a healing tradition with roots in ancient China. For those familiar with Traditional Chinese Medicine (TCM), Kampo formulas all have their historical sources in the ancient Chinese texts, and the choices of herbs can be explained in terms of the Five Elements theory (see Chapter 1). Kampo formulas can also be understood in terms of their interaction with acupuncture, although Kampo does not require the use of acupuncture.

The language used in traditional Oriental medicine sounds "unscientific" to Western ears. However, every Kampo formula listed in this book has been validated in clinical and laboratory studies. The individual herbs have been thoroughly studied from the standpoints of botany, chemistry, and pharmacology. Since 1945, Japanese physicians have systematically harmonized the traditional *sho* with definitions of disease taken from modern medicine. Indeed, one of Kampo's strengths is that it can be used along with Western medicines to good effect.

As a result of the work done in Japan, Kampo has been used in the treatment of hundreds of medically defined conditions—most of which were not even known when the formulas were invented. For example, hay fever was unknown in Japan until 1950. Nonetheless, a Kampo formula invented in the second century A.D., Minor Bupleurum Decoction, offers effective relief from the watery eyes, runny nose, sneezes, and sniffles associated with exposure to airborne pollens.

Another ancient formula, Kudzu Decoction, is useful in treating herpes infections. Herpes can produce an initial outbreak and then remain dormant in nerve tissues for many years before reactivating itself under certain conditions, such as when the body's overall resistance is weakened. Modern medicine tries either to kill or deactivate the virus, or to regulate the process of inflammation with steroids. Both approaches can result in side effects. However, researchers at Japan's Toyama University have found that use of Kudzu Decoction offers a third approach, that of blocking the reactivated virus's ability to destroy cells. While this approach does not kill the virus, it also does not harm the patient, and it does control the infection.

This book is designed to provide a layperson's guide to Kampo. Part One discusses Oriental medicine terminology, how to buy and use Kampo herbs, and a number of herbs and formulas readily available in North America. Part Two shows how these herbs and formulas can be used to treat a host of specific disorders. The appendices provide information on finding Kampo practitioners and products, background information on the herbs, and a glossary.

Despite the fact that Kampo can be readily used with conventional medicine, this ancient system of herbal healing was designed to treat not diseases, but people. The future may bring new bacteria, new viruses, and new threats to health. But the gift of Kampo lies in its ageless ability to improve the condition of the whole person, and it can help anyone achieve a better state of health than he or she has ever experienced before.

Part One

Understanding Kampo

Kampo is a unique, ancient system of herbal medicine that has been reborn in modern Japan. Kampo is the synthesis of Eastern and Western healing traditions, equally understandable in terms of anatomy, chemistry, and physiology as it is in terms of vital energy, energy channels, and symbolic organ systems. Kampo is a person-oriented system that prescribes herbs and herbal combinations to address specific symptoms and symptom patterns.

Kampo differs from other Oriental healing traditions in several important ways. Many approaches to Oriental medicine demand total commitment to a way of thinking about the human body that is completely foreign to Westerners, a mode of thought that requires letting go of scientific concepts about anatomy, physiology, sickness, and health. Other approaches put the responsibility for healthy living solely on the individual, in which illness is a consequence of a personal failure of attitude, willpower, or self-control. In addition to these philosophical problems, the use of Oriental medicine is frequently accompanied by pain. This pain accompanies moxibustion, or the application of burning herbs, and some types of thick-needle acupuncture.

None of these problems exist in Kampo. Over the course of 1,200 years, the masters of Japanese herbalism simplified the principles of Oriental medicine to four basic patterns used to describe any disease: yin and yang, hot and cold, excess and deficiency, interior and exterior. These four patterns can be confirmed in terms of balances of energy (qi), blood, and fluids.

Different diseases, as they are understood in Western medicine, can produce the same symptom patterns in different people, while the same disease can produce different symptom patterns in different people. For every combination of imbalances in the four basic patterns, Kampo has a precise formulation of herbs to bring the person back into balance. A Kampo formula is tailored to the patient, not the disease, and each formula is designed not just to relieve symptoms but to bring the whole person back to health. Kampo considers both physical and emotional conditions to be a reflection of balance in the four basic patterns. Therefore, no imbalance is the result of a failure of self-discipline or "bad attitude."

Kampo medicine is oral medicine. To benefit from Kampo, one need only to take herbal teas or easy-to-use pills, powders, and tonics. Although Kampo is faithful to the ancient formulas of Chinese medicine and can be used knowledgeably with either acupuncture, moxibustion, or therapeutic massage, no other technique is required to enhance Kampo's healing effects. Kampo itself is pain-free.

Every Kampo formula is exactly the same combination of herbs devised by a venerated master herbalist in Chinese, Japanese, or Korean history. Only one combination of herbs listed in this book has been in use for less than 200 years. On the other hand, while this system of medicine contains almost exclusively ancient formulas, it does not include every ancient formula. Kampo formulas are treatments proven over hundreds, and most cases thousands, of years.

Furthermore, every Kampo formula is also validated in terms of scientific medicine. The pioneering work done by the twentieth-century Japanese physician Keisetsu Otsuka linked the four basic patterns associated with Kampo herbs to hundreds of diseases recognized in scientifically defined medicine. The research he started continues today. This work means that Kampo herbs and formulas can be applied to diseases as the West conceives them.

Chapter 1 discusses the history and theory of Kampo. Those already familiar with Oriental medicine will see how Kampo is completely faithful to Traditional Chinese Medicine and its variations practiced in Japan and Korea. For those who are not familiar with Oriental medicine, this chapter will provide a new framework for understanding health and herbalism. Chapter 2 will explain how to buy and use Kampo herbs and herbal products. Chapter 3 will provide descriptions of the Kampo herbs used in this book, including both the traditional ways in which these herbs have been used and the scientific research that confirms their healing powers. Chapter 4 provides the same information for Kampo formulas.

CHAPTER 1

What Is Kampo?

The word *Kampo* is the Japanese pronunciation for a combination of two Chinese characters: *Kan,* or *Han,* which means "from China," and *po,* or *ho,* which means "way." This chapter will discuss how the Chinese way of herbal treatment that eventually became Kampo rests on the work done in the second century A.D. by the revered herbalist Zhang Zhongjing. By Zhang's time, Oriental medicine was already 3,000 years old, and herbalism continued to evolve in both China and Japan as time progressed.

After looking at the history of Kampo, this chapter will explain the theories behind this ancient system of medicine, theories tied into an Oriental approach to medicine much different from that of conventional medicine in the modern West. Western medicine is a disease-based system, in which doctors look for definitive causes of illness. On the other hand, Oriental medicine is a patient-based system, in which doctors look for recognized patterns of disharmony. Despite their differences, these two systems can be used to complement each other. Kampo works well with other treatments, as discussed at the end of the chapter.

THE HISTORY OF KAMPO

To understand the history of Kampo, one must look at two related healing methods—Traditional Chinese Medicine, the root from which Kampo sprang, and Kampo itself.

The Development of Traditional Chinese Medicine

In Chinese legend, herbal medicine was established by the god of husbandry, Shen Nung, while the principles of herbal medicine were recorded as a conversation between the Yellow Emperor and his minister, Chi Po. They spoke of medical philosophy in a part of the book later known as the *Basic Questions (Su Wen),* and of medical practice in part of a book later known as the *Magic Pivot.* Japanese scholars believe that the Yellow Emperor and Chi Po, were, like Shen Nung, mythical figures from Chinese literature.[1] Whether or not they were real historical figures, the writings attributed to them became the world's first medical textbook.

Although this textbook, *The Yellow Emperor's Canon of Internal Medicine (Huang ti nei ching su wen),*[2] was perhaps the earliest textbook on herbal healing, it was almost exclusively concerned with acupuncture. It listed only twenty-eight herbs combined into twelve herbal formulas, none of which is still in use today. These formulas were categorized by the tastes of the substances in them, with the note that "Pungent [taste] disperses, sour retains, sweet moderates, bitter strengthens, and salty softens."

In 168 B.C., shortly after the writing of *The Yellow Emperor's Canon,* China also produced the first book about healing herbs, *Formulas for Fifty-Two Ailments* (*Wu shi er bing fang*). These formulas were very simple and were not given names, although instructions were very specific for formulating teas, pills, and drafts, liquids into which herbs were (sometimes surreptitiously) added. The formulas were mostly described in terms of magic. The idea was that to overcome the malevolent forces that caused illness, herbal medicines had to be imbued with magic through various means.

This combination of magic and medicine eventually came to be called *fang ji.* It included not only the early elements of herbal medicine, but also magic, astrology, and geomancy. Over time, practitioners of *fang ji* were accorded wealth and prominence for their ability to treat disease.

Nonetheless, *fang ji* was not adequate for every medical need. Herbalist Zhang Zhongjing lived in a time of plague. About A.D. 190, a devastating epidemic killed many members of his family. "My relatives were plenty," he wrote, "their number more than two hundred. However, from the beginning of the Chien An era to now, two-thirds of them have died from the *shang han* [infectious cold]."

Zhang was understandably distraught with the doctors of his day. "They do little but vie for fame and power and delight themselves with improving their physical appearance," he wrote, "and they do not thoroughly study the medical classics before they begin to practice, but merely follow their teachers with no attempt to change the age-old formulas."[3]

In response to his great loss, Zhang Zhongjing sought to replace magic with medicine: "I pitied those who were ill and could not be cured. So I studied the medicine of the old classics and collected many prescriptions, and compiled the book *Shang han za bing lun*"[4] (*Discussion of Cold-Induced Disorders and Miscellaneous Diseases*). This book later became revered in Japan as the *Sho Kan Ron,* the ancestor to all of Kampo's herbal manuals. Zhang taught that herbal medicines should conform to people, instead of the other way around. His central idea was that if the fundamental disharmonies causing diseases in individuals were carefully studied, then knowledge of the specific combinations of herbs useful as medicine would naturally follow. Conversely, if physicians thoroughly understood herbs, then each combination of herbs could be precisely matched to the type of imbalance it was meant to treat. (For more information on Zhang's theory of disease, see page 9.)

Zhang's idea worked. Matching herbs to symptoms proved so reliable that in time the name of the formula used for treatment became another name for the diagnosis. For example, instead of saying that a person was suffering a bitter taste in the mouth, dry throat, red eyes, cough, and congestion, one could also say that the person was suffering a Minor Bupleurum Decoction disorder, the name of the formula used to treat this set of symptoms.

Even though much time has passed since the writing of the *Sho Kan Ron*, 20 percent of the herbal medicines used in China and an even greater percentage of the herbal medicines used in Japan still follow recipes exactly as recorded in the *Sho Kan Ron*. The lasting usefulness of this book is not only its foundation of person-centered principles of medicine, but also its establishment of the diagnostic principles of cold and heat, yang and yin (see pages 8 and 9).

The *Sho Kan Ron* was only the first of a series of works on Kampo medicine that have proven useful even into modern times. In the third century A.D., the *Sho Kan Ron* was edited by the celebrated Chinese herbalist Wu Shu-He into two parts: *Discussion of Cold-Induced Disorders* (*Shang han lun*) and *Essentials from the Golden Cabinet (Jin gui yao lue)*. Wang Shu-He added details to the patterns of diagnosis, gave each herbal formula a name, and added details concerning the dosages and methods of preparation for the herbs used in each formula.

Third-century herbalist Ge Hong took the principle of person-centered herbalism a step further. He wrote a volume of simple and inexpensive, yet highly effective, herbal formulas called *Emergency Formulas to Keep Up One's Sleeve* (*Bei ji zhou hou fang*). This book is the source of the main asthma treatment Kampo offers today. In the succeeding seven centuries, Chinese herbalism progressed with publication of *Thousand Ducat Formulas* (*Qian jin yao fang*) and *Supplement to the Thousand Ducat Formulas* (*Qian jin yi fang*) by Sun Si-Miao, and *Arcane Essentials from the Imperial Library* (*Wai tai bi yao*) by Wang Tao. Wang was the first herbalist to include formulas from non-Chinese, possibly Korean, sources. Several dozen formulas recorded in these texts are still in general use.

As the centuries progressed, the Chinese herbalism texts became increasingly voluminous and disorganized. The *Imperial Grace Formulary of the Tai Ping Era* (*Tai ping hui min he ji ju fang*), written between A.D. 982 and 992, contained 16,834 formulas! By the year 1000, so many formulas had been developed that the links between people and treatments became difficult to follow. Books written after Zhang Zhongjing usually failed to note which of up to twenty formulas was best for treating a given condition. Even more confusing was the fact that nuances of diagnosis described by later writers required additions to, and substitutions for, ingredients in the original formulas. These additions and substitutions could be made from over 5,000 available herbs. As confusing as all this was, over the next 500 years Chinese herbalists did devise a theory of Eight Indicators, a theory that is used in Kampo today, and a theory of five Paired Organs, which can be used to check a Kampo diagnosis (see pages 8 and 10).

Efforts to clarify China's herbal knowledge were unsuccessful. In the twelfth century, the scholar Cheng Wu-Ji wrote *A Clarification of the Theory of Cold-Induced Disorders* (*Shang han ming li lun*), which devised seven categories, or *qi fang*, for Kampo formulas. Cheng did make major advances in herbal treatment. In reconsidering the already-ancient *Theory of Cold-Induced Disorders*, he more completely discussed the importance of a disease-causing influence's strength, the location of the disease in the body, the patterns of disease progression, the importance of the patient's constitutional strength, and the effective timing of herbal treatment.

On the other hand, Cheng did not manage to relate these important ideas to particular formulas. His classification system for formulas was less than logical or consistent. For example, one of his observations is regarded throughout Oriental medicine to have no logical basis but is nonetheless quoted today: "To induce sweating do not use an even number of herbs, to drain downward do not use an odd number of herbs."[5,6] Even in twentieth-century North America, there is a persistent misunderstanding that the use of odd or even numbers of herbs is significant.

The disorganization of herbal knowledge during this period led the herbalists to complain. Xu Yin-Song protested, "Nowadays people are unable to differentiate the pulses [an important part of Chinese diagnosis], nor do they recognize the origins of disease. They base decisions on their feelings and use many medicinal substances. This is like hunting for rabbits by sending out many men and horses to surround the area in the hope that, by luck, one of them will stumble upon the rabbit. Treating [illness] like this is really negligent."[7]

Traditional Chinese Medicine (TCM) has continued to develop through the present day, providing the primary health care system for more than 1.5 billion people. Since 1976, TCM practitioners in the People's Republic of China have sought to apply herbal medicine—in combination with the ancient healing techniques of acupuncture, moxibustion (the use of burning herbs), and *tui nei* massage—to the treatment of modern illnesses. TCM combines both ancient techniques and scientific methods in the search for practical health care. TCM, though, presents an excess of riches in some ways. Despite TCM's great usefulness, the Japanese have found that they could simplify it into a uniquely Japanese system of medicine now known as Kampo.

Japan Simplifies TCM: The Development of Kampo

Japanese medicine, like Chinese medicine, once relied on prayers, incantations, and shamanistic practices.[8,9] Sometime after A.D. 593, the Empress Suiko sent armies to invade Korea, where Chinese healing methods were already in use. Reports of Chinese medicine's usefulness so impressed the empress that she sent two emissaries to China to study

Kampo. Knowledge of Kampo later spread to the Buddhist monasteries of Japan during the Nara Period (710–794), when a Japanese monk, traveling in China, fell ill and recovered after being treated with Kampo. Other emissaries also went to China and brought back news of its herbal healing formulas. During the Heian Period (794–1192), the scholar Yasuyori Tamba revised the oldest Japanese medicinal text, *The Way of Medicine* (the *Issinho*), to include all the herbal formulas discovered in China. The resulting work was copied in thirty volumes.

This enormous amount of information about herbal formulas, however, posed the same problems for the Japanese as it did for the Chinese. Gradually, the Japanese began not only to imitate Chinese herbal medicine but to simplify it. Practitioners of Kampo dropped the 16,834 formulas of the *Imperial Grace Formulary,* in favor of the more ancient *Pharmacopoeia of Heavenly Husbandry* (*Shen nung pen ts'ao*). This storehouse of herbal knowledge was edited to 365 formulas, one for each day of the year. It included 120 *Joyaku* (Upper Class Medicine), remedies designed to increase longevity when taken regularly over a long period of time, with no side effects. There were 120 *Chuyaku* (Middle Class Medicine), formulas designed to regenerate energy and keep the body healthy. These medicines sometimes produced side effects and were to be used with caution. Finally there were 125 *Shimoyaku* (Lower Class Medicine), remedies for serious ailments that usually produced side effects and could not be used for too long.[10] From early on, Kampo theorists wanted to find remedies that would heal gently, with the fewest possible side effects.

Part of the motivation for simplifying the Chinese herbal tradition was material necessity. During most of the reign of the Tokugawa shoguns (1603–1867), Japan was a secluded society. Trade with other countries was almost completely cut off, and herbs from China and other foreign sources were almost completely unavailable.

Another motivation for simplifying Chinese herbalism came from the religious devotion of the Buddhist monks. For centuries, monks were the only source of Kampo medicine for the common people. Chinese medicine used a vast array of animal products, such as tiger bone, rhinoceros horn, and whole wasps. But Buddhism gave the monks, and the Japanese people in general, a deep distaste for animal products acquired by unnecessary slaughter. Therefore, except for a few formulas that used shells, fossilized bone, or the byproducts of animals commonly raised for food, Japanese herbalism became almost entirely plant-based.

At one point, the simplification of Kampo reached its limits. In *Myriad Diseases—One Toxin,* Todo Yoshimasu (1702–1773) asserted that all diseases stem from the presence of toxins. Once the body was able to rid itself of the poisons, a cure would follow, and one removed them by simply learning the formulas in the *Sho Kan Ron*. Eventually, Yoshimasu invented a method of treatment called *Meigen* that—in the belief that "like cures like"—used very high concentrations of toxins. However, many patients died, and this method was eventually discarded.

One school of Kampo practitioners, the followers of the sixteenth-century master Dosan Manase, kept some of the Five Element and energy circuit ideas that had been developed in China (see page 10). The Koho school of Kampo in the seventeenth century, on the other hand, rejected these key concepts of Chinese medicine to create an elegant but austere theory of herbal medicine that was uniquely Japanese. These physicians returned to the *Sho Kan Ron,* and subsequently simplified even this quite basic text. For example, Zhang had identified five categories of pathogens, or root causes of disease: wind, cold, heat, dampness, and improper diet or overwork. The Koho master Geni Nagoya (1628–1696) chose to group the four then-known environmental causes of disease into a single category, cold. Nagoya also discarded elaborate theories of yin and yang, using them only as diagnostic indicators. Kampo as it is most frequently practiced today still derives from the teachings of the Koho masters.

The recent explosion in Kampo's popularity among the Japanese (see page 11) has resulted from the rediscovery of its usefulness in treating a broad range of medical conditions. However, Kampo was unused and almost forgotten in Japan for nearly a century. This happened as the Imperial Court decided to focus on innovations in surgical medicine. Although Japan had had a tradition of surgical treatment from the time of Toyo Yamawaki (1705–1762), the Court recognized that Japan's willingness to use anesthesia, antiseptics, and modern surgical techniques imported from the West—methods rejected by Japan's Asian neighbors—would give Japan an important advantage in war preparations. By 1940, no medical school in Japan taught Kampo, and the older system officially had fallen by the wayside.

THE THEORY OF KAMPO

Kampo uses eight unifying principles of diagnosis that came to it from ancient Chinese medicine. The six concepts most used in Kampo medicine—cold and heat, deficiency and excess, and interior and exterior—are intuitive and easy to understand. The other two concepts, yang and yin, at least sound familiar to most people in the West. These eight unifying principles are known collectively as the Eight Indicators, and they are used to describe patterns of symptoms that individuals suffer during the course of disease. As unusual as this diagnostic approach may seem, the basic idea of Kampo is quite simple: Combinations of herbs can correct combinations of imbalances within the body, thereby relieving the combination of symptoms that the patient experiences.

Compared with the elegant theoretical system of TCM, Kampo medicine is a greatly simplified approach to both diagnosis and treatment. Kampo does only enough examination to identify and double-check the combination of herbs that will bring the pattern of symptoms back into balance. TCM practitioners perform a more intricate examination of the patient's diagnostic signs and use the traditional herbal formulas as a starting point, rather than as an endpoint, for prescribing treatment. TCM practitioners give the herbs needed to repair the symptom pattern, plus additional herbs for nuances of the patient's condition they notice in a more involved diagnostic process.

The advantage of the Japanese approach, however, is that always using the same combinations of herbs contained in centuries-old traditional formulas allows predictable results. Doctors can understand the formulas in the same way they understand synthetic drugs. The simplified system of diagnosis also allows the symptom patterns of Kampo to be linked to Western categories of disease, something that is not easily accomplished in TCM. In this way Kampo medicine allows the patient to benefit from the best of both Eastern and Western medicine.

This section first considers the Four Examinations by which Kampo makes a person-centered diagnosis. It then discusses the Eight Indicators as they are used in Japanese herbal medicine today. Finally, this section explains the concepts Kampo borrows from TCM to confirm a diagnosis.

The Four Examinations

The process of diagnosis in Kampo consists of the Four Examinations: examining the patient by sight, examining the patient by sound and smell, inquiring about symptoms, and touching the patient through a process known as palpation. Experienced practitioners of Kampo or TCM can learn much about a patient at a glance. The visual examination notes general appearance (body build, cleanliness, dress, overall nutritional status, posture, stature), appearance of the skin and nails, mobility, muscular development, psychological disposition, and abnormalities in the circulation of blood or fluids (bruises, puffiness, swelling). The hearing examination notes the patient's breathing, abdominal noises, quality and volume of voice, and expressions of pain or discomfort. The third examination, inquiry, is a process of sympathetic questioning in which the practitioner elicits a complete history of the illness. The Kampo physician also probes the patient's prior medical history and family medical history to learn if there are any recurrent illnesses, genetic susceptibilities to disease, or sensitivities to medication. The final step of Kampo medicine is palpation. TCM accomplishes this fourth step of examination by reading the pulse. Japanese medicine also incorporates pulse reading, but places a much greater emphasis on abdominal palpation. Feeling the tone and tenderness of the abdominal wall yields diagnostic clues.

The essence of Kampo diagnosis is embodied in the charge given every student of Kampo medicine: "Listen to your patients, they are telling you their diagnosis." This does not mean, however, that Kampo practitioners must limit themselves to sight, sound, inquiry, and palpation. Since all practitioners of Kampo in Japan (and a growing number of Kampo practitioners in North America) today are trained in Western medicine as well as traditional herbalism, a Kampo physician may use blood tests, ultrasound, X-ray, or other strictly modern techniques to augment the diagnosis. In fact, combining traditional and modern diagnostic techniques is the most effective way to use Kampo. Certain kinds of cancer, for instance, produce no symptoms that are recognized by Western medicine until they are too advanced for treatment. Kampo diagnosis notes symptoms, ignored in Western medicine, that indicate an early development of these kinds of cancer. Western diagnosis can be used to confirm Kampo diagnosis. While the tools of treatment are likely to be those used in Western medicine, diagnosing the disease in time is made possible by Kampo.

The Eight Indicators

The Four Examinations give information about the Eight Indicators used to measure health. Like the Four Examinations, the Eight Indicators came to Kampo from Chinese medicine. In 1116, the Chinese master herbalist Kou Zong-Shi recorded this system of simplified diagnostic categories. He made a list of four pairs of indicators to create a logical framework into which to place the various aspects and stages of disease. The pairs are:

- Cold and heat
- Deficiency and excess
- Interior and exterior
- Yang and yin

Collectively, these indicators form a precise pattern calling for a specific treatment, or, in Japanese, the *sho*. Diagnosis using all eight indicators is not necessary in choosing a formula that will restore health. The full set of indicators, however, serves as a check of the diagnosis, so that the formula given will not have unexpected side effects. In modern Kampo practice, the scientific understanding of the disease process, coupled with knowledge of how the chemical components of herbs work in the body, also serves to make sure the herbs and formulas chosen are the right ones.

Cold and Heat

Although the concepts of cold and heat (in Japanese, *kan* and *netsu*) are intuitive and easily understood, their full meaning in Kampo cannot be directly translated into English. Cold and heat refer not only to a sensation of temperature, but also to the under- or over-activity of bodily processes. Cold and heat can coexist, as in the case of a menopausal patient who has both hot flashes and cold feet. Cold is thought to be more characteristic of women and heat more characteristic of men, not because of any idea of masculine or feminine "energy," but because the curvatures of a woman's anatomy expose her body to cold. Japanese physicians find cold symptoms in many of the diseases Western medicine considers diseases of deficiency, such as hypothyroidism (low thyroid hormones) or hypotension (low blood pressure).

In Japan, due to the pervasive and lasting influence of the Kampo master Geni Nagoya, many people go to the doctor having no complaint other than that they are "cold." The Kampo physician then uses the Four Examinations to characterize the patient's symptoms of cold and heat in a meaningful way (see Table 1.1). In the process of examination, the practitioner looks for symptoms of the body's use of heat to drive out cold through fever, sweating, or inflammation.

The opposite of cold is heat, but in Japanese medicine heat takes on a special meaning. "Natural" heat, such as feeling hot on a summer day or having a fever after getting an infection, is of less concern than "unnatural" heat, which affects some parts of the body but not others, or which is not tied to other symptoms. The most common form of unnatural heat is *nobose,* which is roughly translated as hot flushes. This is a rush of heat to the head with an uncomfortable sensation of heat, congestion, pressure, or muscular tension. This heat can also cause dizziness, dry mouth, redness in the face, ringing in the ears, and a draining of heat away from the lower half of the body, leaving cold hands and feet. Hot flushes are important in the diagnosis of conditions as diverse as anxiety, constipation, depression, hyperthyroidism, insomnia, migraine, fevers, and burns.

TABLE 1.1. COLD AND HOT SYMPTOMS

Cold Symptoms	Hot Symptoms
Desire for warmth	Intense dislike of heat
Chilly body	Hot body
No thirst, or craving for hot liquids	Continuous thirst, craving for cold drinks
Chills	Fever
Pale face or "cold" eyes	Red face and eyes
Diarrhea	Constipation
Large volumes of clear urine	Small quantities of dark urine
Little perspiration	Copious perspiration
Poor digestion and weak appetite	Burning digestion
Desire for sleep	Insomnia
Prolapsed organs and loss of muscle tone	Inflammation and infection

Excess and Deficiency

Usually consideration of cold and heat alone is not quite enough to choose the right herbal remedy. The next pair of indicators to be considered are excess and deficiency, which measure the *taishitsu,* or constitutional state (see Table 1.2). Excess and deficiency measure the person's degree of vitality and ability to withstand disease. Persons with signs of excess react vigorously to disease, with a state of elevated physiological functioning. They are susceptible to diseases of excess, such as high blood pressure or insomnia. They are treated with formulas that "drain" the energy imbalance caused by disease. Persons with signs of deficiency show a weak healing response, with a state of diminished physiological functioning. They are susceptible to the opposites of the diseases of excess, such as low blood pressure and drowsiness. They are treated with formulas that energize the body's response to disease.

Internal and External Used With Yang and Yin

The last four of the Eight Indicators are used more in explaining a diagnosis than in making a diagnosis in Kampo today. The indicators interior and exterior refer to the "location" of a disease process in the body. In ancient Kampo theory, diseases were thought to first invade the "exterior" defenses of the body and work their way progressively to the "interior" defenses.

TABLE 1.2. EXCESS AND DEFICIENCY SYMPTOMS

Symptoms of Excess	Symptoms of Deficiency
Athletic, heavyset	Thin
Firm body fat	Loose body fat
Good muscle tone and elasticity	Poor muscle tone and elasticity
Well tolerant of both heat and cold	Sensitive to extremes of summer heat and winter cold
Assertive, positive communication	Passive, negative communication
Vigorous physical movement	Disinclined to physical movement
No adverse effects from skipping a meal	Feels weak after skipping a meal
Constipation causes discomfort	Constipation for several days does not produce discomfort
Loud voice	Soft voice
Thick, elastic abdominal wall	Thin, soft abdominal wall

The master herbalist Zhang Zhongjing described the progress of disease in six stages. In the first three stages of disease, the body used yang, or outwardly directed, energies to fight the pathogen. At the beginning of a disease, the body is capable of its greatest defense. This stage is known as the Greater Yang. If the disease is not overcome, the body has less and less energy with which to defend itself. The second stage of disease is accordingly called the Lesser Yang, and the next stage is known as the Shadow Yang, in which the body's defensive energy is only a "shadow" of its former strength.

Eventually, the body no longer has enough energy to combat the pathogen, and it must concentrate instead on containing its vital energy. The energy of containment is yin, and so the names of the next three stages are the Greater Yin, Lesser Yin, and Absolute Yin.

Treatments of the Yang and Yin stages of disease run along a continuum of cold and heat, deficiency and excess, and interior and exterior. In the Greater Yang stage, for instance, both the person and the disease-causing pathogen are strong. The treatment strategy in the Greater Yang is to augment the body's response to disease with treatments that increase heat and accelerate bodily processes, such as herbs that purge the digestive tract or increase sweating. In the Greater Yin stage, on the other hand, the body tries a different strategy against a persistent disease, that of starving out the pathogen. The treatment strategy is to augment the body's ability to "hold its own" without stimulating bodily processes that would injure weakened organs. The theory of the Yin stages served as a clue to modern Japanese scientists that centuries-old formulas would be helpful in the treatment of chronic viral infections. In the case of HIV, for instance, the Kampo formula that keeps HIV from multiplying does so without stimulating the immune system (and giving the virus more opportunity to multiply).

Blood, Fluid, and the Vital Energy Called Qi

Examination of the Eight Indicators is enough to find the right herb or formula to treat any condition. However, Kampo also borrows three concepts from TCM to make a second check of the diagnosis. In everyday spoken Japanese, the word *sho* not only means a pattern of symptoms, but also a factual proof. Three more concepts from TCM—blood, fluid, and vital energy—complete the factual proof of the doctor's diagnosis. In this section they are discussed in the order in which they are used in Kampo today, rather than the order in which they are found in theoretical discussions of TCM.

Since every function of the body depends on the proper circulation of blood, Kampo can describe every condition in terms of blood imbalances (*ketsu sho*). Problems arise when blood is "static" (*oketsu*) or "vacant" (*kekkyo*).

Static blood is blood that is no longer free-flowing and has lost its physiological function. It may result from narrowed arteries, blood clots, or tumors. Like a clog in a drainage pipe, static blood can create all kinds of problems in the housekeeping of the body. Its signs are abnormal red, purple, blue, or black coloration of the skin; venous abnormalities (spider veins, varicose veins, large veins in the tongue); and pain in a fixed location. Over a period of years, static blood can "solidify" to form solid tumors. The early signs of static blood, however, warn of upcoming problems.

Since most Kampo practitioners also have some training in Western medical techniques, signs of static blood are a signal for further diagnosis. Static blood signs may warn of defects in its clotting mechanisms, internal bleeding, lesions, and increased vascular permeability due to drug allergies. There may be artherosclerosis, high cholesterol, chronic hepatitis, or menstrual disorders.

Vacant blood is blood that is inadequate to supply the affected organs. The signs of vacant blood are blurred vision, dizziness, dry or chapped skin, insomnia and problems in concentration, pallor (pale complexion, white nails), or irregular menstruation. These signs may stem from an insufficient volume of blood, but there also may be a shortage of red blood cells or hemoglobin. Treatment of vacant blood, like all other conditions, may use Kampo herbs and formulas and/or standard medical means.

Fluid imbalances (*suidoku*) are also useful indicators of disease. Perspiration can be an especially important diagnostic sign, since it tells which of the six Yang and Yin stages the disease has passed. Sweating is more characteristic of the early, Yang stages than the later, Yin stages. Unusual sweating can also be a sign of blood loss, immune deficiency, or an imbalance in the nervous system. Edema, or swelling, is a warning sign of diseases of the heart, kidneys, or liver that may require medical attention. Especially in women, edema causes weight gain, and other symptoms such as bloating, breast pain, joint pain, puffy face, and headache. The other fluid imbalance that is important in Japanese medicine is fluid stagnation. Affecting a single organ system, fluid stagnation is an over-concentration of watery fluids that imperils normal function. Asthma, for example, is a condition of fluid stagnation in the lungs. Congestive heart disease is a condition of fluid stagnation throughout the circulatory system. Fluid stagnation causes its sufferer to be sensitive to the cold, and worsens during exposure to the cold.

The other concept that Kampo borrows from TCM is that of the vital energy known as *qi* (pronounced "kee" in Japanese and "chee" in Chinese). Qi is the body's vital force through which all the organs act in harmony to contain the self and respond to the environment. In the original theory, TCM conceived a somewhat complicated system of five Paired Organs that control and supply each other. In this system, which is known in Japanese medicine as the *go-gyo*, five elements represent the movement of energy on both the cosmic and microscopic levels. These Five Elements—Wood, Fire, Earth, Metal, and Water—both create and restrain each other in recognizable patterns, such as Earth creating Metal through the action of Heat. In the human body, each element is processed by one of the five organ systems: spleen/stomach, lung/large intestine, kidney/bladder, liver/gallbladder, and heart/small intestine. The energy associated with the organ pair's activity then circulates up and down the body in precisely defined energy channels, or meridians.

The importance of qi in modern Kampo is not as an explanation of how the body reacts to the Five Elements, but as a concept that unifies a pattern of symptoms. The "liver" channel, for instance, circulates energy over the breasts and the middle of the eyes to the crown of the head. An energy disturbance in this channel, therefore, can manifest itself in the liver, breasts, eyes, or crown of the head. Yellow eyes, for example, are symptomatic of the liver disorder known as hepatitis. Breast pain may occur at the same time as headache in premenstrual syndrome. Especially in the early diagnosis of cancer, recognizing combinations of symptoms along the energy meridians makes Kampo a useful complement to traditional treatment.

Kampo differs from TCM in its understanding of one of the five organ pairs. In TCM, the "spleen" is thought to be the yang organ which digests food, for which the stomach expends yin energy to contain. Science identifies no such function for the spleen. Japanese practitioners are likely to diagnosis "spleen" abnormalities in terms of weak gastrointestinal function (*icho kyojaku*). When the digestion process is weak, Kampo medications (all of which are taken orally) cannot be absorbed. Noting and treating weak gastrointestinal function is an essential step in treatment with Kampo.

TRADITIONAL MEDICINE IN THE MODERN WORLD: IS KAMPO SCIENTIFIC?

After the opening of Japan to trade in 1856, official Japanese medicine was overwhelmed by the process of adopting Western treatment methods, such as surgical and microbiological techniques, vitamin therapy, and antibiotics. Despite this, interest in Kampo survived. In 1927, Kyushin Yumoto wrote *Superior Chinese Medicine* (*Nokan Igaku*). Kampo practitioners came out into the open and in 1928 formed an association for traditional medicine that later began publishing a newsletter called *Kampo and Kampo Medicine* (*Kampo To Kan'yaku*).

One of Yumoto's students was another physician trained in Western medicine, Keisetsu Otsuka. Otsuka recorded his experiences with Kampo in *Thirty Years of Kampo: Selected Case Studies of an Herbal Doctor.* In this book, Otsuka recorded 374 case studies in which Kampo was applied to medical conditions as defined by Western medicine. First published in 1959 in Japanese, the book was translated into both Chinese and English, and became one of the most significant Kampo manuals.

One of Otsuka's students was a Taiwanese pharmacologist trained in scientific medicine, Hong-Yen Hsu. Hong-Yen Hsu emigrated to the United States after 1945, and established the Oriental Healing Arts Institute (OHAI). OHAI printed the works of Keisetsu Otsuka and other Japanese herbal physicians, and established Kampo as a healing art in the United States. Since the founding of OHAI, several American herb manufacturers have started lines of Kampo formulas, and Kampo medicine has become available at thousands of locations in the United States.

Kampo's revival has resulted in its widespread acceptance and use in Japan. The Japan Society for Oriental Medicine, founded in 1950, sponsored scientific testing of Kampo formulas for medical use. By 1967, the Japanese Ministry of Health had been persuaded that four Kampo formulas were worthy of modern use, and included them on a reimbursement list under the national health insurance plan. By 1976, forty-two formulas had been approved by the Japanese equivalent of the Food and Drug Administration, and by 1996, 148 formulas were approved.[11] Today, almost 77 percent of all Japanese physicians, who have every method of modern medicine at their disposal, use Kampo.[12] Tsumura and Company, a Kampo manufacturer, found that nearly 60 percent of Japanese doctors considered Kampo to be their first choice for some diseases.[13] Unlike TCM formulas, which tend to be quite complex, Japanese formulas use fixed combinations of herbs in standard amounts. This makes Japanese Kampo somewhat less person-centered than TCM, but it offers greater confidence in using herbal treatments and synthetic drugs together.

Kampo's popularity does not stem from its status as a traditional Japanese medicine. In 1976, only 19.2 percent of all Japanese doctors used Kampo.[14] The reason Kampo medicine is experiencing a renaissance in Japan is that doctors have discovered that person-centered medicine provides options in treating disease that disease-centered medicine does not. Of equal importance are the hundreds of studies that have confirmed Kampo's scientific validity.

Kampo is not used in Japan as an emergency treatment (although it is in China). Neither is it used instead of major surgery. In cases where standard medications deliver a predictable result without side effects, Japanese doctors prefer synthetic drugs to Kampo. These doctors, however, note seven situations for which Kampo is especially suitable:[15]

- *Disorders and symptoms in the elderly.* The elderly often have disorders affecting several organs, and the cause of symptoms may not be clear. Also, side effects may appear more readily when prescription drugs are taken by older people. In the elderly, individual differences are especially significant, and in Japanese culture, Kampo allows the physician to assure the patient that individual differences are being respected. In the West, Kampo medicine allows the physician to account for individual differences when planning a treatment program.
- *Disorders involving abnormalities of the immune system.* Among the most exciting applications of Kampo lie in treating abnormalities of the immune system. Clinical studies have proven that Kampo formulas are effective in treating allergy, asthma, lupus, and rheumatoid arthritis. Kampo formulas are also effective in treating viral infections of the immune system.
- *Psychosomatic and psychiatric complaints.* Kampo is a valuable method of treating psychosomatic and psychiatric complaints in that it neither depresses nor overstimulates the central nervous system. Kampo formulas do not induce drowsiness, tremors, or fatigue, nor do they trigger nightmares, hallucinations, or manic behavior. Kampo seeks to treat body and mind together. A "bad attitude" is considered merely to be a reflection of a basic physical imbalance, and treatment is not impeded, nor judgment made, by the expectations of the patient.
- *Subjective symptoms, or "diseases that are not diseases" (jitsuyo kanpo kyoho).* Some conditions, such as menopausal discomforts and chronic fatigue syndrome, are expressed through very different symptoms in different individuals. Since Kampo is a person-based rather than disease-based diagnostic system, its remedies are often more effective for these disorders.
- *Combination therapy to enhance the effects of conventional treatment.* There are cases in which Kampo strengthens the body's response to prescription medications. In the treatment of lupus with prednisolone, for example, use of the formula Ginseng Decoction to Nourish the Nutritive Qi allows the lupus patient to use a reduced dosage of prednisolone, and thus avoid side effects.
- *Combination therapy to prevent side effects of conventional treatment.* Chemotherapy drugs are widely used in cancer treatment. While these compounds fight the disease, they also usually result in anorexia, nausea, vomiting, blood-cell problems, anemia, kidney damage, and loss of hair. The formula Ten-Significant Tonic Decoction greatly reduces these devastating side effects, and also increases the likelihood of remission.
- *Alternative therapy for persons who have allergic and other adverse reactions to standard treatment.* In Japan, Kampo is used in the treatment of persons with rheumatoid arthritis who are at risk of gastrointestinal disorders when given steroid anti-inflammatory drugs. American clinical tests have proven Kampo's effectiveness in this regard.

How often are people in Japan treated with Kampo? Almost 90 percent of patients with hepatitis, chronic liver disease, or liver cancer are treated with Kampo. Nearly half of all people with colds and respiratory tract infections are treated with Kampo. More than one-third of all cases of mental illness and over one-fourth of all cases of allergy, asthma, and bowel irregularity are treated with Kampo herbal formulas.[16]

How often are people in North America treated with Kampo? In addition to people who receive Kampo treatment from a growing number of Japanese-trained TCM practitioners, as many as five million people a year are treated by members of the American Association of Acupuncture and Oriental Medicine (see Appendix A). Kampo formulas have been proven effective in studies at medical schools all over the United States, from the Columbia College of Physicians and Surgeons at Columbia University to the University of California at Berkeley, and at McGill University in Canada.

Still, many experts express reservations about Kampo. These scientists generally believe that the processes of disease and healing work in the body at a chemical level. In this view, single, identifiable chemicals that can be isolated from plant sources—and synthesized in the laboratory—are the only important agents in medicine. As one noted American herbal scientist put it, "Chinese traditional medicine today continues to be a curiosity rather than a science because no one has applied [a] method of selecting the effective ingredient from the host of inactive ones in most Chinese medicines."[17]

Although Japanese herbal medicine carefully verifies the role of each herb in a traditional formula, there are advantages to the chemical approach. Chemicals made in the lab or factory can be packaged in standardized and predictable doses. On the other hand, chemicals found in herbs differ in strength and concentration depending on the effects of soil and weather on the growth of the plant, and the time of year (and day) the plant was harvested. And although we do not often think of individual differences between plants, individual plants may be genetically unique. Also, while the herbs used in Kampo can't be patented, processes for extracting chemicals from them can. Slight changes to the chemicals found in healing plants can also lead to profitable patents.

So what is wrong with the chemical approach? The European scientific community involved with medicinal plant research has come to realize that the effects of any herb cannot be explained by just one chemical constituent. The healing effects of herbs are more likely to involve a combined effect of several or even dozens of different compounds working together. Some of these compounds probably act as support substances that reduce the toxicity of the active compounds. Other compounds in herbs may act as preservatives.[18]

Scientists are beginning to examine the relationships among the various chemicals in a given plant. The non-Kampo herb St. John's wort, for instance, was for years commonly reduced and standardized to a single chemical, hypericin, which was found in laboratory tests to have antidepressant and antiviral effects. Later studies, however, found that using the whole plant is more effective than using hypericin extract alone.[19]

What science is beginning to recognize is that whole plants are more than the sum of their chemical parts. Perhaps future years of careful laboratory work will enable scientific skeptics to accept the theoretical basis of Kampo, which maintains that herbal formulas are more than the sum of the herbs they contain. In the meantime, Kampo continues to demonstrate its proven healing power.

This chapter has provided a great deal of information about Kampo, from its origins to its theories to its methods of diagnosis. Now it is time to take a closer look at the individual herbs used in Kampo.

CHAPTER 2

Buying and Using Kampo Herbs

A person in Japan who wants to undergo Kampo treatment can go to either a pharmacist or to a regular doctor who uses Kampo. But for someone who is not in Japan, the question remains: How does one buy and use Kampo herbs here?

It is strongly recommended that, except for the most commonplace of disorders, Kampo be used under the supervision of a professional health care provider. Finding expert supervision is especially important for someone who is already taking either prescription or over-the-counter medications, since Kampo herbs can interact with such drugs—and with alcohol, for that matter. It is equally important for someone who has a preexisting condition that might react negatively to a specific herb. For example, liver disease often affects the body's ability to clear medicinal substances, including herbs, from the system, and certain herbs can stimulate sex hormone production, which is undesirable in dealing with such hormone-sensitive conditions as prostate or breast cancer.

Since Kampo is not widely practiced in North America, a regular doctor is not likely to be familiar with this system. However, there are doctors, such as naturopaths or nutritionists, who may be willing to work with patients who want to use herbal medicine. It is also possible to find a qualified herbalist or TCM practitioner who is familiar with Kampo (see Appendix A). If adverse effects develop, discontinue use and see a health care provider.

The herbs and formulas discussed in this book have been recommended on the basis of both their effectiveness and their availability (with a few exceptions) in North America. This chapter will first look at where Kampo herbs can be found and what to look for when buying them. It will then discuss how herbs are handled by Kampo manufacturers before giving the best way to make tea. Dosages of individual herbs are given in Part Two, while the issue of formula dosage is dealt with in Chapter 4.

SHOPPING FOR KAMPO HERBS

Finding the herbs used in Kampo is not as difficult a task as one may think. There are several places to look:

- *Health food stores.* Many of these stores carry a fairly wide selection of herbs, including a number of the herbs and formulas used in Kampo. Remember that labeling laws in the United States do not allow an herb's uses to be listed on the package, although usages can be listed in Canada. Also, the person behind the counter may or may not be familiar with herbal medicine.
- *Herb shops.* Most of these stores carry a wide selection of both packaged and loose herbs, and the proprietor is usually knowledgeable about the products he or she sells.
- *Asian markets.* In regions with a large Japanese or Chinese population, there may be food markets that carry Japanese or Chinese specialties, and that also sells traditional herbal medicines.
- *Mail-order catalogs.* Like marketers of other alternative health products, some Kampo distributors operate mail-order services (see Appendix A). There are also online services through which products can be ordered. This form of shopping is very convenient, especially for Kampo formulas. It is important to deal with a reputable company, though, because the product cannot be inspected before purchase.

For someone who has not taken medicinal herbs before, it is not uncommon to be a little intimidated by what is, for many North Americans, a whole new mode of treatment. The process of purchasing and using herbs, though, becomes much more comfortable over time. It is important to know that the same herb can come in different forms:

- *Dry, loose herbs, either ground or whole.* These are made into teas. See Appendix B for what to look for in each herb.
- *Fluid extracts.* These are water-based extracts of individual herbs. They are usually made in a 1:1 ratio, that is, with equal parts of herb juice and water.
- *Patent (over-the-counter) medicines.* These are basically concentrated bottled formulas. Appendix A lists brand names of patent medicines and the traditional formulas to which they correspond.
- *Pills, tablets, and capsules.* A few Kampo formulas (identified in Chapter 4) are taken in solid rather than liquid form. Other formulas are made into teas and then air- or freeze-dried before being turned into convenient tablet

forms. Single-herb products are also available in pill, tablet, or capsule form.

- *Premixed formulas.* This is the form of Kampo most likely to be dispensed by a TCM practitioner (see Chapter 4). The patient is given bags of herbs that are used to brew formulas in tea form, usually with specific instructions.
- *Tea bags.* Many single herbs are available in ready-to-use tea bags, although it may be necessary to use more than one bag per cup to get a medicinally effective dose.
- *Tinctures.* These are alcohol-based extractions of single herbs. Sometimes an herb's healing compounds are more readily available when extracted by alcohol. They are usually made in a 1:5 ratio, that is, one part herb to five parts alcohol. Tinctures are always taken with a small amount of water, since straight tinctures can burn the tongue. Small amounts of tincture are measured in drops, while larger amounts are measured in teaspoons. Glycerin-based extracts can be given to small children instead of tinctures.
- *Syrups.* These are solutions made with herbs, water, and sugar.

QUALITY CONTROL OF KAMPO MEDICINES

Good manufacturing practices (GMP) are important in ensuring the highest possible quality in herbal products, and Japanese manufacturers have set the world's standards in this regard. The first step in GMP is knowing the producer. Commercial buyers rely on growers to apply organic methods of cultivation and to harvest herbs at the appropriate stage of growth, season, temperature, and time of day. Long-term relationships of mutual trust between growers in China and buyers in Japan and the United States are the norm in the Kampo industry.

The second step in GMP is confirming the identity of the herb purchased. The buyer's experience in how an herb should look, smell, and taste is an essential part of this process. This step also usually entails microscopic examination of a sample of the herb to ensure that it is the species of plant required. In some cases, the buyer may prepare a chemical extract to ascertain that the herb contains minimum amounts of those plant chemicals known to have healing effects. In other cases, the medicinal value of the herb will be verified by measurements of ash or water content. Japanese manufacturers also routinely test for the presence of heavy metals, especially arsenic, in order to exclude such contaminants.

The third step in GMP is sanitary storage. Bacteria, insects, and molds must be excluded from the storage space.

Most Americans who use Kampo find the twenty minutes to three hours per day required to prepare teas inconvenient, so Kampo practitioners in the United States increasingly rely on patent (over-the-counter) medicines to ensure that their patients take the formulas in a timely fashion. Quality inspection continues at each stage of the manufacturing process: chopping, blending, extracting, granulating, bottling, and labeling. In Japan, extracts are produced by concentrating and drying on an industrial scale, using the liquid from Kampo teas made by traditional formulas. Liquid patent (over-the-counter) medicines are usually reduced from between $^1/_{10}$ and $^1/_{100}$ of their original volume.

To create dried forms of patent medicines, batches of herbal teas are concentrated to a very small volume. The reduced mixtures are then mixed with a starch filler allowing them to be fashioned into noodlelike strands that are cut into granules, or dried and crushed into powders. At least one American Kampo manufacturer modifies this process by freeze-drying the formula.

In practice, many Japanese Kampo patent medicine manufacturers reduce the dosages of herbs recommended by Kampo's ancient source texts. Most American manufacturers, however, use the original dosages (see Appendix A).

The best method of quality assurance for the individual user of herbal medicines is to find a trustworthy herb dealer. The information in Appendix B on how to recognize quality in the individual herbs is useful. For some herbal extracts, getting the compound specified in Part Two is important. When buying gentian, for example, be sure to purchase the capsules as directed to avoid this herb's extremely bitter taste when taken in other forms. In a few cases, the extract should be standardized to contain a specific amount of compound. For example, solid hawthorn extract should be standardized to contain 10 percent proanthocyanidins.

MEASURING HERBS AND MAKING TEA

Measuring Kampo herbs is simple. Chapter 3 gives both teaspoon/tablespoon and metric measurements. While some herbs are coarsely ground and others are finely ground, there is no need to make adjustments when measuring.

It is not difficult to make Kampo teas. However, their effectiveness depends on proper preparation, so attention to detail is important. First, always make herbal teas in a nonmetallic pot, although the water can be boiled in a metal tea kettle before being poured into the brewing vessel. Metals, particularly aluminum and iron, can react with herbs to cause unknown chemical reactions. The pot must have a tight-fitting lid and be clean.

In most of North America, tap water is good enough for tea. In areas where the tap water has a high mineral content, substitute bottled water. If the amount of water used is not specified, the rule is to cover the herbs with about one-half inch of water before heating. Usually this is $1^1/_4$ cups of water for every ounce of herbs. Before beginning the heating process, allow the herbs to soak in the water for ten to fifteen minutes.

The rule for heating teas is "start fast, end slow." Bring the water to a boil using high heat, then simmer. Most formulas are heated for between twenty and thirty minutes, or until the volume of liquid in the pot reaches the level prescribed by the herbalist. Although formulas from the *Sho Kan Ron* (see Chapter 1) specify the starting and ending amounts of liquid, most modern herbalists do not adhere closely to recommended volumes as long as the tea is taken in the recommended number of doses.

It is important not to lift the lid of the pot too often during the tea-making process, since many herbs contain aromatic oils that can escape if they are boiled in an open pot. If the tea is overcooked or burnt, discard the herbs. *Never* add water to cook again.

Certain herbs and other healing substances require special handling when used to make teas. Some, such as abalone shell and dragon bone, should be boiled for between thirty and forty-five minutes to ensure that their active ingredients enter the tea. Aconite is preboiled to make doubly sure its toxic ingredients do *not* enter the tea. Other herbs, such as artemisia and peppermint, should be added at the end of the tea-making process, approximately five minutes before the water is taken off the heat. These herbs contain aromatic oils that may escape during a long boil. Viscous or "sticky" substances, such as gelatin, are added to the strained tea after the other herbs have been boiled. This prevents their sticking to the bottom of the pot and burning during the making of the tea. Ginseng, because of its expense and rarity, is often boiled separately to obtain maximum effect. It may be sliced thin and then boiled in a double-boiler for two to three hours to ensure that all the active ingredients are released. (Specific tea-making instructions for individual herbs are included in Chapter 3.)

This chapter has provided some tips on shopping for and measuring herbs. The next chapter discusses each specific herb in detail.

CHAPTER 3

The Medicines of Kampo

Chapter 1 described how Kampo evolved into an elegant diagnosis system that identifies various symptom patterns, which can then be treated with combinations of herbs, while single herbs are used to treat single symptoms. Unlike Western medicines, which are, generally, measured doses of single ingredients, herbs are blends of various compounds that work together to balance the body's various systems while rejuvenating those systems that need help. This allows the Kampo practitioner to make a fairly precise match between the patient's symptoms and the applicable herbs, which both reduces side effects and increases effectiveness.

THE KAMPO VIEW OF HERBS

In Kampo, the primary characteristic of each herb is its *energy*, or the effect it has on the body's basic life-sustaining functions. This is known in the West as its "metabolism" and in Kampo as "qi." Cold or cool herbs slow a person's metabolism, which relieves hot symptoms. Warm or hot herbs accelerate the metabolism, which relieves cold symptoms. Neutral herbs are used to treat either hot or cold symptoms. Some herbs are neither hot nor cold, but are used to redirect energy up or down in the body.

Hot and cold are two of Kampo's eight diagnostic principles, known as the Eight Indicators (see Chapter 1). In addition to hot and cold, herbs can be evaluated in terms of the other six indicators: interior and exterior, excess and deficiency, and yin and yang. Herbs that influence the body's exterior are used to treat symptoms associated with the skin, muscles, and joints. The exterior is associated with excess because that is where the body takes a vigorous stand against disease—for example, the fever and mucus production seen in the flu. Herbs that influence the body's interior are used to treat symptoms associated with the deeper defense levels, involving more of the immune system and circulation through more of the body. The interior is associated with deficiency because the body's defense becomes weaker, or more deficient, as the disease disturbs more and more organ systems. This process first exhausts the body's yang energies, which contain disease, and then exhausts the yin energies, which contain the body's fluids. Herbs can also be thought of as either yang or yin, which are roughly analogous to invigorating the exterior or pacifying a pathogenic influence on the interior, respectively. In addition, herbs can be evaluated in terms of blood, water, and qi, fluids disturbed by the presence of disease.

CONVENTIONAL MEDICINE AND KAMPO HERBS

Although every herb used in Kampo can be explained in the traditional terms used in Oriental medicine, it is not necessary to understand the traditional diagnostic system in order to use the appropriate herbs for healing. A generation of scientific researchers in Japan, the United States, and other countries has verified the ability of Kampo herbs to heal.

Mainstream science has confirmed what Oriental medicine calls the energy characteristics of herbs by studying their effects in the body at a molecular level. For example, analysis has shown that hot herbs induce the body to produce large amounts of a substance called superoxide, a free radical needed to activate certain parts of the immune system. At the same time, cold herbs induce the body to produce large quantities of superoxide dismutases, substances that inhibit free radicals. That prevents excessive stimulation of the immune system, which can result in inflammation and tissue damage.[1] Similar research has confirmed the effectiveness of herbs in terms of yang/yin, interior/exterior, and excess/deficiency. Therefore, Kampo herbs can be understood in terms of disease as defined by Western medicine. In fact, Kampo herbs are often valuable additions, or adjuncts, to a standard treatment plan because they can complement various Western treatments.

A GUIDE TO THE ENTRIES IN THIS CHAPTER

This chapter lists the herbs used in Kampo. It is meant to provide a guide to those herbs used in Part Two, which discusses the individual disorders, and those herbs that are used in Kampo formulas, which are discussed in Chapter 4. (See Appendix A for herb sources.)

Each entry in this chapter starts with a description of the plant. This is followed by some brief notes concerning the herb's use in treating conditions diagnosed in terms of Kampo. (To better understand the terminology used in these notes, see Chapter 1; the organs referred to in these notes are the symbolic organs of Kampo, not organs as defined in conventional medicine.) Scientific investigations of each herb's healing properties are then summarized. Finally, some considerations for use are given, such as the different forms in which an herb might be available. These considerations also include tea-making information, such as the amounts of herb and water used (1 cup of water equals 250 milliliters), steeping time, and daily frequency. (For more information on the tea-making process itself, or on the different types of herbal products available, see Chapter 2.) Specific dosages, including how many cups of tea should be taken each day, are given in Part Two. In a few cases, Kampo herbs are used in different applications, such as poultices. Instructions for such applications are also given in each applicable entry.

Kampo medicines are less likely to cause side effects than Western medications, especially when whole herbs are used in formulas. The fact that the whole herb is used means that compounds generally thought of as "extraneous material" in Western medicine are present to keep the active ingredients from producing toxic consequences. However, any substance that is strong enough to heal may be also strong enough to harm when used improperly or when used for too long a period, and there are Kampo products that can be toxic under certain circumstances. This issue is addressed in each applicable entry, as are those situations that would preclude the herb's use, such as pregnancy or a possibly harmful drug interaction. It is always important to consult a health care provider if there is *any* question as to whether or not a Kampo medication is appropriate in any specific case.

In addition to the herbs themselves, several other traditional medicinal substances are discussed. Finally, this chapter lists several purely modern herbal extracts made from traditional medicinal plants. These extracts are included because of their ready availability and extraordinary usefulness in treating some diseases. (For botanical and other information about each herb, see Appendix B.)

HERBS USED IN KAMPO

The following list is composed of plants that are used in Kampo. Each plant is listed under its English name, followed by its Japanese name.

Aconite / Bushi

Description and Parts Used

Aconite is a flower found in Asia, Europe, and North America. Also known as wolfbane (see "Aconite's Hunting History") and blue monkshood, aconite is related to the garden peony (see page 78) and the ranunculus.

Where aconite is grown is critical to its usefulness as medicine. Aconite grown at an elevation of at least 2,500 feet produces the medically important chemicals known as aconitines. Aconite grown at sea level does not.

In Kampo, aconite is never used until it has been processed. Thick, lengthwise sections of the root are boiled from four to six hours or steamed from six to eight hours to remove toxins. Steam-processed aconite is black and has a dark, oily luster. Water-processed aconite is translucent white with a yellowish tinge, and is moist to the touch.

Aconite's Hunting History

According to Greek mythology, Cerberus, the three-headed dog that guarded the gates of Hades, once spat on aconite, making it a powerful poison. For thousands of years, hunters have used the roots of European aconite—a different species than the aconite that is used in Kampo—to poison the tips of arrows used in hunting wolves, giving it the name *wolfbane*.

Uses in Kampo

According to the Japanese master herbalist Todo Yoshimasu, aconite relieves chills, warms cold hands and feet, and stops pain in the fingers, toes, and joints. Aconite warms the body's energy channels to alleviate pain. It helps move emotional energy through the liver's energy channel, which passes over the middle of the breasts and eyes. Aconite dispels cold blocking the organs, sinews, bones, and blood vessels.

Aconite also balances irregularities in the fluid metabolism of the body. It restrains what Oriental medicine calls the "leakage" of fluids that results in diarrhea. Aconite is particularly useful for diarrhea characterized by undigested food particles in the stool, and that is accompanied by chills, cold hands and feet, and weakness.

Scientific Findings and Clinical Experience

In the doses normally prescribed in Kampo medicine, aconite stimulates the vagus nerve, resulting in a reduced heart rate and dilation of the blood vessels leading to the heart. At the same time, it reduces transmission along the nerves that quicken pulse in times of stress. This makes aconite useful in treating congestive heart failure, as it increases cardiac output, or the amount of blood pumped each minute. It also relieves shortness of breath and edema, the fluid accumulation caused by the heart's inability to move fluid within the body.[1] (In overdose, aconite has the opposite effect, stimulating the heart and sometimes leading to ventricular fibrillation, in which the heart beats irregularly.)

Aconite contains a potent painkiller called mesaconitine, which in pure form is a more potent pain reliever than morphine. It raises the threshold of pain and helps the body attune to both relaxation and stress. In laboratory studies, mesaconitine manipulates the brain's production of norepinephrine, one of the chemicals that "excites" the nervous system. During periods of stress, mesaconitine increases the brain's production of norepinephrine, while during periods of relaxation, it decreases norepinephrine production.[2] Whole processed aconite is about as effective in relieving pain as indomethacin.[3] Aconite also relieves pain by acting as an antihistamine, blocking the effects of histamine that would otherwise produce painful soft-tissue swelling.[4]

Considerations for Use

Never use any aconite product, externally or internally, except under professional supervision. Although Oriental herbal formulas utilize carefully processed forms of the relatively nontoxic species of aconite, *Aconitum carmichaeli*, all aconite products are potentially toxic. Use the exact dosage provided by the herbalist. Never use European aconite (*Aconitum napellus*) internally, and never buy any aconite product from a retailer who does not know the difference between Asian and European aconite.

When making a tea with aconite, either by itself or in formulas, boil the aconite for thirty to sixty minutes before adding any other ingredients. This reduces any potential toxins in the aconite. Aconite in teas usually causes a temporary loss of sensation in the mouth and tongue. This is not a sign to discontinue the formula. Fever, on the other hand, is an indication of overdosage and *is* a sign to discontinue the formula.

A toxic overdose of processed Japanese aconite is 0.5 to 2.0 ounces (15 to 60 grams), or fifteen to sixty times the amount that would be prescribed by an herbalist. The antidote for Japanese aconite is lidocaine, used to stabilize the heart rhythm. Emergency care providers may also administer calcium. There is no antidote for European aconite.

Acorus / Shobu

Description and Parts Used

Acorus, which is similar in appearance to the iris, prefers the wet soil found beside lakes and rivers, and in marshy places. The rhizomes, which have an aromatic, spicy fragrance, are the part of the plant used in Kampo. Acorus is the Japanese relative of the American herb calamus, also known as sweet flag.

Uses in Kampo

Acorus is a warming, bitter herb used to open what are described in Oriental medicine as the "orifices" of the heart, allowing the free flow of emotions. It also "benefits wisdom," or enhances the voluntary control of the body, which makes it useful in the treatment of coma, epilepsy, and poor memory. Acorus also dissolves phlegm, both the "substantial," or physically detectable, phlegm that causes respiratory congestion and the "nonsubstantial," or physically undetectable, phlegm that keeps energy from circulating properly, causing numbness and pain. This herb moves the dampness caused by "cold," or infection, that results in inflammation in the ears, back, sides, or joints, and soothes and "transforms turbid dampness," which relieves bloat and gas from overeating. In addition, acorus vitalizes the senses, which keeps nonsubstantial phlegm from accumulating and causing deafness, dizziness, dulled sensation, or stupor.

Scientific Findings and Clinical Experience

"Opening the orifices of the heart" and "benefiting wisdom" have been the basis for modern Chinese herbal medicine's use of acorus to treat a broad range of brain conditions. It works by protecting brain tissue from free radicals, toxic substances that are formed from oxygen. Any of several conditions that result in inadequate oxygen supply to the brain can result in free-radical damage. These conditions include atherosclerosis, stroke, or a temporary strokelike condition known as transient ischemia. The damage actually occurs when the flow of oxygen to brain tissue is restored, because the previously oxygen-deprived cells are temporarily unable to use all the oxygen available to them.

Free-radical damage can occur months or years after the oxygen deprivation preceding it. For this reason, acorus is helpful even if taken years after the onset of the condition that reduced the oxygen supply. Tissue damage in the brain can lead to memory loss or seizures. Acorus also helps prevent this reaction and treats memory loss and seizures. It is most effective when given *before* circulation is restored, that is, in the first few days to a month after a head injury or stroke.

Acorus is particularly effective in preventing damage to the part of the brain known as the amygdala. When the amygdala is damaged, the sight and scent of food do not motivate eating. In experimental studies, acorus cures appetite loss caused by brain damage. Extensive animal testing of acorus-containing preparations shows that such preparations help repair damage to memory caused by defects in the amygdala.[1]

Acorus also affects the brain during withdrawal from cocaine, heroin, and morphine. During the first one to ten days of withdrawal, the addict experiences intense drug cravings, and nausea and vomiting. Acorus can blunt gastric upset during the acute phase of drug withdrawal, although it has no effect on the cravings themselves. However, acorus has effect on long-term drug cravings in the later stages of withdrawal. In this phase the brain can be stimulated by nondrug opiates, such as those found in wheat products, beef, and milk in particular, and those the body produces during meditation. Acorus seems to accentuate the process by which the brain recognizes these nondrug opiates.

Acorus quells the nausea of drug withdrawal through its ability to prevent the secretion of histamine. This chemical causes swelling, and its attendant inflammation and pain. The antihistamine in acorus, known as alpha-asarone, can also reduce allergic, arthritic, and asthmatic inflammation. Scientists have also identified other compounds in acorus that act on body chemicals other than histamine to stop bronchial constriction during asthmatic attacks.[2]

Considerations for Use

Acorus is most commonly supplied by TCM practitioners, and is usually sold in the United States as *Chang Pu* or *Shi Chang Pu*. The herb is given in the form of teas, powders, and tinctures, typically in a dosage corresponding to 1 to 2 grams (about the size of an eraser on a pencil) of the raw herb. Small chunks of dried or "rock" acorus are used in formulas (see Chapter 4) for the treatment of anorexia, cocaine addiction, memory loss, and seizure disorders, while slices of rhizome are used in the treatment of allergy, arthritis, and inner ear infection. Use the herb in teas as directed by the herbalist.

Calamus, the American relative of acorus, contains the potentially cancer-causing chemical beta-asarone. Calamus has been banned for use in the United States. Although acorus is legal in North America, many other countries ban the use of both acorus and calamus in herbal medicine. Acorus should *never* be used without professional supervision.

Agrimony / Senkakuso

Description and Parts Used

Agrimony has paired leaves, green above and silvery beneath, growing along a three-foot stem. It is harvested in the summer, when it produces yellow flowers clustered at the top. All of the above-ground parts of the plant are used in Kampo. Agrimony is also known as cocklebur.

Uses in Kampo

Kampo uses agrimony for its restraining qualities. It stops bleeding and restrains blood leaking from the nose, gums, bladder, or uterus. It is also used when the patient is vomiting or coughing blood. In addition, agrimony is used to restrain diarrhea and dysentery, and to kill parasites, in particular tapeworm and trichomonas vaginitis, a sexually transmitted disease that causes discharge and intense itching.

Scientific Findings and Clinical Experience

Agrimony has been used for thousands of years to stop wound bleeding and to encourage clot formation. Agrimony acts by "tanning" skin cells, making them impermeable to bleeding. This action also prevents bacteria from entering the wound. Agrimony also "tans" cells in the interior of the body, which makes it effective against diarrhea, gastroenteritis, and sore throat, especially in small children. In China, agrimony powder is commonly used to stop bleeding due to trauma or surgery.

Agrimony not only affects bleeding, it also affects blood pressure. In small doses, it tightens blood vessels and thereby increases blood pressure. In large doses, it relaxes blood vessels and lowers blood pressure.

Agrimony contains the chemical agrimophol, which expels parasites. Agrimophol causes the parasite to lose its hold on the body, so that it can be evacuated through the stool or urine. This chemical kills the organisms that cause river blindness, a tropical disease in which parasites infest the eye, and many common bacteria, including *E. coli* and *Staphylococcus*, as well as the deadly bacteria dysentery and typhoid.

New applications for agrimony continue to be found. Animal experiments indicate that agrimony infusions can prevent the development of type 1 diabetes. Agrimony reduces the increase in blood sugar that occurs when insulin is deficient, and counters the excessive thirst that accompanies this disease.[1]

Agrimony also affects the immune system. It stimulates the body to produce immune bodies known as B cells. These cells produce complex chemicals known as antigens that attack invading infectious microbes. Certain kinds of cancer, including chronic leukemia, multiple myeloma, and ovarian cancer, deplete the body's supply of B-cells. Recovery from these kinds of cancer is helped by taking agrimony. In addition, agrimony is helpful in preventing some cases of male breast cancer (see "Breast Cancer in Men" on page 169.)

Considerations for Use

To make agrimony tea, simmer 1.5 teaspoons (1.5 grams) of finely chopped herb in 1 cup of water for five minutes, and strain. Agrimony's low toxicity makes it particularly suitable for children's illnesses.

Because of its effects on the immune system, persons with rheumatoid arthritis, myasthenia gravis, or one of many other autoimmune diseases (including Grave's disease, Hashimoto's hypothyroiditis, lupus, and Sjögren's syndrome) should avoid agrimony.

Akebia (Mu Tong) / Mokutsu

Description and Parts Used

Akebia is a gracefully branching, red-flowered, five-leaved plant. Its name originally meant "open-ended wood." The part of akebia used in Kampo is the stem, which Chinese herbalists call *mu tong*. In Chinese formulas, wild ginger or clematis may be substituted for akebia.

Uses in Kampo

Akebia moves fluids in the body, acting as a diuretic. Akebia also lubricates the joints and the nine orifices: the eyes, ears, nose, mouth, anus, and urethra. This allows the easy passage of the fluids, solids, and phlegm these orifices conduct. Traditional Japanese medicine used akebia in the treatment of gonorrhea, urinary tract infection, swelling due to poor circulation, and jaundice. Stewed akebia and pork knuckle is a Japanese home remedy to stimulate milk production in nursing mothers.

Scientific Findings and Clinical Experience

Akebia stops the process of inflammation by deactivating hormones that allow the capillaries to transport fluids into tissues, since fluid swells soft tissues.[1] Akebia extracts stimulate urination and sedate the central nervous system. They have weak fever-reducing and pain-relieving actions, and stimulate movement of the muscles lining the intestines, which tends to relieve constipation.[2]

Considerations for Use

Akebia is used in Kampo formulas, rather than by itself. Used by itself, this herb can cause excessive urination and dehydration. Akebia should not be used during pregnancy. Formulas that contain akebia (see Chapter 4) usually include herbs that prevent excessive urination.

Alisma / Takusha

Description and Parts Used

Alisma is an aquatic plant also known as the water plantain. Kampo formulas use thick cross sections of the root.

Alisma is a diuretic, but its strength depends on the season in which it is harvested: Winter-harvested alisma is the most potently diuretic, spring-harvested the least. How the herb is preserved is also important. Using wine or bran as a preservative conserves alisma's diuretic effect, while using brine destroys the effect. That is because alisma contains large amounts of potassium, which the body excretes unless the potassium is balanced with sodium from salt, such as that found in brine.

Uses in Kampo

According to the Kampo text *Essentials from the Golden Cabinet,* alisma stimulates deficient kidneys to promote the flow of water. This effect is often referred to as "leaching out dampness," and prevents stagnation of fluids associated with problems such as diarrhea, edema (swelling), and urinary difficulty. This action also dispels damp-heat infections of the vagina and urinary tract.

Ancient Japanese herbalists recommended alisma in the treatment of diseases related to fluid imbalances in the ear, such as dizziness and tinnitus, or ringing in the ears. The effect was understood as quenching kidney fire, which rises to the ear.

Scientific Findings and Clinical Experience

Alisma increases the excretion of sodium, chloride, and urea, lowering both blood pressure and blood-sugar levels.[1,2] It is a rich source of potassium. The herb also lowers cholesterol levels, although not triglyceride levels. In addition, alisma contains chemicals that stimulate immune-system cells to eat disease-causing bacteria and yeasts, particularly candida.[3]

Considerations for Use

Kampo generally uses alisma in formulas (see Chapter 4). In TCM, alisma is not recommended for men prior to attempts to conceive a child, since it is thought to lead to a loss of *jing,* or essence, being passed to the child.

Aloe / Rokai

Description and Parts Used

Aloe, or aloe vera, is a prickly, gray-green succulent native to Africa but cultivated around the world for centuries. It is a perennial with leaves up to two feet long and spikes of yellow or orange flowers. The leaf contains a clear gel that is used topically, while the dried yellow sap taken from the leaf base, known as aloe bitters, is used internally.

Uses in Kampo

Aloe has been used in Kampo medicine since the fourth century B.C.[1] Kampo uses aloe bitters to guide out accumulation, which makes this herb useful in treating constipation, dizziness, red eyes, and irritability due to fever and accumulated heat. Aloe is used to treat liver fire, the cumulative result of dietary or emotional excesses that causes headache, tension below the rib cage, and ringing in the ear. Aloe bitters are also used to kill parasites, especially roundworms in children, and to strengthen digestion.

Scientific Findings and Clinical Experience

Aloe's traditional reputation as a wound and burn healer has been verified by modern research. In animal studies, aloe vera sap activates macrophages, immune-system cells that fight bacterial infection, which allows burns to heal cleanly.[2,3] The sap also stimulates surface blood circulation, which accelerates wound healing. Clinical studies have confirmed that burns and cuts treated with aloe vera gel heal more quickly.[4,5] Aloe has also been shown to rejuvenate sun-aged skin,[6] and to help heal frostbite by increasing the effectiveness of pentoxifylline (Trental), a prescription drug.[7]

Aloe is effective against eczema and psoriasis. A potent anti-inflammatory chemical in aloe is as effective as hydrocortisone in treating skin irritation without hydrocortisone's detrimental effects on the immune system,[8] and aloe gel can be used with hydrocortisone to increase the latter's effectiveness.[9] In a study involving sixty volunteers, daily use of aloe vera gel cured more than 80 percent of the volunteers' psoriasis problems, compared with 7 percent for those treated with the inert placebo substance.[10]

Aloe's positive effects on the immune system make it an important weapon in the fight against cancer. Alo A, one of aloe's active substances, stimulates various components of the immune system.[11-13] This stops both inflammation[14] and the growth of tumors.[15] In a skin cancer study involving animals, aloe gel and vitamin E cream together produced remission approximately 33 percent of the time, compared with 3 percent when no treatment was given.[16] In addition, certain compounds in aloe seem to prevent cancer-causing substances from entering liver tissue. By keeping potential carcinogens from entering the liver, rather than changing the chemistry of the liver itself (like many other cancer treatments), aloe compounds do not cause the liver to create new carcinogens while it deactivates others.[17]

Some clinics have used aloe vera to increase the effectiveness of cancer treatment with the chemotherapy agents cyclophosphamide and 5-fluorouracil,[18] and several studies indicate that aloe vera gel can protect both the immune system and the skin from the effects of radiation treatment.[19,20] In addition, at least one study suggests that aloe juice can reduce the likelihood of lung cancer in smokers.[21]

Aloe has been used to fight viral infections. In a Chinese trial, aloe vera injections appeared to reduce liver damage in 87 percent of hepatitis A patients,[22] and research at the University of Maryland has found that one of aloe's compounds, aloe-emodin, kills the viruses that cause herpes and shingles, as well as some flu viruses.[23]

Aloe has also proven useful in managing blood sugar, cholesterol, and triglycerides. In one five-year study, 3,167 diabetic patients with atherosclerotic heart disease were given 120 grams of parboiled aloe leaves for lunch and dinner each day. The patients showed marked decreases in levels of cholesterol, triglycerides, and sugar.[24] In another test, one in which diabetic patients were given a spoonful of aloe extract with water at every meal for fourteen weeks, the average fasting blood-sugar level fell from a very high 273 milligrams per deciliter to a slightly elevated 151 milligrams per deciliter.[25] Aloe seems to act by stimulating the pancreas to secrete insulin. For this reason, it is potentially helpful only for diabetics who do not have to take insulin. However, one of aloe's strengths is that it does not cause weight gain, a common side effect of some diabetes medications.[26]

Aloe bitters are effective against constipation. When compared with other herbal stimulant laxatives, aloe draws less fluid into the large intestine from the rest of the body, and thus is less likely to cause dehydration or electrolyte disturbances.[27] However, aloe will have little or no laxative effect when taken with antibiotics, as the drugs will kill the friendly intestinal bacteria that make this herb effective.[28]

Aloe has a variety of other uses. Alo A soothes peptic-ulcer inflammation caused by excess acid and stomach-irritating drugs,[29] although it is not effective against ulcers in which stress is a prominent factor.[30] Another compound, aloin, helps prevent alcoholic intoxication, probably by preventing the passage of alcohol from the intestines into the bloodstream.[31,32] Finally, tests at the University of Missouri indicate that aloe vera gel and zinc acetate together form an effective contraceptive gel. The zinc protects the female partner from viral infection, while the aloe serves as a contraceptive.[33]

Considerations for Use

Use aloe gels for skin problems, bitters for constipation, and juice for other disorders, as directed in Part Two. Aloe is also used in formulas (see Chapter 4). Aloe vera gels, either commercially produced or taken from one's own plants, may be applied liberally to the skin as desired. Leaves up to one foot long may be removed from the plant without causing damage. The best time of day for cutting aloe leaves is the midafternoon, when the plant has moved a maximum amount of sap into the leaf.

Any laxative, herbal or otherwise, affects the rate at which other orally administered drugs are absorbed into the bloodstream. Therefore, prescription medication and laxatives should be taken at different times. Long-term use (more than two weeks) of aloe is not recommended because the fluid drawn into the stool can result in depletion of electrolytes, especially potassium, and especially when taken with diuretic drugs.

Aloe should not be taken *internally* during pregnancy or menstruation, or in cases of rectal bleeding, although it may be used externally under these conditions. Scientists have debated whether or not aloe-emodin, aloe's laxative compound, can damage colon cells. The most recent finding is that when taken as directed, aloe poses no risk of causing cancer or genetic damage.[34] Among persons who abuse aloe and similar laxative herbs over a period of at least a year, *and* develop other colon changes, about 3 percent will develop colorectal cancer.[35] This compares with the approximately 4 percent of the population at large who will develop colorectal cancer at some point in their lives. Stopping aloe use before twenty weeks have passed gives the body a chance to reverse its effects. Aloe juice does not carry the risks of aloe bitters.

Amaranth (Achyranthis) / Dogoshitsu (tuniuxi root) / Goshitsu (achyranthis root)

Description and Parts Used

Amaranth provides both a medicinal root and a nutritious grain, and several different species are used in Kampo (see Appendix B). Amaranth root is sold either raw or soaked in sake. The raw root is used in formulas that activate blood circulation, while the sake-soaked root is used in formulas that treat lower body pains, and strengthen bones and tendons. The sake-soaked root is also used in kidney and liver tonics.

Uses in Kampo

In traditional Japanese herbalism, amaranth tonifies the kidney and liver. This dispels stagnant blood and drains pus. Amaranth also induces the downward flow of blood. This action restrains reckless blood that moves upward in the body to cause nosebleed, toothache, and bleeding gums.

As amaranth brings the functions of the kidney and liver back into balance, it benefits the knees and lower back by relieving pain caused by qi deficiency, or energy deficiency. By invigorating the blood, amaranth breaks loose the static blood that causes menstrual problems and vaginal discharges following childbirth. Stimulating blood flow corrects conditions secondary to menstrual irregularity: blurred vision, cramping, headache, and muscle tension, among others. It also clears up vaginal discharges due to infection and urinary problems.

Scientific Findings and Clinical Experience

The chemical ecdysterone, found in amaranth, strengthens the heartbeat and prevents high blood-sugar levels in laboratory tests.[1] Amaranth also causes blood vessels near the surface of the body to dilate, which reduces blood pressure. In animal tests, amaranth extracts have both a contraceptive and an abortion-producing effect.[2]

Considerations for Use

Make amaranth tea by simmering 2 to 4 tablespoons (15 to 30 grams) of the dried herb (which may be labeled *Niu Xi* or *Tu Niu Xi* in herb shops) in 1 cup of water for fifteen to twenty minutes. Strain before drinking. Amaranth is also used in several formulas (see Chapter 4).

Since amaranth can induce abortion in laboratory animals, it should not be used during pregnancy. Similarly, it should not be used by women who wish to conceive. This restriction does not apply to amaranth cereal.

American Ginseng / Seiyojin

Description and Parts Used

In appearance, American ginseng is a smaller version of its more-famous Chinese cousin (see page 57), with its saw-toothed leaves, red berries, and thick, fleshy root. The root, coarsely chopped, is the part used in Kampo. A good-quality root has first a sweet and then a bitter flavor as it is chewed. For most applications, wildcrafted American ginseng is more effective than field-grown ginseng. (To find out how Oriental medicine learned about American ginseng, see "Ginseng Among the Native Americans.")

Uses in Kampo

In Kampo, American ginseng is employed as a tonic to reinforce the body's yin, or constraining functions, and to treat fever. It is especially useful for treating disorders of the lungs, characterized by wheezing and coughing of blood-streaked sputum. It also aids in recovery after fever by treating irritability, weakness, and thirst.

In the practice of TCM in the United States, American ginseng is a very important cooling herb. According to the theory underlying both TCM and Kampo, years of abuse of the body through continual consumption of fatty and spicy foods and through inability to express emotions accumulates in the liver. Eventually the liver is so overburdened with food and emotional energy that it catches "fire." The fire spreads everywhere the liver's energy channel crosses the body. It produces headache, eye inflammation, and breast pain, and predisposes the other parts of the body it crosses to accidental injury. American ginseng "quenches" liver fire. Unlike the better-known Korean or red ginseng, American ginseng cools the body and can be taken on a regular basis through the summer months.

Scientific Findings and Clinical Experience

Like other forms of ginseng, American ginseng traditionally has been applied to restoring health after long periods of illness or prolonged stress. Although this use of the herb has not been validated in scientific testing, anecdotal reports of recovery of health and strength date back 300 years in both China and North America.

Compounds in American ginseng prevent memory deficits in laboratory test animals by increasing the brain's production of acetylcholine. Acetylcholine is an important neurotransmitter, or a chemical that transmits messages between neurons. These ginseng compounds do not, as do most medical treatments for memory loss, stop the action of enzymes that break down acetylcholine to provide needed building blocks for brain tissue.[1]

American ginseng contains compounds that regulate the strength of heartbeat. When there is excess potassium these compounds, called saponins, slow the rate at which heart muscle fibers contract. When there is a potassium deficiency, saponins increase the strength with which heart muscle fibers contract.[2] Other studies have also confirmed the herb's effects on blood pressure.[3]

Ginseng Among the Native Americans

Ginseng has been enormously popular in China for thousands of years. By the beginning of the sixteenth century, supplies of wild ginseng were growing scarce, so the Chinese were forced to look for other sources. Amazingly, an almost identical plant grew in North America, and Native Americans had also put it to medicinal use.

In 1709, Petrus Jartoux, a Jesuit missionary to China, received four pieces of ginseng after accompanying a mapping expedition. He found himself so reinvigorated by the herb after his exhausting journey that he published his observations in the *Philosophical Transactions of the Royal Society of London.* Father Jartoux noted that he thought that the plant could be found in the cold, damp forests of French Canada, similar to the areas of China where it grew wild. Another Jesuit missionary who was working among the Mohawk tribe in Quebec, Père Lafitau, read Father Jartoux's account in 1714. Lafitau promptly located the same plant, called *gar-ent-oguen* or "man plant" by the Iroquois.

This plant turned out to have the same medicinal qualities as Chinese ginseng. Not only did the Iroquois use the same plant, but they used it for the same purposes as the Chinese. By 1748, the Jesuits were selling tons of Canadian ginseng in China for the then-unimaginable price of five dollars a pound.

Ginseng was used throughout North America. The Cherokee tribe of North Carolina called ginseng "the plant of life" and used the root for cramps, dysmenorrhea, and the pain that we would now identify as premenstrual syndrome. The Potawatomi used ginseng to mask the unpleasant tastes of other medicines. The Alabamans took ginseng for stomach pains and nausea, and used it to pack wounds to stop bleeding. The Creeks used ginseng for bronchial disease, cough, croup, and fever. The Menominee used ginseng as the Chinese did, to stimulate mental capacity and as a general tonic.

But one of the most unusual uses of ginseng came from the Pawnee, who combined ginseng with two other herbs into a love potion. Possession of this medicine served to attract all persons to the holder, regardless of animosities. If the hair of a desired woman was added to the mixture, she was said to be incapable of resistance.

American ginseng does not lower blood pressure during acute stress. However, over the span of one to three months, it regulates the body's production of stress hormones. Then, the next time the individual is exposed to stress, stress reactions are greatly reduced.

Various Native American groups used American ginseng in the treatment of female infertility, although no clinical studies have confirmed the usefulness of the herb for this purpose. However, it is known that American ginseng shares compounds with Chinese ginseng that stimulate the pituitary gland to in turn stimulate growth of the uterine lining.[4]

American ginseng is also being tested as a source of compounds for use in the treatment of leukemia.[5]

Considerations for Use

Make American ginseng tea (available as *Xi Yang Shen* or Wild American Ginseng) by simmering 1 to 3 tablespoons (3 to 9 grams) of the herb in 3 cups of water for forty-five minutes, and straining. American ginseng is also available in tincture form, and is used in formulas (see Chapter 4). This herb should not be used when the stomach does not produce enough acid to properly digest food.

Anemarrhena / Chimo

Description and Parts Used

Anemarrhena is a perennial lily with thin leaves up to twenty-eight inches long and clusters of small white or light purple flowers. Native to northern China, anemarrhena grows wild on exposed slopes and hills. The thick rhizome is used in Kampo.

Uses in Kampo

Japanese herbalists prescribe anemarrhena to treat heat in the hands and feet, and fever with discomfort. Anemarrhena clears heat and drains fire, relieving high fever, irritability, and thirst. The herb also treats cough due to heat in the lungs accompanied by the expectoration of thick, yellow sputum.

An important kidney disorder for which both Kampo and TCM use anemarrhena is "wasting and thirsting" disorder, better known in the West as diabetes. Many diabetics have found that anemarrhena preparations lower blood-sugar levels when mainstream medications have failed.

Scientific Findings and Clinical Experience

Anemarrhena is an antidiabetic herb. Laboratory experiments with test animals in Japan indicate that the herb can lower blood-sugar levels by increasing production of glycogen, the main form of stored carbohydrate in the body.[1] Glycogen is made from glucose, or blood sugar, so the more glycogen the body produces, the less glucose there is in the bloodstream.

Anemarrhena is also an antibiotic herb. Anemarrhena teas inhibit the bacteria that cause cholera, salmonella poisoning, and staph infections, among others.[2] This makes it useful in treatment of the diarrhea caused by food poisoning.

Considerations for Use

Anemarrhena appears in many formulas (see Chapter 4).

Angelica Dahurica (Wild Angelica) / Byakushi

Description and Parts Used

Angelica dahurica is a three- to seven-foot sturdy shrub topped with flowers similar to those found on Queen Anne's lace. It has a hollow stem with three-branched leaves. Although angelica dahurica is used more extensively in traditional Japanese medicine than in other Asian herbal systems, it does not grow wild in Japan and must be imported from China.

The herb is harvested between summer and autumn, when the leaves turn yellow. The root is cut lengthwise into thin slices when used in teas.

Uses in Kampo

Kampo uses angelica dahurica to treat menstrual cramps and gastrointestinal spasms. Japanese herbalists also prescribed angelica dahurica for headaches caused by "stagnant pathogens," or digestive-tract diseases that neither improve nor worsen, and for painful swellings in the face, including swollen sinuses. If a sore has not yet discharged, this herb will help reduce the swelling. If pus has formed or the sore has ulcerated, angelica helps discharge pus. It also stops vaginal discharge.

Scientific Findings and Clinical Experience

Angelica dahurica is useful in cases of heart attack. It contains several compounds similar to the heart drug warfarin sodium (Coumadin), one of which opens the coronary vessels and increases circulation to the heart.

Other chemicals in angelica fight weight gain, one of the more troubling side effects of oral medications for diabetes. Most of the older oral medications for diabetes act by stimulating the pancreas to make insulin. Insulin not only transports glucose into all the cells of the body, it also transports fat into fat cells. Chemicals found in angelica dahurica stop this process and thus prevent weight gain.[1] This also makes angelica useful in treating weight gain in people who show early signs of diabetes, possibly delaying or preventing full-blown symptoms.

Angelica is a potent bactericide. This herb can stop the growth of *E. coli,* a common cause of diarrhea. Angelica dahurica also kills the bacteria that cause dysentery and typhoid fever,[2] as well as the microorganisms that cause shigella and salmonella.[3]

Considerations for Use

To make angelica dahurica tea, simmer 1 to 3 tablespoons (3 to 9 grams) of the herb in 3 cups of water for forty-five minutes, and strain. This herb has a very distinctive aftertaste: acrid, bitter, and lastingly pungent. To avoid the taste, use the freeze-dried root in gel-cap form. Angelica is also used in several formulas (see Chapter 4).

Angelica dahurica should not be used during pregnancy.

Apricot Seed / Kyonin

Description and Parts Used

Kampo teas use whole or broken kernels taken from the pit of the apricot, the common fruit.

Uses in Kampo

Both Japanese and Chinese herbalists use apricot seed to expel fluid and mucus that have become stagnant in the throat or chest. According to the classic Kampo texts, apricot seed treats cough, shortness of breath, pain and distention over the stomach, chest pain, and edema, or swelling, throughout the body.

Scientific Findings and Clinical Experience

Once inside the human digestive tract, apricot seed releases hydrogen cyanide, or cyanic acid. This small amount of cyanic acid stimulates the brain's respiratory center and produces a tranquilizing effect. It also produces the antiasthmatic effects this herb exerts in Kampo formulas.[1]

Some apricot seed extracts may help protect cells against the cancer-causing effects of toxic chemicals, including benzopyrenes and acrylamides.[2] Other studies indicate that apricot seeds contain compounds that act like human follicle-stimulating hormone (FSH), which encourages the ovary to produce estrogen.

Considerations for Use

Apricot seeds appear in formulas dispensed by Kampo and TCM practitioners. Dosages usually range from 1 to 3 tablespoons (3 to 9 grams), as measured by the herbalist. Apricot seed teas should always be strained before drinking.

Never eat apricot seeds! Eating apricot seeds can result in dizziness, nausea, vomiting, and headache, which can progress to breathing difficulties, spasms, dilated pupils, cardiac arrhythmias, coma, and even death. Lethal doses range from 50.0 to 60.0 grams. (The lethal dose is 10.0 grams for small children, so store apricot seeds carefully if there are children in the household.) Emergency treatment for apricot-seed poisoning usually requires activated charcoal and syrup of ipecac. The bark and root of the tree itself form Kampo's traditional antidote. In formulas, other herbs counteract apricot seed's toxicity (see Chapter 4).

Amygdaline from apricot seeds is the basis of the discredited cancer cure laetrile. Although apricot seed may contain some compounds useful in the prevention of cancer, no scientific studies show that it is useful in treating cancer once it has appeared.

Arisaema / Tennansho

Description and Parts Used

Arisaema, also known as wild turnip, is a perennial herb found in eastern Asia. It reaches a height of three feet, and has star-shaped leaves with pitcherlike green or purple-white flower bracts.

The root of the herb is dug in autumn and dried for medicinal use. The mealy, milk-white corm of arisaema is odorless, but when chewed, it causes an intensely acrid and persistent impression on the lips and tongue, like that of a severe scald.

Uses in Kampo

Kampo medicine uses arisaema to dry dampness and expel phlegm. (To find out how this usage was almost lost, see "Arisaema, the Lost Herb".) Arisaema is particularly useful for stubborn chest congestion. It also expels "wind-phlegm," an energy imbalance that upsets the nervous system, which manifests itself as dizziness, numbness in the hands or feet, muscle spasms, or seizures. Japanese herbalists recommend arisaema for relief of intensely sore throat, bleeding, and swelling of throat and tongue.

Arisaema, the Lost Herb

Arisaema is unique in Kampo in that its use was lost for approximately 1,000 years. The herbal source book, *The Materia Medica of Shen Nung,* written in A.D. 200, listed arisaema. When the book was recopied in the tenth century, the scribes incorrectly copied the characters for arisaema, and the reference to the herb in Kampo medicine was lost. The respect for the source books of Kampo was so great that only in 1993 did arisaema reappear in historical reference books about Kampo, when Chinese scholars found the transcription error.[1]

Scientific Findings and Clinical Experience

In one Chinese study, treatment with arisaema improved outcomes in 78 percent of cervical cancer cases.[1] In another Chinese study, 105 women with stage II or stage III cervical cancer (in a five-stage system) were given a combination of arisaema and radiation therapy. In twenty cases the cancer disappeared, and in another forty-six the cancer did not spread.[2]

Considerations for Use

Raw, unprocessed arisaema is potentially toxic. In this fom, it is used only as a topical ointment for the relief of inward-sinking abscesses, swelling and pain after trauma, and swollen joints. The root is always peeled before use. When raw arisaema is included in formulas for internal use, it is used in very small amounts (300 to 1,000 milligrams) and balanced by fresh ginger, which reduces its toxicity. The antidote for numbness of the tongue after taking arisaema is granulated sugar.

Traditional Chinese herb shops sell arisaema that has been processed with pig bile. If dietary restrictions preclude pork consumption, ask the herbalist about alternative treatments. Also, arisaema is incompatible with ginseng (see page 57), and will nullify any benefits received from ginseng treatment.

Artemisia / INCHINKO

Description and Parts Used

Artemisia, more commonly known as wormwood, is a bushy perennial that grows from two to four feet high and bears tiny, yellow-green flowers from July to October. Kampo uses broken pieces taken from the top of the plant. Unfortunately, a misunderstanding about wormwood's chemical properties has led some to condemn artemisia as a dangerous drug—see "Misunderstood Artemisia."

Uses in Kampo

Artemisia is a bitter, cooling, drying herb that promotes the flow of fluids within the body. Kampo practioners use artemisia to treat jaundice, gallbladder inflammation, infectious hepatitis, skin diseases with itching and burning, and fever. It relieves jaundice by clearing damp heat, or infection, from the liver and gallbladder. Artemisia also clears heat and releases the exterior of the body to deal with symptoms such as fever and chills, bitter taste in the mouth, stifling sensation in the chest, pain in the side, dizziness, nausea, and loss of appetite.

Artemisia increases a woman's chances of conception. Kampo uses tea prepared from the charred herb to prevent threatened miscarriage when there is vaginal bleeding.

Misunderstood Artemisia

Several herb handbooks warn that artemisia may have intoxicating effects similar to those produced by marijuana. Whether one considers this to be desirable or undesirable, it is simply not true.

This misunderstanding stems from the use of a form of artemisia known as absinthe, a fashionable drink in the nineteenth century. The herb became associated with the death of Poe and the suicide of Van Gogh. It was immortalized in a painting by Degas, which shows a haunting portrait of two absinthe drinkers: hollow-eyed, oblivious to all but the intoxicating beverage. However, the absinthe drinkers in the picture were merely models who later appeared in festive scenes by Renoir.

Thujone, the intoxicating chemical in artemisia, and tetrahydrocannabinol (THC), the active ingredient of marijuana, have similar molecules, and both attach to the same receptor sites in the brain. However, the thujone content of alcoholic beverages containing artemisia is less than one twentieth of the amount needed for intoxication. Any high from artemisia comes from the alcohol in which it is dissolved.

Scientific Findings and Clinical Experience

Artemisia is a proven cholagogue, that is, it stimulates the gallbladder to release bile.[1] Noted American Kampo authorities Dan Bensky and Andrew Gamble cite two studies on artemisia's usefulness in treating infectious hepatitis. In one study, thirty-two patients with infectious hepatitis were treated with from 30 to 45 grams of artemisia three times a day. In all cases fever subsided quickly, jaundice disappeared, and the liver returned to normal size. The average length of treatment was seven days, and there were no reports of side effects or relapses. In the other study, thirteen patients with infectious hepatitis were treated with a combination of artemisia, licorice, jujube fruit (see pages 63 and 66), and sugar. In this study, patients recovered from fever in about three days and appetite loss in little over four days, and saw their jaundice disappear in about seven and a half days. Liver size returned to normal in ten days.[2]

Artemisia is an important treatment for malaria, a disease common in tropical areas. It contains a chemical, artemisine, that acts against *Plasmodium falciparum,* a serious form of malaria for which artemisine is one of a very few treatments. Artemisine is also effective against the organisms that cause river blindness.[3] Finally artemisia treats urinary tract infection caused by *Klebsiella.*[4]

Considerations for Use

To make artemisia tea, simmer 1/2 to 1 teaspoon (0.75 to 1.5 grams) of the herb in 1 cup of water for ten minutes, strain, and drink. Do not use more than 3 teaspoons in any one day, unless directed to do so by an experienced herbal practitioner. Take before meals for hepatitis treatment or to stimulate appetite, and after meals to stimulate the gallbladder. Artemisia is also available in tincture form.

Asiasarum / SAISHIN

Description and Parts Used

Asiasarum is also known as asarum and Chinese wild ginger. The plant bears large, heart-shaped leaves atop trailing stems, and flowers growing from the nodes between the leaves and the stem. Good quality asiasarum makes the tongue numb.

Uses in Kampo

The Japanese name for asiasarum literally means "thin pungent one." The Japanese herbal classics describe asiasarum as an herb that induces sweating to release pathogens that have become stagnant in the chest and diaphragm. Acrid and pungent asiasarum disperses and unblocks the qi, or energy, of the nasal orifices to relieve various types of nasal congestion. Kampo also uses the extremely pungent asiasarum to stimulate circulation to the periphery of the body in order to expel pathogens. All of these effects together account for asiasarum's traditional use as a smelling salt.

Asiasarum exerts most of its effects on the upper half of the body. For this reason, it is useful for arthritic inflammation of the neck and shoulders, colds, cough, earaches, flu, headaches, lung congestion, nasal congestion, and toothaches. A massage with asiasarum oil is the standard remedy in Japan for arthritic spine and joint problems.

Scientific Findings and Clinical Experience

Asiasarum has several different effects. Several plant chemicals isolated from asiasarum have been shown to be potently antiallergenic in animal studies.[1] In other studies, asiasarum has shown itself to be a good antibiotic, effective against *Salmonella, Shigella,* and *Streptococcus.*[2] In Japan, asiasarum, when combined with other herbs, is a common remedy for allergies, colds, and flu, and is used to stimulate respiration in cases of fainting or mild shock. Asiasarum also has anesthetic effects. Putting asiasarum powder on inflamed gums relieves gum pain and toothache for about ninety minutes.[3] Asiasarum also lowers body temperature, whether or not there is fever. Finally asiasarum treats premenstrual back pain that occurs in the small of the back and is worse on taking a deep breath.[4]

Japanese researchers have found that asiasarum has potent applications in the treatment of many purely modern diseases. Asiasarum stimulates the immune system's production of B cells, which are depleted in chronic lymphocytic leukemia, multiple myeloma, and ovarian carcinoma. It also stimulates the activity of the "germ-eating" cells known as macrophages, which are suppressed by all forms of cancer that originate in bone, as well as by carcinomas of the bladder, breast, kidney, lung, prostate, and thyroid that have spread to bone. It affects still other immune-system cells known as T cells, which are suppressed in all forms of carcinoma once it has spread.

Considerations for Use

Asiasarum is used in Kampo formulas (see Chapter 4). While this is a potentially toxic herb, formulas always combine asiasarum in small doses and with other herbs to reduce its potential for harm. This herb is also available as a painkilling massage oil, which should *not* be taken internally.

Asparagus Root / Tenmondo

Description and Parts Used

Asparagus root is the winter-dug tuber of the garden plant, asparagus. Good quality root is a translucent yellow-white. The species of asparagus used in Japan and China is not the same as the species of asparagus grown in North and South America, Australia, and Europe, but both varieties of the plant have the same medicinal uses.

Uses in Kampo

The primary use of asparagus root in Kampo is to "nourish the kidneys." Asparagus root is a gentle diuretic that is especially appropriate for diabetics. In formulas, it relieves fevers and "dry" respiratory symptoms, such as dry mouth, unproductive cough, and chest congestion with phlegm that is hard to cough up.

Scientific Findings and Clinical Experience

Herbalists Dan Bensky and Andrew Gamble report that asparagus root teas have an antibiotic effect on many kinds of bacteria, including three strains of *Streptococcus* and the common skin infection *Staphylococcus aureus.* They also report that asparagus root extracts stop the growth of human leukemia cells in laboratory conditions.[1] *The German Commission E Monographs,* a scientific reference work on medicinal herbs, reports that asparagus root is useful for preventing kidney gravel, or small stones.

Considerations for Use

To make asparagus root tea, simmer 1 teaspoon (1.5 grams) of chopped root in 1 cup of water for forty-five minutes, then strain. Drink between meals. When taking asparagus tea, be sure to maintain adequate potassium supplies by taking the commercial preparation Slo-K or by eating fruits and vegetables. Asparagus stems eaten as a vegetable also have a mild diuretic effect.

Asparagus root is also used in Kampo formulas (see Chapter 4). Do not use formulas containing this herb if there is loss of appetite or diarrhea, or if there are aches and pains from influenza.

Astragalus / Ogi

Description and Parts Used

Astragalus, also known as milk vetch root and locoweed, is a bushy member of the legume family. Its hairy stems grow to a height of sixteen inches. Kampo uses long, thin, diagonal sections of astragalus root that show the exterior at each end. The root should be long, thick, and firm, and have a sweet taste.

Uses in Kampo

Ancient Japanese herbalists used astragalus to treat fluid in the skin associated with the initial stages of infection in the Lesser Yang (one of Kampo's stages of disease), in which disease has "settled" in the body, as well as fluid accumulations associated with the condition we know as eczema. Astragalus augments the protective qi, or energy, and stabilizes the exterior of the body, where its outer defenses lie. This action reduces excessive sweating, or, alternatively, produces therapeutic sweating when other herbs do not work. After severe loss of blood, astragalus tonifies the qi and blood. It also tonifies the digestive processes and augments the qi. This action treats lack of appetite, fatigue, and diarrhea. The herb raises energies from the lower parts of the torso. This action treats prolapsed uterus, rectum, or stomach, and also uterine bleeding.

Astragalus drains swelling in paralyzed limbs, and promotes both urination and the discharge of pus. It heals stubborn abscesses, facial swelling, loss of feeling in the arms and legs, and painful obstructions in the muscles.

Astragalus treats "wasting and thirsting disorder," better known as diabetes. It is especially useful against skin ulcers caused by diabetes.

Scientific Findings and Clinical Experience

Astragalus's traditional use as a diabetes treatment has been confirmed by modern research. In one study persons with various conditions, including an eye disease called diabetic retinopathy, were given 2 to 3 grams (approximately a tablespoon) of a 50-50 mixture of astragalus and another herb called rehmannia (see page 84) three times a day for three months. Improvements in blood flow through the eye were noted in 82 percent of participants. Fasting blood sugar was kept below 150 milligrams / deciliter for 77 percent of participants, without the use of other medications.[1]

Astragalus shows great promise in the treatment of various heart problems. Chinese clinical studies have found that this herb improves circulation after a heart attack by increasing the action of the left ventricle, the heart's main pumping chamber.[2] When taken with the herbs coptis and scutellaria (see pages 42 and 88), astragalus makes the blood more fluid, which helps prevent coronary arteries from becoming clogged by clots. In this regard, it is as effective as aspirin.[3] Clinical testing has also shown that astragalus increases the effectiveness of lidocaine, a drug given to prevent a weak, erratic heartbeat called ventricular fibrillation.[4] The herb also protects heart tissues from damage after blood returns to them after heart attack or bypass surgery.[5]

Chinese researchers have had good preliminary results using astragalus compounds called astragalosides in treating congestive heart failure. Patients treated via injection regain an average of approximately 20 percent of their heart function in two weeks of treatment.[6] Whether similar benefits can be obtained from orally administered astragalus products is not yet known.

Other Chinese doctors have found that astragalus offers more effective relief than the drug nifedipine (Procardia) for angina pain. More than 80 percent of angina patients improved on astragalus treatment without the dizziness, giddiness, heartburn, or headache that nifedipine can cause.[7] Animal studies suggest that astragalus can help prevent the development of cholesterol plaques after an arterial wall has been damaged, which can keep the coronary arteries from becoming too narrow.[8] And astragalus also is useful in the treatment of viral myocarditis, a flulike infection that affects the heart.[9,10]

Astragalus can also be used in cancer treatment. Interleukin-2 (IL-2), a substance produced by the immune system, has been isolated, synthesized, and used to treat colorectal cancer, lymphoma, melanoma, and kidney cancer. IL-2 is extremely toxic when concentrated, but the simultaneous use of IL-2 and astragalus increases the drug's effectiveness. This allows the use of a lower, less toxic dosage of IL-2. Chinese studies have also found that astragalus increases the activity of LAK killer cells, another immune-system component, against some types of melanoma.[11]

Chinese studies of the treatment of small cell lung cancer with standard chemotherapy drugs—carmustine (BCNU, BiCNU), cyclophosphamide (Cytoxan, NEOSAR), methotrexate (Methotrexate Sodium), and vincristine (Oncovin)—combined with astragalus and ginseng (see page 57) produced dramatic increases in longevity. In one study, lung cancer patients survived as long as seventeen years on the combination therapy.[12]

Not every astragalus formula is effective in preventing side effects of every kind of chemotherapy. For example, animal studies indicate that a mixture of astragalus and ligustrum (see page 68) does not prevent depletion of red blood cells during chemotherapy with cyclophosphamide,[13] although it does prevent red cell depletion during mitomycin-C therapy.[14] Astragalus alone, however, is effective in preventing depletion of white blood cells during chemotherapy. A clinical study involving 115 patients receiving various forms of chemotherapy found that 83 percent had higher white blood cell counts when given astragalus.[15]

Astragalus is effective against a number of viral infections. Chinese studies have shown that the herb reduces the incidence of, and shortens the duration of, the common cold,[16] and can be used to treat chronic hepatitis B.[17] It also stimulates beneficial components of the immune system in patients with lupus, namely the natural killer (NK) cells, without stimulating the detrimental components in rheumatoid arthritis, namely the B cells.[18] Astragalus increases interferon production, which stimulates the creation of proteins that prevent viral infection.[19] In addition, astragalus stimulates the immune system in patients with AIDS.

Although astragalus is often an immune stimulant, it is an immune suppressant in the treatment of myasthenia gravis, a disease in which the body's immune system attacks the connection between the muscles and the nerves. In one study, astragalus significantly reduced patients' nicotinic acetylcholine receptor antibodies, a measure of the disease's severity, when compared with antibody levels in a control group of patients.[20]

Astragalus has other uses as well. Not only does astragalus make synthetic IL-2 more effective when used in cancer chemotherapy, it also increases the body's own production of IL-2.[21] Such a production increase after burn injuries reduces stress on the immune system.[22] In ancient Chinese medicine, astragalus seed was used to treat male infertility, and tests have shown that the herb does increase sperm motility.[23] Finally, laboratory tests show that astragalus decreases memory loss after alcohol consumption.[24]

Considerations for Use

To make astragalus tea, simmer 1 to 3 teaspoons (4 to 6 grams) of the herb in 3 cups of water for forty-five minutes. Strain and drink 1 cup at a time. This herb is also freeze-dried in capsules, and as a fluid extract, powdered solid extract, and tincture. Complications accompanying chemotherapy require very large doses of astragalus; see **Chemotherapy, Side effects** in Part Two. Astragalus is also used in formulas (see Chapter 4).

Even in large doses, astragalus is nontoxic. Laboratory animals fed astragalus have been able to eat up to 10 percent of their body weight in astragalus without ill effects.[25] However, do not use this herb if fever or skin infection is present.

Atractylodis, Red / Sojutsu

Description and Parts Used

Oriental medicine uses two varieties of atractylodis, red and white (see below). Adding to the confusion, red atractylodis is also known as black atractylodis (see Appendix B).

Red atractylodis is the rhizome of lance-leafed atractylodis, a plant grown primarily in northern China. Red atractylodis is harvested in the fall. Cross sections of the root are aromatic and dark red.

Uses in Kampo

Red atractylodis clears damp heat, or infection pouring downward in the body. This action stops vaginal discharge and soothes sore, swollen joints. The herb also expels dampness from the hands and feet, relieving pain. Red atractylodis induces sweating and releases the exterior of the body, where the outer defenses are. Thus, it is used in the early stages of infection for headache, body aches, and absence of sweating.

Red atractylodis dries dampness and strengthens the digestion. Symptoms treated by red atractylodis include reduced appetite, diarrhea, a feeling of fullness similar to that from overeating, fatigue, nausea, and vomiting.

Finally, atractylodis is a key herb in Kampo for the treatment of visual disorders. Red atractylodis is used for night blindness or diminished vision with eye pain. Red atractylodis with black sesame seeds is used for cataracts, glaucoma, and night blindness.

Scientific Findings and Clinical Experience

Red atractylodis produces dramatic drops in blood-sugar levels in laboratory models of diabetes. In diabetic rabbits, ten days of treatment with red atractylodis lowered blood-sugar levels from an average of 401 milligrams per deciliter to 160 milligrams per deciliter.[1]

Considerations for Use

If buying red atractylodis at a Chinese herb market, be sure to get *Cang Zhu,* not *Bai Zhu.* To make tea, steep 1 tablespoon (3 to 4 grams) of the sliced root in 1 cup of water for fifteen minutes. This herb is also used in formulas (see Chapter 4).

Do not use red atractylodis in cases of diarrhea combined with excessive sweating.

Atractylodis, White / Byakujutsu

Description and Parts Used

White atractylodis is an erect perennial herb that grows to a height of six feet. It has alternate leaves and purple flowers. Rare in the wild, it is cultivated in China, Japan, and Korea. White atractylodis's pungent yet sweet root is unearthed in the autumn for use in herbal preparations.

White atractylodis is the herb sold in Chinese herb stores as *bai zhu.* This species of atractylodis has large, firm, solid, aromatic roots with a yellowish cross section. In contrast, the root of red atractylodis is an even red color (see above).

Uses in Kampo

White atractylodis is used raw to promote urination, dry-fried to strengthen the digestive system and as an energy tonic, and scorched to stop diarrhea. It moves fluid from inflamed, arthritic joints. This movement also prevents coughing, dribbling, excessive vaginal discharge, and hood vertigo, a condition in which the patient feels both dizzy and as if a tight band is tied across his or her forehead.

White atractylodis stabilizes the exterior, or the body's outer defenses, and stops sweating. This action is especially effective against cold sweats associated with nervous tension or long illness. The herb also "calms the fetus," making the baby kick less.

Scientific Findings and Clinical Experience

In doses of 30 grams, white atractylodis increases the volume of urination from 200 to 600 percent and encourages the excretion of sodium. In animal studies, this effect lasts six or seven hours. This herb protects the liver from damage by the dry-cleaning agent carbon tetrachloride.[1]

White atractylodis increases the time blood takes to clot.[2] This effect is important to persons who have had or who are at risk for heart attack, since heart attacks are caused by blood clots in the coronary arteries. However, it is probably unwise to combine this herb with warfarin sodium (Coumadin).

White atractylodis helps stop the spread of many forms of cancer by halting the production of fibrin. This substance serves as a net on which tumors "string" new blood vessels. The herb also stimulates the immune system to destroy circulating cancer cells. It is a key component in Ten-Significant Tonic Decoction (see Chapter 4), an important cancer-fighting formula.

Considerations for Use

White atractylodis should never be used when there is high fever, excessive urination, or dehydration, or after heatstroke. It should also not be used by heart patients who are taking Coumadin. It is generally used in formulas.

Bamboo Shavings / Chikujo

Description and Parts Used

The bamboo plant, which grows throughout Asia, is actually a species of grass that has long, jointed, hollow stems and long, thin, graceful leaves. Bamboo shavings are soft, yellowish-green cuttings taken from the stem.

Uses in Kampo

Bamboo shavings are used, singly and in formulas with other herbs, to treat conditions as different as bronchitis, belching, chronic hepatitis, and gallstones. The common action of bamboo in all these conditions is its ability to break up phlegm and cool the body. This includes breaking up nonsubstantial phlegm, the type that cannot be detected physically. Such phlegm causes energy blockages in the central nervous system that can lead to epilepsy and insomnia. By cooling the blood, bamboo shaving tea stops nosebleed. This herb helps break thick sputum that results in a stifling sensation in the chest. It also stops vomiting, especially vomiting of bitter or sour material accompanied by bad breath.

Kampo uses bamboo more often to address individual symptoms of disease than as part of an herbal formula to change patterns that lead to disease. Bamboo is usually augmented with only one or two other herbs taken as a tea. For example, bamboo is combined with codonopsis and licorice for hiccups, especially when there is a feeling of fullness or bloating in the stomach; ginger juice, to increase ginger's ability to stop vomiting; scutellaria and snake gourd fruit for cough with fever; whole bitter orange fruit and pinellia for insomnia, as well as for irritability and palpitations caused by nervous tension.

Scientific Findings and Clinical Experience

Powdered bamboo shavings stop the growth of *E. coli, Salmonella,* and *Staphylococcus.*[1] Therefore, this herb is used to control diarrhea resulting from food poisoning.

Bamboo serves as an excellent illustration of the value of unprocessed herbs. Japanese and Chinese herbal medicine have used bamboo for thousands of years in the treatment of coughs and colds. Recent research, however, shows that the antiviral agents of bamboo come not from the bamboo but from a bamboo fungus, *Shiraia bambusicola.* Had bamboo been processed and refined into its identifiable chemicals, the antiviral effect of the herb would have been lost.[2]

Considerations for Use

To use bamboo shaving tea, simmer 1/8 ounce (2 to 3 grams) of bamboo shavings in 1 cup of water for fifteen minutes, and strain before drinking. Bamboo shavings are usually tied into bundles in the size needed for making a single dose of tea.

Do not take bamboo if either nausea or vomiting are present *without fever.* Persons who have lupus should also avoid bamboo.

Barley Sprouts / BAKUGA

Description and Parts Used

Barley sprouts are fully sprouted barley seeds. Good sprouts are large and yellow. They may be boiled whole and eaten as is, or dried, ground into a powder, and added to teas.

Uses in Kampo

As it is used in Kampo, barley neither heats nor cools, but regulates the flow of energy through the body. Barley reduces food stagnation and strengthens the stomach by smoothing the flow of liver energy. This action relieves indigestion caused by the accumulation of undigested starchy foods and, in infants, poorly digested milk. By smoothing the flow of the liver's energy, barley relieves belching, loss of appetite, and a stifling feeling in the upper stomach or under the ribs. Barley is also used to stop excessive milk production.

Scientific Findings and Clinical Experience

Barley was traditionally used for contraception. Actually, it is an abortion stimulant that activates the contractions of childbirth. A very large dose, however, is needed before this effect is seen.[1]

Considerations for Use

To use barley sprouts, mix 1 to 3 tablespoons (6 to 15 grams) of the powder in 1 cup of water. Avoid barley during pregnancy.

Benincasa / TOKANIN

Description and Parts Used

Benincasa, also known as petha, wax gourd, and winter melon, is a climbing vine with three-lobed leaves and large, yellow flowers. Kampo uses the seeds found in the fruit. Good quality seeds are full, round, and white.

Uses in Kampo

Kampo uses benincasa seeds to treat swellings due to irregularities in the circulatory system. Benincasa is a cold and sweet herb that clears heat, moistens the lungs, relieves inflammation (especially of the bladder), and encourages urination.

Kampo herbalists employ benincasa by itself to treat abdominal fullness, bladder infections, cough with hot phlegm, boils, pelvic cysts and tumors, thirst, and vaginal discharge. Modern Kampo practitioners also use it to help men recover from vasectomies.

Scientific Findings and Clinical Experience

Japanese research has shown that benincasa contains immune-stimulant carbohydrates that are released when the herb is boiled.[1] These carbohydrates seem to have tumor-fighting qualities that extend the life of laboratory animals suffering fibrosarcoma, a form of connective tissue cancer.

Other studies indicate that benincasa lowers blood-sugar levels in people with type 2 diabetes, the type of diabetes that usually develops later in life.[2]

Considerations for Use

To make benincasa tea, simmer approximately 1½ to 2 tablespoons (4 to 6 grams) of whole benincasa seeds in 3 cups of water. Strain and drink lukewarm, 1 cup at a time.

Use benincasa with caution if diarrhea is present.

Biota / HAKUSHININ

Description and Parts Used

Biota consists of the leafy twigs of the arborvitae, a shrub resembling the juniper. Biota is cultivated throughout China for medicinal use: raw or charred in teas and formulas, powdered for treating burns.

Uses in Kampo

Biota is thought to correct an imbalance of the body's fire and water. In this condition, the heart lacks energy to contain its fire, and so sends energy upward in the body, where it causes a red tongue. It also fails to contain the emotions. The kidneys are unable to send water upward to the heart to quench the fire, or downward to moisten the intestines.

Bitter, cold, and astringent, biota cools the blood and stops bleeding. Historically, it has been used for bleeding gums, coughing or vomiting of blood, blood in the stool or urine, and uterine bleeding.

Today, Kampo uses biota to promote healing of small- to moderate-sized burns. It also stops coughing and expels phlegm. Biota is especially useful when there is blood-streaked sputum that is difficult to expectorate.

Scientific Findings and Clinical Experience

In modern times, biota is used for the treatment of age-related memory loss, including Alzheimer's disease and accompanying symptoms of depression. Although biota is considered by Kampo practitioners as the most important herb for this purpose, its exact mechanisms of action have not been scientifically established. It is known that the herb activates short-term memory, which is usually the area most affected, rather than long-term memory. In the laboratory, biota, in combination with ginseng and schisandra (see pages 57 and 87), reverses alcohol damage in brain cells.[1]

Biota is used in the treatment of other conditions. It shortens the time needed for blood to clot.[2] Biota stops bleeding from ulcers in an average of 3.5 days. Alcohol extracts of biota stop the growth of the bacteria that cause tuberculosis, pneumonia, and ear infections.[3] In addition, biota appears to be effective against hair loss. In thirteen cases, hair regrew after application of biota tincture. The more often the herb was applied, the more thickly the hair grew.[4] Kampo's view of biota's energy properties suggests that it would be more effective for correcting hair loss that is accompanied by nervous tension.

Considerations for Use

Biota is sold in Chinese herb shops as *Bai Zi Ren.* Make the tea by simmering about $^1/_4$ to a little over $^1/_2$ ounce (2 to 6 tablespoons, or 6 to 18 grams) of the dried herb in 3 cups of water for forty-five minutes. Strain and drink 1 cup at a time.

Do not use biota over the long term, since dizziness, nausea, or vomiting may result. The most effective way of taking biota is to use the formula Biota Seed Pill to Nourish the Heart (see Chapter 4).

Bitter Melon / RAKANKA

Description and Parts Used

Bitter melon, also known as balsam pear and bitter gourd, is a climbing vine that reaches a height of six feet. It has deeply lobed leaves, yellow flowers, and orange-yellow fruit. Native to southern Asia and an important ingredient in Asian cuisine, bitter melon is cultivated in warm-weather regions throughout the world. The fruit, which looks like a cucumber with warts, is the part used in Kampo.

Uses in Kampo

Kampo uses bitter melon as a moistening and cooling herb. It is used in cases in which the body's yin, or ability to hold fluids, is depleted. In recent years Japanese physicians have used bitter melon extracts to treat the "yin" stages of chronic diseases such as diabetes and chronic infection with herpes or HIV.

Scientific Findings and Clinical Experience

Bitter melon is widely used in the treatment of diabetes, and has been shown in clinical and laboratory tests to lower sugar levels in both blood and urine.[1] One of the chemical components of bitter melon, polypeptide-p, lowers blood-sugar levels in persons with type 1 diabetes. Since, unlike insulin, polypeptide-p does not stimulate the movement of fat into fat cells, it has been considered as a replacement for at least some of the injected insulin these persons must take each day, although the herb cannot completely replace insulin. When used to treat this type of diabetes, polypeptide-p is effective only as an injection.

Another of the chemical constituents of bitter melon is charantin, which can be used to treat type 2 diabetes. Dose for dose, it is more effective than tolbutamide, a commonly prescribed drug. Like tolbutamide, charantin stimulates the pancreas to produce more insulin.[2]

Bitter melon is effective against the herpesvirus. Bitter melon extracts are two to three times more effective than the popular prescription drug acyclovir at killing strains of the virus that are *not* resistant to acyclovir. In treating acyclovir-resistant strains, bitter melon is 100 to 1,000 times more effective.[3]

This herb is also useful in the treatment of HIV. Researchers at New York University School of Medicine, working with HIV type 1, have found that bitter melon compounds are capable of inhibiting both infection of immune-system cells and replication of the virus in cells that are already infected.[4] Other studies have found that a chemical in bitter melon increases the effectiveness of drugs such as dexamethasone (Decadron) and indomethacin (Indocin),[5] and that bitter melon acts very rapidly.[6]

Considerations for Use

Bitter melon can be taken in juice or whole fruit form and is also available as a tincture. Do not use the tincture for control of diabetes, as this form does not lower blood-sugar levels.[7] Bitter melon juice is drinkable but quite bitter. Unfortunately, attempts to sweeten the juice would counteract its use in diabetic control, although sweeteners can be used if the herb is being taken for other purposes.

For diabetics, it is likely that long-term results would be better if bitter melon is combined with the non-Kampo herb gurmar (*Gymnema sylvestre*). This herb protects insulin-producing cells in the pancreas and reduces the taste buds' sensation of sweetness, which leads to a reduced craving for sweets. Bitter melon promotes insulin secretion. When taken together, the two herbs have a greater impact on diabetes than if taken separately. Consult a Kampo or TCM practitioner.

In rare instances, diabetics who use bitter melon every day over a period of years develop liver disease that leads to atherosclerosis, or hardening of the arteries. Although researchers have not found any evidence that bitter melon damages liver tissues, they have noted elevations in liver enzymes in laboratory animals given bitter melon extracts on a regular basis.[8] As a safety measure, bitter melon should be avoided altogether by persons who have cirrhosis or a history of hepatitis, or by individuals with HIV or AIDS and a history of liver infection. All other persons who use the herb should do so for four weeks, then discontinue usage for four weeks.

Bitter Orange (Whole Bitter Orange) / Kijutsu

Description and Parts Used

Bitter orange is the whole, unripe fruit of the mandarin orange. Smaller fruits are preferred.

Uses in Kampo

Like the better known chen-pi, or bitter orange peel, cooling whole bitter orange treats abnormal energies or pathogens that lie stagnant within the body. It also treats pain and a blocked feeling in the chest or abdomen. Whole bitter orange moves fluid from inflamed muscles in order to reduce swelling. Various formulas use both the whole fruit and the peel alone to relieve "surface heat," expressed as a sore throat or skin rash.

Scientific Findings and Clinical Experience

Modern medicine has explored processes corresponding to Kampo's use of bitter orange in moving stagnant qi, or energy. One chemical compound found in the herb, synephrine, stimulates the nerves that cause blood vessels to constrict. This action is gentle but effective against *low* blood pressure caused by arterial failure.[1]

Another compound found in bitter orange, natsudaidain, affects the heart. Small doses of natsudaidain increase the heart rate, while large doses slow it down. The larger doses of bitter orange that slow the heart rate do not reduce circulation to the brain and kidneys, however. While natsudaidain is slowing the heart rate, it makes the heart muscle beat more forcefully. At the same time, circulation to the legs is reduced. This action shunts blood to vital tissues in the top half of the body. In laboratory experiments, natsudaidain has all of these effects without the potentially dangerous side effects of some prescription drugs used to stimulate the heart. For this reason, bitter orange is being investigated as a remedy for congestive heart failure.

Bitter orange has other beneficial effects. Tinctures of the herb prevent a wide variety of allergic reactions, particularly when the tincture is made from very young fruit. Bitter orange acts on the uterus and the intestines. In small doses, bitter orange inhibits contractions of these organs, while in large doses, it stimulates contractions.[2]

Considerations for Use

Unripe bitter orange fruit is suitable for persons of overall robust health. For others, the milder-acting ripe orange is a better choice. Bitter orange is also used in a number of formulas (see Chapter 4).

Most people have no difficulty eating ripe oranges whole (with peel). A single ripe orange provides a medicinally effective dose of its medicinally active ingredients. On the other hand, most people will find bitter orange to be more palatable when taken as a tea. A single, small slice of orange (including the peel), weighing as little as $^1/_8$ ounce (2 to 3 grams), brewed in 1 cup of hot water for ten to fifteen minutes is adequate. Tinctures may also be used.

Bitter Orange Peel / Chinpi

Description and Parts Used

Bitter orange peel is the fresh peel of the chen-pi or Mandarin orange. Bitter orange peel comes in large pieces, and is thin-skinned, pliable, red, oily, aromatic. The first taste of the herb is slightly sweet, but the aftertaste is bitter and then pungent. When bitter orange peel is aged, it is called red tangerine peel. The chen-pi orange is prey to a mold, and the moldy peel is also used in Kampo (see page 34).

Uses in Kampo

Bitter orange peel is a warming herb. It moves congested water and phlegm, normalizes the flow of energy through the body, releases pathogens that have become stagnant, and soothes the stomach. It relieves a stuffy chest when the patient has copious, sticky sputum. Various Kampo formulas use both the peel and the whole fruit to relieve surface heat expressed as sore throat and skin rash.

Bitter orange peel regulates the body's flow of energy and improves the transport function of the digestive organs. It is used to relieve symptoms such as bloating, belching, nausea, and vomiting. Bitter orange stimulates the circulation of energy in the body, while directing the body's energies downward.

Kampo practitioners make a tea of bitter orange peel and licorice for the treatment of mastitis, a combination that usually relieves symptoms in two to three days. The treatment is less effective for long-term infections.

Scientific Findings and Clinical Experience

Bitter orange peel has the same active compounds as whole bitter orange. In addition, the peel contains compounds that raise blood pressure when the heart is contracting while not affecting pressure when the heart rests between beats, an action that increases the heart's output.[1]

Unlike whole bitter orange, bitter orange peel contains concentrated amounts of the flavonoids hesperetin and diosmetin, which are useful in the treatment of circulatory problems in the legs, such as leg pains and nighttime leg cramps.

Bitter orange peel teas relax the body's smooth muscles. This may account for the herb's effect on the digestive system, relaxing the muscles that hold food in place in the digestive tract.[2]

Bitter orange is also used in traditional medicine as a female contraceptive. A substance called cirantin, which is concentrated in the peel, keeps the unfertilized egg from being released into the fallopian tube.

Considerations for Use

To make orange peel tea, simmer 1 teaspoon (2 to 3 grams) of powdered bitter orange peel in 1 cup of water for ten to fifteen minutes. Strain and drink, cold or lukewarm, thirty minutes before meals. For allergies, tinctures can be used. Bitter orange peel is also used in a number of formulas (see Chapter 4).

Traditional medicine urges caution in using this herb when "red" symptoms are present, such as red tongue, redness in the face with fever and cough, and spitting of blood.

Black Cardamom / Yakuchinin

Description and Parts Used

Black cardamom is variously known as alpinia oxyphylla fruit, bitter-seeded cardamom, and black cardamom. There is also another herb that is known simply as cardamom (see page 37). Black cardomom has an appearance very similar to that of ginger, which is in the same plant family. Black cardamom sends up a single, central, green stalk with long, green leaves growing in pairs on opposite sides of the stem. A flower spike appears at the top of the central stem and produces the seed, which is used in Kampo. Good-quality seeds are large, full, and intensely aromatic.

Uses in Kampo

Black cardamom is an herb first mentioned in the Chinese work, *Omissions from the Classic Materia Medica,* in the eighth century. This seed, whose name is translated literally as "benefit intelligence nut" from Chinese, was considered to be a vital addition to the classical pharmacy for formulas that help the body retain its essence, which corresponds to the modern idea of DNA.

Essence was thought to reside in the kidneys. Black cardamom warms the kidneys, astringing them from losses of urine and essence. Black cardamom treats frequent urination, urinary incontinence, and dribbling of urine, as well as spermatorrhea, or the loss of sperm through nocturnal emission.

Black cardamom also warms the digestive system and prevents diarrhea, excessive salivation, and a thick, unpleasant taste in the mouth.

Scientific Findings and Clinical Experience

Black cardamom has a tonic effect on the heart,[1] probably by acting as a calcium channel blocker,[2] or a substance that keeps calcium from stimulating the heart muscle to contract too forcefully.

Considerations for Use

Black cardamom is used in the herbal formula Shut the Sluice Pill (see Chapter 4). Women who have pelvic inflammatory disease with vaginal discharge should not use this herb.

Black Cohosh / Shoma

Description and Parts Used

Black cohosh is a perennial herb that bears a three- to nine-foot spike covered with creamy white flowers. This shade-loving plant is found in the woodlands of the Atlantic seaboard states and eastern Canada. The rhizome and roots of a number of closely related species are used in Oriental medicine (see Appendix B).

It makes a difference medicinally whether black cohosh is taken from the wild, grown in a garden, or mass-produced in tissue culture in a laboratory. Black cohosh produces more of its medically active substance when the plant is under stress, such as that caused by insect injury, bright summer sun, and fungal infection.[1]

Uses in Kampo

Traditional Japanese medicine used black cohosh as a cold herb to relieve symptoms of heat on the surface of the body, especially measles and chickenpox. Historically, Japanese herbalists have used black cohosh to treat acne related to the menstrual cycle, bad breath, mastitis, skin eruptions and swellings, sore throat, and stomatitis, an inflammation of the mouth.

Kampo formulas (see Chapter 4), using higher doses of black cohosh than in single-herb forms, detoxify and enable energy to rise in the body. Rising energy restores form to organs that have collapsed. These formulas treat uterine prolapse and hemorrhoids.

Scientific Findings and Clinical Experience

Black cohosh was long thought to be a source of phytoestrogens, plant compounds that mimic the action of estrogen in the body. However, recent research indicates that it is not, at least in animal studies.[2] Instead, black cohosh contains at least three classes of compounds that act in two ways. One, they bind to receptor sites in the reproductive tract, the brain, and other organs that otherwise would receive estrogen. This reduces overall estrogen activity when estrogen levels are high. Two, these compounds block the formation of luteinizing hormone (LH), which stimulates a surge of estrogen production in the first fourteen days of the menstrual period.[3] This stimulates estrogen production when estrogen levels are low. Thus, black cohosh's dual action allows it to stabilize the body's estrogen usage.

Black cohosh's ability to provide balance allows it to prevent the hot flashes, and nervousness, and depressed moods associated with menopause, and to relieve vaginal dryness after menopause.[4] This makes black cohosh ideal for estrogen replacement therapy (see pages 263 and 264), especially when compared with synthetic hormone replacement therapies. Black cohosh is likewise capable of regulating estrogen production before menopause, and is especially useful for treating blurred vision and migraine associated with premenstrual syndrome.

Black cohosh also increases male fertility. One of the chemical constituents of black cohosh, ferulic acid, increases the motility and viability of sperm cells by protecting their cell walls.[5] Purified ferulic acid is available as a health food supplement, but black cohosh, when used in formulas, has a more comprehensive effect.

American herbalists frequently combine black cohosh, a Kampo herb, with goldenseal, an American herb, to treat ringing in the ears. Black cohosh relieves dizziness, and goldenseal relieves inner ear inflammation.

Considerations for Use

Black cohosh is available in a number of forms, including dried and fluid extracts (the dried form standardized for 27-deoxyacteine), dried root in capsules, and tinctures.

Black cohosh's estrogen-simulating compounds require the action of digestive bacteria to enter the human bloodstream in a useful form. Oral antibiotics kill colon bacteria. For this reason, black cohosh is less likely to be effective when taken simultaneously with oral antibiotics. It should be avoided altogether during pregnancy or lactation.

Bletilla / Byakukyu

Description and Parts Used

Bletilla is the rhizome of the bletilla orchid, which is dug in the summer and fall. It is native to the warm, humid regions of southern and eastern China. A quality rhizome is solid, thick, and white, and has no odor.

Uses in Kampo

Gently cooling bletilla stops loss of blood. It is used in formulas mainly for bleeding from the lungs and stomach, coughing or vomiting of blood, and nosebleed. Bletilla also reduces swelling and "generates flesh," which means that it assists in recovery from abrasions, blisters, burns, cuts, and scratches. Bletilla power is applied topically to ulcers, sores, and chapped skin.

Scientific Findings and Clinical Experience

Bletilla promotes platelet aggregation, an important step in the clotting of blood.[1] In a clinical study involving sixty-nine patients with bleeding ulcers, bletilla stopped bleeding in an average of 6.5 days. Bletilla has also been used in treating perforated ulcers, with a success rate of approximately 70 percent.[2]

Bletilla is useful against *Mycobacterium tuberculosis,* the bacterium that causes tuberculosis. In one study, sixty patients who had not responded to other therapies were given bletilla. Of this group, forty-two were clinically cured and thirteen showed significant improvement. Twenty-one patients with chronic dilation of the bronchial tubes, a condition known as bronchiectasis, received long-term bletilla therapy. They all showed significant reductions in sputum production and coughing, as well as control over the spitting and coughing of blood.[3]

Considerations for Use

Bletilla should always be used under professional supervision.

Blue Citrus (Qing Pi) / Jyohi

Description and Parts Used

Blue citrus is the moldy peel of the chen-pi orange. Peel that has not been affected by mold is called bitter orange peel (see page 32).

Uses in Kampo

Blue citrus is used to neither heat nor cool the body, but instead is used to break up stagnant energy associated with the liver, which stores energy related to emotions. Constrained liver energy causes symptoms such as hernia, and distention and pain in the breasts or chest.

Blue citrus also breaks up clumps of stagnant food that results in pain or a stifling feeling in the area above the navel. Blue citrus is usually used for severe food stagnation, when stagnant qi interferes with blood circulation. In addition, blue citrus dries dampness and transforms phlegm, particularly in cases of malaria.

Scientific Findings and Clinical Experience

Blue citrus increases gastric secretion, stimulates the movement of food through the digestive tract, stops vomiting, arrests hiccups, and dispels abdominal distention.[1]

Considerations for Use

Make blue citrus tea by simmering approximately 1 tablespoon of the dried herb in 1 cup of water. Limit steeping time to ten minutes in order to preserve the herb's essential oils. Take the tea thirty minutes before meals.

Use blue citrus with caution in cases of prolonged or systemic illness.

Boneset

See **Eupatorium.**

Boswellia

See **Frankincense.**

Broomrape

See **Cistanche.**

Brucea / ATANSHI

Description and Parts Used

Brucea is the ripe, autumn-harvested fruit of the Java brucea tree, which is native to southeastern China. The fruit is hard, solid, and white, with an oily texture.

Uses in Kampo

Kampo uses warming brucea for stagnant cold of the digestive tract, a condition corresponding to a long-term intestinal infection. The herb is also used to treat the internal heat and external cold caused by malaria. Topically, brucea ointments are used to treat corns and warts.

Scientific Findings and Clinical Experience

A five-year clinical study of cervical cancer patients in China found that brucea teas kill squamous cell cancers of the cervix. In the study, many women achieved five-year remissions.[1] This herb is most suitable for precancerous conditions, such as cervical dysplasia or papilloma.

Laboratory studies have also shown that brucea is an antibiotic. It kills the amoeba that causes dysentery, *Entamoeba histolytica,* and some of the parasites that cause malaria. About 95 percent of those patients with amoebic dysentery who are treated with brucea do not suffer relapses.[2]

Considerations for Use

Brucea is sold in Chinese herb shops as *ya dan zi.* It is too bitter to be taken as a tea, and thus is sold in capsule form.

Bupleurum / SAIKO

Description and Parts Used

Bupleurum, also known as hare's ear root and thorowax root, is a perennial in the same family as carrots and parsley. It grows up to three feet high, with sickle-shaped leaves and clusters of small yellow flowers at the top of the plant. The root is harvested in the spring and autumn.

Identifying the kinds of bupleurum available in herb shops requires learning a little terminology. *Bupleurum chinensis* is known as "northern bupleurum." Because it is harvested in the autumn and is relatively hard, it is also known as "autumnal bupleurum" or "hard bupleurum." Northern bupleurum is more effective in resolving the early stages of infection and in reducing fever. *Bupleurum scorzoneraefolium,* harvested in the spring, is "southern bupleurum," also known as "soft bupleurum" or "fine bupleurum." Southern bupleurum is included in formulas used to treat what Oriental medicine calls "liver" diseases, expressed as painful menstruation and emotional disturbance.

Uses in Kampo

Chinese medicine has used bupleurum for more than 2,000 years to correct disharmony between the liver, which is believed to store emotions, and the spleen, which is believed to digest and transform food. Liver disharmonies manifest themselves as abdominal pain, bloating, indigestion, and nausea, which are also symptoms of a disorder known to Western medicine as viral hepatitis.

Bupleurum is also thought to be a cold herb that quenched fires of the liver, the organ associated with sexual and emotional tensions. Formulas use bupleurum and peony (see page 78) to release pent-up anger. Just as it relaxes emotional tensions stored in the liver, bupleurum also cools the fiery heat of infection. Bupleurum is used to treat bleeding associated with urinary tract infection, convulsions, digestive disturbances, lumps and tumors, menstrual irregularity, muscle tension, and skin ailments. It relieves a symptom pattern that includes bitter taste in the mouth, irritability, pain in the side, a stifling sensation of the chest, and vomiting.

Scientific Findings and Clinical Experience

Bupleurum protects the liver in a number of ways. The herb contains chemicals called saikosides that defend this vital organ from damage caused by drugs and environmental toxins. Bupleurum prevents fatty liver and lowers levels of the liver enzymes involved in cell death. Bupleurum also slows the tissue changes caused by chronic hepatitis.[1] Through its action on the liver, bupleurum may indirectly reduce serum cholesterol and triglyceride levels.[2]

Many practitioners note that bupleurum can bring down fevers caused by almost any condition. It is commonly prescribed for children and pregnant women, especially in cases of common cold and flu. In a study reported by physician-herbalists Bensky and Gamble, bupleurum lowered fevers in 98 percent of 143 patients suffering upper respiratory infections. Of the patients in the study, 88 percent were fever-free within twenty-four hours.[3]

Bupleurum is an important herb for the relief of arthritic inflammation. Bupleurum's saikosides, along with other chemicals, stimulate the pituitary gland into directing the adrenal glands to produce glucocorticoids, which reduce inflammation.[4,5] Bupleurum also increases the effectiveness of glucocorticoid drugs, such as prednisone, used in the treatment of rheumatoid arthritis.

According to the *Japanese Pharmacopeia,* bupleurum serves many other functions. It aids fat metabolism, calms the central nervous system, strengthens the immune response to cancer and viral infection, inhibits inflammatory reactions, and prevents muscle spasms. Bupleurum stops the effects of allergies by blocking 5HT. This substance makes the walls of capillaries more permeable, which leads to soft-tissue swelling.[6] In the eye, this action also prevents capillary damage that results in macular degeneration, and the accumulation of debris that causes floaters. The herb contains a substance called rutin, which helps restrain cancer cells from multiplying indefinitely. Laboratory testing has found that a compound in bupleurum inactivates herpes simplex and measles viruses.[7] Studies have also found that other bupleurum compounds relieve peptic ulcer.[8]

Considerations for Use

Make bupleurum tea by simmering $^1/_2$ ounce of the dried herb in 3 cups of hot water for forty-five minutes. Drink 1 cup at a time. Bupleurum is also available in the form of saikosaponin extract.

Like many other herbs, bupleurum requires the help of friendly bacteria living in the human intestine to be therapeutically useful. These bacteria transform the compounds in the herb into bodily chemicals that relieve inflammation.[9] Therefore, bupleurum should not be used at the same time as antibiotics, which often kill off these bacteria.

Used by itself, bupleurum occasionally causes mild stomach upset. If this happens, reduce the dose. This should not occur if a formula that contains bupleurum (see Chapter 4) is taken. Do not use if fever is present.

Burdock (Arctium Lappa) / Goboshi

Description and Parts Used

Burdock, a relative of the sunflower, grows to a height of five feet and bears reddish purple flower heads covered with spiny bracts. In summer, the grayish red seeds are harvested, and the roots of two-year-old plants are dug. Although native to Asia and Europe, burdock is now grown in temperate-zone gardens around the world.

Uses in Kampo

Burdock seed is a cold, pungent, and sweet herb that detoxifies tissues by encouraging the circulation of qi, or energy. The seeds dispel heat, relieve swellings, normalize breathing, and vent rashes. Externally, burdock-seed poultices are particularly useful for swellings caused by toxins, such as carbuncles and mumps. Internally, they are used to treat dry constipation, and in formulas for cough, rashes, and sore throat (see Chapter 4).

Burdock root is used in other herbal traditions and is used in modern Kampo. However, it is not used in traditional Kampo.

Scientific Findings and Clinical Experience

Burdock is widely regarded in alternative medicine as an important liver detoxification agent and anticancer herb. In the liver, it neutralizes free radicals, substances that damage cells by disrupting the cells' chemistry.[1] Recent studies have shown that burdock induces differentiation in cancer cells,[2] which makes the cancer less aggressive. Burdock also contains factors that stop the cancer-causing effects of environmental toxins.[3]

Herbal practitioners in Japan and Europe have long used burdock as a treatment for chronic skin diseases, especially eczema. European herbalists use burdock root, which seems to work by preventing the body's own immune system from attacking the skin.[4] Japanese herbalists use burdock seed, which kills streptococcal bacteria and many disease-causing fungi that infect cracked skin.[5]

Burdock seeds also provide a valuable supplemental food for diabetics. A chemical extract made from burdock has shown prolonged blood sugar-lowering effects in animal tests. It works by filling the intestines with fiber, which prevents the absorption of sugars. Burdock fibers also prevent the absorption of toxic compounds from food.[6] These fibers are digested in the intestine with the help of bacteria,[7] but only after they have passed into the large intestine. Since most food absorption occurs in the small intestine, toxic compounds are less likely to enter the body.

Kampo practitioners report informally that burdock inhibits the growth of the HIV virus and the bacteria that cause pneumonia and staph infections in AIDS patients. Other practitioners report that the herb promotes lymphatic circulation. This treats lumps and growths of all kinds in the breast, and reduces the severity of lymphadema after breast surgery.

Considerations for Use

Look for burdock-seed cereals, available as *gobo* or *goboshi* in Japanese groceries. A dosage of as little as 1 to 3 tablespoons a day has a therapeutic effect. However, it may be taken in any amount, or as much as is permitted by a specific meal plan. Although burdock root is not traditionally used in Kampo, it may also be beneficial. The root is available in various forms, including dried root and fluid, powdered, or solid extract. Make the dried root into tea by simmering 1 tablespoon (3 grams) of root in 1 cup of water for two to five minutes. Drink the tea without straining.

Do not use burdock seeds on open sores, or if there is diarrhea.

Caltrop / Byakushitsuri

Description and Parts Used

Caltrop, also known as puncture-vine fruit and tribulus, is the grayish white, thorny fruit of a plant native to central China and Japan, and to the Carolinas in the United States. The plant creeps across the ground, with sprawling stems one to three feet long. Each stem supports eight to ten pairs of leaflets, each with one leaf smaller than the other, alternating on opposite sides of the stem. The fruit is covered with a set of irregular horns on one side, and two spines near the middle.

Uses in Kampo

Caltrop's principal use in Kampo is to calm the liver. This action reduces symptoms associated with emotional stress, such as headache (especially when associated with premenstrual syndrome), vertigo, or dizziness. This herb stops itching, especially that associated with hives, and helps the skin recover pigmentation lost in vitiligo.

Caltrop also stimulates the flow of energy along the liver energy channels, which cross the breasts. TCM offers this as an explanation for the fact that caltrop stimulates milk production in nursing mothers.

Scientific Findings and Clinical Experience

Caltrop teas lower blood pressure and stimulate urination. The herb may improve vision, particularly when there are problems with the circulation of fluids in the lens, such as that caused by diabetes.[1]

Considerations for Use

To make caltrop tea, simmer $^1/_4$ ounce (6 grams) of the whole fruit in 1 cup of water for fifteen minutes, and strain before drinking. Use caltrop with caution during pregnancy or after loss of blood.

Cardamom / SHUKUSHA

Description and Parts Used

Cardamom is a medicinal herb native to tropical China and Vietnam. It is closely related to, but not identical to, the cardamom grown in India and Sri Lanka as a spice. Cardamom is a perennial that grows to a height of fifteen feet with mauve-streaked, white flowers and very long, lance-shaped leaves. Kampo formulas call for whole seed pods (broken when the tea is made) that are gathered between October and December when the hull is yellow-green. The seeds themselves are reddish-black. Kampo also uses black cardamom (see page 33).

Uses in Kampo

Cardamom is a gently warming, fragrant herb used for dispelling wetness. It also dispels stagnant qi, or energy, and normalizes the flow of energy through the center of the body. This action relieves pain in the middle of the torso, along with symptoms that include chest pain, constipation, gas, diarrhea, indigestion, stomachache, and vomiting. Cardamom is also useful in cases of decreased urination, such as that seen in urinary tract infections.

In addition, cardamom is used to prevent tonics from causing "stagnation," or incomplete digestion, which is marked by diarrhea.

Scientific Findings and Clinical Experience

Cardamom inhibits the production of prostaglandins, substances that can cause constriction of the blood vessels, asthmatic reactions, blood clots, and peptic ulcers. The herb is especially effective in ulcer treatment when used as part of the formula Minor Construct the Middle Decoction (see Chapter 4).[1] Cardamom also increases the effectiveness of streptomycin against tuberculosis,[2] and is useful in treating malaria.[3]

Considerations for Use

The cardamom used in Kampo is not the same herb used in cooking, but the spice cardamom has the same effects as the medicinal herb,[4] provided the spice is fresh. Kampo practitioners usually keep the seed pods intact until just before dispensing the herb in order to maximize freshness.

To make cardamom tea, simmer 1 to 3 teaspoons of cardamom powder or 1 to 2 tablespoons of seeds in 1 cup of water for no more than ten minutes. Strain before use. This herb is also available in tincture form.

Carthamus / KOKA

Description and Parts Used

Carthamus is an herb native to Iran but spread by commerce to the Far East and North America. It is also known as safflower, and is used to produce cooking oil. An annual herb growing a height of three feet, carthamus has long, spiny leaves with six oval leaflets, and groups of yellow flowers arising from the joint between the leaf and the stem. The flowers are used in Kampo.

Uses in Kampo

Carthamus flower is a bitter, pungent, and warming herb that activates blood circulation. This vitalizes the blood and regulates menstruation. It is used in formulas (see Chapter 4) to treat abdominal and joint pain, and accumulations of blood caused by traumatic injuries.

Scientific Findings and Clinical Experience

Herbalist James Duke notes that carthamus dilates blood vessels that supply the scalp, encouraging the flow of nutrients and oxygen to hair follicles. He recommends adding carthamus powder to shampoo.[1] While this approach will be ineffective against male pattern baldness, it may help reduce hair loss caused by conditions of nervous tension.

Carthamus may prevent skin cancer. In laboratory tests, carthamus tinctures stopped the formation of skin tumors induced by chemical agents.[2] Carthamus reduces the likelihood that cancerous tumors will spread by breaking down fibrin, a protein that supplies a net on which a tumor can grow its own blood vessels. Destroying fibrin prevents the tumor from gaining its own blood supply.[3]

The treatment of atherosclerosis and arteriosclerosis is a modern use of this traditional herb. Chinese physicians report that carthamus prevents the formation of blood clots, and increases the time it takes clots to form. Carthamus is widely used in China to treat coronary heart disease.[4]

Considerations for Use

Since carthamus has a stimulating effect on the uterus, it should not be used internally during pregnancy.[5]

Cassia

See **Cinnamon.**

Chebula / Kashi

Description and Parts Used

Chebula is a Burmese plant botanically related to the chaparral found in North America. Now cultivated in Yunnan province in extreme southern China, chebula provides a shiny, hard, yellowish-brown fruit that is ground for use in decoctions. The fruit is also known as tribulus.

Uses in Kampo

Kampo uses chebula to stop "leaking," a condition that shows itself as chronic diarrhea and dysentery. Since chebula is neither hot nor cold, Kampo uses it for symptom patterns in which diarrhea appears. Chebula also stops "leakage" in the lungs expressed through coughing and raspy voice. Kampo uses it in combination with other herbs to break up phlegm.

Modern TCM uses chebula for treating "rebellious qi," or energy, moving in the wrong direction, that results in headaches, eye problems, and jittery nerves. TCM also uses it for treating itchy skin.

Scientific Research and Clinical Experience

Chinese laboratory studies found that chebula teas have a potent antibiotic effect on *Shigella,* a waterborne organism that causes many cases of travelers' diarrhea.[1]

Considerations for Use

Chebula is used in True Man's Decoction to Nourish the Organs (see Chapter 4). The astringent action of chebula on diarrhea is due to its water-soluble tannins. When the tannins are removed from the herb, it becomes a laxative. Therefore, it is important to carefully strain the formula, since ingesting the herb itself could have a laxative effect.

Chen-pi

See **Bitter Orange Peel.**

Chinese Angelica

See **Tang-Kuei.**

Chinese Date

See **Jujube Fruit.**

Chinese Prickly Ash

See **Zanthoxylum.**

Chinese Rose

See **Rose Hips.**

Chinese Senega Root / Onji

Description and Parts Used

Chinese senega root is also known as polygala. The name of the plant in Japanese originally meant "profound will." Kampo uses the white root.

Uses in Kampo

Chinese senega root is a warming, bitter herb used in Kampo to move moisture and to nurture the emotional organ, the heart. By moving moisture, this herb expels phlegm from the lungs, which alleviates coughs with copious sputum, especially sputum that is difficult to expectorate. Chinese senega root also reduces abscesses and dissipates swellings, especially those of the breasts.

In terms of ancient Kampo, Chinese senega root expels phlegm obstructing the "orifices of the heart," which manifested itself as emotional and mental disorientation and seizures. This herb, especially when used in formulas (see Chapter 4), calms the spirit and quiets the heart, relieving insomnia, palpitations, anxiety, and disorientation. It is considered most effective in cases related to brooding or pent-up emotions.

Scientific Findings and Clinical Experience

Chinese senega root contains a chemical called tenuigenin that irritates the stomach lining, causing a reflex action that stimulates bronchial secretion. Tenuigenin also stimulates uterine contractions, and kills some kinds of bacteria.[1]

Other compounds in Chinese senega root have a profound effect on the rate at which the body absorbs ethanol, the alcohol in alcoholic beverages. In animal studies, these compounds block as much as 90 percent of the ethanol that otherwise would have been absorbed into the body. Japanese researchers are developing products based on this herb to prevent alcohol intoxication.[2]

Considerations for Use

To make Chinese senega root tea, simmer 1 to 3 teaspoons of the dried herb in 1 cup of water for forty-five minutes. Take the tea on an empty stomach. This herb is also available in tincture form.

Do not use Chinese senega root if gastritis or ulcers are present, or during pregnancy.

Chrysanthemum / Kikuka (cultivated chrysanthemum) / Nogikuka (wild chrysanthemum)

Description and Parts Used

It is fitting that the chrysanthemum, Japan's national flower, is used in Kampo. The wild chrysanthemum is a sprawling, leafy plant with clusters of daisylike flowers at its crown.

Uses in Kampo

Chrysanthemum is used for its effects on the eyes. The herb corrects imbalances in liver and kidney function that cause blurred vision, dizziness, dry red eyes, excessive tearing, or spots in front of the eyes.

Chrysanthemum also treats headaches accompanying infection, carbuncles, furuncles, and vertigo. Wild chrysanthemum is thought to be more useful than the cultivated type for treatment of sores and abscesses, especially those of the head and back.

Scientific Findings and Clinical Experience

Various forms of chrysanthemum are used in Kampo to inhibit platelet activating factor, a hormone that triggers asthmatic attacks. The herb also kills the bacteria that cause staph infections.[1]

Considerations for Use

Make a chrysanthemum compress by placing 1 to 2 tablespoons (6 to 12 grams) of dried petals in 3 cups of water. The water should be brought to just below the boiling point before the petals are added, and the mixture steeped off the heat for no more than ten minutes. Strain, and place the petals in a clean cloth. Apply the cloth to the forehead. The compress's effectiveness is enhanced by combining chrysanthemum with an equal amount of prunella (see page 82), also steeped in hot water for ten minutes before straining. In addition, chrysanthemum is used in formulas (see Chapter 4).

Cinnamon / KEISHI

Description and Parts Used

Cinnamon, used in cooking throughout the world, comes from a tropical evergreen tree that reaches a height of between thirty and sixty feet. The tree grows in low-lying rain forests found in India, Sri Lanka, the Philippines, and the West Indies. Kampo uses its reddish brown, soft bark and young twigs, both of which are cut and allowed to ferment in the field before being gathered for drying.

Uses in Kampo

Cinnamon, a warming herb, is used in Kampo to prevent symptoms of misplaced qi, or energy, rising in the body. Cinnamon "leads fire back to its source," that is, it corrects upward-floating energies not restrained by the internal organs. It stops fever, headaches, pain, and inflammation caused by sinusitis and colds, and redness in the face after embarrassment or irritation. In addition to redirecting excessive energy in the upper half of the body, the herb vitalizes deficient energy or cold in the lower half of the body. Cinnamon warms what is called the "gate of vitality" at the kidneys, which reverses aversion to cold, weak back, cold limbs, impotence, and frequent urination. It also energizes the kidneys to "steam up" fluids from the lower parts of the body to the upper parts. This restores waning energies in the digestive system that otherwise would cause abdominal pain and cold, reduced appetite, and diarrhea.

TCM uses cinnamon to correct deficient transmission of energy through the energy channels. It does this by warming the channels and dispersing deep cold. Disorders associated with this problem include cold in the blood, which causes menstrual problems. Other disorders include abscesses and sores that do not heal, as well as chronic cold boils, or skin ulcerations in which the affected skin bulges inward rather than outward.

Cinnamon is also used in formulas to balance disproportionate heat in the top and bottom halves of the body. This includes conditions in which the upper part of the body is hot—dry mouth, sore throat, toothache—and the lower part of the body is cold—lower back pain, coldness in the legs and feet, diarrhea.

While culinary cinnamon is usually made from the bark, Kampo formulas (see Chapter 4) more typically use the twigs. Traditional herbalists believed the twigs have a more potent ability to stimulate sweating, which opens the pores in order to release invading pathogens in the early stages of infection. The twigs also have a more potent warming effect on the body's internal organs.

Scientific Findings and Clinical Experience

Modern medicine has confirmed cinnamon's role in Kampo. In large doses, cinnamon increases the heart rate, and stimulates both perspiration and intestinal motion. After an excitation phase, there is a sedation phase characterized by sleepiness. The sedation phase corresponds to ancient advice to get under covers and go to sleep after taking Kampo formulas containing cinnamon.

Perhaps the most common medicinal application of cinnamon is in the relief of intestinal gas. Both teas and tinctures are equally effective in quelling flatulence. Cinnamon oil, applied topically, is also a long-time remedy for wasp stings. It works by blocking the creation of body chemicals that cause inflammation. And before the twentieth century, cinnamon tinctures were the standard remedy for uterine bleeding, such as that caused by fibroids.

Cinnamon has a wide range of other uses. Certain forms of cinnamon have been found to inhibit a substance in the blood called thromboxane A_2. Thromboxane causes platelets, little cells in the blood, to clump together. These clumps clog arteries and increase the risk of heart attack.[1] Another compound found in cinnamon, propanoic acid, stops the formation of stomach ulcers without interfering with the production of gastric acid. This is important because a lack of gastric acid can lead to indigestion.[2]

Whole cinnamon is an effective treatment for drug-resistant (fluconazole-resistant) yeast infections. It is useful as a treatment for thrush,[3] an oral yeast infection, as well as the gum disease gingivitis.[4] Cinnamon bark oil treats fungal infections of the respiratory tract,[5] including infections caused by *Candida, Histoplasma,* and *Aspergillus niger,* the last of which can cause extremely serious sinus infections.

Like bamboo (see page 29), cinnamon hosts fungi which themselves have medical uses. Cinnamon bark can contain the fungus *Antrodia cinnamomea,* producer of a substance that kills leukemia cells in animal tests. Two other chemicals extracted from cinnamon itself, camphornin and cinnamonin, stop the growth of liver cancer and melanoma cells in the laboratory.[6] Compounds in cinnamon are known to deactivate plasmin, a substance that allows cancer cells to infiltrate surrounding tissue. In addition, cinnamon stimulates the body's production of tumor necrosis factor, an immune-system chemical that fights cancer.

Some Chinese Kampo practitioners inject cinnamon oil into acupuncture points used in treating asthma. There are reports that these injections, which must be performed by a physician, give some asthmatics up to a month's relief.

Liberal use of cinnamon in teas and as a dietary supplement has a salutary effect on AIDS and HIV. Cinnamon contains compounds that stimulate macrophages, immune-system cells that engulf and destroy infectious microorganisms, but not T cells, which host HIV. Cinnamon also stimulates testosterone production, which prevents muscle wasting.

Considerations for Use

The simplest way to use cinnamon is as a tea. Simmer 1 scant teaspoon of ground cinnamon in 1 cup of water for ten minutes. Be sure to use recently purchased cinnamon, since the herb can lose its potency in storage. Cinnamon is also available in oil form.

Individuals with prostate problems should avoid cinnamon.

Cistanche / Nikujuyo

Description and Parts Used

Cistanche, also known as broomrape, is a low-growing herb from Inner Mongolia and Tibet. The root—soft, thick, and densely scaled—is harvested in the early spring, just as the sprouts are emerging.

Uses in Kampo

Cistanche, a warming herb, is one of Kampo's most important herbs in the treatment of impotence. This herb is thought to nourish the "essence," a quality roughly corresponding to the strength of the DNA a father provides his child. It also strengthens the reproductive organs. This action treats cold pains in the lower back and knees, impotence, spermatorrhea (the involuntary flow of sperm), urinary incontinence, and dribbling after urination. Cistanche also warms the womb, which makes it useful in treating female infertility, excessive uterine bleeding, and vaginal discharge.

In addition, cistanche lubricates the intestines. This action is especially important for elderly people, who may experience a loss of fluids that leads to severe constipation.

Scientific Findings and Clinical Experience

Japanese studies have found that cistanche is a potent antioxidant.[1] This may enhance the chemical reactions within the penis that allow an erection to occur.

Considerations for Use

Cistanche is available in freeze-dried form under its Chinese name, *Rou Cong Rong.*

Cistanche should not be used when there is diarrhea due to digestive weakness, as shown by undigested food in the stool. Also, the herb may activate the immune function of the thymus, and as such, it may boost immune response in the elderly. For most people, increased immune response is beneficial. However, individuals with myasthenia gravis should avoid cistanche.[2]

Clematis / Ireisen

Description and Parts Used

Clematis is a vigorous climbing vine used ornamentally in temperate climates around the world. It grows up to 100 feet in length, and has lance-shaped leaves, small flowers, and fluffy seed heads. Kampo uses the autumn-harvested root, which has black bark and a white center.

Uses in Kampo

Neither heating nor cooling, clematis acts to alleviate pain by unblocking the body's energy channels. As the flow of energy through the body is increased, muscular tension is relieved.

Clematis root is a home remedy for fish bones stuck in the throat. When mixed with vinegar and brown sugar, the herb dissolves small bones.

Scientific Findings and Clinical Experience

Laboratory tests have confirmed that clematis raises the threshold of pain.[1] The herb acts as a counterirritant, sensitizing nerve pathways to the minor pain induced by the herb while desensitizing other nerve pathways to more severe, chronic pain. Clematis has been used as an analgesic in treating arthritis. It cools and soothes arthritic pain and swelling.[2] In addition, Chinese studies have found an 80 percent cure rate when clematis was used in treating 33 cases of filariasis, a nematode infection of the lungs that can be spread from dogs to people.[3]

Considerations for Use

Clematis, sold as *Wei Ling Xian,* can be taken in either tea or capsule form. To make the tea, simmer $1\frac{1}{2}$ to 3 tablespoons (6 to 12 grams) of *roasted* clematis in 1 cup of water for ten minutes. Strain before drinking.

Some TCM practitioners advise avoiding consumption of pork or beef while taking clematis root.

Cloud Fungus

See **PSK** under Modern Japanese Herbal Preparations.

Cloves / Choko

Description and Parts Used

The cloves used in Kampo are whole flower buds picked from the plant as they change color from green to red. Kampo medications usually use the male flowers, since their medicinal action is faster than that of the females. Cloves should be fragrant, full, large, oily, and dark red. When added to water, they should not float. The original meaning of the Japanese word for cloves was "spike fragrance."

Uses in Kampo

Cloves warm the middle of the body and direct rebellious qi—qi going in the wrong direction—downward. This action relieves cold that has entered the stomach to cause abdominal pain, diarrhea, hiccups, loss of appetite, or vomiting. Cloves also warm the kidneys and clear vaginal discharges.

Scientific Findings and Clinical Experience

Cloves and clove oil have been used around the world for generations to relieve pain from toothache and dental treatment. Clove teas are also exceptionally effective against persistent fungal infections, such as athlete's foot. Clove oil kills bacteria that cause pseudomonas (*Pseudomonas aeruginosa*), shigella (all species), staph infections (*Staphylococcus aureus*), and strep infections (*Streptococcus pneumoniae*).[1] It increases the effectiveness of acyclovir, a drug used to treat both herpes and chronic fatigue syndrome.[2] This herb also stimulates a mucus-clearing cough, and relieves inflammation of the mouth and throat.

Considerations for Use

Use cloves in the form of clove oil, available from pharmacies and drugstores.

Cocklebur

See **Agrimony.**

Codonopsis / Tojin

Description and Parts Used

Codonopsis is a twining perennial. It reaches a length of five feet, and has oval leaves and purple-veined green flowers. Kampo uses the long, sweet taproot.

Uses in Kampo

Codonopsis holds an important place in Kampo and TCM as a remedy for what is called "false fire syndrome." Usually caused by inappropriate acupuncture or excessive use of ginseng (see page 57), this syndrome is expressed in a symptom pattern of uncharacteristic aggressiveness combined with cloudiness in the urine, headaches, high blood pressure, and/or tight muscles. As a cooling herb, codonopsis is also used in any illness in which spleen qi deficiency, a deficiency of digestive energies, is thought to be the underlying cause.

Scientific Findings and Clinical Experience

Codonopsis has been used for centuries to treat appetite loss, diarrhea, and vomiting. Laboratory studies suggest that codonopsis extracts act by reducing the secretion of pepsin in the stomach, and by slowing the rate at which the stomach passes food to the intestines. In animal studies, codonopsis can prevent the formation of peptic ulcers induced by stress.[1] Codonopsis also eases asthma attacks by reducing the production of hormones that cause constriction of the bronchial passages.[2] With these healing properties, this herb is especially useful for asthma or peptic ulcers that are compounded by loss of appetite, diarrhea, or vomiting.

Codonopsis also plays a valuable role in radiation therapy. A Chinese study involving seventy-six cancer patients found that codonopsis teas could delay radiation's effects on healthy cells. Treatment with the herb increased the ability of interleukin-2, an immune-system chemical, to fight colorectal cancer, lymphoma, melanoma, and kidney cancer (renal cell carcinoma).[3] In addition, codonopsis restrains the immune system in lupus, a disease in which the immune system attacks the DNA found in the body's own skin cells.[4]

Considerations for Use

To make codonopsis tea, simmer 1 tablespoon (3 grams) of the dried herb in 1 cup of water for forty-five minutes, and strain before use. Codonopsis is also available in tablet (*Dang Shen*) and tincture forms.

Codonopsis is a relatively inexpensive herb that is often substituted for ginseng (see page 57) in herbal tonics labeled as "ginseng."

Coix / Yokuinin

Description and Parts Used

Coix is an Oriental grain that bears six to fifteen seed heads, similar to wheat's single seed head, on alternating sides of a single stalk. Grown throughout China as a food crop, coix is harvested at the end of autumn when its seeds have ripened. Quality coix seed is full, large, round, and white.

Coix can be puffed to make it more suitable for treating water accumulation in the digestive tract, that is, bloating or diarrhea. Raw, unpuffed coix is used in cancer treatment.

Uses in Kampo

Historically, Japanese herbalists have prescribed large doses of coix for the treatment of tumors. They also use it as a treatment for diarrhea and plantar warts. In addition, coix is used to clear damp heat, or infection, characterized by a greasy tongue coating and digestive problems; clear heat and expel pus, externally for carbuncles and internally for lung abscesses; and expel fluid causing joint pain and immobility. Coix is also used to promote urination and leach out dampness. This action treats edema, difficult urination, and swelling in the legs. The herb is a standard mastitis remedy in Japan.

Scientific Findings and Clinical Experience

Recent scientific studies have identified chemical compounds in coix that, as long recognized in traditional medicine, fight tumors caused by viruses. The seeds also contain fatty acids that activate the body's natural killer cells, an important part of the immune system, to fight cancer.[1]

Coix is a traditional Kampo remedy for tumors and skin growths of all kinds, including plantar warts, painful warts on the soles of the feet that are caused by a virus. Japanese studies have found that coix stops viral infection by stimulating the immune system to destroy infected cells.[2] A study of seven healthy volunteers who took two capsules of coix three times a day for four weeks found that the herb stimulated production of helper T cells, which stimulate other immune-system cells to attack the virus.[3]

The fatty acids in coix are also believed to help stop the formation of atherosclerotic plaques when high cholesterol levels are present.[4] It is likely that coix inhibits the production of cholesterol in the liver, although it may increase the production of triglycerides.[5] For this reason, coix is only useful as part of a total treatment plan for atherosclerosis, in which a low-carbohydrate diet helps maintain low triglycerides levels in the blood.

Considerations for Use

Coix, a food as well as an herb, can be taken on a long-term basis. Coix cereal is available in Japanese groceries as *hatomugi.* Since coix promotes urination, it should not be used during pregnancy.

Coltsfoot / Kantoka

Description and Parts Used

Coltsfoot is an herb that looks like the dandelion (see page 45). Native to Asia and Europe, it has become naturalized in North America, where it is a common sight along roadsides and in open areas. Kampo uses the flower buds.

Uses in Kampo

Coltsfoot is an acrid, sweet, warming herb. It dissolves sputum while moistening the lungs and relieving inflammation. Kampo uses coltsfoot in Arrest Wheezing Decoction (see Chapter 4) to treat asthma, bronchitis with thick sputum or with blood, chronic cough, wheezing, and, especially, lung conditions associated with smoking. Actually, coltsfoot itself has been smoked for more than 2,500 years as a way of obtaining its medicinal effects.

Scientific Findings and Clinical Experience

Small doses of coltsfoot open the bronchial passages, although large doses close them.[1] The herb also contains mucilages that coat the throat, which relieves irritation. In addition, alkaloid compounds in coltsfoot stimulate the medullary center of the brain to raise blood pressure.[2]

Considerations for Use

Make coltsfoot tea by simmering $^1/_2$ to 1 tablespoon (1.5 to 3.0 grams) of chopped coltsfoot in 1 cup of water for between five and twenty minutes. Strain before drinking. Do not use more than 2 tablespoons of coltsfoot in any one day. Coltsfoot teas can relieve coughing with hoarseness as well as acute inflammation of the mouth and throat.

There is controversy about coltsfoot's safety. Both the leaves and the flowers of the wild herb contain pyrrolizidine alkaloids, compounds that can induce liver cancer even in very small amounts. However, the amount of these alkaloids that occur naturally in a standard dose of coltsfoot is less than $^1/_{100}$ of the amount that produces toxicity. Moreover, a genetically engineered variety of coltsfoot that contains none of the offending substances is now available.[3] Therefore, do *not* use any coltsfoot product that is not certified pyrrolizidine-free. In particular, do not use tinctures. When made with wild coltsfoot, such tinctures contain ten times the concentration of alkaloids as teas made with the same amount of herb. In addition, wild coltsfoot tinctures can aggravate high blood pressure.

Coptis / Oren

Description and Parts Used

Coptis, a low-growing relative of the peony (see page 78), is native to the mountains of China. Kampo uses the root, which is dug in the autumn and sliced.

Coptis is sometimes fried before use in formulas (see Chapter 4). It is dry-fried to increase its cooling properties for use in detoxifying formulas. It is fried in ginger juice (see page 56) for use in antivomiting formulas. It is fried with evodia (see page 50) for formulas used to relieve vomiting, diarrhea, or belching. However, frying or roasting coptis does reduce its ability to kill germs.

Uses in Kampo

Coptis is an intensely bitter herb that puts out the fire of liver infection. Like its American relative goldenseal, coptis detoxifies, dries dampness, and purges inflammation. It is used for symptoms such as delirium, disorientation, high fever, irritability, and rapid pulse. It also treats excessive heat with toxicity, as indicated by abscesses, boils, carbuncles, painful, red eyes, or sore throat. Coptis cools the blood when there is blood in the urine, stool, or vomit, or in cases of bleeding gums or nosebleed.

Coptis drains dampness from the stomach, which relieves heartburn, diarrhea, and/or acidic vomiting. The herb is also used to help the kidneys and heart communicate with each other, thus relieving insomnia and irritability.

Scientific Findings and Clinical Experience

One of the principal active chemicals in coptis is berberine, an extremely effective antibiotic. It kills a vast variety of germs—among them *Plasmodium* (malaria), pseudomonas, salmonella, shigella, staph, strep, vibrio, various kinds of fungi, and leishmania[1]—and is very active against a number of others. This makes it effective against strep throat and sinusitis, among other infectious diseases. Berberine is more potent than the sulfa drugs, and has been proven effective against some bacteria that have acquired the ability to resist antibiotics. Unfortunately, berberine slows down the body's ability to expel germs in the intestine. For this reason, coptis is not useful in stopping diarrhea caused by bacterial infection.

However, as often is the case, the herb itself is more effective than any single chemical that is derived from it. Unlike berberine, coptis is effective against the organisms that cause giardiasis and trichomonas infections of the urinary tract.[2] And the whole herb is very effective against the bacteria that cause tuberculosis. In one study, thirty patients who were spitting blood with cough and fever took coptis capsules for three months. All saw their symptoms disappear.[3]

Clinical studies have shown coptis extracts to be effective against diphtheria, inner ear infections, and scarlet fever. Coptis tea kills *Helicobacter pylori,* a bacterium implicated in both ulcers and chronic gastritis.[4] The tea has also been shown to kill *Candida albicans,* the organism responsible for yeast infections.[5] Coptis has been used to treat anal fissures and inflammatory bowel disease.

When used externally, coptis solutions are useful in treating the eye disorders acute conjunctivitis and superficial keratitis, as well as osteomyelitis, a bone infection of the fingers.[6] Coptis ointments reduce the incidence of infection in first- and second-degree burns.[7]

Coptis has other benefits besides its germ-fighting abilities. Studies indicate that berberine can lower blood-sugar levels in diabetic animals.[8] The herb stimulates the gallbladder to produce bile, and reduces the viscosity of the bile flowing into the bile ducts. This helps the gallbladder to drain more quickly, thus avoiding gallstone formation. In experiments, coptis reduces blood-cholesterol levels, and produces chemicals that hinder the development of arteriosclerosis.[9]

Finally, coptis is a useful cancer treatment. When added to bath water, it increases the skin's ability to absorb 5-fluorouracil (Efudex, Fluoroplex),[10] a drug used to treat both actinic keratosis, a precancerous skin condition, and basal cell carcinoma, a form of skin cancer. In addition, the chemical berberine stops the multiplication of human liver cancer cells.[11]

Considerations for Use

Coptis is an extremely bitter herb. Although TCM practitioners frequently give coptis in the form of teas, many people find the taste intolerable. Instead, tinctures can be used, or the dried herb can be taken in capsule form.

When using coptis, dosage is important. Small amounts stimulate the brain and result in alertness, while the use of large amounts result in drowsiness. Similarly, small doses of coptis increase blood pressure, but large doses lower it. In addition, coptis should not be used for more than two weeks at a time, as it can harm the friendly bacteria that live in the intestines. It is also important to keep in mind that berberine's effectiveness can be limited by vitamin B_6 and the amino acid histidine. When taking coptis for infections, temporarily discontinue vitamin and protein supplements. Avoid this herb altogether during pregnancy.

Coptis is used in poultice form for boils. To make a poultice, mix 1 tablespoon of the powder with an equal amount of water or egg white to form a paste. Apply to the boil and cover with an absorbent bandage. Coptis compresses are used with topical forms of the chemotherapy drug 5-fluorouracil. To make a compress, add 30 drops of tincture to $^1/_4$ cup of warm water, and soak a clean cloth in the mixture. Fifteen minutes before applying the drug, lay the coptis-soaked cloth on the affected skin. Dry, and immediately apply 5-fluorouracil.

Cordyceps

See Other Traditional Healing Substances.

Cornelian Cherry / Sanshuyu

Description and Parts Used

Cornelian cherry is the fruit of the Japanese dogwood. Kampo formulas (see Chapter 4) call for dried whole fruit preserved in brine.

Uses in Kampo

Cornelian cherry stabilizes the kidneys and activates the urinary tract so that it can retain fluids. This inhibits excessive urination. Since the kidney controls fluid balances throughout the body, Cornelian cherry's action on the kidney adjusts fluid balances in the inner ear, relieving vertigo, and in the lens of the eye, treating blurry vision. This action also works against impotence and lower back pain. In Japan, Cornelian cherry is famous for its ability to stop headaches and ringing in the ears suffered by elderly people.

Cornelian cherry warms the body. It warms the stomach to stimulate digestion, and it warms the knees and lower back to assuage pain and paralysis caused by damp and cold.

In formulas, Cornelian cherry stabilizes the menses. This stops excessive uterine bleeding and prolonged menstruation. By acting on the liver, Cornelian cherry calms irritability associated with premenstrual syndrome.

Scientific Findings and Clinical Experience

Cornelian cherry contains the chemicals morroniside and 7-O-methylmorroniside. These compounds increase urine flow and lower blood pressure.[1]

Considerations for Use

Cornelian cherry is most commonly used in formulas (see Chapter 4).

Corydalis / Engosaku

Description and Parts Used

Corydalis is a low-growing plant with narrow leaves and pink flowers that is native to northern China, Japan, and Siberia. This opium-poppy relative survives the harsh conditions of northeast Asia by storing most of its energy reserves in its hard, bright-yellow tuber. The root is unearthed in autumn, dried, and then sliced into cross sections for use in Kampo.

Uses in Kampo

Corydalis is a warming, bitter herb that activates energy circulation while it vitalizes the blood. Corydalis relieves pain caused by stagnant blood in traumatic injuries, menstrual cramps, and other forms of abdominal pain. Oriental medicine also uses corydalis to treat energy stagnation due to constrained liver energy, which results in pent-up emotions.

Scientific Findings and Clinical Experience

Before 1950, both Oriental and Western medicine used corydalis extracts to treat epilepsy and Parkinson's disease. The herb contains tetrahydropalmatine, which is hypnotic, sedative, and tranquilizing.[1]

Corydalis's soothing qualities make it useful in the treatment of insomnia and anxiety. Its alkaloids increase the sleep-inducing effect of barbiturates, and are about 40 percent as effective as morphine in inducing sleep. American herbalists blend corydalis with California poppy (*Eschscholzia californica*) to treat nervousness, insomnia, agitation, and anxiety.[2]

Corydalis is also useful in treating painful abdominal conditions. In formulas (see Chapter 4), it can ease the pain associated with dysmennorhea, although menstrual flow may be reduced.[3] Corydalis is used in a Chinese herbal formula that has been shown to relieve symptoms of stomach ulcer associated with the bacterium *Helicobacter pylori* 80 percent of the time.[4] Alcohol extracts of corydalis also have been tested in the prevention of cataracts associated with diabetes.[5] In addition, corydalis is a key component in some Kampo formulas used to treat cancer, since it helps keep tumors from developing their own networks of blood vessels.

Considerations for Use

Corydalis is used as powder mixed with food.

Do not use corydalis during pregnancy. In formulas meant for expectant mothers, stephania (see page 90), which has many of the same pain-relieving effects as corydalis, is substituted. Continuous use of corydalis results in tolerance, and may also lead to a cross-tolerance to morphine.[6] Anyone who uses any type of a sleeping aid, especially a barbiturate, should be careful of the additive effects of sleeping pills and corydalis.

Cuscuta / Toshishi

Description and Parts Used

Kampo formulas use cuscuta seed, which is sometimes pressed into a bar.

Uses in Kampo

Cuscuta is an acrid, sweet, warming herb that energizes the kidneys to send fluids upward in the body. Cuscuta is used for this purpose in the formula Restore the Right Kidney Pill (see Chapter 4) to treat blurred vision, frequent urination, impotence, tinnitus, and weak back and knees.

Cuscuta has a special effect on hair. It is the primary ingredient in Seven-Treasure Pill for Beautiful Whiskers, a formula used to treat premature graying of the hair in both men and women.

Scientific Findings and Clinical Experience

Cuscuta improves both the immune response and the way blood sugar is used in the body.[1] Its centuries-old application as a hair darkener has not yet been scientifically explained.

Considerations for Use

Do not use cuscuta, or formulas containing it, if either constipation or dark, scanty urine is present.

Dan Shen / Tanjin

Description and Parts Used

Dan shen is a hardy perennial mint cultivated in Inner Mongolia and Manchuria. It grows to a height of thirty-two inches, and has toothed oval leaves and clusters of purple flowers. The root, which is harvested from late autumn to early spring, is used in Kampo. It is coarse and purplish black inside, with small white spots.

Uses in Kampo

Kampo employs dan shen as a bitter and cold herb to energize blood circulation. Dan shen dispels stagnant blood, soothes the heart, and regulates menstruation. It is used by itself in the treatment of static blood causing tumors and skin eruptions accompanied by fever. Chinese Kampo practitioners consider dan shen to be especially useful in treating liver energy, or emotional energy, constrained by "accumulated blood," in which failure to menstruate builds a blood dam that blocks the free flow of emotions from the liver. Dan shen is usually included in Augmented Ophiopogonis Decoction (see Chapter 4) to treat this symptom pattern.

TCM also uses dan shen in the treatment of hepatitis, inner ear infections, mastitis, surgical infections, tonsillitis, and skin infections and diseases, including psoriasis, shingles, and Recklinghausen's neurofibromatosis, a condition marked by thousands of small benign tumors in the skin.[1]

Scientific Findings and Clinical Experience

Dan shen is an important herb in the treatment of circulatory problems. Dan shen extracts relax the smooth muscles that support the coronary arteries and increase circulation to the heart. The herb contains a substance called tanshinone IIA[2] that slows down the transmission of nerve impulses within the heart, reducing the heart's rate while increasing its output. Both dan shen extracts and pure tanshinone IIA prevent the formation of clots in the bloodstream. Lastly, the herb reduces cholesterol and triglyceride levels in blood plasma. In clinical studies, researchers in China have reported the following results:

- Among 323 angina patients in Shanghai, 57 percent had electrocardiograms (EKGs) that showed improvement after the patients took dan shen pills. The herb was used for periods ranging from one month to nine months. Some patients had lowered cholesterol levels, and some patients who had problems with high blood pressure saw their pressure readings drop as they continued to take the herb.[3]
- In a study of sixty-five patients who had suffered strokes caused by cerebral atherosclerosis, or arteries narrowed by cholesterol in the brain, nine patients recovered completely from paralysis and language difficulties, and forty-eight showed significant improvement, while only eight showed no progress. These patients were given dan shen by intramuscular injection.[4]
- In a study of 113 patients with phlebitis, a painful vein inflammation, twenty-eight were completely cured after taking dan shen tea.[5]

The way dan shen affects the circulatory system seems to be due to its ability to change the rate at which the body absorbs and uses copper.[6] When copper is bound by compounds in dan shen, the body cannot make fibrin, a protein "rope" on which new blood vessels are suspended. Many diseases involve excessive blood-vessel production. In diabetic retinopathy and macular degeneration, stopping such production stops bleeding and forestalls optic damage. In chronic fatigue syndrome, forestalling blood-vessel production helps maintain blood pressure, which ensures that the brain receives enough oxygen for normal function. In cancer, disabling a tumor's ability to make its own blood supply greatly reduces its ability to spread.

Considerations for Use

Make dan shen tea by simmering $^1/_2$ ounce (15 grams) of powdered root in 3 cups of boiling water for twenty minutes. Strain and drink, 1 cup at a time, at room temperature.

Dan shen tincture is used for angina and other circulatory problems. This tincture should only be taken under professional supervision.

Dan shen is useful for short-term treatment of skipped periods or uterine fibroids.[7] On the other hand, long-term use of dan shen can be harmful, since it stimulates estrogen production.[8] Use dan shen for such conditions only under the supervision of a knowledgeable practitioner and for no more than twenty-eight days.

Dandelion / HOKOEI

Description and Parts Used

Known best in North America as a weed marring freshly cut lawns, dandelion grows wild in most of the world and is cultivated as an herb in China, France, and Germany. Young leaves are picked in the spring for tonic salads, and in the summer for the manufacture of medicinal teas and tinctures. The roots of two-year-old plants are dug in the fall.

Uses in Kampo

Kampo uses dandelion to clear energies derived from hostile, pent-up emotions, which are associated with the liver. Dandelion clears the liver's energy channel, thus soothing painful, red, or swollen eyes. It also breaks up "clumps" of energy that manifest themselves as lumps and nodules at other points on the liver channel, especially the breasts. Dandelion promotes urination and stimulates lactation.

Scientific Findings and Clinical Experience

Dandelion leaves are a powerful diuretic, although their exact mode of action is still not understood. Unlike many conventional diuretics, which cause a loss of potassium, dandelion leaves are rich in potassium, causing a net gain of this vital mineral.[1] Because of its diuretic effect, dandelion relieves fluid retention after excessive salt consumption or as a part of premenstrual syndrome. And by increasing potassium levels, the herb reduces muscle spasms and nighttime leg cramps.

Dandelion contains not only more potassium than any other herb, but more iron and vitamins as well. It also has more carotenoids, the natural source of vitamin A, than carrots. Due to its high nutritive content, it has been used for generations to treat anemia due to deficiencies of folic acid, iron, and vitamin B_{12}.

German research has shown that dandelion root is a mild bitter, or appetite stimulant. Dandelion root also has a significant cleansing effect on the liver and stimulates the production of bile.[2] This effect on bile production allows the herb to perform two tasks. One, it can regulate bowel function, and is noted for its ability to relieve constipation without causing diarrhea. Two, it can correct gallbladder problems and spasms of the bile duct, although it is not recommended when there are gallstones, as such usage could increase pain.

Dandelion is also useful in the treatment of chronic, nonspecific irritable bowel syndrome. Bulgarian studies of an herbal combination that included dandelion found that more than 95 per cent of patients with large-intestine pain were pain-free after fifteen days of treatment. The combination also improved bowel regularity.[3]

European herbalists frequently prescribe dandelion tincture as a weight-loss aid. Dandelion is particularly effective in removing water weight through its diuretic effect. It may also help the liver regulate blood sugars in a way that reduces appetite without inducing hypoglycemia, or low blood sugar.[4] In one study, animals that were given daily doses of dandelion extract for a month lost up to 30 percent of their body mass.[5]

Dandelion has other uses. In a study of 472 herbs, Chinese scientists found that dandelion was among the ten most effective in controlling herpes simplex, the type of infection responsible for cold sores and genital herpes.[6] In addition, dandelion is a traditional hangover remedy. Although this use has not been scientifically verified, it is likely that dandelion stimulates the liver to break down acetaldehyde, an alcohol byproduct that triggers headache and indigestion. It is also possible that the herb's ability to stimulate the excretion of acetaldehyde byproducts, without upsetting the body's mineral balance, relieves stress on inflamed tissues.

Considerations for Use

To make dandelion tea, simmer between 1 scant teaspoon and 1 scant tablespoon (1 to 3 grams) of the dried herb in 1 cup of water for ten minutes. Strain before use. Dandelion is also available in tincture, tablet, and fluid extract forms. Take all forms on an empty stomach.

Dendrobium / SEKKOKU

Description and Parts Used

Dendrobium is a Chinese orchid. Kampo formulas call for dendrobium stem and leaf, which are usually tied into small bundles. Dendrobium has many of the same qualities as ophiopogon (see page 77), although dendrobium offers greater relief for stomach pain.

Uses in Kampo

Dendrobium is a slightly cold and sweet moistening herb used to treat dry mouth, thirst, and stomach pain after prolonged fevers and sunstroke. Dendrobium relieves mouth sores activated by exposure to sun and heat, such as those caused by herpes. The herb is also used to strengthen the lower back and brighten the vision, especially in cases of cataract.

Scientific Findings and Clinical Experience

Two toxic compounds found in minute quantities in the outside layers of dendrobium stem are under study for their ability to stop protein formation in the HIV virus. If the virus cannot form protein it cannot create a protective coat, which keeps it from leaving infected cells to infect healthy cells.[1] Dendrobium also contains compounds that stop toxins called free radicals from causing cataracts.[2]

Considerations for Use

Dendrobium can be made into tea, or taken as a tincture. In either case, its use should be supervised by an herbalist. This herb is also used in formulas (see Chapter 4).

Dioscorea / SANYAKU

Description and Parts Used

Dioscorea, also known as the wild or medicinal yam, is native to moist tropical zones around the world. In the tropics, dioscorea vines can climb to a height of twenty feet, bearing heart-shaped leaves and green, tiny flowers. Herbal formulas call for thick, diagonal slices of peeled rhizome. Powdered dioscorea serves as a thickening agent for many foods. In addition, the herb is a traditional beauty aid (see "Beauty Served by Dioscorea").

Beauty Served by Dioscorea

Throughout history, dioscorea has been recognized as a beautifying herb. The *Rokkasen* (Six Major Poets) records the story of Ono no Komachi, who was the most beautiful woman in the world. The key to her beauty was her diet—she lived on wild game, barley gruel, and dioscorea. When barley and yam are eaten together, their fibers swell with the water of the gruel and give the diner a feeling of fullness. This prevents overeating, which helped Komachi stay slim. The fibers of dioscorea then clean the intestines, which allows circulation of fluids. This gave Komachi her clear and beautiful skin.[1]

The fabled yam also provided the source for one of the twentieth century's most influential medical revolutions, the Pill. For decades, mass production of the hormones used in birth control pills was stymied by a lack of the chemical "raw material." This compound, diosgenin, was eventually found in the wild yam. While earlier processes used tons of animal ovaries to produce grams of hormone, scientists quickly learned that an acre of yams could produce 500 pounds of diosgenin, and the contraceptive revolution ensued.

Although the yam provided the raw materials for the Pill, diosgenin itself has no hormonal activity. Nor can the human body convert it into something that does. Therefore, be warned: Do *not* use dioscorea as a contraceptive!

Uses in Kampo

Kampo uses dioscorea as a natural laxative, and as a qi, or energy, tonic for the spleen, or the body's digestive function. As a smoothing and regulating herb for the body's energies, dioscorea is used to treat coughs, diabetes, frequent urination, spermatorrhea (the involuntary flow of semen), night sweats, and general weakness.

Kampo digestive formulas combine dioscorea with ginseng (see page 57), while formulas for kidney diseases such as diabetes combine dioscorea with hoelen (see page 61). See Chapter 4 for formula information.

Scientific Findings and Clinical Experience

Dioscorea has long been used in the treatment of both type 1 and type 2 dependent diabetes. In animal studies, alcohol extracts of dioscorea have dramatic effects on blood-sugar levels. Dioscorea reduced sugar levels by 50 percent in both diabetic and normal test animals.[1] Dioscorea even reduces sugar levels in type 1 diabetes.[2]

In North and Central America, dioscorea is a traditional relaxing remedy for painful menstruation and ovarian pain. The action of the herb is not related to estrogen balance, but rather to its anti-inflammatory action. This action also allows dioscorea to relax stiff muscles while it reduces arthritic inflammation and pain. Saponins, the anti-inflammatory substances in dioscorea, are water-soluble, and thus alcohol tinctures will not help ease arthritic inflammation. Alcohol tinctures of dioscorea, however, have antiasthmatic, antitussive, and expectorant effects.[3]

Considerations for Use

Dioscorea is best used as a tincture. Dioscorea is effective even in very low doses and has virtually no toxicity.

Some patent (over-the-counter) medicines sold as "dioscorea creams" contain synthetic progesterone, the same compound used in the Pill. Almost always, this progesterone is not listed on the label. Be sure to verify that any product purchased is made from herbal ingredients.

Dong Quai

See **Tang-Kuei.**

Dracaena Lily / Kekketsu

Description and Parts Used

In Japan and China, "dragon's blood" is harvested from the dracaena lily. Dragon's blood is an iron-black substance that the plant oozes in the late summer and which turns blood-red when powdered.

Uses in Kampo

Kampo and other traditional Asian herbal systems use dragon's blood to treat conditions under the doctrine of similars, that is, they use a blood-colored substance to treat diseases involving bleeding. Dracaena lily dispels static blood and relieves pain caused by bruises, contusions, falls, fractures, and sprains. Applied to the skin, it stops bleeding and helps heal skin ulcers. In China, it is sometimes combined with equal quantities of frankincense and myrrh (see pages 97 and 99) to relieve pain from minor traumatic injuries, or with pollen to treat chronically ulcerated skin.

Scientific Research and Clinical Experience

Herbalists Dan Bensky and Andrew Gamble report that dracaena lily teas have an antibiotic effect on many kinds of skin fungal infections. They also report that dracaena can occasionally cause strong allergic reactions.[1]

Considerations for Use

Draecena lily is used in Trauma Pill (see Chapter 4).

Drynaria Rhizome / Kotsusaiho

Description and Parts Used

Drynaria is a fernlike woodland plant that grows in southeastern China and Taiwan. Kampo uses the large, brown rhizome.

Uses in Kampo

In Chinese, drynaria rhizome is called *gu sui bu*, or "mender of shattered bones." Historically, it has been used to mend sinews and bones damaged by falls, fractures, contusions, and sprains. It is especially useful for torn ligaments and simple fractures.

Drynaria rhizome regulates outwardly directed, or yang, energies in the body. It also tonifies the kidneys, which in Oriental medicine are responsible for symptoms such as pain or weakness in the lower back and knees, the ringing in the ears known as tinnitus, hearing loss, toothache, and bleeding gums. As a kidney tonic, drynaria rhizome also stimulates the growth of hair.

Scientific Findings and Clinical Experience

Drynaria rhizome reverses side effects of streptomycin treatment, especially headache, dizziness, and numbness of the lips and tongue. It has also been proven effective in treating tinnitus and hearing loss.[1]

Considerations for Use

Drynaria tinctures are used topically for male pattern baldness. Drynaria rhizome stimulates blood circulation, so individuals who are taking blood-thinning medications should use it with caution.

Ephedra / Mao

Description and Parts Used

Ephedra is a shrub with long, narrow, sprawling stems and very small leaves. At a mature height of only twenty inches, the herb is well suited to the cold, windy deserts of its native northern China and Inner Mongolia. Also known as ma huang, ephedra has been used since very ancient times—there are reports of its being found with a body that was buried in Mesopotamia 40,000 years ago. Although all parts of the plant are used in Kampo, it is the top that is used in the treatment of asthma, ephedra's most notable use.

Uses in Kampo

Ephedra is an essential herb in Kampo. Warming and pungent, ephedra stops the progress of a pathogen while it is still in the body's most superficial layers, or exterior—the skin, joints, and muscles. The confrontation of the infection and the defensive energies of the body create pain. Ephedra opens the "interstices" of the skin to give the pathogen a route of escape, and to give the body a route by which to flush the pathogen out through perspiration. This action stops patterns of chills and fever, as well as headache, caused by "tight" skin.

In addition to helping the body fight off the initial stages of infection, ephedra also regulates the flow of qi, or energy, through the lungs. It stops cough and wheezing due to the obstruction of lung energy by invading "cold" influences. It redirects the upward-flowing energies that cause cough to a downward direction, supplying the body with air. It also encourages the flow of fluids downward. This drains off fluids in the top half of the body that cause swelling and pain, especially in the initial stages of infection.

Scientific Findings and Clinical Experience

Ephedrine, a chemical found in ephedra, acts in many of the same ways as the hormone epinephrine, also known as adrenalin. The herb increases blood pressure and heart rate, and relaxes bronchial muscles to open air passageways. Ephedrine also stimulates perspiration and lowers body temperature.

Ephedrine travels in the body in ways that epinephrine cannot. Ephedrine crosses the blood-brain barrier, rapidly entering nerve tissue, and increases the activity of the brain centers that control breathing and blood-vessel contraction. This allows the herb to relieve symptoms associated with allergy, asthma, colds, and flu.

Ephedra compounds have been extensively researched for use in the treatment of obesity. In one tightly controlled Danish study, 25 men and 145 women followed a low-calorie diet (provided by the testing laboratory) and took either an inert placebo or 20 milligrams of ephedrine plus 200 milligrams of caffeine per day. At the end of eight weeks, those taking the placebo had lost an average of eighteen pounds, while those taking the ephedrine lost an average of twenty pounds. While the difference in total pounds lost was not great, the ratio of fat to lean tissue lost was much better for the ephedrine group. After six months, weight loss averaged thirty-five pounds for the test group compared with twenty-nine pounds for the placebo group.[1] In very-low-calorie diets given to obese women, ephedrine did not increase weight loss, but preserved muscle tissue by stimulating the muscles' use of protein.[2]

Smokers who quit often gain weight because of what scientists believe is a steady and sustained fall in the production of hormones that stimulate the burning of fat in heat-generating brown fat cells.[3] Ephedrine and ephedra stimulate the production of these hormones. This process is assisted by substances called methylxanthines, such as caffeine in coffee and tea, and theophylline in tea. In animal testing, a combination of ephedrine, methylxanthines, and aspirin has been shown to completely prevent weight gain due to dietary excess, genetics, and adrenal dysfunction.[4]

Although virtually every study has noted that ephedrine can cause hand tremors and insomnia during the early stages of weight loss, almost every study has also noted that these symptoms disappeared upon discontinuation of the drug.

Considerations for Use

Ephedra is taken as powder mixed with food or tincture, or in tea form. To make ephedra tea, simmer 1 tablespoon of dried herb in 1 cup of water for forty-five minutes. Strain and drink between meals. Asthmatics may supplement other medications with ephedra tincture. This herb is also used in formulas (Chapter 4).

Ephedra should not be used by persons taking a monoamine oxidase (MAO) inhibitor, a class of drugs prescribed for depression, or by those who have high blood pressure, anxiety, glaucoma, or a prostate disorder. Ephedra affects different people in different ways. The same dosage of the same preparation of ephedra may raise blood pressure in some individuals, have no effect in others, and even lower pressure in still others. The most modest effect on blood pressure occurs when ephedra is taken orally, as in traditional Kampo teas.[5] In overdose, ephedra can cause insomnia and tremors. Ephedra is not addictive, but when it is taken for a long time, larger and larger doses are necessary to get the same effect.[6] And in rare instances, overuse of ephedra combined with vigorous exercise and inadequate water intake results in kidney stones. Be sure to drink eight glasses of water daily when taking any ephedra product.

When using ephedra as a weight-loss aid, it is important to remember that caffeine or ephedrine alone will not stimulate weight loss—calorie restriction is a must. Although research studies have used isolated components of ephedra, it is preferable to use the whole herb, since the herb contains compounds that can offset the side effects of ephedrine.

Several states have laws regulating the sale and use of ephedra. The legal situation concerning this herb is constantly changing, so it is important to learn the laws of one's own state before using ephedra products. To learn why this herb has been banned in some places, see "The Truth About Ephedra."

The Truth About Ephedra

Ephedra has been used for thousands of years by people all over the world. However, the drug's safety has been called into question because of at least one death associated with herbal stimulants purported to contain ephedra. It is a sad example of what can happen when a chemical derivative is used in place of the whole herb.

In ancient legend, the first person to discover ephedra was an elderly Aryan who had, in accordance with his tribe's custom, been exiled after he became too old to hunt. Wandering alone, he found the "thousand boughs" of ephedra, and learned that it produced both energy and a mild euphoria. Feeling stronger and happier, this herbal pioneer created soma, or ephedra juice, the drink of perpetual youth. Eventually, Aryans both young and old used soma to enhance their hunting skills. The herb was later adopted by both the Chinese and the Romans.

Chinese medicine applied ephedra to the treatment of colds and congestion. *The Herbal Classic of the Divine Plowman* listed ephedra among the "middle class" herbs, effective herbs that could cure disease but could also cause some undesirable side effects. Both Chinese medicine and Kampo used ephedra with caution in persons with yin constitutions. In Western terms, such persons have high blood pressure, hyperthyroidism, prostate disease, or glaucoma. Chinese medicine and Kampo also recognized that the nodes joining the leaf segments are the toxic parts of the plant. For hundreds of years, Kampo herbalists have removed them during processing.

The problems with ephedra have arisen through Western efforts to extract individual chemicals from the herb rather than using the herb as a whole. The chemical ephedrine, for instance, relieves asthma but also induces high blood pressure. The whole herb ephedra contains pseudoephedrine, which slows the heart rate and lowers blood pressure, offsetting any toxic effects of ephedrine.

Unfortunately, chemical compounds like those found in ephedra have appeared in "herbal" combinations sold under such names as Cloud 9, Herbal Ecstasy, and Ultimate Xphoria. These combinations are meant to create an herbal high. In search of such an experience, one college student took eight pills of Ultimate Xphoria, and subsequently died.

These stimulants are *not* ephedra. Ephedra's euphoriant effect is attributable to a chemical also known as cathine. In a chemical analysis of Ultimate Xphoria, however, cathine was almost totally absent. Thus one might take an herbal pill, feel stimulated but not "high," and take some more, putting greater and greater stress on one's internal organs.

Obviously, no one should take substances such as Ultimate Xphoria. Anyone with a medical condition for which ephedra would be appropriate should take the herb, by itself or in a recognized Kampo formula, *after* being examined for precluding conditions, such as high blood pressure. An herbalist or Kampo practitioner can help determine how this herb may best be used.

Epimedium / Inyokaku

Description and Parts Used

Epimedium is a low-growing herb in the same family as coptis (see page 42). Its yellow-green leaves are usually steeped in wine before being fashioned into pills.

Uses in Kampo

Epimedium is a kidney tonic. It is used to treat a variety of diseases Kampo associates with deficient kidney energy, including memory problems, frequent urination, impotence, lower back and knee pain, and spermatorrhea (involuntary flow of semen). In addition, epimedium is a liver tonic that regulates ascending energies from the liver. In this capacity, it is used to treat lower back pain, dizziness, and menstrual irregularities. This heating herb also expels cold from the joints, and relieves spasms and cramps in the hands and feet.

Scientific Findings and Clinical Experience

There are many herbs with estrogenlike effects. Epimedium is an unusual herb in that it has testosteronelike effects. It stimulates sexual activity in both men and women, increases sperm production, stimulates the sensory nerves, and increases sexual desire. It also increases blood flow to the penis. Epimedium mildly stimulates tissue growth in the prostate, testes, and the ring muscle controlling the anus.

Epimedium has strong effects on the cardiovascular system. It increases blood flow to the heart by causing the coronary blood vessels to dilate. This action lowers blood pressure and is long-lasting, although the body can develop a tolerance to the herb after long-term use.[1] It also prevents a protein called fibrin from being deposited on capillary walls. This prevents loss of sexual function in men with atherosclerosis.

In laboratory tests, epimedium has an inhibitory effect on the polio virus and the staph bacterium *Staphylococcus aureus,* which is associated with ear infections.[2] The herb kills HIV and the bacteria that cause staph infections, gonorrhea, and pneumonia. Epimedium also stimulates the activity of germ-eating immune-system cells called macrophages.

Epimedium is useful in cancer treatment. It binds with copper, which keeps that element from being used in a process by which cancer cells can form their own blood vessels. Without a blood supply, tumors cannot grow and spread.

Considerations for Use

Epimedium should be taken as directed by an herbalist. It is a relatively nontoxic herb, but can have side effects with prolonged use, such as dizziness, vomiting, dry mouth, thirst, or nosebleed. If any of these symptoms appear, discontinue usage. Extreme overdoses can result in exaggerated reflexes, spasms, and respiratory arrest. Individuals with prostate disorders should avoid epimedium.

Epsom Salts

See **Mirabilite** under Other Traditional Healing Substances.

Eucommia / Tochu

Description and Parts Used

Eucommia is a tree native to the temperate zones of China that reaches a height of up to seventy-five feet. A single tree has both male and female flowers, the male flowers in loose clusters and the female flowers appearing singly in the points of the leaves. The bark is used in Kampo. Eucommia leaf, better known as *tochu-cha,* is a popular beverage in Japan.

Uses in Kampo

Kampo uses eucommia bark as a tonic for the kidney and liver. As an acrid, sweet, and warming herb, it is included in most formulas for weakness and pain in the lower back and knees, and for bone and joint problems, urinary incontinence, and the prevention of miscarriage. Kampo also uses formulas containing eucommia to calm a "kicking" fetus during pregnancy. The most commonly used eucommia-containing formula in Kampo is Major Ledebouriella Decoction (see Chapter 4).

Scientific Findings and Clinical Experience

Eucommia bark extract is used to treat high blood pressure.[1] The herb lowers blood pressure by dilating the peripheral blood vessels, or those vessels that extend beyond major vessels such as the aorta. (In high doses, though, eucommia constricts blood vessels.) Eucommia also stimulates urination, thereby indirectly lowering blood pressure.

Laboratory studies show that eucommia extracts activate germ-destroying factors in the immune system.[2] Additional studies in Japan have found that substances extracted from eucommia bark can keep HIV from entering healthy cells, and at a dosage that is less than 1 percent of the dosage that damages healthy cells.[3]

Japanese scientists have also found that eucommia teas can protect cells against substances, called mutagens, that cause genetic mutations, which in turn can both hasten the aging process and lead to tumor formation. One study found that the herb can reduce tissue damage after radiation exposure.[4] Eucommia has also been found to enhance the antiaging effects of ginseng (see page 57) when used in teas in a ratio of one part ginseng to three parts eucommia. This herbal combination stimulates the production of collagen,[5] which reduces skin wrinkling and joint damage. And a small study indicated that eucommia may protect the body against mutagens in food. The women in this study passed fewer mutagens in their urine when they took eucommia teas daily. When they discontinued the tea, their mutagen levels rose.[6]

Considerations for Use

The classical Kampo texts warn that eucommia should be used with caution when there is fever.

Eupatorium / Hairan

Description and Parts Used

Eupatorium is a plant in the same family as the sunflower, native to central China and Japan and closely related to a species of eupatorium found in North America. Growing to a height of five feet, it bears tapering lance-shaped leaves and multiple purple or white flowers. The above-ground parts of the plant are used in Kampo.

Uses in Kampo

Eupatorium, "aromatically transforms dampness," stimulating fluids to rise to their proper place in the body. This herb is particularly useful for encouraging the circulation of lymph—what Chinese medicine calls the "middle burner"—and relieving a stifling sensation in the chest that may be accompanied by lack of appetite, nausea, and a white, moist tongue coating. Eupatorium is used for "damp" diseases in both winter and summer, relieving both winter coughs and summer colds.

Scientific Findings and Clinical Experience

German clinical studies have shown that hot infusions of eupatorium relieve nasal congestion and scratchy throat caused by the common cold.[1] The herb is particularly useful in combination with the non-Kampo herb echinacea, increasing echinacea's immune-stimulant effect by 50 percent.[2] In some studies, eupatorium has been found to be as much as ten times as effective as echinacea in stimulating the human immune system.[3]

Eupatorium is also useful in maintaining the strength of the immune system in people with cancer. Eupatorium stimulates the activity of B cells, which are depleted in chronic leukemia, multiple myeloma, and ovarian carcinoma, and also stimulates T cells, which are depleted in Hodgkin's disease, Kaposi's sarcoma, and all forms of carcinoma once they have spread. The herb can prevent the pain of kidney stones, provided it is taken when pain is first noticed. Eupatorium also soothes the pain of urinary tract infections, particularly when there is scarring of the urinary tract.

Considerations for Use

Make an infusion from 1 ounce (30 grams) of *dried* eupatorium in 3 cups of boiling water. Allow the mixture to stand off the heat for thirty minutes, then strain. Drink 1 cup at a time. Eupatorium is also available in tincture form.

Fresh eupatorium should *never* be used to make herbal teas. The fresh herb contains tremetrol, which can cause nausea, stomachache, or vomiting.

Evodia / Goshuyu

Description and Parts Used

Evodia grows throughout southern China, and has been introduced to southern Japan. The fruit, the part used in Kampo, is picked from August to October, when it is brownish green and not completely ripe. The fruit should be full, round, and aromatic.

Uses in Kampo

Evodia warms the middle and disperses cold. It is used to relieve constrained liver qi, which produces headaches, pain in the pit of the stomach with nausea, drooling, inability to taste, and hernia. Evodia redirects rebellious qi, or qi moving upward in the digestive tract when it should be moving downward, and stops vomiting. This action stops heartburn and flank pain. It also stops diarrhea and warms the digestive organs.

One of the most important uses of evodia in TCM is to

lead fire downward from sores in the mouth and on the tongue. For this purpose, evodia is powdered, mixed with vinegar, and placed on the center of the soles of the feet.

Scientific Findings and Clinical Experience

Evodia is an effective painkiller. It also has strong antibiotic activity against the organisms that cause cholera and against the parasite *Hirudo.*[1]

Modern practitioners of traditional medicine in China have found that evodia plasters applied to soles of the feet can, surprisingly, lower blood pressure.[2] Evodia plasters applied to the navel have been especially helpful in relieving irritable bowel syndrome.[3]

Considerations for Use

Evodia is used in formulas (see Chapter 4).

Do not use evodia in cases of pregnancy. Uterine contractions caused by evodia can be blocked by indomethacin or mepacrine.[4]

Fennel Seed / SHOUIKYO

Description and Parts Used

The herb used in Kampo is the seed of the fennel used in cooking. Fennel seed is yellow-green and aromatic, dried on the plant and harvested in autumn when the fruit has ripened.

Uses in Kampo

Kampo uses fennel to balance the nutritive qi, or the body's sustaining energies. Fennel seed regulates the nutritive qi and harmonizes the digestive and propulsive functions of the stomach. It relieves abdominal pain, indigestion, anorexia, and vomiting.

Scientific Findings and Clinical Experience

Fennel seed and fennel seed oil reduce the amount of time required to empty the digestive tract. They also stop intestinal spasms and encourage the passage of gas.

Fennel seed teas reduce symptoms of hernia, frequently eliminating the need for surgery. In one clinical study, a six-week course of treatment with fennel seed teas cured fifty-nine out of sixty-four cases of vaginal hydrocele, in which a loop of intestine presses against the vagina.[1]

Fennel seed has other uses as well. It increases the effectiveness of streptomycin against tuberculosis, although it has no effect on the bacteria themselves.[2] And European herbalists have prescribed fennel seed for centuries to stimulate milk production in nursing mothers.

Considerations for Use

Make fennel seed tea by crushing 1 or 2 tablespoons (2.5 to 5.0 grams) of fennel seeds and simmering them in 1 cup of water for ten to fifteen minutes. Drink the tea between or after meals. In order to release their essential oils, the seeds must be crushed immediately before use. The tea can also be given to children. In addition, fennel seed is used in formulas (see Chapter 4).

Use fennel seed tea rather than fennel seed oil. Pure essential oil of fennel seed *increases* rather than decreases intestinal irritation. In addition, avoid fennel seed when an estrogen-sensitive disorder is present, such as breast or uterine cancer, fibroids, ovarian cysts, or fibrocystic breast disease. Fennel increases estrogen production.

Forsythia / RENGYO

Description and Parts Used

Forsythia is a shrub native to China and Japan. It reaches a height of ten feet, and bears toothed leaves, bright yellow flowers, and a fibrous fruit. Kampo uses half-shells of the fruit, which is picked just before it ripens, while it is still blue-green. "Old" forsythia fruits have already ripened and have a yellow skin. The green fruit is considered the best.

Uses in Kampo

Ancient Oriental herbalists used forsythia to treat infectious scabies as well as pimples and other skin diseases. Herbalists also used forsythia to treat breast tumors, heat rash, and swollen lymph glands. Forsythia has been a key ingredient in formulas (see Chapter 4) used to treat epidemics from the eleventh century until today.

These uses stem from forsythia's ability to detoxify the blood, clear fever and inflammation, and discharge substantial phlegm, or phlegm that has a tangible form. Cooling Forsythia is one of Kampo's most effective medicines for treating inflammations of the gums, mouth, tongue, and throat.

Scientific Findings and Clinical Experience

Forsythia has been shown to have antibacterial actions against *E. coli* and *Salmonella,* and against the bacteria that cause diphtheria, plague, staph infections, tuberculosis, and pneumonia.[1]

Forsythia also helps relieve allergies. It contains a substance called forsythiaside that inhibits the enzymes responsible for inflammation and swelling.[2] Combined with forsythia's antibacterial action, this allows the herb to provide relief for strep throat.

Considerations for Use

To make forsythia tea, simmer 2 teaspoons (2 to 3 grams) of the dried herb in 1 cup of water for forty-five minutes, then strain and drink. Or make a day's dose of the tea all at once by tripling the amounts of forsythia to 2 tablespoons (6 to 9 grams) and using 3 cups of water. If used within twenty-four hours, forsythia tea does not need refrigeration. This herb is also available in tablet form, sold in Chinese herb shops as *Wien Qiao.* Use forsythia for allergy treatment only under the supervision of an herbalist.

Foxglove

See **Rehmannia.**

Fritillaria (Cirrhosa) / Senbaimo

Description and Parts Used

Fritillaria cirrhosa is the bulb of a Chinese lily. The bulb is gathered in the late summer or autumn. It should not be confused with another form of fritillaria (see below).

Uses in Kampo

Fritillaria cirrhosa clears heat and dissipates nodules, sores, swellings, and lung abscesses. Fritillaria also transforms phlegm and stops coughing. It is most effective for a pattern of symptoms including difficult expectoration, reduced appetite, and a stifling sensation in the chest and upper abdomen.

Scientific Findings and Clinical Experience

Injections of fritillaria cirrhosa into laboratory animals create a profound and prolonged decrease in blood pressure. The herb stimulates uterine contractions but inhibits intestinal movement.[1] Kampo physicians in China use fritillaria cirrhosa in the treatment of thyroid cancer.

Considerations for Use

Fritillaria cirrhosa is available as Fritillaria and Pinellia Syrup (*Qing Chi Hua Tan Tang*). Avoid if weakness from a chronic health problem is present. It is also used in formulas (see Chapter 4).

Fritillaria (Thunberg Fritillaria Bulb) / Setsubaimo

Description and Parts Used

Thunberg fritillaria bulb is a lily that is gathered in the early summer after the above-ground parts of the plant have withered. Kampo uses thick slices of the rhizome.

Specifying the species of fritillaria is important, because another variety of fritillaria used in Oriental medicine (see above) is toxic without careful processing.

Uses in Kampo

Thunberg fritillaria is a cold, bitter herb that clears heat and dissipates nodules. It purges heat in the chest, dissolves thick phlegm, and fights inflammation. Formulas containing Thunberg fritillaria are used to treat coughs with colored mucus, tubercular lung abscesses, sore throat, and swollen glands.

Scientific Findings and Clinical Experience

Thunberg fritillaria dilates the bronchial tubes, relieves cough, and stops salivation. Scientists have found that this species of fritillaria acts in a manner similar to the drug dexamethasone, which is used to treat nasal allergy and inflammation, and lupus.[1]

Chinese clinics use thunberg fritillaria combined with platycodon (see page 81) to treat breast tumors and cysts.

Considerations for Use

Thunberg fritillaria is available as Fritillaria and Pinellia Syrup.

There are disagreements among Kampo practitioners whether this species of fritillaria is toxic, but as a safety measure, unprocessed fritillaria should never be taken internally. Since fritillaria stimulates uterine contractions,[2] avoid it during pregnancy.

Galangal / Koryokyo

Description and Parts Used

The galangal plant, which grows in humid, tropical climates around the world, is in the same family as ginger, cardamom, and turmeric. The rhizome is harvested in late summer and early autumn from plants that are four to six years old.

Uses in Kampo

Galangal warms the middle of the body. It alleviates abdominal pain, as well as vomiting, hiccups, and diarrhea.

Scientific Findings and Clinical Experience

In laboratory studies, galangal teas kill the bacteria that cause anthrax, strep infections, and staph infections.[1] Other studies have shown that galangal stops the production of hormonelike substances called prostaglandins that cause swelling, inflammation, and pain, particularly in allergic reactions to chemotherapy agents.[2]

Considerations for Use

Make galangal tea by simmering $^1/_2$ teaspoon (0.5 to 1.0 grams) of the dried herb in 1 cup of water for five minutes. Drink thirty minutes before eating. Galangal is also used in Calm the Middle Powder (see Chapter 4).

Store galangal in a cool, dark place. Do not store it in a plastic container.

Gambir / Chotoko

Description and Parts Used

Gambir is a glossy, purplish red vine that grows in tropical regions. It has alternate leaves and "hooks" that look like anchors at every leaf node. Kampo uses the stems with the hooks attached—the more hooks, the better. In the traditional method of preparation, the herb is boiled, mixed with rice husks, and allowed to dry in the sun.

Uses in Kampo

For several centuries Japanese herbalists have recognized

gambir as a sedative and antispasmodic that is useful in the treatment of convulsions, dizziness, headaches, high blood pressure, migraine headaches, seizures, and vertigo. TCM's depiction of how gambir works in the body is especially vivid. TCM says that gambir calms "internal wind," that is, symptoms that seem to "blow" from place to place in the body, by sedating "the exuberance of the liver," that is, emotions spilling over into misplaced actions, such as convulsions and seizures.

Scientific Findings and Clinical Experience

Kampo uses gambir in formulas for the treatment of childhood epilepsy (see Chapter 4). Research in Japan shows that gambir, in combination with gastrodia (see page 55), prevents seizures by destroying free radicals, substances that can cause cellular damage. These herbs also keep free radicals from activating lipid peroxides, compounds that destroy cell walls.[1]

In pregnant women, gambir is used to reduce fetal movement in the eighth month, and to relieve postpartum spasms.

Considerations for Use

Although gambir can be used by itself, the herb is almost always combined with gastrodia—see Gastrodia and Uncaria Decoction in Chapter 4.

Gardenia / Sanshishi

Description and Parts Used

The gardenia is an evergreen shrub native to southeastern China. Although it has been adapted to gardens around the world, it prefers warm, humid climates. Gardenia grows up to ten feet tall and produces white flowers in the spring. Kampo uses the fruit, which is harvested September through November when it turns reddish yellow.

Uses in Kampo

Gardenia is cold, sour, and astringent. Kampo medicines employ gardenia to purge infectious inflammation, clear fever, and detoxify the blood. Gardenia is used in formulas (see Chapter 4) to treat weeping skin ailments, pelvic inflammatory disease, urinary tract and vaginal infections, bleeding, jaundice, liver and gallbladder disorders, high fevers, and red eyes.

Kampo uses gardenia in several forms. The whole fruit is used in teas to clear heat and remove irritability in symptom patterns that include delirious speech, fever, insomnia, irritability, nervous unrest, and/or a stifling sensation in the chest. The whole fruit also treats infections of the nose or eyes and sores in the mouth or facial region. Kampo practitioners powder gardenia fruit and mix it with egg white and vinegar to reduce swelling and move static blood caused by traumatic injury.

Both traditional Japanese herbalism and TCM use charred gardenia fruit to cool the blood and stop bleeding. This form of the herb treats blood in the stool or urine, bloody vomit, or nosebleed.

Scientific Findings and Clinical Experience

Modern medicine has found additional applications for gardenia. One of the chemicals found in gardenia fruit, crocetin, stops the formation of substances called free radicals that can harm liver cells.[1] Crocetin also stops inflammation caused by bruises and contusions.[2] Laboratory studies show that gardenia stimulates blood flow to the internal organs in the early stages of pancreatitis, increasing the pancreas's oxygen supply and reducing the rate of cell death.[3]

This herb stimulates the digestive system. Gardenia teas and some of the chemicals found in gardenia can stimulate the gallbladder to secrete bile within twenty to forty minutes. Gardenia teas also stimulate the secretion of gastric juices and increase the activity of the muscles in the stomach that pass food down to the intestine.

Gardenia is also effective against infections. In tropical medicine, gardenia teas inhibit ringworm, a fungal infection of the skin, and the organisms that cause schistosomiasis, a parasitic disease.[4] Gardenia also provides long-lasting relief for fevers caused by infection.[5]

Considerations for Use

The most common way to use gardenia is to use formulas or make teas from crushed or whole fruits. Make the tea by steeping 1 tablespoon of gardenia fruit in 1 cup of water for forty-five minutes. Strain before drinking. "Whole" gardenia fruits are split on the half shell so the herb's active compounds can enter the tea.

Gardenia fruit may interfere with normal digestive function by causing diarrhea. In cases where this may be a problem, the herb is dry-fried until it is yellow, and then crushed before making the tea.

Several compounds in gardenia, particularly gardenic acid, can induce abortion in the early stages of pregnancy.[6] This effect may not occur with the use of formulas containing gardenia, but women who wish to become pregnant should avoid this herb altogether.

Garlic / Taisan

Description and Parts Used

Garlic is a pungent herb used around the world in cooking and natural medicine. It is a bulbous perennial with a single stalk that grows to a height of from one to three feet, with green-white or sometimes pale pink flowers. The plant was originally found in Central Asia, where it is the most important herb in Unani, or Persian, traditional herbal medicine.

Uses in Kampo

Traditional Japanese medicine has long used garlic to kill intestinal parasites and prevent influenza. Kampo also uses garlic to treat ringworm of the scalp and food poisoning that results from shellfish consumption. The followers of Kampo master Todo Yoshimasu (see Chapter 1) used garlic to counter reactions to "toxins" that resulted in consumption (what is now called tuberculosis), coughing spells, diarrhea, and dysentery.

Scientific Findings and Clinical Experience

Garlic has been shown to have a wide variety of medicinal uses. This includes an ability to combat the two biggest killers in North America, heart disease and cancer, as well as infection-fighting properties.

Garlic fights heart disease in two ways. First, it prevents lipid peroxidation, a kind of rancidity that affects cholesterol.[1] Peroxidation is part of the process by which cholesterol plaques are deposited in the walls of blood vessels, narrowing them and leaving them vulnerable to blockage by blood clots. Garlic can also reduce cholesterol levels, as shown by dozens of studies. In one twelve-week study, fifty men with high cholesterol levels were given one capsule a day containing either 900 milligrams of garlic or an inert placebo and another capsule containing either 12 grams of fish oil (which contains circulation-regulating essential fatty acids) or a placebo. Total cholesterol levels went down by an average of 11 percent in participants who were given only garlic, compared with 12 percent in those who took both garlic and fish oil, and 8 percent in those who took only fish oil. Garlic also reduced amounts of low-density lipoprotein (LDL), or "bad" cholesterol.[2]

Garlic also acts against heart disease by stimulating fibrinolysis, a process by which blood clots are dissolved.[3] Ajoene, a compound isolated from garlic, keeps small blood cells called platelets from forming clots.[4] Ajoene is unstable in the human body, but tends to build up when garlic is taken in small doses over a period of weeks. Taking a single, large dose of garlic does not affect clotting capacity.[5]

Atherosclerosis and blood clots in the brain can cause stroke, so it is not surprising that garlic can reduce the risk of stroke. In addition, garlic may reduce brain damage after stroke. Animal studies show that garlic extracts reduce the formation of substances that can cause the tiny capillaries in the brain to flood brain tissue with fluids.[6] Garlic extract also contains compounds that protect brain tissue from cell-damaging free radicals.[7]

Garlic can lower blood-sugar levels in diabetics. It ties up chemical receptors that otherwise would deactivate insulin, the hormone that controls sugar usage, and also stimulates the pancreas to secrete insulin. It does so without stimulating weight gain, a common side effect of many diabetes medications.[8]

Garlic helps strengthen the immune system. In one study, participants who ate 600 milligrams of garlic powder every day for three months showed significant increases in the immune-system cells that act against infectious bacteria.[9] In a study involving AIDS patients, consumption of between 5 and 10 grams (equivalent to two large cloves) of garlic extract each day for twelve weeks resulted in an increase in natural killer (NK) cell activity by as much as 2,100 percent.[10] This action makes garlic useful in conditions that require strong immune defenses, such as cancer and infections.

Garlic has been known for many years to reduce the risk of cancer. The use of garlic is associated with lower rates of cancer of the breast, colon, larynx, and stomach (and the esophagous in men).[11] The herb contains compounds that prevent a tumor from developing its own blood supply, tumor formation after exposure to carcinogenic chemicals, and the spread of tumors once they have started.[12,13] Other chemicals reduce the production of cell-damaging free radicals in liver and lung tissue.[14] Garlic has been found to prevent the growth of the bacterium *Helicobacter pylori,* thought to be associated with stomach cancer,[15] and laboratory studies have confirmed that a stable component of garlic oil, S-allylmercaptocysteine (SAMC), stops the proliferation of hormone-sensitive breast and prostate cancer cells.[16]

Garlic works well with other anticancer treatments. Garlic powder, usually taken in tablet form, increases the effectiveness of selenium supplements meant to prevent the growth and spread of breast cancer.[17] Animal studies find that garlic protects tissues from the effects of whole-body radiation.[18] However, garlic is not appropriate for persons undergoing treatment with recombinant tumor necrosis factor (rhTNF), as the herb reduces the activity of rhTNF.[19]

Garlic is effective against colds and other infections. Garlic is a prime ingredient in the kosher cold remedy, chicken soup. It activates "germ-eating" macrophages, or immune-system cells,[20] which inhibits other viruses that may cause upper respiratory infection. Garlic also controls colds contracted at high altitude, such as those caught on ski vacations or during air travel.[21] Garlic applied to the ear canal is a traditional remedy for earaches. Tests have found that garlic treatment stopped the growth of *Aspergillus* and *Candida,* two fungi that sometimes cause ear inflammation.[22]

Garlic has other uses as well. Studies have found garlic to be the most effective treatment available for infection with the parasite that causes sleeping sickness, a disease that occurs in Africa.[23] In addition, Eastern European studies have found that taking ground garlic for several months is an effective antidote for chronic lead poisoning and other forms of heavy-metal poisoning.

Considerations for Use

The most beneficial way to take garlic is to use 2 to 3 cloves per day in food preparation, preferably raw. Garlic tablets, including deodorized garlic tablets, can be used to lower cholesterol levels. If taken for its ajoene content—to prevent atherosclerosis, reduce the risk of cancer, or correct heavy metal toxicity—garlic is best taken in the form of tablets that have been enterically coated so that the ajoene does not break down in the digestive tract.

To make garlic oil for use in ear infections, use one part minced garlic in five parts olive oil. The oil can be refrigerated for up to two weeks.

There are conditions in which the medicinal use of garlic

is not advised. Persons who are taking blood-thinning drugs such as warfarin sodium (Coumadin) should avoid garlic because the herb adds to the drug's effects. Also, garlic will counteract the effects of *Bifidus* and *Lactobacillus* cultures taken to restore normal digestion.

Gastrodia / Tenma

Description and Parts Used

Gastrodia is the rootstock of the gastrodia orchid, found in China. Its Chinese name, *tian ma,* means "heavenly hemp." Kampo uses broad, thin slices of the solid, translucent, yellowish white rhizome.

Uses in Kampo

Gastrodia is Oriental medicine's chief herb for settling internal wind, which manifests itself as dizziness, epileptic seizures, headache, high blood pressure, joint pain, muddled speech, muscle spasms, and vertigo. Since gastrodia is an energy-neutral herb, it is useful in formulas used both to sedate the nervous system and to relieve emotional tensions stored in the liver (see Chapter 4). Relieving the emotional stresses stored in the liver prevents headaches (especially migraine headaches and headaches that seem to center in the eyes), breast pain, and high blood pressure.

Scientific Findings and Clinical Experience

In laboratory tests using gastrodia injections, this herb increases blood flow to the heart muscle and increases the heart's resistance to oxygen deprivation. Gastrodia also encourages deep sleep and relaxes the central nervous system.[1] Gastrodia is especially effective in relieving facial muscle spasms and nerve pain.

Kampo medicine uses gastrodia together with gambir (see page 52) in many formulas for the treatment of epilepsy. Research in Japan shows that these two herbs prevent seizures through their action as free-radical scavengers, or destroyers of chemicals that damage cells. Gastrodia and gambir increase the brain's production of its own free-radical scavenger, superoxide dismutase. These herbs also prevent the action of free radicals that would activate lipid peroxides, compounds that destroy cell walls.[2] Gastrodia's antioxidant action also makes it useful for protecting brain tissue in Alzheimer's disease.

Gastrodia can also help protect the brain after a stroke occurs. In stroke, brain cells often do not die when a blood clot cuts off their oxygen supply. Instead, they adapt to low oxygen conditions and are only damaged when the circulation of oxygen-laden blood is restored to them. The cells are overwhelmed with oxygen, some of which oxidizes, or burns, the cells' membranes. Compounds in gastrodia stop this form of free-radical destruction.

Considerations for Use

Although gastrodia can be used by itself, the herb is almost always combined with gambir—see Gastrodia and Uncaria Decoction in Chapter 4.

Gastrodia is an extremely expensive herb. When using a patent (over-the-counter) medicine that includes gastrodia, check the list of ingredients to make sure the manufacturer did not substitute the cheaper dendrobium (see page 46).

Gentian / Ryutan

Description and Parts Used

Gentian, a perennial plant that grows up to three feet tall, is widely cultivated in China, and is harvested from the wild in Spain and the Balkans. It bears alternating leaves on a single stem that is topped with five-petalled yellow flowers. The root is used in Kampo.

In both Chinese and Korean, the terms for gentian can be literally translated as "dragon gallbladder herb." This attests to gentian's ability to treat fiery inflammations of the gallbladder that cause intense discomfort.

Uses in Kampo

Kampo uses the extreme cooling action of gentian to pacify fire associated with the liver and gallbladder. Gentian drains damp heat, or infection, from the upper parts of the gallbladder's energy channel, where it causes sore throat, swollen eyes, swollen and painful ears, or sudden deafness. The herb drains damp heat from the lower parts of the gallbladder's energy channel, where it creates symptoms such as jaundice, pain, swelling or dampness in the genital area, or foul-smelling vaginal discharge with itching. Gentian also constrains upward-reaching liver "fire" that causes headache or red eyes, and relieves liver syndromes that result in convulsions, fever, spasms, or pain in the sides.

Scientific Findings and Clinical Experience

Gentian helps ease not only gallbladder problems but also indigestion. The bitter taste of gentian triggers a reflex reaction that stimulates the production of saliva and gastric juices. Gentian also stimulates the production of bile. Increasing the production of digestive juices stimulates both digestion and appetite.

Gentian has other uses. Gentianine, a compound found in gentian, relieves both pain and fever, and is about twice as potent as aspirin.[1] In addition, laboratory studies have confirmed the value of gentian in the treatment of eye disease, especially in preventing retinal changes seen in diabetics.[2] And in China, gentian has been used with a minimal dose of the steroid drug prednisone to more than double the chances of achieving remission in lupus patients.[3]

Considerations for Use

A familiar form of gentian is the drink called Angostura Bitters, also called "gentian bitters." In Europe and particularly in Germany, gentian bitters are taken before fatty meals as an aid to digestion. This herb is also available in capsule form, which eliminates the extremely bitter taste, and is used in Kampo formulas (see Chapter 4).

Avoid gentian in cases of diarrhea caused by poor digestion, as shown by undigested food in the stool.

Giant Peony

See **Moutan.**

Ginger / Kankyo (dried) / Shokyo (fresh)

Description and Parts Used

Ginger is the most widely used and widely available herbal remedy on the planet. Billions of people use ginger daily as food and medicine. A tropical perennial growing to a height of two feet, ginger has lance-shaped leaves and bears stalks of white or yellow flowers.

Ginger has long been the subject of fable and literature. For centuries, Europeans obtained ginger from Arab spice traders, who protected their sources by inventing stories of ginger fields located in lands stalked by a fierce people called troglodytes. And Shakespeare wrote in *Love's Labour Lost*, "... had I but one penny in the world thou shouldst have it to buy ginger-bread."

Uses in Kampo

Ginger is used either fresh or dried in nearly two thirds of all traditional Chinese and Japanese formulas (see Chapter 4). Fresh ginger is used to relieve dryness and heat, while dried ginger is used to relieve dampness and chill. In TCM, ginger is said to "rescue devastated yang," a condition in which invading cold or infection has reached the interior of the body. Ginger warms the energy channels and stops bleeding, especially uterine bleeding. It is a detoxifier, and is always included in formulas with potentially toxic herbs such as aconite and pinellia (see pages 18 and 80).

Scientific Findings and Clinical Experience

Scientists have found evidence to support ginger's wide range of medicinal actions. These actions include the lowering of cholesterol levels; providing relief for allergies and asthma, arthritis, colds, and nausea; and protecting the body against toxins and parasites.

Ginger inhibits cholesterol production in the liver, where most of the body's cholesterol supply is produced.[1] This helps prevent atherosclerosis, in which cholesterol-laden plaques form in the arteries. A heart attack or stroke may occur if a blood clot becomes stuck in arteries narrowed by atherosclerosis, and ginger can help prevent clot formation. Studies confirm that compounds found in ginger decrease the activity of platelet-activating factor (PAF), a blood clotting agent.[2,3]

Moreover, ginger's ability to reduce PAF activity makes this herb effective against allergies and asthma. PAF, which stimulates the inflammation seen in allergy and the bronchial constriction seen in asthma, becomes more active when fat is consumed. Dried ginger can offset this effect.[4,5] In Indian tests, the consumption of 5 grams of dried ginger per day for seven days reversed blood-fat increases caused by the daily consumption of 100 grams of butter.[6]

Laboratory studies have confirmed ginger oil's usefulness in treating arthritis.[7] A three-year study of fifty-six persons with rheumatoid arthritis found that about 75 percent of the patients achieved relief from pain and swelling by taking powdered ginger, and without the side effects of conventional drugs.[8] Ginger relieves the pain of rheumatoid arthritis by stopping the body's production of inflammation-promoting substances.

Ginger's effectiveness against infection has also been confirmed by science. One ginger compound kills cold viruses at a concentration of less than one part per million, a concentration comparable to that found in raw ginger.[9] This makes the unprocessed herb an effective treatment for colds. Ginger has also been found to inhibit the production of immune-system compounds called cytokines, an action that reduces inflammation.[10]

Japanese scientists have isolated several antiulcer compounds from dried ginger.[11] Ginger protects the lining of the stomach from alcohol damage,[12] which can aggravate existing ulcers and promote the development of new ones.

Mothers-to-be may find ginger especially useful. Some babies are born breech, that is, feet first instead of head first. Chinese researchers report that simply applying a ginger paste to a specific acupuncture point results in a 77-percent correction of breech births, compared to 52 percent in a control group who had their babies turned manually.[13] Ginger is also an age-old remedy for morning sickness.

In fact, one of ginger's best-known properties is its ability to quell nausea. Ginger has been found to be more effective in relieving motion sickness symptoms than Dramamine,[14,15] a popular nonprescription remedy. Ginger also eases nausea caused by treatment with 8-MOP, a drug taken by patients undergoing photopheresis, a light-activated chemotherapy.[16]

Ginger protects the body from a variety of noxious substances. The herb is a proven scavenger of free radicals, substances that cause cellular damage.[17,18] When used in Kampo formulas, ginger protects the body from the cancer-inducing effects of valproic acid (Depakote), a common treatment for seizure disorders.[19]

Ginger also protects against foodborne infection. It contains a chemical called zingibain that dissolve parasites and their eggs.[20] In Japan, ginger's antiparasitic effect is put to use in sushi preparation. Sushi is traditionally eaten with pickled ginger, and ginger extracts have been shown to kill the anisakid worm, a parasite sometimes carried in raw fish, within sixteen hours.[21] In addition, ginger tea effectively treats schistosomiasis, a parasitic disease increasingly prevalent among tourists returning to the United States.[22,23]

Considerations for Use

Make ginger tea by simmering $^1/_4$ teaspoon (0.5 to 1.0 gram) of ground ginger in 1 cup of water for five minutes. Be sure to use recently purchased ginger, as ground ginger can lose its potency over time. Otherwise, use freeze-dried ginger in capsule form. For asthma, ginger hexanol extract is the preferred form.

Although there are warnings in Chinese medicine about ginger use during pregnancy, ginger used in moderation—$^1/_2$ teaspoon (1 gram) two to three times per day—poses no risk to the baby's health.[24] Recent studies indicate that eating as much as 2 to 3 tablespoons of raw ginger or 5 to 8 tablespoons of cooked ginger (15 or 40 grams, respectively) daily will not stimulate uterine contraction.[25]

To make a painkilling ginger compress, grate 1 or 2 fresh ginger roots into thin strips 2 to 4 inches (5 to 10 centimeters) long, and place the grated ginger in a muslin cloth. Tie the cloth to make a bag, leaving room for air and water to circulate. Drop the bag into boiling water just removed from the heat, and allow it to simmer for seven to ten minutes. The resulting liquid should have a golden tint and a distinctive ginger aroma. While the liquid is still hot but not scalding, dip a terrycloth towel into the liquid and apply to the affected area for between fifteen and twenty minutes. Repeat every four to six hours until the pain subsides.

Ginkgo Nut / Ginkyo

Description and Parts Used

The long-lived ginkgo tree is a native of Japan that is grown around the world for its hardiness and beauty of its fan-shaped leaves. Although ginkgo leaf (see page 100) is used in Kampo, most traditional ginkgo remedies use ginkgo nut, or "silver nut," rather than the leaf. Ginkgo extract cannot be substituted for ginkgo nut.

Uses in Kampo

In Kampo medicine, ginkgo nut is a sweet and bitter, energy-neutral herb that strengthens the lungs, relieves wheezing and coughing, loosens phlegm, and helps the reproductive system contain fluids. Whole nuts are traditionally used to treat asthma, tuberculosis, frequent urination, and vaginal discharge. Ginkgo nuts are also dyed red and used as a food in both Japan and China.

Scientific Findings and Clinical Experience

Ginkgo-nut teas prevent asthmatic attacks by deactivating platelet activating factor (PAF). PAF acts as a "green light" to the body's immune system for asthmatic reactions. PAF causes red blood to form clumps. These clumps produce the hormone serotonin, which causes the smooth muscles lining the air passages in the lungs (bronchioles) to contract. While the smooth muscles supporting the lungs and the blood vessels stiffen, PAF makes the walls of the blood vessels become more permeable. This "ooziness" allows inflammation-causing hormones to pass through.

The compound in ginkgo nuts that counteracts PAF, Ginkgolide B, can prevent and treat asthmatic attack and hives. Ginkgolide B acts by blocking PAF out of PAF's receptor sites on blood cells.[1]

Ginkgolic acid, also found in ginkgo nuts, kills salmonella, staph, and tuberculosis bacteria in the laboratory, although these findings have not been duplicated in clinical trials with human patients. In addition, ginkgo-nut teas can cause uterine contractions.

Considerations for Use

Ginkgo nuts are generally used as part of a formula, Arrest Wheezing Decoction (see Chapter 4).

Long-term overdoses of ginkgo-nut teas can cause skin disorders and shedding of the mucous membranes. Short-term overdoses can cause headache, fever, tremors, irritability, or shortness of breath. The antidote is 60 grams of boiled raw licorice or 30 grams of boiled ginkgo shells. This reaction can be avoided by including the hard shells and thin linings of the nuts when using the herb.[2] And since ginkgo nut can stimulate uterine contractions, it should be avoided during pregnancy.

Ginseng / Ninjin

Description and Parts Used

Ginseng is a low-growing perennial plant native to the cool-summer regions of China, North Korea, and Siberia. Very seldom found in the wild, it is a labor-intensive crop that takes at least four years to mature. The root of the plant is dug in the fall, washed, steamed, and dried for use in Kampo.

Ginseng has a tremendous range of beneficial effects. Because of its high cost, a large number of other "ginsengs" are available: Alaskan, American, Brazilian, Indian, Siberian. These other "ginsengs" have medicinal value, but none as great as Korean or red ginseng, *Panax ginseng*. (See American ginseng, page 23, and Siberian ginseng, page 105. Also see "Ginseng Among the Native Americans" on page 23.)

Uses in Kampo

Ginseng is the most famous of the Kampo herbs and the most important of the qi, or energy, tonics. Warming and sweet, ginseng nourishes the digestive organs and the lungs, aids upward circulation of energy in the body, improves the defensive qi (*wei qi*), and calms the mind. Ginseng's uses in traditional Japanese herbalism include providing aid for both digestion and recovery from prolonged illness, expulsion of food pathogens, and diarrhea control. Ginseng also supplements body fluids, stops severe thirst, relieves cold in the hands and feet, and quells symptoms of anxiety.

Ginseng is described in Kampo as one of the "Four Gentlemen" or "Four Emperors," herbs that act harmoniously as a group and are not given to extreme effects. (Also see white atractylodis, hoelen, and licorice, pages 29, 61, and 66.) This title was modeled after the Confucian term for a person who exhibits ideal behavior.[1] Ginseng appears not only in Four-Gentlemen Decoction, but in dozens of other formulas as well (see Chapter 4).

Scientific Findings and Clinical Experience

Ginseng's traditional and best-known use as a male aphrodisiac has been confirmed by research.[2] It stimulates a part of the brain called the hypothalamus to secrete substances that stimulate cell growth and healing in the sex organs. The herb also promotes better blood circulation within the penis. In addition, ginseng can be used to treat male infertility. An Italian study of sixty men found that ginseng use increased testosterone levels, as well as the number and motility of sperm cells.[3]

Ginseng is also effective against cancer. Kampo employs it in a number of formulas used in cancer treatment, especially Ten-Significant Tonic Decoction. A Korean clinical trial showed that regular consumption of ginseng lowered the risk of developing various types of cancer by between 85 percent for ovarian cancer to 45 percent for lung cancer, although it did not lower the risk for several other types, including cancer of the breast and bladder.[4]

Polyacetylinic alcohol, a compound found in ginseng, retards cell reproduction in tumors and increases the effectiveness of the drug mitomycin in the treatment of stomach cancer.[5] Other compounds called ginsenosides have been found to induce cell differentiation, a prelude to natural cell death, in human leukemia cells.[6] Ginseng also protects cells in the digestive tract from injury during radiation therapy.[7]

Ginseng treatments increase the body's resistance to lung cancer.[8] Experiments in China found that when ginseng therapy was combined with traditional radiation and chemotherapy for small cell lung cancer, longevity was extended by between three and seventeen years.[9]

Although ginseng therapy does not shrink melanoma tumors, it keeps them from developing a blood supply for further growth.[10] In animal studies, a compound found in ginseng called ginsan retards the growth of melanoma at dosages far lower than that which would cause a toxic reaction.[11]

Ginseng may prevent liver damage in people exposed to various drugs and toxins. These include dexamethasone, a drug used during the lupus treatment,[12] and carbon tetrachloride, a common dry cleaning agent.[13]

Ginseng is a useful treatment for both heart attack and stroke. Tests have shown that ginseng slows the heart rate and reduces the heart's demand for oxygen.[14] It also increases the effectiveness of the drug digoxin in the treatment of heart failure without causing additional side effects.[15] At the same time, ginseng increases the strength with which the heart muscle can contract and protects the heart from myopathy, a weakness or wasting of the muscle.[16] Ginseng protects nerve tissue from reperfusion damage, which occurs when blood circulation returns to an area after a heart attack or stroke.[17] It also protects nerve tissue from free radicals, substances that can destroy cells.[18]

Heart attack and stroke can occur as the result of high blood pressure or high cholesterol levels. Ginseng compounds relax the linings of blood vessels, which prevents high blood pressure.[19] And studies indicate that ginseng reduces levels of total cholesterol, LDL or "bad" cholesterol, and triglycerides.[20]

Other chronic disorders respond well to ginseng. People with type 2 diabetes often find that after two weeks of taking ginseng tea, their blood-sugar levels go down by between 40 and 50 milligrams per deciliter. Ginseng can reduce insulin requirements and prolong insulin's effect.[21] In addition, studies have found that a combination of ginseng and the non-Kampo herb echinacea increased the activity of natural killer cells, an important immune-system component, in chronic fatigue syndrome (CFS) patients.[22] Ginseng has also been found to improve almost all indicators of psychological health in CFS patients, especially levels of attention and concentration.[23]

Studies have found that injected ginseng compounds increase the body's production of adrenocoricotropic hormone (ACTH) and certain steroid hormones, such as adrenalin.[24] This stimulates the natural function of the body's stress-response system, which keeps the adrenal glands from "burning out" during prolonged periods of stress. In animal studies, the herb has been found to increase learning ability under stress. It also reduces digestive upsets caused by emotional stress and inhibits ulcer formation.[25]

Ginseng both relieves pain and increases the effectiveness of other painkillers, especially aspirin, and does so without inducing drowsiness.[26] Ginseng compounds may reduce the stress of *anticipated* pain.[27]

This important herb has many other uses. Ginseng, in combination with biota and schisandra (see pages 30 and 87), reverses alcohol damage to brain cells in laboratory tests,[28] and may be useful in the treatment of fetal alcohol syndrome.[29] Ginseng therapy may prevent the onset of nervous unrest during treatment with morphine.[30] In addition, it may help in withdrawal from methamphetamines[31] and cocaine.[32] Ginseng extracts reduce susceptibility to the life-threatening allergic reaction known as anaphylactic shock, which is marked by breathing difficulties and extremely low blood pressure.[33]

Considerations for Use

The most potent ginseng is "wild mountain root," imported from Jilin province in China. This grade is also called *"jilin* root" or *"ji lin shen."* It is expensive but worth the cost in treating serious ailments. "Ginseng whiskers" is a less expensive form of the herb that is recommended over "sugar root," which is a still less expensive ginseng-flavored rock candy. Also, field-grown ginseng is thought to be less potent than ginseng gathered in the wild.

To make ginseng tea, buy whole roots and cut them into thin slices, 1 tablespoon or less (2 to 4 grams) at a time. Simmer in 1 cup of boiling water for forty-five minutes. Because it is an expensive herb, ginseng is often brewed in a ginseng cooker, available from Chinese herb stores and East Earth Trade Winds (see Appendix A). By tradition, avoid green tea and arisaema (see pages 59 and 25) when using ginseng, since both may reduce ginseng's efficacy.

Ginseng is also available in extract or tincture form. Ginseng teas are less convenient than extracts, but more therapeutically active. If using an extract or tincture, be aware that strengths vary greatly by manufacturer, and that some formulations include the less-expensive codonopsis, coptis, or Siberian ginseng (see pages 41, 42, and 105).

Consumption of extremely large amounts of tincture, on the order of 100 milliliters or more, may result in headache. This is an early sign of overdose, and means that the dose should be reduced. Gross overdoses of ginseng extract—40 to 100 times the prescribed amount—can cause rash and itching all over the body, dizziness, fever, headache, and hemorrhage. Take small amounts of ginseng regularly for best results.

Herb users in the warmer climates of the southern United States, particularly those in the Gulf Coast states, may find ginseng that is not used as part of a balanced formula to be excessively warming during the hottest summer weather. Ginseng use during extreme heat may result in mild fever or sleeplessness. American ginseng (see page 23) is a cooling alternative.

Green Tea / Ocha

Description and Parts Used

A native of the rainy forests of Southeast Asia, the tea plant is cultivated in Burma, China, India, Japan, Sri Lanka, and Africa. The evergreen leaves are limp and downy when young, thick and rounded when mature. In the wild, this small tree is very branchy. Cultivated tea plants are regularly pruned and kept to a height of about five feet to make harvesting easy. Only leaf buds and young leaves are harvested, by hand, to make tea.

Green tea is the unfermented form of the familiar beverage. Unfermented tea contains proteins—15 to 20 percent by dry weight—and natural sugars—5 percent by dry weight. It also contains B vitamins, vitamin C and its cofactors, and caffeine, among other substances. Although all of these constituents are not lost in the fermenting process that makes the more aromatic (and for North Americans, more familiar) black tea, green tea is a better source of the chemicals that give the herb its healthful properties.

Uses in Kampo

Green tea is cold and bitter. It clears heat from the eyes and refreshes the spirit. When taken with herbal formulas, green tea prevents side effects caused by warming or drying herbs.

Green tea is used widely in Asian households to treat burns. The tannins in green tea "tan" the skin, encouraging the formation of a protective layer across the burn.

Scientific Findings and Clinical Experience

Refreshing green tea contains the chemicals theophylline and caffeine. These chemicals stimulate the central nervous system, increasing alertness and reducing fatigue, and induce chemical changes that increase heart rate. Theophylline accounts for green tea's diuretic properties. It keeps the kidneys from reabsorbing sodium and chlorine, which increases the amount of fluid excreted. This stops short-term weight gain resulting from consumption of salty foods.[1] Theophylline also increases blood flow to the kidneys.

Theophylline is extracted from the leaves and used to relax the smooth muscles supporting the bronchial tubes, an important step in treating asthma and bronchitis. Drinking green or black tea provides theophylline in doses large enough to affect asthma.[2]

Up to 30 percent of the weight of a leaf of green tea consists of potent antispoilage chemicals called phenols that allow green tea to play a number of roles.[3,4] Green tea protects red blood cells and liver cells from free radicals, substances produced as the body uses oxygen that can damage cells. And another free-radical scavenger found in green tea, epigallocatechin gallate, prevents damage in the lens of the eye that could lead to cataracts.[5]

Green tea also benefits the circulatory system. It lowers blood cholesterol without side effects,[6] and lowers blood pressure using a mechanism employed by modern drugs called ACE inhibitors.[7] Green tea extracts prevent blood from becoming too thick in animals fed a high-fat diet.[8] In diabetics, green tea extracts suppress the formation of sticky blood proteins called glycosylation products, which can cause small blood vessels to thicken and leak.[9] Green tea also keeps sugar out of the bloodstream in the first place by inhibiting sugar-extracting enzymes in the mouth and intestines.[10]

Green tea contains chemicals called catechins that kill many foodborne bacteria, especially *Clostridium*,[11] which is associated with colon cancer. In animal studies, this action prevents the growth of colorectal tumors.[12] Catechins also prevent *Streptococcus mutans* from forming dental plaque.[13] (This explains why Asians cleaned their teeth with whisks of green tea leaves before the invention of toothpaste.) Green tea's antimicrobial effects make it useful in other conditions as well, such as ear infections and eczema.

Green tea is useful in treating other forms of cancer besides colorectal cancer. It deactivates plasmin, a chemical that allows cancer cells to spread. This herb provides protection from the effects of repeated exposure to gamma radiation, which prevents thyroid cancer. Green tea catechins prevent the cancer therapy drug mitomycin from causing changes in the bone marrow that lead to leukopenia, a dangerous complication of cancer treatment. Green tea compounds also reduce the effects of estrogen within the body. This action is beneficial in some forms of breast cancer, and in other conditions as well.

Green tea extract helps ward off the flu by preventing influenza A viruses from replicating. This effect holds even when the extract is given at $^1/_{100}$ the concentration of amantadine, the only other effective flu-treatment therapy. Green tea extracts also protect against infection with the influenza B virus, against which amantadine is not effective.[14]

Considerations for Use

Use 1 teaspoon (2.5 grams) of green tea for each cup of tea made. This is considerably more than the amount contained in commercial tea bags, which sometimes hold as little as 0.5 grams of tea or even less. Brew the tea ten minutes and no longer. After brewing, drink with or without straining the tea, as desired. Green tea is also available in the form of catechin extract. As many as ten 240-milligram capsules (equivalent to forty cups of tea) can be taken each day, with increasing therapeutic benefit, but some people will experience nervousness and nausea at that dose.

As little as one or two cups of green tea beverage taken daily has a beneficial effect. Animal studies suggest that very large amounts of green tea, as much as half an ounce eaten rather than brewed into beverages, could be ingested without toxic effects.

Some herbal formulas, particularly those for the early stages of cold and flu, act at a molecular level by producing free radicals. Green tea stops the reactions that form free radicals. Take green tea to avoid coming down with colds or flu, but if the flu does strike, discontinue green tea use until symptoms subside.

Do not take green tea within one hour of taking herbal teas or patent (over-the-counter) medicines. This avoids diluting the decoction in the stomach or interfering with the medication. Finally, do not drink *green* tea if using ginseng regularly. Green tea can reduce the effectiveness of ginseng. Black tea is not known to have this effect.

Hawthorn / Sanzashi

Description and Parts Used

The hawthorn, a member of the rose family, is a deciduous, thorny tree that grows to a height of twenty-five feet. It bears small, white, five-petalled blossoms in the late spring that give way to red berries in the late summer. There is considerable debate among researchers concerning which parts of the plant have the greatest medicinal value. Fresh and dried berries, fresh and dried flowering tops, dried flowers, dried leaves, and dried flowers and leaves combined are all used.

Many species of hawthorn are used in herbal medicine. *Crataegus laevigata* (Poiret) DeCandolle (*Crataegus oxyacantha*) and *Crataegus monogyna* (Poiret) are commonly used in Europe and the United States. Oriental herbalists employ *Crataegus sinaica* Boiss, also known as Japanese hawthorn.

Uses in Kampo

In Kampo, the sweet and sour, warming hawthorn fruit is used to treat food stagnation caused by the overconsumption of meat. Hawthorn fruit not only disperses accumulated food, it also dispels stagnant blood, which causes menstrual pain, soft uterine tumors, and hernia. In this regard, it is similar to gardenia and peony (see pages 53 and 78).

Scientific Findings and Clinical Experience

A large body of scientific research has shown that the fruits, leaves, and flowers of various hawthorn species dilate the blood vessels, lower blood pressure, and dissolve cholesterol deposits.[1] Laboratory studies indicate that the herb may have even broader circulatory benefits, including effects on blood sugar and blood viscosity, or stickiness.[2]

Studies also show that substances found in hawthorn interact with key enzymes in the heart to change the way in which heart muscle contracts.[3,4] Hawthorn increases circulation within and around the heart, and compensates for mild cases of cardiac deficiency.[5] Increased heart circulation eases the pain of angina, which is caused by spasms of the coronary arteries. German studies have confirmed hawthorn's benefit for angina patients when the herb was taken for at least eight weeks.[6]

Hawthorn is an effective treatment for atherosclerosis, in which cholesterol gathers in plaques on blood-vessel walls. Atherosclerosis impairs circulation, and hawthorn fights this process in two ways. It increases the rate at which the liver converts LDL cholesterol, the "bad," artery-clogging kind, into HDL cholesterol, the "good," artery-clearing kind.[7] Indian scientists have found that *Crataegus laevigata* tincture increases the rate at which the liver uses cholesterol to create bile, which enters the intestines and eventually leaves the body.[8] Hawthorn also fights atherosclerosis by providing antioxidants, which prevent plaque formation, when an extract of *Crataegus monogyna* is used.[9,10]

Impaired circulation is also a factor in Alzheimer's disease and other forms of age-related memory loss. Oriental medicine has long used hawthorn to treat such conditions, and research has identified two ways in which the herb works. One is through its effect on cholesterol, since fewer and smaller plaques in the arteries supplying the brain means that more blood reaches the brain's tissues. The other way is through its high content of both vitamin C and substances that assist vitamin C, known as cofactors. These substances strengthen tiny blood vessels called capillaries in the brain, especially when these vessels are under stress from high blood pressure or microscopic blood clots. Open capillaries result in more nutrients and oxygen for the brain.

Another brain disorder helped by hawthorn is Attention Deficit Disorder/Attention Deficit Hyperactivity Disorder (ADD/ADHD). Hawthorn extracts relieve restlessness, acting out, and anxiety in children. The herb not only increases circulation to the brain, it also stops inflammatory responses caused by allergies. Allergies give the brain of an ADD or ADHD patient more information than it can process efficiently. Extracts of *Crataegus laevigata* have a sedative effect on the central nervous system.[11]

Hawthorn also plays an important role in immune stimulation. Animal studies show that an extract of *Crataegus sinaica* berry and leaf activates the part of the immune system that protects the body against infection by causing antibodies to bind to invading germs.[12] Hawthorn fruit preparations show significant action against pseudomonas (*Pseudomonas aeruginosa*) and shigella (*Shigella* spp.).[13]

Hawthorn is a good treatment for rheumatoid arthritis. Substances in the berries called anthocyanidins and proanthocyanidins help stabilize the collagen in cartilage, which reduces joint damage. Hawthorn-flower extracts prevent the formation of thromboxane A_2, a hormone involved in inflammatory processes.[14] The most effective species is *Crataegus levigata*. Hawthorn is also effective against osteoarthritis, the kind caused by wear and tear.[15]

Hawthorn's immune-stimulating effects make it useful in cancer treatment. Hawthorn contains rutin, which accelerates cell death of leukemia and Burkitt's lymphoma cells. It also contains compounds that deactivate plasmin, a chemical that allows cancerous tumors to spread through the body. In one laboratory study, hawthorn extract stopped 93 percent of the growth in cultures of human larynx cancer cells. In the future, extracts of the hawthorn species *Crataegus monogyna* may be used to treat laryngeal cancer.[16]

Hawthorn has several other uses. Animal studies have shown that hawthorn extracts protect heart, liver, and pancreas tissue from the effects of a glucocorticoid drug called isoproterenol sulfate,[17] commonly prescribed for asthma. Hawthorn extracts may also reverse tissue damage in asthma patients caused by hydrocortisone and steroid drugs. The anthocyanidins and proanthocyanidins help maintain healthy capillaries.[18,19] This makes hawthorn a useful treatment for bleeding gums and other conditions related to capillary health.

Considerations for Use

Make hawthorn tea by simmering from $^2/_3$ teaspoon to 1 scant teaspoon (1 to 1.5 grams) in $^2/_3$ cup of water for fifteen minutes. Strain before drinking. Hawthorn is also available as dried herb in capsules, fluid extract, solid extract (standardized to contain 10 percent proanthocyanidins), or tincture.

It is important to take products made from the species of hawthorn and part of the plant most beneficial for each specific health condition. For example, when buying hawthorn extracts for treatment of ADD/ADHD, be sure the label states that the source plant is *Crataegus laevigata* or *Crataegus oxyacantha*. An herbalist or Kampo practitioner can help determine which product is best in each case.

Some herbs should not be used in cases where immune-system stimulation is not desirable, such as in cases of lupus or HIV infection, because they stimulate the production of more immune-system cells. Hawthorn can be used when such conditions are present because it only affects existing immune-system cells.

Many people will find hawthorn fruit to have a laxative effect. Hawthorn leaf and flower teas are preferable if the herb is to be used by itself. And while hawthorn and other natural sources of vitamin C can be extremely helpful for Alzheimer's patients, they should *not* be used when there is a danger of increasing aluminum absorption, such as when certain types of antacids are used. This is especially crucial for Alzheimer's patients (see the Part Two entry). In this instance, a synthetic source of vitamin C is preferable, as synthetic ascorbic acid does not increase aluminum absorption.

Hemp

See **Marijuana Seed.**

Hoelen / Bukuryo

Description and Parts Used

Hoelen, also known as poria, is a mushroom that grows underground on the roots of pines and other trees around the world. In many parts of the world, hoelen is used as a food rather than as a medicine. This was true in the nineteenth century, when hoelen was known as tuckahoe in the eastern and southern United States. A single mushroom could grow to weigh between fifteen and twenty pounds, and since large mushrooms could be ground into bread flour, the herb became better known as Tuckahoe bread. It should be noted that relatively few specimens reach this size.

Good quality hoelen is solid and heavy. The outer skin should have thick wrinkles and a lustrous, red color. When hoelen is cut, the cross section should be white.

Uses in Kampo

Hoelen is a versatile, moisture-moving mushroom that can be combined with other herbs to heat or cool the body, or to relieve exterior or interior complaints (see Chapter 4). Hoelen is used to promote urination and to relieve diseases that are thought to be accumulations of moisture, such as diarrhea, lung congestion, swollen joints, and vertigo. Hoelen is also a sedative, quieting the heart and calming the spirit, and as such is used to treat irritability, reddening of the face, and short temper.

Scientific Findings and Clinical Experience

Hoelen has a long history of use in China for the treatment of senile amnesia and dementia. A factor in both disorders is the brain damage that occurs when oxygen supply is restored to the brain after a stroke or other blockage. This increases the production of substances called free radicals, which attack the cell membranes. Recent studies show that hoelen stops this process.[1]

Hoelen has also been shown to relieve a chronic kidney inflammation called glomerulonephritis. This occurs when the body produces antibodies to its own tissues, such as in lupus and rheumatoid arthritis. Sometimes, these antibodies accumulate in the kidney, which becomes clogged and loses its ability to retain essential products. Proteins begin to leak out into the urine, a process that can quickly progress to kidney failure. One of hoelen's main constituents, pachyman, can halt this process by preventing the accumulation of antibodies. With pachyman treatment, it is not necessary to counteract kidney inflammation with steroid drugs, which can have side effects such as fatigue, puffiness, weight gain, and behavioral changes.[2]

Another chemical in hoelen, poriatin, is an immune suppressant, which makes the herb valuable in treating rheumatoid arthritis and lupus directly. While pachyman keeps errant immune-system cells from accumulating in the kidney, poriatin acts to stop the disease at an even earlier stage, by preventing the formation of antibodies in the first place.[3,4] It also stops the production of cytokines, chemical messengers that immune-system cells use to coordinate attacks on tissues.[5] In addition, poriatin stops the activity of related chemical messengers, such as the interleukins and tumor necrosis factor.

While hoelen does stop runaway immune responses, it

does not leave the body defenseless. Pachyman stimulates the immune system's "search-and-destroy" cells, the macrophages, which attack both infectious microbes and tumor cells.[6] A chemically altered form of pachyman, carboxymethylpachymaran, also retards tumor-cell growth. In addition, this substance has been reported to produce an immediate cure in nearly half of all viral hepatitis patients.[7]

Hoelen is a unique immune-suppressing, rather than immune-stimulating, treatment of Kaposi's sarcoma in AIDS. Hoelen mushroom suppresses the formation of T cells, [8,9] giving HIV fewer host cells to infect. At the same time hoelen stimulates the activity of macrophages to destroy Kaposi's sarcoma cells.[10]

Considerations for Use

Dried or fresh hoelen can be taken daily in food. Hoelen tea can be brewed for twenty minutes from bags containing 1.5 grams of hoelen each, or the herb can be taken in tincture form. Improvement in chronic conditions may take three to four months of consistent use. Only one case of hoelen side effects appears in medical literature, in which an allergic reaction resulted in hives and stomach upset.

Since hoelen benefits persons with autoimmune kidney disease through several different mechanisms, taking the whole mushroom is preferable to taking chemical extracts of individual components. However, persons who have long-term systemic illnesses that cause excessive urination should avoid this herb.

Houttynia / Juyaku

Description and Parts Used

In Oriental medicine, houttynia is known as the "fishy smelling herb." The leaves, stems, and roots of this vine, which is native to south China, are used together in Kampo.

Uses in Kampo

Houttynia drains heat, relieves toxicity, and expels pus. It is applied to sores, external and internal, that are associated with fever or pus. Houttynia also drains damp heat, or infection, and encourages urination. Kampo uses houttynia in the treatment of lung abscesses, chronic bronchitis, and pneumonia, as well as chronic cervical and uterine infections, cystitis, dysentery, inner ear infections, leptospirosis, mastitis, pelvic inflammatory disease, and urinary infection.

Scientific Findings and Clinical Experience

Houttynia's diuretic effect comes from quercitrin, which increases blood flow to the kidney and stimulates urination.[1]

As little as one part of houttynia diluted in 40,000 parts of water can kill the bacteria that cause staph infections, pneumonia, and typhoid fever, as well as the bacterium *E. coli,* by stimulating the germ-eating activity of white blood cells. Houttynia is also antiviral, killing herpesvirus and the viruses that cause influenza. It also slows stomach cancer development.[2]

Considerations for Use

Use houttynia as directed by an herbalist. It is sold in Chinese herb shops as *Yu Xing Cao.* According to Kampo authorities, this herb should not be used for "yin" furuncles, that is, skin infections which leave an indentation on the skin.

Jack-in-the-Pulpit

See **Arisaema.**

Japanese Hawthorn

See **Hawthorn.**

Japanese Honeysuckle

See **Lonicera.**

Japanese Lily

See **Ophiopogon.**

Japanese Mint / Keigai

Description and Parts Used

Japanese mint, also known as schizonepeta, is native to China and Japan, and widely cultivated in the Far East. Unlike most other members of the mint family, which tend to hug the ground, Japanese mint grows to a height of twenty-five feet on square, upright stems that bear lancelike leaves and whorls of small flowers. The above-ground parts of the plant are used in Kampo.

Uses in Kampo

In *Formulas from the Discussion Illuminating the Yellow Emperor's Basic Questions* by Liu-Wuan Su, written in 1172, Japanese mint was identified as an excellent agent for the release of cold in the early stages of infection. It opens the pores and allows the body to expel invading pathogens. Opening the pores also relieves pain, so Japanese mint is also used in skin rubs and ointments. In addition, this herb is useful for carbuncles or boils when they first appear, especially when they are accompanied by chills and fever.

Japanese mint alleviates itching and vents rashes, and is an auxiliary herb in combinations that stop bleeding from the intestines or uterus. In the eighteenth and nineteenth centuries, it was employed as an herbal contraceptive, although with limited success.

Scientific Findings and Clinical Experience

Scientific investigation has confirmed that Japanese mint heals skin infections by stimulating circulation within the skin[1] and by causing perspiration.[2] The herb can also, when charred, shorten blood clotting time.

Considerations for Use

Make Japanese mint tea by placing 1 to 3 tablespoons (3 to 9 grams) of the herb in 3 cups of boiling water. Remove from the heat and allow to steep no more than ten minutes. Strain before drinking. Although Japanese mint may be used by itself, it is most often taken with another Japanese herb, ledebouriella (see page 65), in the form of Ledebouriella Powder That Sagely Unblocks (see Chapter 4).

As an eruptive herb, Japanese mint tea is indicated only for the early stages of rashes, measles, carbuncles, and sores. Do not use it on open sores.

Japanese Watermelon / SUIKA

Description and Parts Used

Japanese watermelon is related to the watermelon grown in North America, but belongs to a different species—*Citrullus vulgaris* instead of *Citrullus colocynthis.* Like North American watermelons, Japanese watermelon sends out creeping, vine-like stems up to fifty feet (sixteen meters) from its central stem and taproot. The stems bear alternating indented leaves. The fruit of Japanese watermelon is similar to the North American and Israeli field varieties of watermelon, but are usually smaller and more nearly spherical in shape.

Uses in Kampo

Japanese watermelon is an energy-moving herb that generates fluids and clears summerheat, the fever and inflammation resulting from infectious diseases caught during the summer months, especially hepatitis. It also promotes urination and clears jaundice. The herb is used to treat hepatitis and symptoms that include significant thirst and dark, scanty urine.

Scientific Findings and Clinical Experience

Japanese watermelon has a diuretic effect. This is probably because of the fruit's high concentrations of the amino acids citrulline and arginine, which stimulate the creation of urea by the liver.[1] The kidneys eliminate urea as rapidly as it is produced, so the production of urea increases frequency and quantity of urination.

Considerations for Use

Kampo uses Japanese watermelon in the formula Clear Summerheat and Augment the Qi Decoction (see Chapter 4).

Job's Tears

See **Coix.**

Jujube Fruit / TAISO

Description and Parts Used

The jujube "date" comes from a plant that is more closely related to trees of the rainy Pacific Northwest than to the date palm of the Arabian deserts. Jujube is a spiny deciduous tree that reaches a height of twenty-five feet with toothed leaves and clustered flowers that bear the black or reddish-brown dates.

Uses in Kampo

Jujube is the "servant" herb of Kampo, aiding the circulation of other herbs in formulas through the bloodstream to the gallbladder, heart, liver, and spleen (see Chapter 4). It also makes teas of other herbs sweeter and more palatable by reducing the body's physiological response to sweetness, so that bitterness is not as readily noticed.[1]

The classic Kampo texts describe jujube as an energizing tonic for the digestive system, since it eases abdominal pain, relieves severe cramps, and stops palpitations that seem to rise upward in the body. The herb is an ingredient in almost all Kampo formulas used for treating digestive upset.

Kampo texts also refer to jujube as a source of nourishment for the blood and calm for the spirit. Kampo has used jujube for centuries to restore intellectual abilities lost in old age. It is also used to correct wan appearance, irritability, and mood swings.

Scientific Findings and Clinical Experience

Research has revealed that jujube is particularly effective in quelling digestive upset caused by viral hepatitis. Clinical tests show jujube fruit, peanuts, and brown sugar used together stop destruction of liver tissues by viral hepatitis, as shown by lowered levels of liver enzymes.[2] In laboratory tests and clinical studies, jujube protects the liver from both the toxic effects of carbon tetrachloride and from oxidation by free radicals, harmful substances that damage cells.[3] Kampo practitioners report that jujube cures allergic purpura, a condition producing skin rash and hemorrhage under the skin. Jujube is effective for this condition, and for other allergies and asthma, because it contains a substance called cAMP, which blocks histamine production.[4]

Jujube is also a rich source of vitamin C, with 1.0 percent ascorbic acid in the immature fruit.[5]

Considerations for Use

Jujube fruit requires no special preparation—simply eat the *pitted* dates. The fruit is very nontoxic, so its use cannot result in an overdose. Still, since jujube creates a sense of fullness, avoid it in cases of food stagnation or bloating, or if intestinal parasites are present.

Kelp / KONBU

Description and Parts Used

The term "kelp" covers a number of brownish-green seaweed species. Seaweeds used as kelp may grow from a few feet to over a hundred feet in length, but those most commonly used in Kampo are harvested when they are three feet long. The entire plant is used. Kelp is harvested year-round in the North Atlantic and Mediterranean, and off the Japanese coasts.

Kelp is an important part of the diet in Japan, Norway, and Scotland. For vegans—vegetarians who eat no animal products at all—it supplies vitamin B_{12}.[1]

Uses in Kampo

In Kampo, kelp is an energy-neutral herb that reduces and softens "substantial phlegm," the sticky secretions of mucus that interfere with breathing and the accumulations of lymph that cause swelling in the neck. Kelp gently stimulates urination and relieves swelling throughout the body, although it is usually combined with other herbs to relieve swelling because its effects are extremely mild.

Scientific Findings and Clinical Experience

Kelp is a gentle laxative. Up to 45 percent of its weight consists of algin, a complex carbohydrate that swells in water.[2] Algin forms a gel within the intestines, which coats and soothes the intestinal lining and softens the stool.

It is kelp's bulk-producing effect that contributes to the low rates of breast cancer in Japan. Because kelp decreases transit time, or the time it takes food to get from one end of the digestive system to the other, its use lowers the risk that estrogens present in the stool will be absorbed back into the bloodstream.[3] Lowered estrogen levels are associated with lower rates of cancer, including breast and colorectal cancer.

In a similar manner, kelp may also protect the body against heavy metal poisoning. A compound in kelp called fucoidan forms an insoluble complex with cobalt, iron, manganese, or zinc, minerals that, while vital to health in small amounts, can be toxic in large amounts.[4] Kelp may also prevent absorption of radioactive strontium 90, possibly because of its high iodine content.[5]

Other compounds in a specific species of kelp, bladderwrack, have been found to kill the HIV virus without injuring healthy cells. These substances are present in both fresh and powdered kelp.[6]

Kelp's effects on the circulatory system are useful in the treatment of atherosclerosis and metastatic cancer. Kelp contains compound that prevent the formation of blood clots in narrowed blood vessels. These compounds act by breaking down fibrin, a protein that the body uses to "string" the framework of new blood vessels. When cancerous tumors cannot develop their own blood supply, they are unable to grow and spread.[7]

Animal studies have found several species of kelp to be useful in diabetes treatment. These species contain substances that can lower blood-sugar levels by between 18 and 50 percent.[8] Some diabetics have experienced about a 50-percent drop in blood sugar (from 200 to 300 milligrams per deciliter down to from 100 to 150 milligrams per deciliter) for up to twenty-four hours after eating kelp.

Kelp can, as part of a low-calorie diet, help stimulate weight loss. An Italian study found that dieters who ate kelp lost weight at twice the rate of those who did not. These results were confirmed by scientists at Oita School of Medicine in Japan. There, kelp was found to stimulate the satiety center in the brain when used as part of a very-low-calorie diet—only 370 calories a day.[9] In addition, bladderwrack has long been used to reduce cellulite deposits, or unsightly lumps of fat on the thighs. It is believed that this plant stimulates thyroid function, which increases the rate at which the body uses energy and, as a consequence, decreases fat deposits. Numerous users report success, although no studies have been done in this area.

Since iodine is a critical element in many thyroid hormones, it has long been thought that increasing available iodine with kelp would stimulate thyroid hormone production. However, scientists have since learned that too much iodine can actually inhibit thyroid activity. Studies of Japanese coastal cities in which large amounts of kelp are eaten revealed that kelp is associated with very high rates of low-level hypothyroidism, or low thyroid activity.[10] It is as if constant consumption of kelp first stimulates and then depletes thyroid function. For this reason, kelp is no longer recommended for hypothyroid conditions.

Considerations for Use

Kelp can be eaten as an occasional diet item in any quantity desired. It should not be eaten every day, though, to avoid consuming too much iodine. Limit consumption to once a week.

Kudzu / KAKKON

Description and Parts Used

The creeping kudzu vine is used in Japan both as food and medicine. The common term "kudzu" in English corresponds to the Japanese term for kudzu starch, used in thickening soups and making noodles.

Kudzu is used in Kampo both raw and roasted. Raw kudzu powders are used to treat fevers and symptoms of infection, while roasted kudzu powders are used in the treatment of diarrhea. Among American practitioners of TCM, kudzu is usually called "peuraria."

Uses in Kampo

Kampo's primary use of kudzu is to release muscles tightened in the early stages of infection. Kudzu, a cooling herb, also clears heat, which eases headache as well as stiffness in the upper back and neck.

In addition, kudzu nourishes the fluids to alleviate thirst. It vents measles, hastening recovery in cases where there is incomplete coverage by the rash. The herb also stops diarrhea caused by food- or waterborne infection and treats symptoms of high blood pressure, such as headache, dizziness, ringing in the ears, or tingling sensations.

Scientific Findings and Clinical Experience

Kudzu is an effective anticancer herb because of its effects on estrogen. Many kinds of cancer are stimulated by the hormone estrogen, including those of the breast, uterus, and skin. Like many other plants in the legume family, kudzu contains several chemicals that are very similar to estrogen. This activity has been traced to a chemical called formononetin. Formononetin has no effect on the body by itself, but is changed by the friendly bacteria in the digestive tract into an estrogenlike compound called daidzein. Daidzein binds to cells that ordinarily would be bound by estrogen. Therefore, daidzein locks out estrogen from activator sites on breast cancer cells, but does not itself stimulate the cancer cells to reproduce.[1]

Daidzein is also effective against other types of cancer. In cancer, cells do not mature and allow other cells to replace them—they are said to not differentiate from a reproductively active state. Daizein has been shown to be very potent in forcing differentiation of human leukemia in two studies,[2,3] and also in forcing differentiation of melanoma cells even at very low concentrations.[4]

Studies in Japan, the United States, and Finland have shown that the isoflavones, the chemical family that includes formononetin, are clearly associated with reduced rates of breast and uterine cancer.[5] While kudzu has not been linked to the prevention of prostate cancer, studies have shown that more of the isoflavones found in kudzu and soy appear in urine samples from Japanese men than in urine from American men. Perhaps not coincidentally, Japanese men have lower rates of prostate cancer than American men.[6]

Isoflavones, such as those found in kudzu, are not limited to fighting cancer. The isoflavones found in kudzu and other legumes increase blood flow to the brain, decrease the amount of oxygen needed by the heart, and even prevent the muscle spasms of premenstrual syndrome.[7]

Kudzu improves coronary circulation and lowers the heart's need for oxygen. Substances in the herb relax the muscles lining the left coronary vessel and lower the heart rate. Another compound is a beta-blocker, which reduces a racing pulse induced by stress.

Kudzu improves blood circulation to the brain by lowering resistance to blood flow within the cerebral vessels. This may explain kudzu's usefulness in treating the early stages of deafness and atrophy of the optic nerve.[8,9] Kudzu is most appropriate for treatment of nerve damage in persons with a long history of high blood pressure.

Kudzu's ability to relieve muscle aches and fever make it a soothing treatment for colds and flu. Over 2,000 years ago, the venerated Chinese herbalist Zhang Zhongjing described kudzu as opening the "interstices" of the skin to allow the body to purge itself of pathogenic influences, which were thought to be trapped by tight muscles. This is scientifically explained by kudzu's ability to increase circulation, since a better blood supply tends to reduce pain and stiffness. The herb may also act directly on the viral infections that produce muscle pain.

Chinese physicians have used kudzu as a cure for alcoholism for over 2,000 years. The tea that is used is called *xing-jiu-ling,* literally translated as "sober up." A biochemist at Harvard Medical School, Wing-Ming Keung, compiled studies of over 300 cases in Hong Kong. In all of the cases he reviewed, kudzu tonics were considered effective for controlling and suppressing the patient's appetite for alcohol without side effects. Kudzu usually reduced alcohol cravings within a week, and in over 80 percent of the cases, alcohol cravings were completely gone within two to four weeks of treatment.

Researchers at Indiana University have discovered two compounds in kudzu that alter the enzymes which break down alcohol in the liver.[10] As a result, an alcohol byproduct called acetaldehyde builds up. When this happens, nausea, facial redness, and general discomfort usually ensue. These compounds work in the same way as the prescription drug Antabuse. The kudzu compounds, however, do not induce nausea to as great an extent as disulfiram (Antabuse), although both treatments increase the discomfort of intoxication.

Considerations for Use

To make kudzu tea, place 2 heaping teaspoons (5 grams) of powdered kudzu in 1 cup of warm water. Drink without straining. Kudzu is also available in tablet form. Kudzu extracts are usually standardized so that a 10-milligram tablet extract is equivalent to 5 grams of the herb. This herb is also used in formulas, most notably Kudzu Decoction (Chapter 4). Kudzu is an extraordinarily nontoxic herb. Taking as much as 3 ounces (about 100 grams) in a single dose has no side effects.

It is important to remember that kudzu's estrogenlike effects only occur once the friendly intestinal bacteria process the herb. For this reason, antibiotic use will nullify the effect of kudzu use, including the use of Kampo formulas, as these drugs may harm the intestinal bacteria.

Although the matter has not been researched, it is possible that in the treatment of alcohol abuse persons of East Asian ancestry will have the greatest response to kudzu. In Eastern Asia, especially in Korea, as much as 80 percent of the population lacks the enzyme that processes acetaldehyde, the byproduct of alcohol consumption. Since alcohol tolerance is genetically lower among such persons, kudzu will have a more dramatic effect.

Ledebouriella / Bofu

Description and Parts Used

Ledebouriella, a native of Inner Mongolia, is similar in appearance to its relative, parsley. Kampo uses the coarse, yellow-cored taproot.

Uses in Kampo

The Chinese name for ledebouriella, *fang feng,* literally means "guard against wind." Kampo medicine traditionally used ledebouriella to fight "wind" as a pernicious influence. Ledebouriella releases the exterior to expel wind causing headache, chills, and body aches in the early stages of infection. Ledebouriella also expels "wind dampness," which causes stiff joints, and relieves "intestinal wind," which causes recurrent, painful diarrhea with bright-red blood in the stool.

The eighteenth-century Japanese herbalist Todo Yoshimasu prescribed ledebouriella for painful or numb joints, migraine headaches, red eyes, stiff back and neck muscles, spasms in the hands and feet, and inability to turn the head.

Scientific Findings and Clinical Experience

Ledebouriella inhibits the actions of some flu viruses, as well as those of the bacteria that cause shigella, pseudomonas, and staph infections. Ledebouriella has a mild fever-relieving effect when given orally, and raises the threshold of pain. It also has been used as an effective antidote for arsenic poisoning.[1]

Ledebouriella-based formulas are used to treat arthritis and obesity, and to relieve the diarrhea associated with morphine withdrawal.

Considerations for Use

In modern Kampo, ledebouriella is almost always used as part of a formula (see Chapter 4). Ginger (see page 56), used in cooking or as a medicine, counteracts the effects of ledebouriella. Therefore, do not use ginger when taking a ledebouriella-based formula.

Licorice / KANZO

Description and Parts Used

Next to ginger, licorice is the world's most widely used herbal remedy. The licorice plant is a woody-stemmed perennial that grows to a height of six feet. It bears clusters of creamy white flowers similar in appearance to those of its relative, the lupine. In the autumn, roots of three- to four-year-old plants are dug for medicinal use. After drying, the root is either used as is, or processed further by being either dry-fried or honey-fried. When buying licorice, it is important to buy roots that include the thin, reddish-brown bark. The bark should have no wrinkles, and the interior of the root should be powdery but firm.

Kampo, along with TCM and Korean herbal medicine, uses a species of licorice that grows in Inner Mongolia called *Glycyrrhiza uralensis* Fischer. European herbalists use a closely related but different species of licorice, *Glycyrrhiza glabra* L. North America is home to yet another medicinally useful species, *Glycyrrhiza lepidota* (Nutt.) Parsh.

Uses in Kampo

Licorice is the "emergency herb" of Kampo because it is used to treat acute symptoms in the early stages of infection. It can tonify the digestive tract to stop loose stools or moisten the lungs to stop coughing, regardless of whether the symptoms are associated with overstimulation (heat) or understimulation (cold). Since it is neither hot nor cold, raw licorice can be used with all other herbs to harmonize their effects; to supplement energy; and to reduce fever, inflammation, and spasms. As a result, it appears in dozens of Kampo formulas (see Chapter 4).

Licorice is a unique herb in that it is believed to activate all of the energy channels in the body. Licorice moderates spasms and alleviates pain, especially in the abdomen or legs. This versatile herb is also used to clear heat and relieve fire toxicity expressed as carbuncles, sores, or sore throat. Licorice can be used internally or topically for this purpose.

Licorice's penetrating sweet flavor, fifty times sweeter than table sugar, is used to mask unpleasant flavors of other herbs. The sweet flavor of licorice is enhanced by honey frying, in which the licorice is fried in honey until it turns a bright orange.

Scientific Findings and Clinical Experience

Licorice has been found to act against viruses, ulcers, and inflammations. It also protects the body against cancer-causing toxins.

Some Japanese physicians have experimented with this herb as a means of keeping HIV infection from progressing to AIDS.[1] When the licorice compound glycyrrhizin was given intravenously to AIDS patients, the patients became HIV-negative after three treatments. The researchers thought that acted by keeping the HIV virus from multiplying.[2] In another study, forty-two hemophilia patients with HIV-1 infection received glycyrrhizin along with two amino acids. The patients did not become HIV-negative, but they did experience relief from oral yeast infection, lymph node swelling, and rash. Immune and liver function also improved.[3]

Licorice is extensively used in modern Japanese medicine to treat hepatitis B. Glycyrrhizin "locks" the hepatitis B virus into cells to keep the infection from spreading. This chemical consistently improves liver function and occasionally brings about total recovery from hepatitis B.[4] Minor Bupleurum Combination, a formula that uses licorice, is also effective against hepatitis B, particularly in children.[5] Glycyrrhizin has been used with interferon, an immune-system component, in the treatment of hepatitis C, resulting in complete recovery about 40 percent of the time.[6]

Licorice, particularly when used in the formula Minor Bluegreen Dragon Decoction, contains chemicals called saponins that affect several other viruses, particularly influenza virus A. Licorice saponins both encourage the multiplication of phagocytes, immune-system cells that digest germs and virus-infected tissues, and assist in the process.[7] Laboratory tests show that licorice kills a number of viruses, including those that cause measles, herpes, and Newcastle disease (a disease passed from chickens to people) without harming human cell function.[8]

Another disorder that can be helped by licorice is chronic fatigue syndrome (CFS), which is marked by overwhelming fatigue. More than 95 percent of CFS patients have a condition in which low blood pressure results in oxygen starvation of brain cells, causing depression and fatigue.[9] This condition stems from adrenal-hormone deficiencies that cause the body to lose both sodium and water, resulting in drops in both blood volume and blood pressure.[10] Licorice can reverse this process. Glycyrrhizinic acid, a chemical in licorice related to glycyrrhizin, blocks the activity of an enzyme that otherwise would destroy the adrenal hormone cortisol. Proper cortisol levels in the bloodstream cause the kidneys to retain more sodium, and thus more water. This leads to higher blood pressure.[11]

Glycyrrhizinic acid was the first compound proven to promote the healing of ulcers. Unlike many ulcer drugs, glycyrrhizinic acid does not reduce acid production in the stomach, which would result in incomplete digestion. Instead, it increases the stomach's defense mechanisms by fortifying the stomach's protective mucous coating. Glycyrrhizinic acid also increases circulation to the cells lining the intestinal wall, boosting their supply of nutrients and oxygen.[12]

Since glycyrrhizinic acid can cause retention of sodium and water, deglycyrrhizinated licorice (DGL), which has no known side effects, is available. DGL inhibits gastric-juice secretion and protects the lining of the stomach from aspirin damage.[13] In one study of 874 patients with duodenal ulcers, DGL was compared with three conventional treatments, antacids and two prescription drugs. There were no differences in cure rates, but the DGL patients had a lower rate of ulcer recurrence.[14] In another study, DGL was given to forty patients who had suffered more than six ulcer attacks during the previous year. Half of the patients received 3,000 milligrams per day for eight weeks. The other half received 4,500 milligrams per day for sixteen weeks. All forty patients showed improvement, but the higher dosage produced greater relief from pain and vomiting.[15]

Licorice also soothes inflammatory conditions, such as asthma. Glycyrrhizin stops the production of free radicals. These harmful substances cause the release of hormones that stimulate inflammation and swelling of the bronchial passageways. The herb also stimulates the secretion of mucus in the windpipe, which relieves dry cough. In addition, licorice increases the effectiveness of steroid drugs used to treat asthma. Scientists have confirmed that compounds in licorice increase the half-life of cortisol, thus increasing the drug's control over asthmatic inflammation. Clinical studies have also shown that glycyrrhizin supplements prednisolone therapy, allowing the patient to take smaller doses of the drug with fewer side effects.[16]

Licorice can reduce allergic hypersensitivity reactions by tightening the walls of capillaries, making them less capable of allowing fluids to flow into tissues. This reduces swelling. In this way, licorice prevents the massive inflow of fluids into the lungs seen in extreme allergic hypersensitivity reactions. These reactions can lead to a life-threatening condition called anaphylactic shock.

Rheumatoid arthritis is another inflammatory condition helped by licorice. In this case, glycyrrhizin not only stops free-radical production, it also slows the rate at which the liver breaks down antiarthritic hormones, both those produced naturally and those taken in drug form. As in the case of asthma, licorice also allows arthritis patients to take smaller doses of prednisolone (Blephamide, Pediapred, Prelone).[17] Kampo formulas used for arthritis treatment frequently combine licorice with bupleurum (see page 35). Bupleurum stimulates production of glucocorticoid hormones[18] at the same time licorice is preventing their breakdown. Licorice also eases inflammatory skin conditions, such as eczema.

Licorice can protect the body against a number of cancer-causing toxins. It prevents the formation of skin tumors in response to noxious chemicals. Glycyrrhetic acid protects against tumor formation. It also inhibits the cancer-causing effects of pollutants such as benzopyrenes and a chemical called aflatoxin that is found in improperly stored food grains.[19] Licorice also protects the body against some arsenic compounds, urethane, caffeine, and nicotine. Kampo uses licorice and ginger in formulas to counteract potentially toxic herbs, such as aconite (see pages 56 and 18).

Licorice has other benefits. In various studies, it has increased the effectiveness of standard tuberculosis treatments, reduced the steroid dosages needed to treat Addison's disease, increased the effectiveness of cortisone, and cured a disease called congenital paramyotonia, in which the muscles become paralyzed when exposed to cold.[20]

Considerations for Use

Make licorice tea by simmering 1 teaspoon (3 grams) of the herb in 1 cup of water for fifteen minutes. Strain and drink. Licorice is also available as glycyrrhizin extract and, for peptic ulcers only, as DGL. To be effective, DGL must be taken in a chewable form, since the mixture of saliva and DGL releases factors that stimulate the growth of cells lining the digestive tract.

Too much of a good thing is possible in licorice. Licorice used *by itself* can have potent side effects, including water retention, swelling, high blood pressure, and irregular heart rhythms. Symptoms of licorice overconsumption are similar to those of severe allergy, except they are not relieved by antihistamines.[21] However, these complications do not appear unless very large quantities of licorice are consumed, on the order of 50 grams per day.[22] Avoid these side effects by carefully following the dosage and time limits discussed in the applicable Part Two entries, by using formulas instead of the herb by itself where advisable (see a Kampo practitioner), and by including potassium-rich fruits and vegetables in the diet, such as bananas and apricots.

Persons with high blood pressure should avoid licorice, as should those with estrogen-sensitive disorders, such as fibrocystic breast disease, breast cancer, or uterine cancer, because licorice promotes the conversion of testosterone into estrogen.[23] In addition, licorice is a primary ingredient in smokeless or chewing tobacco. Excessive use of smokeless tobacco can have all the effects of excessive licorice use, especially high blood pressure.[24]

Ligusticum / KOHON

Description and Parts Used

Ligusticum is an Asian perennial that reaches a height of six feet. It bears toothed leaves and greenish-yellow flowers. The root is dug for medicinal use in autumn, after the leaves have fallen.

Uses in Kampo

Ligusticum is another herb with a long history of medicinal use, appearing in *The Divine Husbandman's Classic of the Materia Medica* in the first century B.C. Ligusticum expels invading cold and relieves pain, especially headache. It is especially useful for pain that travels from the center of the head down to the cheeks and teeth. Ligusticum also treats acute lower back pain.

Scientific Findings and Clinical Experience

Scientific studies have confirmed that ligusticum has a gentle antiviral action, and can be used to treat secondary bacterial and yeast conditions that occur after a viral infection. The active constituent of ligusticum is Z-ligustilide, which scientists have found to be about half as effective as the drug ribavirin (Virazole).[1]

Like ribavirin, ligusticum is effective against both influenza A and B. Ribavirin, however, has to be applied as an aerosol to coat the linings of the mouth, nose, and throat in order to prevent infection. Ligusticum may be taken as a mouthwash or gargle. Ligusticum washes are also effective against respiratory syncytial virus, the germ that causes viral pneumonia.

Some species of ligusticum are useful in preventing leukopenia, a reduction in the amount of white blood cells, when used with the chemotherapy drug mitomycin. Ligusticum extracts help the body maintain its white blood cell count, and also activate both T and natural killer cells.[2]

Considerations for Use

Ligusticum is best taken as a tincture. It also appears in a number of formulas (see Chapter 4).

Ligusticum is an extremely drying herb. It should not be used in cases of what Kampo calls "blood deficiency," as shown by female infertility, irregularities of the skin and nails, menstrual irregularities, or pallor.

Ligustrum / Joteishi

Description and Parts Used

Ligustrum, also known as privet, is a member of the olive family that is common in southeastern China. The tree produces firm, round, grayish black fruits that bear a resemblance to olives. The fruits are harvested for medicinal use in the fall and winter.

Uses in Kampo

Kampo uses ligustrum to treat hot symptoms resulting from a deficiency of yin, or containing, energies. It tonifies the kidneys and liver to prevent dizziness, premature graying of the hair, soreness of the lower back, and tinnitus, all of which can be associated with sexual excess. In fact, a literal translation of the plant's name from the original Japanese is "female chastity seed." Ligustrum also increases visual acuity in persons with kidney or liver problems.

Scientific Findings and Clinical Experience

Ligustrum is remarkably nontoxic, and this quality is of greatest value in the herb's use as a cancer treatment. Animal studies at Loma Linda University in California show that as little as 500 micrograms—one-half of a thousandth of a gram—of ligustrum deters kidney cancer, with a cure rate of 100 percent if given while the tumors are small.[1]

Chinese studies have found that ligustrum lowers both cholesterol and triglyceride levels in test animals. It also reduces the rate at which atherosclerotic plaques form in the blood-vessel linings,[2] and prevents leakage from capillaries.

Considerations for Use

Make ligustrum tea by steeping 1 tablespoon (2 to 3 grams) of dried herb in 1 cup of hot water for forty-five minutes. Strain before drinking.

In Kampo, persons who have yang deficiency, or a lack of active emotional or physical energy, should avoid ligustrum. It should also be avoided in cases of diarrhea caused by incomplete digestion of food, as shown by undigested food in the stool.

Lily Bulb / Byakugo

Description and Parts Used

Lily bulb is the corm of a Chinese garden lily, *Lilium brownii.* Grown throughout China, lily bulb is harvested in autumn or winter when the above-ground parts of the plant have been killed by frost. Lily bulb should be yellowish white, with uniform scales on its surface.

Uses in Kampo

Kampo included lily bulb in formulas recorded in *The Divine Husbandman's Classic of the Materia Medica,* written over 2,000 years ago. Kampo uses lily to encourage the flow of fluids to the lungs, where it relieves cough and then stops sore throat. Ancient Chinese herbalists thought that lily bulb "protected the metal," stabilizing the lungs (the Metal organ in Chinese medical theory; see Chapter 1) and also clearing the heart of random emotions. This changed the outward, or physical, body by stopping insomnia, irritability, and restlessness.

Scientific Findings and Clinical Experience

Scientific study has confirmed that lily bulb contains antihistamines,[1] which makes it useful for respiratory problems.

Considerations for Use

Lily bulb is used in the formula Lily Bulb Decoction to Preserve the Metal (see Chapter 4).

Lindera / Uyaku

Description and Parts Used

Lindera is the powdery brown root of the lindera shrub, native to the Hunan province of southern China. Almost-oval leaves grow on opposite sides of lindera's multiple stems, and flowers and fruit grow from the nodes between the leaves and stems.

Uses in Kampo

Kampo's primary application of lindera is in stopping frequent urination and urinary incontinence, particularly in the formula Shut the Sluice Pill (see Chapter 4). Lindera tonifies the energy of the kidneys to propel urine through the bladder, thus avoiding urine retention. Lindera also helps essential energy, or qi, circulate through the body in ways to avoid both "clumping" of qi and pain in the abdomen, chest, and flanks. Kampo physicians also use lindera to dispel accumulated cold that manifests itself as lower abdominal pain, hernia, or menstrual pain.

Scientific Findings and Clinical Experience

Kampo practitioners have long known that dusting lindera powder on the skin dilates blood vessels, increases blood flow, and relaxes stiff muscles. Laboratory studies in Taiwan offer an explanation of how lindera normalizes the flow of qi, and consequently of blood, through the body. The herb contains a compound, dicentrine, that blocks the effects of adrenaline on the circulatory system. Dicentrine increases the flow of blood through tissues without changing heart rate or output.[1] Unlike the major classes of prescription treatments for high blood pressure, dicentrine does not affect nerves to the smooth muscles surrounding bronchial passageways or nerves involved in male erection. It has no calcium-channel blocking qualities that increase risk of heart attack, and it does not change the production of blood-pressure regulating hormones by the kidneys.

In tests of 472 herbs, scientists in the People's Republic of China found that lindera is also one of Kampo's ten most effective herbs for the treatment of herpes infections of the eyes.[2] Japanese scientists have isolated a chemical unique to lindera that keeps melanoma cells from manufacturing the pigment melanin.[3]

Considerations for Use

Lindera is available as a fluid extract called *Wu Yao.*

Prolonged use of relaxing lindera encourages weight gain. Also, Kampo masters warn that lindera is not to be used when there is "interior heat," that is, advanced infection.

Lithospermum / Shiso

Description and Parts Used

Lithospermum is a Kampo herb from two different parts of the Orient that is used in two different forms. One variety is native to Tibet and is known as "soft purple herb" for its soft root. Another variety is native to southeastern China and is known as "hard purple herb" for its hard root. Kampo uses the "hard purple" root.

Uses in Kampo

In Kampo, lithospermum is a cooling herb that relieves fire from toxic infections, especially infections that result in deep purple rashes. It clears the damp heat of yeast or fungal infections of the skin and vagina, and moistens the intestines, relieving constipation.

Scientific Findings and Clinical Experience

Lithospermum kills microbes and strengthens the immune system. Japanese studies have found that lithospermum kills Epstein-Barr virus, which is associated with chronic fatigue syndrome.[1] Lithospermum ointments, available at Chinese herb retailers, relieve skin inflammation caused by bacterial or fungal infections.

Another Japanese study found that lithospermum reverses immune suppression caused by the cancer treatment mitomycin (Mutamycin). The herb stimulates the body's production of natural killer cells and increases the activity of macrophages, "germ-eating" immune-system cells.[2] Not only does lithospermum reduce the side effects seen in this form of cancer treatment, it also inhibits tumors from developing their own blood supplies and spreading through the body.

European scientists have found that lithospermum prevents the formation of kidney stones. This action is believed to be due to the presence of saponins, soaplike compounds that disinfect the kidney and urethra.[3]

Considerations for Use

Lithospermum is available in tincture form, which may be labeled "stone seed." It is difficult to overdose on this herb; animal studies suggest that a 110-pound (50-kilogram) adult would experience blood in the urine, diarrhea, and fever after taking 500 grams, or 50 to 150 times the recommended dose. Even when taken in gross overdose, the symptoms caused by lithospermum go away if the herb is discontinued for a few days.

Lobelia / Hanpenren

Description and Parts Used

Lobelia is a fall wildflower common throughout China and, like many other Oriental medicinal herbs, in the eastern United States. Reaching a height of two feet, it bears white flowers alternating on a central flower stem. Traditional American herbal medicine uses seeds from the seedpods of *Lobelia inflata,* so named for the pods' tendency to swell and open. Kampo medicine uses the leaves, roots, and stems of a very closely related species, *Lobelia chinensis,* in the same way American herbal medicine uses lobelia seed.

Uses in Kampo

Kampo has used lobelia for thousands of years. Lobelia reduces swelling and encourages urination. TCM also uses this herb for cooling the blood and reducing the toxicity of insect stings and snakebites. In addition, lobelia cools the blood in what are called "fire toxin" patterns, such as tonsillitis. Modern TCM uses lobelia for the treatment of ascites in the later stages of schistosomiasis, a parasitic disease.

Scientific Findings and Clinical Experience

Herbalists agree that lobelia is an effective asthma treatment. Lobelia contains three chemicals that are powerful expectorants with a long history of use. Lobeline, the principal chemical, first stimulates and then relaxes the central nervous system as the dosage is increased. It promotes the release of hormones that relax the smooth muscles lining the bronchial passageways.[1] Lobelia is currently used in anti-smoking gums, since lobeline calms nicotine cravings.

Considerations for Use

Lobelia leaf is available in tincture and fluid extract form, or freeze-dried in capsules. Overdoses of lobelia produce low blood pressure, as shown by rapid heartbeat and sweating. If either of these symptoms occurs, contact a physician immediately. Less serious side effects of the herb include constipation and stomach upset. If these symptoms occur, discontinue use of the herb.

Locoweed

See **Astragalus.**

Longan / Ryuganniku

Description and Parts Used

Longan is a popular fruit in Japan. Native to southeastern China and Taiwan, the longan tree bears clusters of large, soft, sweet, yellowish brown fruits anytime from June to October. The fresh fruit is used both medicinally and as a food.

Uses in Kampo

In Chinese Kampo, longan is used as a tonic for the heart and spleen. It is thought to calm the spirit, relieving dizziness, forgetfulness, heart palpitations, and insomnia, especially when these problems arise from excessive concentration or overwork. It is usually combined with acorus for forgetfulness in old age and with tang-kuei (see pages 19 and 91) for insomnia.

Scientific Findings and Clinical Experience

Herbalists Dan Bensky and Andrew Gamble note that concentrated longan teas kill most disease-causing fungi.[1]

Considerations for Use

Longan is an important component of Restore the Spleen Decoction, in which it is thought to "anchor the spirit" in cases of depression (see Chapter 4).

Lonicera / Kinginka

Description and Parts Used

Lonicera consists of the flower buds of the Japanese honeysuckle. Kampo uses unopened yellow buds with an intense aroma, harvested just before they would open, in late spring. The vine grows throughout China, especially in Hunan province.

Uses in Kampo

Kampo's primary use of lonicera is to clear heat and relieve toxicity. Lonicera treats hot, painful sores and swellings in various stages of development along the liver's energy channel, especially the breast, throat, and eyes. It expels heat in the early stages of headache and sore throat. It also clears the heat of dysentery and urinary tract infection.

Scientific Findings and Clinical Experience

Lonicera contains compounds that neutralize staph infections (*Staphylococcus albus, Staphylococcus aureus*) and the influenza virus.[1] Lonicera also lowers serum cholesterol, by stopping the absorption of cholesterol from food in the colon.[2]

In the People's Republic of China, lonicera is used with astragalus and ophiopogon (see pages 27 and 77) to treat viral myocarditis, an inflammation of the heart muscle.[3] Adding apricot seed and scutellaria to the formula creates a treatment for bronchial pneumonia in infants.[4] Taiwanese researchers have found that lonicera compounds called caffeoylquinates inhibit the replication of the HIV virus, although they also impair reproduction of healthy human cells.[5]

Considerations for Use

Lonicera is available in capsule form as honeysuckle flower or *Jin Yin Hua.* This herb is also used in formulas (Chapter 4).

Traditionally, lonicera is not used when there is chronic diarrhea or sores oozing a clear exudate.

Lophatherum / Tanchikuyo

Description and Parts Used

Lophatherum is a grass that grows throughout southeastern China. It is gathered in late spring or early summer before its flowers have bloomed. Kampo uses the stem and leaves.

Uses in Kampo

Lophatherum is a cold, pungent, sweet, descending herb. It is used when there is a fever-producing disease characterized by heat penetrating inward and downward, causing scanty, concentrated urine. This herb's sweet taste makes it useful in tonics for persons recovering from illness.

Scientific Findings and Clinical Experience

Lophatherum is a weak diuretic that acts by increasing the excretion of salt into the urine. It also contains antifever compounds.

Considerations for Use

Lophatherum is used in formulas (see Chapter 4).

Loranthus (Mulberry Mistletoe) / SOKISEI

Description and Parts Used

Loranthus is the stem of the mulberry mistletoe, also known as European mistletoe. It is a parasitic evergreen shrub that forms bunches as much as ten feet (three meters) across on the limbs of host firs, oaks, and pines. It is not the same herb as American mistletoe. Loranthus has feathery leaves, yellow flowers in clusters of three, and round, sticky, white berries. American mistletoe has white flowers and leaves that are more rounded.

Uses in Kampo

Loranthus is an energy-regulating tonic for the liver and kidneys. Kampo uses it to strengthen the sinews and bones, and to relieve soreness and pain in the lower back and knees. It is an effective treatment for joint problems and numbness. Loranthus nourishes the blood and stops bleeding during pregnancy.

Kampo includes loranthus in formulas (see Chapter 4) designed for a symptom pattern that includes dizziness, headache, insomnia or dream-disturbed sleep, numbness, tinnitus, twitching and spasms in the hands and feet, and vertigo. In these formulas, loranthus acts by stimulating circulation.

Scientific Findings and Clinical Experience

Loranthus was introduced into the treatment of cancer in 1917. Today, extracts from the plant, usually given as an injection, are widely used as a supplemental treatment in cancer therapy in Europe. The herb's most important active agents are the lectins, which poison cancer cells and stimulate the immune system. German laboratory studies have found that lectins condition tumors to become sensitive to the immune system. Tumors that are ordinarily immune to natural killer (NK) cells are conditioned by loranthus treatment to allow NK cells to "lock onto" and destroy cancer cells.[1] Loranthus extracts increase the activity of NK cells by as much as five- to tenfold.[2] The extracts also stimulate the movement of immune-system cells called T cells that "patrol" the body seeking cancer and infection.[3] In addition, these extracts also increase the production of beneficial free radicals that fight a wide range of cancers.[4]

A Swiss study of fourteen breast cancer patients showed that a standardized extract of loranthus, Iscador, increased the rate at which breast cells were able to repair their DNA. Repairing DNA prevents mutations that can result in the formation of cancerous cells. At the beginning of the study, the rate at which the cancer patients' cells repaired damage to DNA was only 16 percent of that in healthy individuals. After just nine days of treatment, the rate increased to nearly 50 percent.[5]

In animal studies, loranthus extracts prevent the spread of melanoma to lung tissue by approximately 80 percent. However, the extract must be used *before* the cancer spreads to the lung.[6]

Animal studies have also confirmed that loranthus lectins reduce the risk of leukopenia, or white blood cell deficiency, during chemotherapy with cyclophosphamide (Cytoxon). Loranthus also prolongs survival time and reduces risk of leukopenia after exposure to or treatment with radiation.[7]

Considerations for Use

Loranthus is used in formulas (see Chapter 4). Do not use American mistletoe instead of loranthus, since the two herbs often have opposite effects. And do not eat the berries, which can be very toxic, especially for infants.

In addition, Modern European medicine uses loranthus extensively, in the form of lectin extracts given by injection. A typical course of treatment lasts several months to several years, with injections given three to seven times a week. Such extracts are marketed as Novapharm in Austria, Vysorel in Germany, and Iscador in many other countries, and are approved for use throughout Europe (see Appendix A for more information). These products must be used only under professional supervision, and as part of an overall treatment plan.

Commercial mistletoe extracts have minimal side effects, but in rare cases allergic symptoms, including reactions leading to shock, have been reported. An injection usually produces an increase in body temperature and flulike symptoms that indicate the herb is taking effect. The injection site can become inflamed, and abdominal pain with nausea may occur. Individuals who are taking a monoamine oxidase (MAO) inhibitor should not receive lectin injections.

Lotus / GUSETSU (ROOT) / KAYO (LEAF) / RENBO (SEED RECEPTACLE WITHOUT SEEDS) / RENNIKU (STAMEN) / RENSHI (SEED) / RENSHIN (SPROUT)

Description and Parts Used

The lotus flower, an emblem of the mystique of Japan, grows in shallow fresh waters in temperate climates around the world. The lotus is a water lily that anchors itself with a taproot extending to underwater sediment and puts out large, fan-shaped leaves that hold its flowering stem above the water. The lotus native to Japan, China, and India has blue or lavender petals, while the lotus native to North America has yellow or white petals. Most of the lotus used in Kampo is grown in Fujian or Hunan provinces in China.

Even in a scientific age, the lotus continues to puzzle. Australian scientists have found that the lotus is a "warm-blooded" plant, maintaining its body temperature during nighttime chill. Scientists at a Japanese manufacturer of Kampo drugs have raised seedlings from lotus seeds that had been sealed in a jar for over 1,000 years.

In the *Odyssey*, Homer tells about a magical lotus fruit

that caused those who ate it to forget country, home, and friends. Thus, the expression "lotus-eater" came to mean a dreamy, lazy person who has lost contact with reality. The "lotus" eaten in ancient Greece, however, was a prickly, shrubby, dry-land plant closely related to the jujube.

Uses in Kampo

The various parts of the lotus plant have different healing applications in Kampo. Lotus seed nourishes the heart, thought to be the reservoir of thought, and calms the spirit, relieving anxiety, irritability, and insomnia. Lotus seed is also used to stop diarrhea, and to prevent premature ejaculation in men or excessive uterine bleeding and vaginal discharge in women. Kampo uses the nodes of the lotus rhizome to stop bleeding and break up blood stasis, or accumulations of blood that no longer deliver qi (energy) as they should, particularly bleeding or stasis associated with the liver, lungs, or stomach.

Kampo uses the seed receptacle without seeds to stop uterine bleeding, prevent miscarriage, and cure diarrhea caused by eating spoiled food in the summer. Kampo uses lotus sprouts to treat insomnia or irritability due to fire in the heart, and also to bind the male "essence" by preventing nocturnal emission and premature ejaculation.

Lotus leaf treats summer diseases. It is used for symptom patterns that include fever, irritability, and sweatiness, especially with diarrhea. Like the seed and seed receptacle, the leaf stops bleeding, especially the vomiting of blood. Kampo practitioners sometimes apply fresh lotus-leaf compresses to the skin to stop bleeding or oozing of clear discharge.

The stamens, or male organs, of the lotus flower are used as a "similar" to treat male sexual dysfunction, on the principle that plants or plant parts shaped like parts of the human body cure that part of the body. Kampo uses lotus stamen in formulas to help the kidney consolidate its "essence," or reproductive information. Kampo employs lotus stamen and seed together to reduce nocturnal emission, since the storage of semen over long periods of time is thought to enable the conception of healthier children.

Scientific Research and Clinical Experience

Japanese and Chinese research scientists have built a considerable body of research on the healing properties of lotus. Japanese scientists have found that the lotus plant is a source of two chemicals, asimilobine and lirinidine, that act in the same way as fluoxetine (Prozac), keeping the brain from destroying the mood-elevating chemical serotonin.[1] Lotus root counteracts fever and inflammation from yeast infection.[2] It contains steroid compounds that experiments show are as powerful as the prescription drugs dexamethasone and phenylbutazone in relieving arthritic inflammation.[3] It also contains other compounds that counteract drug-induced depression.[4] Lotus-root tinctures lower blood-sugar levels about two-thirds as much as equivalent dosages of tolbutamide, a commonly prescribed antidiabetic drug.[5] Modern Kampo physicians are investigating the use of lotus seed receptacle as a treatment for cervical cancer.

Considerations for Use

The form of lotus that Kampo uses the most is Clear Summerheat and Augment the Qi Decoction (see Chapter 4), which is particularly useful for summer colds.

Lycium / JIKOPPI

Description and Parts Used

Lycium is a Tibetan herb that resembles the American prickly ash. Lycium grows up to twelve feet tall, and bears alternating, semioval leaves and bright berries. Fresh and dried fruit as well as fresh and dried root are used in Kampo. The Japanese word for lycium originally meant "earth bone bark."

Uses in Kampo

In TCM, lycium fruit is used to treat deficiencies of the kidney and liver, which together provide vital energy to the eyes. Lycium fruit relieves blurred vision and other forms of diminished visual acuity. Since the herb is neither cold nor hot, it also can be used to treat abdominal pain, sore back and legs, impotence, and sinus or chest congestion caused by either cold or hot conditions. Chinese herbalists used lycium to treat "wasting and thirsting disorder," known in modern times as diabetes.

The ancient masters of Kampo thought lycium bark drained "fire" floating upward through the kidney channel, relieving toothache. The bark also clears heat and stops coughing. In addition, it cools the blood, relieving bloody urination, nosebleed, and vomiting of blood. Lycium drains fire caused by yin deficiency, which expresses itself as low-grade fevers, irritability, night sweats, and thirst.

Scientific Findings and Clinical Experience

Lycium is a significant antidiabetic herb. When taken orally, it lowers levels of blood sugar and cholesterol, and lowers blood pressure as well.[1] Lycium's effect on blood sugar may be attributed to its protective effect on the liver.[2] Lycium extracts have also been found to protect red blood cells from the action of toxins called free radicals.[3] This reduces the likelihood of atherosclerosis induced by prolonged, uncontrolled high blood-sugar levels. When used to treat high blood pressure, lycium does not cause orthostatic hypotension, or the tendency to faint when rising from a seated position.

Lycium is also effective against cancer. In one Chinese study, lycium extracts were found to induce remission in seventy-five patients with melanoma or cancer of the colon, lung, or kidney.[4] In another Chinese study, lycium extracts had no effect on lung cancer when used by themselves, but sensitized cancerous tissues in the lung to make radiation treatment more effective.[5]

Lycium has other uses as well. Concentrated lycium teas are effective in reducing pain and inflammation caused by gingivitis. Lycium also stops malarial fevers. In one test, giving patients a combination of lycium and green tea (see page 59) two to three hours before the onset of fever had a significant effect in 145 of 150 cases.[6]

Considerations for Use

Make lycium tea by simmering 1 tablespoon (2 to 3 grams) of the whole fruits in 1 cup of water for fifteen to twenty minutes. Strain before drinking. Or use the concentrate, marketed as *Gou Qi Zi.*

Since lycium is a cooling herb, do not use it in the early stages of infection, which are traditionally thought of as those stages when fever is needed as part of the body's immune defense. Also avoid lycium if diarrhea is present.

Ma Huang

See **Ephedra.**

Magnolia / Koboku (bark) / Shini (flower)

Description and Parts Used

The magnolia tree Kampo uses for its bark is the same magnolia that grows in the southeastern United States. Magnolia bark is harvested between April and June from trees that are between fifteen and twenty years old. The bark is thick, fine-textured, oily, and aromatic, with a dark purple inner surface.

The magnolia tree Kampo uses for its flower does not grow wild in the United States. Kampo uses green flower buds picked in the early spring before they open. Most of the magnolia bark and flowers used in Kampo are taken from trees in the Chinese province of Sichuan.

Uses in Kampo

Magnolia bark promotes the movement of energy throughout the body, transforming dampness and resolving stagnation. The herb is used when "dampness distresses the digestive organs," causing bloating, rumbling, and gas, or when food "stagnates" to produce symptoms such as a bloated feeling, distention of the chest and/or abdomen, loss of appetite, diarrhea, or vomiting. Magnolia bark is an important herb for eliminating discomfort caused by dietary excess, and is included in formulas used to treat gastrointestinal problems (see Chapter 4).

Magnolia bark also warms and transforms phlegm and directs rebellious qi—qi that is going the wrong way—downward in the body. These actions stop coughing, wheezing, and stifling sensations in the chest.

Magnolia flower is put to the same uses as magnolia bark, but acts more gently. It is an acrid but aromatic warming herb. Kampo uses magnolia flower instead of magnolia bark when respiratory congestion is higher in the body, particularly when there is a stifling sensation in the chest. The flower is a fast-acting remedy for any kind of nasal or sinus congestion. Kampo also makes occasional use of flowers taken from the species (*Magnolia officinalis*) normally used for its bark. These flowers relieve stomachache related to emotional tension.

Scientific Findings and Clinical Experience

The bitter taste of magnolia bark can stimulate salivation, secretion of stomach juices, and movement of the intestinal muscles. Two compounds found in magnolia bark, magnocurarine and tubocurarine, block impulses in nerve fibers leading to the muscles. This enables these compounds to relax skeletal muscles. The herb can also increase uterine contractions.

Magnolia bark benefits the circulatory system. Magnocurarine and tubocurarine lower blood pressure.[1] Another bark component, magnolol, is 1,000 times more effective than vitamin E in preventing free-radical reactions that cause cholesterol plaques to be deposited in coronary artery tissue.[2]

Magnolia bark acts against various types of infections, including streptococcal infections, staph infections, shigella, viral hepatitis, and amoebic infections.[3]

Considerations for Use

Since the flower has a hairy surface, it should be rubbed with a clean cloth or wrapped in cheesecloth before being used in tea. This herb is available as Magnolia Flower Combination.

Maitake

See Modern Japanese Herbal Preparations.

Marijuana Seed / Mashinin

Description and Parts Used

Marijuana is a woody annual native to India, Iran, and China, and naturalized throughout the world. The seed, called "hemp seed" in Japanese herbal preparations and "linum" in Chinese preparations, appears in numerous Kampo products.

Federal law prohibits use of all parts of the marijuana plant except seed that has been heated to 220°F (105°C), which makes it sterile. Heat-treated marijuana seed is imported from China.

Uses in Kampo

In Kampo, marijuana seed is used to relieve constipation and irregularity. The classic texts of Oriental medicine praise its ability to aid blood circulation and to lubricate the gastrointestinal tract. Ancient Japanese herbalists prescribed marijuana seed for inflammation of the large intestine with stagnant stools, and painful urination or red urine with fever. In Kampo, marijuana seed is almost never used by itself, but rather in formulas such as Hemp Seed Pill (see Chapter 4).

Scientific Findings and Clinical Experience

Marijuana seed is a mild purgative that stimulates the intestinal mucous membrane, which increases secretions and movement within the bowel. None of the Asian texts mentions a hallucinogenic effect from the seed.[1]

Marijuana seed has also been used to lower high blood

pressure. In one study, patients who took marijuana seed for between five and six weeks showed a reduction in blood pressure without side effects.[2] The effect is related to the seed's high content of essential omega-3 fatty acids.

Considerations for Use

Marijuana seed will not produce a "high," but will cause a positive urine test for THC, the high-producing component, although sophisticated testing methods can distinguish use of marijuana seed from that of other plant parts.

Milk Vetch

See **Astragalus.**

Mint

See **Japanese Mint.**

Mistletoe, Mulberry

See **Loranthus.**

Morinda / HAGEKITEN

Description and Parts Used

Morinda is a deciduous creeping vine with twining stems and white flowers. Native to China, the plant is cultivated for export in Guangdong, Guangxi, and Fujian provinces. Growers harvest its large, thick, intertwined, purple roots in the spring and fall for use in Kampo. When boiled, the roots yield a characteristic yellow pigment.

Uses in Kampo

Kampo employs morinda as an energizing tonic for the kidneys. This action dispels reactions to cold in the environment (such as weather changes and allergens), increases mental power, and strengthens bones. It also quiets and soothes the five Paired Organs (see Chapter 1).

Morinda is an energy-generating herb used in the treatment of impotence, pain and weakness of the lower back and legs, bone degeneration, broken bones, torn ligaments, and joint pain. It is particularly useful for quelling pains that seem to migrate through the body.

Scientific Findings and Clinical Experience

Morinda helps promote male sexual health. Laboratory studies have found that morinda is an antidepressant herb with the unique property of increasing, rather than diminishing, male sexual function. Chinese scientists have identified the antidepressant compounds in morinda as inulin and nystose, two sugars, and succinic acid, a compound created from simple sugars.[1]

American studies have found morinda to be effective in lowering high blood pressure.[2] Many prescription treatments for high blood pressure have the undesired side effect of interfering with erections. Like the beta-blocker drugs, morinda lowers blood pressure by relaxing tension in the tissues that line the arteries. Unlike the beta-blockers, morinda also relaxes the arteries that fill the chambers of the penis with blood. Because morinda does not stimulate the veins that transport blood out of the erect penis, erections are both strengthened and prolonged.

Morinda also helps smooth out irregular menstrual periods. The scientific reasons for this action are not clear, although Kampo practitioners have prescribed morinda for almost 2,000 years in such cases. They most commonly prescribe the herb to women who also have either cold or pain in the back or pelvic region, along with frequent urination or urinary incontinence.

Morinda is an exceptionally rich source of vitamin C and its helpers, or cofactors, which help maintain the structural integrity of tiny blood vessels called capillaries. The herb can also stimulate the formation of white blood cells to fight infection.[3]

Considerations for Use

To make morinda tea, simmer 2 to 5 tablespoons (6 to 15 grams) of the coarsely chopped herb in 3 cups of water for forty-five minutes. Strain before drinking. Morinda is also available in freeze-dried form.

Although TCM uses morinda in cases of frequent urination or urinary incontinence, TCM practitioners warn that the herb should be avoided if there is dribbling or difficult urination.

Monkshood, Blue

See **Aconite.**

Motherwort / YAKUMOSO

Description and Parts Used

Motherwort, a member of the mint family native to Central Asia, is now naturalized to North Africa and Europe. It bears toothed, palm-shaped leaves and pink, lipped flowers. Motherwort is also cultivated as a garden plant. The above-ground parts are used in Kampo.

Uses in Kampo

In Kampo, motherwort is known as "benefit mother herb." A slightly cold herb, it invigorates the blood and regulates the menses. Kampo physicians use motherwort for female infertility, immobile abdominal masses, irregular menstruation, and postpartum abdominal pain. Motherwort also promotes urination and reduces acute swelling. Kampo physicians find the herb especially useful for treating swelling when there is also urine in the blood.

Scientific Findings and Clinical Experience

Scientific study has confirmed motherwort's usefulness for

gynecological problems. This herb relieves headache, dizziness, and increased appetite associated with premenstrual syndrome. It is especially useful for women who have overactive thyroids (hyperthyroidism).[1]

The Latin name for motherwort, "lion heart," belies its centuries of use as a remedy for weak heart. Motherwort strengthens heartbeat but does not increase pulse rate. Instead, it sedates and relaxes the coronary artery, resulting in increased circulation to the heart. *The German Commission E Monographs,* a well-respected herbal reference work, prescribes motherwort for irregularities of the heart caused by adrenal overstimulation and hyperthyroidism.[2]

Considerations for Use

Motherwort is usually taken as a tea. Simmer 2 teaspoons (3 grams) of chopped herb in 1 cup of water for ten minutes, strain, and drink. This herb is also available in tincture form, and is used in formulas (see Chapter 4).

Moutan (Giant Peony) / Botanpi

Description and Parts Used

The moutan, or giant peony, is found throughout China, but especially in northeastern China and Inner Mongolia. The root bark is harvested in October or November from plants that are between three and five years old. Moutan is closely related to the wild white peony (*Paeonia lactiflora*) and the European peony (*Paeonia officinalis*) (see page 78). Moutan is used in its raw form to clear what Kampo calls "static blood," and in charred form to stop bleeding.

Uses in Kampo

Moutan is Kampo's principal herb for treating gynecological problems associated with stagnant blood—which results in abdominal masses, failure to menstruate, and lumps—because it activates blood circulation. It also treats bruises caused by traumatic injuries. TCM uses moutan to clear fire ascending through the liver's energy channels, which relieves headache, eye pain, flank pain, and flushing associated with painful menstruation.

Moutan also clears blood heat, sedates, and soothes inflammation. In this capacity, Kampo uses this cold, bitter, acrid herb for premenstrual syndrome, as well as mouth sores, skin eruptions, and edema, or swelling, in the form of Warm the Menses Decoction (see Chapter 4).

Scientific Findings and Clinical Experience

Research supports Kampo's use of moutan for problems associated with the menstrual cycle. The herb acts by reducing inflammation, which relieves pain and water retention. This ability has been linked to one of moutan's main chemical components, paenol. In addition, moutan has analgesic, sedative, and anticonvulsant effects, and it lowers body temperature.[1]

Moutan also has the ability to reduce high blood pressure. In one clinical study, twenty patients were given moutan for thirty-three days. This treatment resulted in across-the-board reductions of diastolic blood pressure—the pressure exerted when the heart is at rest—by 10 to 20 mm Hg.[2] This ability seems to be related to chemicals called acetophenones, which stimulate circulation by reducing the blood's tendency to clot.[3] Paeonol, the anti-inflammatory chemical, protects the heart tissue from free radicals, byproducts of normal oxygen use that can damage cells.[4] Paeonol may also interrupt the process by which cholesterol is deposited in the artery linings. This prevents the arteries from becoming narrow and stiff, which can lead to high blood pressure. Interestingly, moutan also appears in formulas used to correct *low* blood pressure.

Moutan is an antimicrobial agent, effective against *E. coli,* typhoid and paratyphoid bacteria, staph infection (*Staphylococcus aureus*), strep infection (*Streptococcus hemolyticus*), pneumonia bacteria, and cholera bacteria.

Considerations for Use

Because moutan stimulates blood flow, avoid it during pregnancy, or if there is excessive menstrual flow. Moutan is used in Cinnamon Twig and Poria Pill (see Chapter 4), which is used to stop bleeding during pregnancy. However, this formula contains other herbs that keep moutan from increasing circulation to the womb.

It is also important to avoid foods seasoned with garlic while taking moutan, since garlic, like moutan, stimulates blood flow and contains potent anticoagulant factors (see page 53).

Mu Tong

See **Akebia.**

Mulberry Root / Sohakuhi

Description and Parts Used

Mulberry root is bark shaved from the root of the white mulberry tree, native throughout China. The leaf of the mulberry is notable for being the only food of silkworms. The Kampo preparation of the root, also known as morus, is white and powdery.

Uses in Kampo

Mulberry root is a cold and sweet herb used to move moisture, which relieves cough and asthma. Mulberry, in the form of Arrest Wheezing Decoction (see Chapter 4), also aids in the downward circulation of moisture to treat facial edema, inadequate urination, high blood pressure, headaches, and red eyes.

Scientific Findings and Clinical Experience

Mulberry root has been shown to affect the body's moisture content. It acts as a diuretic by stimulating the movement of salt into the urine, which indirectly lowers blood pressure.[1] Because of differences in soil mineral content, mulberry root grown in Japan has a greater effect on blood pressure than that grown in China.

Some studies have found mulberry root to be a potent antidiabetic. Both whole-herb teas and a protein found in the root, moran A, greatly lower blood-sugar levels in both diabetic and normal laboratory animals.[2]

Mulberry bark contains compounds that inhibit the bacteria that cause strep, staph, and tubercular infections.[3] It is also a mild tranquilizer.[4]

Interestingly, even rotten mulberry root has health benefits. The rotten herb seems to kill human disease fungi similar to the fungi that rot the root itself.[5]

Considerations for Use

Since mulberry root is a diuretic, it should not be used when there is already excessive urination. The herb's diuretic effect usually lasts five or six hours.

Mustard Seed

See **White Mustard Seed.**

Notopterygium / Kyokatsu

Description and Parts Used

Notopterygium, although it is also known as notch-leafed fern, is really not a fern at all. Rather, it is a member of the same family as carrot and fennel. Like many other Kampo herbs, notopterygium is grown commercially in China's Sichuan province. Kampo uses the irregularly-shaped root, which shows many red spots when sliced.

Uses in Kampo

In Kampo, notopterygium is prescribed for diseases of the Lesser Yang stage of disease (see Chapter 1), marked by chills, numbness, and pain on the surface of the body. Notopterygium, a warming herb, also relieves pain and stiffness in the joints and muscles, painful and inflamed eyes, cloudy vision, and itchy skin.

The most common combination of symptoms for which notopterygium is used includes joint pain, a general feeling of heaviness, drowsiness, and headaches that center around the eyes. These symptoms are corrected by the formula Ligusticum Chuanxiong Powder to Be Taken With Green Tea (see Chapter 4).

Scientific Findings and Clinical Experience

Notopterygium prevents painful inflammation by tightening the walls of the capillaries. This keeps fluids from pouring into the tissues, which reduces swelling.[1]

Considerations for Use

An overdose—more than about $^1/_2$ ounce, or 15 grams—of notopterygium may cause nausea and vomiting. Most Kampo formulas use 4 grams or less.

Freeze-dried notopterygium water extracts have been found to cause cell mutations in laboratory mice, although there is no evidence the herb has any mutagenic or carcinogenic effect in humans.[2] As a safety measure, never use notopterygium by itself, and never use any formula containing this herb for more than six weeks. Women who are or could become pregnant should avoid both the herb and any formulas that use it.

Nutmeg / Nikuzuku

Description and Parts Used

Nutmeg is a tropical tree that is native to Indonesia. It grows to a height of forty feet, and bears aromatic leaves and clusters of small, yellow flowers. The flowers yield nuts, which are gathered when ripe for use in Kampo and as the source of the common spice.

Uses in Kampo

Kampo uses nutmeg as a remedy for gastrointestinal complaints. It binds the intestines and arrests chronic diarrhea, particularly when used in the formula True Man's Decoction to Nourish the Organs (see Chapter 4). In Chinese Kampo, nutmeg is thought to "warm the middle burner," moving energy and relieving pain in the abdomen. By redirecting digestive energies, nutmeg also acts to stop vomiting. In addition, nutmeg is used to stimulate appetite in persons who have suffered long illnesses.

Nutmeg plasters are used to treat a variety of skin diseases, including eczema and ringworm, and as a counterirritant in the treatment of arthritis. In Ayurvedic medicine, India's version of herbalism, nutmeg is a male aphrodisiac.

Scientific Findings and Clinical Experience

Nutmeg contains a chemical called myristicin, which is responsible for its medicinal effects. Myristicin is an anti-inflammatory compound approximately as effective as the over-the-counter pain reliever indomethacin.[1] Nutmeg is known to prevent tissue destruction in the intestines caused by *E. coli*,[2] and contains substances that fight bacteria and yeasts.[3] Nutmeg also protects the body against chemically induced cancers.[4] Preliminary testing with rabbits indicates that nutmeg extracts could reduce total cholesterol while increasing the amount of HDL, or "good," cholesterol.[5]

At one time nutmeg was widely believed to have a psychoactive effect comparable to marijuana's,[6] since in large doses myristicin can induce delirium. However, the effects are variable and accompanied by side effects.

Considerations for Use

Kampo formulas use whole nutmeg. Roasting nutmeg increases its warming effect and makes it more useful in diarrhea treatment.

Ophiopogon / Bakumondo

Description and Parts Used

Ophiopogon is a Japanese lily that has the appearance of a winter grass, green with long, flowing leaves. Kampo uses the tuber, which is aromatic, chewy, soft, sweet, thick, and yellowish white in color. It is usually fried in wine when used as a tonic. In some parts of China, the lily liriope is substituted for ophiopogon.

Uses in Kampo

Ophiopogon is a sedative for the heart, which in Kampo is the seat of the emotions. When the heart is disturbed the person becomes irritable, especially at night.

Ophiopogon is also a moisturizer. It moistens the lungs and stops cough due to thick sputum, and generates fluids to relieve dry tongue and mouth. It also moisturizes the intestines to relieve constipation after fever. Symptoms eased by ophiopogon include dry cough, thirst, nervous unrest, scanty urine, sore throat, and mouth sores. Kampo practitioners use this herb to treat chronic bronchitis and diabetes.

Scientific Findings and Clinical Experience

Ophiopogon has a number of effects on the cardiovascular system. It increases coronary blood flow, increases the vigor of heart muscle fibers, helps the heart deal with oxygen deprivation, and slowly elevates blood pressure.[1]

Considerations for Use

Ophiopogon is used in formulas (see Chapter 4). Do not use this herb if diarrhea is present.

Opium Poppy Husk / Ozokukoku

Description and Parts Used

Opium poppy husk is the hard, thick, yellowish white fruit of the opium plant. It is *not* a source of the substance that is processed into codeine, heroin, or morphine.

The analgesic and sedative properties of opium have been well known around the world for thousands of years. The effects of opium on the mind were known in ancient Sumeria, and references to opium poppy juice are mentioned in the writings of the Greek physician Theophrastus in the third century B.C. In 1680 the English physician Sydenham wrote, "Among the remedies which it has pleased Almighty God to give to man to relieve his sufferings, none is so universal and so efficacious as opium."

Uses in Kampo

In Kampo medicine, opium poppy husk binds up the intestines to prevent chronic diarrhea and dysentery, contains lung qi, or energy, to prevent coughs, and alleviates pain of any kind. It also stabilizes what TCM calls the "lower burner," or the part of the body below the navel, to prevent overly frequent urination. Opium poppy husk is usually combined with schisandra to treat persistent cough, and with coptis (see pages 87 and 42) to treat chronic diarrhea. It is also used in the formula True Man's Decoction to Nourish the Organs (see Chapter 4).

Scientific Findings and Clinical Experience

Unrefined opium poppy latex and opium poppy husk contain more than twenty distinct medicinally active chemicals. This family of chemicals, referred to as opioids, includes opium. The opioid drugs have a unique ability to mimic mood-altering drugs naturally produced in the central nervous system. The morphine in opium reacts with specialized nerve cells to slow breathing, reduce movement through the gastrointestinal tract, and induce a feeling of euphoria, or well-being. These are the same effects produced by body chemicals called endorphins. Morphine eases pain by reducing the negative perception of pain. Pain is still felt, but it is not perceived as unpleasant.

Other compounds in opium react with other nerve cells to create unpleasant feelings of disorientation and depersonalization, mimicking body chemicals known as the dynorphins. Still other compounds in opium react with other nerve cells in the same way as the body's own enkephalines to induce pain relief and insensitivity to changes in temperature. Fortunately, the opium compounds imitating the unpleasant effects of dynorphins and enkaphalines exist in very low concentrations, and the predominant sensation produced is euphoria.

In small doses, opium slows respiration and suppresses cough. It has no effect on the cardiovascular system as long as the user remains lying down. It decreases secretion and movement through the stomach and intestines, and slows the rate at which the bladder empties itself. It greatly increases pressure in the bile duct. Opium suppresses the action of the immune system, especially of the natural killer (NK) cells, although it may increase the activity of the microbe-eating macrophages.

Considerations for Use

The amount of opium and opioid drugs found in opium poppy husk is very small. It is essentially impossible to overdose on opium poppy husk. The dose of opium available from the raw herb used in Kampo is less than that available from other over-the-counter products containing opium.

Nonetheless, opium poppy husk and formulas containing it should be avoided by persons with gallbladder problems, obstruction of the bile duct, or a tendency to retain urine, and by pregnant women. Chronic use of opium poppy husk can cause constipation. Opioid drugs can pass through the placenta to the unborn child. If opium is taken shortly before birth, the child may experience depressed breathing.

Peach Seed / Tonin

Description and Parts Used

Peach seed, which is also called persica, consists of the kernels taken from peach pits. In Kampo, the kernel skins are removed.

Uses in Kampo

The bittersweet peach seed, which is neither cooling nor warming, activates blood circulation and vitalizes the blood. Traditional Chinese and Japanese herbalists still use peach seed in combinations with other herbs to treat pain and distention in the lower abdomen, especially pain associated with premenstrual syndrome, and also that associated with appendicitis, cysts, dry constipation, and tumors.

Scientific Findings and Clinical Experience

Peach seed tincture has a gentle anticoagulant effect. This action may be similar to the effect of taking aspirin to prevent heart attack, without some of the side effects that continued use of aspirin has on the immune system. Unlike some blood-thinning agents, peach seed does not create a bleeding risk. Instead, it is useful in correcting platelet aggregation defects that can cause bleeding.[1]

Considerations for Use

Peach seed is available in capsule form under the name *Xao Ren*. This herb is also used in Kampo formulas (see Chapter 4).

Peony / BYAKUSHAKU

Description and Parts Used

Peony is the common name for the white peony root, taken from the well-known flower. Kampo also uses the giant peony, known as moutan (see page 75).

Uses in Kampo

Peony root is Kampo's basic herb for detoxifiying the blood. This herb curbs rising liver energy, which stops headache and dizziness. This action also relieves painful spasms in the abdomen, cramps in the hands and feet, and abdominal pain associated with diarrhea or dysentery. Peony helps the body contain energies that would rise to the surface to cause spontaneous sweating or night sweats. The herb also nourishes the blood and regulates the menses. This action treats menstrual dysfunction, vaginal discharge, and uterine bleeding. In addition, peony stops nocturnal emission.

Scientific Findings and Clinical Experience

Kampo's uses of peony have been confirmed by scientific investigation. Peony dilates blood vessels, including those leading to the heart. This action increases circulation. Peony increases the white blood cell count, which enhances the immune response, and has antispasmodic, sedative, pain-relieving, and fever-lowering properties.[1]

The two compounds of greatest interest in peony are paeonol and paeoniflorin. Both compounds inhibit platelet aggregation, a necessary step in reactions leading to allergic inflammation and bronchial constriction in asthma.[2] Paeonol, a proven antibacterial agent, is a useful muscle relaxant. Paeoniflorin is broken down by friendly intestinal bacteria into substances that have potent effects on the central nervous system, especially in terms of controlling epilepsy.[3] The use of paeoniflorin is also being explored as a treatment for age-related memory loss and senile dementia.[4]

Peony, when used as part of the formula Ten-Significant Tonic Decoction, also has anticancer effects (see Chapter 4).

Considerations for Use

Antibiotics use can reduce peony's effectiveness, since these drugs can disrupt the friendly intestinal bacteria needed to break down paeoniflorin. Persons who have been weak for a long period of time and have poor digestion should avoid peony. This herb should also be avoided by persons who have an estrogen-sensitive disorder, such as breast cancer or ovarian cysts, as peony can have estrogenlike effects, and can interfere with certain cancer medications.[5]

Peppermint / HAKKA

Description and Parts Used

Peppermint is a square-stemmed annual that yields the popular flavoring agent. It grows from thirty-two to thirty-six inches high, and has aromatic, serrated leaves. The finest quality peppermint is grown in the northwestern United States. Kampo does not always use the same plant identified in the West as "peppermint," but both plants have the same actions and contain the same chemical compounds.

Peppermint teas are used around the world to calm queasy stomachs and to quell indigestion. Peppermint leaves contain a volatile oil that is 50 to 75 percent menthol. This oil is the basis of most medicinal preparations that use peppermint.

Uses in Kampo

Although peppermint has been used as a flavoring for centuries, it has been used as a medicine for even longer than that. Mint is used in Kampo and TCM in the same way peppermint is used in Western herbalism. In Oriental medicine, the herb is understood to have a variety of actions. It is used to clear the head and eyes, and benefit the throat. This action soothes sore throat, red eyes, and headache. Kampo most commonly uses the formula Ledebouriella Powder That Sagely Unblocks (see Chapter 4) for these problems. Peppermint disperses heat—called "wind-heat"—that causes fever, headache, and cough. The herb also releases pent-up emotions, known as "constrained liver qi." This action relieves symptoms such as pressure in the chest or side, emotional instability, and emotional and cognitive disturbances associated with premenstrual syndrome. In addition, peppermint is used to vent rashes. Peppermint is used in the early stages of rashes, such as that associated with measles, to induce the rash to come to the surface of the skin. This hastens recovery.

Scientific Findings and Clinical Experience

Peppermint has gastrointestinal effects that go beyond simple indigestion relief. Irritable bowel syndrome is a condition in which the intestines pass food through the colon before it is fully digested. This causes cramps and diarrhea. Peppermint oil blocks the contractions of the smooth muscles lining the intestines, reversing some of the symptoms of irritable bowel syndrome.[1] This oil is also effective in relieving digestive disturbances caused by chronic hepatitis. In addition, British physicians have found a 40-percent reduction in the incidence of spasms caused by barium enemas when peppermint oil is used.[2]

Peppermint oil is also effective against food poisoning, as shown by its amazing ability to stop the growth of *Salmonella.* Japanese experiments with a number of foods stored at 86°F (30°C) for two days showed that peppermint oil stopped the growth of *Salmonella* and slowed the growth of *Listeria,* another harmful microbe.[3]

Peppermint oil can relieve headache when applied to the skin. Researchers at Christian-Albrechts University in Germany found that peppermint oil applied to the forehead produces the same pain-relieving effect as 1,000 milligrams of acetaminophen, or two 500-milligram Tylenol tablets. In most subjects, regardless of age, duration of the headache, or gender, peppermint was just as effective at relieving pain as Tylenol.[4]

Injectable peppermint formulations have been found to increase the activity of estrogen, and to increase the abortion-inducing activity of progesterone, found in contraceptive pills given to terminate pregnancy in the first one to ten days after conception in laboratory animals.[5] Oral peppermint preparations do not have this effect.

Considerations for Use

Make peppermint tea by pouring 1 cup of boiling water over 1 tablespoon (1.5 grams) of chopped herb. Brew for five to ten minutes, strain, and drink. Since peppermint tea increases bile production, do *not* take this herb during an acute gallstone attack. This herb is also available as oil in capsules and as specially coated tablets that are meant to pass through the stomach and break down in the small intestine.

To use peppermint oil for headaches, apply a light coating of oil across the entire forehead and to the neck, if there is pain in the back of the head. Apply only enough oil to moisten the area, as extra oil that does not adhere to the skin has no effect. Massaging the skin of the forehead or neck is not necessary, although it may help. Peppermint oil will smudge makeup.

Perilla / Shisoyo (leaf) / Soshi (seed)

Description and Parts Used

Perilla is a large-leafed mint grown throughout the Orient. English-language practitioners of Japanese herbal medicine often refer to perilla as the beefsteak plant, referring to the size and shape of its leaf. Kampo uses the leaf, seed, and stem of the plant, all harvested in the summer. Japanese cooking uses perilla as a seafood condiment. The herb helps prevent digestive upset and skin reactions caused by allergies to fish and shellfish.

Uses in Kampo

The master herbalist Todo Yoshimasu described perilla as a gentle, warming regulator of qi, or energy. It relieves discomfort in the stomach and chest, and dispels pathogens from the surface of the body. The leaf "releases the exterior" of the body to help immune reactions in the early stages of infection, the stem allows the chest to expand, and the seed directs energies downward in the body, correcting coughing, vomiting, sinus congestion, and headache.

In teas, perilla leaf has a mucilaginous, coating quality that soothes sore throat caused by frequent coughing. Perilla leaf quells bloating, diarrhea, nausea, and vomiting, and stops morning sickness during pregnancy.

Scientific Findings and Clinical Experience

Japanese researchers are investigating the role of perilla oil, extracted from the seed, in regulating the growth and proliferation of fat cells. They have found that including perilla oil in the diet activates a process that keeps the fat cells from living indefinitely after their normal life cycle. Perilla oil does this without interfering with genes regulating the early stages of the fat cell's growth, which allows the body to keep a normal complement of fat cells for necessary fat reserves.[1]

Japanese researchers have also found that perilla leaf suppresses excessive production of tumor necrosis factor-alpha (TNF-alpha). TNF activates the immune system to respond to and ultimately remove inflammation (although it also can contribute to inflammation in autoimmune disorders).[2] This effect is due to several different compounds, all of which can be extracted from the herb in traditional tea form.

The perilla plant is one of many plant sources of perillyl alcohol. Scientists at two American institutions have found that this substance has the potential to stop the development of colon cancer,[3] and act as a chemotherapy agent for breast, pancreatic, and prostate cancer.[4]

Considerations for Use

Kampo medicine uses perilla in formulas (see Chapter 4). Kampo teaches that perilla seeds are not to be taken when there is diarrhea.

Phellodendron / Obaku

Description and Parts Used

Phellodendron is a tree found throughout northeastern China. Kampo uses the cork, or inner bark, taken from ten-year-old plants. Phellodendron is also known as yellow fir, amur cork-tree bark, or simply "cork." This herb is related to coptis (see page 42).

Uses in Kampo

The cork of the phellodendron tree has been used in China for thousands of years to treat fever. Japan's eighteenth-century compendium of medicine, *Ippondo-Yakusen,* prescribed phellodendron as a worm remedy, and to treat inflammation of the digestive system, diarrhea accompanied by fever, "hotness" of the eyes due to fever-producing diseases, and fever accompanying pelvic inflammation.

Phellodendron drains damp heat, or infection, that is flowing downward in the body. It is used to treat thick, yellow vaginal discharges, foul-smelling diarrhea, and dysentery. Phellodendron also treats damp heat that has entered the leg, with symptoms such as red, swollen, and painful feet, legs, or knees.

Phellodendron quenches kidney fire, or inflammation, that is rising upward in the body. It relieves night sweats and afternoon fevers, as well as nocturnal emission and spermatorrhea. Phellodendron also drains fire toxins from sores and damp skin lesions.

Scientific Findings and Clinical Experience

Phellodendron contains a combination of chemicals that is especially useful in controlling diarrhea. One chemical, berberine, kills a vast variety of germs, including cholera, gonorrhea, shigella, staph, strep, salmonella, various kinds of fungi, *Plasmodium* (malaria), and leishmania.[1] In many cases, berberine kills microbes that have become resistant to antibiotics.

In addition to berberine, phellodendron contains as-yet-unidentified compounds that deactivate the stomach's "trigger zone" for digestive problems.[2] These compounds reduce the production of stomach acid. This short-circuits a chain reaction that leads to vomiting and diarrhea.

Pharmacological studies have shown that phellodendron also acts on the central nervous system to lower blood pressure, stimulate pancreatic secretions, and regulate the motion of the muscles lining the intestinal tract.[3]

Considerations for Use

Phellodendron is usually taken with coptis in formulas (see Chapter 4). Although there are no reports of allergy to multiple-herb formulas containing phellodendron, there are reports of persons developing rashes when taking phellodendron by itself.

Pinellia / Hange

Description and Parts Used

Pinellia is the rhizome of the "half summer" plant, a graceful herb with drooping stems and elongated leaves in the same family as Siberian ginseng (see page 105). Native to the Chinese provinces of Hubei and Sichuan, it is harvested from July to September.

Raw pinellia is toxic and only used externally. Chinese herbs stores almost never sell this form of the herb, known as *ban xia.* Pinellia is processed in two different ways for internal use. It is deep fried with ginger, vinegar, or alum to make the preparation known as *fa ban xia,* which is what customers actually get when they ask for *ban xia.* Pinellia is also deep fried in ginger juice to create a preparation known as *jiang ban xia.*

Uses in Kampo

Pinellia root is a warming, pungent herb used to move stagnant fluids and to stop vomiting. It is also used to treat chest pain, sore throat, cough, and stomach rumbles. In fact, pinellia is one of the most important herbs in the treatment of digestive disturbances. Pinellia acts by causing "rebellious" energy to descend in the body. This action keeps the lungs from producing sputum, and stops nausea and vomiting.

Pinellia also dissipates nodules and reduces congestion. Pinellia removes phlegm lingering in the chest or obstructions caused by phlegm anywhere in the body. It also dissolves what Kampo calls "phlegm nodules" in the neck, such as goiter and scrofula.

Scientific Findings and Clinical Experience

Pinellia stops nausea and vomiting by acting on the nervous system to prevent the vomiting reflex. It slows down nerve impulses that are necessary for vomiting, and also slows down impulses that control the heartbeat. Thus, pinellia acts like a beta-blocker drug in that it reduces heart rate and lowers blood pressure, especially in persons who are emotionally distressed.

Pinellia can act as a stimulant. It is somewhat unusual among Oriental herbs in that it contains nicotine, large amounts of the amino acids arginine and glutamic acid, and cholesterol. While arginine stimulates replication of the herpesvirus, glutamic acid can be used to make another amino acid, glutamine, that inhibits alcohol consumption in alcoholics. Taking small amounts of pinellia will not affect blood-cholesterol levels, but the nicotine will have a noticeable effect on the nervous system. Pinellia's stimulant qualities allow it to act as an antidote for strychnine poisoning by restoring the central nervous system's ability to initiate muscle movements.[1]

Pinellia is a long-term antihistamine, which makes it useful for many respiratory disorders. Histamine constricts the bronchial passageways. This makes breathing difficult, and induces inflammation and swelling. Pinellia blocks the nerve signals that start the secretion of histamine, easing bronchitis when used in formulas (see Chapter 4). Pinellia teas are also appropriate for the treatment of pneumosilicosis, or black lung disease, a chronic disorder that generally affects coal miners. Pinellia slows the course of the disease, with early usage producing the best results.[2] In addition, pinellia is an antibiotic. Pinellia tincture ear drops usually stop oozing inner ear infections in one to two days.

Pinellia is used in many formulas, including Pinellia and Magnolia Bark Decoction, which provides relief to persons suffering from anxiety or depression, and Pinellia Decoction to Drain the Epigastrium, which is a useful adjunct to chemotherapy or radiation treatment (see Chapter 4).

Considerations for Use

Pinellia has a potent ability to stimulate the body during infection. In fact, pinellia is so stimulating that it is potentially toxic. In Kampo formulas, pinellia is always processed to remove toxicity. This herb should always be used under the supervision of a Kampo or TCM practitioner.

Pinellia is never used when there is any kind of bleeding. This herb generally does not pose a problem, though, when used in Kampo formulas, since other ingredients offset this effect. Pinellia is also to be used with caution when there is fever. Discontinue any formula containing pinellia if preexisting fevers worsen, since that is a sign that the wrong formula has been chosen.

Pinellia root contains compounds that make the glaucoma medication pilocarpine less effective. Persons who take pilocarpine should not take pinellia by itself. Formulas in which pinellia is the main ingredient are safe for their intended short-term use when used with this drug.

Plantain (Psyllium Seed) / SHAZENSHI

Description and Parts Used

Kampo uses whole seeds, gathered in summer and autumn when the seeds have ripened. Ground plantain seed, also known as plantago or psyllium seed, is the main ingredient of dozens of over-the-counter bulk-forming laxatives.

Uses in Kampo

Plantain is a cold, sweet herb that promotes the descent of fluids in the body. By promoting urination, plantain relieves any type of edema or painful urinary dysfunction caused by yeast infections of the urinary tract. By releasing moisture through urination, it helps solidify the stool and relieve diarrhea. By accumulating moisture within the colon, it helps relieve constipation. And by softening the stool, it helps ease the discomfort of hemorrhoids.

Plantain expels phlegm and stops coughing, especially for respiratory infections that produce large amounts of sputum. This herb is also useful for eye problems, such as cataracts, dry eyes, red eyes, and sensitivity to light.

Scientific Findings and Clinical Experience

Plantain seed powder can lower blood levels of glucose and cholesterol by keeping these substances from being absorbed out of the intestine.

In China, plantain seed tea is injected directly into joints to prevent dislocation. This therapy is especially useful in stopping repeated dislocations of the temporomandibular, or jaw, joint.[1] It works by lubricating the joint, which blocks the pain that keeps the patient from using the joint.

Considerations for Use

Virtually all of the mucilage in plantain seed is contained in the seed coat, so the herb is effective whether added whole to teas or consumed as a powder. To make plantain tea, place 2 teaspoons (10 grams) of seed in a muslin cloth. Tie the cloth so that the seeds will not leak out. Place the teabag in 1 cup of boiling water, then simmer over low heat for forty-five minutes. Remove the bag, and drink the tea while still warm. To make a cold decoction, place 1 teaspoon (5 grams) of ground plantain seed in $^{1}/_{2}$ cup of cold water. Allow the mixture to stand for fifteen minutes, then drink *without* straining the seeds out of the mixture. Immediately after taking plantain, drink another cup of fluid. This herb is also used in formulas (see Chapter 4).

Plantain in the quantities used in Kampo teas does not interfere with other means of managing diabetes. However, diabetics who use large quantities of plantain-powder products may find that their absorbed-sugar levels can go down to the point that they may need to reduce their dosage of insulin.

Platycodon / KIKYO

Description and Parts Used

Platycodon is an herb found throughout eastern China and in Japan. Like many other Oriental herbs, it is also native to the southeastern United States. The plant grows to a height of three feet and is supported by a single taproot. It sends up a single flowering spike at the head of a central stem bearing alternating, simple leaves. The distinguishing characteristic of platycodon is its swollen flower, the source of another common name, balloon flower.

Kampo uses the root of the plant. The root should be bitter, firm, large, thick, and white.

Uses in Kampo

Platycodon opens up lung qi, or energy. This action expels phlegm and stops coughing. Platycodon also promotes the discharge of pus, especially pus associated with abscesses in the throat; see Ledebouriella Decoction That Sagely Unblocks in Chapter 4.

Along with apricot seed (see page 25), platycodon is an herb for singers and speakers. It treats hoarseness, laryngitis, and loss of voice. Platycodon is most useful for vocal problems related to general stress and fatigue, while apricot seed is more likely to be used for those problems associated with infection.

Scientific Findings and Clinical Experience

Platycodon works on dry cough by increasing secretions in the lungs and throat. In animal studies, platycodon teas have lowered blood-cholesterol levels by stimulating the liver to turn cholesterol into the bile, and have reduced blood-sugar levels. Platycodon is a mild tranquilizer,[1] and it increases the activity of macrophages and neutrophils, cells that eat bacteria.

Considerations for Use

Use platycodon with caution if peptic ulcers are present. Platycodon contains a chemical called platycodin that can stimulate bleeding. For the same reason, persons who are taking an anticoagulant, such as warfarin sodium (Coumadin), should not use this herb. In Kampo formulas, platycodon is balanced with other herbs to reduce this effect. One of the herbs used is licorice (see page 66), which soothes peptic ulcers.

Polygonum / Kashuu

Description and Parts Used

Polygonum is a long vine with tiny leaves on dozens of alternating small branches. It has a nutlike tuber. Polygonum grows in Guangdong and Sichuan provinces in southeastern China, and is also found in the wild in North Carolina. The Japanese name for this herb literally means "vine to pass through the night." The herb is also known as Chinese cornbind and fleeceflower vine. The stems, which are used in Kampo, should be coarse, firm, and purplish brown.

Uses in Kampo

Polygonum, an energy-neutral herb, unblocks the body's energy channels. This action relieves general numbness, pain, soreness, and weakness. Polygonum also nourishes the "heart," the seat of the emotions, and calms the spirit. This action is particularly useful for dream-disturbed sleep.

Scientific Findings and Clinical Experience

In laboratory tests, polygonum extracts reduce blood levels of cholesterol and triglycerides.[1] One chemical found in this herb prevented cholesterol from forming blood-vessel plaques in test animals fed large amounts of cholesterol.[2]

Polygonum also stops cancer invasion, the process by which tumor cells infiltrate neighboring tissues. Cancer cells secrete a substance called plasmin. Particularly in breast cancer, plasmin destroys the membranes connecting adjacent, healthy cells, allowing the cancerous tumor access to the bloodstream. Polygonum thwarts the action of plasmin, and reduces the rate at which cancers can spread.[3]

Considerations for Use

Polygonum is used in formulas (see Chapter 4). It produces no known side effects. This herb, usually sold as *Ho She Won*, is particularly useful in cases of repeated nightmares.

Polyporus / Chorei

Description and Parts Used

Polyporus is the stem of the polypore mushroom, a native of southeastern China. It has a shiny, red skin and a powdery, white center, and produces many caps from a single stem. Unlike hoelen (see page 61), with which it is often confused, this mushroom is always taken from the wild in either spring or autumn. Polyporus is also sold as umbrella polyphore.

Uses in Kampo

Polyporus is an energy-neutral herb that helps move fluids downward in the body. It is a diuretic that disperses moisture and relieves thirst, and is used in formulas that purge damp heat, or infection with inflammation, from the urinary tract (see Chapter 4). It is also employed in formulas to relieve difficult urination, edema, abdominal bloating, kidney inflammation and stones, diarrhea, vaginal discharge, and thirst.

Scientific Findings and Clinical Experience

Polyporus is used with dan shen (see page 44) to treat hepatitis B. In one Chinese study, three months of treatment with either herb normalized levels of ALT, an enzyme that indicates liver-damage levels, in about 50 percent of the patients. That figure increased to 80 percent when the two herbs were used together. After nine months, two-thirds of the patients treated with both herbs showed signs of remission. Only 50 percent of the patients treated with polyporus alone, and 25 percent of the patients treated with dan shen, showed such signs.[1]

The addition of polyporus to the diet has been found in Japanese research to lower blood-cholesterol levels significantly.[2] Studies of closely related mushrooms indicate that polyporus stimulates bile production.[3] Cholesterol is used to create bile, and bile is eventually excreted from the body, thus reducing cholesterol levels.

Polyporus also shows promise as a cancer-fighting agent. In animal studies, polyporus used by itself is almost as effective in extending the lives of liver cancer patients as the standard chemotherapy agent mitomycin-C. Each substance when used by itself increases life expectancy about 70 percent. When used together, polyporus and mitomycin extend life expectancy about 120 percent.[4] Doctors think that polyporus acts to increase the activity of macrophages, cells that eat cancer cells, in the liver.[5] Laboratory studies of the crude drug *chorei*, or powdered polyporus, show that it causes cell differentiation—which leads to cell death—in leukemia cells.[6]

In addition, polyporus has been used with some success to restore hair loss due to male pattern baldness. However, the polyporus extract used to grow hair has only been tested on mice.[7]

Considerations for Use

Polyporus is used in Kampo formulas (see Chapter 4).

Poria

See **Hoelen.**

Privet

See **Ligustrum.**

Prunella / Kagoso

Description and Parts Used

Prunella is a creeping perennial plant in the mint family. Native to Asia and Europe, prunella grows in meadows and along roadsides, thriving in sunny areas. The plant bears pointed oval leaves and blue or pink flowers. The aboveground parts of the plant are harvested in summer, when the plant is in bloom.

Uses in Kampo

In TCM, prunella is used to treat disturbances of the liver, which usually reflect the harmful effects of pent-up emotions. Prunella addresses symptoms that occur on the liver's energy channel, including dizziness, headache, red or swollen eyes, and especially eye pain that increases in the evening. It is also used for hernia and swollen lymph glands.

Scientific Findings and Clinical Experience

Scientific study has shown prunella to be an effective treatment for viral infections. A study of 472 Chinese medicinal plants found that prunella was among the ten most effective in the treatment of herpes simplex I. In seventy-eight cases of herpetic keratitis, an eye problem caused by the herpesvirus, thirty-eight patients treated with prunella eye drops were cured and thirty-seven improved, while only three did not benefit from the herb.[1]

A study of 204 Japanese medicinal plants found that prunella made one of the strongest showings in terms of anti-HIV properties. At a dosage of 16 micrograms per milliliter, prunella extracts completely eradicated HIV under laboratory conditions.[2] Canadian scientists have confirmed that prunella extracts block cell-to-cell transmission of the virus and interfere with the virus's ability to bind with T cells, immune-system cells that are destroyed by HIV infection.[3] Scientists at the University of California at Davis have identified the complex sugar in the herb that accounts for its actions against HIV.[4]

Considerations for Use

To make prunella tea, simmer 1 ounce (30 grams) of the dried herb in 3 cups of water for forty-five minutes. Strain before drinking between meals.

Do not use prunella if diarrhea, nausea, stomachache, or vomiting is present.

Psoralea / HOKOTSUSHI

Description and Parts Used

Psoralea is a climbing bean found throughout China. Psoralea seeds, which are harvested in the fall when they have ripened, should be large, solid, and black. Unlike garden beans, psoralea seeds are pungent and bitter.

Uses in Kampo

Psoralea, a bitter yet warming herb, stabilizes the essence of the kidneys (what conventional medicine calls DNA) and decreases urine output. This action stops excessive or frequent urination, incontinence, and spermatorrhea. Psoralea also tonifies the kidneys, and relieves impotence, premature ejaculation, and weaknesses in the lower back and extremities.

In ancient Kampo, psoralea was said to help the kidneys "grasp qi," which otherwise would cause wheezing in the lungs. Psoralea also warms the digestive tract. This action stops diarrhea, gurgling noises, and abdominal pain.

Scientific Findings and Clinical Experience

Psoralea is used to treat several skin and hair conditions. As a treatment for eczema, it offers a cure rate of about 25 percent. Psoralen, a chemical found in psoralea, makes the skin more sensitive to ultraviolet light, and eczema treatments require that the herb be used with either sun lamps or natural sunlight in order to be effective. Psoralea plus ultraviolet light was a startlingly effective treatment for baldness in one study. Of the forty-five participants, eighteen regained their hair completely and another fifteen showed significant hair gain.[1] Psoralea is an important ingredient in Seven-Treasure Pill for Beautiful Whiskers (see Chapter 4), which is used to treat hair loss.

Psoralea is also useful in the treatment of vitiligo, in which patches of skin lose their pigmentation. In one study, forty-nine patients underwent six months of psoralea treatment. Of these patients, 14 percent were cured and another 19 percent regained pigmentation on at least two thirds of the affected skin.

Psoralea acts as an antiseptic against staph infections, including penicillin-resistant versions. In addition, psoralea contains corylifolinin, a substance that opens the coronary arteries and stimulates heart contractions.

Psoralea contains bavachinin, corylfolinin, and psoralen, all of which inhibit osteosarcoma and lung cancer.[2]

Considerations for Use

Psoralea is available as a freeze-dried herb in capsules under the names Psoralea Seed capsule, Scruffy Pea, and *Bu Gu Zhi.*

Psoralea is unusual in that it can sensitize the skin to both healing and harmful ultraviolet rays from the sun. Unless this herb is being used to treat a light-sensitive disorder, use sunscreen or avoid sun exposure when taking it.

Psyllium Seed

See **Plantain.**

Qing Pi

See **Blue Citrus.**

Red Atractylodis

See **Atractylodis, Red.**

Red Peony

See **Peony.**

Red Sage

See **Dan Shen.**

Red Tangerine Peel

See **Bitter Orange Peel.**

Reed Root / Rokon

Description and Parts Used

Reed root is a Chinese grass that has been introduced to, and overrun, vast areas of the American South, where it is known as Johnson grass. In Kampo, the plant's densely branching rhizome has been used since the fifth century A.D.

Uses in Kampo

As a cooling, sweet herb, reed root clears heat and generates fluids. It relieves fever, irritability, and thirst. It is especially useful for clearing heat from the lungs, and is included in formulas to treat cough and expectoration of thick, yellow sputum.

Reed root is also used to clear heat from the stomach, expressed as belching or vomiting. It clears heat from the body through the urine, relieving dark or scanty urine or blood in the urine. Finally, reed root encourages rashes to surface, bringing fevers "to a head." This allows the patient to progress to the next stage of recovery.

Scientific Findings and Clinical Experience

Chinese clinical studies have found that reed root is useful in treating pulmonary abscesses. In the laboratory, this herb acts as an antibiotic against *Streptococcus.*[1]

Considerations for Use

Persons who have been diagnosed as energy deficient by a practitioner of Oriental medicine, especially if incomplete digestion is present, should avoid reed root. Kampo uses this herb in formulas (see Chapter 4).

Rehmannia / Jukujio (cooked) / Shojio (raw)

Description and Parts Used

Rehmannia is a perennial herb that grows on sunny slopes in northern and northeastern China. This low-growing perennial reaches a height of one to two feet, and has sticky leaves resembling those of spinach. It bears flower stalks topped with purple flowers. The root is harvested in the fall, after the plant has flowered.

Rehmannia is sometimes confused with the foxglove plant, also called digitalis, the leaves of which are powdered to form the base of the heart drug digoxin. Rehmannia is a different species in the same genus. Different parts of each herb are used in medicine, and the two frequently confused plants have different applications.

Rehmannia root comes in two forms, raw and cooked. The reddish-yellow unprocessed or raw rehmannia is a cold and bittersweet herb used to clear heat from the blood and treat sore throat, thirst, mouth sores, and bloody discharges. The black sun-dried or cooked rehmannia is a warm and sweet herb used to nourish the blood. Cooked rehmannia is used to treat anemia, infertility, diabetes, thirst, loss of hearing, weak knees, and lower back pain.

Uses in Kampo

The primary use of rehmannia in Kampo is to clear heat. Kampo uses rehmannia when heat has overwhelmed the exterior energies of the body and entered what is called the "nutritive" level, causing high fever, thirst, hemorrhage, and a scarlet tongue. Rehmannia generates fluids and cools heart fire, expressed as mouth and tongue sores, irritability, insomnia, and facial flush.

Kampo also uses rehmannia to treat kidney diseases. These conditions include "wasting and thirsting disorder," also known as diabetes, as well as night sweats, nocturnal emission, lower back pain, dizziness, ringing in the ears, hearing loss, and premature graying of the hair.

Scientific Findings and Clinical Experience

Rehmannia teas have been used successfully in treating eczema. Rehmannia also is reported to alleviate joint pain and swelling, along with nodules and rash, caused by rheumatoid arthritis.

Rehmannia has a protective effect on the liver. Teas made with raw rehmannia root have protected animals from liver damage caused by carbon tetrachloride, a common dry cleaning agent. In a hospital test, fifty volunteers with infectious hepatitis took injections of rehmannia and licorice (see page 66). Forty-two of the patients showed improvement within ten days.[1]

Although rehmannia is an important herb in Oriental medicine for the treatment of diabetes, clinical studies to confirm this effect have been equivocal. Japanese studies found rehmannia to be weakly hypoglycemic.[2]

The effect of a traditional herbal formula based on rehmannia, however, is much better documented. Eight-Ingredient Pill With Rehmannia has become one of the most popular herbal treatments for diabetes in Japan. The formula lowers blood sugar, aids insulin regulation, and halts the progress of diabetic nerve damage in type 1 diabetes (see Chapter 4). Herbal combinations based on rehmannia can lower blood-sugar levels as much as 50 milligrams per deciliter in the course of two weeks' use.

Another formula, Six-Ingredient Pill With Rehmannia, has become popular in the treatment of developmental disorders in children, including attention deficit disorder/attention deficit hyperactivity disorder (ADD/ADHD). In the United States, herbal practitioners have reported success using this formula to treat delayed development in children with cerebral palsy or ADD.[3]

Considerations for Use

Rehmannia teas can cause diarrhea or nighttime urination. For example, about 10 percent of eczema patients who take rehmannia experience diarrhea. Kampo formulas that contain this herb are better choices.

Reishi

See Modern Japanese Herbal Preparations.

Rhubarb Root / DAIO

Description and Parts Used

Kampo uses a variety of rhubarb that is more vigorous than the European and North American garden vegetable. In the perpetually cool climates of Tibet and parts of China, rhubarb is a thick-rooted perennial that grows to a height of ten feet. It bears large, palm-shaped leaves and clusters of small red flowers. The literal meaning of the name for rhubarb root in Japanese and Chinese is "big yellow." Rhubarb root is gathered in September or October after the stem and leaves have withered and turned yellow, from plants that are at least three years old.

Uses in Kampo

Aged rhubarb root is a fast-acting laxative described in the classical literature of Kampo as an "attacking" purgative that has the power to "flush" pathogens from the body. Rhubarb drains heat from the body through the stool, purging heat accumulations that can cause fever, thirst, and profuse sweating. Rhubarb also purges accumulations causing pain and swelling in the abdomen, and dispels static blood causing skipped menstrual periods, immobile abdominal masses, and pain due to traumatic injury.

In addition, rhubarb is also used to drain heat from the blood. It eliminates blood in the stool from bleeding hemorrhoids, and checks what is called "reckless movement of hot blood that overflows," exhibited as bloody vomit or nosebleed accompanied by constipation.

Scientific Findings and Clinical Experience

Rhubarb, like aloe (see page 21), exerts its laxative effects through anthracene compounds formed in the root as it is cured and aged. These compounds do not act directly on the body, but first must be broken down into substances called emodins by friendly intestinal bacteria. The emodins act on the lining of the intestinal wall by stimulating forward-moving contractions while inhibiting backward-moving contractions, thus purging the intestinal contents. Since rhubarb is a potent purgative, Kampo usually combines it with several other herbs to moderate its effects.

Rhubarb is useful for stopping gastrointestinal spasms. The herb is four times more potent than papaverine, a drug isolated from opium. In addition, rhubarb stimulates gallbladder output, which aids digestion.

Emodins and rheins, another family of rhubarb compounds, may stop the growth of breast cancer, liver cancer, and melanoma. These substances halt the process by which a cancerous tumor develops its own blood supply prior to spreading throughout the body. Rheins further reduce the activity of cancer cells by reducing the rates at which they can create proteins and use glucose as a cellular fuel.[1] Emodins stimulate the production of white blood cells, which fight cancer. In one study involving sixty-seven patients, emodin treatment increased white blood cell counts by more than 1,000 cells per cubic millimeter of blood.[2]

Boiling rhubarb changes rheins into a form called rhein anthroquinones, anticancer chemicals that can be more readily absorbed through the large intestine. Mixing rhubarb with licorice (see page 66) increases the rate at which the large intestine can absorb these cancer-fighting substances.[3] Kampo formulas used to treat what are called "blood stagnation" tumors are made with vinegar rather than water, which further increases the rate at which the intestine can absorb rhein anthroquinones.

The most effective form of rhubarb for cancer treatment, however, is not its traditional form, rhubarb tea. The problem with using rhubarb for cancer treatment is that very large amounts of rhubarb yield very small amounts of rheins and emodins. For this reason, an effective dose of rhubarb for cancer treatment is at least 100 times the effective dose for constipation treatment—an amount that is certain to disrupt the digestive process, despite the fact that longer boiling times do reduce rhubarb's laxative effect. Rheins and emodins are available in purified, injectable forms for medical use. Rhubarb products meant to be taken by mouth, though, are useful when used as part of an overall cancer-treatment program.

Rhubarb is also effective against trichomonas, a sexually transmitted microbe that can cause vaginal infections. Rhubarb, a diuretic as well as a laxative, alkalinizes urine to a pH as high as 8.4. This creates unfavorable conditions for the growth of trichomonas, which prefers pH levels of between 5.5 and 5.8.[4] Animal studies find that rhubarb's antitrichomonal effect is canceled out by compounds that produce cell-damaging substances called free radicals. This suggests that nutritional therapy with antioxidants increases the effectiveness of herbal therapy with rhubarb for trichomonas vaginitis.[5]

There are some reports that rhubarb lowers blood pressure and blood-cholesterol levels.[6]

Considerations for Use

Rhubarb tea offers quick relief of constipation. Simmer 1 to 4 teaspoons (3 to 12 grams) of rhubarb root in 1 cup of water for from fifteen to a maximum of forty-five minutes, strain, and drink. Rhubarb tea can be flavored with cinnamon or peppermint (see pages 39 and 78).

If friendly bacteria are not present in the colon, either through antibiotics use or because of a poor diet, rhubarb does not have a laxative effect. And, if rhubarb is boiled for more than two hours, the laxative compounds are destroyed before they are taken into the body. Instead, potentially *constipating* rhubarb tannins are boiled out of the root. Rhubarb is also available in injectable form and in two non-Kampo formulations, Essiac and Hoxie teas, and is included in Kampo formulas (see Chapter 4).

Using rhubarb root over a period of years causes undesirable changes to liver, thyroid, and stomach tissues. However, before tissue damage occurred, an individual would experience noticeable adverse effects, such as nausea, vomiting, diarrhea, and abdominal pain. Do not use any laxative, herbal or synthetic, on a steady basis. Do not use rhubarb if abdominal pain, rectal bleeding, or diarrhea is present. Avoid rhubarb during menstruation, and consult a health care provider prior to use if pregnant or nursing. Discontinue use in the event of diarrhea or watery stools.

Rose Hips / Gekkika (combination of hips and petals)

Description and Parts Used

Rose hips, the fruits of the rosebush, ripen and turn red after the petals have fallen off the flower. Most rose hips used in herbal medicine are taken from an ancient European variety of rose, the dog rose. These plants can be quite long-lived—there are European roses that have been in continuous production for more than 600 years. Kampo uses a combination of the hips and the petals.

Uses in Kampo

In Kampo, gently warming rose hips are used to invigorate the blood. In particular, they are used to regulate the menses, thus relieving static-blood patterns that include absent or scanty menstruation, and/or abdominal or chest pain and swelling. Rose hips are also used to treat swollen lymph glands. Rose hips are combined with brown sugar to make a sweetened rose hip tea, especially for treating abdominal pain, emotional stress, and constipation.

Scientific Findings and Clinical Experience

Rose hips are a traditional Japanese remedy for memory loss due to aging. They contain both vitamin C and the vitamin C cofactors needed to increase capillary circulation within the brain. This action increases the supply of oxygen and glucose to brain tissue. It also increases supplies of acetylcholine, a brain chemical vital to memory.

Traditional Kampo medicine had no concept of vitamins, but the usefulness of rose hips as a source of vitamin C bears mentioning. Rose hips contain up to 2 percent vitamin C, four times more than that found in oranges. The vitamin content depends on the form in which the hips are stored. Studies have shown that rose powder completely loses its vitamin C content in six months. Rose hips cut in half, however, retain most of their vitamin C content for at least eighteen months. In addition, the red and yellow pigments of the rose are derived from beta-carotene, a precursor to vitamin A.

Considerations for Use

Rose hips can be used in the form of rose-hip vitamin C. Commercial herbal teas can also be used, many of which combine rose hips with hibiscus blossoms. In some parts of the United States, rose hips are also available in the form of rose jam.

Safflower

See **Carthamus.**

Salvia

See **Dan Shen.**

Saussurea / Mokko

Description and Parts Used

Saussurea, the root of a woody herb in the sunflower family, is also known as costus root and aucklandia. Saussurea has been used in Oriental medicine since the time of the *Divine Husbandman's Classic of the Materia Medica,* written in the first century B.C.

Uses in Kampo

Kampo uses the bitter but warming saussurea to normalize the flow of qi, or energy. Stagnant qi in the digestive organs can result in lack of appetite, abdominal pain, nausea, vomiting, and a feeling of fullness in the epigastrium, or the pit of the stomach. Stagnant qi in the liver and gallbladder can result in pain in the sides.

Saussurea has strong antiseptic qualities useful for bronchial, intestinal, and vaginal infections. The herb is used to treat abdominal and chest pains, bronchial asthma, weak digestion, peptic ulcers, and premature contractions during pregnancy.

Scientific Findings and Clinical Experience

Scientists have found evidence of saussurea's benefits for the digestive and respiratory systems. The herb increases the rate at which the stomach empties its contents into the intestines.[1] Chemical extracts from saussurea stop the formation of peptic ulcers induced by stress.[2] Saussurea contains substances that stop allergy-induced bronchial spasms in laboratory tests. The herb also dilates the bronchial tubes and lowers blood pressure.[3]

Saussurea also increases the ability of liver cells to withstand infection from viral hepatitis B. In the future, medications made from saussurea for treatment of hepatitis B will consist of the isolated extracts of costunolide and dehydrocostus lactone from the herb.[4]

Considerations for Use

This herb is used in Kampo formulas (see Chapter 4).

Scallion / Sohaku

Description and Parts Used

The scallion used in Kampo is the bulb of the spring onion. It is a popular food item in cuisines around the world.

Uses in Kampo

Kampo uses scallion to disperse cold in the form of either abdominal pain or nasal congestion, release tight muscles in the exterior of the body and induce sweating, and relieve toxicity causing clumps or nodules under the skin.

Scientific Findings and Clinical Experience

Scallion and miso soup was first acknowledged as a medically potent "herbal" preparation in *Emergency Formulas to Keep Up One's Sleeve,* a compendium of Kampo knowledge written by Ge Hong in A.D. 341. Modern textbooks of herbal medicine in China often list this soup as the first remedy their students learn. Kampo has used scallion in soup for over 1,500 years to treat upper respiratory infection.

Scallions, like onions, have many of the same heart-protective effects as garlic (see page 53) when taken in a dosage of approximately 1 ounce (30 grams) per day, either raw or in cooking. The key element in scallions that relieves heart and artery disease, however, is sulfur. Scallions grown in soils deficient in sulfur to have an exceptionally mild taste do not contain the compounds that counteract atherosclerosis and clot formation.[1]

Considerations for Use

Scallions are used in Unblock the Orifices and Invigorate the Blood Decoction (see Chapter 4).

Schisandra / Gomishi

Description and Parts Used

Schisandra is an aromatic woody vine native to both northeastern China and the eastern United States. Reaching a length of up to twenty-five feet, it bears oval leaves, pink flowers, and spikes of red berries. The berries are dried for use in Kampo.

Uses in Kampo

The Japanese name for schisandra literally means "five tastes," referring to the fact that schisandra is sweet, salty, bitter, sour, and pungent. This quality allows it to act on any energy state of the body.

In traditional Japanese herbalism, schisandra was used mainly to treat coughing and "hood vertigo," a sensation of constriction that feels like a band around the head. Schisandra can inhibit sweating and generate fluids, an action that stops "cold sweat" due to emotional stress and offsets dehydration induced by diabetes. This herb also quiets the spirit and calms the heart, which relieves insomnia, irritability, nightmares, and palpitations. In addition, schisandra can tonify the kidneys and bind essence. This action stops nocturnal emission, spermatorrhea, frequent urination, and vaginal discharge.

In addition to its use in Kampo formulas (see Chapter 4), schisandra can be combined with a number of other herbs for specific uses.

Scientific Findings and Clinical Experience

Schisandra is one of Kampo's most useful herbs for the treatment of liver ailments. It protects the liver from chemical damage, particularly damage from chemicals that have to be activated by the liver to become poisonous, such as carbon tetrachloride.[1] Laboratory studies show that schisandra extracts increase the liver's ability to make the enzyme glutathione peroxidase, which deactivates several kinds of free radicals, or substances that attack the outer membranes of liver cells.[2] Glutathione peroxidase also helps offset damage done to the liver by chronic viral hepatitis and HIV.[3]

One schisandra extract, produced in Japan as gomisin A, blocks the immune system's production of inflammation-causing substances.[4] In animal studies, the extract is life-saving if given when massive doses of bacterial toxins are present. This is because gomisin A prevents liver inflammation and tissue destruction, and does so without harming the immune system.[5]

Gomisin A also stimulates liver regeneration. Animal studies show that this compound stimulates growth of healthy liver tissue by increasing the production of ornithine decarboxylase, an enzyme critical to the early stages of tissue recovery.[6] This can hasten recovery from liver surgery. In addition, animal studies have found that gomisin A is one of three schisandra compounds that prevent the development of skin cancer after chemical injury.[7]

Schisandra is used to treat insomnia. Animals studies have found that this herb increases sleeping time when used with the sleep-inducing drug phenobarbital.[8] Schisandra also increases the effectiveness of benzodiazepam tranquilizers, such as Librium and Valium, allowing patients to take lower doses of these potentially addictive drugs. The herb itself can be used to treat insomnia, headache, dizziness, and palpitations associated with emotional stress.[9]

Schisandra has other uses. Animal studies show that schisandra, when used with biota and Korean or red ginseng (see pages 30 and 57), prevents memory loss following excessive alcohol consumption. This combination does not, however, accelerate recovery from intoxication.[10] Schisandra stimulates the central nervous system to maintain breathing, which makes the herb useful as an antidote to morphine overdose. It also increases visual acuity and field of vision, as well as tactile sensitivity.[11]

Considerations for Use

To make schisandra tea, simmer $^1/_2$ teaspoon to 1 tablespoon (1.5 to 9 grams) of chopped berries in 1 to 2 cups of water for forty-five minutes. Strain before drinking between meals. It is also available freeze-dried in capsules, which are sold as Hoelen & Schisandra.

It is essentially impossible to overdose on schisandra in tea form. A toxic dose for a 150-pound (70-kilogram) person would be $1^1/_2$ pounds (750 grams) of berries. However, schisandra does increase the flow of bile.[12] Therefore, individuals with gallstones or blockages of the bile ducts should not use this herb. Schisandra also stimulates the uterus and induces labor, so it should be avoided during pregnancy.

Scrophularia / Genjin

Description and Parts Used

Scrophularia is an upright perennial herb found throughout China. It has a square stem, oval leaves, small round brown flowers in clusters, and green seed capsules. Kampo uses the above-ground parts of the plant. Its English name is derived from the similarity in appearance between its root and scrofula, a once-common tubercular condition in which lymph nodes in the neck swell to form hard, protruding lumps. Scrophularia is prepared in salt before it is used to treat diseases caused by fluid imbalance.

Uses in Kampo

Kampo medicine uses scrophularia to clear heat and to maintain fluid balance within the body. Scrophularia is indicated when a fever has reached the "blood level" and has begun to cause bleeding, dry mouth, fever, and a purplish tongue. This herb also maintains fluid in the intestines, which relieves constipation (see Increase Fluids Decoction in Chapter 4). In Kampo medicine as well as in European herbalism, scrophularia was used to soften hardness and dissipate nodules, especially those in the neck that give this herb its English name.

Scientific Findings and Clinical Experience

Scientific study has revealed that scrophularia has a strong antibiotic effect, especially against *Pseudomonas aeruginosa.* Scrophularia teas are also known to prevent high blood pressure caused by fluid imbalance.

Considerations for Use

To make scrophularia tea, simmer 1 to 2 (grams) teaspoons of powdered root in 1 cup of water for thirty minutes, and strain. Scrophularia is sold in Chinese herb shops as *Xuan Shen.*

Scutellaria / Ogon

Description and Parts Used

Scutellaria, also known as skullcap and scute, is a perennial herb native to the region of Lake Baikal in eastern Siberia and to northern China. It thrives on open grasslands at elevations below 2,000 feet in the wild, and is cultivated both as a medicinal herb and as an ornamental plant. Scutellaria grows to a height of between one and four feet, and bears lance-shaped leaves and purple flowers. The root is used in Kampo.

Scutellaria has held a central place in Oriental medicine for at least 2,000 years. When a northwestern Chinese tomb built in the second century A.D. was excavated, workers found ninety-two wooden tablets containing herbal formulas, many of which listed scutellaria.

Scutellaria is processed in different ways according to how it is used in treatment. It is dry-fired to reduce its cooling properties and help it enter the blood. It is sautéed in wine to enhance its ability to treat damp heat, which causes stuffy chest and coughs. And it is charred for preparations to stop nosebleed, vomiting or coughing of blood, or blood in the stool.

Uses in Kampo

Scutellaria is an important herb for clearing heat and drying dampness from the stomach and intestines. Scutellaria is used to treat symptoms that include diarrhea, fever, a stifling sensation in the chest, and thirst without the ability to drink.

Scutellaria is also useful in treating excessive internal heat, which causes the blood to move "recklessly." It calms the fetus, pacifying the womb when the fetus is restless or kicking excessively.

Scutellaria sedates energy that ascends from the liver, which can cause headache, irritability, red eyes, redness in the face, and a bitter taste in the mouth. This herb also drains fire from what is called "the upper burner," or the head and chest. This condition can cause high fever, irritability, thirst, and cough with thick, yellow sputum.

Scientific Findings and Clinical Experience

Scutellaria has been extensively researched. Its proven properties include, among other things, the ability to fight infections and cancer, and to promote circulatory health.

Scutellaria inhibits infections with *Staphylococcus aureus, Streptococcus pneumoniae, Pseudomonas aeruginosa, Corynebacterium diphtheriae* (diptheria), and *Neisseria meningitidis* (gonorrhea). In one study, penicillin-resistant staph infections remained sensitive to scutellaria.[1] Tinctures of this herb are effective against fungal infections of the skin and tongue.[2]

Scutellaria acts against a number of viruses, including HIV-1. It contains a compound called baicalin. Baicalin inhibits reverse transcriptase, a chemical the virus needs to replicate, and also inhibits formation of the protein bridges HIV uses to enter cells.[3] Scutellaria's usefulness in treating HIV is enhanced by the fact that the herb does not directly stimulate the immune system, since such stimulation increases the number of cells that can be infected by the virus. Instead, scutellaria acts against the virus itself. (Scutellaria *injections* can have a pronounced immune-suppressant effect, lowering white blood cell counts significantly.)

Another scutellaria compound shuts down the replication process in influenza viruses A and B, as long as it is administered between eighteen and fifty-four hours *before* infection.[4,5] This makes scutellaria effective for flu prevention, but not for treatment.

Scutellaria has also been enlisted in the war against cancer. Baicalin is effective against the human T cell leukemia virus and Epstein-Barr virus.[6] The latter is associated both with some forms of cancer and with chronic fatigue syndrome. Russian clinics have had success in using scutellaria to increase the effectiveness of the chemotherapy agents flurouracil and cyclophosphane in patients with lymphosarcoma.[7] For many years, Chinese medicine has relied on scutellaria for the treatment of liver, lung, and colorectal tumors. Chinese physicians consider this herb to be particularly effective against the cancer-causing effects of fungal toxins formed in food, such as aflatoxin.

Scutellaria can play an important role in circulatory health. In laboratory studies, this herb lowers blood-cholesterol levels in animals fed a high-fat diet, and stimulates the gallbladder to release bile.[8] Bile flushes cholesterol out of the liver and into the intestines, where it may be excreted. A scutellaria compound called baicalin inhibits the growth of scar tissue on the arterial linings.[9] This reduces the risk that high cholesterol levels will result in the formation of atherosclerotic plaques on artery walls. Scutellaria also dilates blood vessels and stimulates urination to lower blood pressure.[10]

Scutellaria can also ease a number of inflammatory conditions. Baicalin interferes with a complex set of hormonal reactions that both activate arthritic inflammation[11] and constrict the bronchial tubes to cause asthma. Equally important, laboratory studies show that scutellaria prevents DNA damage from dexamethasone, a prescription drug widely used to treat both conditions.[12] Other substances in scutellaria prevent histamine and similar compounds from provoking hay fever attacks, in a manner similar to that of the prescription drug cromolyn sodium.[13]

Scutellaria has other properties. A Chinese study looked at the use of a multiherb combination that contains scutellaria as an alternative to ritalin treatment in what the Chinese label "minimal brain dysfunction in children," known in North America as attention deficit hyperactivity disorder (ADHD). This treatment was slightly less effective than ritalin, but children in the herbal treatment group showed fewer incidents of bedwetting, and gains of between four and ten points on intelligence tests.[14] Methanol scutellaria extracts stimulate the growth of collagen in the gums. This action reverses gingivitis.[15] And scutellaria helps fight stress.

Finally, scutellaria's power as a free-radical scavenger has many applications. Baicalin protects liver tissue from the free radical-generating effect of iron overload.[16] Scutellaria blocks the action of aldose reductase, a substance that causes diabetic cataracts,[17] and prevents the formation of cataracts associated with cholesterol oxidation.[18] Scutellaria has a high zinc content,[19] which helps the tissues of the eye use vitamin A.

Considerations for Use

Make scutellaria tea by simmering $^1/_2$ to 1 teaspoon (1 to 2 grams) of the chopped dried herb in 1 cup of water for fifteen minutes. Strain before use. This herb is also available in capsule, fluid and powdered solid extract, and tincture form, and is used in Kampo formulas (see Chapter 4).

Do not use scutellaria if "cold" diarrhea is present, that is, diarrhea caused by foodborne infection or that which occurs after excessive consumption of cold drinks.

Shiitake

See Modern Japanese Herbal Preparations.

Siberian Ginseng

See Modern Japanese Herbal Preparations.

Skullcap

See **Scutellaria.**

Snake Gourd (Trichosanth) Fruit / Karo

Description and Parts Used

Snake gourd fruit is the whole fruit of a vine also known as trichosanth, grown throughout eastern Asia wherever the summers are warm and humid. The fruit should be large, intact, and orange-yellow, with a sugary taste. The root and the seed are also used (see below and page 30).

Uses in Kampo

Snake gourd fruit, a sweet and cold herb, expands the chest. It releases phlegm and dissipates nodules, lung abscesses, and breast abscesses.

Scientific Findings and Clinical Experience

Snake gourd fruit inhibits the growth of *E. coli, Pseudomonas,* shigella (*Shigella sonnei*), and many common fungal infections of the skin. There have been preliminary studies of this herb's usefulness in liver cancer treatment.[1]

Considerations for Use

Persons who are experiencing indigestion should not use snake gourd fruit.

Snake Gourd (Trichosanth) Root / Tenkafun

Description and Parts Used

Snake gourd root is the white, firm, powdery root of the trichosanth vine, grown throughout eastern Asia wherever the summers are warm and humid. The word for snake gourd root is literally translated as "heavenly flower powder." The fruit and the seed are also used (see above and page 30).

Uses in Kampo

Kampo uses snake gourd root to "quench uprushing fire." This bitter, cold, sour, and sweet herb clears and dissolves heat phlegm that rises in the body to produce abscesses, swellings, and tumors.

Snake gourd root is thought to generate fluids lost in "wasting and thirsting disorder," or diabetes. Snake gourd seed also relieves toxicity and expels pus, especially from breast abscesses. After cooling, teas made with this herb can be applied topically to such abscesses.

Scientific Findings and Clinical Experience

Chemical extracts of snake gourd root have a variety of pharmaceutical applications. The herb is an expectorant and a potent laxative. It dilates the coronary vessels and increases the heart's tolerance for oxygen deprivation.[1] Laboratory tests of snake gourd root extracts also show some effectiveness against penicillin-resistant gonorrhea.

Trichosanthin, a chemical extracted from snake gourd root, is effective against twelve different forms of lymphoma and leukemia. It works by shutting down the metabolic machinery of cancerous cells without affecting healthy ones.[2,3]

Trichosanthin is also effective against HIV. This substance inhibits the virus's ability to multiply without harming the body's cells.[4] Trichosanthin is the basis of Compound Q, a nutritional supplement. There are informal reports that Compound Q has *reversed* HIV infection in approximately 20 percent of the volunteers who have tried it.

Snake gourd root extracts have a stimulant effect on the uterus similar to that of oxytocin, a drug used to induce labor. In China, snake gourd root extracts are given intravenously to end abnormal pregnancies such as choriocarcinoma and hydatidform mole, two tumorous conditions, and ectopic pregnancy, in which the fetus becomes implanted in the fallopian tube instead of the uterus. Such pregnancies, which cannot be carried to term, can endanger the mother's life. Injections of trichosanthin are approximately 99 percent effective when used for this purpose.[5]

Finally, although snake gourd root is traditionally used in the treatment of diabetes, alcohol extracts of the herb have no effect on blood-glucose levels, and water-based teas actually *raise* serum glucose levels.[6]

Considerations for Use

Kampo uses snake gourd root in formulas (see Chapter 4).

Avoid snake gourd root, and formulas based on it, during pregnancy. An overdose may not only induce abortion but may also lead to kidney malfunction and tissue destruction.[7]

Snake Gourd (Trichosanth) Seed

See **Benincasa.**

Snakeroot, Black

See **Black Cohosh.**

Snow Fungus

See Modern Japanese Herbal Preparations.

Solomon's Seal / Gyokuchiku

Description and Parts Used

Solomon's seal, also known as jade bamboo, is a lily grown in northern China and Japan. It is in the same plant family as Siberian Solomon's seal (*Polygonatum sibiricum,* also known as *huang jing*).

Uses in Kampo

Solomon's seal is a sweet tonic used to generate fluids. It also relieves nervous unrest and thirst. The herb is used in cases of dry cough, insatiable hunger, and general weakness after a long, consumptive illness.

Kampo uses Solomon's seal to relieve conditions caused by insufficient fluids leading to pain and spasms in the sinews.

Scientific Findings and Clinical Experience

In China, Solomon's seal is used to treat heart failure in patients allergic to digoxin. It also decreases the Smölyogi effect, the drastic drop in blood-sugar levels that occurs from one to two hours after consuming a high-sugar meal or snack.[1]

Considerations for Use

Solomon's seal is used in formulas (see Chapter 4). Do not use if bloating is present.

Stephania / Kanboi

Description and Parts Used

Stephania is a twining tropical vine in the same family as calumba, an African herb used for anorexia and digestive complaints. Kampo formulas made in Japan use sinomenium, the root of a Japanese plant also known as moonseed. Kampo formulas made in China use stephania, or *han fang ji* (Chinese *fang ji*), in the same way as sinomenium. Chinese herbalists refer to sinomenium as Japanese *fang ji* or *qing teng.* Adding to the confusion, another Chinese herb, aristolochia, is also referred to as *fang ji,* or *guang fang ji.*

Uses in Kampo

Stephania stimulates urination and reduces edema, or swelling, especially in the legs and feet. It is also used to treat gurgling intestinal sounds, fullness in the abdomen, and ascites, or fluid accumulation in the abdomen. Stephania alleviates pain and fever, and hot, red, painful, swollen joints.

Scientific Findings and Clinical Experience

Stephania acts in a way similar to morphine but is much less potent, with an analgesic effect about $^{1}/_{25}$ that of morphine. Japanese folk medicine uses stephania to prevent swelling in traumatic joint injuries. Laboratory tests confirm this effect.[1]

Considerations for Use

Because of the considerable confusion surrounding this herb, take it only as an ingredient in Kampo formulas (see Chapter 4). It does not matter if the formula contains stephania or sinomenium; either formulation will be effective.

Do not use stephania if diarrhea is present.

Sweet Flag

See **Acorus.**

Szechuan Pepper

See **Zanthoxylum.**

Tang-Kuei (Chinese Angelica) / Toki

Description and Parts Used

Tang-kuei, also known as dong quai, is the dried and sliced root of Chinese angelica, a plant native to China and Japan. When grown under cultivation, Chinese angelica is a sturdy perennial reaching a height of up to six feet. The plant bears bright green leaves and clusters of white flowers.

Uses in Kampo

Tang-kuei is Kampo's most important herb for stimulating blood circulation. It invigorates the blood and dispels cold. This action activates blood that collects in the tissues after traumatic injury, and helps circulate toxins out of boils and carbuncles. The herb moistens the intestines and unlocks the bowels. This action relieves constipation caused by intestinal dryness. Tang-kuei also reduces swelling, expels pus, alleviates pain, and assists in the recovery from abrasions, blisters, and cuts. Finally, this herb tonifies the blood and regulates the menses. This action relieves patterns of blood deficiency causing symptoms such as skipped menstrual cycles, painful or difficult menstruation, blurred vision, palpitations, and ringing in the ears.

Scientific Findings and Clinical Experience

One of tang-kuei's best-known uses is that of a regulator for the female reproductive system. It contains compounds that stimulate the uterus, as well as compounds that relax the uterus. A Kampo formula based on this herb, Tang-Kuei and Peony Powder (see Chapter 4), is used to treat a number of disorders affected by estrogen, the main female hormone.

Tang-kuei also aids the male reproductive system by increasing male fertility. One of the chemicals in tang-kuei, ferulic acid, increases the motility and viability of sperm cells by protecting their walls from the action of cell-harming free radicals.[1] There is some evidence, however, that ferulic acid *increases* the risk of free-radical damage to sperm cells in men undergoing chemotherapy with bleomycin.[2]

Kampo's view of tang-kuei as an important blood herb has been verified by scientific study. Tang-kuei teas lower blood pressure and prolong the resting period between heartbeats. They also dilate the coronary blood vessels to increase coronary blood flow. Tang-kuei inhibits the release of the chemical in the blood that promotes the formation of clots and starts inflammatory reactions. This action helps keep microscopic blood vessels in the eye from leaking, stops swelling in allergic reactions, and keeps cancerous tumors from developing their own blood supplies. The herb is a rich source of vitamin B_{12} and other nutrients necessary for blood cell production in bone marrow, which makes it useful in the treatment of pernicious anemia. In animal studies, the addition of tang-kuei to the diet has reduced the formation of atherosclerotic plaques, or cholesterol deposits that develop on artery walls.[3] Tang-kuei is also used to treat the blood-vessel disorders thrombophlebitis, in which clots form in the veins, and constrictive aortitis, a narrowing of the aorta, the body's main artery, by inflammation.

Tang-kuei is a traditional treatment for skin conditions, including eczema, psoriasis, a loss of pigmentation called vitiligo, and Recklinghausen's neurofibramatosis, a condition in which thousands of benign tumors form in the skin.[4] It does not stimulate the growth of healthy skin cells; actually, in overdose, it may kill healthy cells.[5] Rather, tang-kuei compounds called coumarins stimulate circulation to the skin, while other compounds in the herb block the production of inflammation-generating substances called prostaglandins that would normally be transported to the skin by this increased circulation.[6] Tang-kuei also inhibits the formation of immune-system elements called antibodies at the very beginning of the inflammation process.[7]

Tang-kuei serves other purposes. It has been used in the treatment of arthritis, chronic kidney inflammation, and neuralgia, or pain that follows the course of a nerve.

Considerations for Use

Make tang-kuei tea by simmering 1 or 2 teaspoons of the herb in 1 cup of water for forty-five minutes. Strain before drinking, and take between meals. This herb is also available as dried root, fluid extract, freeze-dried root, powdered solid extract, or tincture.

The tang-kuei compounds that stimulate the uterus are water-soluble, and absorbed into the body from all forms except tinctures. The relaxing compounds are soluble in alcohol, and are absorbed into the body from tinctures. Thus, the form of tang-kuei used is an important consideration in treatment. Avoid taking tang-kuei *tea* and other water-based preparations during pregnancy. On the other hand, do not use tang-kuei *tincture* to treat insufficient menstrual flow, as it will further decrease flow. Also avoid tang-kuei for thirty days after the first symptoms of a herpes infection or recurrence, as this herb inhibits the body's defenses against the virus.[8]

Tuckahoe

See **Hoelen.**

Turmeric / Ukon (rhizome) / Kyoo (root)

Description and Parts Used

Turmeric is a perennial plant found in India and throughout southern and eastern Asia. It grows to a height of three feet and bears pairs of lance-shaped leaves on alternate sides of the stem, which sprouts from a knobbed rhizome. The root of the plant is used both as a spice and in Kampo.

Fresh turmeric "root," actually the rhizome, is bright orange inside. Kampo also uses the lateral root branches, which are brownish yellow inside.

Uses in Kampo

Turmeric root branches have been used in Kampo at least since the middle of the seventh century A.D. An acrid, bitter, and warming herb, it invigorates the blood. This action unblocks delayed menstruation, and relieves swelling and pain caused by traumatic injury. Turmeric root is thought to invigorate the flow of vital energy, or qi, especially through the shoulders. By stimulating the flow of energy, this herb quells wind disorders, in which painful symptoms seem to migrate from one site to another throughout the body.

Turmeric rhizome has been used in Kampo even longer, since at least the sixth century. Like the root, the rhizome stimulates the circulation of both blood and energy throughout the body. By breaking up static blood, turmeric rhizome relieves the pain of traumatic injury and hastens the healing of chronic sores. It promotes the flow of energy not only to the shoulders, but also to the abdomen, chest, flank, and womb. Under the principle of similars, or "like heals like," Kampo medicine uses the bright orange rhizome to treat the "bright orange condition" of jaundice. Finally, turmeric rhizome clears the heart, the seat of the emotions. By clearing the channels of the heart of energy debris or nonsubstantial phlegm, turmeric rhizome quells agitation, anxiety, mental derangement, and seizures.

Very few Kampo formulas include turmeric. Instead, it is used in combination with one or two other herbs for the relief of specific conditions. Kampo practitioners combine turmeric rhizome with amaranth and moutan for nosebleed, purplish skin blotches, and spitting of blood; with bupleurum for pain and swelling in the flanks, irregular menstrual periods, and dysmenorrhea, especially when accompanied by symptoms of constrained emotion; and with dan shen for chest pains with fever. Turmeric root is combined with cinnamon for difficult menstruation and postpartum abdominal pain, and with both astragalus and cinnamon for what Kampo calls "painful obstruction" of energy, resulting in shoulder pain.

Scientific Findings and Clinical Experience

The most prominent compound in both turmeric rhizome and turmeric root is curcumin. Curcumin's medical effectiveness has been recognized in dozens of pharmacological and medical journals. Laboratory tests also show curcumin to have an extraordinary range of benefits, including the ability to fight cancer and heart disease.

Curcumin is a powerful cancer preventative. It inhibits the action of p450, a liver enzyme that causes some environmental toxins to be processed in ways that make them carcinogenic.[1] Curcumin affects cancers associated with tobacco use by absorbing nitric oxide, a chemical produced in the lungs when they are exposed to tobacco, which prevents reactions associated with cancer and inflammation.[2] It also stops the cellular reaction in both the lungs and the mouth that activates cancer-causing agents in both cigarette smoke and smokeless tobacco.[3]

Curcumin helps prevent colorectal cancer. It works in the same manner as do nonsteroidal anti-inflammatory drugs (NSAIDs),[4] by suppressing the genes necessary for both the start and the spread of cancer.[5] Curcumin suppresses two genes necessary for colorectal cancer development.[6] And it prevents damage caused by aflatoxin, a poison produced during improper storage of grains and peanuts.[7]

Curcumin can also help cancer patients by curtailing the activity of platelet activating factor (PAF). PAF is necessary for the formation of new blood vessels, which tumors need to grow and spread.

Curcumin can be beneficial in the treatment of specific cancers. Curcumin causes the death of cancerous cells arising from several different types of tissue.[8] In the laboratory, the chemical kills cultures of human leukemia cells.[9] It reduces the development of chemically-induced mouth and tongue cancers by as much as 90 percent.[10] It affects skin cancer by counteracting cancer-causing effects of ultraviolet light when applied to the skin before exposure,[11] and by stopping chemically induced skin cancers.[12] In clinical trials, curcumin improves melanoma survival rates by preventing melanoma cells from creating protein[13] and by inhibiting their spread to the lungs.[14]

Curcumin can aid cancer recovery by stimulating the immune system. In cases of chronic leukemia, multiple myeloma, and ovarian cancer, it stimulates the production of B cells. In cases of Hodgkin's disease, Kaposi's sarcoma, and any form of cancer that has spread, it stimulates the production of T cells. Curcumin also works well with some cancer treatments, preventing lung damage caused by the chemotherapy drug cyclophosphamide[15] and by whole-body radiation.[16]

Curcumin is beneficial in the treatment of heart problems. It helps relax blood vessels to lower blood pressure.[17] Curcumin lowers the risk of heart attack during treatment with the steroid drug isoproterenol,[18] and reduces tissue damage during an attack.[19]

Curcumin also improves heart health, and circulatory health in general, by inhibiting atherosclerosis. PAF seals the leaks in blood vessels, in part by stimulating the production of fibrous tissue. This can lead to the development of a cholesterol-laden plaque at the site. Curcumin deactivates PAF. Moreover, it fights cell-damaging free radicals more actively than vitamin E, a noted free-radical scavenger.[20] In addition, curcumin helps prevent atherosclerosis in diabetics, and also stops the loss of protein through the kidneys in poorly controlled cases of diabetes.[21]

Turmeric can relieve inflammatory conditions. By stopping the release of PAF, it stops the reactions that induce an asthmatic attack.[22] Curcumin also relieves the discomfort caused by bursitis and carpal tunnel syndrome by deactivating immune-system cells that may cause inflammation, without harming the body's ability to defend itself.[23] Clinical studies have confirmed that the volatile oil in turmeric can ease acute pain caused by arthritis, eczema, gastritis, psoriasis, or tendinitis. Its effectiveness is equal to that of steroid preparations such as hydrocortisone and phenylbutazone,[24,25] but without their side effects.

Curcumin may also help patients with HIV infection. It can help prevent HIV from progressing to AIDS by acting as a protease inhibitor, or a substance that keeps the virus from entering the cell's DNA.[26] It counteracts integrase, an enzyme HIV needs to attach itself to human DNA.[27] It also reduces some of the tissue destruction seen in AIDS by deactivating tumor necrosis factor.[28]

Curcumin provides other health benefits. It increases the production of enzymes that digest sugar and fat,[29] and stops cholesterol from crystallizing into gallstones.[30] It increases the blood's oxygen-carrying capacity by protecting hemoglobin, the chemical that transports oxygen throughout the body.[31] It increases the production of IgG antibodies, the largest class of infection-fighting antibodies.[32] It helps reverse liver damage caused by excessive iron consumption. Finally, curcumin acts against gum inflammation by halting the action of a gene that creates gum-irritating chemicals.[33]

Considerations for Use

Many of the disorders in Part Two call for curcumin extract. To use turmeric itself in tea form, simmer $^3/_4$ ounce (20 grams) of turmeric in 2 cups of water until the volume of the mixture is reduced to $1^1/_2$ cups. Do not strain the mixture before using. Turmeric is also available in powder and tincture form.

To make a turmeric poultice, place 1 teaspoon (3 grams) of turmeric powder mixed with 1 teaspoon of water, and apply in a clean cloth placed over the affected area.

Persons with congestive heart disease for which doctors have not been able to identify a cause should avoid curcumin. There is evidence that this condition results from the overactivity of a gene called p53 that can, when damaged, weaken the heart.[34] Curcumin protects gene p53, and therefore may indirectly contribute to the destruction of healthy heart tissue.

Tea

See **Green Tea.**

Viola / Shikajicho

Description and Parts Used

Viola is a perennial flower found in Japan and northern China. Like its relative the garden pansy, viola bears purple, white, and yellow blossoms, and grows to a height of no more than one foot. Kampo uses the entire plant, dug either in spring when the flowers are blooming or in autumn when the fruits have ripened.

Uses in Kampo

Kampo medicine uses viola to clear heat and relieve fire toxicity. This reduces hot swellings, especially red, swollen eyes, and also relieves swollen throat and mumps. Washes made from viola are used topically to treat abscesses and sores, especially on the head and neck.

Scientific Findings and Clinical Experience

Viola's traditional use as a treatment for painful abscesses and sores is confirmed by scientific study. Viola contains soothing mucilages as well as salicylic acid, the precursor of aspirin. It protects the skin from drying out as it relieves pain. Science has also confirmed viola's ability to "move water" in persons suffering fluid retention or swollen joints. The herb seems to increase the water excretion without changing mineral balance, promoting the loss of chlorides but not that of sodium or potassium. This action conserves the minerals essential to normal muscle function, especially that of heart muscle.

Viola is reported to keep HIV from "erupting" from infected cells.[1,2] It also contains compounds that inhibit the reproduction of the bacteria that cause tuberculosis, a common complication of AIDS. The herb has the added advantage of being extremely nontoxic. This is especially beneficial for people with AIDS, who must often take a number of drugs that cause various toxic side effects.

Considerations for Use

To make viola tea, simmer 1 ounce (30 grams) of the herb in 1 quart (1 liter) of water for forty-five minutes. Strain before dividing the tea into 1-cup doses.

Treatment for HIV and AIDS requires the species of viola used in Kampo rather than that used in American and European herbalism, *Viola yedoensis* instead of *Viola tricolor.* If taking prepared tablets or extracts of viola as an AIDS preventative, make sure the herb used is *Viola yedoensis.* It is sold in bulk in Chinese herb shops as *Zi Hua Di Ding.*

Vitex / Mankeishi

Description and Parts Used

Vitex is an aromatic, deciduous tree native to the western Asia mainland and to China. It grows to a height of twenty-one feet, and bears palm-shaped leaves and small, lilaclike flowers. The ripe yellow-red berries are harvested in the fall for use in Kampo.

Vitex was known to the Greeks in the time of Homer, more than 1,000 years before it was used in China. Homer's sixth century B.C. epic, the *Iliad,* mentions vitex as a symbol of chastity capable of protecting people against evil. As the herb's nickname "chaste tree" implies, vitex was thought to reduce the libido. Vitex berries were chewed by monks to stop unwanted sexual desire.

Uses in Kampo

In China, herbalists began using vitex in the sixth century A.D. to relieve headache, eye pain, and painful, red, or swollen eyes. The herb was thought to harmonize the energies circulating on the liver channel, which could be upset by emotional disturbance or by pent-up emotions.

Scientific Findings and Clinical Experience

Vitex is especially beneficial for women. Breast pain, menopausal and menstrual symptoms, and premenstrual syndrome are often caused by hormonal imbalances during the luteal phase of the menstrual cycle, the phase that occurs after the release of an egg from the ovary. Sometimes the corpus luteum, the yellowish ovarian scar that forms after the egg is released, produces inadequate amounts of estrogen and progesterone or excessive amounts of testosterone. Vitex stimulates the production of estrogen and progesterone, while it counteracts the production of testosterone. A German study found that the European form of vitex, agnus castus, can reestablish the luteal phase of the period in women whose periods are abnormally short.[1]

Vitex's hormonal effects also allow it to be used in cases of ovarian cysts and endometriosis, a condition in which the endometrial tissue normally found within the uterus escapes into the abdominal cavity, causing pain and menstrual difficulties. Moreover, the suppression of testosterone allows vitex to be used by men with prostate problems, including prostate cancer, as these conditions are often aggravated by testosterone.

Vitex can also help women who cannot nurse adequately. After a woman gives birth, levels of both estrogen and progesterone fall, and levels of a third hormone, prolactin—which stimulates the production of milk—often fluctuate greatly. Vitex keeps prolactin at relatively constant levels, allowing a predictable flow of breast milk.[2]

Considerations for Use

Vitex also is available in tincture and extract (both solid and fluid) form. In using this herb, it is important to remember that for long-term relief it is necessary to continue taking the herb for three to six months after symptoms disappear.[3] Vitex must be used with caution, since it has been known to stimulate the release of multiple eggs from the ovary, potentially resulting in multiple births.[4] Men seeking to become fathers should not take vitex. Animal studies indicate that the seeds can completely halt sperm production, reduce testosterone production, and cause the testicles to atrophy.[5]

Water Plantain

See **Alisma.**

Watermelon

See **Japanese Watermelon.**

Wheat / Fushobaku

Description and Parts Used

Wheat, a major food grain around the world, is a grasslike plant that bears seeds atop a stalk two to four feet tall. The wheat used in Kampo is "green wheat," or wheat berries that are not quite ripe. Wheat is used raw, or is dry-fried until aromatic.

Uses in Kampo

Wheat is useful in the treatment of heating due to deficiency, that is, the body's inability to produce fluids for perspiration. Wheat is said to nourish the qi and yin of the heart, that is, wheat energizes the containing, or yin, energies of the heart to hold emotions properly. As part of the Kampo formula Licorice, Wheat, and Jujube Decoction, wheat is also used to prevent bedwetting in children (see Chapter 4). Modern doctors in China use this formula as a safe treatment for hot flashes during menopause, premenstrual, and postpartum palpitations and sweating. The combination also relieves chronic low-grade fevers and prevents emotional outbursts.

Scientific Findings and Clinical Experience

Wheat has actions surprisingly similar to those of opium. Opiumlike alkaloids in wheat bind to the same receptor sites in the brain as opium, morphine, and heroin. This accounts for the calming effect of some so-called "comfort foods," as well as psychological reactions in some persons especially sensitive to wheat gluten, a protein found in wheat.[1] Some schizophrenics can be treated without medication when they follow a wheat-free diet.

Considerations for Use

Wheat is used in several Kampo formulas.

White Atractylodis

See **Atractylodis, White.**

White Mustard Seed / Hakugaishi

Description and Parts Used

White mustard, a biennial herb, sends up a central stalk from a taproot. Rounded, almost oval leaves grow on alternating sides of stems that branch out from the stalk. The plant produces yellow flowers on small stems that extend from the top of the stalk.

White mustard seed—which has medicinal qualities separate from those of black mustard seed—is gathered from July to September, when the fruit has ripened. Kampo uses whole seed to make teas and ground seed mixed with vinegar to make plasters.

Uses in Kampo

Kampo medicine uses white mustard seed to dry fluids, transform phlegm, calm wheezing, and direct rebellious qi—qi moving in the wrong direction—downward. White mustard seed is used for rheumatic conditions, urinary infections, and flu, as well as inflammations of the nerves and the membranes surrounding the lungs.

Scientific Findings and Clinical Experience

Some TCM practitioners inject mustard seed preparations into the acupuncture points used in the treatment of chronic bronchitis and colds. This approach is reported to be extremely effective in treating wheezing and difficulty in coughing up phlegm. However, a more traditional approach uses a mustard seed plaster. Both white and black mustard seeds make effective plasters, but the essential oils in white mustard seed do not evaporate in a hot plaster.

Both mustard seed plasters and mustard seed teas kill many kinds of fungi that infect the skin.

Considerations for Use

To make a plaster, mix two handfuls of ground mustard seed with enough lukewarm water or vinegar to make a thick slurry, and heat. It is important to not let the mixture reach a temperature of more than 140°F (60°C), or the enzyme that makes the plaster work will be deactivated. When the mixture is warm, spread it on a piece of clean cloth and place the plaster, cloth side down, on the chest. Leave the plaster on until there is a strong burning sensation, usually about five minutes. The plaster *must* be removed in fifteen to, at the very most, thirty minutes.

Mustard seed plasters should not be applied to any part of the body where there is insufficient blood circulation. They should not be used by people who have circulatory problems, or placed on varicose veins.

Wild Angelica

See **Angelica Dahurica.**

Wild Yam

See **Dioscorea.**

Wolfbane

See **Aconite.**

Wolfberry

See **Lycium.**

Zanthoxylum / SHOKUSHO

Description and Parts Used

Zanthoxylum, or Szechuan pepper, is not in the same family as the hot peppers used in Southwestern and Mexican cuisine. Rather, it is the fruit of the Chinese prickly ash, a shrub grown throughout China, especially in Szechuan province. The "Chinese" prickly ash is also found in the southeastern United States. The shiny red fruits are gathered in the late summer and fall for culinary and medicinal use.

Uses in Kampo

Zanthoxylum has been used in many cultures for centuries to kill intestinal parasites and to protect against parasitic infection, and is used for this purpose in Kampo. Zanthoxylum is also used to warm the middle in order to eliminate digestive symptoms of cold, such as diarrhea and vomiting. In addition, this herb is used as an aphrodisiac.

Brown sugar and zanthoxylum taken together is a Japanese home remedy for ending the flow of breast milk after a child is weaned. The effect takes one to two days.

In TCM, Szechuan pepper seeds (called *jaio mu* or "pepper eyes") have their own applications. Szechuan pepper seeds move water and calm wheezing. They are used for edema with fullness and swelling or wheezing with cough and congestion.

Scientific Findings and Clinical Experience

The chemical constituents of zanthoxylum and related peppers that give them their heat also kill foodborne bacteria and parasites. Pepper extracts kill foodborne *Clostridium, Listeria,* and *Streptococcus* on contact.[1] Zanthoxylum is especially effective against roundworms. Zanthoxylum in sesame oil arrests pain from roundworms within thirty minutes, although it is not effective in long-standing cases.[2] Powdered pepper enemas eliminate pinworms in children, and powdered zanthoxylum in capsules is useful against schistosomiasis, a waterborne infection common in tropical areas, because it increases appetite and lessens tissue destruction. Zanthoxylum extracts can be used externally to treat scabies, a parasitic infestation of the skin.

Zanthoxylum is effective in Major Construct the Middle Decoction (see Chapter 4) against abdominal pain from a number of sources, including ulcers, gallbladder disease, and intestinal spasm. This effect, however, is temporary.

Some zanthoxylum species contain compounds that cause sickle cells to change back to normal cells. Although tests of this herb on sickle cells are equivocal, sickle cell anemia patients who use it report that it reduces pain.[3]

Some persons report an increase in sexual desire after eating zanthoxylum in food.

Considerations for Use

Zanthoxylum plasters can be applied over areas of pain. Grind a handful of pepper pods, taking care not to get the powder under fingernails or in the eyes, and mix with enough warm (not hot) water to make paste. Put the paste in gauze and place over the affected area. Leave the plaster on the skin until there is a feeling of heat, about five to ten minutes.

Zizyphus / Sansonin

Description and Parts Used

Zizyphus, also known as sour jujube, is a large shrub native to the Chinese provinces of Hebei, Henan, Liaoning, and Shaanxi. It is not the same herb as the jujube fruit (see page 63). The zizyphus fruit is large, full, and purplish red.

Uses in Kampo

Zizyphus is used primarily to treat abnormal sweating. It also nourishes the heart, which quiets the spirit and alleviates insomnia, irritability, and palpitations caused by anxiety.

Scientific Findings and Clinical Experience

Zizyphus lowers blood pressure and can have a hypnotic effect. As a sedative, zizyphus is effective and extremely non-toxic.[1]

Considerations for Use

Zizyphus is used in the formula Restore the Spleen Decoction (see Chapter 4). Do not use zizyphus if fever or severe diarrhea is present.

OTHER TRADITIONAL HEALING SUBSTANCES

The following is a list of substances, other than herbs, that have been traditionally used in Kampo medicines. Scientific research has not been done on all of these substances. Each substance is listed under its English name, followed by its Japanese name.

Abalone Shell / Sekketsumei

Description

Abalone shell is the large, multicolored, shiny shell of the Pacific abalone, used in Japan for both food and medicine. Good quality abalone shell is thick.

Uses in Kampo and Scientific Findings

In traditional Japanese medicine, abalone shell was added to formulas to move fire downward in the body. It relieved symptoms such as dizziness, headache, and red eyes caused by the rising of pent-up emotions.

Today, abalone shell is included in Kampo formulas used to treat various eye problems, including bloodshot eyes, blurred vision, light sensitivity, and spots, called floaters, before the eyes.

Considerations for Use

Abalone shell is used in Gastrodia and Uncaria Decoction (see Chapter 4). When this formula is used in tea form, the abalone shell should be boiled for between thirty and forty-five minutes before the other ingredients are added.

Cordyceps / Tochukaso

Description

Cordyceps is the "winter bug summer herb," an antlered fungus that grows in insect larvae, usually before the insect's cocoon is formed. It is a short, stick-like fungus with a fat, full, round, yellow-white cross-section. It is gathered in the early summer. Although this fungus is found throughout Japan and in China and the Atlantic seaboard of the United States, it is very difficult to collect from the wild and is usually grown in laboratory tissue cultures.

Medicinal mushroom expert Christopher Hobbs writes that in ancient China, cordyceps was used exclusively in the Emperor's palace because it was very scarce. It was prepared by stuffing it into the stomach of a duck, and then slowly roasting the duck over a low flame. Then the cordyceps was removed, and the duck was eaten for eight to ten days.[1]

Uses in Kampo and Scientific Findings

Kampo's primary use of cordyceps is as an energy tonic for the kidneys. Cordyceps increases the kidneys' yang, or externally directed energy, to treat impotence and lower back pain. It also helps the kidneys steam water to the lungs, transforming phlegm and stopping bleeding during chronic cough caused by asthma or tuberculosis.

Modern medical research has discovered many applications for this ancient fungus. Cordyceps both stimulates the immune system in cases of immune deficiency and curbs the immune system in cases of immune excess. Laboratory studies have found that complex sugars in cordyceps stimulate the germ-engulfing activity of macrophages, particularly in the peritoneum, or the membrane lining the abdominal cavity.[2] Other laboratory studies have found that in lupus, a condition of immune excess, cordyceps extends life expectancy of skin cells and protects cell DNA from antibodies.[3] Cordyceps extracts stimulate natural killer (NK) cells to fight lymphoma, and reactivate B cells, the immune system's first line of defense, after treatment with the immune-suppressant chemotherapy drug cyclophosphamide.[4]

Cordyceps also has a pronounced effect on the cardiovascular system. Cordyceps tinctures increase the heart's strength while slowing the pulse,[5,6] and raise HDL ("good") cholesterol levels while lowering total cholesterol and LDL ("bad") cholesterol levels.[7]

Several clinical studies of cordyceps have found that it helps the circulatory system move fluids out of regions of the body in which they have accumulated in cases of chronic hepatitis[8] and kidney failure.[9] It also helps a majority of cases of tinnitus caused by fluid accumulation in the inner ear, although it is not helpful in cases when tinnitus is accompanied by a long history of auditory nerve disorder.[10]

Finally, cordyceps is a clinically proven aphrodisiac. In a clinical study of 155 cases of sexual dysfunction, 64 percent of patients reported increased sexual interest and activity after forty days' treatment (compared to 31 percent of patients given a placebo). Doctors found that the patients who improved when treated with cordyceps had increased levels of estrogen and testosterone in their bloodstreams.[11] Follow-up studies with laboratory animals found that cordyceps also stimulates sperm production.[12]

Considerations for Use

Cordyceps can be used in its natural form, but it is more common to take cordyceps in capsule or prepared tea form. Avoid if a hormone-sensitive disorder is present.

Dragon Bone / Ryukotsu

Description

Dragon bone is fossilized mastodon bone. As such, it is a mineral and not an animal-based substance.

Uses in Kampo and Scientific Findings

Dragon bone is one of the most important mineral compounds used in Kampo. It is a cold medication that regulates excess energy, particularly when expressed as anger or manic behavior.

In the classic Japanese Kampo texts, dragon bone is prescribed chiefly for palpitations in the abdomen. Japanese herbalists prescribe dragon bone to control nocturnal emission and correct a cold sensation in the tip of the penis.

Dragon bone is also used to calm liver wind. This is pain or irritation moving along the liver's energy channel, which passes over the breasts and eyes. This action prevents irritability, restlessness, dizziness, vertigo, blurred vision, and bad temper, particularly if these symptoms are associated with breast pain or menstrual irregularity. Dragon bone also prevents the leakage of fluids, including night sweats, cold sweats associated with emotional stress, vaginal discharge, and uterine bleeding or nocturnal emission. Finally, this substance is used to treat chronic sores. For this purpose, dragon bone is powdered and applied to the skin.

Considerations for Use

Dragon bone is used in formulas (see Chapter 4). When formulas are used in tea form, the dragon bone should be boiled for between thirty and forty-five minutes before the other ingredients are added. Tradition holds that fish should not be eaten while taking medicines made with dragon bone.

Frankincense / Nyuko

Description

Frankincense, or mastic, is the gum collected from the frankincense, or olibanum, tree. Along with myrrh (see page 99), frankincense was traded for centuries in the Middle East, as seen by biblical references to this substance. Frankincense is aromatic, granular, and translucent. In North America, this substance is known as boswellia.

Uses in Kampo and Scientific Findings

Kampo uses frankincense to invigorate the blood and move essential energy, or qi. Frankincense moves qi away from sites of traumatic injury, as well as from carbuncles, sores, and swellings, to relieve pain. It relaxes sinews to quell spasms. Frankincense also generates tissue growth to promote healing of carbuncles, skin sores, sore throat, and traumatic injury.

Ayurvedic medicine, the traditional herbal medicine of India, has used frankincense to treat osteoarthritis for centuries. However, newer extracts of boswellic acids, this substance's main active ingredients, get better results. Laboratory studies have shown that boswellic acids deactivate the hormonal triggers for inflammation and pain in osteoarthritis. These acids stimulate the growth of cartilage and increase blood supply to inflamed joints.[1] Clinical studies using frankincense have yielded good results in both osteoarthritis and rheumatoid arthritis.[2]

Considerations for Use

Frankincense is used in the formula Trauma Pill (see Chapter 4). Since this substance stimulates blood circulation, do not use it during pregnancy.

Gelatin / Akyo

Description

In Oriental medicine, gelatin is processed from donkey hide. This yields a product similar to the food gelatin used in North America.

Uses in Kampo and Scientific Findings

Gelatin is energy-neutral, and can thus be combined with either hot or cold herbs. It nourishes the blood to relieve dizziness and palpitations, moisturizes the lung and colon, and helps the inner organs contain fluids. Gelatin is also used to stop leakages of blood. It is used in formulas for anemia, bleeding beneath the skin or broken blood vessels in the skin, blood in the stool, irregular menstruation, and uterine or urinary bleeding (see Chapter 4).

From a scientific viewpoint, gelatin has several properties. Its primary action is to stimulate hematopoiesis, the production of red blood cells and hemoglobin in the bone marrow. Gelatin not only stimulates the bone marrow, it also increases the rate at which the bones use calcium. This can prevent osteoporosis.[1] Gelatin also helps muscle tissue to regenerate after injury.[2]

Gelatin contains a compound, dermatan sulfate, that breaks up blood clots. This compound has been isolated for pharmaceutical use.[3]

Considerations for Use

Regular food gelatin *cannot* be substituted for donkey-hide gelatin in formulas. For those that wish to avoid the use of animal products, there are many alternatives to formulas that use donkey-hide gelatin. See a Kampo or TCM practitioner for advice.

Do not use donkey-hide gelatin in the early stages of infection, as it is thought to restrain fluids that otherwise would be sweated out during fevers.

Gypsum / Sekko

Description

Gypsum is the mineral calcium sulfate. Its name in Japanese literally means "stone paste."

Uses in Kampo and Scientific Findings

Gypsum is a cold and sedating mineral. Kampo uses it to quell high fevers with irritability, intense thirst, and profuse sweating without chills. Although Kampo has used gypsum successfully for centuries to lower fevers, laboratory experiments have not yet explained its action. In addition, gypsum is used to treat delirium and distress. It is applied topically to eczema, burns, and ulcerated sores, and may also be taken internally for these conditions.

Kampo frequently uses gypsum in formulas containing ephedra (see page 47) to counter the excessive sweating this herb may produce, and to increase ephedra's diuretic effects. Formulas that contain gypsum are used to treat high fever, sunstroke, nervous unrest, thirst, lung infections, and sore throat (see Chapter 4).

Considerations for Use

When formulas containing gypsum are used in tea form, the gypsum should be boiled for between thirty and forty-five minutes before the other ingredients are added. Do not use formulas containing gypsum if nausea or vomiting is present.

Kaolin (Halloysite) / Shakusekishi

Description

Kaolin is a medicinal red clay found in China and in many other locations throughout the world. The literal translation of the Chinese words for kaolin is "crimson stone resin," which refers to both the clay's color and its gelatinous texture.

Uses in Kampo and Scientific Findings

Warming yet astringent kaolin binds the intestines and stops diarrhea, and contains the blood in its channels. A kaolin-based formula, Peach Blossom Decoction, is used to treat bleeding hemorrhoids (see Chapter 4). Kaolin is used in teas to stop intestinal or uterine bleeding, and bleeding from excessive menstruation or rectal prolapse, a condition in which the rectum falls out of its normal position. Kaolin is used topically to stop bleeding from traumatic wounds and to heal chronic ulcers.[1] It is also applied as a warm paste to relieve breast pain caused by fibrocystic breast disease.

Considerations for Use

Use kaolin with caution during pregnancy. Do not use this substance at all in cases of diarrhea due to infection or pelvic inflammatory disease.[2]

Magnetite / Jiseki

Description

Magnetite is a powder made of iron oxide and clay. It is usually prepared by being dipped in vinegar and then fired under intense heat. The resulting product is shiny and either dark gray or black, and it strongly attracts iron.

Uses in Kampo and Scientific Findings

Magnetite, a bitter and cold mineral, is thought to stop bleeding and settle "reflux of qi," a condition in which the energies of the digestive tract move upward instead of downward, causing acid reflux, belching, heartburn, hiccups, and vomiting. Kampo adds magnetite powder to formulas, such as Pill for Deafness That Is Kind to the Left Kidney, used to treat blurred vision, hearing loss, insomnia, irritability, tinnitus that sounds likes swarming insects, and vertigo (see Chapter 4). Magnetite is used in place of other minerals, such as cinnabar, that have similar properties but are toxic.

Considerations for Use

Persons with weak digestion should avoid magnetite. Both women past menopause and men should not use this substance for more than one month, since iron can accumulate in—and interfere with the function of—the liver, pancreas, heart, and bone marrow.

Malt Sugar / Koi

Description

Malt sugar—which is quite different from table sugar—is made by powdering sprouted barley, and then adding germ from unsprouted seeds (see page 30). Wheat, rice, or bamboo sprouts may also be used.

Uses in Kampo and Scientific Findings

According to the classic Kampo texts, malt sugar strengthens and tones the middle of the body, stops coughing, promotes phlegm secretion, and nourishes and moistens the heart, lungs, liver, stomach, and intestines. Malt sugar settles stomach qi, or energy, and prevents bloating, belching, hiccups, indigestion, and stomachache. It is used in formulas that address these symptoms (see Chapter 4).

Young barley leaves contain an antioxidant that is a more powerful free-radical scavenger than vitamin E, which is one of the most powerful scavengers known.[1] This allows malt sugar to slow down the process of atherosclerosis, in which cholesterol is deposited on artery walls.

Considerations for Use

Because malt sugar generates fluids in the digestive tract and lungs, avoid it in cases of vomiting or congestion. Also, avoid this substance during pregnancy, as malt sugar made from barley contains compounds known to cause abortion.

Mirabilite (Epsom Salts) / Bosho

Description

Mirabilite is the mineral magnesium sulfate, also known as Epsom salts, Glauber's salt, and mirabilitum. Good quality mirabilite is crystalline and clear.

Uses in Kampo and Scientific Findings

Mirabilite is cold. This allows it to clear heat and reduce swelling of red, swollen, painful eyes; swollen, ulcerated mouth or throat; and red, swollen skin lesions, including breast lesions.

Japanese master herbalist Todo Yoshimasu prescribed mirabilite as a laxative and purgative to relieve hardness of the area above the stomach, severe pain upon pressure in the lower left abdomen, dry stools, stagnant food in the digestive tract, and illnesses caused by stagnant pathogens. Mirabilite is not a stimulant laxative. Rather, it acts as a salt, drawing water into the colon and thus easing defecation.

Mirabilite may also be involved in a reflex action in which its bitter taste stimulates the flow of saliva, gastric juices, and bile in a manner similar to that of gentian (see page 55). The exact nature of mirabilite's effect on the nervous system is as yet unspecified.[1]

Considerations for Use

Mirabilite is used in formulas (see Chapter 4). Women who are pregnant, have given birth within the past six weeks, or are menstruating should not use mirabilite. Individuals with high fever or severe inflammation should also avoid this substance.

Musk / Jako

Description

Musk, a glandular secretion obtained from deer, is well-known throughout the world as a perfume component. The musk used medicinally in Kampo is harvested from wild deer in Tibet or from domesticated deer raised in the Chinese provinces of Anhui, Shaanzi, and Sichuan.

Uses in Kampo and Scientific Findings

Musk is a medicinal compound of extraordinary usefulness. The primary use of musk is as an intensely aromatic substance that opens the orifices, allowing the free flow of energy throughout the body. This action affects a wide range of diseases that impair the consciousness or the conscious control of the body, such as seizures and tetanus.

Musk is also used in Kampo to invigorate the blood. This action alleviates pain, breaks up clumps, and reduces swelling. It is particularly applicable to carbuncles and sores or to fixed immovable masses, such as cysts. Musk also invigorates the flow of qi throughout the body when energy flow is interrupted by painful obstruction or traumatic injury.

Considerations for Use

Musk is used in Kampo formulas (see Chapter 4), and is usually identified in medicines as "secretio moschus." Since the musk deer is an endangered species, musk collected in the wild is extremely expensive, and musk dosages are usually measured in hundredths of a gram. Almost all patent (over-the-counter) medicines will substitute a synthetic musk or musk gathered from domesticated deer.

Myrrh / Motsuyaku

Description

Myrrh is a resin harvested from the myrrh tree, grown in East Africa and the Arabian peninsula. Myrrh is aromatic and has a reddish brown color. In some Chinese preparations, the myrrh is heated in vinegar before being added to the formula.

Uses in Kampo and Scientific Findings

Like frankincense (see page 97), myrrh is a bitter, energy-neutral herb used to vitalize the blood. By activating blood circulation, myrrh relieves pain from hard abdominal masses, carbuncles, difficult menstruation, sores, swellings, and trauma, and alleviates chest pain. Myrrh also helps regenerate tissues damaged by traumatic injury. It is used topically to promote the healing of chronic sores.

European herbalism uses tincture of myrrh as an antiseptic gargle and rinse. Unlike other mouthwashes that coagulate the cells lining the mouth and throat to form a protective barrier against bacteria, myrrh only acts to prevent soreness and inflammation, and leaves the linings of the mouth and throat intact.[1]

Considerations for Use

Myrrh is available in tincture form, and is used in the formula Trauma Pill (see Chapter 4).

Oyster Shell / Borei

Description

Oyster shell is taken from oysters of various species harvested off the coasts of Japan and China. The shell should be large, white on the outside, and shiny on the inside.

Crushed oyster shell is used raw as a sedative or cooked to prevent leakage of fluids.

Uses in Kampo and Scientific Findings

Oyster shell is a cooling sedative that calms uprushing qi, or energy. It clears fevers, neutralizes excess stomach acid, and reduces perspiration. It can be combined with dragon bone to treat insomnia, epilepsy, and manic behavior. Japanese herbalists prescribe oyster shell formulas to treat palpitations as well as tumors in the chest and abdomen.

Up to 95 percent of the chemical content of oyster shell is calcium carbonate, the same chemical compound found in limestone. Modern Japanese medicine uses oyster shell to promote bone growth after breaks and fractures, and to compensate for calcium deficiency in pregnant women.[1]

Even the oyster's most well-known product has medicinal value. Ground pearls, known as margarita, are cooked with bean curd water for two hours before being ground into a powder. This powder is then mixed with honey to calm persons who are easily frightened, and made into an eyewash to treat blurred vision.

Considerations for Use

Oyster shell is always used in formulas (see Chapter 4). When formulas containing this substance are used in tea form, the oyster shell should be boiled for between thirty and forty-five minutes before the other ingredients are added. Oysters harvested from polluted waters can be contaminated with lead or other heavy metals. Keep these toxins from leaching out into the tea by making sure that acids, such as vinegar or orange juice, do not get into the formula.

Talc / Kasseki

Description

Talc is magnesium silicate. The literal translation of the Chinese word for talc is "slippery rock."

Talc, applied externally, is used as a household remedy for diaper rash and prickly heat. In Kampo, talc is used internally in combination with various herbs.

Uses in Kampo and Scientific Findings

Talc is a bland, cold, and sweet mineral that promotes the downward circulation of fluids in the body, and clears heat from the bladder and stomach. It is especially beneficial for the urinary tract in that it soothes the tract, promotes urination, stops bleeding from inflammation, and aids the movement of kidney gravel and stones. Talc is used in formulas, such as Ledebouriella Powder That Sagely Unblocks (see Chapter 4), to treat blood in the urine, insufficient or painful urination, thirst, and urinary gravel or stones. Talc also protects the lining of the stomach, and prevents diarrhea and vomiting. In addition, it inhibits the absorption of poisons from the gastrointestinal tract.[1]

Considerations for Use

Talc should not be used by persons who are urinating excessively. TCM also suggests that talc products should not be used *internally* by men seeking to become fathers. Talc encourages spermatorrhea, or the abnormal flow of semen, which is thought to reduce the life essence (*jing*) transmissible to the child.

MODERN JAPANESE HERBAL PREPARATIONS

The following is a list of preparations that have been created in recent years from medicinal substances, mostly mushrooms, long known to Japanese herbalists and physicians. Many of these medicinal substances represent twentieth-century refinements of traditional healing compounds. Since they target specific symptoms and specific diseases, they are not part of Kampo's person-centered medicine. Used properly, however, they are powerful healing agents.

Ginkgo

Description

Ginkgo extract is taken from ginkgo leaf, the fan-shaped leaf of the ginkgo tree. This ancient plant is grown around the world for its hardiness and beauty. Ginkgo nut (see page 57), the seed of the ginkgo, is also used in Kampo.

Scientific Research and Clinical Experience

Scientific studies have confirmed ginkgo's traditional use in the treatment of asthma and bronchial congestion. Ginkgo acts against these conditions by inhibiting a chemical called platelet activating factor (PAF).[1] This action keeps the smooth muscles that line the lungs' air passages from contracting. It also stops inflammation-causing hormones from passing through blood-vessel walls into the tissues.

PAF is also known to be a factor in heart attack, stroke, and poor circulation in the legs (a painful condition called intermittent claudication), all of which respond to ginkgo treatment.[2] The underlying factor in these conditions is atherosclerosis. When a blood vessel is damaged, PAF causes a leak-sealing clot to develop in the vessel wall and stimulates the production of fibrous tissues that cover the injury site. This starts a process by which cholesterol gathers into a vessel-narrowing plaque. By deactivating PAF, ginkgo reduces the rate at which fibrous tissues are produced. The herb also helps keep immune-system cells called macrophages from gathering at the site[3] and pumping cholesterol into the arterial wall.[4] In Germany, where ginkgo is prescribed for intermittent claudication, treatment usually brings relief in six weeks.

Strokes can happen when a blood clot becomes stuck in a narrowed blood vessel in the brain. By inhibiting plaque development, ginkgo can protect against stroke. The herb is also helpful after a stroke. Much of the damage done by a stroke is caused by the formation of cell-damaging free radicals when circulation and oxygen are restored. Over time, ginkgo increases the production of free-radical fighters.[5–7]

This ability also allows ginkgo to stop nerve damage after compression spinal injuries.[8]

Impotence is another disorder often caused by circulatory malfunction. In one study, the use of 240 milligrams of ginkgo extract per day resulted in recovery of potency within six months.[9] Ginkgo causes the blood vessels to relax, resulting in a greater blood supply to the penis and stronger erections.[10]

Ginkgo's most exciting application may be in the treatment of Alzheimer's disease. This ailment is at least partly caused by an inadequate supply of glucose, or blood sugar, to the brain, which may alter functions of brain cells and their supporting structures. Ginkgo can both speed up the process by which the brain uses glucose and increase blood flow to the brain. The herb also improves the brain's use of a chemical called acetylcholine (see "Ginkgo—The Memory Herb and Alzheimer's Disease" on page 149).

German researchers studied the use of ginkgo to treat elderly persons with either Alzheimer's disease or mental debility caused by atherosclerosis. Four weeks of ginkgo therapy reduced dementia, increased coping skills in daily life, and relieved depression.[11] Actually, ginkgo can be used to treat depression in general by increasing the flow of oxygen to the brain. This is particularly true in elderly patients when the herb is combined with prescription drugs.[12,13] Other experiments show that ginkgo combined with ginger (see page 56) reduces anxiety.[14]

Another brain disorder that can be treated with ginkgo is attention deficit disorder (ADD) in adults. ADD is marked by forgetfulness and an inability to concentrate. Clinical studies suggest that in ADD, portions of the brain essential to planning and concentrating are not as active as other parts of the brain.[15] Ginkgo allows more oxygen to reach underactive parts of the brain. Studies have found evidence that ginkgo does enhance brain function in healthy adults.[16] Many students report that studying is easier after taking a single 600-milligram dose.

Gingko has also shown itself to play a valuable role in cancer treatment. It improves oxygen delivery throughout the body, and high oxygen levels prevent a tumor from developing its own blood supply. Ginkgo deactivates PAF, which also keeps tumors from developing a blood supply.[17] Additionally, ginkgo contains quercetin, which accelerates cell death of leukemia and Burkitt's lymphoma cells.[18,19] Quercetin slows the growth of colon, lung, and liver cancers,[20,21] and that of estrogen-activated cancers, including bladder cancer,[22] breast cancer,[23] and ovarian cancer (when simultaneously treated with cisplatin).[24]

Various eye and ear problems can be treated with ginkgo. Diabetic retinopathy affects the retina, the "screen" in the back of the eye. In this disorder, capillaries that nourish the retina leak fluid or blood, causing cell damage. Ginkgo prevents damage caused by the high blood-sugar levels seen in diabetes.[25,26] In addition, type 2 diabetes causes excessive production of a substance that encourages the growth of fragile capillaries. Quercetin inhibits production of this substance.[27]

Another serious eye disorder is macular degeneration, which is associated with excessive capillary growth in the macula, the part of the retina responsible for fine vision. As in diabetic retinopathy, these capillaries leak, damaging the tissues. Gingko can stop this process by deactivating PAF, which is essential for the growth of new capillaries. The herb increases circulation within the eye, which supplies more oxygen to the retina. Ginkgo also increases circulation to the lens and acts as a free-radical scavenger, which reduces cataract formation.[28] In addition, the herb prevents destruction of the ocular nerve in glaucoma.

Ginkgo has been used in clinical trials to treat sudden hearing loss. In one study, up to 40 percent of patients regained their hearing after ten days of ginkgo treatment.[29] This herb is also effective against tinnitus, or a constant ringing in the ears, if treatment begins within six to eight weeks of onset.[30,31]

Gingko has other uses. There are studies that support its use in treating multiple sclerosis.[32–34] These studies indicate that ginkgo is more helpful when used long-term to prevent relapses than in treatment of acute relapse symptoms. Ginkgo can also moderate the body's stress response by interrupting production of hormones that are secreted under stressful conditions.[35] Ginkgo can protect the body *after* radiation exposure occurs, either through accident[36] or through radiation therapy. Finally, there is evidence that ginkgo can halt a condition known as sinus tachycardia, in which the pulse races.[37]

Considerations for Use

Ginkgo is available in tablet form. These tablets contain a concentrated extract of the medicinally important compounds in the herb. This form of ginkgo is more effective for disorders involving mental function when the entire day's dose is taken at once. Quercetin, a compound found in ginkgo, is available in tablet form, although commercially available quercetin is taken from other sources.

Is ginkgo leaf tea a natural alternative to ginkgo leaf extracts? The answer usually given is no, because ginkgo tablets contain fifty times the concentration of ginkgolides than ginkgo leaf. However, daily use of $^1/_3$ ounce (10 grams) of ginkgo leaf in tea would yield enough active ginkgo compounds to have the wide range of beneficial effects listed above.[38]

Perhaps one in one hundred people who use ginkgo will experience stomach upset. If stomach upset or nausea recurs, discontinue usage. Individuals who develop headaches about an hour after taking ginkgo, and who normally do not have headaches, should also discontinue usage. Finnish doctors report that a few persons taking ginkgo experienced orthostatic hypotension, a sudden loss of blood pressure when moving from a seated to a standing position, after using ginkgo for a few days.[39] Again, if this happens, discontinue use. In addition, there have been two isolated reports in the medical literature of "spontaneous" bleeding under the skin associated with chronic ginkgo use.[40] To avoid this extremely remote possibility, take a "vacation" from ginkgo every six months for six weeks.

LEM

Description

Lentinula edodes mycelium (LEM) is a chemical isolated from *Lentinula edodes*, better known as the shiitake mushroom. It is a protein-bound sugar that is soluble in water, and contains vitamins B_1 and B_2.[1] LEM is, along with lentinan, one of the shiitake extracts most widely used in medical treatment (see right and page 105).

Scientific Findings and Clinical Experience

LEM has been the subject of intense research efforts. Hundreds of clinical trials have documented the usefulness of LEM in the treatment of HIV, high cholesterol, and liver disorders.

Of the two most common shiitake extracts, LEM and lentinan, LEM is the more strongly antiviral. In the laboratory, it has been shown to inhibit HIV infection in cultures of human T cells, the immune-system components destroyed by HIV.[2] Other studies have found that LEM prevents the progression of HIV to AIDS by stopping cell-to-cell transmission of the virus.[3] LEM also increases the effectiveness of the drug AZT against viral replication in laboratory tests,[4] probably by stimulating the production of an immune-system chemical called interleukin-1.

LEM lowers levels of cholesterol in the blood through the action of a chemical called eritadenine. Adding eritadenine in amounts as low as 0.005 percent of the total to the diet of laboratory animals—equivalent to adding one one-hundredth of an ounce to every pound of food—lowered total cholesterol levels by 25 percent within one week.[5] This cholesterol-lowering activity is more pronounced when the animals are fed a diet high in fat.[6] Additional studies have found that LEM and other shiitake extracts can lower both cholesterol levels and blood pressure.[7] These extracts can also accelerate the accumulation of "bad" LDL cholesterol in the liver, which transforms it into "good" HDL cholesterol.[8]

LEM is especially beneficial to liver health. Clinical studies have shown that this extract can help the liver produce antibodies to hepatitis B,[9] a strain of hepatitis that increases the patient's risk of developing liver cancer. Therefore, LEM can fight liver cancer before it develops. And in animal studies, injections of LEM slowed the growth of cancerous liver tumors.[10]

Considerations for Use

LEM powder is readily available from natural food stores and herb shops. It is remarkably nontoxic. In more than twenty years of use in Japan, no evidence of acute toxicity has ever been noticed in LEM users, even when used in massive doses. LEM can occasionally cause mild diarrhea or skin rashes. Should these symptoms occur, consult a health care provider.

Lentinan

Description

Lentinan, like LEM, is an extract of the shiitake mushroom (see left and page 105). Chemically, it is in the shape of a helix, similar to the DNA helix. This is thought to account for lentinan's healing properties. It is water-soluble and is not destroyed by heat, acids, or alkalis.[1]

Scientific Findings and Clinical Experience

Lentinan provides powerful immune system support. This allows it to fight AIDS, various cancers, and other serious conditions, as well as the common cold.

In AIDS treatment, lentinan stimulates the production and activation of various immune-system components, including antibodies, interferon, natural killer (NK) cells, and macrophages. It is particularly active in augmenting helper T cells, the cells that direct the immune system's attack and are themselves destroyed by HIV. There are reports that lentinan has been helpful in treating persons with low T-cell counts who do not have other AIDS symptoms.[2] In one case in which an HIV-positive patient was treated with lentinan, the count rose from 1,250 T cells per milliliter of blood to 2,045 per milliliter in thirty days, and then to 2,542 per milliliter after sixty days.[3]

Even though lentinan's ability to stimulate the immune system is potent, this extract is not recommended for patients with HIV infections that have not progressed to AIDS. HIV is capable of mutating into drug-resistant forms. Since the cells that HIV infects are the same cells stimulated to reproduce by lentinan, use of this extract can actually provide the virus with more cells to infect, which gives it more opportunities to transform itself into an untreatable strain.

Japanese physicians have long used lentinan in cancer treatment. Lentinan does not act directly on cancer cells. Instead, it activates the immune system's lymphokine-activated killer cells and NK cells to attack various types of cancers, including carcinoma,[4] hepatoma,[5] and sarcoma.[6,7] Lentinan counteracts the formation of prostaglandins. These substances can cause inflammation, which restrains the immune system's T cells from reaching maturity.

Stomach, or gastric, cancer is unusually difficult to treat because its early symptoms are often so vague that the cancer is usually quite advanced by the time it is found. Japanese physicians have found that lentinan stimulates the capacity of specialized blood cells to produce immune-system chemicals, mainly interleukin and tumor necrosis factor, that prevent cancer's growth and spread. Lentinan is especially useful when surgery is not feasible.[8,9]

Japanese physicians also use lentinan to treat breast cancer in women who have had mastectomies without followup radiation therapy.[10] When chemotherapy is used, lentinan prevents immune-system damage if given *before* treatment begins.[11] In addition, Japanese animal studies have shown that lentinan increases the effectiveness of cancer treatment with a specific type of interleukin called interleukin-2. When used together, the two treatments prevented the spread of breast cancer to the lung.[12]

Even when cancer has spread to the lung, lentinan can increase survival time. In a group of sixteen patients with advanced cancer, Japanese medical researchers injected lentinan directly into malignant areas. All the patients eventually died, but the average survival time of patients who responded to the treatment was 129 days, compared with 49 days for those who were not given the drug.[13]

Japanese physicians also report that lentinan is a useful treatment for low natural killer cell syndrome (LNKS), a disease that causes disabling fatigue. This disease appears to be identical to chronic fatigue syndrome as it is diagnosed in the West. Lentinan treatment has been successful in reversing symptoms, including remittent fever, persistent fatigue, and low NK cell activity.

Lentinan may be useful in treating drug-resistant tuberculosis. One study looked at three patients with tuberculosis of the lung who had shed disease-resistant bacteria for ten years. Treatment with lentinan stopped the shedding of new bacteria,[14] a finding confirmed in several animal studies.[15]

Considerations for Use

Lentinan's actions are highly dose-dependent. Given by injection twice a week, 1 *milligram* of lentinan is enough to have a therapeutic effect, while injecting more than 10 milligrams of lentinan per week can suppress the immune system. Use of lentinan in this form requires that the provider pay careful attention to the individual's condition and circumstances.

Large quantities of lentinan are required when the drug is taken in the form of capsules, which are actually air-dried or freeze-dried shiitake teas. The precise dosage must be determined by the provider. Still larger amounts of shiitake mushroom are needed to receive a therapeutic amount of lentinan. Therefore, it is best to use lentinan capsules or injections.

Maitake

Description

Maitake is a Japanese mushroom closely related to polyporus (see page 82). The word *maitake* is literally translated from Japanese as "dancing mushroom," so named because in ancient times people who found maitake could exchange it for its weight in silver, leading to their dancing in celebration. Maitake is recognized by its small, overlapping tongue- or fan-shaped caps, usually fused together at the base of tree stumps or on tree roots.

Scientific Findings and Clinical Experience

Maitake has proven itself to be an effective cancer fighter. In laboratory tests, powdered maitake increased the activity of three types of immune cells—macrophages, natural killer (NK) cells, and T cells—by 140, 186, and 160 percent, respectively. It reduced tumor formation by 86 percent in mice that were given maitake when compared with mice that did not receive maitake.[1] A Chinese clinical study established that maitake treatment reduces the rate of recurrence of bladder cancer after surgery from 65 to 33 percent.[2] Researchers have found that maitake, when combined with the standard chemotherapy drug mitomycin (Mutamycin), inhibits the growth of breast cancer cells—even after the tumors are well-formed—and prevents the spread of such cells to the liver.

The anticancer compounds in maitake, known as the Maitake D-fraction,[3] have shown positive results in American studies on breast and colorectal cancer.[4] Chinese doctors also report positive results in sixty-three patients who had liver, lung, or stomach cancers, or leukemia.[5] And two American doctors have used Maitake D-fraction in treating Kaposi's sarcoma, a form of cancer usually seen in people with AIDS.[6]

Maitake protects the liver. Chinese doctors conducted a controlled trial with thirty-two patients who had chronic hepatitis B. The recovery rate was 72 percent in the maitake treatment group, compared with 57 percent in the control group. Hepatitis antigens disappeared in more than 40 percent of the maitake patients, meaning the virus had been purged from their bodies.[7]

Laboratory studies also show that maitake protects liver tissue from hepatitis[8] caused by carbon tetrachloride and paracematol. These compounds go through a two-step process in the liver, in which they are first activated into toxic forms and then deactivated into harmless forms. Since maitake helps the liver handle chemical poisons in both steps, it protects this vital organ against a very broad range of chemicals. Maitake, along with LEM (see page 102), is one of the most effective herbal ways of preventing drug-induced hepatitis.[9]

Methanol extracts of maitake mushroom quickly lower blood pressure in laboratory animals, although the effect does not last very long.[10] A small-scale clinical study conducted by the Ayurvedic Medicine Center of New York found that a proprietary formula called Grifron lowered systolic blood pressure an average of 14 mm Hg and diastolic blood pressure an average of 8 mm Hg.[11] (Systolic pressure occurs when the heart contracts, diastolic when it relaxes.) Simply eating maitake or drinking maitake tea does not have this effect.

Maitake also lowers blood-sugar levels in people with type 2 diabetes.[12] There have been cases in which taking Maitake D-fraction daily have lowered blood sugar levels from a very dangerous 400 milligrams per deciliter to a moderate 155 milligrams per deciliter in four weeks. The compound seems to work by decreasing insulin resistance.

Finally, maitake provides nutritional support by enhancing the intestine's ability to absorb micronutrients, or those nutrients needed in very small amounts. This is especially true of copper,[13] since increasing copper absorption also increases the absorption of zinc.

Considerations for Use

Maitake is available fresh or dried for use in food or tea, or as

Maitake D-fraction. It is best used as an adjunct treatment for chronic conditions.

Maitake has been used in multiple sclerosis (MS) patients to increase production of a family of immune-system chemicals called the interferons,[14] some of which have been shown to stabilize MS patients.[15] However, one form of interferon stimulated by maitake, gamma-interferon,[16] helps destroy nerve tissue. Therefore, persons with MS should avoid maitake until this remedy has been more thoroughly tested.

PSK

Description

PSK, also known as krestin, is an extract from the kawaratake mushroom. Kawaratake, whose name in Japanese literally means "mushroom on the river bank," is common in the woods of Japan, China, and the United States. It sports a fan-shaped fruiting body that resembles a turkey tail in shades of blue, brown, gray, or white, giving it the common name "turkey-tail mushroom" in English. In Japan, the mushroom is the source of *polysaccharide Kureha,* or PSK, the most widely sold health food in the country.

Scientific Findings and Clinical Experience

PSK's effectiveness against cancer is so widely recognized in Japan that in one year, purchases of PSK accounted for over 25 percent of the nation's entire expenditures on cancer treatment.[1] It is especially beneficial when used with standard chemotherapy or radiation therapy.

PSK stops the spread of tumors by disabling the enzymes that allow tumor cells to break out of the matrix that hold healthy cells in their proper places. This is especially useful in increasing the effectiveness of radiation therapy for uterine cancer. For example, in a study of patients with fairly advanced uterine and cervical cancer at the National Cancer Center Hospital in Tokyo, some patients took 3 to 6 grams of PSK every day in conjunction with radiation therapy, while others received radiation alone. After radiation, 36 percent of the patients who took PSK had no observable cancer cells, but that was true of only 11 percent of those who did not take PSK. The two-year survival rate was 94 percent for patients who took PSK and 74 percent for those who did not. The five-year survival rates were 79 percent and 48 percent, respectively.[2]

Doctors have seen an increase in survival rates when PSK is used with either radiation therapy or chemotherapy in cases of lung cancer. In one study of 185 patients with advanced (Stage III) lung cancer, the five-year survival rate for people who received both radiation therapy and PSK exceeded that of those who received radiation alone by 400 percent.[3] In another study involving 169 patients, PSK extended longevity in patients who received chemotherapy by an average of seven weeks.[4]

PSK also helps people with colorectal cancer. It checked the disease's progress and increased survival rates in one trial involving 124 patients, all of whom were also treated with mitomycin (Mutamycin). PSK reduced the depth to which the cancer invaded the intestinal wall, and curtailed spread to both lymph nodes and blood vessels.[5] In laboratory studies, PSK increases the effectiveness of the chemotherapy agent 5-fluorouracil.[6] It reduces the rate of cancer growth in the cecum, the place where the large intestine begins, and reduces the rate at which cancer enters the lymph system. PSK increases the effectiveness of immune-system components called T cells against colorectal tumors,[7] and has also been found to prevent the spread of colon cancer to the liver.[8] In one eighteen-year study, PSK reduced the spread of colon cancer to the peritoneum (the membrane lining the intestinal cavity) and the lungs in 60 percent of the patients who took it.[9]

PSK has other uses as well. It protects immune cells in the linings of artery walls from the action of harmful chemicals called free radicals. This prevents the immune cells from attracting low-density lipoprotein (LDL), the "bad" cholesterol that gathers into artery-clogging plaques.[10] In addition, PSK increases resistance to viral skin infections in people with eczema.[11]

Considerations for Use

PSK is available in dried extract form.

Reishi

Description

In Japan, reishi is known as the "phantom mushroom" because of the difficulty in finding it. Although over 99 percent of all wild reishi mushrooms are found growing on old Japanese plum trees, fewer than ten mushrooms will be found on 100,000 trees. Japanese farmers now grow reishi indoors. This art was perfected by Shigeaki Mori, who developed an elaborate, two-year-long method of culturing wild reishi spores on plum-tree sawdust.[1]

Reishi has been used in folk medicine in Japan and China for over 4,000 years, especially in the treatment of liver diseases. In *Ben Cao Gang Mu (Omissions From the Materia Medica),* one of China's most famous natural history books, reishi is said to "lighten [spiritual] weight and increase longevity."[2] Reishi was thought to release trapped emotional energy from the liver so that the individual could turn to higher, more spiritual pursuits.

Scientific Findings and Clinical Experience

Treatment with reishi is beneficial in a number of disorders, both common, such as allergy and asthma, and uncommon, such as altitude sickness and mushroom poisoning.

Reishi contains antihistamine compounds.[3] They block the histamine-induced inflammation and swelling seen in respiratory allergies, and reduce the severity of stomach upset associated with food allergies. Reishi's antihistamines ease asthma by preventing the inflammatory reactions that constrict the airways within the lungs and make breathing difficult. (These antihistamines also ease inflammation associated with uterine fibroids.) In addition, reishi stimulates the maturation of immune cells known as macrophages, which engulf and digest infectious bacteria. This prevents secondary infections from developing into cases of chronic bronchitis. These mature macrophages are also active against yeasts, which makes reishi a valuable treatment for yeast infections.[4]

Reishi is effective against leukemia. Animal studies show that reishi extract causes leukemia cells to become differentiated, which checks their ability to reproduce wildly. Instead, they behave in the same manner as ordinary cells, maturing into forms that reproduce normally at the end of a regular life cycle.[5] It is also effective against other forms of cancer.

Chinese physicians claim reishi is especially beneficial for hepatitis patients who have not suffered severe loss of liver function.[6] In TCM theory, persons whose "liver" symptoms are compounded by emotional stress or ongoing tension are most helped by reishi. Reishi can also help persons with fatty deposits or irritation within the liver caused by overindulgence in alcohol or fatty foods.

Reishi helps ease altitude sickness among Himalayan mountain climbers[7] by maintaining good circulatory health at reduced atmospheric pressures. It also serves as a useful antidote. Reishi teas, given over a period of two to three days, accelerate recovery from mushroom poisoning.[8] Reishi also helps overcome the nervous excitement that results from excessive caffeine consumption.[9] Reishi's effects on the brain have led to its use in cases of age-related intellectual decline, such as that associated with Alzheimer's disease and cerebral atherosclerosis. Reports of the successful use of reishi for this purpose remain anecdotal, but are numerous. Finally, reishi is used to treat myotonia dystrophica, a hereditary disease that causes the muscles to atrophy,[10] and to remove wrinkles,[11] age spots, and freckles.

Considerations for Use

Reishi is probably the most widely available medicinal mushroom in the world. It is available not only as a foodstuff, but also in the form of tea, syrup, tablets, or tinctures. Use two 1-gram tea bags to make each cup of tea. Fresh reishi is available in different colors, each with a different taste and healing purpose. Consult a Kampo or TCM practitioner for advice on which type is the best in any given situation.

Shiitake

Description

Shiitake is a mushroom that grows on the Japanese shiia tree. Used as a food for thousands of years in the Orient, it has become popular in the United States as a tasty alternative to the blander mushroom varieties more commonly sold in supermarkets.

In or shortly before the year A.D. 200, the Japanese Emperor Chuai was offered the shiitake by the Kyusuyu, an aboriginal people of Japan. Shiitake was used even earlier in China, where it was known as *hoang-mo.* Kampo, however, overlooked the use of shiitake until well into the twentieth century. Shiitake is the basis of several extracts, including LEM and lentinan (see page 102).

Scientific Findings and Clinical Experience

The primary use of shiitake mushroom is in lowering levels of both total cholesterol and low-density lipoprotein (LDL), the "bad" cholesterol that builds up within arteries. In animal studies using eritadenine, a chemical found in shiitake, cholesterol levels were reduced by 25 percent in one week. This effect is more pronounced in subjects on high-fat diets than those on low-fat diets. Japanese scientists have found that shiitake compounds accelerate the accumulation of LDL in the liver, which transforms it into "good" HDL cholesterol.[1]

Shiitake has other uses. It stimulates the immune system. This allows it to fight yeast infections common in diabetes[2] and to increase production of an immune-system component called interferon, which is thought to rein in the blood-vessel overgrowth seen in macular degeneration. Shiitake also helps stop the formation and spread of stomach cancer.

Considerations for Use

Shiitake can be eaten in food. It is also available in tablet, syrup, and tincture forms.

Some people use shiitake as a cancer preventative. It blocks the formation of cancer-causing dietary nitrites, chemicals found in meats and many preserved products. However, persons with bladder cancer should not use *raw* shiitake, as it contains a chemical known to cause this disease.

Siberian Ginseng (Eleuthero)

Description

As its name suggests, Siberian ginseng is a hardy shrub native to the southeastern part of Siberia, just north of China's Amur River. Siberian ginseng also grows in China, Japan, and Korea. A deciduous plant, it grows to a height of ten feet and bears three- to seven-toothed leaflets on each stem. The dried root is used in Kampo. Siberian ginseng is in the same family as, but is not identical to, Korean or red ginseng (see page 57).

Scientific Findings and Clinical Experience

Siberian ginseng has come into worldwide use only in the twentieth century, but few herbs have been as extensively researched. In the 1950s, the Russians began searching for inexpensive alternatives to red ginseng in the prevention of respiratory diseases during the Far North's long winters. What they found was an herb that can prevent colds and flu, but can also fight cancer.

Siberian ginseng has a proven ability to prevent upper respiratory infections. Russian studies involving tens of thousands of participants found that taking Siberian ginseng for eight to ten weeks *before* the beginning of the cold and flu season reduces the incidence of these diseases by more than

95 percent.[1] This herb stimulates the activity of several immune-system components: B and T cells, which direct the immune response to infection; macrophages, "germ-eating" cells that attack bacteria; and interferons, which interfere with every stage of viral infection.[2] Siberian ginseng's ability to reduce inflammation also makes it useful in the early stages of Ménière's disease.[3]

Siberian ginseng also helps people cope with stress. It is used to treat problems with concentration and sensitivity to environmental stresses, such as noise, drafts, and changes in weather. This helps people who suffer from clinical depression. It also eases depression directly by balancing serotonin, dopamine, epinephrine, and norepinephrine, brain chemicals that determine mood.[4] The herb's stress-fighting and depression-relieving capacities make it useful in the treatment of attention deficit disorder. In men, Siberian ginseng stimulates the body's production of testosterone, which makes it a valuable aid in impotence treatment. This herb's infection-fighting, stress-reducing, and testosterone-increasing activities combine to make it an ideal training aid for athletes (see "Siberian Ginseng Goes to the Gym").

The most exciting research on Siberian ginseng, however, has been done on its ability to fight cancer. Siberian ginseng stimulates B cells, which are depleted in chronic leukemia, multiple myeloma, and ovarian carcinoma. It also stimulates T cells, which are depleted in Hodgkin's disease, Kaposi's sarcoma, and all forms of carcinoma once they have spread.

Siberian Ginseng Goes to the Gym

Athletes around the world have adopted Siberian ginseng as a training aid. Athletes use it to increase performance, bolster the immune system against the demands made on it during exercise, reduce fatigue after workouts, and reduce the effects of stress.

The Russians were the first to use Siberian ginseng as a training aid. A Russian scientist named I.I. Brekhman conducted years of painstaking studies on dozens of native Russian plants, trying to find a replacement for red ginseng as a cold and flu fighter. Brekhman wanted an herb that would raise an individual's resistance to stress and normalize physical function, and do so without causing side effects. All of these qualities are present in Siberian ginseng, which Brekhman and his colleagues found to have an impressive range of benefits.[1]

In time, the herb was investigated as a legal stimulant for the Soviet Union's international athletes. The Soviet (and later, Russian) Olympic team has publicly acknowledged its use of Siberian ginseng since the Munich Olympics of 1972, and the herb was credited by team nutrition and pharmacology adviser Sergei Portugalov for Russia's unexpected capture of eleven gold medals at the Lillihammer Winter Olympics in 1994. Chess players, cosmonauts, musicians, and high-level Russian military officers started using Siberian ginseng, while its use in athletics went global. Basketball player Charles Barkley, for instance, is reported to drink thirty bottles of Siberian ginseng tonic a week.[2]

Unfortunately, scientific studies of Siberian ginseng's usefulness in athletic performance have yielded results that are difficult to interpret. For instance, in a study conducted at Old Dominion University, athletes who were given Siberian ginseng had consistently higher maximum heart rates and higher rates of oxygen consumption than athletes who were given an inactive placebo. Athletes taking the herb also did not become exhausted as quickly. Runners had higher concentrations of lactic acid in their muscles after their races, which is an indication of greater muscular activity. These complicated measurements could only be conducted on sixteen athletes, however, so the study failed to capture statistically significant differences in performance.[3] Other studies have also shown positive but not statistically significant benefits from Siberian ginseng.[4,5]

If the effects of Siberian ginseng are not direct, could they be indirect? The answer seems to be that Siberian ginseng keeps athletes from getting sick and prevents them from becoming run down through heavy training. It also speeds their return to physiological normalcy following strenuous workouts. Siberian ginseng can, when used over the long term, improve an athlete's overall training program, promote more consistent training, and quicken reflexes and lower race times.

Followers of competitive sports know that simple respiratory infections can dash the competitive hopes of the even the most superbly trained athletes. Athletes are easy prey for germs. Intense or prolonged endurance exercise—sometimes even a single workout or race—causes large increases in hormones that can decrease the activity of the immune system, specifically the T and natural killer (NK) cells. The NK cells form an important line of defense against infectious agents, especially against viruses and bacteria that attack the upper respiratory system. Data show that Siberian ginseng, when taken as a preventative, can reduce athletes' rates of infection by 35 percent. Siberian ginseng spurs the bone marrow and the immune system to greater activity. Some researchers believe that Siberian ginseng increases the synthesis of interferon, a powerful chemical that boosts immune-system activity. Other researchers believe that the herb stimulates the activity of germ-eating macrophages. Unfortunately, the effectiveness of Siberian ginseng's infection-fighting components fades fairly quickly, so it must be taken continuously.

Siberian ginseng also reduces fatigue after workouts. It reduces the "burn" after exercise, thus reducing muscle soreness without the side effects of aspirin and other painkillers. By raising the amount of energy available to the muscles very quickly, Siberian ginseng allows athletes to train consistently and to perform several hard workouts in a short time.

Finally, Siberian ginseng's stress-lowering effect is important to athletes because it moderates the production of cortisol. Overtrained athletes often have high levels of cortisol, which is a catabolic, or protein-destroying, stress hormone. Siberian ginseng deactivates cortisol before the hormone can cause tissue damage.

Considerations for Use

Make Siberian ginseng tea by placing 1 teaspoon (2 to 3 grams) of powdered herb in 1 cup of hot water, and steeping for five to ten minutes. Alternatively, use pure eleuthero extracts as directed by the manufacturer. Remember to dilute extracts with a small amount—up to $^1/_4$ cup—of water before drinking. Do *not* use sugar-sweetened ginseng drinks.

If using bottled ginseng tonics, make sure the product contains real Siberian ginseng (*Eleutherococcus senticosus*), and not other herbs which may be spuriously labeled as "ginseng." Siberian ginseng extracts are a complex mixture of at least forty-three active and inactive compounds.[5] For this reason, it is difficult to know if any specific formulation contains the most useful compounds. That is why this herb is best taken in tea form.

Persons who have myasthenia gravis or rheumatoid arthritis and diseases related to it, such as lupus, psoriatric arthritis, and Sjögren's syndrome, should avoid Siberian ginseng. This herb stimulates the immune system to produce B cells, a process which aggravates these conditions. Also avoid Siberian ginseng if a prostate problem exists, including cancer or tumors secondary to prostate cancer, since this herb contains compounds that stimulate testosterone production.[6]

Snow Fungus

Description

Snow fungus is a white, nearly translucent, "trembling" fungus that grows on a great variety of trees throughout Asia and in warmer climates worldwide. The fungus is sometimes called "wood ear" for its appearance on the decaying logs on which it grows. Good quality snow fungus has a pale, yellowish white color and a mucilagelike texture.

Chinese and Japanese herbalists have used snow fungus for more than 2,000 years to enhance beauty, stimulate sexual activity, lower fevers, and heal ulcers. Snow fungus was thought to "moisten" the lungs and protect them from damage. Kampo uses snow fungus to lubricate the lungs and intestines, relieving coughs or constipation, and to increase semen production, stimulate saliva secretion, strengthen vital energy, and nourish the brain. Traditionally, Chinese and Japanese physicians combined snow fungus with glehnia roots, lily bulbs, and rock candy for tuberculosis or the coughing up of blood; with jujube (see page 000) and pork for debility after a long illness; and with prince root and rock candy for shortness of breath.

Scientific Findings and Clinical Experience

Scientific studies have found that snow fungus's mucilagelike compounds, which are called polysaccharides, fit like keys into receptor sites, or "locks," on certain cells in the immune system. This activates the cells to fight infections or tumors. These polysaccharides increase the production of interferon[1] and interleukin-2,[2] two important immune-system chemicals, and stimulate the production of germ-eating cells called macrophages.[3] Snow fungus also increases the activity of natural killer cells and enhances the effectiveness of antibodies.[4]

Chinese and Japanese physicians use snow fungus to treat infections. A Chinese clinical study found that both snow fungus and its spores increase the activities of macrophages, an action that boosts resistance to chronic bronchitis.[5] Chinese physicians report that treating chronic hepatitis B with snow fungus powders results in a cure rate of between 50 and 75 percent after three months of treatment, and more than 90 percent after thirty-six months of treatment.[6]

Snow fungus reduces the rate at which cancers spread. Cancerous tumors must establish their own blood-vessel systems to get the nutrients and oxygen they require to multiply and spread. Compounds in snow fungus counteract a blood chemical called platelet activating factor, or PAF. This makes the blood less likely to clot and spin a fibrin "net" on which the tumor's new blood vessels can form.

Snow fungus can be used in treatment plans for specific types of cancer. Laboratory tests have demonstrated that fungus extracts kill cervical cancer cells,[7] as well those from other types of tumors. Snow fungus is known to sensitize the cervix and uterus to radiation treatment, making the radiation more effective. The most valuable medical use of snow fungus, however, is to prevent leukopenia, or deficient white blood cell counts, in patients undergoing chemotherapy or radiation treatment.[8]

In Japan, snow fungus is used to prevent atherosclerosis—the process by which cholesterol gathers into plaques within the arteries—by lowering total blood-cholesterol levels. Powdered snow fungus is added to what are sold as "cholesterol-controlling" foods and drinks. To date, however, only one preliminary study has confirmed the fungus's value for this purpose.[9]

In addition, snow fungus is supposed to remove facial freckles if eaten regularly. This application has not been scientifically confirmed.

Considerations for Use

Snow fungus, like all the other "jelly fungi," has no known toxicity and can be taken as either food or medicine. Snow fungus is prepared by covering the dried fruiting body of the fungus with water and allowing it to stand for a couple of hours, and then simmering it over low heat for twenty minutes until it reaches a pastelike consistency. The paste can then be added to soups or combined with sugar to make a medicinal candy. It must be used for at least four weeks to be effective.

Snow fungus is also available as a patent (over-the-counter) medicine called *Yin Mi Pian*.

Soy Isoflavones

Description

The soybean contains several medicinally useful chemicals, including isoflavones and lecithin (see this page). The two most beneficial of the isoflavones are daidzein and genistein (and the closely related compounds daidzin and genistin).

Scientific Findings and Clinical Experience

Soy isoflavones are useful cancer fighters. Chemically, they are similar to the human hormone estrogen. This similarity allows isoflavones to attach to estrogen receptors in human cells, blocking entry for the hormone. Isoflavones are just different enough, however, to not stimulate cells like estrogen does. This keeps estrogen away from cells that are sensitive to estrogen, especially cancerous cells in the bladder, breast, colon, prostate, and skin.

Daidzein is an estrogen-blocking isoflavone, which is created by helpful intestinal bacteria from the soy chemical formononetin. Daidzein locks out estrogen from breast cancer cells without stimulating the cells to reproduce.[1] It also fights cancer by causing tumor cells, which are immature, to differentiate, or mature into forms that die and are replaced. Daidzein has been shown to be very potent in forcing differentiation of human leukemia cells[2,3] and of melanoma cells even when absorbed in very low concentrations.[4]

Genistein is the most extensively researched anticancer chemical in the Japanese diet. Although the chemical is most often associated with Japanese dietary patterns, it has been most extensively researched in Finland. Finnish researchers conducted decades of exacting studies to explain why the people of Japan enjoy lower rates of breast, ovarian, prostate, and other cancers, and found genistein to be the common denominator.[5]

Genistein is especially valuable in reversing cancer risk associated with certain kinds of excess weight in women. Women who are physically inactive and have genetic tendencies for diabetes often develop insulin resistance, in which the body is forced to produce more and more insulin to transport glucose to the cells where it is needed. Insulin also enables the transport of fat into fat cells, and fatty tissue produces estrogen. Insulin furthermore activates estrogen and progesterone receptors,[6] which stimulates the growth of cells, including estrogen-activated cancer cells. Since genistein blocks estrogen from its receptors on cells, it helps fight the effects of excess estrogen production.

Genistein counteracts cancer development on several levels. It deactives a harmful protein called tyrosine protein kinase, a key player in stimulating cell growth. This keeps cancer cells from multiplying.[7] Genistein also affects other key enzymes involved in the cancer formation process.[8] Like daidzein, genistein causes cancer cells to differentiate,[9] stopping wild multiplication. In addition, genistein stops the process by which tumors develop their own systems of blood vessels.[10] This action deprives cancer cells of nutrients and oxygen, keeping them at a very small size.

Considerations for Use

The easiest way to get soy isoflavones is by taking soy germ or soy isoflavone extract. Soy germ should preferably be added to cereals or smoothies.

Soy isoflavones are also present in soy products such as cooked soybeans, miso, or tofu (soy bean curd), and in the herb kudzu (see page 64).

Soy Lecithin

Description

Soy lecithin, like soy isoflavones (see this page) is an extract of the soybean. It contains soy chemicals called phospholipids, which are responsible for soy lecithin's medicinal effects.

Scientific Findings and Clinical Experience

Numerous clinical and laboratory studies have shown that soy lecithin can protect the liver from damage caused by alcohol, tetrachlorides found in cleaning solvents, acetaminophen (tylenol), and galactosamine, a protein that can irritate the liver. In laboratory studies of chronic hepatitis, soy lecithin has shown an ability to protect the liver against fatty deposits and fibrosis, the development of nonfunctional fibrous tissue. Soy lecithin works on the liver cells' membranes, helping the membranes to renew and repair themselves.

Soy lecithin can also reduce blood-cholesterol levels. This occurs through a complex process, in which the partially digested lecithin is chemically reassembled in the intestinal wall into a form that attracts cholesterol. The lecithin then steers the larger, low-density lipoprotein (LDL), or "bad" cholesterol, to the liver, where it is broken down into the smaller high density lipoprotein (HDL), or "good" cholesterol. In addition, soy lecithin contains a compound that prevents destruction of oxygen-deprived brain tissue.

Considerations for Use

Take soy phospholipids, which are identified individually on the label as 3-sn-phosphatidylcholine, phosphatidylethanolamine, and phosphatidylinositic acid, or as "total phospholipids."

Although soy lecithin helps reverse alcoholic cirrhosis of the liver, it is important to curtail or stop alcohol use when using this substance. Mild diarrhea may occur when soy lecithin is first used.

CHAPTER 4

The Formulas of Kampo

Chapter 3 explained how the individual herbs and other healing substances used in Kampo work, in terms of the principles of both Kampo and conventional medicine. This chapter will take a look at the combinations of herbs, called formulas, that Kampo has devised to treat certain symptom patterns, including a look at formula dosage.

KAMPO FORMULAS: PATTERNS OF SYMPTOMS, PATTERNS OF HERBS

Formulas are herbs in harmony. Over the centuries, Kampo has learned how to match combinations of herbs to combinations of symptoms. Since this process involves selecting the formula that matches a person, rather than a disease, the same formula may be applied to many different disease conditions as they are understood in conventional medicine. Conversely, two persons with the same disease may benefit from different formulas.

The reason for this is that, in the Japanese tradition of herbal healing, formulas fit symptom patterns like a lock and key. Every healing tea is made with exactly the same herbs and exactly the same amounts of herbs brewed in the same amount of water as was used by the ancient masters of Kampo. Kampo uses the least number and smallest amount of herbs needed to treat any symptom pattern. This differs from TCM, in which formulas are made up as they are needed, drawing on the herbalist's extensive knowledge of the principles of herbal medicine. This allows the TCM practitioner to treat symptom patterns that are not included in the classics of Kampo literature, but also makes it impossible to compare the treatment the patient receives with either the Kampo classics or the principles of conventional medicine.

Combining herbs also restrains and reinforces their effects. The results of taking a single herb may be too drastic or too weak to affect a symptom pattern. This herb can be combined with other herbs to strengthen or soften it. Combining herbs augments desirable effects and counteracts side effects.

An oft-cited example of this principle is the use of ephedra, a well-known herb Kampo uses to treat asthma. Used by itself, ephedra stops wheezing. Combined with apricot seed, ephedra both stops wheezing and settles cough. Combined with cinnamon, ephedra induces sweating that breaks a fever. Combined with gypsum, ephedra stops sweating and cold chills. Combined with atractylodis, ephedra stimulates urination and indirectly reduces swelling.[1]

CONVENTIONAL MEDICINE AND KAMPO FORMULAS

The healing effects of herbal combinations have been known in Kampo for centuries, but they are also being confirmed by modern science. Japanese researchers have found that boiling ephedra with licorice, for example, releases 50 percent more of the asthma-stopping chemical ephedrine than boiling the same amount of ephedra in the same amount of water by itself. Boiling ephedra, apricot seed, gypsum, and licorice together has a greater healing effect on asthma than boiling each substance separately and then combining the teas.

The effectiveness of a formula depends not only on which herbs are used, but also on how much of the herbs are used. Japanese scientists looked for an anti-inflammatory chemical called glycyrrhetic acid in a simple formula made from licorice and peony root. Licorice supplies the acid. Used short-term, this chemical stops inflammation, but if it builds up in the bloodstream, it can cause side effects. Peony did not seem to have any direct effect on the healing process, so scientists wondered if including it was a mistake.

The classic formula calls for 6 grams of licorice and 6 grams of peony root. When the scientists boiled the licorice without any peony at all, they measured a small amount of glycyrrhetic acid that broke down slowly. When they boiled the licorice with 4 grams of peony, they measured even less glycyrrhetic acid, but it broke down quickly. When they boiled the licorice with 6 grams of peony, they measured the greatest amount of the acid (thus giving the greatest amount of relief), that broke down the most quickly of all (thus avoiding side effects).[2,3] Changing the proportions of herbs changes their effectiveness, so Japanese herbalists stick to tried-and-true formulas.

HOW TO TAKE KAMPO FORMULAS

The Japanese names of many formulas end in *-to* (in Chinese, *-tang*), which literally means "soup." The classics of Kampo prescribed precise lists of ingredients for each herbal "soup," specifying which herbs go into the soup and exactly how much each herb is to be used. As long as the right formula is selected for the symptom pattern, no changes need to be made for dosage. Adults and children have different symptom patterns, so they receive different formulas. Heavyset and thin persons also have different symptom patterns, so they receive different formulas. The dosage of the formula, however, is always the same. The only rule is to take all of the "soup."

Making a tea is always the most effective way to take a formula. The active principles of herbs are always best absorbed from teas. Every Kampo formula is available in this form. The herbs are chosen and weighed by the herbalist, who also provides specific tea-making instructions with the herbs. No measurements, other than using the specified amount of water, are necessary.

However, many people find the traditional way of taking Kampo teas too time-consuming, and turn to over-the-counter extracts and tablets (see Chapter 2). Not every formula can be made into a pill or a tincture. Some formulas, particularly those made with mint, depend on the release of aromatic essences that cannot be included in pill form. Other formulas need larger amounts of ginger or licorice than can be put in a pill to avoid stomach upset. For these reasons, not every formula is available as a pill or extract, although most formulas are (see Appendix A).

In taking over-the-counter Kampo preparations, dosage does make a difference. Different manufacturers use different processes. One manufacturer may reduce the tea 10 times, another 100. Teas can be freeze-dried to make a slurry from which to form pills, or gently boiled to a solid mass. Dosages are different for formulas made by different manufacturers, but the amount the patient should take is stated on the label.

Labels are sometimes confusing to first-time users of Kampo since they give a range of dosages, such as "take 2 to 3 pills daily," rather than an exact dosage. What "2 to 3 pills daily" means in practical terms is that two pills is the minimum anyone can take to improve symptoms, but taking more than three pills provides no additional benefit. In Japan, makers of Kampo formulas have recognized that literally thousands of chemical reactions in the digestive process can affect the way Kampo is absorbed, but that the total difference in absorption from person to person is usually less than 30 percent.[4] To allow for individual differences, they first choose a dosage that exactly matches the dosage in the traditional formula (in this example, $2^1/_2$ pills), and then allow for the possibility that sometimes the digestive system does not absorb quite as much of the herbs as effective treatment requires.

When Kampo doesn't work, the problem is usually the way the herbs are taken. Take formulas on an empty stomach, and with a small amount ($^1/_2$ cup, or 150 milliliters) of warm water. Taking the medication with water ensures that it arrives in the digestive tract. Taking the medication on an empty stomach ensures that it does not chemically react to food.

Just as in conventional medicine, however, sometimes Kampo patients get the wrong formula. If a mistake has been made in the choice of herb, taking a small amount of the herb or drug will produce only small side effects. Taking a large amount of a new herb or medication will produce larger side effects. To stay on the side of safety, use the lower recommended dose for at least three days. Then, if there are no problems, increase the amount. (This principle does not apply to teas given by a Kampo practitioner, only to over-the-counter Kampo products.) As an additional safeguard against side effects caused by taking the wrong formula, the lowest recommended dosage is best for:

- Persons who are allergy-prone or who have digestive problems.
- Children, the elderly, and persons of low body weight.
- Persons who have chronic diseases in addition to the symptoms treated by the formula.

Persons in these categories are usually better off taking minimum dosages of any medication, whether herbal or conventional.

Additionally, it is best to take less than the minimum recommended dosage of any formula during a healing crisis. Part of the process of bringing the body back into balance may involve purging toxins, a process marked by diarrhea, nausea, or vomiting. (The formulas that have the highest potential to induce a cleansing reaction contain rhubarb root.) Take one-quarter of the usual dose of patent medicine (or take one-half of the tea) while the cleansing reaction is happening. If the right formula is being used, the healing crisis should pass in two to three days, and the usual dosage then can be resumed. If the cleansing process does not end within three days, discontinue the formula and consult the herbalist who provided it. Probably the formula is a slight mismatch to symptoms, and the herbalist can provide a formula that is a better match to symptoms and does not cause further cleansing.

As with any form of medicine, always consult a health care practitioner if there is any question about dosage or whether a specific formula is appropriate in each specific case.

A GUIDE TO THE ENTRIES IN THIS CHAPTER

Each entry in this chapter contains a list of herbs and the symptom pattern they are used to treat. Formulas are not only explained in traditional terms of heat and cold, excess and deficiency, interior and exterior, yin and yang, blood, water, and qi (see Chapter 1), but also in terms of tested and true clinical and scientific experience. Kampo formulas are often described in terms of government officials in Oriental feudal society. The chief herb in the formula acts against the principal symptom pattern. The deputy aids the chief, or fights a coexisting symptom pattern. The assistant may, depending on the formula, reinforce the effects of the chief or deputy herbs, or moderate toxicity of those herbs. The envoy directs the formula's effects to the proper energy channels, and harmonizes the actions of the other herbs.

The traditional explanations of how formulas work paint a picture of the disease process. Knowing these explanations is a way to understand patterns of symptoms intuitively. (A number of the traditional explanations refer to the TCM theory of Paired Organs; see Chapter 1.) Scientific explanation is a way to control disease with confidence. It is important to remember that while formula research is ongoing, the herbs themselves have been more extensively researched than the formulas; see Chapter 3 for information on herbal research. Finally, each entry lists the conditions most commonly treated with the formula and any specific cases in which the formula should not be used. If a formula is not available in an over-the-counter form, that fact is also noted.

FORMULAS USED IN KAMPO

Each of the following formulas is listed under at least one disorder in Part Two. Note, however, that a formula is not necessarily listed in Part Two under all those disorders for which it may possibly be used. Each formula is listed under its English name, followed by its Japanese name.

WHERE TO FIND KAMPO FORMULAS

Kampo formulas can be obtained from TCM herbalists and/or Kampo practitioners. In addition, most of these formulas are available as over-the-counter products. See Appendix A for names of manufacturers and their corresponding commercial Kampo remedies.

Arrest Wheezing Decoction / TEI-ZEN-TO

This formula contains apricot seed, coltsfoot, ephedra, ginkgo nut, licorice, mulberry root, perilla seed, pinellia, and scutellaria.

It is designed for a symptom pattern marked by wheezing with coughing and expectoration of much thick, yellow sputum; simultaneous fever and chills; and labored breathing.

In the classical understanding of this formula, ephedra stops wheezing and releases the body's exterior, enabling both expectoration and perspiration. Ginkgo nut also stops wheezing, but counteracts any excessive stimulation caused by ephedra. The deputy herb apricot seed reinforces the action of ephedra, helping the air passageways expand, while the deputies coltsfoot, perilla seed, and pinellia direct the body's circulation of energy downward. Mulberry root and scutellaria drain heat, reflecting the modern understanding of these herbs as antibacterials, while the envoy herb licorice harmonizes the actions of the other herbs in the formula.

The medically defined conditions most commonly treated with this formula include asthma and chronic bronchitis, especially in smokers.

Prolonged overdosage of Arrest Wheezing Decoction in tea form can cause skin disorders and shedding of the mucous membranes. Short-term overdoses can cause headache, fever, tremors, irritability, or shortness of breath. The antidote is a tea made by boiling 60 grams of raw licorice or 30 grams of ginkgo nut shells in 3 cups of water, strained before drinking. This reaction can be avoided by including the hard shells and thin linings of the ginkgo nuts when making the tea.[1] To avoid both the ginkgo problem and the ill effects of eating apricot seeds, use this formula in patent-medicine form. Use of the formula should be avoided altogether by asthmatics who are experiencing diarrhea. In addition, use with caution if fever is present, and discontinue if preexisting fevers worsen.

Astragalus Decoction to Construct the Middle / OGI-KENCHU-TO

This formula contains astragalus, cinnamon twig, fresh ginger, honey-fried licorice, jujube fruit, malt sugar, and peony. It is a variation of Minor Construct the Middle Decoction (see page 128).

This formula is designed for a symptom pattern that includes low-grade fever or chills; soreness; discomfort in the hands and feet; intermittent, spastic abdominal pain that responds favorably to warmth and pressure; and a desire for hot beverages.

Kampo ascribes this pattern to a shortage of energy, or qi, in the middle of the body. This happens when the nutritional energies the body extracts from food are out of balance with the defensive energies of the immune system. Cinnamon twig warms the abdomen and peony reestablishes a balance of yin and yang. Malt sugar stops abdominal pain while licorice stops the spasms. Ginger and jujube help to balance digestive and defensive energies. Astragalus stops sudden sweating, aids in recovery from shortness of breath, and strengthens the pulse.

The medically defined conditions most commonly treated with this formula include chronic allergies in children and peptic ulcers.

Augmented Four-Substance Decoction / KAMI-SHIMOTSU-TO

This formula contains amaranth, anemarrhena, white atractylodis, raw coptis, eucommia, red ginseng, ligusticum, ophiopogon, phellodendron, white peony, cooked rehmannia, schisandra, and tang-kuei.

It is designed for a symptom pattern that includes blurred vision, dizziness, lusterless complexion, and generalized muscle tension accompanying amenorrhena, or failure to menstruate. This is nearly the same symptom pattern addressed by Four-Substance Decoction (see page 121), from which this formula was derived, except that Augmented Four-Substance Decoction is also used when there is weakness in the arms and legs. In addition, Kampo employs the augmented formula, which has been in use since the sixteenth century, for any kind of atrophy in men or women that creates weakness in the limbs and difficulties in motion.

Peony and rehmannia help the body create blood, and ligusticum and tang-kuei help that blood to circulate. The other herbs support the actions of the main herbs.

The medically defined conditions most commonly treated with this formula include blurred vision, high blood pressure, migraines, menstrual problems, and multiple sclerosis.

Augmented Rambling Powder / KAMI-SHOYO-SAN

This formula contains white atractylodis, bupleurum, gardenia, hoelen, honey-fried licorice, moutan, white peony, and tang-kuei. It is a variation of Rambling Powder (see page 132).

In general, this formula treats a symptom pattern that includes alternating fever and chills, a bitter taste in the mouth, dry mouth and throat, fatigue, headache, reduced appetite, and, in women, distended breasts or irregular menstruation. Specifically, the formula treats short temper, sudden-onset fever and sweating, excessive menstrual flow, and uterine bleeding.

Ancient Kampo held that the vital energies of emotion were stored in the liver. When they built up beyond the liver's capacity to contain them, they caused the body or the mind to "shake," especially on the energy channel supplied by the liver, that is, the external genitalia, the breasts, the centers of the eyes, and the crown of the head. Bupleurum was used to unlock these emotional energies. Peony and tang-kuei restored normal circulation after emotional energy was redirected. The other five herbs of this formula augmented the effects of the primary herbs (hence the name, Augmented Rambling Powder), and could be extended even more by nibbling a mint leaf or small, thin slice of ginger after taking the decoction.

Modern research has found that Augmented Rambling Powder lowers estrogen levels.[1] This makes it effective against disorders affected by estrogen, such as breast cancer, and other disorders of the breast and female reproductive tract. The formula can be used to increase the effectiveness of estrogen-binding drugs, such as tamoxifen (Nolvadex). Augmented Rambling Powder reduces tenderness in the breasts and lower abdomen, irritability, water retention, headache, and digestive disturbance before and at the beginning of the period.

For several generations, Chinese doctors have used this formula to treat macular degeneration, an eye disease that often results in blindness, and atrophy of the optic nerve caused by "toxin accumulation." Recent Japanese research has found that the formula acts against macular degeneration by reducing the tendency of the tiny blood vessels serving the retina to secrete collagen, a protein that indirectly clouds the field of vision.[2]

The medically defined conditions most commonly treated with this formula include bloodshot eyes; breast and uterine cancer; melanoma; endometriosis, in which the tissue that lines the uterus starts growing elsewhere in the body; fibrocystic breast disease, in which the breasts develop benign growths; fibroids, or benign uterine tumors; menstrual problems and menopause; ovarian cysts; premenstrual syndrome; and macular degeneration.

Because gardenia contains a compound that can cause early-pregnancy abortion, this formula should not be used by women who are trying to become pregnant.

Biota Seed Pill to Nourish the Heart / HAKUSHI-YOSHIN-TO

This formula contains acorus, biota seed, hoelen, honey-fried licorice, lycium fruit, ophiopogon, cooked rehmannia, scrophularia, and tang-kuei. It is a variation of Emperor of Heaven's Special Pill to Tonify the Heart (see page 118).

Biota Seed Pill is designed for a symptom pattern that includes constipation with dry stool, fatigue, forgetfulness, inability to think or concentrate for even a very short time, insomnia or very restless sleep, irritability, palpitations with anxiety, and red tongue.

In ancient times, this formula was thought to correct an imbalance of the body's fire and water. The heart lacked energy to contain its fire, and so it would fail to contain the emotions and would send energy upward, causing the tongue to turn red and, more importantly, leading to disordered behavior. The kidneys were unable to send water upward to the heart in order to quench the fire, or downward to moisten the intestines. The "essence," or uniqueness, of the individual escaped downward from the kidneys, however, and was gradually lost.

What Kampo calls "heart" energy is what Western medicine recognizes as mental and emotional capacity. Thus, the medically defined conditions most commonly treated with this formula include Alzheimer's disease, depression, and memory loss.

Bupleurum and Cinnamon Twig Decoction / SAIKO-KEISHI-TO

This formula contains bupleurum, cinnamon twig, fresh ginger, ginseng, jujube fruit, licorice, peony, pinellia, and scutellaria.

It is designed for a symptom pattern that includes bitter or sour taste in the mouth, dizziness, dry throat, a feeling of fullness in the chest, fever and chills, heartburn, irritability, nausea, reduced appetite, vomiting, and joint pain with a "crackling" sensation.

In Kampo, "crackling" pain results when a pathogen is trapped beneath the outer muscles and skin after it has been in the body for several weeks or months. Attempts to expel the pathogen can generate heat, but the expenditure of energy can also result in chills. Bupleurum and scutellaria drain heat from the site of "battle" between the body and the pathogen without driving fever deeper in the body. Ginseng, jujube, and licorice support the body's energy and keep the pathogen from going deeper, while the other herbs normalize the flow of energy and fluids throughout the body to prevent heartburn, irritability, and vomiting, which occur when the energy of battle is misdirected upward.

The medically defined conditions most commonly treated with this formula include joint and muscle pain caused by colds and flu, and irritability and digestive problems associated with premenstrual syndrome. Use with caution if fever is present, and discontinue if preexisting fevers worsen.

Bupleurum and Kudzu Decoction to Release the Muscle Layer From *Medical Revelations* / IGO SAIKATSU KAIKITO

This formula combines anemarrhena, bupleurum, fritillaria cirrhosa, gypsum, kudzu, licorice, moutan, raw rehmannia, red peony, and scutellaria. It was, as its name suggests, first recorded in the book *Medical Revelations*, written by herbalist Cheng Guo-Peng in 1732.

This formula is used to treat fevers that occur without chills, headache, or thirst. The theory behind its creation was that pathogenic influences can sometimes become trapped in the "layer" of the body beneath the muscles and the skin. The body vigorously defends itself against the invading infection, generating heat. Bupleurum and kudzu open the "layers" to allow the body to purge the pathogen through perspiration. Gypsum and scutellaria remove excess heat to the blood, the circulation of which is stimulated by rehmannia. Anemarrhena clears heat and drains fire, relieving high fever, irritability, and thirst, and also treats cough due to heat in the lungs with the expectoration of thick, yellow sputum. Fritillaria stops coughing. It also transforms "phlegm," an energy congestion that causes pain, which frees the blockage. Moutan and red peony clear misdirected upward-moving energies that could cause tension or eye pain, while licorice harmonizes the effects of all the other herbs in the formula.

Kampo uses this formula to lower fevers. It also helps rebalance cognitive symptoms that may appear during long fevers, such as loss of attention or slurred speech. Kampo does not use this formula to treat pain.

The medically defined condition most commonly treated with this formula is insomnia, specifically that which occurs after an upper respiratory infection or a bout of the flu.

When this formula is used in tea form, the gypsum should be boiled for between thirty and forty-five minutes before the other ingredients are added. The formula should not be used if nausea or vomiting is present.

Bupleurum, Cinnamon Twig, and Ginger Decoction / SAIKO-KEISHI-KANKYO-TO

This formula combines bupleurum, cinnamon, ginger, honey-fried licorice, oyster shell, scutellaria, and snake gourd (trichosanth) root. It is an ancient variation on Minor Bupleurum Decoction (see page 128), which was invented in the second century A.D. by Kampo master Zhang Zhongjing.

This formula is designed to treat a symptom pattern that includes alternating fever and chills, a feeling of fullness over the stomach, sweating on the head, thirst, and urinary difficulty.

Kampo designed this formula to treat infections that have stayed in the body long enough to have worn down the body's immune resistance. The principal two herbs in this formula, bupleurum, and scutellaria, drain heat from the "battleground" where the invading pathogen is fought—the liver and gallbladder. The herbs open a route through which the body can rid itself of the infection. Both herbs cool the body, which prevents fever from affecting "deeper" organs, or those that control the body's yin, or containing, energies.

Snake gourd root relieves thirst caused by fever. Pinellia breaks up phlegm. Oyster shell sedates and calms the body, and especially keeps the emotional energies normally contained in the liver from overheating and aggravating fever. Ginger counteracts any potential toxicity from pinellia, while licorice harmonizes the effects of all the herbs together.

The medically defined conditions most commonly treated with this formula include sweating, swelling, thirst, and urinary difficulty during premenstrual syndrome. It is also used to treat chills caused by malaria.

When this formula is used in tea form, the oyster shell should be boiled for between thirty and forty-five minutes before the other ingredients are added. This formula should be avoided during pregnancy.

Bupleurum Decoction to Clear the Liver / SAIKO-SEIKAN-TO

This formula contains bupleurum, burdock, forsythia, gardenia, ledebouriella, licorice, ligusticum, red peony, raw rehmannia, scutellaria, snake gourd (trichosanth) root, and tang-kuei.

It is designed for a symptom pattern that includes bad breath, the coughing up of thick sputum, flushed cheeks, severe headache, hearing loss, insomnia, irritability, and dark urine associated with pelvic infection or inflammation, or with menstrual irregularity.

This formula is a gentle variation on Gentiana Longdancao Decoction to Drain the Liver (see page 122). Unlike the gentian formula—which has a potent action on infections, and the fevers and irritation they cause, by moving them down through the urinary tract—the bupleurum decoction deals with symptoms that move up in the body to cause sores on the head. It can relieve "clumps" of fire in the upper parts of the body to stop headache, redness in the face, ringing in the ears, and irritability. Bupleurum especially disperses heat associated with emotional tension, or liver energy in Oriental medicine. While bupleurum stops upward-moving fire, the formula uses gardenia and scutellaria in smaller amounts to stop downward-moving fire. Other herbs in the formula promote urination, which also carries away body heat.

The medically defined condition most commonly treated with this formula is insomnia generated by constant emotional stress. Chinese physicians also use this formula to treat other conditions, including children's inner ear infections; eczema; herpesvirus infections, including shingles (herpes zoster); pelvic inflammatory disease, in which the fallopian tubes become inflamed; yeast infections; eye diseases, including acute glaucoma, central retinitis, conjunctivitis, corneal ulcers, and uveitis when accompanied by emotional stress; the testicular inflammations epididymitis and orchitis; gallstones; hyperthyroidism; and intercostal neuralgia, or nerve pain between the ribs.

This formula should be avoided during pregnancy.

Bupleurum Plus Dragon Bone and Oyster Shell Decoction / SAIKO-KA-RYUKOTSU-BOREI-TO

This formula contains bupleurum, cinnamon bark, dragon bone, fresh ginger, ginseng, hoelen, jujube fruit, pinellia, oyster shell, rhubarb root, and scutellaria. Traditionally, it also included minium (lead oxide), but this toxic substance is no longer included by manufacturers in either Japan or the United States.

This formula is designed for a symptom pattern that includes constipation, delirious speech, inability to rotate the trunk, sensation of fullness in the chest, and a feeling of heaviness throughout the body.

Traditional Kampo viewed the chief ingredients of the formula—bupleurum, cinnamon bark, and scutellaria—as being able to collect or "bottle up" the pathogenic influence that caused the symptoms. The heavy compounds in the formula—dragon bone, oyster shell, and, in the original formulation, lead—were thought to weigh down and calm the floating spirit. Ginseng and hoelen restored the circulation of fluids, relieving any sense of heaviness throughout the rest of the body. The other herbs were thought to provide support.

Bupleurum Plus Dragon Bone and Oyster Shell Decoction is used to treat nervous persons who suffer from arteriosclerosis, in which cholesterol deposits form in the middle of the artery wall. The formula increases the ratio of high density lipoprotein (HDL), or artery-clearing "good" cholesterol, to low-density lipoprotein (LDL), or artery-blocking "bad" cholesterol,[1] while reducing the nervous tension that may contribute to high blood pressure.

In Japan, this formula is used to treat migraines caused by environmental stresses, such as weather changes, noise, allergens, and drafts. Clinical tests show that it acts in the brain by destroying toxins called free radicals. These free radicals play a role in the formation of a hormone called $5HT_1$, which causes constriction of the cerebral vein and results in excruciating pain.[2] This formula's ability to support brain function also allows it to help people with Alzheimer's disease, anxiety, depression, and memory loss.

Kampo physicians use this formula to treat anxiety, insomnia, palpitations, and other signs of nervous tension in persons of robust constitution, and arteriosclerosis in persons suffering from these symptoms. The formula is also used by Kampo practitioners in China to treat A-V block, in which stimulating nerve impulses do not reach the heart; gastritis; hyperthyroidism; a hearing disorder called Ménière's disease; postconcussion syndrome; schizophrenia; spasm of the sternocleidomastoid muscle, a muscle that allows the spine to flex; and symptoms of menopause.

When this formula is used in tea form, the dragon bone and oyster shell should be boiled for between thirty and forty-five minutes before the other ingredients are added. Use with caution if fever is present, and discontinue if preexisting fevers worsen.

Calm the Middle Powder / ANCHU-SAN

This formula contains cardamom, cinnamon twig, corydalis, fennel seed, galangal, licorice, and oyster shell. Chinese-made patent medicines based on this formula often add hoelen.

Like Minor Construct the Middle Decoction (see page 128), a closely related formula, this formula "constructs," or builds up, energy in the middle of the body in a "minor," or gentle, manner.

It is designed for a symptom pattern that includes intermittent, spasmodic abdominal pain when the stomach is empty. There may also be dry mouth and throat, slight fever, and nonspecific discomfort in the hands and feet. The patient is usually thin and has poor muscle tone.

The chief ingredient in this formula, cinnamon twig, disperses cold from the stomach, whether in the form of excessive consumption of cold or raw foods, excessive consumption of fatty foods, food poisoning, or consumption of indigestible foods. Cardamom and galangal amplify the warming effect of cinnamon. Corydalis activates the circulation of energy, and thereby stops abdominal pain. Licorice works with fennel seed to stop spasmodic abdominal pain and gas.

The corydalis in this formula may prevent the spread of certain kinds of cancers.

The medically defined condition most commonly treated with this formula is irritable bowel syndrome. Kampo practitioners also use it to treat other conditions, including inflammatory bowel disease, chronic hepatitis, ulcers, chronic kidney inflammation, fevers of unknown origin, gastritis, leukemia, pernicious anemia, and hypoglycemia, or low blood-sugar levels.

When this formula is used in tea form, the oyster shell should be boiled for between thirty and forty-five minutes before the other ingredients are added.

Calm the Stomach Powder / HEII-SAN

This formula contains white atractylodis, bitter orange peel, honey-fried licorice, and magnolia bark.

It is designed for a symptom pattern that includes acid regurgitation, belching, distention and fullness in the pit of the stomach and abdomen, heavy sensation in the limbs, increased desire for sleep, loose stools or diarrhea, loss of appetite, loss of the sense of taste, nausea, and vomiting. All four herbs in the formula act directly on these symptoms.

The medical conditions most commonly treated with this formula include chronic fatigue with loss of appetite and constant desire to sleep, and peptic ulcer. Kampo practitioners also use it to treat gastroenteritis, or inflammation of the stomach and intestines, and to induce labor.

Since this formula can induce labor, it should not be used during pregnancy.

Capital Qi Pill / TOKI-GAN

This formula contains alisma, Cornelian cherry, dioscorea,

hoelen, moutan, cooked rehmannia, and schisandra. It is Six-Ingredient Pill with Rhemannia (see page 134) modified by the addition of schisandra.

This formula is designed for a symptom pattern of chronic wheezing in which the person is always short of breath and wheezing begins after very little exertion.

Schisandra, the principal herb, relieves wheezing. The other herbs in the formula act in groups of three to reinforce this effect. Rehmannia and its deputies, Cornelian cherry and dioscorea, stabilize the body's "essence," protecting the reproductive system from damage by the other three herbs, alisma, hoelen, and moutan, which drain fluids out of the body. Together, these seven herbs treat a symptom pattern that can include soreness and weakness in the lower back, dizziness, diminished hearing, ringing in the ears, chronic sore throat, and toothache, all aggravating asthma.

The medically defined condition most commonly treated with this formula is asthma brought on by physical exertion. Because the diuretic trio of alisma, hoelen, and schisandra reduces sweating, Capital Qi Pill is also used to treat night sweats caused by Hodgkin's disease.

Cimicifuga and Kudzu Decoction / SHOMA-KAKKON-TO

This formula contains black cohosh (also known by its botanical name, cimicifuga), kudzu, honey-fried licorice, and red peony.

It is designed for a symptom pattern that includes rashes which do not spread evenly, such as those caused by measles; cough; fever and chills; generalized body ache; headache; red eyes; sneezing; and tearing.

Black cohosh is the traditional Japanese remedy for rashes, while kudzu treats muscle pain and tightness. Red peony restores normal circulation of blood and other fluids, relieving bloodshot eyes. Licorice harmonizes the effects of the other herbs.

The medically defined condition most commonly treated with this formula is bloodshot eyes caused by allergy. Kampo practitioners also use it to treat other conditions, including influenza, measles, and scarlet fever.

Cinnamon and Peony Decoction / KEISHI-KA-SHAKUYAKU-TO

This formula contains cinnamon twig, fresh ginger, jujube fruit, honey-fried licorice, and peony. It is Cinnamon Twig Decoction (see page 116) modified by doubling the dosage of peony. Traditionally, this formula was used when its symptom pattern had been misdiagnosed, and the patient was mistakenly treated with purgatives.

Cinnamon and Peony Decoction is designed for a symptom pattern that includes aversion to wind, chills, dry heaves, fever that is not relieved by sweating, headache, and stiffness in the neck and shoulders. Unlike some symptom patterns that include fever, there is no unusual thirst in this pattern.

The medically defined conditions most commonly treated with this formula include nasal allergy compounded by a feeling of fullness in the chest, and colds that have caused chest congestion. Additionally, Kampo practitioners use the formula to treat "weak" constipation, in which a long-term illness has sapped the patient's energy and taken away the ability to pass stools.

Cinnamon Twig and Poria Pill / KEISHI-BUKURYO-GAN

This formula contains cinnamon twig, hoelen (also known as poria), moutan, peach seed, and peony.

It is designed for a symptom pattern of mild, persistent bleeding of purple or dark blood during pregnancy, accompanied by abdominal pain that increases with pressure. It also is used for abdominal spasms, immobile masses in the lower abdomen with pain and tenderness, and menstrual irregularity.

Cinnamon Twig and Poria Pill is an unusual formula in that it stops uterine bleeding by increasing, rather than decreasing, blood circulation. The idea was that if blood was obstructed from its normal pathways, it could have two undesirable effects. Blood stasis could cause abdominal spasms and tension, amenorrhea, dysmenorrhea, and uterine masses, and blood trapped behind the stasis could "leak," causing uterine bleeding.

Cinnamon and hoelen reduce the stasis of blood by stimulating circulation. Hoelen encourages blood to flow downward in the body, encouraging normal circulation to the heart. Since the heart was thought to house the spirit, hoelen lifted the spirits of the patient. Peony, usually white peony, stopped spasms and relieved abdominal pain. Moutan and peach seed reduce fixed uterine masses and aid in upward circulation of blood. Because the herbs are bitter, the formula was usually taken as a pill made with honey. Chinese authors of Kampo reference works regard the honey itself as an "herbal" agent, ensuring that the herbs reach their desired locations in the body.

Modern Japanese doctors use this formula to treat "blood effusion," marked by acne and feelings of blood rushing to the head, red face, or coughing with copious phlegm. They use the formula to treat acne in both men and women, but especially that accompanying menstrual irregularities. The formula is also used to treat "blood effusive chills," colds in which there is a feeling of blood rushing to the head with red face and cough with copious phlegm. Japanese physicians only give the formula to persons who have a robust, or *jitsu-sho,* constitution.

Research has confirmed the traditional use of Cinnamon Twig and Poria Pill for disorders of the female reproductive tract. Laboratory studies have found that it reduces bloodstream estrogen levels by inhibiting the production of DNA in the ovaries.[1] Estrogen inhibition reduces the growth of breast cancers that respond to estrogen, and makes tamoxifen, a drug often used in these types of tumors, more effective. Estrogen inhibition may also have an effect on some forms of melanoma and on uterine cancer. In endometriosis, a disorder in which the tissue that lines the uterus settles elsewhere in the body, estrogen inhibition reduces the rate at which this tissue grows. It similarly slows the development of ovarian cysts and uterine fibroids. The formula has been found in laboratory studies to stop the growth of uterine fibroids without interfering with the menstrual cycle or causing weight gain.[2]

Cinnamon Twig and Poria Pill is also useful in treating reproductive problems in men, especially those caused by variocele, or varicose veins that affect the spermatic cord. The formula improves circulation in the lower abdominal region and reduces blood retention. In Japanese clinical studies, it causes a remission from variocele in about 80 percent of cases, and also increases sperm count and sperm motility.[3] Traditionally, this formula is given to men who are "warm-natured," that is, those who prefer cold temperatures to warm temperatures, and who have a tendency to muscle strain. Such men are subject to variocele.

Cinnamon Twig and Poria Pill shows promise in treating the skin disorder scleroderma. Japanese scientists have found that the formula stops collagen formation in scleroderma cells but not in normal cells.[4] The formula also prevents free-radical damage to brain tissue deprived of oxygen, as in cerebral arteriosclerosis or stroke.[5]

The medically defined conditions most commonly treated with this formula include acne, colds, breast cancer and fibrocystic breast disease, uterine cancer and fibroids, ovarian cysts, melanoma, endometriosis and menstrual problems, and both female and male infertility.

Cinnamon Twig Decoction / KEISHI-TO

This formula contains cinnamon twig, fresh ginger, jujube fruit, honey-fried licorice, and peony. It contains the core ingredients for a large number of formulas that add from one to three other herbs to treat individual variations in symptom patterns. Among the formulas that use Cinnamon Twig Decoction for their base are Cinnamon and Peony Decoction, Cinnamon Twig Decoction Plus Dragon Bone and Oyster Shell, and Cinnamon Twig Decoction Plus Kudzu (see 115 and right).

Cinnamon Twig Decoction is designed for a symptom pattern that includes aversion to wind, chills, dry heaves, fever that is not relieved by sweating, headache, and stiffness in the neck and shoulders. Unlike some symptom patterns that include fever, there is no unusual thirst.

Traditional Kampo regarded the chief herb of the formula, cinnamon, as a means of releasing cold that had invaded the muscle layer of the body. The deputy herb, peony, combines with cinnamon to release tight muscles, and also provides nutritive energy. Ginger eases nausea and vomiting, while jujube fruit and licorice harmonize the other herbs.

The medically defined conditions most commonly treated with this formula include allergies (including hives), eczema, and upper respiratory tract infections. Kampo practitioners also use it to treat angioedema (giant hives), and blood-vessel spasms in the brain that can cause either migraine or a temporary strokelike condition called transient ischemic attack. It is also used to accelerate recovery from childbirth.

Cinnamon Twig Decoction Plus Dragon Bone and Oyster Shell / KEISHI-KA-RYUKOTSU-BOREI-TO

This formula contains cinnamon twig, dragon bone, fresh ginger, jujube fruit, licorice, oyster shell, and peony. It is a variation of Cinnamon Twig Decoction (see left).

This formula was traditionally used to treat excessive sexual desire in women, and dizziness, hair loss, insomnia, lack of sensation in the glans penis, and watery diarrhea in men.

This formula corrects deficiencies and imbalances of both yin (holding energies) and yang (exerting energies). In the associated symptom pattern, the body has too little yin energy overall but too much yin above the kidneys. This excess holding energy creates high blood pressure, hot flashes, blushing, emotional outbursts, or even seizures. The yin deficiency below the kidneys leads to excessive urination and a failure of the penis to contain blood (what Western medicine calls impotence). At a deeper level, this formula addresses a lack of communication between the kidneys, which carry the person's genetic heritage, and the heart, which is the seat of emotional experience.

The medically defined condition most commonly treated with this formula today is hair loss in men, especially when accompanied by "kidney" symptoms such as lower back pain, insomnia, watery diarrhea, dizziness, and lack of sensation in the penis. This formula tends to restore hair lost on the sides of the head, but not on the top. The formula can be used by both men and women in robust health who have insomnia accompanied by depression, dream-filled sleep, feelings of frustration, and palpitations.

When this formula is used in tea form, the dragon bone and oyster shell should be boiled for between thirty and forty-five minutes before the other ingredients are added.

Cinnamon Twig Decoction Plus Kudzu / KEISHI-KAKKON-TO

This formula contains cinnamon twig, fresh ginger, jujube fruit, kudzu, honey-fried licorice, and peony. It is a modification of Cinnamon Twig Decoction (see left); kudzu is added to treat patients for whom muscular stiffness is the most troubling symptom.

This formula is designed for a symptom pattern that occurs in the early stages of upper respiratory infection, including sensitivity to wind, stiff neck and upper back, and sweating.

The medically defined conditions most commonly treated with this formula include headache with stiffness in the neck or back.

Cinnamon Twig, Licorice, Dragon Bone, and Oyster Shell Decoction / KEISHI-KANZO-RYUKOTSU-BOREI-TO

This formula contains cinnamon twig, dragon bone, honey-fried licorice, and oyster shell. It is not available as a patent medicine, but is widely available as a prescription from practitioners of Kampo and TCM. The Chinese name is *gui zhi gan cao long gu mu li.*

Kampo originally used this formula to counteract the effects of improper acupuncture resulting in "false fire syndrome," in which the "heart" became deprived of yin and was no longer able to contain the emotions. This formula is also used for any disorder in which the "spirit drifts upward," causing irritability, palpitation, restlessness, and spontaneous utterances, such as unintentional speech, moaning, or crying. Cinnamon restores the yang, or outwardly directed, energies of the body, allowing actions and emotions that should be expressed outwardly to leave the body in normal channels. The heavy ingredients of the formula, dragon bone and oyster shell, weigh down the spirit so it stays in the heart, where it will not produce nervous symptoms.

Kampo uses this formula primarily to treat misplaced energies of the yang layers of the body (see Chapter 1), especially irritability with spontaneous sweating. Chinese patent medicines based on the formula usually quintuple the doses of dragon bone and oyster to increase the formula's calming effect.

The medically defined conditions most commonly treated with this formula include headache, diarrhea, impotence, menstrual problems, sinusitis, hair loss, and seizures.

When this formula is used in tea form, the dragon bone and oyster shell should be boiled for between thirty and forty-five minutes before the other ingredients are added.

Clear Summerheat and Augment the Qi Decoction / SEISHO-EKKI-TO

This formula contains American ginseng, anemarrhena, dry-fried coptis, dendrobium, Japanese watermelon rind, licorice, lophatherum, lotus (hooks from the stem), ophiopogon, and a thin rice porridge. As the inclusion of American ginseng (a recent introduction to Kampo) suggests, this formula was only recorded in 1852 by the Chinese Kampo master Wang Meng-Ying.

This formula is designed for a symptom pattern that includes apathy, fever, profuse sweating, scanty and dark urine, shortness of breath, and thirst.

Traditional Japanese medicine thought of summerheat as an external force that could enter the interior of the body and then "steam" outward through the pores of the skin. Summerheat caused loss of fluids, which led to intense thirst and a desire to curl up rather than extend the body normally.

The chief herb in this formula is American ginseng. Like Korean or red ginseng, American ginseng builds up body energy (qi), generates fluids, and nourishes the containing, or yin, energies of the body. Unlike Korean ginseng, American ginseng does so without overheating the body, and instead helps clear heat from summertime infection from the body. Watermelon rind also clears heat and is aided by lotus. Anemarrhena and lopthatherum stop irritability and thirst. Coptis is a cold herb that can put out "fires," keeping the underlying condition from worsening while the other herbs act.

The medically defined conditions most commonly treated with this formula include fevers, heat exhaustion, and infections of the upper respiratory tract. Kampo physicians have experimented with this formula in the treatment of HIV, since it contains the HIV-fighter dendrobium (see Chapter 3), and does not include any herbs which are known to directly stimulate the immune system.

This formula should not be used for fevers and upper respiratory infection accompanied by an upset stomach.

Coptis Decoction to Relieve Toxicity / OREN-GEDOKU-TO

This formula contains dry-fried coptis, gardenia, phellodendron, and scutellaria. It is designed for a symptom pattern that includes dark urine, high fever, and irritability.

The traditional understanding of this formula was that the coptis in it removed fire from the heart, and in so doing relieved symptoms of infection, or toxicity, throughout the body. Scutellaria was thought to remove heat from the upper reaches of the lymphatic system, called the upper burner, and phellodendron was thought to remove heat from the lower part of the body, or the lower burner. Gardenia drained heat from the body through the urine. Once heat was removed from the body, toxins were thought to disappear.

Coptis Decoction to Relieve Toxicity has numerous applications in modern Japanese medicine. It is used to treat insomnia in persons with "blood effusive" symptoms: redness in the face, a feeling of blood rushing to head, high blood pressure, and possibly chronic constipation. It lowers blood pressure and reduces the likelihood of the formation of blood clots, and increases blood flow to the brain.[1] It is more effective than conventional antibiotics in treating bacterial infections that cause acne.[2] It is a proven destroyer of free radicals, harmful chemicals that damage cells. This protects brain tissue and memory from the effects of inadequate oxygen supply after stroke,[3] and makes the formula useful in Alzheimer's disease and certain forms of depression. This formula is used to treat arteriosclerosis, commonly called hardening of the arteries; conjuctivitis, infection of the eye's surface and/or the inner eyelid; and gingivitis, or gum inflammation. It protects the lining of the stomach,[4] and kills *Helicobacter pylori,* a bacterium that converts nitrates in food to cancer-causing chemicals[5] and which has been linked to peptic-ulcer formation. It treats yeast infections aggravated by diabetes, especially thrush and esophageal infections causing heartburn.[6] The formula contains berberine, which prevents the multiplication of cancerous cells in digestive tract cancers.[7,8] It is also used by Kampo practitioners to treat anxiety resulting in delirious speech with "hot symptoms," such as bleeding from the nose or gums, fever, headaches, and redness in the neck and face. In addition, it is used for boils and other toxic swellings, dysentery due to hepatitis, and nosebleed.

Because gardenia contains a compound that can cause early-pregnancy abortion, this formula should not be used by women who are trying to become pregnant.

Drive Out Stasis From the Mansion of Blood Decoction / KEPPU-CHIKUO-TO

This formula contains raw amaranth, whole bitter orange, bupleurum, carthamus, licorice, ligusticum, peach seed, platycodon, red peony, cooked rehmannia, and tang-kuei. This formula's vivid name is a direct translation from the Chinese, and is the one most commonly used in English. At one time, the "mansion" was an area above the diaphragm. In a larger sense, the mansion of blood includes the vessels in which blood gathers and moves.

This formula is designed for a symptom pattern that includes a choking sensation when drinking, chronic hiccups, dark or purplish lips or facial complexion, depression, dry heaves, evening fever, insomnia, irritability, mood swings, chest pain, restless sleep, and chronic, piercing headache.

In this symptom pattern, blood does not flow downward from the diaphragm. At the same time, emotional energies become bottled up within the liver, amplifying the imbalance. Clearing energies cannot rise from the kidneys to the head, and the result is a stubborn headache. Since the flows of both blood and energy are obstructed, the headache is in a fixed position and is especially resistant to painkillers. In the worst cases, these obstructions press against the stomach, forcing food upward. As a result, there may be vomiting or hiccups. The herbs in the formula act to clear these obstructions.

The medically defined conditions most commonly treated with this formula include depression accompanied by extreme psychosomatic symptoms, or symptoms of psychological origin, generally those found in the traditional pattern. It is particularly useful for depression accompanied by migraine headaches. Kampo practitioners also use this formula to treat hives; high blood pressure; costochondritis, an inflammation of the rib cage; postconcussion headache; menopausal symptoms; trigeminal and intercostal neuralgia, nerve pain in the face and between the ribs; and a number of heart conditions, including cor pulmonale, coronary artery disease, and rheumatic valvular heart disease.

Eight-Ingredient Pill With Rehmannia (Rehmannia-Eight Combination) / HACHIMI-JIO-GAN

This formula contains alisma, honey-fried astragalus, Cornelian cherry, dioscorea, hoelen, moutan, cooked rehmannia, and schisandra.

Eight-Ingredient Pill with Rehmannia was formulated in the nineteenth century to address the same symptom pattern as the centuries-older Six-Ingredient Pill with Rehmannia (see page 134): dizziness, light-headedness, night sweats, ringing in the ears or diminished hearing, and soreness and weakness in the lower back. Unlike the six-ingredient formula, this formula is especially designed to reduce sweating.

In this formula, schisandra keeps the patient from breaking out in a cold sweat, while alisma relieves fluid accumulations in the inner ear. The other six herbs work in the same way as in Six-Ingredient Pill with Rhemannia.

Recent research has shown that Eight-Ingredient Pill with Rehmannia has applications far beyond the symptom pattern for which it was designed, especially in the treatment of diabetes. In fact, it has become one of the most popular herbal diabetes treatments in Japan. The formula aids insulin regulation, and halts the progress of diabetic nerve damage in insulin-dependent diabetes. It smoothes out the effects of insulin by giving the patient tighter control of blood-sugar levels. This prevents eye and circulation problems,[1] although the formula will not reduce the amount of insulin needed.

The formula has long been recognized for its ability to prevent the formation of diabetic cataracts. It acts by inhibiting the enzyme aldose reductase, which converts the glucose forced into the lens by high blood-sugar levels into sorbitol, a potent toxin.[2] It also restores the proper balance of sodium, potassium, and calcium, which helps keep the lens transparent.[3] Laboratory tests indicate that the use of Eight-Ingredient Pill With Rehmannia can delay the development of cataracts by ten to fifteen years. The formula is also useful for relieving symptoms caused by Alzheimer's disease, other forms of memory loss, arteriosclerosis, hyperthyroidism, and prostate problems, although it should be used with caution in the treatment of enlarged prostate (see **Prostate Enlargement, Benign** in Part Two). This formula should be avoided altogether in cases of prostate cancer, as it increases testosterone production.[4]

Emperor of Heaven's Special Pill to Tonify the Heart / TEN'NOHOSHIN-TAN

This formula contains asparagus root, biota, dan shen, red ginseng, hoelen, Japanese mint, ophiopogon, platycodon, cooked rehmannia, schisandra, scrophularia, tang-kuei, and zizyphus. Codonopsis is often substituted for Korean or red ginseng. Traditionally, herbalists fashioned these herbs into pills and then rolled the pills in a dusting of cinnabar, or mercuric oxide, powder. Patent medicines based on this formula for sale in North America do not use the potentially toxic cinnabar.

This formula gets its name from the seventeenth-century author of *Secret Investigations Into Obtaining Health,* who wrote that it came to him in a dream from the emperor of heaven.

It is designed for a symptom pattern that includes insomnia, irritability, poor concentration, short-term memory loss, racing pulse, and "dry" symptoms, such as constipation and dry throat.

Kampo explains this formula, which has been used for more than 300 years, in terms of bolstering the essence of the individual. When essence has become depleted by excessive thinking, deliberation, or too much reading, the body can no longer provide energy that moves upward from the kidneys to the heart, which in Kampo is the emotional center. Deficiencies of essence can result in wind, in which symptoms move from one part of the body to another, and memory falters. All of the herbs in the formula address this deficiency in essence.

The medically defined conditions most commonly treated with this formula include insomnia, memory loss, and constipation.

Do not use this formula if there is loss of appetite or diarrhea, or if there are aches and pains from influenza.

Ephedra Decoction (Four Emperors Combination) / MAO-TO

This formula contains apricot seed, cinnamon bark, ephedra, and honey-fried licorice. It is designed for a symptom pattern that includes fever and chills, with chills predominating; generalized body aches; headache; and wheezing.

The ancient sages of Kampo described the action of this formula as enabling the qi, or vital energy, to break out of an energy prison built by an invading pernicious influence. The pernicious influence, which Westerners would understand as an allergen or pathogen, kept the protective energies of the body bottled up below the skin, so the skin itself became clammy and cold to the touch. Cold closed the pores and prevented sweating. Imbalance in defensive energies caused imbalance in digestive energies, producing generalized body aches. The blockade of energy in the exterior of the body caused energy to build up in the lungs, which used this energy to tighten airways, resulting in wheezing.

In the traditional understanding of this formula, the chief herb, ephedra, encourages sweating and stops wheezing. Warming cinnamon also encourages sweating, and facilitates the flow of energy through the lung. This opens airways and provides the pathogenic influence with a way out of the body. Licorice keeps ephedra and cinnamon from causing the patient to sweat too heavily.

Research shows that Ephedra Decoction not only treats the symptoms of colds, but can keep colds from spreading when used at the earliest stages of infection.[1] Research has also found that this formula can prevent skin injury caused by ultraviolet radiation from the sun.[2,3]

The medically defined conditions most commonly treated with this formula include asthma, bronchitis, colds, and flu. Many Kampo practitioners in the United States consider this formula to be essential for treating asthma, although Japanese physicians are more likely to use variations of the formula which correct more specific symptoms (see **Asthma** in Part Two). Kampo physicians in both countries use this formula in the early stages of rheumatoid arthritis to relieve swelling and pain, especially if symptoms are worse in cold weather.

There is evidence that Ephedra Decoction can be used to treat tonsillitis and stomatitis, or inflammation of the mouth. Kampo practitioners also use this formula to treat lobar pneumonia and a kidney inflammation called acute glomerulonephritis.

To avoid ill effects from eating apricot seeds, use this formula in patent-medicine form.

Ephedra, Apricot Kernel, Gypsum, and Licorice Decoction / MA-KYO-KAN-SEKI-TO

This formula contains, as the name suggests, apricot seed, ephedra, gypsum, and licorice. This is a gentler version of Ephedra Decoction (see left), in which warming cinnamon is replaced by cooling gypsum.

This formula is designed for a symptom pattern that includes cough, fever (with or without sweating), labored breathing, nasal flaring and pain, rapid pulse, sneezing, and thirst.

The medically defined conditions most commonly treated with this formula include asthma and infections of the upper respiratory tract. Kampo practitioners also use it to treat various other types of respiratory problems, including pneumonia, diphtheria, and pertussis, or whooping cough.

When this formula is used in tea form, the gypsum should be boiled for between thirty and forty-five minutes before the other ingredients are added. Actually, it is a good idea to use this formula in patent-medicine form, so as to avoid ill effects from eating apricot seeds (see Chapter 3). Do not use this formula if nausea or vomiting is present.

Ephedra, Asiasarum, and Prepared Aconite Decoction / MAO-BUSHIN-SASHIN-TO

This formula contains asiasarum, ephedra, and prepared aconite. It is designed for a symptom pattern that includes exhaustion, fever without sweating, and a sensation of severe cold or chills. These chills are relieved by adding layers of clothing or lying under covers.

Many Kampo formulas treat disease by "sweating out" the outside pernicious influence causing disease. This formula is designed to rout disease without overheating the body, especially in cases in which the patient's energies have become seriously depleted, and in which diverting energy into fever would harm the inner organs. Ephedra disperses exterior cold that keeps the pathogen inside the body, as it gives the body a passageway through which to expel the infection. Aconite stimulates the body's outward-directed, yang energies, and accelerates the elimination of the pathogen. Asiasarum disperses interior cold that also keeps the pathogen inside the body, and directs the other herbs to the energy channels most affected by long-term disease.

Despite the fact that this formula was created almost 2,000 years ago, it is effective against such modern conditions as allergy to cedar pollen.[1] The formula is most effective when used at the beginning and end of the season, and it cannot overcome the effect of direct exposure to massive amounts of cedar pollen. Still, for millions of sufferers of cedar pollen allergies in Japan and the United States, this formula promises allergy relief without the side effect of drowsiness and without prescription drug interactions. The formula also restores the energy sapped from the body by allergy or asthma, which corrects laryngitis, sore throat, and chronic wheezing.

If taking this formula as a tea, boil the aconite for thirty to sixty minutes before adding any other ingredients to reduce any potential toxins in the aconite. Both teas and patent medicines may cause a loss of sensation in the mouth and tongue, which is not a sign to discontinue the formula. Fever, on the other hand, is a sign to discontinue the formula.

Evodia Decoction / GOSHUYU-TO

This formula contains evodia, fresh ginger, ginseng, and jujube fruit. It is designed for three different symptom patterns: diarrhea and vomiting with cold hands and feet, dry heaves or spitting of clear fluids with headache at the crown of the head, and vomiting immediately after eating with acid regurgitation.

Evodia and ginger stop vomiting. Ginseng strengthens digestion, while jujube fruit makes the formula more palatable.

The medically defined condition most commonly treated with this formula is migraine, especially since migraine is often accompanied by vomiting. Kampo practitioners in China also use it to treat other conditions, including inflammations of the gallbladder, stomach, and intestines; high blood pressure; a hearing problem called Ménière's disease; morning sickness; and trigeminal neuralgia, or facial nerve pain.

Five-Accumulation Powder / GOSHAKU-SAN

The formula contains angelica dahurica, red atractylodis, bitter orange, bitter orange peel, cinnamon bark, ephedra, dried ginger, hoelen, licorice, ligusticum, magnolia bark, peony, pinellia, platycodon, and tang-kuei. What Kampo calls the five accumulations—of blood, cold, dampness, qi, and phlegm—are relieved by this formula.

It is designed for a symptom pattern that includes abdominal pain, aversion to food, body aches, diarrhea with rumbling noises, feelings of fullness in the abdomen and chest, fever and chills without sweating, headache, stiffness in the back and neck, and vomiting.

Two of the chief herbs, angelica dahurica and ephedra, release cold from the exterior of the body. The other two chief herbs, cinnamon bark and ginger, expel cold from the interior. Other herbs in the formula treat accumulations of blood, dampness, energy, or phlegm.

The medically defined condition most commonly treated with this formula is diarrhea. Kampo practitioners also use it to treat other conditions, including mild gastritis and upper respiratory tract infection. It is particularly useful for treating colds in people who are especially fatigued by catching cold, and whose neck muscles tighten during colds. Use with caution if fever is present, and discontinue if preexisting fevers worsen.

Five-Ingredient Powder With Poria / GOREI-SAN

This formula contains alisma, white atractylodis, cinnamon bark, hoelen (also known as poria), and polyporus.

This formula is used for three overlapping symptom patterns. In the first, there is fever, headache, irritability, strong thirst but with vomiting immediately after drinking, and difficulty in urination. In the second, there is diarrhea, excessive fluid accumulation, generalized sensation of heaviness throughout the body, and vomiting. In the third, there is cough, shortness of breath, vertigo, and vomiting of frothy saliva.

In the understanding of traditional Kampo, the first symptom pattern indicates the existence of excessive fluids. The outside pernicious influence, or pathogen, has penetrated to the level of the bladder, disrupting its functions and causing urinary difficulty and water retention. When fluids cannot be transported down through the bladder, they are vomited up. In TCM, this is known as water rebellion disorder.

The second group of symptoms are caused by digestion deficiencies, which lead to difficulties in water transport. Water and dampness overflow into the muscles and accumulate under the skin, producing edema and a feeling of heaviness. The body's failure to transport water also affects the lymphatic system, and thus disease can progress deeper into the body. The normal energy flows through the stomach and intestines are reversed, giving rise to spontaneous vomiting and diarrhea. In TCM, this is known as sudden turmoil disorder.

The third group of symptoms is caused by a congestion of fluids in the lymphatic system. Congestion causes a throbbing sensation below the navel. As in the first set of symptoms, stagnation caused by congested fluids can force an upward rebellion in the form of frothy vomiting. Since the yang, or outwardly directed, energies that power the muscles are also trapped in the lower half of the body, the muscles that hold the body upright are inadequately powered, resulting in vertigo. If so much fluid accumulates that it encroaches on the lungs, the result may be shortness of breath or coughing.

Alisma is chief herb in this formula. Cold and sweet, alisma puts out heat in the bladder (which can result from the body's reaction to a "cold" infectious agent reaching the bladder). Hoelen promotes urination and activates the yang, defensive energies of the body to expel the infectious agent. White atractylodis helps the digestive system process fluids, and cinnamon twig "provides wood for the fire under the cauldron of the kidneys"[1] to make "steam" and raise fluids in the body. Cinnamon twig also dispels pathogenic influences from the exterior of the body (see Chapter 1).

In scientific terms, this formula acts by decreasing the number of adhesion cells in the kidneys,[2] which stimulates urination, and by reducing the amount of fluid eliminated through the intestines.

Five-Ingredient Powder With Poria is used to treat glaucoma. In a Chinese study, fifty-five glaucoma patients were given the formula, and 63 percent of them experienced reductions in eye pressure within the first month of use.[3] The formula also relieves Ménière's disease, a hearing disorder associated with tinnitus and dizziness, caused by trauma or fever. In addition, this formula is part of a combination formula called *sairei-to.*

The medically defined conditions most commonly treated with this formula include diarrhea with vomiting and difficulty in urination, glaucoma, and Ménière's disease. Kampo practitioners also use Five-Ingredient Powder With Poria to treat various stomach disorders; abdominal fluid accumulations associated with liver cirrhosis; genitourinary infections; hepatitis; hydrocele, or fluid in the scrotum; kidney inflammation; and neurogenic bladder syndrome, in which nerve damage impairs bladder function.

Four-Gentleman Decoction / Shikunshi-to

This formula contains white atractylodis, ginseng, hoelen, and honey-fried licorice. Many Chinese-made patent medicines substitute the cheaper codonopsis for ginseng, although American- and Japanese-made patent medicines usually do not. The patent medicines in Appendix A all contain ginseng.

In Confucian cultures, it was common to refer to things that were important and that could be grouped together harmoniously as "gentlemen," after the Confucian term for a person who exhibits ideal behavior. The four herbs in this formula are mild and blend well together, and are therefore called the "four gentlemen" of Kampo.

This formula is designed for a symptom pattern that fits the classic *kyo-sho,* or deficient constitution: pale complexion, loose stools, low and soft voice, reduced appetite, and limb weakness.

Kampo designed Four-Gentleman Decoction for digestive deficiencies caused by poor diet, excessive worry and deliberation, and overwork. When the digestive function is deficient, the transformation of food into blood and energy (qi) is impaired. This deficiency manifests itself in acquiescent rather than assertive behavior, soft voice, and pale complexion. When the digestive system lacks the energy to transport food, the result is loose stools or diarrhea. Since (in the Chinese understanding of Kampo) the digestive function governs the limbs, the arms and legs become weak.

The chief herb in this formula for remedying these symptoms is ginseng. Warming and sweet, ginseng is a digestive tonic. Warming and bitter atractylodis also stimulates digestion and gives momentum to the movement of fluids through the proper courses in the digestive system. Hoelen also removes fluids, and assists ginseng and atractylodis. Licorice warms the digestive system and prevent accumulations of fluids from reaching the immune system (known in TCM as the triple burner).

The medically defined conditions most commonly treated with this formula include irritable bowel syndrome and peptic ulcers caused by improper eating habits, excessive alcohol consumption, excessive deliberation or worry, or overwork. Kampo practitioners also use the formula to treat chronic stomach inflammation, diabetes, and uterine fibroids, and to reduce recovery time after surgery. Laboratory studies in Japan have determined that Four-Gentleman Decoction effectively prevents plaque buildup and gingivitis,[1] although it is not appropriate for every symptom pattern involving bleeding gums (see **Bleeding Gums** in Part Two).

Four-Substance Decoction / Shimotsu-to

This formula contains ligusticum, peony, cooked rehmannia, and tang-kuei. It is designed for a symptom pattern, generally seen in women, that includes blurred vision, dizziness, lusterless nails, pallid complexion, and pain around the navel and in the lower abdomen. The patient menstruates irregularly, with little flow, or may not menstruate at all. Historically, the formula is also used to treat hard abdominal masses and restless fetus disorder, in which the baby kicks excessively.

Two of the herbs in this formula, peony and rehmannia, were traditionally known as "blood of the blood" herbs, that is, they help the body create blood. To keep that blood from accumulating as a hard mass if a menstrual period was missed, two herbs that stimulate blood circulation, ligusticum and tang-kuei, were added to the formula.

This formula is an excellent example of TCM's understanding of the treatment of "liver" problems. A normal menstrual cycle depends on the liver to provide and shut off the supply of blood at appropriate times. When the liver sends too little blood into circulation, the menses become scanty or the period is missed. Blood that does not move well becomes static around the navel and in the lower abdomen, causing pain. A deficient liver is also unable to send energy along its energy channel, which supplies the eye. The result is blurred vision and eyestrain. The health of the liver is also reflected in the nails; when liver blood is deficient, the nails become dry, lusterless, and soft.

The medically defined condition most commonly treated with this formula is irregular menstruation. Kampo practitioners also use it to treat other conditions, including hives, insufficient lactation, neurogenic or "nervous" headache, and threatened miscarriage.

Frigid Extremities Decoction / Shigyaku-to

This formula contains prepared aconite, fresh ginger, and honey-fried licorice. The original formula in the *Sho Kan Ron,* one of Kampo's classic texts, called for raw, unprocessed aconite. However, modern Kampo practitioners always use steam-treated aconite.

This formula is designed for a symptom pattern that includes extremely cold hands and feet; abdominal pain; aversion to cold; constant desire to sleep, and to sleep with the knees drawn up; diarrhea with undigested food particles; and a lack of thirst.

Aconite is used to jolt the body's energy processes when they are worn down by long illness. Ginger and licorice moderate and soften the effects of aconite, which can be toxic when used by itself. This formula is reserved for chronic conditions in which the body's internal energy is severely compromised.

The medically defined conditions most commonly treated with this formula include depression with persistent upset stomach, diarrhea, some symptoms of hypothyroidism, and nosebleed. Kampo practitioners use it in heart attack aftercare and to treat inadequate blood supply to the heart. It is also used in stomach and intestinal inflammation that results in diarrhea and vomiting, underactivity of either the pituitary gland or the adrenal glands, and intractable arthritis.

If taking this formula as a tea, boil the aconite for thirty to sixty minutes before adding any other ingredients to reduce any potential toxins in the aconite. Both teas and patent medicines may cause a loss of sensation in the mouth and tongue, which is not a sign to discontinue the formula. Fever, on the other hand, is a sign to discontinue the formula.

Frigid Extremities Powder / SHIGYAKU-SAN

This formula contains bitter orange, bupleurum, honey-fried licorice, and peony. It is a gentler version of Frigid Extremities Decoction (see page 121).

Frigid Extremities Powder is designed for a symptom pattern that includes, as one might expect, coldness in the fingers and toes, and sometimes a sensation of fullness in the chest.

In ancient times it was thought that "a clear yang firms up the four limbs." Yang energy was derived from food, and deficiencies in the energy of the hands and feet were thought to be sometimes caused by digestive problems. Therefore, this formula was, and is, used to treat digestive diseases, such as gallstones and peptic ulcer, especially if the patient also has cold hands or feet.

The medically defined conditions most commonly treated with this formula include gallstones and ulcers. TCM practitioners also use it to treat gallbladder, stomach, or breast inflammations; fibrocystic breast disease, in which benign lumps develop; and hepatitis.

Gastrodia and Uncaria Decoction / TENMA-KOTO-IN

This formula contains abalone shell, amaranth, eucommia, gambir (also known as uncaria), gardenia, gastrodia, hoelen, loranthus, motherwort, polygonum, and scutellaria.

This formula is designed for a symptom pattern that includes dizziness, headache, insomnia or dream-disturbed sleep, numbness, twitching and spasms in the hands and feet, and tinnitus, or a constant ringing in the ears.

Abalone shell, gastrodia, and gambir were thought to extinguish "liver wind," or the energy currents stimulated by pent-up emotions. Gardenia and scutellaria were used to treat fire from infection, and the other herbs in the formula were included to stimulate circulation. The effects of gambir and gastrodia are discussed in their respective Chapter 3 entries.

The medically defined condition most commonly treated with this formula is blurred vision caused by high blood pressure. Kampo practitioners also use it to treat other disorders, including seizure disorders. This formula is most useful in borderline cases of seizure disorder, in which the neurologist allows a patient to accept or decline stronger medications. Prescription drugs often have to build up in the bloodstream to become effective, and easily become ineffective or toxic if even slightly too much or too little of the drug is taken. For this reason, one should *never* abruptly discontinue prescription seizure medication without a doctor's supervision. And because gardenia contains a compound that can cause early-pregnancy abortion, this formula should not be used by women who are trying to become pregnant.

When this formula is used in tea form, the abalone shell should be boiled for between thirty and forty-five minutes before the other ingredients are added.

Gentiana Longdancao Decoction to Drain the Liver / RYUTAN-SHAKAN-TO

This formula contains akebia, alisma, bupleurum, gardenia, gentian, plantain (psyllium seed), raw rehmannia, scutellaria, and tang-kuei. Bupleurum Decoction to Clear the Liver (see page 113) is a variation on this formula.

Gentiana Longdancao Decoction is designed for a symptom pattern that includes bitter taste in the mouth, dizziness, headache, hearing loss, irritability, red and sore eyes, short temper, and swelling in the ears. It is also used to treat difficult or painful urination with a sensation of heat in the urethra. In women, the syndrome treated by this formula often includes a shortened menstrual period with unusually dark blood, and vaginal discharge and irritation.

"Draining the liver" refers to reducing excess heat in the energy channels dominated by the liver and gallbladder. The liver channel passes over the external genitalia and the breasts, and over the eyes. The gallbladder channel is paired with the liver channel, starting at the eyes and crossing the head. When heat is constrained in these channels, it causes fever, inflammation, and swelling. The chief herb used to drain the liver is the formula's namesake, gentian. Gentian is assisted by gardenia and scutellaria, which also stimulate the movement of fluids. Bupleurum is thought to release heat caused by the accumulation of emotional energy. The other herbs in the formula drain heat by stimulating urination, or they protect the body's ability to produce fluids from the overly aggressive action of gentian, gardenia, or scutellaria.

The medically defined conditions most commonly treated with this formula include children's inner ear infections; eczema; herpesvirus infections, including shingles (herpes zoster); pelvic inflammatory disease, in which the fallopian tubes become inflamed; yeast infections; eye diseases, including acute glaucoma, central retinitis, conjunctivitis, corneal ulcers, and uveitis when accompanied by emotional stress; the testicular inflammations epididymitis and orchitis; gallstones; hyperthyroidism; and intercostal neuralgia, or nerve pain between the ribs.

Because gardenia contains a compound that can cause early-pregnancy abortion, this formula should not be used by women who are trying to become pregnant.

Ginseng Decoction to Nourish the Nutritive Qi / NINJIN-YOEI-TO

This formula contains astragalus, white atractylodis, bitter orange peel, Chinese senega root, cinnamon bark, ginseng, hoelen, honey-fried licorice, peony, cooked rehmannia, schisandra, and tang-kuei. It is a variation of Restore the Spleen Decoction (see page 133).

This formula addresses a symptom pattern that includes anxiety, dream-disturbed sleep, forgetfulness, palpitations, and withdrawal from social activity. It also addresses physical symptoms caused by insufficient fluids, such as dry mouth and skin, and sores that will not heal, as well as loss of appetite; fatigue; shortness of breath, especially upon exertion; and a feeling of warmth on the body's surface.

The spleen, which in Oriental medicine is the organ that houses intelligence, was thought to provide energy to the heart, the organ that houses the emotions. When excessive deliberation taxed the spleen's energy, the heart was also deprived of energy, and emotional symptoms resulted. This formula supports the spleen's function.

In Japan, Ginseng Decoction to Restore the Nutritive Qi is used to increase the effectiveness of prednisolone (Pediapred, Prelone),[1] a steroid drug used to treat asthma, cancer symptoms, and lupus, among other diseases.

The medically defined conditions most commonly treated with this formula include anemia, dry mouth and throat, dry skin, forgetfulness, hair loss, jaundice, shortness of breath, sores that will not heal, and tired limbs as symptoms accompanying a wide range of diseases.

Guide Out the Red Powder / DO-SEIKI-SAN

This formula contains akebia, licorice, lophatherum, and raw rehmannia. It is designed for a symptom pattern that includes "red" symptoms, such as irritability with a sensation of heat in the chest, red face and tongue, sores around the mouth, thirst with a desire to drink cold beverages, and dark, painful, rough, or scanty urination.

Kampo practitioners before the modern era thought that this formula worked by cooling the blood and stimulating urination. Rehmannia was thought to enter the heart to cool the blood and to enter the kidneys to generate fluids, which controlled the fire in the heart. Akebia cleared heat from the heart's energy channels and also promoted urination through its stimulation of the small intestine's energy channel. Lophatherum was thought to clear heat from the heart caused by emotional irritability. Licorice soothed rough urination.

The medically defined conditions most commonly treated with this formula include diseases marked by blood in the urine. This includes kidney stones and kidney cancer, for which the formula offers symptomatic relief without affecting the underlying disease. Kampo practitioners also use it to treat nightmares, a mouth inflammation called stomatitis, and the urinary tract disorders cystitis and glomerulonephritis.

Hemp Seed Pill / MASHININ-GAN

This formula contains apricot seed, bitter orange, magnolia bark, marijuana (hemp) seed, peony, and rhubarb root. It is designed for a symptom pattern that includes constipation with hard stool that is difficult to expel, and frequent urination.

The chief herb in this formula is marijuana seed, which is used in Kampo formulas to moisten the intestines and thus relieve dry constipation. The other herbs support the functions of marijuana seed. Apricot moves energy downward in the body. Bitter orange breaks up accumulation, especially in the intestines. Magnolia bark also disperses the accumulated bolus of food. Rhubarb is a purgative. Kampo herbalists traditionally used honey to bind the herbs in Hemp Seed Pill together, and honey was also thought to moisten the intestines.

The medically defined condition most commonly treated with this formula is habitual, postpartum, or postsurgical constipation. Kampo practitioners also use it to treat hemorrhoids.

Under federal law, the inclusion of heat-sterilized marijuana seed (often labeled *linum* or *mai zi ren*) in traditional remedies is legal. Marijuana seed will not produce a "high," but will cause a positive urine test for THC, the high-producing component, although sophisticated testing methods can distinguish use of marijuana seed from that of other plant parts.

To avoid ill effects from eating apricot seeds (see Chapter 3), use this formula in patent-medicine form.

Honey-Fried Licorice Decoction / SHA-KANZO-TO

This formula contains cinnamon twig, gelatin, fresh ginger, ginseng, jujube fruit, honey-fried licorice, marijuana seed, ophiopogon, and raw rehmannia. Traditionally, this formula is taken with at least half a shot glass, or 10 milliliters, of sake or other clear wine.

It is designed for a symptom pattern that includes constipation, dry mouth and throat, emaciation, insomnia, irritability, palpitations upon anxiety, shortness of breath, and weak pulse.

Traditionally, this formula was thought to correct a condition in which the heart was undernourished and could no longer provide a place in which the spirit might reside, leading to insomnia and irritability. Insufficient fluids led to constipation, dry mouth and throat, and an emaciated appearance. The chief herb in this formula, honey-fried licorice, was thought to nourish the heart and boost the energy of the body as a whole. Ginseng regulated the flow and production of energy in the organs and calmed the spirit, which relieved anxiety and palpitations. The other herbs in the formula stimulated the flow and formation of blood and other fluids.

The medically defined condition most commonly treated with this formula is chronic fatigue with "dry" symptoms: dry skin, feverish sensations in the hands and feet, anxiety, insomnia, irritability, and weight loss caused by hyperthyroidism. Kampo practitioners also use it to treat other conditions, including emphysema, heart valve problems and other heart disorders, listlessness and fatigue, and pulmonary tuberculosis.

Under federal law, the inclusion of heat-sterilized marijuana seed (often labeled *linum* or *mai zi ren*) in traditional remedies is legal. Marijuana seed will not produce a "high," but will cause a positive urine test for THC, the high-producing component, although sophisticated testing methods can distinguish use of marijuana seed from that of other plant parts.

Kidney Qi Pill From *The Golden Cabinet* / KINKI-JINKI-GAN

This formula contains alisma, cinnamon twig, Cornelian cherry, dioscorea, hoelen, moutan, prepared aconite, and raw rehmannia. *The Golden Cabinet* is a fourth-century document that explains the formulas of Zhang Zhongjing, among the first of China's master herbalists.

This formula is designed for a symptom pattern thought in Oriental medicine to be a result of deficient kidney function. It includes lower back pain and a cold sensation in the lower half of the body, either excessive urination or difficult urination occurring with fluid accumulation throughout the body, tension in the lower abdomen, and weakness in the lower extremities.

The chief herb in this formula is rehmannia, a tonic that helps the kidneys retain fluid. This prevents what the historical herbalists of Kampo called "wasting and thirsting," or what Western medicine would identify as diabetes. At the same time, Cornelian cherry and dioscorea harmonize the kidneys' bolstered yin energy with the body's other energies. These herbs ensure the normal flow of fluids, and make it possible for the formula's heating herbs, cinnamon and prepared aconite, to deal with chronically "cold," or rheumatic, joints and with asthma.

The medically defined condition most commonly treated with this formula is leg or lower back pain in persons with both arthritis and diabetes. Kampo practitioners also use it to treat other conditions, including beriberi, asthma, chronic kidney disorders, hypothyroidism, and hyperaldosteronism, or excessive production of the hormone aldosterone by the adrenal glands.

If taking this formula as a tea, boil the aconite for thirty to sixty minutes before adding any other ingredients to reduce any potential toxins in the aconite. Both teas and patent medicines may cause a loss of sensation in the mouth and tongue, which is not a sign to discontinue the formula. Fever, on the other hand, is a sign to discontinue the formula. Kidney Qi Pill should not be used by persons who are taking antiseizure medications. The formula removes both fluid and minerals from circulation, which can cause bloodstream levels of prescription medications to become too concentrated.

Kudzu Decoction / KAKKON-TO

This formula contains cinnamon twig, ephedra, fresh ginger, jujube fruit, kudzu, licorice, and peony. It is designed for a symptom pattern that includes stiffness in the neck and upper back, and fever and chills without sweating.

Kudzu relieves tightness in the neck and back, and the other herbs in the formula increase circulation and induce sweating.

The symptom pattern for Kudzu Decoction matches the early stages of herpesvirus infection. This makes the formula a useful treatment for this often stubborn virus, which comes in two forms, HSV-1 and HSV-2, and can form painful lesions on the skin, mouth, eyes, or genitals. The immune system vanquishes most viral infections, such as colds, within a few days to a few weeks. Herpesvirus, however, can remain without symptoms in nerve tissues for many years, only to become reactivated when the body's overall resistance is weakened, when the infected area is exposed to ultraviolet light, or when the tissue containing the virus is damaged. The resulting illness can cause serious complications, and even result in death among young children and adults who have compromised immune systems. Even with treatment, damage is almost inevitable once the virus has entered nerve tissue.

The virus's long latent period makes treating herpes with conventional drugs difficult. Indirect approaches, in which the immune system is stimulated, can also be dangerous when the person is also infected with HIV, as the HIV virus can mutate to untreatable forms when it is exposed to large numbers of immune cells.

Researchers at Toyama University in Japan saw the connection between herpesvirus infection and the symptom pattern for Kudzu Decoction, and studied the use of this formula as a herpes treatment. Their research shows that the formula neither kills the virus directly nor activates the body's immune system. Instead, Kudzu Decoction blocks the tissue-damaging effects of the reactivated virus.[1] In this way, Kampo treats one disease without creating a worse condition in its place.

The medically defined conditions most commonly treated with this formula, besides herpes, include alcoholism, nasal allergy or colds accompanied by stiff neck and upper back, diarrhea in children and that caused by food allergies, inner ear infection, and sinusitis. Kampo practitioners also use it to treat brain inflammation, hives, polio (which is still a threat in extremely poor countries), and cervical myositis, a muscle inflammation in the neck. Kudzu Decoction also protects eczema-damaged skin from the effects of herpes infection.[2]

Ledebouriella Powder That Sagely Unblocks / BOFU-TSUSHO-SAN

This formula contains white atractylodis, ephedra, forsythia, gardenia, gypsum, Japanese mint, ledebouriella, licorice, ligusticum, mirabilite, peony, peppermint, platycodon, scutellaria, talc, tang-kuei, and wine-treated rhubarb root. Traditionally, the formula is taken with three thin slices of fresh ginger.

This formula acts "sagely" by inducing sweating without injuring the body's exterior, and by purging the intestines without injuring the interior. It is designed for a pattern that includes several of the following symptoms: constipation, dark urine, difficult urination, difficulty in swallowing, dizziness, dry mouth, light-headedness, nasal congestion with thick discharge, rapid pulse, red and sore eyes, a stifling sensation in the chest, strong fever and chills, and a tendency to become flushed in the face when excited or embarrassed.

The chief herbs in the formula, ephedra and ledebouriella, disperse cold, or pathogenic influences, from the body's exterior by inducing sweating. Mirabilite and rhubarb root are powerful laxatives that dispel heat through the stool. Japanese mint and peppermint assist ephedra and ledebouriella in relaxing the exterior, while gardenia and talc dispel heat from infection through the urine. The other herbs in the formula regulate the function of the digestive tract, except for platycodon, which soothes the throat to allow swallowing, and ginger, which keeps the other ingredients from causing stomach upset.

Many modern Japanese practitioners use this formula in the treatment of obesity, a usage confirmed by laboratory research. The formula activates special fat cells, called brown cells, that burn fat to maintain body temperature. This reduces both total body weight and the percentage of body fat without changes in the number of calories consumed.[1]

Kampo practitioners also use this formula to treat other conditions, including acne, carbuncles, dermatitis, food poisoning, hives, and influenza.

When this formula is used in tea form, the gypsum should be boiled for between thirty and forty-five minutes before the other ingredients are added. Because gardenia contains a compound that can cause early-pregnancy abortion, this formula should not be used by women who are trying to become pregnant. Do not use this formula if nausea or vomiting is present.

Licorice, Wheat, and Jujube Decoction / KAN-KYO-NINJIN-HANGE-GAN

This formula contains jujube fruit, licorice, and wheat berries. It is designed for a symptom pattern that includes disorientation, frequent attacks of sadness with crying spells, inability to control oneself, restless sleep, and frequent bouts of yawning. In the syndrome's early stages, the dominant symptoms are disorientation, impulsiveness, and fitful sleep. As the condition progresses, what Oriental medicine calls the "lost soul" produces attacks of unusual behavior related to a loss of self-control, such as crying or yawning.

This syndrome is attributed to anxiety, excessive worry, or pensiveness, all of which can disrupt the normal flow of energy. Jujube fruit and wheat are calming herbs,[1] and licorice settles stomach upset. Throughout the Orient, this exceptionally nontoxic formula is given to women and children who experience frequent sobbing and loss of emotional control, and who display a demeanor of social detachment.[2]

The medically defined condition most commonly treated with this formula is bedwetting in children. It is also given to infants who wake crying at night.

Licorice, Wheat, and Jujube Decoction is unusual in that it can be made at home from readily available ingredients. Place $^1/_2$ ounce (15 grams) of wheat berries, slightly more than $^1/_4$ ounce (9 grams) of licorice root, and 10 pitted jujube dates in 3 cups (750 milliliters) of water, and simmer for forty-five minutes. Strain and drink. The wheat berries and jujube can also be eaten after being puréed into a porridge.

Ligusticum Chuanxiong Powder to Be Taken With Green Tea / SENKYU-CHACHO-SAN

This formula contains angelica dahurica, asiasarum, Japanese mint, ledebouriella, licorice, ligusticum, notopterygium, and peppermint. As its name suggests, it is taken with a cup of green tea.

This formula is used for a symptom pattern that includes headache in any part of the head, especially when accompanied by dizziness, fever and chills, or nasal congestion.

The chief herb in this formula is Japanese mint, which relieves headache, especially headache caused by what we would now call allergy. Ligusticum, angelica dahurica, and notopterygium relieve headache caused by energy imbalances in the qi channels. The other herbs in the formula relieve generalized body aches. Cold green tea, taken with the formula, clears heat from the eyes and prevents the formula's drying herbs from causing side effects.

The medically defined condition most commonly treated with this formula is headache, especially that caused by allergies. Kampo practitioners also use this formula to treat other conditions, including colds, sinusitis, head pains after concussion, migraine headaches, nasal allergies, and tension headaches.

Do not use this formula for more than six weeks.

Lily Bulb Decoction to Preserve the Metal / HYAKU-GOKOKIN-TO

This formula contains lily bulb combined with fritillaria cirrhosa, licorice, ophiopogon, white peony, platycodon, both cooked and raw rehmannia, scrophularia, and tang-kuei. Kampo named this formula after its ability to preserve and stabilize the energy of the lungs, associated with metal (see Chapter 1), and for its chief herb, lily bulb.

This formula is designed for a symptom pattern that includes coughing with blood-streaked sputum, wheezing, dry sore throat, and feverish hands and feet.

The formula employs lily bulb, ophiopogon, raw and cooked rehmannia, and scrophularia to relieve heat. By calming the emotions, peony prevents wheezing. The other herbs in the formula also stop coughing and increase circulation to the lungs.

The medically defined conditions most commonly treated with this formula include black lung disease, chronic bronchitis, strep throat, and primary tuberculosis.

Lonicera and Forsythia Powder (Honeysuckle and Forsythia Powder) / GINGYO-SAN

This formula contains burdock seed, forsythia, Japanese mint, honey-fried licorice, lonicera (honeysuckle), lophatherum, peppermint, platycodon, reed rhizome, and prepared soybeans. Kampo herbalists use raw soybeans to provide a medium in which the formula can ferment.

The formula is designed for a symptom pattern that includes cough, headache, slight fever with no chills, racing pulse, sore throat, and thirst.

This formula uses lonicera (honeysuckle) and forsythia especially to control early-stage abscesses and sores which are painful, red, and swollen, and are accompanied by symptoms of an exterior condition. The other herbs treat fever and chills, pain and stiffness of the head and neck, soreness and pain of the extremities, and snoring.

This formula is a traditional remedy for sore throat pain. Laboratory tests have shown that it kills *Streptococcus,* the germ that causes strep throat.[1] One of the herbs, platycodon, is an immune stimulant that increases the activity of macrophages and neutrophils, cells that eat bacteria. Platycodon does this without increasing the number of these cells. This makes the formula safe for persons with HIV, since the presence of more immune-system cells gives the virus more chances to multiply and mutate.[2]

The medically defined condition most commonly treated with this formula is strep throat. Kampo practitioners also use the formula to treat other conditions, including acne, acute bronchitis, influenza, sinusitis, measles, and mumps. When other treatments are unavailable, Chinese doctors use this formula to treat the early stages of encephalitis and meningitis.

Major Bupleurum Decoction / DAIO-SAIKO-TO

This formula contains bitter orange, bupleurum, fresh ginger, jujube fruit, peony, pinellia, rhubarb root, and scutellaria. A "major" bupleurum decoction treats a more advanced stage of disease than a "minor" bupleurum decoction. Both Major and Minor Bupleurum Decoctions (see page 128) treat diseases that have defeated the body's initial level of immune defense.

Major Bupleurum Decoction is designed for a symptom pattern that includes bitter taste in the mouth, burning diarrhea or no bowel movements at all, continuous vomiting, despondency, fever and chills, and nausea.

Traditional Kampo understood this formula as acting by venting excess energy from the body. The chief herb, bupleurum, and its deputy, scutellaria, removed heat from the liver and gallbladder. Bitter orange broke up stagnant energy in the chest, while rhubarb root drained excess heat from the intestines and relieved pain in the abdomen. Peony "softened the liver," removing emotional tension, and ginger and jujube fruit protected the body's nutritive energy.

In medical terms, the conditions Kampo physicians most commonly treat with this formula include diabetes, gallstones, high cholesterol, and migraine. For diabetics, Major Bupleurum Decoction is helpful because it reduces the rate at which glucose enters the bloodstream after meals and increases the efficiency of insulin.[1] It is especially useful when diabetes has been complicated by long-term gastrointestinal disorders.

This formula reduces the concentration of cholesterol in the bile, which inhibits gallstone formation.[2] Recent studies have found that this formula is also useful for persons who have problems with both excess weight and high cholesterol. Three months of treatment usually raises levels of high-density lipoprotein (HDL), the artery-clearing "good" cholesterol, and lowers levels of low-density lipoprotein (LDL), the artery-clogging "bad" cholesterol. This treatment also prevents the free-radical reactions that can lead to arteriosclerosis, in which cholesterol is deposited within the artery walls.[3]

Major Bupleurum Decoction's ability to fight free radicals allows it to reduce nerve damage after heart attack and stroke. This damage is done by free radicals that are formed as blood circulation is restored to the heart or brain.[4]

Kampo practitioners also use Major Bupleurum Decoction to treat other conditions, including dysentery and food poisoning; malignant high blood pressure, an extremely dangerous form of the disorder; hepatitis; malarial fevers; trigeminal neuralgia, or facial nerve pain; an abdominal-cavity infection called peritonitis; and inflammations of the pancreas, gallbladder, stomach or intestines, or of the membranes lining the chest cavity, called the pleura. Use with caution if fever is present, and discontinue if preexisting fevers worsen.

Major Construct the Middle Decoction / DAI-KENCHU-TO

This formula contains fresh ginger, ginseng, malt sugar, and zanthoxylum. The last item (also known as hot Szechuan pepper) is used, surprisingly, to reduce stomach pain. This action is reflected in its name: "major," or strong, and "construct the middle," which means increasing energy to the middle of the body.

This formula is designed for a symptom pattern that includes abdominal pain so intense that the person cannot tolerate being touched, with a strong sensation of cold in the epigastrium, or pit of the stomach, and vomiting to the point of being unable to eat.

The herbs in this formula are used to stop a condition traditional Japanese medicine described as "uprushing cold energy." Uprushing energy, as the name suggests, expresses itself as vomiting. When extremely hot herbs, such as zanthoxylum and its deputy, ginger, are given, the stomach's energy resumes its normal, downward course. The other substances, ginseng and malt sugar, support the function of zanthoxylum and ginger.

Major Construct the Middle Decoction is the most commonly used remedy in Japan for food allergy that causes cramping and diarrhea. It is also effective for nasal allergy, reported to be effective in treating eighty of ninety-three cases in one Chinese study.[1]

The medically defined condition most commonly treated with this formula is allergy, both nasal and digestive. This includes food allergy symptoms that are sometimes mistaken for eczema. Do not use if fever is present.

Major Ledebouriella Decoction / DAI-BOFU-TO

This formula contains raw amaranth, astragalus, white atractylodis, eucommia, ginseng, ledebouriella, honey-fried licorice, ligusticum, notopterygium, peony, prepared aconite, cooked rehmannia, and tang-kuei.

This formula was originally prescribed for "crane's-knee wind," a condition in which one or both knees become enlarged, swollen, and painful, with atrophy above or below the knee. It was also prescribed for "dysenteric wind," in which the legs are so painful and weakened after a dysenteric disorder that it is difficult to walk. The herbs in this formula work in tandem to expel "cold" from, and provide energy to, the bones, joints, sinews, and lymphatic system.

The medically defined conditions most commonly treated with this formula include dysenteric disorders that occur during withdrawal from morphine.[1] It is also used to treat arthritic conditions of the knees.

If taking this formula as a tea, boil the aconite for thirty to sixty minutes before adding any other ingredients to reduce any potential toxins in the aconite. Both teas and patent medicines may cause a loss of sensation in the mouth and tongue, which is not a sign to discontinue the formula. Fever, on the other hand, is a sign to discontinue the formula. Do not use this formula for more than six weeks.

Major Order the Qi Decoction / DAI-JOKI-TO

This formula contains bitter orange, magnolia bark, mirabilite, and rhubarb root. It is designed for a symptom pattern of severe constipation and flatulence. There may also be abdominal pain that increases upon pressure and, in the most extreme cases, delirious speech and profuse sweating from the palms and soles.

Kampo sees this symptom pattern as a condition of excess and heat. Rhubarb root purges excess heat from the intestines, and its propulsive action is aided by the cold, salty mirabilite. Bitter orange reduces sharp pains caused by constipation, while magnolia bark reduces the feeling of abdominal fullness.

The medically defined condition most commonly treated with this formula is constipation, particularly postoperative constipation. Kampo practitioners also use it to treat other conditions, including appendicitis, children's pneumonia, the early stages of dysentery, roundworm, uncomplicated intestinal obstruction, and pancreatitis, or inflammation of the pancreas.

Minor Bluegreen Dragon Decoction / SHO-SEIRYU-TO

This formula contains asiasarum, cinnamon twig, ephedra, fresh ginger, honey-fried licorice, peony, pinellia, and schisandra. In Chinese folk religion, the bluegreen dragon was the spirit of the east, a wood spirit. A major bluegreen dragon produced downpours of rain, while a minor bluegreen dragon produced billowing waves on the sea. Thus, this formula was named after the minor bluegreen dragon for its ability to produce waves of movement in the chest that relieve congestion.

This formula is designed for a symptom pattern that includes chills; copious amounts of white, stringy sputum that is difficult to cough up; coughing; fever without sweating; generalized body aches; a sensation of heaviness; wheezing; and possibly difficulty in breathing when the patient is lying down.

The chief herbs in this formula, ephedra and cinnamon bark, release cold from the exterior of the body and transform congested fluids, which eases congestion, in the interior. Their deputies, asiasarum and ginger, warm the interior, transform congested fluids, and help the chief herbs loosen tight muscle layers. The assistant herbs prevent excessive action of the chief and deputy herbs: schisandra prevents leakage of lung energy, peony nourishes the blood, and pinellia harmonizes the stomach. Licorice balances the effects of the acrid and sour herbs in the formula, and generally increases energy.

Laboratory studies show that Minor Bluegreen Dragon Decoction effectively prevents influenza A infection when taken from four to seven days before infection. It does not act directly on the virus, but rather stimulates the immune system to better handle the virus.[1]

Studies have also shown this formula to be a useful allergy medicine. Several tests, including a double-blind test with 200 participants in Japan, found that Minor Bluegreen Dragon Decoction is effective against allergic inflammations of the nose and eyes.[2,3] As an antihistamine, the formula acts against the chemical histamine, responsible for most of the discomfort associated with allergies. Unlike other antihistamines, it does not cause drowsiness or cardiac complications when used with other medications.[4]

The medically defined conditions most commonly treated with this formula include allergies, acute bronchitis, bronchial asthma, and flu. It is especially useful for colds in infants and young children with coughs, phlegm, and profuse, watery nasal discharge. Use with caution if fever is present, and discontinue if preexisting fevers worsen.

Minor Bupleurum Decoction / SHO-SAIKO-TO

This formula contains bupleurum, fresh ginger, ginseng, jujube fruit, honey-fried licorice, pinellia, and scutellaria. A "minor" bupleurum decoction treats a less advanced stage of disease than a "major" bupleurum decoction. Both Minor and Major Bupleurum Decoctions (see page 126) treat diseases that have defeated the body's initial level of immune defense. Minor Bupleurum Decoction is one of the most extensively researched Kampo formulas.

Like Bupleurum and Cinnamon Twig Decoction (see page 112), this formula is designed for a symptom pattern that includes a bitter or sour taste in the mouth, dizziness, dry throat, a feeling of fullness in the chest, fever and chills, heartburn, irritability, nausea, reduced appetite, and vomiting. Unlike Bupleurum and Cinnamon Twig Decoction, Minor Bupleurum Decoction is not used for joint pain.

Traditionally, this formula was used to fight infectious diseases that had weakened the body's defenses, known as lesser yang diseases, from progressing to chronic conditions, known as yang brightness diseases. It was thought to be an exceptionally useful formula in treating chronic conditions that we would now call infections because of its "ascending" action, which drives the pathogen to levels nearer the surface of the body. Most herbs used to treat fevers cool the body with a "descending" action, driving the pathogen to deeper levels.

Not surprisingly, given its traditional usage, Minor Bupleurum Decoction stops the progression of viral infections such as hepatitis and HIV. In Japan, this formula has become the treatment of choice for viral hepatitis, and has a 90 percent success rate. Clinical tests of persons with hepatitis B show that Minor Bupleurum Decoction increases the production of immune system components that both keep the virus from forming protein and attack the virus directly. Chemical analysis has found that the formula's effectiveness is derived from complex molecules found in the whole herbs themselves, and not in simple chemical extracts taken from the herbs.[1]

The value of Minor Bupleurum Decoction in the treatment of liver disease is not limited to viral hepatitis. Tests have shown the formula to be effective in preventing the progression of liver cirrhosis,[2] and in slowing or stopping the development of liver cancer cells.[3] In animal studies, it stops the progression of hyperplastic alveolar nodules, or precancerous cells in the breast, to breast cancer.[4]

Minor Bupleurum Decoction is also effective against other types of viruses. In the laboratory, the formula has produced a 50-percent reduction in the ability of HIV to replicate itself, a figure that jumps to 80 percent for leukemia viruses. It acts by blocking an enzyme known as reverse transcriptase, which the virus uses to convert its genetic information into a form it can use to reproduce.[5] Studies at Columbia University show that the formula is capable of stopping HIV reproduction in 80 percent of patients who have AIDS-related complex (ARC) syndromes, although it is ineffective in stopping the virus in patients who have AIDS.

Minor Bupleurum Decoction is also used in asthma treatment. It stops the formation of hormones that start asthmatic attacks.[6] The formula increases the effectiveness of prednisolone (Pediapred, Prelone), and may make it possible to reduce dosages of prednisolone needed to control asthma or any of several other diseases, including Crohn's disease, hemorrhoids, hyperthyroidism, and multiple sclerosis.[7] The formula also increases the effectiveness of dexamethasone (Decadron),[8] another steroid drug. In addition to modifying some of the reactions of free radicals (cell-harming substances) that contribute to asthma, Minor Bupleurum Decoction reduces the formation of atherosclerotic plaques from cholesterol by attacking free radicals, and increases the ratio of HDL to LDL[9]. In addition, this formula is part of a combination formula called *sairei-to.*

Kampo practitioners also use Minor Bupleurum Decoction to treat other conditions, including influenza; childhood diarrhea; habitual constipation; acute rheumatic fever; renal colic, or excruciating pain associated with kidney stones, and acute pyelonephritis, a bacterial kidney infection; stomach irritation caused by reflux of bile from the small intestine; gallbladder and lymph-node inflammations; mumps; intercostal neuralgia, or nerve pain between the ribs; malaria; postpartum fever; and pulmonary tuberculosis.

Avoid Minor Bupleurum Decoction if fever or skin infection is present. Taken long-term in patent medicine form, this formula can cause headache, dizziness, and bleeding gums. These side effects can be avoided if the formula is prepared as a tea. This formula also worsens side effects of treatment with alpha-interferon, an immune-system chemical used in the treatment of various disorders, including multiple sclerosis.[10]

Minor Construct the Middle Decoction / SHO-KENCHU-TO

This formula contains cinnamon twig, fresh ginger, honey-fried licorice, jujube fruit, malt sugar, and peony.

It was developed by revered herbalist Zhang Zhongjing to treat spasmodic abdominal pain resulting from overwork or poor diet. In the symptom pattern, the digestive system is unable to provide nutrients to the body, especially the limbs. The person may therefore crave hot beverages to supply the energy lacking from the digestive process. The heart is also deprived of the energy it needs to contain emotions, and the result may be irritability, nightmares, or bedwetting (in children).

Malt sugar sweetens the formula and stops abdominal pain. Cinnamon activates the lymphatic system and dispels "cold," infectious influences. Peony, as used in this formula, harmonizes the relationship between the energy derived from food and the energy the body uses to protect itself from disease. Licorice reinforces the ability of malt sugar to stop abdominal pain, while ginger and jujube harmonize the actions of the other warm and sweet herbs.

The abdominal pain corrected by this formula occurs when the stomach is full. (For treatment of abdominal pain occurring when the stomach is empty, see Calm the Middle Powder, page 114.) This formula is useful in the treatment of inflammatory bowel disease and peptic ulcer. It is also helpful in cases of childhood bedwetting, especially when the child experiences nightmares, and anemia.

Ophiopogonis Decoction / Bakumondo-to

This formula contains ginseng, jujube fruit, licorice, cooked rice, ophiopogon, and pinellia.

It is designed for a symptom pattern that includes coughing and spitting of saliva, dry and uncomfortable sensation in the throat, dry mouth, red tongue, shortness of breath, and wheezing.

Zhang Zhongjing, the early Chinese master herbalist, devised Ophiopogonis Decoction to treat a condition called "lung atrophy." In Oriental medicine, this condition is actually caused by heat that results from deficiency in the stomach. This heat rises in rebellion and scorches the lungs. When the lungs cannot receive nourishment from the stomach over an extended period of time, the lungs shrivel, or "atrophy." Rebellious energy from the stomach prevents lung energy from descending properly, causing coughing and wheezing. The scorching causes shortness of breath and depletes fluids, leaving only saliva or a thick, sticky sputum that cannot be dislodged from the throat.

Modern science explains how Ophiopogonis Decoction can act on both the stomach and the lungs. Laboratory tests show that it increases the activity of beta-adrenergic nerve fibers,[1] which relax the bronchial tubes, the uterus, and the lower gastrointestinal tract. This action also stimulates the burning of fat. In addition, this formula stimulates the nerves that open breathing passages in the lungs while suppressing the nerve that causes the cough reflex. Unlike other drugs that suppress this reflex, such as codeine, Ophiopogonis Decoction seems to only act on this nerve during a bronchitis or asthmatic attack.[2]

Ophiopogonis Decoction has also been used in clinical tests for the treatment of Sjögren's syndrome, an autoimmune disease in which the body attacks its own moisture-producing glands. The formula increases salivary secretion and prevents oral infections caused by Sjögren's syndrome,[3] and in other situations, such as treatments for cancer and Parkinson's disease, in which salivation is reduced.

In the aftercare of heart attack, Ophiopogonis Decoction increases coronary blood flow, increases the vigor of heart muscle fibers, helps the heart deal with oxygen deprivation, and slowly elevates blood pressure.[4] It is especially appropriate for heart attack patients who are experiencing coughing, sneezing, wheezing, upper respiratory infections, or asthma. This formula also increases the effectiveness of most of the steroid drugs used to treat eczema and multiple sclerosis, as well as the effectiveness of methylprednisone in the treatment of Graves' ophthalmopathy (bulging eyes) in hyperthryroidism.

Kampo practitioners use Ophiopogonis Decoction to treat other conditions, including allergies; Crohn's disease; acute or chronic pharyngitis, or inflammation of the voice box; esophageal reflux and heartburn; stomach inflammation; peptic ulcer; and pulmonary tuberculosis. Use with caution if fever is present, and discontinue if preexisting fevers worsen.

Oyster Shell Powder / Borei-to

This formula contains astragalus, ephedra, oyster shell, and raw wheat berries. It is designed for a symptom pattern that includes being easily startled, general debility, irritability, lethargy, shortness of breath, and spontaneous sweating that worsens at night.

Traditional Kampo understood this formula to work by "anchoring floating yang," or settling displaced emotional energies, primarily through the action of the chief ingredient of the formula, oyster shell. Wheat also exerts a calming effect on the body, and astragalus and ephedra together normalize breathing and control perspiration.

The medically defined condition most commonly treated with this formula is chronic fatigue.

When this formula is used in tea form, the oyster shell should be boiled for between thirty and forty-five minutes before the other ingredients are added.

Peach Blossom Decoction / Toka-to

This formula contains dried ginger, kaolin, and cooked rice. Kaolin, the chief ingredient, gives the formula the color of peach blossoms, which explains the name.

The formula is designed for a symptom pattern that includes abdominal pain which responds favorably to local pressure or warmth, and dark blood or pus in the stool.

Traditional Japanese medicine understood this condition as resulting from an energy deficiency in the digestive tract that kept it from properly digesting food. This deficiency was in turn caused by an energy deficiency in the kidneys, which kept them from either providing fluids or regulating the digestive system's nutritive energy. Ginger is used to expel cold from the digestive tract. Kaolin stops the secretion of blood and pus by the intestines, while rice stabilizes the stomach.

The medically defined condition most commonly treated with this formula is hemorrhoids with blood in the stool or with bleeding noticed after defecation. It is also used in syndromes marked by pus or blood in the stool and abdominal pain, such as Crohn's disease.

Peach Pit Decoction to Order the Qi / TOKAKU-JOKI-TO

This formula contains cinnamon twig, honey-fried licorice, mirabilite, peach seed, and rhubarb root. It is designed for a symptom pattern that includes acute lower abdominal pain and urinary incontinence. Women experiencing this syndrome will have irregular periods. In severe cases, there also may be delirious speech or manic behavior.

The ancient theorists of Kampo believed that this formula broke up accumulations of blood that constrained the flow of the lymphatic system. This buildup of blood caused acute lower abdominal pain. The alterations in the flow of qi, or energy, deprived the bladder of energy, so that it was unable to hold urine, and the person experienced incontinence. The lymphatic blockage also held heat until heat began to rise to the heart, the organ from which mental clarity emanates. Retained heat rose and disturbed the spirit, producing symptoms such as delirious speech, irritability, manic behavior, restlessness, and thirst.

The chief herbs of the formula, peach seed and rhubarb root, purge accumulations of blood and clear unhealthy heat. As a result unhealthy heat no longer has anything to which it can attach, and fever abates. Cinnamon warms the blood vessels with a healthy heat that encourages circulation. Purgative mirabilite softens areas of hardness and also dispels accumulation. Licorice protects the stomach from upset by moderating the harsh qualities of the other herbs in the formula.

Peach Pit Decoction to Order the Qi promotes weight loss by stimulating the body to burn fat. In ancient medical theory, this formula was thought to remove weight gained after an assault by a pathogenic influence, such as weight gain after prolonged illness and activity or after many attempts at dieting.

The medically defined conditions most commonly treated with this formula include obesity, and acne in persons with a strong constitution, a ruddy complexion, and a tendency to be constipated.

Peony and Licorice Decoction / SHAKUYAKU-KANZO-TO

This formula contains honey-fried licorice and peony. It is used to relieve a symptom pattern that includes spasms of the calf muscles with irritability and slight chills. It is also used to treat abdominal spasms and pain in the hands. For centuries, Peony and Licorice Decoction has been used to help children fall asleep—it is one of the oldest Kampo formulas in use.

Chinese herbalists explained the formula in terms of its effect on the liver. Peony alleviated pain caused by rebellious emotions stored in the liver. When these emotions were released, they could cause cramps and pain throughout the body, particularly in the abdomen, calves, and hands. The energy channels of the liver also crossed the breasts and genitals, so misplaced liver energy could also affect these organs as well. Licorice was a digestive tonic.

Modern research supports the traditional view of Peony and Licorice Decoction as a valuable aid to the reproductive system. Scientists have found that this formula increases the body's production of a hormone called DHEA, which is converted into estrogen.[1] This action makes it useful in treating menopausal symptoms. Peony and Licorice Decoction can also increase a woman's chances of becoming pregnant by balancing levels of the various hormones involved in pregnancy.[2] In men, the formula decreases testosterone production.[3] This can reduce prostate tissue growth, which can slow both benign prostate enlargement and the spread of prostate cancer.

The medically defined conditions most commonly treated with this formula include menopause, female infertility, and prostate problems. Kampo practitioners also use it to treat chronic pelvic inflammatory disease and various types of nerve pain.

Because Peony and Licorice Decoction stimulates estrogen production, it should not be used by women with estrogen-sensitive disorders, such as breast or uterine cancer, fibrocystic breast disease, uterine fibroids, or endometriosis.

Pill for Deafness That Is Kind to the Left Kidney / JIRO-SAJI-GAN

This formula contains acorus, alisma, Cornelian cherry, dioscorea, hoelen, magnetite, moutan, cooked rehmannia, and schisandra. It is a variation of Six-Ingredient Pill with Rehmannia (see page 134). To that formula's ingredients, this formula adds the psychoactive herbs acorus and schisandra and the calming substance magnetite to treat a set of related symptoms that include blurred vision, dizziness, hearing loss, insomnia, irritability, and ringing in the ears that worsens at night, especially in the elderly.

This formula is designed for a symptom pattern that includes continuous tinnitus likened to the sound of swarming insects. It is also used for blurry vision, hearing loss, insomnia, irritability, and vertigo. According to *The Yellow Emperor's Classic of Internal Medicine,* an ancient Chinese herbal manual, "The kidney's qi goes through the ear. If the kidney is harmonized, the ear can hear the five tones." In Oriental medicine, the left kidney refers to the yin, or supportive, energies of the kidney, while the right kidney refers to the yang, or circulating, energies of the kidney. When the left kidney qi is depleted, the ear cannot "contain" sounds, and buzzing and ringing sensations ensue.

The medically defined conditions most commonly treated with this formula include hearing problems associated with aging.

Pinellia and Magnolia Bark Decoction / HANGE-KABOKU-TO

This formula contains fresh ginger, hoelen, magnolia bark, perilla leaf, and pinellia.

In master herbalist Zhang Zhongjing's *Essentials from the Golden Cabinet,* this formula was recommended for "women who feel as if a piece of roasted meat were stuck in their throats." The condition, which of course can also be experienced by men, has come to be known in Oriental medicine as "plum-pit qi," better known in English as a lump in the throat. This formula is designed for a symptom pattern that includes a feeling of something caught in the throat that can be neither swallowed nor expectorated, and a heavy or stifling feeling in the chest.

This symptom pattern is thought to result from emotional upset resulting from circumstances that the person figuratively cannot swallow. The body's energy then becomes pent up, and the lungs and stomach lose their natural ability to move energy downward. When energy cannot be moved downward, fluids cannot be transported, and are turned into phlegm. The resulting phlegm clashes with the body's energy and ultimately lodges in the throat.[1] Magnolia turns phlegm back into its fluid form and hoelen causes this fluid to drain downward. The other herbs in the formula also move fluid downward to prevent vomiting.

Today, this formula is most commonly used to provide symptomatic relief for anxiety or depression. Kampo practitioners also use it to treat other conditions, including chronic laryngitis, esophageal spasms, gastrointestinal disorders, hysteria, and tracheitis, or inflammation of the airway. Use with caution if fever is present, and discontinue if preexisting fevers worsen.

Pinellia, Atractylodis Macrocephala, and Gastrodia Decoction / HANGE-BYAKUJUTSU-TENMA-TO

This formula contains white atractylodis, aged bitter orange peel (also called red tangerine peel), fresh ginger, gastrodia, hoelen, jujube fruit, licorice, and pinellia.

This formula is designed for a symptom pattern that includes severe dizziness and copious sputum, headache, nausea or vomiting, and a stifling sensation in the chest.

The chief herbs of this formula are gastrodia and pinellia. Gastrodia transforms phlegm, reducing congestion, and relieves dizziness, headache, and vertigo. Pinellia dries dampness, transforms phlegm, and directs the energies of the digestive system downward. The assistant herb hoelen strengthens the digestive function and encourages urination. The other assistants, aged bitter orange peel, ginger, and jujube fruit, harmonize the passage of food through the stomach with the body's other digestive functions, while the envoy herb licorice makes the mixture palatable and prevents excessive action of any single herb. White atractylodis supports the functions of the other herbs by strengthening the digestive process and drying up phlegm.

The medically defined condition most commonly treated with this formula is high blood pressure aggravated by emotional tension and stress. Kampo practitioners also use it to treat other conditions, including a hearing disorder called Ménière's disease and orthostatic hypotension, or the tendency to faint when moving from a seated to a standing position. Use with caution if fever is present, and discontinue if preexisting fevers worsen.

Pinellia Decoction to Drain the Epigastrium / HANGE-SHASHIN-TO

This formula contains coptis, dried ginger, ginseng, honey-fried licorice, jujube fruit, pinellia, and scutellaria. It was originally designed to counteract the effects of excessive purging with other Kampo formulas.

This formula is designed for a symptom pattern that includes fullness and tightness of the epigastrium, commonly referred to as the pit of the stomach, with very slight or no pain; intestinal rumbling with diarrhea, dry heaves, or vomiting; and reduced appetite.

Pinellia Decoction to Drain the Epigastrium shows promise in a purely modern application. Researchers at Japan's Hoshi University have found the formula to be effective in preventing damage from radiation burns when taken after radiation exposure.[1] A particularly useful characteristic of this formula for cancer patients is that it relieves diarrhea without affecting intestinal motion,[2] so it does not produce constipation if too much is taken. The formula has also been found to inhibit cAMP, a chemical substance that starts an inflammation-causing chain reaction.[3]

The medically defined conditions most commonly treated with this formula include diarrhea and the side effects of radiation therapy. Use with caution if fever is present, and discontinue if preexisting fevers worsen.

Polyporus Decoction / CHOREI-TO

This formula contains alisma, gelatin, hoelen, kaolin, and polyporus. It is designed for a symptom pattern of urinary difficulty accompanied by fever and thirst with a desire to drink. Secondary symptoms may include cough, diarrhea, insomnia, irritability, or nausea.

According to master Chinese herbalist Zhang Zhongjing, this symptom pattern is caused by injury from cold entering the yang brightness, or lesser yin, stage of disease (see Chapter 1), where it transforms into heat. Heat disturbs the water pathways, resulting in urinary difficulty. Heat also gives rise to fever. When the persons suffering fever give in to the desire to drink, fluids cannot be eliminated through the urine, so they are eliminated through the stool, resulting in diarrhea.

The principal ingredient of the formula, polyporus, reinforces the water pathways and encourages urination. Alisma unblocks the deep parts of the water pathways that involve the kidneys. Kadinum clears heat and relieves urethral pain. Gelatin dries up fluids and prevents excessive urination.

Modern research has confirmed Polyporus Decoction's effectiveness in the treatment of urinary problems. Hospital tests show that over 90 percent of patients with a combination of symptoms modern Japanese doctors call "urethral syndrome"—painful urination and/or a sense of retained urine—found relief when taking this formula, and without side effects.[1] The formula also removes kidney stones, but is very dose-specific. Modern Chinese formulas employ two to three times the amounts of herbs specified in the *Sho Kan Ron*, Japan's standard Kampo text. Clinical tests of Polyporus Decoction show that at low, or Japanese, doses, the formula relieves kidney stones. It does so without forcing the body to excrete citrate, the body's form of vitamin C, unlike most kidney-stone medications. High-dose Polyporus Decoction, however, has no effect on kidney stones.[2]

The medically defined conditions most commonly treated with this formula include urinary tract infections and kidney stones. The formula is also used to treat a range of other conditions in which nausea and vomiting are prominent symptoms.

Prepared Aconite Decoction / Bushi-to

This formula contains white atractylodis, ginseng, hoelen, peony, and prepared aconite.

It is designed for a symptom pattern that includes aching bones and joints, aversion to cold, cold extremities, and fatigue. This formula is a variation of True Warrior Decoction (see page 137), which is used when the primary symptom in the pattern is swelling. Prepared Aconite Decoction, which is used when the primary symptom is pain, contains double the aconite dosage for increased pain relief.

The medically defined conditions most commonly treated with this formula include arthritis, high blood pressure, hypothyroidism, and a hearing disorder called Ménière's disease.

If taking this formula as a tea, boil the aconite for thirty to sixty minutes before adding any other ingredients to reduce any potential toxins in the aconite. Both teas and patent medicines may cause a loss of sensation in the mouth and tongue, which is not a sign to discontinue the formula. Fever, on the other hand, is a sign to discontinue the formula.

Prolong Life Decoction / Zokumei-to

This formula contains apricot seed, cinnamon twig, ephedra, dried ginger, ginseng, gypsum, licorice, ligusticum, and tang-kuei.

It is designed for a symptom pattern that includes paralysis on one side of the body, an asymmetrical facial expression, and slow and slurred speech. In this symptom pattern, the patient is unable to recognize friends or identify sources of pain. There may also be dry stools, low-grade fever, and redness in the face.

This formula has four chief herbs—apricot seed, ephedra, ginger, and ligusticum—all of which stimulate the flow of energy through its proper channels. Deputy herb tang-kuei stimulates the flow of blood, while deputy gypsum removes heat. The third deputy herb, cinnamon bark, stimulates the yang energies, or those that are directed from the body to the environment, such as movement and speech. The envoy licorice harmonizes the overall effect, and ginseng generally energizes the body.

The medically defined condition most commonly treated with this formula is arthritis in which the patient is unable to turn to the side. Kampo practitioners also use the formula to treat facial paralysis, hives, rheumatoid arthritis, and stroke.

When this formula is used in tea form, the gypsum should be boiled for between thirty and forty-five minutes before the other ingredients are added. Actually, to avoid ill effects from eating apricot seeds (see Chapter 3), it is best to use this formula in patent-medicine form. Do not use this formula at all if nausea or vomiting is present.

Rambling Powder / Shoyo-san

This formula contains white atractylodis, bupleurum, hoelen, honey-fried licorice, white peony, and tang-kuei. Traditionally, peppermint leaves and thin slices of roasted ginger were eaten after the tea was drunk. Rambling Powder was named after an ancient Chinese story, "Rambling Without a Destination," in which the author wrote of rising above a constrained worldview. The formula was thought to release pent-up, or constrained, emotional energies and correct their influences on the body.

This formula is designed for a symptom pattern that includes reduced appetite, dizziness, fatigue, headache, and dry mouth and throat.

The traditional explanation of how this formula works is that the liver sometimes sends so much energy to the spleen that it interferes with the digestive process. This in turn reduces the liver's blood supply, so that the liver is unable to release the products of energy produced by pent-up emotions to the right organs at the right time. Bupleurum unlocks this energy, while peony and tang-kuei restore normal circulation. The other herbs support the main three.

Remarkably, even though Kampo's explanation of how this formula works dates from the eleventh century, it roughly corresponds to a more recent understanding of the liver, in which scientists have found that certain herbal compounds block the liver's responses to the stress hormone cortisol.

The medically defined conditions most commonly treated with this formula include fibrocystic breast disease, in which the breasts develop small benign lumps; hepatitis; menopause; pelvic inflammatory disease, an inflammation of the fallopian tubes; peptic ulcer; and fibroids, or benign uterine tumors.

Regulate the Stomach and Order the Qi Decoction / Choi-joki-to

This formula contains licorice, mirabilite, and rhubarb root. It is designed for a symptom pattern that includes mild constipation, bleeding or swollen gums, and/or nosebleed.

Mirabilite and rhubarb root are cooling substances that drain heat, which can rise to affect the gums or nose. Licorice prevents the stomach upset that could be caused by taking too much of the other two ingredients.

The medically defined conditions most commonly treated with this formula include constipation, nosebleed, and bleeding gums.

Restore the Right Kidney Pill / Uki-gan

This formula contains cinnamon bark, Cornelian cherry, cuscuta, dioscorea, eucommia, lycium fruit, prepared aconite, cooked rehmannia, and tang-kuei. Chinese versions of this formula may also include human placenta, although Japanese versions of this formula almost always omit it.

The formula is designed for a symptom pattern that includes aversion to cold, coolness in the hands and feet, exhaustion after a long illness, impotence, knee pain, and lower back pain.

In ancient Kampo, the right kidney was thought to be responsible for circulating fluids throughout the body, and restoring it normalized the kidneys' influence on the rest of the body. Chief herbs aconite and cinnamon bark increase the right kidney's energy flow. Cornelian cherry, cuscuta, dioscorea, lycium, and rehmannia serve as deputy herbs that increase the circulation of blood and other fluids, while eucommia supports overall function. Together, the herbs restore what is called "essence" in older people and in persons suffering from chronic diseases.

The medically defined condition most commonly treated with this formula is impotence that occurs as a complication of long-term disease, such as diabetes.

If taking this formula as a tea, boil the aconite for thirty to sixty minutes before adding any other ingredients to reduce any potential toxins in the aconite. Both teas and patent medicines may cause a loss of sensation in the mouth and tongue, which is not a sign to discontinue the formula. Fever, on the other hand, is a sign to discontinue the formula. Do not use this formula if either constipation or dark, scanty urine is present.

Restore the Spleen Decoction / Kihi-to

This formula contains astragalus, white atractylodis, Chinese senega root, ginseng, hoelen, honey-fried licorice, longan, saussurea, tang-kuei, and zizyphus.

"Restoring the spleen" refers to restoring the ability of the spleen, thought to store intelligence, to circulate nutritive energy to the heart, thought to store emotion. When intelligence overwhelmed emotion, either by excessive contemplation or by overly studious thought, the symptom pattern addressed by this formula appeared. This pattern included anxiety, dream-disturbed sleep, forgetfulness, palpitations (with or without anxiety), and withdrawal from social activity.

The chief herbs in this formula—astragalus, white atractylodis, ginseng, and licorice—have a tonic action on the spleen and build up the body's energy. The deputy herbs longan and tang-kuei anchor the sprit, while hoelen and zizyphus calm the spirit. The other deputy herb, Chinese senega root, calms the spirit by facilitating the flow of energy to the heart. Saussurea supports the functions of the chief and deputy herbs by restoring normal digestion.

The medically defined condition most commonly treated with this formula is depression. Kampo practitioners also use the formula to treat other conditions, including anemia, congestive heart disease, a heartbeat irregularity called supraventricular tachycardia, mood disorders, a muscle-wasting disease called myasthenia gravis, a skin problem called purpura, and uterine bleeding.

Rhubarb and Licorice Decoction / Daio-kanzo-to

This formula contains, as its name suggests, licorice and rhubarb root. It is designed for a symptom pattern that includes severe constipation and vomiting.

Rhubarb root purges the intestines. Licorice prevents stomach upset that could be caused by rhubarb.

The medically defined condition most commonly treated with this formula is constipation.

Rhubarb and Moutan Decoction / Daio-botanpi-to

This formula contains benincasa, mirabilite (added after the herbs have been boiled, when made in tea form), moutan, peach seed, and rhubarb.

Kampo originally designed the formula for lower abdominal distention and pain that increases upon pressure, with the pain usually worse on one side. There also may be sporadic fever and chills with sweating. This formula breaks up accumulations of blood and disperses "clumps" of energy. The unhealthy habits that cause these symptoms have been traditionally linked to poor dietary habits, especially bingeing on greasy foods.

In modern Japan, this formula is used to relieve *oketsu*, or blood stasis syndrome, the loss of various kinds of brain function after stroke. It fights free radicals, toxins that damage cells, and has been shown to be effective in preventing brain damage after stroke and a "ministroke" condition called transient ischemic attack.[1] Japanese physicians also use it to treat infection after vasectomy.

Historical sources say that Rhubarb and Moutan Decoction should never be taken by persons with appendicitis.

Sairei-to

This is a combination of two existing formulas; see **Five-Ingredient Powder With Poria** and **Minor Bupleurum Decoction.**

Settle the Emotions Pill / Teishi-gan

This formula contains acorus, Chinese senega root, ginseng, and hoelen, four herbs widely prescribed in China and Japan for age-related loss of mental function.

This formula is designed for a symptom pattern that

includes poor memory compounded by insomnia, dizziness, hot flashes, or dry mouth. Other symptoms include apprehension, easy fright, or incessant laughter, with anxiety and forgetfulness. This pattern most often occurs in persons who have suffered a severe emotional shock.

The herbs in this formula settle the emotions by increasing the body's general energy level. Ginseng and hoelen, the chief herbs, calm the spirit by augmenting the flow of energy to the heart. Acorus and Chinese senega root clear the senses in order to calm the spirit.

The medically defined conditions most commonly treated with this formula include anxiety, Alzheimer's disease, memory problems, and obsessive-compulsive disorders.

Seven-Treasure Pill for Beautiful Whiskers / SHICHIGYOKU BIZENTAN

The formula contains raw amaranth, cuscuta, hoelen, lycium, psoralea (dry-heated with black sesame seeds), Solomon's seal (steamed with black sesame seeds), and tang-kuei. In ancient China, black whiskers were considered more attractive than gray, and there are seven ingredients in the formula, hence the name. This formula is not available as a patent medicine, but is widely available from Kampo and TCM practitioners. Its Chinese name is *qi bao mei ran dan.*

This formula is designed for a symptom pattern that includes premature graying of the hair, usually with loose teeth, lower back pain, and difficulties in achieving sexual satisfaction.

Kampo associated all of these symptoms with energy deficiencies of the kidneys. Kidney health is expressed in the hair of the head, so graying hair is a sign of kidney deficiency. Soreness and weakness in the lower back, along with sexual difficulties, were also thought to be symptoms of kidney disease. In addition, the kidneys were also thought to generate bone marrow, which holds the teeth in place. The chief herb in the formula, Solomon's seal, is an intensely bitter herb thought to circulate to the bones and sinews. The deputies cuscuta and lycium nourish the kidneys. Amaranth, the other deputy, strengthens the sinews and bones in general, and the lower back and knees in particular. Tang-kuei is a blood stimulant, enabling the blood to send nutrients to the hair. Hoelen and psoralea prevent too much kidney energy from flowing upward at the expense of normal downward flows of kidney energy, as in urination.

Although the formula has not been studied under clinical conditions, Seven-Treasure Pill for Beautiful Whiskers is used widely and successfully in Japan and China to prevent graying of the hair.

Do not use this formula if either constipation or dark, scanty urine is present.

Shut the Sluice Pill / SHUKU-SENGAN

This formula contains black cardamom, dioscorea, and lindera. Like a sluice, this formula stops frequent urination due to failure of bladder control.

It is designed for a symptom pattern that includes frequent, clear, prolonged urination, or urinary incontinence during sleep. This formula is considered too mild for adults, but is successfully used to treat childhood bedwetting.

Traditional Kampo explained how this formula worked in terms of "grasping qi." The writer of *Fine Formulas for Women,* the book in which this formula first appears, thought that sausurrea warmed the kidneys and enabled them to "grasp" fluids, giving them control over urination. Lindera dispersed cold, infectious influences that could affect the kidneys, and dioscorea enabled the digestive system to produce energy to send to the kidneys. This formula is considered too mild for adults, but successfully treats childhood bedwetting.

The medically defined condition most commonly treated with this formula is childhood bedwetting.

Six-Gentleman Decoction / RIKKUNSHI-TO

This formula contains white atractylodis, bitter orange peel, ginseng, hoelen, honey-fried licorice, and pinellia. In Confucian cultures, it was common to refer to things that were important and that could be grouped together harmoniously as "gentlemen," after the Confucian term for a person who exhibits ideal behavior. The six herbs in this formula are mild and blend well together, and therefore are called the "six gentlemen" of Kampo.

This formula is designed for a symptom pattern that fits the classic *kyo-sho,* or deficient constitution: pale complexion, loose stools, low and soft voice, reduced appetite, and limb weakness. Unlike Four-Gentleman Decoction (see page 121), which is used for the same symptoms, this formula also treats vomiting or coughing with copious amounts of stringy, thin, white sputum through the addition of bitter orange peel and hoelen.

The medically defined condition most commonly treated with this formula is peptic ulcer. It has also been shown to reduce memory loss in Alzheimer's disease. Use with caution if fever is present, and discontinue if preexisting fevers worsen.

Six-Ingredient Pill With Rehmannia (Rehmannia-Six Combination) / ROKUMI-JIO-GAN

This formula contains alisma, Cornelian cherry, dioscorea, hoelen, moutan, and cooked rehmannia.

It is designed for a symptom pattern that includes dizziness, light-headedness, night sweats, ringing in the ears or diminished hearing, and soreness and weakness in the lower back.

In TCM, this pattern of symptoms is a classic presentation of deficient yin, or containing, energy of the kidneys and liver. The kidneys govern the bones and are responsible for generating marrow, which gives the bones their resiliency and strength. When the kidneys are weak, there will be a general weakness in the bones closest to the kidneys, that is, the lower back and legs. The kidneys are also responsible for generating the "marrow" that makes up the brain. When the containing energies of the liver are deficient, fire can spread along its energy channel. This can result in fevers, flushes, sore throat, and toothache.

Six-Ingredient Pill with Rehmannia corrects these symptoms with two groups of three herbs. The first group, Cornelian cherry, dioscorea, and cooked rehmannia, enriches the containing energies of the kidney. Cornelian cherry prevents improper dispersion of energies from the liver, and dioscorea strengthens digestion. The second group of herbs, alisma, hoelen, and moutan, drains energies downward. This counters fire rising in the liver and helps food pass in its normal, downward direction through the stomach and intestines.

Modern Kampo medicine is most concerned with this formula's ability to treat the "marrow," which is the brain. It is effective against attention deficit disorder (ADD), a condition that causes learning and behavioral problems. It has been used for over 1,000 years in the treatment of children who experience any of the Five Delays: in standing up, walking, growing hair, developing teeth, or talking. In the United States, herbal practitioners who use Six-Ingredient Pill With Rehmannia offer anecdotal reports of success in treating children who have either cerebral palsy or ADD.[1]

Kampo also uses Rhemannia-Six Combination to treat certain forms of cancer; diabetes; macular degeneration, an eye problem that can lead to blindness; and tinnitus, or ringing in the ears. Kampo practitioners use the formula to treat a wide range of conditions, including high blood pressure, hyperthyroidism, urinary tract infection and inflammation, pulmonary tuberculosis, failure to thrive, several eye disorders, and functional uterine bleeding, or abnormal bleeding that is generally caused by hormonal imbalances.

Because Six-Ingredient Pill With Rehmannia stimulates estrogen production,[2] it should be avoided by women with estrogen-sensitive disorders, such as breast or uterine cancer, fibrocystic breast disease, uterine fibroids, or endometriosis.

Stephania and Astragalus Decoction / BOI-OGI-TO

This formula contains astragalus, white atractylodis, fresh ginger, jujube fruit, honey-fried licorice, and stephania.

It is designed for a symptom pattern that includes sweating, swelling, and a heavy sensation in the body. There may also be difficulty in urination.

The traditional interpretation of this symptom pattern was that a pathogenic influence had become lodged in the body's exterior, or outer layers. The strategy of the formula was to release the exterior, which stopped sweating and swelling, while not destabilizing the immune system. One of the chief herbs in the formula, astragalus, is Kampo's main tool for stimulating the protective qi, or what we would now call the immune function. The other chief herb, stephania, releases the energy channels, thereby relieving pain, and promotes urination. The other herbs in the formula stimulate urination and calm the stomach.

The medically defined conditions most commonly treated with this formula include arteriosclerosis, in which cholesterol gathers within the artery walls, and weight gain caused by fluid retention. Kampo practitioners also use the formula to treat rheumatic heart disease, fluid accumulations in the abdomen, and the kidney inflammations acute glomerulonephritis and chronic nephritis.

Tang-Kuei and Peony Powder / TOKI-SHAKUYAKU-SAN

This formula contains alisma, white atractylodis, hoelen, ligusticum, peony, and tang-kuei. It was designed to treat continuous, mild cramping in the lower abdomen during pregnancy.

Tang-kuei, peony, and ligusticum restore blood circulation to its normal channels and release the pent-up emotional energies from the liver. The other herbs in the formula encourage urination.

In modern Japanese medicine, Tang-kuei and Peony Powder is applied to a wide range of conditions that benefit from reduced estrogen production.[1] It is used to treat acne that occurs in the first fourteen days of the menstrual cycle; to increase the effectiveness of the drug tamoxifen (Nalvodex) in the treatment of breast cancer; and to stop cyclical growth of endometriosis, fibrocystic breast disease, ovarian cysts, and uterine fibroids. Unlike some treatments, this formula does not have a masculinizing effect, since it decreases estrogen production by the ovaries[2] without reducing the ratio of estrogen to testosterone in circulation.[3] In the case of endometriosis, in which the tissue that lines the uterus grows elsewhere in the body, Tang-kuei and Peony Powder reduces the formation of inflammatory compounds in endometrial tissue.[4]

Another modern application of this formula is the treatment of summer colds that cause nasal congestion and chills throughout the body. It is also appropriate for "air conditioning stress," or nasal congestion caused by too many changes from natural to air-conditioned environments in the summer.

Tang-kuei and Peony Powder has been applied to the treatment of the cognitive disorders seen in old age. Tsumura and Company, a Japanese Kampo manufacturer, has sponsored studies that have determined the formula helps sodium, potassium, and calcium move across cell membranes in the brain. These changes in ion, or mineral, balance reduce the production of cell-damaging free radicals.

European studies of Tang-Kuei and Peony Powder indicate that the formula can also stop excessive free-radical production in the cardiovascular system, thus stopping the process of atherosclerosis. In addition, the formula breaks down proteins damaged by free radicals from the stomach, and increases the production of the protein-digesting hormone trypsin in the stomach.[5] Since Alzheimer's disease and related disorders stem from abnormal protein breakdowns, the risk of developing such disorders is reduced when proteins are more completely digested before entering the bloodstream.

The medically defined conditions most commonly treated with this formula include disorders affected by estrogen production, such as breast and uterine diseases, and colds. Kampo practitioners also use this formula to treat beriberi, a kidney inflammation called chronic nephritis, pelvic inflammatory disease, and recurrent miscarriage.

Tang-Kuei, Gentiana Longdancao, and Aloe Pill / Toki-ryukai-gan

This formula contains aloe, raw coptis, gardenia, gentian, musk, phellodendron, rhubarb root, saussurea, scutellaria, and tang-kuei.

Like Gentiana Longdancao Decoction to Drain the Liver (see page 122), this formula is designed for a symptom pattern that includes bitter taste in the mouth, dizziness, headache (including migraine headache), hearing loss, irritability, red and sore eyes, short temper, and swelling in the ears. It is also used to treat difficult or painful urination with a sensation of heat in the urethra. In women, the syndrome treated by this formula often includes vaginal discharge and irritation.

Gentian drains heat from the liver's energy channels. It is assisted by gardenia and scutellaria, which also stimulate the movement of fluids. Aloe eases constipation and "gallbladder fire" that can cause delirious speech, manic behavior, restlessness, and vertigo. The other herbs in the formula drain heat by stimulating urination, or they protect the body's ability to produce fluids from the overly aggressive action of gentian, gardenia, or scutellaria.

This formula is used for more severe forms of the same illnesses treated by Gentiana Longdancao Decoction. These include eczema; herpes, including herpes zoster (shingles); pelvic inflammatory disease, which affects the fallopian tubes; and yeast infections. Kampo practitioners also use it to treat the eye disorders acute glaucoma, central retinitis, conjunctivitis, corneal ulcers, and uveitis; the testicular inflammations epididymitis and orchitis; gallstones; hyperthyroidism; inner ear infections; and intercostal neuralgia, or nerve pain between the ribs.

Because gardenia contains a compound that can cause early-pregnancy abortion, this formula should not be used by women who are trying to become pregnant.

Ten-Significant Tonic Decoction (All-Inclusive Great Tonifying Decoction) / Juzen-taiho-to

This formula contains astragalus, white atractylodis, cinnamon bark, ginseng, hoelen, honey-fried licorice, ligusticum, peony, cooked rehmannia, and tang-kuei. The traditional way to take this formula is with a "chaser" of one or two paper-thin, small slices of fresh or pickled ginger. Chinese-made patent medicines based on this formula often substitute codonopsis for ginseng, but the brands of patent medicines recommended in Appendix A do not.

The formula is designed for a symptom pattern that includes continuous palpitations, easily fatigued extremities, light-headedness, loss of appetite, pallid or sallow complexion, shortness of breath, and vertigo.

In Kampo, the chief herbs of this formula, ginseng and rehmannia, are thought to be warming in nature. Ginseng helped the body overcome cold symptoms, such as easy fatigue, and rehmannia stimulated the production and circulation of blood. The deputy herbs, white atractylodis and hoelen, were thought to help the body leach out fluid accumulation, and the other deputy herbs, peony and tang-kuei, reinforced the action of rehmannia. Cinnamon bark, ginger, licorice, and ligusticum harmonized the effects of the chief and assistant herbs, and made the entire mixture more palatable and easier to drink.

Even though this formula was invented nearly 900 years ago, clinical research has found many modern applications for it. It is useful as a general tonic for persons with AIDS and chronic fatigue syndrome.[1] It stimulates the production of two important immune-system components, natural killer (NK) cells and a group of chemicals called the interleukins.[2]

In fact, Ten Significant Tonic Decoction's ability to support the immune system makes it the most versatile Kampo formula of all in cancer treatment. Tests at the University of Kansas have found that the formula prolongs survival time and minimizes side effects in a number of ways. Besides preventing nausea, vomiting, and loss of appetite, the formula increases the effectiveness of the chemotherapy drugs cisplatin (Platinol), cyclophosphamide (Cytoxan, NEOSAR), fluorouracil, and mitomycin (Mutamycin). After chemotherapy, it stimulates not only the immune system but also the production of red blood cells, and reduces drug-induced kidney damage. It also prevents damage to the bone marrow, thymus, and spleen during radiation therapy.[3]

The medically defined conditions most commonly treated with this formula include AIDS, chronic fatigue syndrome, and many types of cancer.

This formula stimulates production of B cells, immune-system cells that attack the body's own tissues in rheumatoid arthritis. Individuals who have this condition should avoid the formula.

Tonify the Middle and Augment the Qi Decoction / Hochu-ekki-to

This formula contains astragalus, white atractylodis, bitter orange peel, black cohosh, bupleurum, ginseng, honey-fried licorice, and tang-kuei.

It is designed for a symptom pattern that includes aversion to cold, intermittent fever that worsens upon exertion, spontaneous sweating, and a thirst for warm beverages. There may also be a desire to curl up, laconic speech, loose and watery stools, and shiny but pale complexion.

The ancient sages of Kampo explained this symptom pattern as a deficiency of energy from the incomplete digestion of food, as shown by undigested food in the stool. This, in turn, deprives the body of its outwardly directed, or yang, energies, especially those that move upward in the body. When nutritive energy is deficient, the arms and legs also become soft and weak. The person acquires a tendency to curl up in fetal position. Energies that cannot move upward move downward. This interferes with the normal circulation of fluids, and creates spontaneous sweating and fever that varies according to time of day and worsens on exertion. Because the underlying condition is an energy deficiency, the person craves hot (energizing) beverages, rather than cold.

The chief herb, astragalus, corrects the energy deficiency and helps the yang energies of the digestive system move upward in their proper channels. White atractylodis, ginseng, and licorice also energize the digestive tract. Tang-kuei invigorates the blood to move energy upward in the body, and is assisted in this by black cohosh and bupleurum. Bitter orange makes the entire formula digestible and also helps essential energy move upward.

The principal medical application of this formula in Japan is the treatment of male infertility for which there is no readily discernible cause. In one hospital study, 20 percent of the participating couples achieved conception within twelve weeks, and 51 percent of the men had increased sperm counts.[1] Animal studies indicate that the formula works by stimulating the production of proteins that allow the sperm to reach functional maturity. The formula is particularly effective in alleviating male reproductive problems caused by use of the cancer treatment doxorubicin hydrochloride (Adriamycin).[2]

In addition, Tonify the Middle and Augment the Qi Decoction effectively prevents bacterial infection by activating germ-eating cells called macrophages. In animal tests, this has enabled the immune system to kill *Listeria* infections within sixty minutes after injection.[3] The formula can also activate the immune system to attack certain kinds of cancer by increasing the number of natural killer (NK) cells,[4] and can help the bone marrow recover after cancer treatment with either cyclophosphamide or radiation.[5]

The medically defined conditions most commonly treated with this formula include male infertility and bacterial infections. It is also used for cancer, except for kidney cancer, in which it suppresses key immune-system components.[6] Kampo practitioners also use this formula to treat other conditions, including chronic bronchitis; chronic hepatitis; debility after a severe or prolonged illness; urinary incontinence after childbirth; insufficient lactation; cerebral arteriosclerosis, in which cholesterol plaques calcify in the walls of arteries that supply blood to the brain; corneal ulcers; reduced levels of white blood cells; vaginal discharge; pernicious anemia; prolapse, or a falling out of position, of the rectum or uterus; myasthenia gravis, a serious autoimmune disease; kidney inflammation; recurrent miscarriage; and uterine bleeding.

Trauma Pill / TETSU-DAGAN

This formula contains ephedra, frankincense, ligusticum, myrrh, and tang-kuei. It also includes three items normally not widely used in Japanese medicine: cicada shells, iron filings, and "dragon's blood," a product of the dracaena lily named for its red color.

As its name suggests, this formula is designed for symptoms that follow traumatic injuries, such as bruising, swelling, and pain at a fixed location in the body.

Six of the substances in the formula—cicada shells, dragon's blood, frankincense, ligusticum, myrrh, and tang-kuei—stimulate the flow of blood to and from areas of traumatic injury. This prevents the accumulation of blood that causes bruising and swelling. Ephedra opens the area between the skin and muscles to allow for the free circulation of blood, and helps guide the action of the five blood-stimulating ingredients. Iron filings promote the healing of fractured bones.

Kampo physicians use this formula exclusively for treating traumatic injury from contusions, falls, fractures, and strains.

True Man's Decoction to Nourish the Organs / NINJIN-YOZO-TO

This formula contains white atractylodis, chebula, cinnamon bark, ginseng, honey-fried licorice, nutmeg, opium poppy husk, peony, saussurea, and tang-kuei. It was named after one of the "eight immortals" in Chinese legend, Lü, the pure-yang true man. This formula is not available as a patent medicine, but is widely available from Kampo and TCM practitioners. Its Chinese name is *zhen ren yang zang tang*.

The formula is designed for symptom patterns in which the most prominent feature is chronic diarrhea, sometimes to the point of incontinence. Accompanying symptoms may include persistent abdominal pain that responds favorably to local pressure or warmth, fatigue, lack of strength in the legs, lower back pain, and a pale tongue.

The herbs in this formula are considered to be tonics that dispel cold from the digestive tract and restore the body's fluid metabolism.

The medically defined conditions most commonly treated with this formula include chronic diarrhea in both children and people with AIDS, and in Crohn's disease, which is marked by the development of ulcers in the small and large intestines. The formula is also helpful in chronic fatigue syndrome and incontinence.

True Man's Decoction should be carefully strained before use to avoid a laxative effect. Avoid alcohol, wheat, cold or raw foods, fish, and greasy foods when taking this formula. This formula should not be used by persons with gallbladder problems, obstruction of the bile duct, or a tendency to retain urine, or by pregnant women.

True Warrior Decoction / SHIMBU-TO

This formula contains white atractylodis, fresh ginger, hoelen, peony, and prepared aconite. In Oriental tradition, the "true warrior" is the spirit of the north who manages fire and water. This formula, which was thought to increase yang energy and regulate urination, was named after that spirit.

This formula is designed for a symptom pattern that includes abdominal pain, deep aching, heaviness in the extremities, and urinary difficulty. There may also be cough, dizziness, a heavy sensation in the head, palpitations, a swollen tongue with tooth marks, and vomiting.

The chief herb in this formula is aconite, which energizes the kidneys to resume their function of transforming water. This helps the body use water to moisten tissues, making them healthy and whole, and keeps water from stagnating in the joints and lungs. The deputy herbs, white atractylodis and hoelen, strengthen the digestive system and promote urination. Ginger reinforces the kidney's ability to circulate water away from the lungs and skin.

The medically defined conditions most commonly treated with this formula include anorexia and wasting in advanced cases of AIDS, arthritis, supportive care after radiation treatment, an intestinal disorder called Crohn's disease, a hearing disorder called Ménière's disease, high blood pressure, and hypothyroidism.

If taking this formula as a tea, boil the aconite for thirty to sixty minutes before adding any other ingredients to reduce any potential toxins in the aconite. Both teas and patent medicines may cause a loss of sensation in the mouth and tongue, which is not a sign to discontinue the formula. Fever, on the other hand, is a sign to discontinue the formula.

Two-Cured Decoction / NICHIN-TO

This formula contains hoelen, aged bitter orange peel (also known as red tangerine peel), honey-fried licorice, and pinellia. Traditionally, the patient eats a thin slice of ginger after taking the formula in tea form. The name of this formula refers to the curing, or drying, of its two chief ingredients, bitter orange peel and pinellia, before use.

Two-Cured Decoction is designed for a symptom pattern that includes cough with large amounts of easily expelled phlegm, nausea or vomiting, palpitations, and a stifling sensation in the chest and diaphragm.

The herbs in this formula treat dampness by drying. One of the chief herbs, pinellia, dries dampness, expels phlegm, and causes rebellious stomach qi, or qi that is moving in the wrong direction, to descend. The other chief herb, bitter orange peel, revives the digestive process and directly treats coughing, distention, nausea, and vomiting. Hoelen, the deputy herb, stops diarrhea, and resolves palpitations and vertigo caused by upward-rising phlegm. The assistant herb, honey-fried licorice, restores normal passage of food through the digestive tract. Ginger, the envoy herb, prevents nausea.

Chinese research has found that Two-Cured Decoction reduces estrogen levels in women with breast cancer or fibrocystic breast disease.[1]

The medically defined conditions most commonly treated with this formula include disorders that benefit from reduced estrogen production, such as breast cancer, endometriosis, fibrocystic breast disease, ovarian cysts, premenstrual syndrome, or uterine fibroids.[2] Kampo practitioners also use it to treat other conditions, including chronic bronchitis, chronic gastritis, drooling in children, goiter, a hearing disorder called Ménière's disease, and peptic ulcer. Use with caution if fever is present, and discontinue if preexisting fevers worsen.

Unblock the Orifices and Invigorate the Blood Decoction / TSUKYO-KAKKETSU-TO

This formula contains carthamus, fresh ginger, jujube fruit, ligusticum, musk, peach seed, red peony, and scallion. It is designed for a symptom pattern in which the openings of the head are "blocked" by accumulations of blood, which explains the name. The musk is usually dissolved in sake before being added to the formula at the end of the brewing period.

This formula is a modification of the parent formula Drive Out Stasis in the Mansion of Blood Decoction (see page 118). While the parent formula is designed to correct static blood in the chest, Unblock the Orifices and Invigorate the Blood Decoction is designed to correct static blood above the chest, in the shoulders, face, and head. Static blood above the chest could manifest itself as headache, hair loss, ringing in the ears, purple complexion, bags under the eyes, and "brandy" nose. Obstruction of the normal flow of blood to the heart results in depression and mental fatigue.

The medically defined conditions most commonly treated with this formula include bags under the eyes and headache. Kampo practitioners also use it to treat the manic phase of bipolar disorder, also known as manic-depressive illness; concussion; hives; high blood pressure; various heart disorders, including cor pulmonale, coronary artery disease, and rheumatic valvular heart disease; symptoms related to menopause; migraine; and nerve pain in the face or between the ribs.

Warm the Gallbladder Decoction (Bamboo and Hoelen Decoction) / UNTAN-TO

This formula contains bamboo shavings, bitter orange, bitter orange peel, fresh ginger, hoelen, licorice, and pinellia. "Warming" the gallbladder refers to the treatment of cold, or depletion of the energy channels, of the gallbladder after a serious illness. Depletion of energy in these channels was thought to cause irritability and insomnia.

This formula is designed for a symptom pattern that includes anxiety, dizziness, gnawing hunger of indeterminate origin, insomnia, nausea or vomiting, palpitations, and sometimes seizures with the production of copious sputum.

Bamboo is the chief herb in Kampo for the treatment of gallbladder problems. In this formula, it reverses the flow of rebellious qi, or energy that flows upward to cause most of the symptoms in the pattern. The assistant herbs bitter orange peel and pinellia normalize the flow of energy through the stomach, while the assistants hoelen and licorice strengthen the digestive processes and encourage urination.

Hoelen and licorice also calm the spirit. The envoy herb ginger regulates the relationship between the gallbladder and stomach to stop vomiting. Bitter orange reinforces the formula's antiemetic effect by redirecting "rebellious qi" downward.

The medically defined conditions most commonly treated with this formula include peptic ulcer and insomnia in persons who have ulcers. Kampo practitioners also use the formula to treat chronic bronchitis, chronic gastritis, hepatitis, Ménière's disease, and the early stages of schizophrenia. Use with caution if fever is present, and discontinue if preexisting fevers worsen.

Warm the Menses Decoction / Unkei-to

This formula contains cinnamon twig, gelatin (dissolved into the strained formula), evodia, fresh ginger, ginseng, licorice, ligusticum, moutan, ophiopogon, peony, pinellia, and tang-kuei. "Warming the menses" refers to stimulating the flow of blood through its normal pathways in the womb. This action stimulates the menstrual flow, or, during pregnancy, removes obstruction in the "conception vessel" that supplies nutrients to the fetus.

This formula is designed for a symptom pattern that includes early or late menstruation and mild, persistent uterine bleeding with continuous flow; bleeding between periods; a cold sensation in the lower abdomen; dry lips and mouth; low-grade fever in the late afternoon; and warm palms and soles. Women who have this pattern are often infertile.

All of the substances in this formula regulate and stimulate the flow of blood to the womb. Evodia and cinnamon twig dispel cold and unblock and improve circulation in the blood vessels. Evodia helps the movement of qi, or energy, and alleviates pain. Ligusticum, peony, and tang-kuei nourish the blood, break up static blood, and regulate the menses, while gelatin and ophiopogon help generate fluids. Moutan regulates the menses and clears "heat from deficiency," that is, heat which builds up because the body lacks fluids to carry it away. Ginger, ginseng, licorice, and pinellia harmonize the effects of the other herbs.

As one would expect, the medically defined conditions most commonly treated with Warm the Menses Decoction generally affect the female reproductive tract. They include functional uterine bleeding, or abnormal bleeding generally caused by hormonal imbalances; infertility; irregular menstruation; symptoms related to menopause; benign tumors called uterine fibroids; ovarian polycystic disease, in which a number of cysts develop within the ovaries; and pelvic inflammatory disease, an inflammation of the fallopian tubes. The formula is also used to treat infertility in men who have variocele, or varicose veins that affect the spermatic cord. As a circulatory stimulant, it is used to treat fatigue after colds, and eczema in the hands made worse by exposure to hot water. Use with caution if fever is present, and discontinue if preexisting fevers worsen.

Warming and Clearing Decoction / Unsei-in

This formula contains raw coptis, gardenia, ligusticum, peony, phellodendron, cooked rehmannia, scutellaria, and tang-kuei. "Warming" refers to energizing blood and fluids so that they circulate in their proper courses. "Clearing" refers to stopping the constant spotting of blood or fluids on the outside of the body.

Warming and Clearing Decoction is a modification of Four-Substance Decoction (see page 121). Kampo uses the four-herb combination to treat blurred vision, dizziness, lusterless complexion, and generalized muscle tension during amenorrhea. Warming and Clearing Decoction adds coptis to treat continuous or excess uterine bleeding, and to treat stubborn skin diseases, such as eczema and hives.

The formula is designed for continuous uterine bleeding, or chronic weeping skin diseases such as eczema and hives.

Because gardenia contains a compound that can cause early-pregnancy abortion, this formula should not be used by women who are trying to become pregnant.

White Tiger Decoction / Byakko-to

White Tiger Decoction contains anemarrhena, gypsum, honey-fried licorice, and a rice porridge. In Oriental mythology, the white tiger was the Metal spirit of the west whose appearance in the autumn heralded the end of summer's heat. The use of its name here is a metaphor for the action of the formula, which reduces fever. The pathogenic influences against which the "white tiger" is effective are the four "greats": great fever, great pulse, great sweating, and great thirst.

This formula is designed for a symptom pattern that includes high fever and aversion to heat, marked irritability, profuse sweating, rapid pulse, red face, and severe thirst. Frequently, there is also bleeding from the gums or nose, headache, or toothache.

The chief ingredient in this formula is gypsum, a cooling agent that stops fever and toxic reactions. Its deputy, anemarrhena, is bitter, cold, and moistening. Honey-fried licorice and rice are added to the formula to ensure that the cold actions of the other components do not interfere with normal digestion.

The medically defined conditions most commonly treated with this formula include bags under the eyes, bleeding gums, and nosebleed. Kampo practitioners also use it to treat diabetes, heat stroke, lobar pneumonia, periodontic disease, and early stages of the brain disorders encephalitis and meningitis.

When this formula is used in tea form, the gypsum should be boiled for between thirty and forty-five minutes before the other ingredients are added. Do not use this formula if nausea or vomiting is present.

White Tiger Plus Atractylodis Decoction / Byakko-ka-so-jyutsu-to

This formula contains anemarrhena, red atractylodis, gypsum, honey-fried licorice, and a rice porridge. This formula, a modification of White Tiger Decoction (see page 139), is not available as a patent medicine, but is widely available from Kampo and TCM practitioners. Its Chinese name is *bai hu jia cang zhu tang.*

White Tiger Plus Atractylodis Decoction is designed for a symptom pattern that includes high fever and aversion to heat, marked irritability, profuse sweating, rapid pulse, red face, and severe thirst, plus a generalized sensation of heaviness and pain in the joints.

Cooling gypsum, the chief ingredient, stops fever and toxic reactions. The deputy, anemarrhena, is bitter, cold, and moistening. Honey-fried licorice and rice prevent the cold actions of the other components from interfering with normal digestion. Red atractylodis relieves joint pain.

The medically defined condition most commonly treated with this formula is diabetes with circulatory problems in the lower half of the body.

The gypsum should be boiled for between thirty and forty-five minutes before the other ingredients are added. Do not use this formula if nausea or vomiting is present.

White Tiger Plus Ginseng Decoction / Byakko-ka-ninjin-to

This formula contains anemarrhena, ginseng, gypsum, honey-fried licorice, and a rice porridge. It is a modification of White Tiger Decoction (see page 139) designed for a symptom pattern that includes high fever and aversion to heat, marked irritability, profuse sweating, rapid pulse, red face, and severe thirst, in which severe thirst is the most prominent symptom.

Gypsum, the chief ingredient, is a cooling agent that stops fever and toxic reactions. Deputy anemarrhena is a bitter, cold, and moistening herb. Honey-fried licorice and rice are used to make sure that the cold actions of the other herbs do not interfere with normal digestion. Ginseng relieves thirst.

This formula is used in the treatment of diabetes accompanied by fever, thirst, profuse sweating, and generalized weakness. It acts by counteracting the body's production of glucagon, a hormone that increases blood-sugar levels.[1] Some Japanese physicians also use this formula together with steroid creams to treat skin allergy.

When this formula is used in tea form, the gypsum should be boiled for between thirty and forty-five minutes before the other ingredients are added. Do not use this formula if nausea or vomiting is present.

Yellow Dragon Decoction / Oryu-to

This formula contains bitter orange, fresh ginger, ginseng, jujube fruit, licorice, magnolia bark, mirabilite, platycodon, rhubarb root, and tang-kuei. In Chinese mythology, a yellow dragon was a ruler over earth, the element processed by the "spleen" and stomach (see Chapter 1).

It is designed for a symptom pattern that includes foul-smelling, green, and watery diarrhea; abdominal pain that increases upon pressure; delirious speech; dry tongue and mouth; fever; impaired consciousness, sometimes including hallucinations; lethargy; shortness of breath; and thirst.

The herbs in this formula treat diarrhea by accelerating the passage of the contents of the intestines, which purges the body of unhealthy, foul-smelling stools. Mirabilite and rhubarb root, the chief ingredients, unlock the bowels to drain heat, the root cause of the digestive upset seen in this symptom pattern. The deputy herbs bitter orange and magnolia bark also stimulate bowel movement. Ginseng protects the body's fluid balance, and both jujube fruit and licorice restore digestive function. The other herbs support these functions.

The medically defined condition most commonly treated with this formula is extreme fatigue after diarrhea or dysentery. It is also used to treat chronic fatigue syndrome.

Part Two
Disorders Treated With Kampo

Part One explained how Kampo uses unique combinations of herbs to restore balance to persons with unique experiences of symptoms. It also described the scientific research that has been done on Kampo herbs and formulas. Part Two offers an A-to-Z listing of medical conditions that can be treated with Kampo. One of Kampo's great strengths is that it can be used in the context of both person-oriented Oriental medicine and disorder-oriented Western medicine.

Each entry contains introductory material that explains the disorder from the conventional Western viewpoint and then from the Kampo perspective. One is a logical way to understand disease, the other, an intuitive way. One provides confidence in herbs and formulas, the other provides a picture by which a person can visualize a return to health. The Kampo material does not refer to organs as they are understood in the West, but to the symbolic organ systems discussed in Chapter 1. This is followed by two groupings of treatments, herbs and formulas. Only the best herbs and formulas for each condition have been listed, not all applicable therapies. (For more information on the individual herbs and formulas, see Chapters 3 and 4.) Herbs and formulas that should be avoided by someone with a specific disorder are also listed. Like Part One, Part Two of this book refers to the scientific studies on which it bases it recommendations. These references can be consulted for additional information.

The basic principle of Kampo is "just enough medicine to restore balance." In general, herbs offer symptomatic relief and formulas offer systematic treatment. In cases of a condition that is "almost" under control except for one or two prominent symptoms, consult the list of *herbs.* Most herbs will be effective after three to four weeks' use, although the text lists exceptions.

If a chronic condition exists or if there are multiple symptoms, consult the list of *formulas* for the formula that most closely matches the existing pattern of symptoms. As a rule, if more than two herbs are needed to control symptoms, it is better to take the appropriate formula. Formulas are usually effective in three to four months. Unlike herbs, formulas are designed to correct the underlying disease processes that cause a given pattern of symptoms.

In the long-term treatment of chronic conditions, it is especially important to choose a Kampo drug in consultation with a doctor and a qualified herbalist, or Kampo or Traditional Chinese Medicine (TCM) practitioner. To ensure selection of the most beneficial formula, many vendors of both over-the-counter Kampo formulas and combinations of bulk herbs for teas will insist on confirmation of the diagnosis by a health care professional.

Herbs and formulas can always be described in terms of their actions in the context of conventional Western medicine, such as lowering blood-sugar levels or counteracting specific hormones, or stopping the multiplication of specific germs or types of cancer cells. They also can be described in terms of the outward symptoms used to make Kampo diagnoses. Entries in this section present the level of description needed to choose among treatments. Some treatments are described in terms of the laboratory findings they would change, and others in terms of the outward symptoms they would eliminate.

Herbs and formulas are not "tonics" to be indiscriminately substituted for prescription drugs. In many cases, though, Kampo therapies and specific prescription medications interact positively for increased control of disease. Particularly in the treatment of allergy, asthma, autoimmune diseases (including rheumatoid arthritis and lupus), cancer, and psoriasis, herbs may increase the effectiveness of medical treatments or reduce their side effects. Some prescription drugs have so many side effects that they cannot be used continuously. For these drugs, certain herbs and formulas reduce the likelihood of relapse on the days or weeks the prescription drug is not taken. Always check with a health care professional to make sure that any herb or formula used does not have a negative interaction with a prescription drug being taken for a specific illness.

Herbs and formulas are also useful in disease prevention. Some formulas have proven effectiveness for preventing the progression of chronic diseases. Minor Bupleurum Decoction, for instance, has been shown to stop the progression of chronic viral hepatitis to liver cancer. If there is a medical diagnosis of a specific condition that is expected to progress to a more serious disease, the listed herbs or formulas should be used on a long-term basis. However, it is important to avoid creating other imbalances by taking too much of a single herb or formula. After taking any herb or formula for three months, see a health care professional for reassessment. As symptoms improve, it may be beneficial to continue with the same treatment or to start taking a different herb or formula. It may also be necessary to change or discontinue prescription medication. The doctor may determine that further treatment is not needed, depending on whether or not sufficient improvement has been made.

The traditional and most effective way to take Japanese medicinal herbs and formulas is as herbal teas. Teas offer the broadest range of water-soluble active compounds from herbs. Consistent use of herbs and formulas, however, is more important than traditional use. If the daily preparation of teas is so inconvenient that doses are skipped, herbs can be taken in alternative forms. For descriptions of these forms, and for some general instructions on making herbal teas, see Chapter 2.

Most Kampo formulas are available as concentrated liquid extracts made from prepared teas, or as tablets made from freeze-dried powders of multiple-herb teas. Sources of formulas available as patent (over-the-counter) medicines are listed in Appendix A.

It is important to remember that Kampo works with, rather than against or in place of, conventional medicine. Herbs and formulas that provide relief when taken with a prescription medication will affect the body differently if the prescription is abruptly discontinued. Herbs and formulas stop discomfort and prolong life in serious conditions such as cancer, diabetes, and lupus, but they are most effective when combined with conventional treatment. Kampo does not substitute for healthy lifestyle choices or ongoing medical care.

If there are any questions regarding diagnosis or the appropriateness of an herb or formula, or any general questions about health, a physician should always be consulted.

If There Are Children . . . Or If a Baby Is on the Way

Every entry for a childhood disease clearly marks Kampo remedies that can be given to children. In general, children aged six to twelve may be given one-half of the adult dose, while children aged three to six may be given one-quarter of the adult dose. Every entry notes any exceptions to these dosages. In addition, as is the case with many conventional medicines, a number of Kampo remedies are not suitable for use during pregnancy (although there are formulas especially designed for pregnant women). A pregnant woman should talk to a Kampo or TCM practitioner, as well as her obstetrician, before using Kampo.

ACNE

Acne is the presence of blackheads, whiteheads, or pimples blocking the pores of the skin. It is the most common of all skin problems. An overwhelming majority of Americans experience some degree of acne between puberty and age twenty-four, although it may occur at any stage of life.

Acne is not caused by "dirty" pores. Instead, acne results when the skin produces too much sebum and keratin, substances that can clog pores and trap bacteria inside. Acne only occurs when increased production of the male sex hormone testosterone alters the function of the sebaceous, or sebum-producing, glands. Testosterone stimulates the sebaceous glands to produce greatly increased amounts of oils and waxes. This hormone also stimulates the cells lining the hair shafts to produce keratin, a hard substance that can block the passage of sebum from the pores.

Acne can progress to form nodules, tender accumulations of pus deep in the skin; cysts, nodules that fail to drain; or large, deep pustules that break down soft tissues below the skin. Untreated acne can lead to scarring and pitting.

Acne is most common during those stages of life in which the body creates the most testosterone. During puberty, the bodies of both boys and girls produce more testosterone. This hormone, or more specifically, a byproduct known as dihydrotestosterone,[1] thickens the skin and toughens the underlying tissues. Despite the fact that this process occurs in everyone who passes through puberty, not everyone develops acne, because each person's body chemistry is a little different. Since male sex hormones stimulate sebaceous secretion, acne is more common in boys than in girls.

As hormone levels diminish in both sexes after adolescence, acne also diminishes. Hormonal fluctuations, however, can cause flareups throughout adulthood. In women, these flareups are often triggered by the premenstrual release of progesterone. Since many oral contraceptives contain progesterone, the use of these drugs can also cause outbreaks, as can steroid treatment in men.[2] Other factors that contribute to acne development include heredity, stress, and cosmetics use.

Just as modern medicine sees acne as resulting from an imbalance of the hormone that "heats" sexual desire, Kampo see acne as a condition of heat arising from the blood, the lungs, or the stomach, or from an infection. A condition Japanese doctors call "blood effusion" results when the blood is "stirred," either during the menstrual period or during periods of emotion. Blackheads, whiteheads, and itchy skin result from "lung heat," in which acne accompanies allergies or chronic respiratory infection. Stomach heat and infectious toxins result in painful lesions that appear not only on the face but elsewhere on the body. This form of acne responds to formulas containing the herb coptis (see **Coptis** in Chapter 3).

KAMPO FORMULAS

See Chapter 4 for dosage information and discussions of individual formulas.

Cinnamon Twig and Poria Pill

Used to treat blood effusion.

Coptis Decoction to Relieve Toxicity

Clinical studies have found coptis to be more effective against acne than the antibiotics erythromycin or minocycline.[3]

Caution: Should not be used by women who are trying to become pregnant.

Lonicera and Forsythia Powder (Honeysuckle and Forsythia Powder)

Used to treat acne caused by lung heat.

Peach Pit Decoction to Order the Qi

Used to treat acne in persons with strong constitutions and ruddy complexions who tend to be constipated. Useful for women who have menstrual problems.

Tang-Kuei and Peony Powder

Relieves acne caused by menstrual irregularities. Acts by decreasing estrogen production in the ovaries.[4]

AIDS

AIDS (acquired immune deficiency syndrome) is a disease characterized by a profound defect in the immune system. It develops as the result of infection with the human immunodeficiency virus (HIV). HIV is usually passed through sexual contact or blood-to-blood contact, or from infected mothers to their children.

Doctors diagnose AIDS when a patient's total count of T cells, an important immune-system component, drops to 200 or less (compared with from 1,000 to 1,500 in a healthy person). But doctors also take note of any decrease in the ratio of helper T cells to suppresser T cells. Helper T cells are those cells that help the immune system act against bacteria, viruses, and cancerous cells. Suppresser T cells, on the other hand, suppress the immune system's response to these invaders, a process meant to keep the system from becoming overactive.

The body's response to the initial HIV infection, and to the accompanying loss of immune function, varies from person to person. In some people, the progression from HIV to AIDS follows a recognized pattern. Rashes or mild flulike symptoms are followed by months or years of no symptoms, until some other factor limits immune resistance. At that point, the disease becomes active, producing symptoms that include fever, fatigue, diarrhea, mouth sores, night sweats, and swollen lymph glands. This stage is often called AIDS-related complex (ARC). However, in other people, the disorders seen in full-blown AIDS produce the first symptoms.

The decrease in helper T cells and the increase in suppresser T cells results in an increased susceptibility to infections and cancer. In 50 percent of all AIDS patients, the first symptom is *Pneumocystis carinii* pneumonia. This is a bacterial infection that only takes hold in the body in the absence of an immune defense. Many patients develop Kaposi's sarcoma, a connective tissue cancer almost exclusively associated with AIDS. Other infections commonly experienced by AIDS patients include those caused by cytomegalovirus, Epstein-Barr virus, herpes, salmonella, tuberculosis, and yeasts.

Before 1996, the mortality rate for full-blown AIDS was nearly 100 percent. Since then, innovations in treatment promise to extend the life expectancies of treated patients almost indefinitely. The overwhelming majority of AIDS patients in the world, however, do not have access to these treatments.

Kampo offers ways to fill in the gaps of conventional treatment. Since the virus that causes AIDS was unknown before 1981, traditional Japanese medicine did not have a concept of HIV in particular, nor of viruses in general. However, Kampo medicine did have a concept of diseases of the Lesser Yang (see Chapter 1). This is a condition of stalemate between the destructive energies of infection, which are trying to involve more and more of the body, and the body's defensive energies, which are trying to drive the infection out. Scientists in the United States and Japan have noted that the progression of HIV infection matches the symptom pattern associated with the Lesser Yang.

Scientists have found that the formula most commonly used for diseases of the Lesser Yang, Minor Bupleurum Decoction, has a profound effect on AIDS, including an ability to complement "AIDS cocktails," multidrug therapies that have proved effective against the disease. Systematic testing has revealed that many other traditional herbs and formulas are extremely helpful in treating AIDS. Before using any of these treatments, however, be sure to discuss them with a physician, who can determine if a specific substance's effect is appropriate for any specific stage of the disease.

INDIVIDUAL KAMPO TREATMENTS

See Chapter 3 for discussions of individual herbs, traditional healing substances, and modern herbal preparations, including directions for making tea.

SUGGESTED DOSAGES	COMMENTS
Astragalus (Herb)	
Fluid extract (1:1), ¼–½ tsp (1–2 ml) 3 times daily. or Freeze-dried herb in capsules, 500–1,000 mg 3 times daily. or Powdered solid extract (4:1), 250–500 mg 3 times daily. or Tea, 1 c 3 times daily. or Tincture (1:5), 1–1½ tsp (4–6 ml), 3 times daily. Place in a cup, add 2 tbsp water, and take in a single sip.	Stops opportunistic infection by *Streptococcus.* Kills the virus that causes hepatitis B,[1] which is sometimes transmitted along with HIV. Contains compounds that increase the ability of immune cells called lymphokine-activated killer (LAK) cells to attack cancers, such as Kaposi's sarcoma,[2] and that simulate helper T cell activity. *Caution:* Do not use when fever or skin infection is present.
LEM (Modern Herbal Preparation)	
Powder, as directed on label.	Prevents the progression of HIV to AIDS by stopping cell-to-cell transmission of the virus.[3] *Caution:* Can occasionally cause mild diarrhea or skin rashes. Should these symptoms occur, consult a health care provider.
Lentinan (Modern Herbal Preparation)	
Intramuscular injection (usual form), less than 10 mg, exact dosage based on patient's condition and circumstances. Given under professional supervision. or Powder, dosage to be determined by provider. Much greater dosages required than in injectable form.	Acts on the immune system by stimulating the production of antibodies and interferon, and activating natural killer (NK) cells and macrophages. Particularly active in augmenting helper T cells. Helpful in treating persons with low T-cell counts who do not have other AIDS symptoms.[4]
Maitake (Modern Herbal Preparation)	
Fresh or dried maitake in food, 1–2 tbsp (3–7 g) daily. or Maitake D-fraction in capsule or tablet form, 500 mg 3 times daily before meals. or Tea, 1 c 2–4 times daily.	Contains a carbohydrate-based substance known to kill HIV and to keep HIV from killing T cells.[5]
Prunella (Herb)	
Tea, 1 c 3 times daily between meals.	Blocks cell-to-cell transmission of HIV and interferes with the virus's ability to bind with T cells.[6] *Caution:* Do not use if diarrhea, nausea, stomachache, or vomiting is present.
Scutellaria (Herb)	
Dried herb, 1–2 1,000-mg capsules 3 times daily. or Fluid extract (1:1), ¼–½ tsp (1–2 ml) 3 times daily. or Powdered solid extract (4:1), 250–500 mg 3 times daily. or Tea, 1 c 3 times daily. or Tincture (1:5), 1–1½ tsp (4–6 ml) 3 times daily. Place in a cup, add 2 tbsp water, and take in a single sip.	Contains baicalin, which deactivates reverse transcriptase, an enzyme HIV needs to insert itself into human DNA, without affecting the T cells' ability to replicate.[7] Also prevents many other kinds of infections without involving the overtaxed immune system. *Caution:* Avoid in cases of diarrhea caused by foodborne infection or excessive consumption of cold drinks.

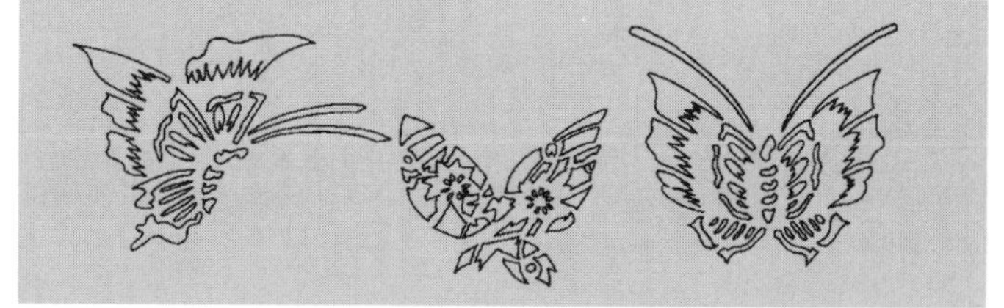

Turmeric (Herb)	
Curcumin, the yellow pigment found in turmeric, 250–500 mg twice daily between meals.	Curcumin stops HIV replication by deactivating the virus's long terminal repeat gene.[8] Also inhibits the activity of HIV integrase, an enzyme that allows the virus to use a human cell for its own replication.[9] Inhibits other factors necessary for HIV replication.[10]

Viola (Herb)	
Use under professional supervision.	Reported to keep HIV from "erupting"out of infected cells.[11,12] Contains compounds that keep germs which cause tuberculosis, a common AIDS complication, from multiplying. Use *Viola yedoensis* instead of *Viola tricolor.* Sold in bulk in Chinese herb shops as *zi hua di ding.*

KAMPO FORMULAS

See Chapter 4 for dosage information and discussions of individual formulas.

Minor Bupleurum Decoction

Can prevent the progression of HIV infection to AIDS[13,14] by activating immune cells that control the virus without activating those that could suppress immune response or cause destruction of healthy tissues. Increases the ability of 3TC (lamivudine) or AZT (zidovudine) plus 3TC, drugs used in AIDS "cocktails," to stop HIV multiplication in T cells.[15] Stops 90% of the activity of reverse transcriptase.[16] Does not interfere with T-cell reproduction.[17] Especially useful for people with AIDS who also have hepatitis (*see* **Hepatitis**).

Caution: Do not use if fever or skin infection is present. Taken long term in patent medicine form, can cause headache, dizziness, and bleeding gums. Side effects can be avoided if the formula is taken as a tea.

Ten-Significant Tonic Decoction (All-Inclusive Great Tonifying Decoction)

Useful as a general tonic for persons with AIDS. Stimulates production of interleukins and NK cells.[18]

True Man's Decoction to Nourish the Organs

Used to treat diarrhea or dysenteric disorders marked by unremitting diarrhea to the point of incontinence. Not available as a patent medicine, but widely available from Kampo and TCM practitioners as *zhen ren yang rang tang.*

Caution: Avoid alcohol, wheat, cold or raw foods, fish, and greasy foods. Should not be used by persons with gallbladder problems, obstruction of the bile duct, or a tendency to retain urine, or by pregnant women.

True Warrior Decoction

Used to treat advanced stages of wasting and anorexia, with coldness in the hands and feet, and such a severe state of weakness that hunger pangs have ceased. May cause a loss of sensation in the mouth and tongue.

Caution: Discontinue the formula if fever occurs.

CONSIDERATIONS

❑ *See also* **HIV Infection.**

ALCOHOLISM

Alcoholism is a condition in which an individual depends on the daily consumption of alcohol to avoid the physical and psychological symptoms of withdrawal. Over time, the individual tends to consume increasing quantities of alcohol, and to become more and more dependent on it.

In the United States, alcoholism affects at least 10 million people and contributes to 200,000 deaths a year. Men are twice as likely to be affected as women, and although most alcoholics are middle-aged, many young people either are or are becoming alcohol-dependent. The total number of people affected, however, is much greater than the number of alcoholics. Alcohol-related automobile fatalities (a factor in half of the annual fatal accidents in the United States), crime, diminished work productivity, and disrupted family life all mark a large-scale social problem.[1]

Alcoholism goes beyond just simple intoxication. Intoxication is associated with discomfort, impaired judgment, poor coordination, and pain. Intoxication is alcohol abuse, but it is not necessarily alcohol dependency. Alcoholism, though, always involves abuse, but does not necessarily involve discomfort, impairment, and pain every time the alcoholic drinks. Some alcoholics can drink quite a bit and still appear sober.

Long-term alcoholism is associated with a number of serious disorders. Its effects on the nervous system make the individual prone to psychological disorders such as depression. Its effects on the liver, digestive organs, and kidneys can lead to diseases of these organs. In addition, it increases a person's risk of developing high blood pressure, impotence, stroke, and several types of cancer.

There are many indications that alcoholism is, at least in part, a genetic condition. The incidence of alcoholism is four to five times higher among biological children of alcoholic parents than among children of nonalcoholic parents.[2] Certain ethnic groups, especially Japanese and Koreans, have low alcoholism rates. Members of these groups do not have a gene that breaks down acetaldehyde, a chemical that is produced when the body processes alcohol, that causes headache, nausea, and redness in the face.[3] Individuals without this gene are much less likely to develop alcohol dependence because they generally cannot tolerate more than one or two drinks. Members of other ethnic groups are genetically able to break down acetaldehyde very efficiently, and thus have a much greater tendency toward alcoholism.

Although Kampo physicians have used herbs to treat alcoholism for over 2,000 years, they used different strategies for treating alcoholism's effects and its causes. Western medicine recognizes alcoholism's health effects in terms of cirrhosis of the liver, but Kampo recognized alcoholism's effects in terms of drying out the blood, which caused problems in the liver and gallbladder. However, Kampo theorists did not develop an understanding of a symptom pattern for alcoholics who have not yet experienced "dry blood," and instead found therapies for alcoholism by trial and error.

Some Kampo treatments work by slowing down the body's processing of acetaldehyde. This increases the discomfort associated with intoxication, which creates an aversion to alcohol. In this respect, they act like the prescription drug Antabuse, but with less severe side effects.

INDIVIDUAL KAMPO TREATMENTS

See Chapter 3 for discussions of individual herbs, traditional healing substances, and modern herbal preparations, including directions for making tea.

SUGGESTED DOSAGES	COMMENTS
Kudzu (Herb)	
Dried extract, 1 10-mg tablet 3 times daily. or Tea, 1 c 3 times daily.	Contains two compounds that alter the liver enzymes which break down alcohol.[4] As a result, produces mild nausea, swelling, redness in the face if taken before drinking alcoholic beverages. If kudzu is not available, use **Kudzu Decoction** (see formulas list).
Reishi (Modern Herbal Preparation)	
Dried extract, 3 1-g tablets 3 times daily. or Syrup, as directed on label. or Tincture (1:5), 1 tbsp (10 ml) 3 times daily. Place in a cup, add 2 tbsp water, and take in a single sip.	Beneficial for patients with alcoholic liver disease who have not yet experienced severe loss of liver function.[5] In Kampo, is most useful in persons whose "liver" symptoms are compounded by emotional stress or ongoing tension. Also useful when excess alcohol use has produced fatty deposits or irritation within the liver.
Soy Lecithin (Modern Herbal Preparation)	
Soy phospholipids, 1,500–3,000 mg daily. Identified individually on the label as 3-sn-phospatidylcholine, phosphatidylethanolamine, and phospatidylinositic acid, or as "total phospholipids."	Protects liver tissue from effects of alcohol by speeding regeneration and stabilization of cell membrane. Acts by stopping free-radical activity that would destroy the membrane and by stimulating collagen creation for repair and support. *Caution:* Mild diarrhea may occur when soy lecithin is first used.

KAMPO FORMULAS

See Chapter 4 for dosage information and discussions of individual formulas.

Kudzu Decoction

The main Kampo treatment for alcoholism. Contains kudzu compounds that slow down the body's processing of acetaldehyde.

CONSIDERATIONS

❏ *See also* **Cirrhosis, Alcoholic** and **Hangover.**

ALLERGIES, FOOD

An allergy is an overreaction by the immune system to a normally harmless substance. Millions of people have allergic reactions to specific foods. Such reactions include various digestive complaints, such as gas, nausea, and diarrhea, and a wide range of other symptoms, including respiratory congestion, swelling, itching, hives, and eye inflammation. Sometimes there is a delay between eating the food and experiencing the reaction, which can make food allergies hard to track. Food allergies can also contribute to chronic health problems, such as asthma. The offending foods can be identified through either an elimination diet (see consideration below) or allergy testing.

Food allergy occurs when the immune system reacts to a normally benign component in certain foods, most commonly corn, fish and shellfish, eggs, chocolate, citrus fruit, nuts, and berries. Some people have an allergic reaction to gluten, which is the major protein component of wheat. This is called *celiac sprue*. Cereal grains that are related to wheat, such as barley, oats, and rye, also contain proteins that can cause sprue.

Several factors can cause the immune system to react to food. One is *leaky gut syndrome*, a disorder in which a digestive-system fault allows relatively large food particles to pass into the bloodstream, where they provoke allergic reactions. Another factor is stress, since some scientists believe that high levels of stress hormones reduce the body's ability to keep large food particles out of the bloodstream. And another possible factor is the overabundance of immune-system cells called helper T cells in the bloodstream,[1,2] since these cells stimulate a strong allergic reaction.

The terms "food allergy" and "food intolerance" are often used interchangeably, but they describe two separate conditions. Food intolerance occurs when the digestive tract lacks the enzymes necessary for proper nutrition. An example of this is *lactase deficiency*, which causes the sufferer to experience abdominal tension, cramping, and diarrhea after eating milk or dairy products. If left unchecked, celiac sprue can also lead to lactose intolerance.

Food allergy or intolerance corresponds to a condition traditional Japanese medicine described as "uprushing cold energy." Uprushing energy, as the name suggests, frequently expresses itself as vomiting, although cold can also stop the normal, downward passage of food through the intestines. This cold does not completely overwhelm the digestive tract, but causes the system to work in fits and starts, experienced as cramps and spasms. Warming herbs enable the stomach's energy to resume its normal, downward course.

INDIVIDUAL KAMPO TREATMENTS

See Chapter 3 for discussions of individual herbs, traditional healing substances, and modern herbal preparations, including directions for making tea.

SUGGESTED DOSAGES	COMMENTS
Ginger (Herb)	
Tea, 1 c 3 times daily.	Settles the stomach and deactivates platelet activating factor, the chemical messenger that starts allergic reactions.

KAMPO FORMULAS

See Chapter 4 for dosage information and discussions of individual formulas.

Kudzu Decoction

Used for diarrhea caused by food allergies.

Major Construct the Middle Decoction

Remedy of choice in Japan for food allergy causing cramping and diarrhea. *Caution:* Avoid if fever is present.

CONSIDERATIONS

❑ Individuals who are not sure what foods are causing the problems should keep a detailed diary of foods eaten each day and symptoms that occur. Once a list of suspect foods has been created, these foods should be eliminated from the diet, one at a time, and then reintroduced, again one at a time, to pinpoint exactly which foods are at fault.

❑ If a doctor has diagnosed celiac sprue, avoid wheat, barley, buckwheat, millet, oats, rye, and triticale, and foods that can contain them, such as beer, canned soup, ice cream, malt, vodka, and whisky.

❑ Persons with lactose intolerance should read labels carefully. Various dairy components, such as milk solids, are added to a wide variety of packaged foods. It may help to try over-the-counter products that contain the enzyme necessary for lactose digestion.

❑ For information on the role of food allergies in other disorders, see the following: asthma, "Managing Asthma With Nutrition," page 156; Crohn's disease, page 194; ear infections, page 203; eczema, "Managing Eczema Through Diet," page 206. *See also* **Diarrhea.**

ALLERGIES, RESPIRATORY

An allergy is a super-sensitive reaction to a normally harmless substance. Both children and adults suffer seasonal allergies to pollens from blooming plants as well as allergies to animal danders, feathers, and a tremendous variety of environmental chemicals.

Respiratory allergies cause sneezing, weeping, coughing, nasal drip, and painful irritation of the eyes, ears, nose, and throat. Secondary symptoms include fatigue, headache, nosebleed, and itchiness. Allergies can also aggravate other health problems, including asthma, eczema, and acne.

The most common seasonal respiratory allergy, hay fever, is a creation of modern air pollution. In 1819, English physician and allergy patient John Bostock was only able to find 28 other cases among 5,000 people. Similarly, records indicate that hay fever was unknown in America before 1850. Now, however, one in six Americans sneezes, wheezes, and tears through the allergy season.[1]

The exact cause of allergies is unknown, although heredity is thought to play a role. In addition, babies who are not breastfed do not receive their mothers' antibodies to various allergy-provoking substances, which may make such children vulnerable to allergy development.

Allergy symptoms are caused by the release of histamine, which can enter circulation in one of two ways. Most frequently, an allergy-causing substance, or antigen, enters the body and triggers the release of antibodies. These antibodies prompt histamine-bearing mast cells to secrete the substance into the bloodstream. The histamine then "docks" at receptor sites on various types of cells. In this way, it signals smooth muscles lining blood vessels to relax, lowering blood pressure (which makes it difficult for the body to circulate fluids away from the lungs), and smooth muscles lining the bronchial passages to contract, increasing air resistance. Histamine also stimulates secretion from the salivary glands and stomach lining, sedates the central nervous system, and causes fluid to flow into the sinuses and nasal passages.

The other way histamine can enter the bloodstream is by the destruction of mast cells. Drugs and chemicals can cause the walls of mast cells to break, spilling histamine into the bloodstream. The same reactions occur, but with greater intensity.

Most drugs for allergy act by blocking the histamine receptor sites. The disadvantage of these drugs is that they can cross from the bloodstream to the brain, causing sleepiness and sedation. Kampo herbs and formulas used to treat allergies shield cells from histamine's effects, but cannot cross the blood-brain barrier.

The scientific explanation of how Kampo treatments work as antihistamines is consistent with Kampo's ancient understanding of allergy. The ancient theorists saw allergy as an invasion of "cold" entering the skin. The body repelled the cold by producing heat, and by opening the pores of the skin to give the pathogen a route of escape. If the pathogenic cold did not flee, then the body produced copious amounts of fluid and phlegm to wash it out of the body.

Since respiratory allergy was extremely rare in ancient Japan, Kampo theorists did not develop an understanding of the energy imbalances that cause chronic allergies. Instead they treated both chronic and seasonal allergies with the same herbs. Many Japanese herbalists today report that a single course of treatment with the right herbs usually leads to remission in cases of chronic allergy. In cases of seasonal allergy, none of these herbs or formulas is intended for year-round constant use. Start them one or two weeks before the beginning of the applicable allergy season, and discontinue them one or two weeks after the end of the season.

INDIVIDUAL KAMPO TREATMENTS

See Chapter 3 for discussions of individual herbs, traditional healing substances, and modern herbal preparations, including directions for making tea.

SUGGESTED DOSAGES	COMMENTS
Acorus (Herb)	
Powders, teas, and tinctures: 1–2 g, measured and dispensed by herbalist.	Contains alpha-asarone, a potent antihistamine.[2]

Bitter Orange, Bitter Orange Peel (Herb)	
Tea, either herb, 1 c 3 times daily. or Tincture (1:5), bitter orange peel, 10 drops 3 times daily. Place in a cup, add 2 tbsp water, and take in a single sip.	Prevents a wide variety of allergic reactions, especially when very young fruits are used. *Caution:* Kampo urges caution in using these herbs if "red" symptoms exist: red tongue, redness in the face with fever and cough, and spitting of blood.

Bupleurum (Herb)	
Saikosaponin extract, 1 300-mg tablet daily. or Tea, 1 c 3 times daily.	Stops swelling or constriction of the bronchial passages by blocking 5HT, a substance that allows passage of body fluids into soft tissues.[3] Also counteracts the production of watery mucus in hay fever. *Caution:* Do not use if fever is present. Occasionally causes mild stomach upset. If this happens, reduce the dose. Do not take antibiotics when taking bupleurum.

Ephedra (Herb)	
Powdered herb in food, 1–3 tbsp (3–9 g) daily. or Tea, 1 c 1–3 times daily. or Tincture (1:5), 15 drops 3 times daily. Place in a cup, add 2 tbsp water, and take in a single sip.	Acts on the sympathetic nervous system. This causes the bronchial passages to dilate, and accelerates and intensifies respiration. *Caution:* Do not use if taking an MAO inhibitor, or if high blood pressure, anxiety, glaucoma, or a prostate disorder is present. Be sure to drink 8 glasses of water daily.

Forsythia (Herb)	
Use only under supervision of an herbalist.	Treats allergic reactions to medication.[4]

Hawthorn (Herb)	
Dried herb in capsules, 3–5 g daily. or Fluid extract (1:1), $\frac{1}{4}$–$\frac{1}{2}$ tsp (1–2 ml) 3 times daily. or Solid extract, 100–250 mg 3 times daily. Should be standardized to contain 10% proanthocyanidins. or Tea, $\frac{2}{3}$ c 3–4 times daily. or Tincture (1:5), 1–1$\frac{1}{2}$ tsp (4–6 ml) 3 times daily. Place in a cup, add 2 tbsp water, and take in a single sip. Can be given to children (see inset on page 142).	Contains antihistamines called histadine decarboxylase blockers.[5]

Jujube Fruit (Herb)	
Pitted fruits, 3–12 daily.	Relieves allergic purpura, a condition producing skin rash and bleeding under the skin.[6]

Magnolia, Scutellaria (Herbs)	
Magnolia Flower Combination, as directed on label, 3 times daily. and Scutellaria tea, 1 c 3 times daily.	Effective against nasal allergies and sinusitis.[7]

Reishi (Modern Herbal Preparation)	
Dried extract, 3 1-g tablets 3 times daily. or Dried mushroom in food, approx. $\frac{1}{4}$–approx. $\frac{1}{2}$ oz (5–10 g) daily. or Syrup, as directed on label. or Tea, 1 c 3 times daily. or Tincture (1:5), 1 tsp (4 ml) 3 times daily. Place in a cup, add 2 tbsp water, and take in a single sip.	Contains antihistamines,[8] as well as compounds that stop platelet activating factor, hormone that causes the bronchial passages to constrict.[9] *Caution:* Do not use in an area where reishi grows wild. Airborne reishi spores can themselves cause allergies.

KAMPO FORMULAS

See Chapter 4 for dosage information and discussions of individual formulas.

Cinnamon and Peony Decoction

Treats nasal allergy compounded by feelings of fullness in the chest.

Cinnamon Twig Decoction

Treats skin or nasal allergies compounded by fever and chills, headache, and stomach upset.

Ephedra Decoction (Four Emperors Combination)

Relaxes the airway, which stops wheezing. A variation, Ephedra, Apricot Kernel, Coix, and Licorice Decoction, is designed to lower fever, in addition to treating other symptoms. Use either formula in patent-medicine form.

Ephedra, Asiasarum, and Prepared Aconite Decoction

Specifically treats nasal congestion caused by allergy to cedar pollen when taken before beginning of cedar pollen season.[10] May cause a loss of sensation in the mouth and tongue.

Caution: Discontinue the formula if fever occurs.

Kudzu Decoction

Treats nasal allergy accompanied by stiff neck and upper back.

Major Construct the Middle Decoction

Extremely effective for nasal allergies.[11]

Ophiopogonis Decoction

Stops "sneezing fits." Also relieves spasmodic cough, flushed face, dry and scratchy throat, feeling of sputum being stuck in the throat, and hoarseness.

Caution: Use with caution if fever is present, and discontinue if preexisting fevers worsen.

CONSIDERATIONS

❑ *See also* **Asthma.**

Alzheimer's Disease

Alzheimer's disease is a degenerative brain disorder that destroys memory, undermines personality, and ultimately causes death. Some health professionals call it the country's "disease of the twenty-first century," because doctors expect the number of Alzheimer's victims to grow as the population ages. About 250,000 cases are diagnosed annually.[1]

Family history and age are the two main risk factors for Alzheimer's disease. Viruses, head injuries, and excessive exposure to certain metals, most notably aluminum, may also play a role. The illness begins slowly, with bouts of forgetfulness, and progresses to a stage in which the patient totally depends on others for all needs, both physical and mental. Diagnosis is based on symptoms and the elimination of other disorders. There is no way to definitively test living persons for Alzheimer's disease.

Almost everything medical science knows about Alzheimer's comes from postmortem examinations. The first such examination was conducted in 1906 by Alois Alzheimer, who observed unusual changes in brain tissue from a woman who had died at the age of fifty-five after developing dementia five years earlier. Alzheimer found that her brain tissue contained nerve cells with tangled fibers and clumps of degenerating nerve endings.

In Alzheimer's disease, brain cells disappear from both the cerebral cortex, a structure in the front of the brain that is the center of intellectual activity, and the hippocampus, a structure deep in the brain involved with memory and reasoning. As the cells malfunction and die, the connections between them are lost. This interferes with the intricate process of cell-to-cell communication.

Researchers have linked the cellular changes seen in Alzheimer's disease to a defect in the apolipoprotein-E, or Apo-E, gene.[2] This gene is responsible for the transport of cholesterol, an essential building material for all cell membranes. Cholesterol, a fat, needs a carrier to circulate through the water-based bloodstream, so the liver attaches it to a water-soluble protein. When the resulting lipoprotein package arrives at a cell, the protein inserts itself into the cell membrane and unloads its cholesterol. The protein is then snapped off and recycled. In the brain tissue of Alzheimer's patients, the faulty Apo-E gene causes the carrier protein to be snapped off at the wrong place.

Immune cells circulating in the brain read the malformed protein as a signal that something is wrong with the cell. The immune system treats this defect as an invading microorganism and sets out to destroy the invader. The problem is compounded when beta amyloid peptide, a potentially toxic substance, is created by the faulty protein break.[3] As beta amyloid disintegrates, it generates free radicals, which in turn destroy cell membranes.[4] The resulting mass of dead cells becomes entangled and forms a beta-amyloid plaque. Spiral filaments of protein form irregular circles around nerve cells and lead to the cells' death and destruction.

Kampo identified a symptom pattern corresponding to Alzheimer's disease in the 1540s. Kampo envisioned this pattern of anxiety, fatigue, inability to think or concentrate for even short periods of time, irritability, memory loss, and palpitations as an imbalance of fire and water. The heart stores the spirit and sends the concentrated energy of the spirit in the form of "fire" to the kidneys. The kidneys are energized by this energy and send water to nourish the heart. Excessive thinking and deliberation disturb the yin, or containing, energy of the kidneys so that they no longer capture the fire of the heart. They do not send the heart water, and the heart is unable to circulate nourishment through the body. Its fire races upward to the head, which is first heated and then burned.

This metaphor predicted what science would learn about how Kampo can help people with Alzheimer's disease. Some Kampo preparations regulate oxygen availability to the brain. When the brain's supply of blood and oxygen is constant, fewer free radicals form and fewer brain cells are damaged. Other Kampo preparations either provide extra nutrients to repair damaged brain tissue or increase the sup-

Ginkgo—The Memory Herb and Alzheimer's Disease

Ginkgo extract helps many diseases of senility, including Alzheimer's disease. Ginkgo extract increases the functional capacity of the brain through its effects on acetylcholine, a chemical that allows the nerve cells responsible for memory and reasoning to communicate with each other. Ginkgo makes the hippocampus, the part of the brain most affected by Alzheimer's disease, more receptive to acetylcholine. It also increases the ability of acetylcholine to transmit messages.[1]

The benefits of ginkgo in treating the early stages of Alzheimer's disease have been demonstrated in two carefully controlled, double-blind studies. In the first study, 216 patients with either Alzheimer's disease or loss of mental function caused by multiple "ministrokes" were given either 240 milligrams of either ginkgo extract or a placebo daily for twenty-four weeks. The data from the 136 patients who completed the study show that ginkgo was very useful in treating both kinds of dementia.[2]

A second study, published in the *Journal of the American Medical Association,* was the first clinical study of ginkgo extract conducted in the United States. In this study, 202 patients with Alzheimer's disease, at six research centers supervised by Harvard Medical School and the New York Institute for Medical Research, were given either 120 milligrams of ginkgo extract or a placebo daily. Ginkgo treatment improved symptoms in 64 percent of the patients. There were no reports of side effects.[3] In addition to treating Alzheimer's disease, ginkgo is useful when symptoms are caused by insufficient blood flow or depression misdiagnosed as Alzheimer's disease. (For more information on ginkgo, *see* **Ginkgo** in Chapter 3.)

ply of glucose (blood sugar) to the brain. Since Kampo provides nutrients and the latest prescription drugs conserve nutrients, Kampo greatly assists the healing process in this difficult-to-treat condition.

INDIVIDUAL KAMPO TREATMENTS

See Chapter 3 for discussions of individual herbs, traditional healing substances, and modern herbal preparations, including directions for making tea.

SUGGESTED DOSAGES	COMMENTS
Ginkgo (Modern Herbal Preparation)	
Ginkgolide extract, up to 500 mg daily in a single dose.[5]	See "Ginkgo—The Memory Herb and Alzheimer's Disease" on page 149. Most manufacturers recommend 160–240 mg daily, but Alzheimer's disease requires higher dosages.[6]
Hawthorn (Herb)	
Dried herb in capsules, 3–5 g daily. or Fluid extract (1:1), $\frac{1}{4}$–$\frac{1}{2}$ tsp (1–2 ml) 3 times daily. or Solid extract, 100–250 mg 3 times daily. Should be standardized to contain 10% proanthocyanidins. or Tea, $\frac{2}{3}$ c 3–4 times daily. or Tincture (1:5), 1–1$\frac{1}{2}$ tsp (4–6 ml) 3 times daily. Place in a cup, add 2 tbsp water, and take in a single sip.	Lowers blood-cholesterol levels by increasing the rate at which cholesterol is broken down. Helps atherosclerotic lesions in the walls of blood vessels to shrink and become smoother, indirectly increasing blood supply to the brain.
Jujube Fruit (Herb)	
Pitted fruits, 10 daily.	Reported to restore memory.[7]
Rose Hips (Herb)	
Natural rose-hip vitamin C, 1,000 mg daily. Rose-hip vitamins have a shelf life of 6 mos. or Tea, 1 c as desired.	Traditional Japanese remedy for memory loss due to aging. Contains both vitamin C and the vitamin C cofactors needed to increase capillary circulation in brain tissue. This increases the supply of oxygen, glucose, and acetylcholine. *Caution:* Should not be used when there is danger of increasing aluminum absorption.
Soy Lecithin (Modern Herbal Preparation)	
Very high doses of soy phospholipids, 15–25 g (15,000–25,000 mg, or 30–50 500-mg capsules). Identified individually on the label as 3-sn-phospatidylcholine, phosphatidylethanolamine, and phospatidylinositic acid, or as "total phospholipids."	Source of phosphatidylcholine, which prevents destruction of brain tissue in conditions of oxygen deprivation. Since soy provides nutrients that the prescription drug tacrine preserves, the two treatments are complementary. May help *mild to moderate* cases. If there is no noticeable improvement within 2 weeks, supplements should be stopped, since soy lecithin at this dosage is expensive and can cause mild diarrhea.

KAMPO FORMULAS

See Chapter 4 for dosage information and discussions of individual formulas.

Biota Seed Pill to Nourish the Heart

Considered most important formula in Kampo for age-related memory loss, although actions are not yet scientifically confirmed. Biota activates recent memory rather than long-term memory.[8]

Bupleurum Plus Dragon Bone and Oyster Shell Decoction

Reduces agitated behavior. Free-radical scavenger, absorbing oxide and hydroxide ions that would destroy nerve tissue.

Caution: Be sure the formula does *not* include the traditional ingredient minium (lead oxide). Use with caution if fever is present, and discontinue if preexisting fevers worsen.

Coptis Decoction to Relieve Toxicity

Potent free-radical scavenger, preventing the damaging effects of both aluminum and D-aspartic acid from the artificial sweetener aspartame.

Eight-Ingredient Pill With Rehmannia (Rehmannia-Eight Combination)

Keeps blood-sugar levels constant. Particularly useful for persons who have both Alzheimer's and diabetes.

Gastrodia and Uncaria Decoction

Contains gastrodia, which increases circulation to the brain. This herb also increases brain's production of its own free-radical scavenger, superoxide dismutase, which prevents free radicals from activating compounds that destroy cell walls.[9]

Settle the Emotions Pill

Contains four herbs widely prescribed in China and Japan for age-related loss of mental function: acorus, ginseng, hoelen, and polygala. Treats poor memory compounded by insomnia, dizziness, hot flashes, or dry mouth.

CONSIDERATIONS

❑ Because of the connection between aluminum and Alzheimer's disease, exposure to this metal should be avoided. Do not use aluminum cookware, and buy bottled, not canned, beverages. Also, read labels carefully when shopping. Aluminum is used in some processed foods, such as processed cheese, pickles, cake mixes, and baking soda. This metal is also found in some antacids, buffered aspirins, antidiarrhea preparations, douches, deodorants, and shampoos.

❑ *See also* **Memory Problems.**

ANEMIA

Anemia is a condition in which the blood is deficient in red blood cells or the hemoglobin (iron-containing) portion of those cells. Red blood cells transport oxygen from the lungs to the tissues of the body, exchanging fresh oxygen for "used" oxygen, or carbon dioxide. The symptoms of anemia result from a failure of the red blood cells to provide oxygen efficiently. Anemia can manifest itself as pallor, breathlessness, weakness, and a tendency to tire easily.

Anemia can be diagnosed from laboratory tests that show a low level of total red blood cells or red blood cells of abnormal shape and size. Some people assume that anemia is always caused by "iron-poor" blood and that they need iron supplements. However, determining the cause of anemia is never a task for self-diagnosis. It is essential that laboratory tests be done, especially those tests that measure iron levels, before trying to correct the problem.

The underlying cause of anemia may be excessive blood loss, excessive red blood cell destruction, or deficient red blood cell production. These conditions can be produced by different factors, including infections, medications, pregnancy, and heavy menstruation. The majority of anemia cases, however, result from deficient red blood cell production caused by nutrient deficiency, and are treated with nutrient supplementation. The three nutrients that are usually responsible are iron, vitamin B_{12}, or folic acid. Iron-deficiency anemia is a form of *microcytic anemia,* in which the red blood cells are very small. Vitamin B_{12}, or pernicious, anemia is a form of *macrocytic anemia,* in which the red blood cells are very large.

Kampo describes anemia as a pattern of constraint imposed on the liver, the organ the body uses to store blood. When the liver cannot export blood, its vital energies build up and cause not just a lack of blood but also disturbances along the liver energy channel, which crosses the breasts and the eyes. Anemia also results from the liver's inability to provide energy to the digestive tract. "Warming" the digestion treats anemia.

INDIVIDUAL KAMPO TREATMENTS

See Chapter 3 for discussions of individual herbs, traditional healing substances, and modern herbal preparations, including directions for making tea.

SUGGESTED DOSAGES	COMMENTS
Dandelion (Herb)	
Tea, 1 c 3 times daily on an empty stomach. or Tincture (1:5), 10–15 drops 3 times daily on an empty stomach. Place in a cup, add 2 tbsp water, and take in a single sip.	Contains more iron, potassium, and vitamins than any other Kampo herb. Treats anemia due to deficiencies of folic acid, iron, or vitamin B_{12}.[1]

KAMPO FORMULAS

See Chapter 4 for dosage information and discussions of individual formulas.

Four-Substance Decoction

Treats all forms of anemia. Increases both the production and the circulation of blood.

Minor Construct the Middle Decoction

Treats anemia brought on by overwork and/or improper eating habits.

Pinellia Decoction to Drain the Epigastrium

Treats anemia due to "cold" in the stomach, which manifests itself as abdominal fullness, diarrhea, reduced appetite, and stomach rumbles.

Caution: Use with caution if fever is present, and discontinue if preexisting fevers worsen.

Rambling Powder

Treats anemia when there is also fever or chills, irregular menstruation, or distended breasts, all symptoms of constrained liver energy.

ANGINA

Angina is a squeezing or pressurelike pain in the chest caused by an insufficient supply of oxygen to the heart muscle. Angina usually precedes a heart attack, although many people have angina for years without experiencing damage to the heart itself. Since physical exertion and stress increase the heart's need for oxygen, they are usually the triggers for an angina attack. Angina pain may radiate to the left shoulder blade, left arm, or jaw. The pain usually lasts from one to twenty minutes.

Angina is almost always caused by atherosclerosis, the buildup of cholesterol that narrows and eventually closes the coronary arteries, the blood vessels leading to the heart. Blockage of the coronary arteries reduces the supply of blood and oxygen to the heart. When the flow of oxygen to the heart is substantially reduced, or when there is an unusually high demand for oxygen in the heart, angina is the result. Angina can also be caused by extremely low blood-sugar levels (hypoglycemia). That is because hypoglycemia can lead to increased production of hormones associated with stress, which can put a strain on the heart.

Angina can be relieved surgically, although that method is not without its problems (see "Angina—Is Surgery Necessary?" on page 152). Nutritional management of angina and coronary artery disease consists of two strategies, removing the dietary factors that cause angina and adding dietary supplements that prevent it. Cholesterol cannot be completely removed as a risk factor, since some cholesterol is absolutely necessary to the normal functioning of every cell in the body. The compounds that energize the formation of cholesterol plaques, however, can be greatly reduced. These compounds include excess amounts of iron and copper, which create harmful substances called free radicals. These free radicals activate immune cells known as macrophages, which form a platform, called a foam cell, on which cholesterol can accumulate and later calcify in the artery wall.

Dietary restriction alone may take two to five years to have an effect, but it is also possible to accelerate the process of healing with Kampo. While modern medicine sees the cause of angina as the circulation of unneeded nutrient *chemicals* through the body, by the nineteenth century Kampo medicine saw the cause of angina as the circulation of unneeded nutrient *energies.* The saying in Kampo was, "When energy circulates, blood will circulate." If the emotional "energies" of the liver were disseminated evenly, and the respiratory energies from the lungs were diffused throughout the body, then blood would flow smoothly and new blood would be produced.

Angina—Is Surgery Necessary?

Medical treatment of angina typically involves an angiogram, followed by angioplasty or coronary artery bypass surgery. An angiogram is an X-ray procedure in which dye is injected into the coronary arteries to locate blockages. These blockages are then most often opened with balloon angioplasty, a surgical procedure in which the diameter of the blocked artery is increased with the aid of a very small balloon attached to a flexible tube. More difficult cases typically involve coronary artery bypass surgery, a procedure in which the coronary artery is bypassed by construction of an alternate route using a portion of vein from the patient's leg.

Several clinical studies have challenged the widespread use of angiograms, angioplasty, and coronary artery bypass surgery by cardiologists. In one study, 134 out 168 candidates for angioplasty or coronary bypass surgery were treated instead with noninvasive therapies and followed for five years. This group of patients experienced fatal heart attacks at the rate of approximately 1 percent annually, compared with annual mortality rates of from 1 to 2 percent for patients treated with angioplasty and from 5 to 10 percent for patients treated with coronary bypass surgery.[1,2] Another study found that patients with healthy hearts but with one, two, or three of the major heart vessels blocked did surprisingly well without surgery. Regardless of the number or severity of the blockages, each group had the same low death rate of 1 percent per year.[3] That same year, the average death rate from bypass surgery was slightly over 10 percent, or about one death in ten operations.[4] In other words, bypass surgery and balloon angioplasty are appropriate only for the most serious cases of angina. Discussing nonsurgical alternatives with a doctor is a good idea for an individual whose condition is not critical.

INDIVIDUAL KAMPO TREATMENTS

See Chapter 3 for discussions of individual herbs, traditional healing substances, and modern herbal preparations, including directions for making tea.

SUGGESTED DOSAGES	COMMENTS
Dan Shen (Herb)	
Tincture. Use only under professional supervision.	Important herb in modern Kampo treatment of angina. Relaxes smooth muscles supporting the coronary arteries and increases circulation to the heart through the action of a calcium channel blocker, tanshinone IIA.[1] Reduces pulse rate, but increases cardiac output. Breaks down fibrin, a protein that forms a "net" on the artery wall on which clots can form, and stops clot formation. *Caution:* Avoid if an estrogen-sensitive disorder is present, such as bladder cancer, melanoma, or disorders of the female reproductive system.
Hawthorn (Herb)	
Dried herb in capsules, 3–5 g daily. or Fluid extract (1:1), $\frac{1}{4}$–$\frac{1}{2}$ tsp (1–2 ml) 3 times daily. or Solid extract, 100–250 mg 3 times daily. Should be standardized to contain 10% proanthocyanidins. or Tea, $\frac{2}{3}$ c 3–4 times daily. or Tincture (1:5), 1–1$\frac{1}{2}$ tsp (4–6 ml) 3 times. Place in a cup, add 2 tbsp water, and take in a single sip.	Treats angina when chest pain occurs upon excitement or exertion but not when the patient is at rest. Dilates coronary blood vessels by relaxing the smooth muscle surrounding them. Interacts with key enzymes in the heart to change the way heart muscle tissue contracts,[2] counteracting the heart muscle's energy-limiting enzyme.[3] To have a positive effect on angina, hawthorn must be taken for at least 8 weeks.[4]

KAMPO FORMULAS

See Chapter 4 for dosage information and discussions of individual formulas.

Drive Out Stasis From the Mansion of Blood Decoction

Supportive therapy for chest pain with cough or hiccups and/or insomnia.

Gastrodia and Uncaria Decoction

Contains gastrodia, which increases blood flow to heart muscle and increases its resistance to oxygen deprivation. This herb also encourages deep sleep and relaxes the central nervous system, which leads to reduced production of the stress hormone adrenaline.[5,6]

Caution: Should not be used by women who are trying to become pregnant.

CONSIDERATIONS

❑ Chelation therapy is used to draw toxic substances out of the body. A chelating agent called ethylenediaminetetraacetic acid (EDTA) can reverse angina; it seems that EDTA's therapeutic effect results from chelating out excess iron and copper.[7] While the evidence supports the use of chelation therapy to reverse atherosclerosis and the angina it causes, the same effect can be achieved over the long term with diet. Avoid taking mineral supplements, especially iron-enriched tonics, and limit or eliminate consumption of red meat, especially liver and other organ meats.

❑ *See also* **Atherosclerosis** and **High Cholesterol**.

ANXIETY

Anxiety is a condition of inappropriate nervousness or fear. It can cause shortness of breath, heart palpitations, and tingling sensations in the face, hands, and feet. While appropriate fear is a rational response to a real danger, anxiety usually lacks a clear or realistic cause. Some level of anxiety is normal and possibly even healthy by helping the body stay alert to danger.[1] But high levels of anxiety for long periods of time are not only unpleasant but can lead to significant health problems, such as chronic fatigue, diabetes, high blood pressure, and increased susceptibility to infection.

Anxiety is classified as *generalized anxiety disorder,* in which symptoms last six months or more; *phobias,* in which anxiety is provoked by a specific situation, such as being at a height; or *panic disorder,* which is marked by panic attacks that occur for no obvious reason. In a panic attack, the person feels overwhelming dread and terror, often accompanied by feelings that he or she is going to die or go crazy. Anxiety is also associated with sleep disturbances, mood swings, forgetfulness, difficulty in concentrating, and fatigue.

Most doctors treat anxiety and panic attacks with benzodiazepam tranquilizers or tricyclic antidepressants. These drugs can cause a number of side effects. In addition, the tranquilizers carry a high potential for addiction, and withdrawal can be emotionally and physically unpleasant. The antidepressants can sometimes cause the individual taking them to go from depression to manic excitement. This can make day-to-day functioning so difficult that the person's anxiety actually becomes worse.

Psychological factors do play a role in anxiety, but this disorder has a nutritional basis as well. The key is a chemical called lactic acid, created when the body burns glucose, or blood sugar, without oxygen. (This occurs for example, when a person exercises so vigorously that he or she cannot catch breath.) Lactic acid is changed into lactate and transported to the liver, where it is changed into harmless pyruvic acid. Persons who tend to suffer panic attacks, however, are unable to convert lactate into pyruvic acid, and so have elevated blood levels of lactate.

Traditional Japanese medicine also described anxiety in nutritional terms. The heart, the seat of the spirit, powered the circulation of nutritive energy throughout the body. Anxiety occurred when the "energy" of the heart or other organs was displaced, either by long-term suppression of emotions or through sudden shock. Unable to channel the emotional energy unleashed by the heart, other organs begin to "shake." The person experienced worry, insomnia, disturbing dreams, shortness of breath, or dizziness, in addition to painful tension in various parts of the body.

Kampo designed anxiety treatments in terms of channeling the heart's energy and increasing qi circulation. In fact, the most basic Kampo treatments for anxiety act by increasing circulation to the brain, rather than by changing the brain's chemistry. Other Kampo treatments for anxiety do change brain chemistry by locking into receptor sites that normally receive tranquilizers, but without occupying other receptor sites that induce drowsiness. Kampo treatments offer relief from the *symptoms* of anxiety without interfering with one's ability to handle stressful conditions.

INDIVIDUAL KAMPO TREATMENTS

See Chapter 3 for discussions of individual herbs, traditional healing substances, and modern herbal preparations, including directions for making tea.

SUGGESTED DOSAGES	COMMENTS
American Ginseng (Herb)	
Tea, 1 c 3 times daily. Available as *Xi Yang Shen* or Wild American Ginseng. or Tincture (1:5), as directed on label. Place in a cup, add 2 tbsp water, and take in a single sip.	Reduces effects of anxiety and stress on immune function.
Corydalis (Herb)	
Powdered herb with food, 2 g twice daily. Must be weighed by an herbalist.	Treats nervousness, insomnia, and agitation without inducing drowsiness.[2] Changes metabolism of a class of brain chemicals known as the enkephalins. Most effective when combined with California poppy; mix available from Kampo or TCM practitioners.
Ginger (Herb), Ginkgo (Modern Herbal Preparation)	
Ginger tea, 1 c 3 times daily. and Ginkgolide extract, 1 40-mg tablet or 1 60-mg tablet daily.	Together these herbs reduce anxiety by increasing flow of oxygen and nutrients to the brain.[3]
Ginseng (Herb)	
Fluid extract or tincture, as directed on label. or Tea, made with Korean or red ginseng, 1 c daily.	Helps prevent symptoms of anxiety during withdrawal from methamphetamines[4] and cocaine.[5] Prevents onset of anxiety and nervous tension during treatment with morphine.[6] Reduces stress of *anticipated* pain.[7] If using ginseng extracts or tinctures (which are not as therapeutically active as teas), be sure the product contains *Panax ginseng.* Note that strength may vary by manufacturer.

HERBS TO AVOID

Individuals who have anxiety should avoid ephedra. For more information regarding this herb, see Chapter 3.

KAMPO FORMULAS

See Chapter 4 for dosage information and discussions of individual formulas.

Bupleurum Plus Dragon Bone and Oyster Shell Decoction

Treats insomnia, palpitations, and short temper caused by anxiety in persons of robust constitution.

Caution: Be sure the formula does *not* include the traditional ingredient minium (lead oxide). Use with caution if fever is present, and discontinue if preexisting fevers worsen.

Coptis Decoction to Relieve Toxicity

Treats anxiety resulting in delirious speech with "hot" symptoms, such as bleeding from the nose or gums, fever, headaches, and redness in the neck and face.

Caution: Should not be used by women who are trying to become pregnant.

Pinellia and Magnolia Bark Decoction

Relieves "lump in the throat" and stomach upset accompanying anxiety. Appropriate for persons of "deficient" constitution, as marked by pale complexion, cold hands and feet, weak muscle tone, soft speech, and a tendency to behave passively.

Caution: Use with caution if fever is present, and discontinue if preexisting fevers worsen.

CONSIDERATIONS

❑ To reduce lactate production, avoid alcohol, caffeine, and sugar. Take calcium, magnesium, and the B-vitamins niacin, pyridoxine, and thiamin. As simple an act as avoiding coffee for one week can bring about significant relief of symptoms.[8]

ARRHYTHMIA

See **Congestive Heart Failure.**

ARTHRITIS

See **Osteoarthritis** and **Rheumatoid Arthritis.**

ASTHMA

The word "asthma" comes from the Greek term meaning "breathlessness." The symptoms of asthma are recurrent attacks of shortness of breath, cough, wheezing, and expectoration of sticky, stringy sputum. These symptoms are followed by a prolonged phase marked by abnormal breath sounds and wheezing. Asthma constricts the muscles lining the small air passages, or bronchi, of the lungs, which keeps air from leaving the lungs. About 10 million Americans have asthma, and the incidence of this disorder is increasing.

Physicians describe asthma as *extrinsic* or *intrinsic.* An extrinsic attack is set off when a very small particle to which the body has been sensitized enters the lungs. This particle, or allergen, activates antibodies to produce massive amounts of immunoglobulin E (IgE). IgE binds to mast cells, specialized immune cells especially numerous in the lungs and nasal passages. When activated by IgE, mast cells explode and release a chemical called histamine into tiny blood vessels called capillaries. This causes fluids to flow out of the capillaries into the smooth muscles lining the bronchial passages. The muscles then tighten, making breathing more difficult.

Histamine plays the same role in intrinsic asthma as in the extrinsic version, but in intrinsic asthma the attack is set off by cold air, emotional upset, exercise, infection, and/or toxic chemicals. Such factors trigger a surge in the production of leukotrienes, chemicals that are a thousand times more potent than histamine in closing airways. In sensitive individuals, leukotriene production is increased even more by the use of aspirin or nonsteroidal anti-inflammatory drugs (NSAIDs).[1,2] In addition, the bodies of intrinsic asthmatics usually make less of the hormones that allow the bronchial muscles to relax.

Among children under sixteen, whom asthma strikes most often, 90 percent of asthma is extrinsic, while among adults, more than 50 percent is intrinsic.[3] The lungs are more susceptible to both forms of asthma for several days after exposure to the air pollutant ozone and for several weeks after a viral infection.[4]

In ancient times in Japan and in other parts of the world, asthma was known but was extremely rare. Kampo medicine described asthma in terms that parallel the modern understanding of the condition. Asthma is an attack of "wind" and "cold" on the exterior of the body. The cold closes the pores of the skin and bottles up energy, especially the energies of the lungs, which are forced to expend their energy in wheezing.

Many of Kampo's formulas for asthma help prescription drugs balance the "energies" of the body. Prescription drugs such as steroids have serious side effects, including changes in the skin and hair, reduced resistance to infection, swelling, and weight gain. Herbal formulas can increase the effectiveness of steroid treatments so that they can be used in lower dosages with fewer side effects.

It is important to remember that Kampo herbs and formulas are most effectively used to prevent asthmatic attacks, and to make prescription drugs for asthma more effective. They are best used with a nutrition management program (see "Managing Asthma With Nutrition" on page 156). Kampo treatments should *not* be used to treat acute asthmatic attacks. See a physician promptly during an acute attack.

INDIVIDUAL KAMPO TREATMENTS

See Chapter 3 for discussions of individual herbs, traditional healing substances, and modern herbal preparations, including directions for making tea.

SUGGESTED DOSAGES	COMMENTS
Acorus (Herb)	
Powders, teas, and tinctures: 1–2 g, measured and dispensed by herbalist.	Contains alpha-asarone, a potent antihistamine, and compounds that act on other chemicals involved in asthma attacks.[5]
Codonopsis (Herb)	
Tablets, 1 g 3 times daily. Available as *Dang Shen.* or Tea, 1 c 3 times daily. or Tincture (1:5), ½–1 tsp (2–4 ml) 3 times daily. Place in a cup, add 2 tbsp water, and take in a single sip.	Reduces, but does not eliminate, the total number of mast cells in the lungs.[6] Also slows production of leukotrienes.

Ephedra (Herb)	
Powdered herb in food, 1–3 tbsp (3–9 g) daily. or Tea, 1 c 1–3 times daily. or Tincture (1:5), 15 drops 3 times daily. Place in a cup, add 2 tbsp water, and take in a single sip. To supplement other medications in acute asthma, 10 drops every 30 mins for up to 3 hours.	Acts on the sympathetic nervous system. This causes the bronchial passages to dilate, and accelerates and intensifies respiration. *Caution:* Do not use if taking an MAO inhibitor, or if high blood pressure, anxiety, glaucoma, or a prostate disorder is present. Be sure to drink 8 glasses of water daily.

Ginger (Herb)	
Hexanol extract, as directed on label 3 times daily. This is the recommended form.[7] or Tea, 1 c 3 times daily.	Deactivates platelet activating factor (PAF), the chemical messenger that starts allergic and asthmatic reactions.

Ginkgo (Herb, Modern Herbal Preparation)	
Ginkgolide extract, 1 40-mg tablet 3 times daily or 1 60-mg tablet twice daily (120 mg total). Increasing dosage to 160 mg (4 40-mg tablets) or 180 mg (3 60-mg tablets) may give increased relief.	Ginkgo nuts have been used in asthma relief for more than 2,000 years (see **Arrest Wheezing Decoction** on formulas list). Extracts also offer control by preventing the release of serotonin, which causes air passages to constrict.[8]

Hawthorn (Herb)	
Dried herb in capsules, 3–5 g daily. or Fluid extract (1:1), ¼–½ tsp (1–2 ml) 3 times daily. or Solid extract, 100–250 mg 3 times daily. Should be standardized to contain 10% proanthocyanidins. or Tea, ⅔ c 3–4 times daily. or Tincture (1:5), 1–1½ tsp (4–6 ml) 3 times daily. Place in a cup, add 2 tbsp water, and take in a single sip. Can be given to children (see inset on page 142).	Prevents tissue damage caused by steroid drugs.[9] Extracts may also reduce tissue damage caused by treatment with hydrocortisone and other steroid drugs.

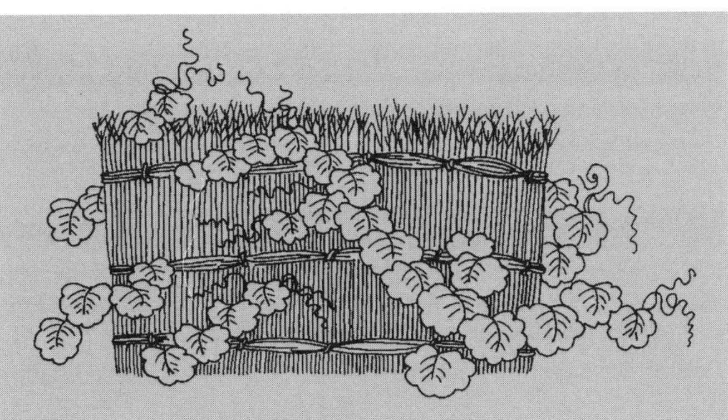

Licorice (Herb)	
Glycyrrhizin extract, 200–800 mg daily, depending on severity of symptoms for up to 6 weeks. Resume after a 2-week break. or Tea, 1 c 1–5 times daily for up to 6 weeks. Resume after a 2-week break.	Contains glycyrrhizin, which stops the free-radical production that provokes release of inflammatory hormones. This action also prevents histamine reactions that could cause stomach upset accompanying an asthmatic attack. Stimulates mucus production in the trachea to relieve dry cough without increasing mucus production in the bronchial tubes. Increases the effectiveness of the asthma drug cortisol in cases of intrinsic asthma. Also supplements prednisolone therapy.[10] Avoid deglycyrrhizinated licorice (DGL). *Caution:* Avoid if high blood pressure is present. Also avoid if an estrogen-sensitive disorder is present, such as bladder cancer, melanoma, or disorders of the female reproductive system.

Lobelia (Herb), St. John's Wort	
Herbal combination, as directed on label.	Lobelia combined with the non-Kampo herb St. John's wort is especially helpful for asthmatics who want to stop smoking.

Reishi (Modern Herbal Preparation)	
Dried extract, 3 1-g tablets 3 times daily. or Syrup, as directed on label. or Tincture (1:5), 1 tbsp (10 ml) 3 times daily. Place in a cup, add 2 tbsp water, and take in a single sip.	Contains antihistamines,[11] which prevent the inflammation that makes breathing difficult. *Caution:* Do not use in an area where reishi grows wild, since airborne reishi spores can cause allergies.

Scutellaria (Herb)	
Dried herb, 1–2 1,000-mg capsules 3 times daily. or Fluid extract (1:1), ¼–½ tsp (1–2 ml) 3 times daily. or Powdered solid extract (4:1), 250–500 mg 3 times daily. or Tea, 1 c 3 times daily. or Tincture (1:5), 1–1½ tsp (4–6 ml) 3 times daily. Place in a cup, add 2 tbsp water, and take in a single sip.	Contains baicalin, which stops hormonal reactions that constrict the bronchial tubes and cause asthma.[12] Baicalin prevents DNA damage from dexamethasone, a drug widely used to treat asthma.[13] *Caution:* Avoid in cases of diarrhea caused by foodborne infection or excessive consumption of cold drinks.

Turmeric (Herb)	
Curcumin, the yellow pigment found in turmeric, 250–500 mg twice daily between meals.	Curcumin is a useful supplemental treatment. It works by stopping the release of PAF.[14]

Managing Asthma With Nutrition

Nutritional management can be extremely useful in the treatment of asthma, especially in children. When making dietary changes, it is important to note the kind of asthma, gender, and age group for which the intervention is most helpful.

Many studies have found a link between asthmatic attacks, which may be immediate or delayed, and food allergy.[1–3] In children, foods that are most likely to trigger immediate attacks are eggs, fish, shellfish, nuts, and peanuts. Foods most commonly associated with delayed attacks include milk, chocolate, wheat, citrus, and food colorings.[4] For more information, *see* **Allergies, Food.**

Hypochlorhydria, or deficient production of gastric acid in the stomach, has been linked to asthma in both children[5] and adults,[6] and with a higher incidence of allergies.[7] In adults, hypochlorhydria is particularly detrimental when combined with leaky gut syndrome, in which the intestinal walls become overly permeable. As a result, large food molecules enter the body and provoke allergic reactions. This condition is marked by frequent diarrhea with food particles in the stool. Asthmatics who have this problem should take special care to identify and avoid allergenic foods.

Naturopaths have used magnesium supplements for more than eighty years to treat asthma.[8] This mineral causes the smooth muscles lining the bronchi to relax.[9] Oral magnesium therapy can raise the body's magnesium stores to an acceptable level in about six weeks.

Omega-3 essential fatty acids can, when combined with reduced sugar and saccharin consumption, reduce the risk of asthma by causing the body to produce a less inflammatory class of leukotrienes.[10] Cold-water fish is a rich source of omega-3, which is also found in oils from borage seed, evening primrose, flaxseed (linseed), and hemp. Eating fish once a week has been found to cut the risk of getting asthma by one-third in children.[11]

The bodies of children with asthma often cannot process an amino acid called tryptophan. The body converts tryptophan into serotonin, a compound that, among many other things, can cause air passages to constrict. Children with this defect can benefit from a low-tryptophan diet,[12] in which tryptophan-rich foods such as turkey and milk are eliminated. Supplementation with vitamin B_6 can also be useful, since this vitamin helps the body break down tryptophan.[13]

When vitamin C intake is low, the risk of asthma is high. Vitamin C can be broken down by environmental toxins.[14,15] Carotenes, catechins, flavonoids, and selenium decrease the vitamin-destroying effect of toxins within the bronchial tubes. Therefore, supplementation with these nutrients may be helpful.

Yeast infection indirectly contributes to asthma. Yeast produces the acid protease,[16] which provokes allergic responses and increases the amount of IgE in circulation. Treating yeast infections (*see* **Yeast Infections**) can ease asthma in many cases.

KAMPO FORMULAS

See Chapter 4 for dosage information and discussions of individual formulas.

Arrest Wheezing Decoction

Treats a symptom pattern of wheezing with coughing and expectoration of large amounts of thick, yellow sputum, simultaneous fever and chills, and labored breathing. Use this formula in patent-medicine form.

Caution: Do not use if diarrhea is present. Use with caution if fever is present, and discontinue if preexisting fevers worsen.

Capital Qi Pill

Relieves asthma brought on by physical exertion.

Ephedra Decoction (Four Emperors Combination)

TCM considers this formula to be especially beneficial in treating children's asthma. Seek the advice of the dispensing herbalist on a suitable child's dosage. A variation, Ephedra, Apricot Kernel, Coix, and Licorice Decoction, is designed to lower fever, in addition to treating other symptoms. Use either formula in patent-medicine form.

Ephedra, Apricot Kernel, Gypsum, and Licorice Decoction

Relieves asthma with nasal allergy or nasal flaring. Offers specific relief for sensitivity to cedar pollen. Use this formula in patent-medicine form.

Caution: Avoid if nausea or vomiting is present.

Ephedra, Asiasarum, and Prepared Aconite Decoction

Treats chronic coughing and wheezing. Useful when there is a sensation of extreme cold and severe chills relieved by covering up, slight fever, no sweating, and exhaustion. May cause a loss of sensation in the mouth and tongue.

Caution: Discontinue the formula if higher fever occurs.

Ginseng Decoction to Nourish the Nutritive Qi

Allows reduction in prednisolone dosage.[15] Is also likely to increase the effectiveness of hydrocortisone, methylprednisone, and prednisone.

Kidney Qi Pill From *The Golden Cabinet*

Traditionally used to treat asthma occurring simultaneously with pain in the lower half of the body. Symptom pattern may include irritability to the point of having difficulty in lying down, and breathing most comfortably while leaning against something. May involve either urinary difficulty with edema or excessive urination, sometimes to the point of incontinence. May cause a loss of sensation in the mouth and tongue.

Caution: Discontinue the formula if fever occurs.

Minor Bluegreen Dragon Decoction

Relieves asthma with copious production of white, stringy sputum.

Caution: Use with caution if fever is present, and discontinue if preexisting fevers worsen.

Minor Bupleurum Decoction

Allows reduction in prednisolone dosage.[16] Is also likely to increase the effectiveness of hydrocortisone, methylprednisone, and prednisone. Stops the chemical reaction that leads to the release of leukotrienes.[17]

Caution: Do not use if fever or skin infection is present. Taken long term in patent medicine form, can cause headache, dizziness, and bleeding gums. Side effects can be avoided if the formula is taken as a tea.

Ophiopogonis Decoction
Treats a symptom pattern of coughing, and spitting of saliva, dry and uncomfortable sensation in the throat, dry mouth, red tongue, shortness of breath, and wheezing.
Caution: Use with caution if fever is present, and discontinue if preexisting fevers worsen.

CONSIDERATIONS

❑ *See also* **Allergies, Respiratory.**

ATHEROSCLEROSIS

Atherosclerosis is the process by which cholesterol is deposited on the inside of blood vessels. This decreases their ability to supply tissues with blood, which can lead to a number of cardiovascular diseases, including stroke, angina, and heart attack. Atherosclerosis is the underlying cause of about 40 percent of all deaths in the United States.

When a blood vessel is injured by mechanical injury, high blood pressure, or infection, a chemical called platelet aggregating factor (PAF) causes red blood cells to clump together to seal the leak in the vessel wall. PAF also stimulates the production of fibrous tissues over the injury site.

Stress hormones cause the production of monocytes, immune cells which become macrophages, capable of consuming dead tissue. The macrophages are sent to the injured vessel to clean up debris. Other hormones increase the number of smooth muscle cells lining the injured part of the vessel wall. When the number of smooth cells increases, more cholesterol is pumped through the lining of the blood vessel. Both muscle cells and macrophages can accumulate cholesterol, leading to the formation of a plaque. The type of cholesterol that accumulates is low-density lipoprotein (LDL), or "bad" cholesterol, as opposed to high-density lipoprotein (HDL), or "good" cholesterol.

The plaque itself can raise blood pressure, causing further injury to the blood vessel, and further plaque formation. A hormonal condition can arise in which more and more macrophages are attracted to the site of the injury, bringing more and more cholesterol to the smooth muscle tissues. If this state of injury and repair persists over a number of years, blood vessels can become completely blocked.

Doctors recommend that atherosclerosis patients eliminate major sources of dietary cholesterol, especially that obtained from organ meat and eggs, as a way of stopping the disease process before it starts. Organ meats are especially damaging, as they are potent sources of iron. Excess iron can create free radicals, substances that activate macrophages, which can then accumulate cholesterol. Cholesterol-reducing drugs, which usually act by modifying the way the liver processes cholesterol, may be used. It is important to remember, though, that the body needs cholesterol to function.[1] Reducing cholesterol levels does not always improve health, since this substance only causes atherosclerosis when the blood vessel lining is damaged. In fact, cholesterol deficiencies can themselves result in other diseases.

Kampo takes a different approach to the problem of atherosclerosis. Modern medicine sees this disease as the circulation of unneeded nutrient *chemicals* through the body, but Kampo sees it as the circulation of unneeded nutrient *energies*. The Kampo maxim is, "When energy circulates, blood will circulate."

Many Kampo treatments for atherosclerosis balance the body's energy levels. For example, ginkgo stabilizes an organ identified in ancient Kampo as the "lower burner" by binding with lower-burner energy. In medical terms, this means that ginkgo keeps PAF from attracting clumps of blood platelets to the site of a plaque. Kampo treatments also balance nutrient levels by reducing excess cholesterol, and they prevent the production of free radicals.

INDIVIDUAL KAMPO TREATMENTS

See Chapter 3 for discussions of individual herbs, traditional healing substances, and modern herbal preparations, including directions for making tea.

SUGGESTED DOSAGES	COMMENTS
Astragalus (Herb)	
Fluid extract (1:1), ¼–½ tsp (1–2 ml) 3 times daily. or Freeze-dried herb in capsules, 500–1,000 mg 3 times daily. or Powdered solid extract (4:1), 250–500 mg 3 times daily. or Tea, 1 c 3 times daily. or Tincture (1:5), 1–1½ tsp (4–6 ml), 3 times daily. Place in a cup, add 2 tbsp water, and take in a single sip.	Keeps macrophages from creating plaques after artery walls are damaged.[2] Reduces blood levels of triglycerides, a form of fat, and total cholesterol without affecting HDL cholesterol.[3] *Caution:* Do not use when fever or skin infection is present.
Coix (Herb)	
Cereal, 1 oz (30 g) daily. Available in Japanese groceries as *hatomugi.*	Contains fatty acids that prevent plaque formation in damaged blood vessels when high cholesterol levels are present.[4] Inhibits cholesterol production in the liver, although it may increase triglyceride production.[5] Only useful when used with a restricted-carbohydrate diet, which helps maintain low triglyceride levels.

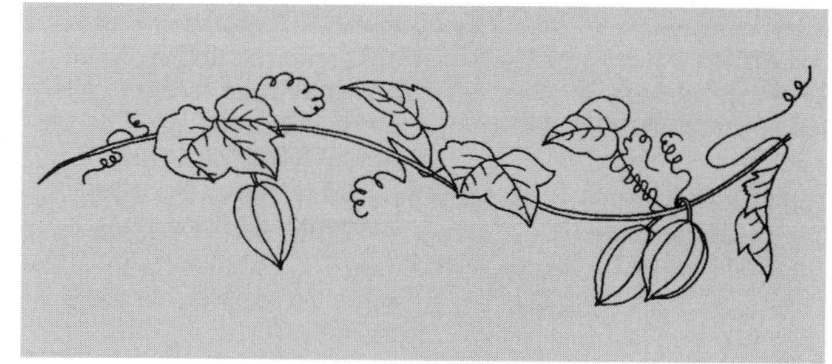

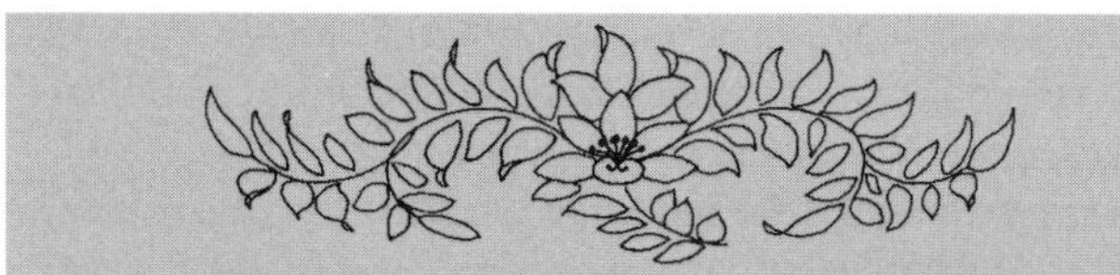

Garlic (Herb)

Enterically coated tablets, as directed on label (usually at least 900 mg daily).

Reduces levels of total and LDL cholesterol.[6] Contains ajoene, which helps prevent blood clot formation.[7] Ajoene builds up slowly over several weeks. A single large dose of garlic is not effective,[8] and only enterically coated tablets are an effective source of ajoene.

Caution: Do not use with the blood-thinner warfarin sodium (Coumadin). Garlic will counteract the effects of *Bifidus* and *Lactobacillus* cultures taken as digestive aids.

Ginger (Herb)

Freeze-dried herb in capsules, 1,000 mg 3 times daily.

or

Tea, 1 c 3 times daily.

Contains compounds that reduce cholesterol levels and decrease PAF activity. Also stimulates uptake of oxygen into muscle tissue.[9]

Ginkgo (Modern Herbal Preparation)

Ginkgolide extract, 1 40-mg tablet 3 times daily or 1 60-mg tablet twice daily (120 mg total). Increasing dosage to 160 mg (4 40-mg tablets) or 180 mg (3 60-mg tablets) may give increased relief.

Deactivates PAF. Neutralizes free radicals, which prevents cholesterol accumulation by macrophages.[10] Stops copper from transforming LDL cholesterol into a macrophage-attracting form.[11]

Hawthorn (Herb)

Dried herb in capsules, 3–5 g daily.

or

Fluid extract (1:1), ¼–½ tsp (1–2 ml) 3 times daily.

or

Solid extract, 100–250 mg 3 times daily. Should be standardized to contain 10% proanthocyanidins.

or

Tea, ⅔ c 3–4 times daily.

or

Tincture (1:5), 1–1½ tsp (4–6 ml) 3 times daily. Place in a cup, add 2 tbsp water, and take in a single sip.

Increases the rate at which the liver converts LDL cholesterol to HDL cholesterol. Provides antioxidants that prevent plaque formation. Tinctures increase rate at which liver uses cholesterol to create bile, thus eliminating cholesterol through the stool. May also reduce triglyceride levels.[12]

Lycium (Herb)

Concentrate, 1 1,000-mg tablet 3 times daily. Available as Longevity Tonic (recommended) or *Gou Qi Zi.*

or

Tea, 1 c 3 times daily.

Helps prevent atherosclerosis in diabetics. Protects red blood cells from free-radical damage,[13] reducing likelihood of atherosclerosis caused by prolonged, uncontrolled high blood-sugar levels.

Caution: Do not use if diarrhea is present.

Peach Seed (Herb)

Dried extract, 1 1,000-mg capsule 3 times daily.

Can be used to provide a 3- to 4-week break from daily aspirin therapy, a treatment that helps prevent clotting but can put a strain on the immune system. Available as *Xao Ren.*

Caution: Do *not* stop aspirin therapy without supervision of a health care provider.

PSK (Modern Herbal Preparation)

Dried extract, 6 1,000-mg tablets daily until cholesterol levels stabilize at the desired level.

Protects macrophages from free-radical damage by activating the enzyme glutathione peroxidase. Effects are greatest when there is adequate selenium in the diet.[14]

Turmeric (Herb)

Curcumin, the yellow pigment found in turmeric, 250–500 mg twice daily between meals.

Deactivates PAF and short-circuits the clotting process. More potent antioxidant than vitamin E.[15] Especially helpful for diabetics.[16]

KAMPO FORMULAS

See Chapter 4 for dosage information and discussions of individual formulas.

Coptis Decoction to Relieve Toxicity

Stimulates bile production, increasing the rate at which cholesterol is removed from circulation. Also produces free-radical scavengers called superoxide dismutases, which stop macrophages from accumulating cholesterol.[17]

Eight-Ingredient Pill With Rehmannia (Rehmannia-Eight Combination)

Relieves atherosclerosis affecting the lower extremities.

CONSIDERATIONS

❑ Onions have many of the same heart-protecting effects as garlic when approximately 1 ounce (30 grams) per day are used in food preparation, either raw or cooked. The key element, however, is the presence of sulfur. Very mild onions, which are grown in sulfur-deficient soils, do not contain the compounds that counteract atherosclerosis and clot formation.[18]

❑ *See also* **High Cholesterol.**

ATTENTION DEFICIT DISORDER/ATTENTION DEFICIT HYPERACTIVITY DISORDER (ADD/ADHD)

Attention Deficit Disorder (ADD) is a condition marked by learning disability, hyperactivity, and/or impaired judgment. The best known form of ADD is Attention Deficit Hyperactivity Disorder (ADHD), which affects children. The hallmark of ADHD is constant motion and disruptive behavior. A less severe form of the condition, ADD without Hyperactivity, also occurs in children. Because adults usually have developed some measure of coping skills, clinicians refer to both ADD and ADHD in adult patients as residual ADD.

Among North American youngsters, ADHD is the most common neurological disorder, affecting about 5 percent of school-aged children.[1] Both ADD and ADHD tend to run in families, and boys with ADHD outnumber girls by at least 3 to 1. Researchers do not know how many adults have residual ADD, but its symptoms are inattention, impulsiveness, and hyperactivity, usually alternating with bouts of depression.

Scientific study suggests that the common factor of ADHD, childhood ADD, and residual ADD is a coordination failure within the brain. In order to sort out and focus on selected stimuli from the environment, certain brain regions must be activated while others are inhibited. The right hemisphere and prefrontal lobes of the brain must be signaled to pay attention.[2] The signal to these parts of the brain must be switched through a tiny area known as the locus ceruleus.[3] The locus ceruleus transmits information through norepinephrine,[4] one of a number of brain messenger chemicals called neurotransmitters. If the locus ceruleus cannot trigger the production of norepinephrine, or the brain's blood vessels cannot carry it, or the prefrontal lobes and right hemisphere are insensitive to it, the result is ADD or ADHD. Sugar consumption blunts the brain's responsiveness to norepinephrine and contributes to the problem.[5]

Physicians most commonly prescribe psychostimulant or antidepressant drugs to deal with all three disorders. Paradoxically, excessive use of stimulant drugs may cause depression and lethargy. Over time, psychostimulant drugs may become ineffective and cause a "rebound" effect, in which anger and frustration suddenly reappear.

Kampo medicine did not have the concepts that modern medicine now uses to explain ADD. However, the Kampo herbs recommended in this book have been found to increase the flow of blood and oxygen to the brain and to balance production of the various neurotransmitters. They help the locus ceruleus communicate with the prefrontal lobes and right hemisphere without overstimulating norepinephrine production or making the control centers of the brain hypersensitive to it. Some Kampo treatments also keep the brain from becoming "overloaded" with sensory information from pain or allergies.

In addition, Japanese doctors for centuries have described the symptoms we associate with childhood ADD in terms of a more comprehensive symptom pattern of delayed development. This pattern consists of the Five Delays, which involve delays in growth of hair on the head, standing up, the development of speech, the development of teeth, and walking. A formula, Six-Ingredient Pill With Rhemannia, is used to treat this pattern.

INDIVIDUAL KAMPO TREATMENTS

See Chapter 3 for discussions of individual herbs, traditional healing substances, and modern herbal preparations, including directions for making tea.

SUGGESTED DOSAGES	COMMENTS
Ginkgo (Modern Herbal Preparation)	
Ginkgolide extract, 1 40-mg tablet 4 times daily or 1 60-mg tablet 3 times daily.	Best herb for adult ADD.
Hawthorn (Herb)	
Dried herb in capsules, 3–5 g. or Fluid extract (1:1), 1/4–1/2 tsp (1–2 ml) 3 times daily. or Solid extract, 100–250 mg 3 times daily. Should be standardized to contain 10% proanthocyanidins. or Tea, 2/3 c 3–4 times daily. or Tincture (1:5), 1–1 1/2 tsp (4–6 ml) 3 times daily. Place in a cup, add 2 tbsp water, and take in a single sip. Can be given to children (see inset on page 142).	Relieves acting out, anxiety, and nervous unrest in children. Also stops inflammatory responses caused by allergy, reducing sensory "overload." Extracts of the species *Crataegus laevigata* (also called *Crataegus oxyacantha*) sedate the central nervous system.[6]
Scutellaria (Herb)	
Dried herb, 1–2 1,000-mg capsules 3 times daily. or Fluid extract (1:1), 1/4–1/2 tsp (1–2 ml) 3 times daily. or Powdered solid extract (4:1), 250–500 mg 3 times daily. or Tea, 1 c 3 times daily. or Tincture (1:5), 1–1 1/2 tsp (4–6 ml) 3 times daily. Place in a cup, add 2 tbsp water, and take in a single sip. Can be given to children (see inset on page 142).	Prevents allergic reactions that can add to sensory overload. Has the added benefit of preventing colds and flu. *Caution:* Avoid in cases of diarrhea caused by foodborne infection or excessive consumption of cold drinks.

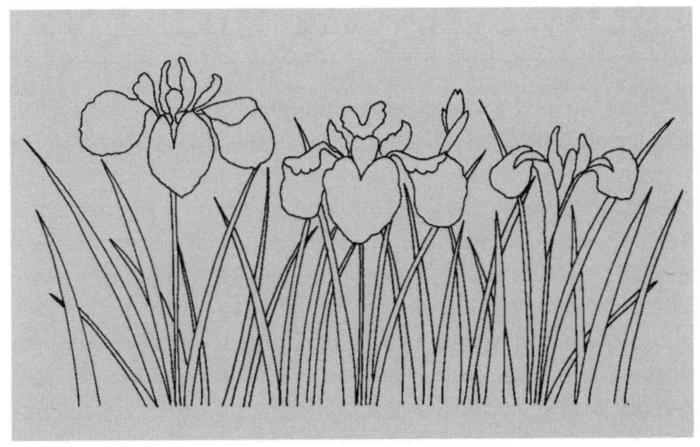

Siberian Ginseng (Modern Herbal Preparation)	
Eleuthero extract, as directed by manufacturer, in 1/4 c water. Be sure to use pure extract, *not* sugar-sweetened ginseng drinks. or Tea, 1 c 3 times daily. Can be given to children (see inset on page 142).	Most appropriate for children with ADD who also have recurrent inner ear infections. Treats difficulty in concentrating and sensitivity to environmental stresses, such as changes in weather, in both children and adults. Relieves depression in adults by balancing effects of various neurotransmitters.[7] *Caution:* Should be avoided by persons with myasthenia gravis; rheumatoid arthritis and diseases related to it, such as lupus, psoriatic arthritis, and Sjögren's syndrome; or prostate cancer.

KAMPO FORMULAS

See Chapter 4 for dosage information and discussions of individual formulas.

Licorice, Wheat, and Jujube Decoction

Stops crying in hyperactive children. Reduces sensory overload by blocking pain; acts by occupying brain receptor sites that receive sedative drugs such as opium[8] without causing addiction. Reduces symptoms of withdrawal from Ritalin. Also relieves sadness and mild depression in adults with ADD.[9] Seek the advice of the dispensing herbalist on a suitable child's dosage. Can be made at home in tea form (see Chapter 4).

Six-Ingredient Pill with Rehmannia (Rehmannia-Six Combination)

Preserves the neurotransmitter acetylcholine in the brain's frontal lobes.[10] Treats any of the Five Delays, and has been used successfully by American herbalists in treating childhood ADD/ADHD.[11] Also effective for adults with ADD, especially those who experience dizziness, lightheadedness, night sweats, ringing in the ears or diminished hearing, and soreness and weakness in the lower back. Seek the advice of the dispensing herbalist on a suitable child's dosage.

Caution: Avoid if an estrogen-sensitive disorder is present, such as bladder cancer, melanoma, or disorders of the female reproductive system.

BASAL CELL CARCINOMA

See **Skin Cancer (Basal Cell Carcinoma).**

BEDWETTING, CHILDREN'S

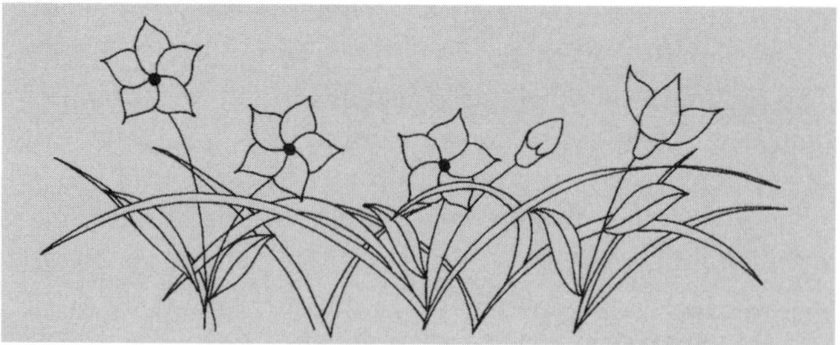

Wetting the bed is an embarrassing problem that affects from 5 to 7 million children in the United States alone. The medical term for bedwetting is *enuresis.* This refers to the involuntary discharge of urine beyond the age when a child should be able to control urination, usually age six or older. The key word is "involuntary." Bedwetting is *not* a behavioral problem. Punishing or ridiculing the child worsens the situation.

Bedwetting tends to run in families. It also seems to occur more often in children born to mothers younger than twenty, and to second- and third-born children.[1] This condition almost always resolves itself as a child matures. However, if not properly handled, it can predispose the child to emotional difficulties.

Current medical research offers several explanations of bedwetting. Recent studies indicate that this problem occurs after the kidneys have been damaged by infection and no longer have as great a reserve capacity.[2,3] This is especially true when a child relapses into bedwetting after having achieved bladder control. Another likely explanation is basically hormonal. Antidiuretic hormone causes the kidneys to retain water. If this hormone is deficient, fluid flows from the kidneys into the bladder. This action pulls sodium into the bladder as well, which draws even more water with it. In addition, since antidiuretic hormone is made in the brain, changes in brain chemistry associated with a stressful or scary situation decrease hormone production. Production can also be decreased by exposure to chemicals or nicotine from secondhand smoke.[4]

There are pharmaceutical treatments for bedwetting. Antidepressants, such as imipramine (Tofranil), are used to stimulate the brain, including the centers that create antidiuretic hormone. Imipramine can cause the child to suffer insomnia and develop a sweet tooth, among other side effects. Desmopressin acetate nasal spray is a synthetic form of antidiuretic hormone. Desmopressin acetate can work very quickly. The effect is canceled out, however, if the child consumes caffeinated drinks, and this drug is expensive. More seriously, it can cause the blood to clot too readily if used within two weeks of an attack of either chicken pox or shingles.[5]

The Kampo theory behind the formulas used to treat bedwetting is that the bladder lacks the energy to hold urine when the kidneys are under attack by infectious agents. If kidney problems are corrected, the healing of bladder problems will follow.

There are settings, such as spending the night at a friend's house or going to camp, when desmopressin therapy is preferable to any herbal intervention. On a long-term basis, however, herbal approaches offer comparable relief with fewer side effects at a lower cost. Kampo treatments are best undertaken with a doctor's help, since the physician can determine the underlying cause of the problem. Also, seek the advice of the dispensing herbalist on a suitable child's dosage for formulas.

INDIVIDUAL KAMPO TREATMENTS

See Chapter 3 for discussions of individual herbs, traditional healing substances, and modern herbal preparations, including directions for making tea.

SUGGESTED DOSAGES	COMMENTS
Scutellaria (Herb)	
Dried herb, 1–2 1,000-mg capsules daily. or Fluid extract (1:1), ¼–½ tsp (1–2 ml) daily. or Powdered solid extract (4:1), 250–500 mg daily. or Tea, 1 c daily.	The herb of choice in children who have had bladder infections. Arrests allergic irritation and fights a very broad range of bacteria and viruses. Particularly useful when combined with the non-Kampo herbs chamomile or passionflower. Give solid forms as soon as the child comes home from school, or liquid forms in the early evening after dinner. Do *not* give to children under age 6. *Caution: Never* use alcohol-based tinctures for bedwetting, since alcohol can aggravate this condition. Avoid in cases of diarrhea caused by foodborne infection or excessive consumption of cold drinks.

KAMPO FORMULAS

See Chapter 4 for dosage information and discussions of individual formulas.

Licorice, Wheat, and Jujube Decoction

Treats bedwetting aggravated by crying spells and depression. Wheat has actions surprisingly similar to those of codeine.[6] Can be made at home in tea form (see Chapter 4).

Minor Construct the Middle Decoction

Stops stomach spasms and increases bladder tone, allowing the child's bladder to hold more urine. Relieves vertical tension in the abdomen and nervous stomach, conditions that accompany stress.

Shut the Sluice Pill

Traditional Japanese "bladder tonic," strengthening bladder yin, or containing energy, so that the bladder can hold urine through the night.

CONSIDERATIONS

❑ To avoid a sodium-potassium imbalance, have the child avoid salty foods. Make sure he or she eats at least one serving of potassium-rich fruits and vegetables, such as bananas, oranges, or tomatoes, every day.
❑ Some parents use a moisture alarm in cases of bedwetting. A moisture sensor sets off the alarm when the child begins to wet the bed, which awakens the child. If the child does not awaken, then the parent must awaken the child. The net effect is that "accidents" will become less frequent and eventually disappear.
❑ *See also* **Bladder Infection.**

BLADDER CANCER

Bladder cancer is the most common cancer of the urinary tract. It usually strikes mature men who have been exposed to cigarette smoke and/or industrial carcinogens. Symptoms include blood in the urine, along with frequent, painful, and/or urgent urination.

Up to 45 percent of all bladder cancers occur among smokers.[1] Other agents that cause this disease include 2-napthylamine, a chemical widely used in the cigarette, dye, and rubber industries. Cyclophosphamide, a drug used to treat other forms of cancer, can cause bladder cancer,[2] as can radiation therapy for cervical cancer. Bladder cancer is also associated with excess consumption of painkillers containing acetaminophen, especially if taken after meals that include charcoal-broiled beef.[3] In addition, recurrent bouts of kidney stones or urinary tract infections have been linked to bladder cancer.

Bladder cancer is classified in stages, from stage 0 through stages A to D, according to how far it has spread. This cancer tends to spread to nearby organs, such as the colon, and the pelvic bones. If bladder cancer is treated before it has spread, the probability of surviving five years is more than 90 percent.[4]

The current understanding of bladder cancer is that it develops through at least a two-stage process within the cell. In the first stage, a cancer-causing agent destroys part of a gene known as gene p16. This "gatekeeper" gene lets the cell know whether the cell is genetically healthy enough to reproduce or if it is so unhealthy that it should be replaced. When gene p16 is damaged, the cell acts as if it were genetically healthy and continues to multiply far in excess of the numbers needed to replace it. Such damage makes the cancer more likely spread.[5]

The body has a second line of defense against genetic damage, gene p53.[6] This gene serves as a "molecular patrolman" by making sure that defective cells do not multiply. Carcinogens, however, can also attack gene p53. This leaves cancer cells free to multiply and spread. In addition, bladder cancers pick up hormonal signals to grow and multiply, especially from estrogen, the primary female hormone.[7] Estrogen also makes cancer-fighting natural killer cells less effective. Fortunately, estrogen's effects occur slowly, so bladder cancer can often be caught in time for effective treatment.

The mainstay of medical treatment for bladder cancer, besides surgery, is the chemotherapy drug cisplatin and its variants. Scientists are striving to develop bladder cancer treatments that are less punishing to healthy tissues. Other chemotherapy agents that are used include doxorubicin hydrochloride (Adriamycin) and fluorouracil (5-FU). Immunotherapy is also used, in which concentrated amounts of the body's own immune-system chemicals are given (such as interleukin-2).[8]

In terms of traditional Japanese medicine, bladder cancer is an exceptionally severe manifestation of "heat." Heat normally rises in the body. When the normal flow of energy through the bladder is interrupted by a pathogenic influence, heat becomes "damp heat," which falls to the lower portions of the body and produces toxins in the bladder.

Although Kampo's explanation of bladder cancer is metaphorical rather than scientific, in the last twenty-five years scientists have proven that the herbs used in Kampo to relieve "heat" do, in fact, have specific anticancer effects. One herbal extract, curcumin, has been shown to reactivate gene p53. Other herbal therapies protect the immune system.

Kampo treatments for bladder cancer are most effective when used in the context of conventional medical treatment (see considerations below). Since different herbs act on different phases of the disease process, consult with a trained health provider.

INDIVIDUAL KAMPO TREATMENTS

See Chapter 3 for discussions of individual herbs, traditional healing substances, and modern herbal preparations, including directions for making tea.

SUGGESTED DOSAGES	COMMENTS
Astragalus (Herb)	
Fluid extract (1:1), 1/4–1/2 tsp (1–2 ml) 3 times daily. or Freeze-dried herb in capsules, 500–1,000 mg 3 times daily. or Powdered solid extract (4:1), 250–500 mg 3 times daily. or Tea, 1 c 3 times daily. or Tincture (1:5), 1–1 1/2 tsp (4–6 ml), 3 times daily. Place in a cup, add 2 tbsp water, and take in a single sip. For dosages used with chemotherapy, *see* **Chemotherapy Side Effects.**	Slows spread of cancers known to respond to gene p53. Contains compounds that increase both the ability of immune cells called lymphokine-activated killer (LAK) cells to attack cancerous tumors[9] and the effectiveness of immunotherapy with a combination of melatonin and interleukin-2. *Caution:* Do not use when fever or skin infection is present.
Ginkgo (Modern Herbal Preparation)	
Ginkgolide extract, 1 40-mg tablet twice daily. or Quercetin extract, 1–2 125-mg capsules 3 times daily between meals.	Contains quercetin, which slows the growth of estrogen-activated cancers.[10] For best results, take quercetin with bromelain, which increases absorption. *Caution:* Do not take quercetin with the prescription drugs Procardia or Seldane.
Maitake (Modern Herbal Preparation)	
Large dosages are required when used in cancer treatment: Fresh or dried maitake in food, 1/2–1 oz (15–30 g) daily. or Maitake D-fraction, 4 500-mg capsules 3 times daily before meals. or Tea, 1 c 8–16 times daily. Lower dosages can be used if the cancer is in remission. See listing on page 144.	General immune stimulant that increases the activity of various immune-system cells and reduces tumor formation.[11] Has been shown to reduce the recurrence rate of bladder cancer after surgery.[12]
Siberian Ginseng (Modern Herbal Preparation)	
Eleuthero extract, as directed on label, in 1/4 c water. Be sure to use pure extract, *not* sugar-sweetened ginseng drinks. or Tea, 1 c up to 3 times daily.	Possibly reduces growth rate of bladder cancer cells. Effective against cancer cells that respond to immunotherapy, possibly including bladder cancer. Contains compounds that stimulate various immune-system components.[13] *Caution:* Should be avoided by persons with myasthenia gravis; rheumatoid arthritis and diseases related to it, such as lupus, psoriatic arthritis, and Sjögren's syndrome; or prostate cancer.
Turmeric (Herb)	
Curcumin, the yellow pigment found in turmeric, 250–500 mg twice daily between meals.	Curcumin activates gene p53.[14] May also suppress genes necessary for bladder cancer growth. Prevents lung damage caused by the chemotherapy drug cyclophosphamide[15] and reduces lung damage after exposure to whole-body radiation.[16]

HERBS TO AVOID

Individuals who have bladder cancer should avoid *raw* shiitake mushroom. Cooked shiitake does not pose a problem. Persons with bladder cancer should also avoid herbs that increase estrogen production: cordyceps, dan shen, fennel, licorice, and peony. For more information, see Chapter 3.

KAMPO FORMULAS

See Chapter 4 for dosage information and discussions of individual formulas.

Coptis Decoction to Relieve Toxicity

This formula was traditionally used to treat "fire toxins," such as those produced in this disorder, as shown by a symptom pattern of high fever, irritability, dry mouth and throat, nosebleed and/or swelling with inflammation. Contains coptis, which stops multiplication of many types of cancer cells, and scutellaria, which prevents chemotherapy damage to the immune system. Can be used under a doctor's supervision after chemotherapy to reduce side effects. Do not use within 48 hours of taking cisplatinol, or the antioxidant properties of the formula will counteract the therapeutic effects of the drug.

FORMULAS TO AVOID

Individuals with bladder cancer should avoid formulas that increase estrogen production: Peony and Licorice Decoction, and Six-Ingredient Pill With Rhemannia (Rhemannia-Six Combination). For more information regarding these formulas, see Chapter 4.

CONSIDERATIONS

❑ To reduce side effects and increase effectiveness when using chemotherapy, *see* **Chemotherapy Side Effects.** To learn about herbal treatments that can prevent a cancer from developing its own blood supply, *see* **Cancer.**

Bladder Infection (Cystitis)

Bladder infections, known medically as *cystitis*, are generally caused by bacteria. Urine, as secreted by the kidneys, is sterile. It can be contaminated when it reaches the urethra, the tube that carries urine from the bladder to outside the body. Bacteria can reach the bladder from the urethra or, much more rarely, through the bloodstream.

Bladder infections cause burning pain during urination and increased frequency of urination, especially at night. There may be the desire to urinate even if the bladder is empty. Infections can also cause cloudy, dark, or foul-smelling urine, along with lower abdominal or back pain, fever, and chills.

Bladder infections occur much more commonly in baby boys than in baby girls, but by age twenty more than 98 percent of these infections occur in women. Ten to 20 percent of all women have at least one bladder infection every year.[1] Pregnancy and menopause are associated with a greater chance of infection, as are prostate infections in men. In both sexes, untreated diabetes and decreased immune function can play a role. Recurring bladder infection is a significant health problem, since most recurrent infections will eventually involve the kidneys.

Bladder infections occur when the natural balance of bacteria in the urethra has been disturbed, either by systemic illness or by use of antibiotics. The body has several defenses against infection. Urine flow tends to wash away bacteria. The surface of the bladder itself has antimicrobial properties. In men, prostate fluid contains many antimicrobial substances. Finally, the acidity or alkalinity (pH) of the urine usually does not favor bacterial growth. (For information on how to affect urine pH, see "Cranberry Juice and Kampo".) Bladder infections typically only take hold when there is some trauma to the urinary tract. This injury can occur during childbirth or intercourse, or it can be caused by structural abnormalities that block the free flow of urine.

The conventional medical treatment for bladder infections is antibiotic therapy. There is a growing concern, however, that antibiotic therapy actually increases the risk of recurrent bladder infections by giving rise to antibiotic-resistant strains of *E. coli*.[2,3] Antibiotic therapy also eliminates the protective shield of normally occurring "friendly" bacteria that line the external opening of the urethra. Antibiotics can cause this shield to be stripped away or be replaced by less effective microorganisms.

In traditional Japanese medicine, bladder infections are a manifestation of "heat." Heat normally rises in the body. When there is excessive water in the body, heat becomes "damp heat," which falls to the lower portions of the body and may express itself as infections of the uterus or bladder. In bladder infection, the body has become unable to circulate water upward, so damp heat is poured downward into the bladder. This infection may be aggravated by damp heat descending from the liver, which is associated with anger, and by heart heat spreading emotional energies downward.

The herbs used in Kampo have specific antibacterial effects, and are most effective when used in the context of conventional medical treatment. Since specific herbs act on specific microorganisms, choosing herbs is best done after a doctor's diagnosis of the infection's cause. Formulas for bladder infections are effective when taken over the long term, sometimes for as long as a year.

INDIVIDUAL KAMPO TREATMENTS

See Chapter 3 for discussions of individual herbs, traditional healing substances, and modern herbal preparations, including directions for making tea.

Cranberry Juice and Kampo

The bacteria that are responsible for bladder infections cannot grow until they attach to the mucosal lining of the bladder or urethra. Anthocyanins, substances found in cranberries, interfere with the bacteria's ability to "stick" to the lining of the bladder, thus preventing infection.[1]

Drunk in large amounts, cranberry juice can also change the acid-base balance of the urine in a way that inhibits bacterial growth. The amount of cranberry juice needed to do this, however, is large—6 cups (1½ liters) per day.[2]

Several clinical studies have shown that cranberry juice successfully treats bladder infections. In one investigation, 16 fluid ounces (approximately 500 milliliters) of cranberry juice taken daily relieved symptoms in 73 percent of the sixteen men and forty-four women participating in the study. Discontinuing the juice, however, caused a relapse in more than 60 percent of the people who had benefited from it.[3]

Cranberry is available as either juice or extract tablets. Drink at least 16 fluid ounces of *unsweetened* juice, or take one or two 250-milligram tablets three times a day. Most commercial cranberry juices are diluted with two parts of water and have added sugar for taste. If pure cranberry juice is hard to find, use artificially sweetened juice on a short-term basis, alternating it with other herbal supplements.

Cranberry changes the environment of the bladder and urinary tract, but does not affect infectious organisms directly. For best results, use a combination of cranberry and the antibacterial herbs of Kampo.

SUGGESTED DOSAGES	COMMENTS
Artemisia (Herb)	
Tea, 1 c 3 times daily. or Tincture (1:5), 20 drops in ¼ c hot water 3 times daily for 21 days. Children aged 6–12 years may be given ½ of the adult dose. Do not give to children under age 6.	Treats infections caused by *Klebsiella*,[4] which causes uncomplicated infections but is extremely difficult to treat with antibiotics.
Astragalus (Herb)	
Tincture (1:5), 20 drops in ¼ c hot water 3 times daily for 21 days. Can be given to children (see inset on page 142).	Treats infection caused by *Proteus*,[5] which secretes enzymes that encourage kidney stone formation. *Caution:* Do not use when fever or skin infection is present.
Cardamom (Herb)	
Tincture (1:5), ¼–½ tsp (1–2 ml) in ¼ c hot water 3 times daily for 21 days.	Treats infection caused by *E. coli*,[6] the growth of which is encouraged by the use of diaphragms or spermicidal foam contraceptives. Also stops urinary incontinence in both men and women.
Coptis (Herb)	
Dried herb, 1 500-mg capsule 3 times daily. or Tincture (1:5), 20 drops 3 times daily. Place in a cup, add 2 tbsp water, and take in a single sip.	Contains berberine, which promotes the release of compounds that activate the immune system.[7] Also activates macrophages, the immune cells most responsible for the destruction of infectious yeasts.[8] Often cures infections with either *E. coli*[9] or *Proteus*.[10] Berberine is more effective if urine is alkaline. Avoid meat or take ¼ tsp (0.5 g) baking soda in ⅓ c (50 ml) of water every time the herb is taken. *Caution:* Do not use during pregnancy or on a daily basis for more than 2 weeks at a time. Do not use with supplements that contain vitamin B_6 or the amino acid histidine.
Eupatorium (Herb)	
Tincture (1:5), 20 drops in ¼ c hot water 3 times daily for 21 days.	Treats infections when kidney stones exist or there is scarring of the urinary tract.
Garlic (Herb)	
Cloves in food, preferably raw, 2–3 daily. The recommended form. or Tablets (including deodorized) as directed on label, at least 900 mg daily. Can be given to children (see inset on page 142). Deodorized garlic is a good choice.	Increases immune system's production of "germ-eating" granulocytes and monocytes.[11] Especially helpful in treating infections caused by *Streptococcus faecalis*[12] in children. *Caution:* Do not use with the blood-thinner warfarin sodium (Coumadin). Garlic will counteract the effects of *Bifidus* and *Lactobacillus* cultures taken as digestive aids.

KAMPO FORMULAS

See Chapter 4 for dosage information and discussions of individual formulas.

Gentiana Longdancao Decoction to Drain the Liver

Traditionally given to women whose infections occur at the same time as emotional distress.[13] Especially appropriate when symptoms include eye irritation, fatigue, irritability, whitish vaginal discharge, painful urination, and swelling or inflammation in the ears.

Caution: Should not be used by women who are trying to become pregnant.

Polyporus Decoction

Prevents formation of kidney stones and stops scarring of the urethra that invites infection. Found to reduce the risk of kidney stone attacks in 70 percent of people who take it for 4 weeks.[14]

CONSIDERATIONS

❑ Women who have recurrent bladder infections usually benefit from the reintroduction of friendly bacteria into the vagina. The best way to do this is by using commercially available *Lactobacillus acidophilus* capsules or tablets, sometimes labeled only as "Acidopholous." Place one or two capsules in the vagina before going to bed every other night for two weeks.

BLEEDING GUMS

Bleeding gums are recognized by blood in the mouth or on the toothbrush after brushing. Although this is not a serious condition in itself, bleeding from the gums is a warning sign of periodontal disease. Periodontal means "located around a tooth," and periodontal diseases are disorders of the gums or any other structures supporting the teeth. Periodontal diseases are the leading cause of adult tooth loss.

Gingivitis is the early stage of periodontal disease. Gingivitis results when plaque—sticky deposits of bacteria, food, and mucus—adhere to the teeth. Plaque accumulations cause the gums to become inflamed and swollen. As the problem develops into *periodontitis*, pockets of bacteria accumulate and produce more plaque, separating the gums from the teeth. Bacterial growth causes the gums to become red, soft, and shiny. At this stage the gums bleed easily, but usually there is no pain. *Pyorrhea* is a more advanced stage of periodontitis. In pyorrhea, the bone beneath the gums begins to erode. Brushing the teeth causes heavy bleeding, and pus may be visible when the gums are pressed. In time, the teeth loosen and fall out.

The Kampo classic *Secrets from the Orchid Chamber* described bleeding gums as a symptom of destructive "heat." In this symptom pattern, an infection in the stomach creates heat. This heat spreads to the kidneys and destabilizes their yin, or holding, energies. Hot energy from the kidneys rise upward in the body outside its usual channel, spreading its heat and inflammation to the teeth. Stomach "fire" joins this energy and loosens the teeth. The fire also fills the energy channels overlying the face, causing frontal headache.

Kampo also treats gum diseases caused by dry mouth,

since saliva rids the mouth of the offending bacteria. Some chronic conditions, such as diabetes, Parkinson's disease, and especially Sjögren's syndrome, cause chronic dry mouth.

For this condition, formulas must be used as *mouthwashes*, rather than as oral medications, to be effective. Use ten drops of any formula-based patent medicine in 1/4 cup of water twice daily.

INDIVIDUAL KAMPO TREATMENTS

See Chapter 3 for discussions of individual herbs, traditional healing substances, and modern herbal preparations, including directions for making tea.

SUGGESTED DOSAGES	COMMENTS
Cinnamon (Herb)	
Oil, 15–30 drops, up to 3 times daily. Place in a cup, add 2 tbsp warm water, and take in a single sip.	Cinnamon fights gingivitis by disabling plaque bacteria's ability to break down the collagen lining the gums.[1,2]
Cloves (Herb)	
Oil, 2–3 drops in 1/4 c (60 ml) warm water used as mouthwash 2–3 times daily.	Oil is 60–95% eugenol, which is thought to give the oil its painkilling properties.[3] Cloves are also strongly antimicrobial. Hawaiian variety acts against the bacteria that cause pyorrhea (*Streptococcus pyogenes*).[4]
Coptis (Herb)	
Tincture (1:5), 2–3 drops in 1/4 c warm water used as mouthwash twice daily.	Contains berberine, which kills the bacteria that cause gingivitis. If coptis is unavailable, substitute tinctures of the non-Kampo herbs goldenseal or Oregon grape root (same cautions apply). *Caution:* Do not use during pregnancy or on a daily basis for more than 2 weeks at a time. Do not use with supplements that contain vitamin B_6 or the amino acid histidine.
Green Tea (Herb)	
Catechin extract, 1 240-mg tablet 3 times daily. or Tea, 2–3 cups daily.	Whisks of green tea were traditionally used in China and Japan as herbal toothbrushes. Kills bacteria that cause plaque[5] as well as many foodborne infections, especially *Clostridium*.[6] To avoid dilution problems, do not take tea within 1 hour of taking other teas or patent medicines.
Hawthorn (Herb)	
Fluid extract (1:1), 2–3 drops in 1/4 c warm water used as mouthwash twice daily.	Maintains integrity of cell walls in gum tissue.
Myrrh (Traditional Healing Substance)	
Tincture (1:5), 10–30 drops up to 3 times a day as needed. Place in a cup, add 2 tbsp water, and use as a mouthwash.	Acts on inflammatory processes to prevent soreness and inflammation while preserving linings of gums and mouth.[7]
Scutellaria (Herb)	
Fluid extract (1:1), 1/4–1/2 tsp (1–2 ml) 3 times daily. or Powdered solid extract (4:1), 250–500 mg 3 times daily.	Extracts, especially methanol extracts, stimulate the growth of collagen in the gums, which reverses gingivitis.[8] *Caution:* Avoid in cases of diarrhea caused by foodborne infection or excessive consumption of cold drinks.
Turmeric (Herb)	
Tea, 1/4 c (50 ml), used as mouthwash 3 times daily. Store in refrigerator. or Tincture (1:5), 1 tsp (4 ml) 3 times daily. Place in a cup, add 2 tbsp water, and take in a single sip.	Halts action of a gene that creates gum-irritating chemicals.[9] Do *not* substitute the turmeric compound curcumin.

KAMPO FORMULAS

See Chapter 4 for dosage information and discussions of individual formulas.

Calm the Stomach Powder

Relieves toothache, particularly when pain extends into the head. Painful areas respond favorably to cold and worsen with heat.

Coptis Decoction to Relieve Toxicity

Most effective of all Kampo formulas tested for ability to prevent plaque formation.[10] Prevents bleeding gums and stops gum infection, and also relieves dry mouth.

Caution: Should not be used by women who are trying to become pregnant.

Four-Gentleman Decoction

Informal tests have found that this formula stops plaque formation.

Ledebouriella Powder That Sagely Unblocks

Stops dry mouth and bitter taste in the mouth. Best formula for treating bleeding gums accompanied by discharge of pus.

Caution: Should not be used by women who are trying to become pregnant, or if nausea or vomiting is present.

Ophiopogonis Decoction

Increases the activity of beta-adrenergic nerve fibers, such as those that stimulate salivation.[11] Increases saliva secretion in persons who have Sjögren's syndrome.[12] Also useful for diabetics who experience an increase in cavities, gum irritation, and plaque.

Caution: Use with caution if fever is present, and discontinue if preexisting fevers worsen.

White Tiger Decoction

Used to treat bleeding gums accompanied by fever or infection.

Caution: Avoid if nausea or vomiting is present.

BOILS

A boil, also known as a furuncle, is a deep-seated infection of an entire hair follicle and the adjacent tissue. A cluster of boils is called a *carbuncle.* A boil usually appears as a small rounded or conical nodule surrounded by redness, progressing to form a localized pus pocket with a white center. The most common sites for boils are hairy parts of the body that are exposed to friction, such as the armpits, buttocks, groin, and neck, although they may appear in other places as well. Boils cause tenderness and pain, and can cause mild fever.

Almost all boils stem from infection with the bacterium *Staphylococcus aureus*, known commonly as "staph." Staph may enter the skin through abrasions caused by friction, moisture, or pressure. Plugging the pores of the skin with cosmetics or petroleum jellies may trap the infection within, giving it an opportunity to multiply. Most boils heal within a week to ten days. Recurrent boils indicate poor nutrition; an underlying disease affecting immune response, such as anemia, diabetes, or HIV; or chronic perspiration in the folds of the skin.[1]

Kampo theory explains boils as external manifestations of toxins and "heat." When the muscles trap an external pathogenic influence that cannot escape through the skin, the infection generates toxins and heat. The heat attempts to burn an escape through the skin, producing boils, carbuncles, and oozing lesions. Kampo also notes a category of "cold" boils, skin ulcerations associated with deficient energy. Cold boils ooze clear fluid, and the affected skin bulges inward rather than outward. Kampo herbs and formulas offer antibiotic relief. In many cases, Kampo herbs can treat strains of staph infection that have become antibiotic-resistant.

If boils do not begin to heal after two or three days of treatment, consult a physician. Unchecked staph infections can spread to adjacent tissues, causing cellulitis, or enter the bloodstream, causing bacteremia. When boils do respond to treatment within two to three days, continue the treatment for seven to fourteen days, and at least two or three days after outward symptoms have disappeared.

INDIVIDUAL KAMPO TREATMENTS

See Chapter 3 for discussions of individual herbs, traditional healing substances, and modern herbal preparations, including directions for making tea.

SUGGESTED DOSAGES	COMMENTS
Cinnamon (Herb)	
Oil, 2–3 drops applied to skin 2–3 times daily.	Treats "cold" boils.
Coptis (Herb)	
Poultice, applied twice daily (see Chapter 3 for directions).	Contains berberine, which is especially toxic to staph.[2] Also promotes the release of compounds that activate the immune system.[3] Unlike other types of poultices, coptis poultices usually will not cause the boil to rupture. If fever is present, use **Coptis Decoction to Relieve Toxicity** (see formulas list). If coptis is unavailable, substitute the non-Kampo herb goldenseal.
Dan Shen (Herb)	
Tea, 1 c 3 times daily.	Treats boils and other forms of skin eruption that occur during menstrual irregularity. *Caution:* Avoid if an estrogen-sensitive disorder is present, such as bladder cancer, melanoma, or disorders of the female reproductive system.
Japanese Mint (Herb)	
Tea, 1 c 2–3 times daily.	Expels pathogens by "promoting eruption." Useful for boils when they first erupt, especially when they are accompanied by chills and fever.
Tang-Kuei (Herb)	
Tea, 1 c 2–3 times daily.	Treats boils that occur at the site of traumatic injury. Also known as dong quai.

KAMPO FORMULAS

See Chapter 4 for dosage information and discussions of individual formulas.

Coptis Decoction to Relieve Toxicity

Used instead of coptis when symptoms include fever. More effective than many antibiotics in treating skin infection.[4]

Caution: Should not be used by women who are trying to become pregnant.

Trauma Pill

Treats "cold" boils.

CONSIDERATIONS

❑ Healing is accelerated when the patient eliminates all factors that can depress the immune system, such as prescription or illicit steroid use and overconsumption of either sugary foods or alcohol. Proper personal hygiene is also very important.

BONE CANCER

Bone cancer is not one disease but a collection of several classes of related diseases. The two most common forms of *primary* bone cancer, or that which originates in the bone, are multiple myeloma and osteosarcoma. *Secondary* bone cancer is cancer that originates elsewhere in the body. Bone cancer's most notable symptom is pain.

Multiple myeloma is the most common form of primary bone cancer. It usually affects older people. This disease attacks the tissues that create B cells, which in turn create antibodies that fight disease. Although an epidemic of multiple myeloma was observed among radiation-exposure survivors about twenty years after World War II, the most likely cause of this disease today is chronic overstimulation of the B cells. These cells are activated by petroleum products and by chemicals used in farming, leatherworking, and woodworking.

Since multiple myeloma depletes the body's supply of B cells, one of the main problems in managing the disease is reduced resistance to infection. Multiple myeloma patients are particularly susceptible to infections in the urinary tract, lungs, and sinuses.

While radiation therapy is used to reduce localized bone pain, chemotherapy is the main treatment option for multiple myeloma. Usually steroid drugs, such as dexamethasone and prednisone, are used. When used in combination, they can extend remission time.[1] These drugs can also, ironically, destroy bone. Even more importantly, they depress the immune system, which is already depressed by the disease itself.

Prednisone can also be given along with interferon, a chemical produced by the immune system. This therapy is generally given after the myeloma has been stabilized by other forms of chemotherapy,[2] and has been shown to increase life expectancy. Doctors almost always prescribe interferon to be given in the evening, so that its flulike side effects will not appear until after the patient has had a chance to get some sleep.

Osteosarcoma is the other major form of primary bone cancer. Doctors are not sure what causes this disease. But since it most often affects adolescents, it may be related to the rapid bone growth that occurs in childhood. It is classified into stages, I through IV, according to its size and extent of spread. This form of cancer does not damage the immune system the way multiple myeloma does, and so is less complicated to manage. However, it can spread to the lungs. Doctors usually treat osteosarcoma with surgery and chemotherapy using either cisplatin or cyclophosphamide.

Probably the largest number of bone cancer patients have secondary tumors. Cancers of the bladder, breast, kidney, lung, ovary, and prostate can all spread to bone through the bloodstream. Even after these cancers establish themselves in bone, they retain the characteristics they had in their organ of origin. Estrogen-stimulated breast cancer, for example, is still stimulated by estrogen when it spreads to bone tissue. The same is true of testosterone-stimulated prostate cancer. Other characteristics carry over as well, including destruction of gene p53, a gene responsible for stopping the multiplication of cancer cells.

Kampo regards bone health as one of the best indicators of a person's long-term overall condition. Daily and monthly changes in the balance of yang and yin are reflected in the muscles and skin, but energy imbalances register in the bones very slowly.

Persons who develop bone cancer have yang, vigorous constitutions. They are usually strongly built with a lean physique. Their excess energy manifests itself in a number of external symptoms. There may be greenish fatty spots on the skin on the outside of the ankle. The inside of the wrist may also show a greenish tint. The toenails and the fingertips may become white, and there may be calcifications, or hard bumps under the skin, on the face or head, especially the scalp.

Japanese doctors often recognize bone cancer through these symptom patterns. The medical use of Kampo in treating bone cancer is based on painstaking scientific research, mostly conducted since 1980, that has tested hundreds of herbs and formulas.

Kampo cannot replace medical treatment for bone cancer. However, Kampo remedies can make conventional treatment of this disease both more effective and more bearable (see considerations below). Kampo also provides other benefits. These include increasing the body's natural production of interferon, stimulating the immune system in general, preventing the spread of osteosarcoma to the lungs, and reducing pain. For maximum benefit, choose among the herbs in the appropriate categories after talking to a health care provider. Especially in treating childhood bone cancer, always work with a Kampo or TCM practitioner along with the physician; the dosages provided in this entry are meant for adults. In cases of secondary bone cancer, see the primary-cancer entry, such as breast or prostate cancer, for additional information and treatments.

INDIVIDUAL KAMPO TREATMENTS

See Chapter 3 for discussions of individual herbs, traditional healing substances, and modern herbal preparations, including directions for making tea.

Treatments That Increase the Body's Production of Interferon

SUGGESTED DOSAGES	COMMENTS
Bupleurum (Herb)	
Saikosaponin extract, 1 300-mg tablet daily. or Tea, 1 c 3 times daily.	Also inhibits cyclic AMP, a chemical that causes inflammation; prevents muscle spasms and steroid-induced side effects; and relaxes smooth muscles. Blunts pain and swelling by blocking 5HT, a substance that allows passage of body fluids into soft tissues.[3] Especially useful when symptoms include fever without sweating. *Caution:* Occasionally causes mild stomach upset. If this happens, reduce the dose. Do not take antibiotics when taking bupleurum.
Lentinan (Modern Herbal Preparation)	
Intramuscular injection (usual form), 0.5–50 mg effective daily dose, depending on patient's condition and circumstances. Smaller, more frequent doses more effective than larger, less frequent doses. Given under professional supervision. or Powder, dosage to be determined by provider. Much greater dosages required than in injectable form.	Also activates several types of immune-system cells: T cells,[4] plus lymphokine-activated killer cells (LAK) and natural killer (NK) cells against osteosarcoma.[5,6] May prevent spread of osteosarcoma to the lung.[7]

Siberian Ginseng (Modern Herbal Preparation)	
Eleuthero extract, as directed by manufacturer, in $\frac{1}{4}$ c water. Be sure to use pure extract, *not* sugar-sweetened ginseng drinks. or Tea, 1 c 3 times daily.	Is also a natural complement to lentinan in that it activates B cells to their maximum effectiveness.[8] *Caution:* Should be avoided by persons with myasthenia gravis; rheumatoid arthritis and diseases related to it, such as lupus, psoriatic arthritis, and Sjögren's syndrome; or prostate cancer.

Treatments That Stimulate the Immune System

Astragalus (Herb)	
Fluid extract (1:1), $\frac{1}{4}$–$\frac{1}{2}$ tsp (1–2 ml) 3 times daily. or Freeze-dried herb in capsules, 500–1,000 mg 3 times daily. or Powdered solid extract (4:1), 250–500 mg 3 times daily. or Tea, 1 c 3 times daily. or Tincture (1:5), 1–1$\frac{1}{2}$ tsp (4–6 ml), 3 times daily. Place in a cup, add 2 tbsp water, and take in a single sip. For dosages used with chemotherapy, *see* **Chemotherapy Side Effects.**	Contains compounds that both stimulate T cells, which are depleted in secondary bone cancer, and increase the ability of LAK cells to attack cancerous tumors.[9] *Caution:* Do not use when fever or skin infection is present.

Maitake (Modern Herbal Preparation)	
Large dosages are required when used in cancer treatment: Fresh or dried maitake in food, $\frac{1}{2}$–1 oz (15–30 g) daily. or Maitake D-fraction, 4 500-mg capsules 3 times daily before meals. or Tea, 1c 8–16 times daily. Lower dosages can be used if the cancer is in remission. See listing on page 144.	Increases the activity of various immune-system cells and reduces tumor formation.[10]

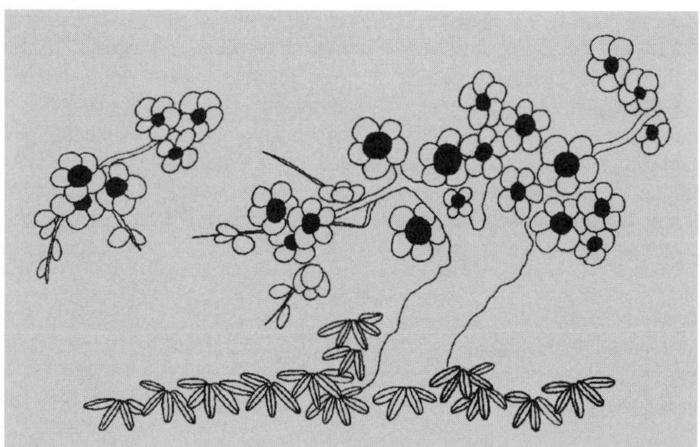

Scutellaria (Herb)	
Dried herb, 1–2 1,000-mg capsules 3 times daily. or Fluid extract (1:1), $\frac{1}{4}$–$\frac{1}{2}$ tsp (1–2 ml) 3 times daily. or Powdered solid extract (4:1), 250–500 mg 3 times daily. or Tea, 1 c 3 times daily. or Tincture (1:5), 1–1$\frac{1}{2}$ tsp (4–6 ml) 3 times daily. Place in a cup, add 2 tbsp water, and take in a single sip.	Contains compounds that kill a number of disease-causing viruses and bacteria which commonly affect persons with multiple myeloma. Also prevents influenza A or B infection. Other compounds inhibit spread of bone cancer. *Caution:* Avoid in cases of diarrhea caused by foodborne infection or excessive consumption of cold drinks.

Treatments That Prevent Spread of Osteosarcoma to the Lungs

Psoralea (Herb)	
Freeze-dried herb, 1 1,000-mg capsule 3 times daily.	Contains bavachinin, corylfolinin, and psoralen, all of which inhibit osteosarcoma and lung cancer.[11] Sold as Psoralea Seed capsule, Scruffy Pea, or *Bu Gu Zhi.* *Caution:* Use sunscreen or avoid exposure to sunlight.

KAMPO FORMULAS

See Chapter 4 for dosage information and discussions of individual formulas.

Formulas That Reduce Pain

Ophiopogonis Decoction

Also increases the effectiveness of hydrocortisone, methylprednisone, prednisone, and prednisolone.[12] Is particularly appropriate for persons also experiencing coughing, wheezing, and involuntary spitting of saliva.

Caution: Use with caution if fever is present, and discontinue if preexisting fevers worsen.

CONSIDERATIONS

❑ To reduce side effects and increase effectiveness when using chemotherapy, *see* **Chemotherapy Side Effects.** To reduce side effects when using radiation therapy for pain relief in cases of multiple myeloma, *see* **Radiation Therapy Side Effects.** To learn about herbal treatments that can prevent myeloma from dissolving bone[13] or a cancer from developing its own blood supply, *see* **Cancer.**

❑ Individuals who have multiple myeloma and subsequent infection should *see* **Bladder Infection, Bronchitis and Pneumonia,** or **Sinusitis.**

BREAST CANCER

Breast cancer is the most common form of cancer among women, affecting as many as one woman out of every nine at some point in life. Breast cancer also occurs among men, although at a much lower rate (see "Breast Cancer in Men"). Symptoms include a lump or thickening in the breast; a clear, bloody, or yellow discharge from the nipple; and, in rare instances, breast pain. Cancerous breast lumps are firm and do not shrink and expand with the menstrual cycle. While most lumps are not cancerous, all breast abnormalities should be brought to a doctor's attention.

Major risk factors for breast cancer include age, family history, smoking,[1] and, in postmenopausal women, obesity. Alcohol consumption and radiation exposure are other factors, and environmental toxins may also play a role.

In women who do not smoke, the most important risk factor is lifetime exposure to the female hormone estrogen. The growth of approximately 75 percent of all breast cancers is accelerated by higher estrogen levels in the bloodstream. Such cancers are *estrogen-dependent.* Lifetime estrogen exposure is increased by early start of menstruation, late menopause, use of estrogen replacement therapy, and late or no childbearing. Estrogen exposure can be reduced by eating properly (see "Lowering Estrogen Levels Through Diet" on page 207).

Breast cancer is classified according to a multistage system that measures tumor size, the amount of lymph-node involvement, and the absence or presence of spread to other organs such as the bones, lungs, and liver. The main treatment is surgery. This ranges from lumpectomy, in which the lump itself is removed with a small amount of surrounding tissue, through more extensive operations to radical mastectomy, in which the breast, parts of the chest muscle, and armpit lymph nodes are removed. After surgery, a woman may receive radiation therapy or various forms of chemotherapy.

One of the most useful treatments is hormonal therapy. Estrogen interacts with an anticancer gene known as gene p53. This gene is a "molecular patrolman" that makes sure genetically defective cells do not multiply. Estrogen, however, promotes so much cellular growth within the breast that gene p53 is unable to keep track of all the defective cells. Removing estrogen reduces the rate of cell growth so that this gene can do its job.[2]

Unfortunately, gene p53 can itself be damaged, which makes it ineffective. Defects in this gene carry a high risk of cancer in both breasts,[3] and are prominent in breast cancer that spreads to the lungs.[4] This gene is so important, in fact, that measuring the amount of the gene in a breast biopsy is a better predictor of future health than the size or spread of the tumor.[5]

Hormonal therapy uses drugs that act like estrogen within the body. They attach to cells at the same places estrogen does, but stimulate less cell growth. This gives gene p53 less work to do. Tamoxifen is a drug widely used after surgery for this purpose. However, while tamoxifen reduces the risk of breast cancer, it increases the risk of uterine cancer.[6]

Breast cancer was historically unknown in Kampo, but the ancient theorists did have a concept of how tumors and other breast diseases develop. Breast disease usually arose from a combination of constraints on the liver and deficiencies of blood. When the liver was constrained, usually as a result of emotional tension or bad diet, it could not send its energy upward through the body. Neither could the liver release blood to circulate energy in the rest of the body. Energy gradually built up along the energy channels controlled by the liver, both of which pass directly over the breast. This energy could be transformed into clumps. These clumps, or tumors, could be energized to break out of the breast. At the same time, the liver did not release enough blood to carry the defensive energies of the body to protect the breast.

There are Kampo herbs and formulas that block estrogen without side effects, and that offset the side effects of chemotherapy and radiation therapy (see considerations below). Herbs also provide other benefits, including activation of gene p53. Always use Kampo as part of a medically directed overall treatment plan for breast cancer.

Breast Cancer in Men

Breast cancer strikes men only 1 percent as often as it strikes women. Because it is not often suspected as a cause of symptoms, it is often discovered at an advanced stage. Risk factors for male breast cancer include diseases in which the body produces too much estrogen, family history, radiation exposure, and exposure to the tropical disease organism *Schistosoma.*[1] In general, the same treatments are used as in female breast cancer, except that in men spread of the disease may be treated by removal of the testes to eliminate the hormones that stimulate cancer growth.

Men who have breast cancer should take any of the herbs or formulas recommended for women that reduce estrogen production. Both men and women who have been exposed to the tropical disease schistosomiasis will benefit from the use of agrimony, as this disease can contribute to the development of both breast tumors and benign calcified cysts that appear as cancers on mammograms.[2] Agrimony contains compounds that interrupt the life cycle of the parasite. It also stimulates B cells, immune-system cells that produce antibodies against cancer and various forms of infection. Take 1 cup of agrimony tea (see Chapter 3 for tea-making directions) two to three times daily for up to three months.

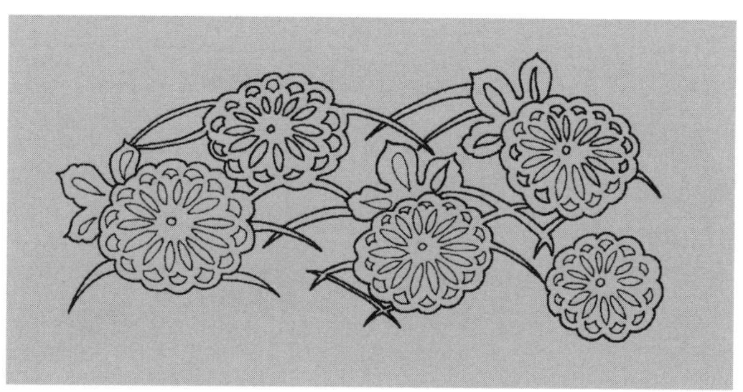

INDIVIDUAL KAMPO TREATMENTS

See Chapter 3 for discussions of individual herbs, traditional healing substances, and modern herbal preparations, including directions for making tea.

SUGGESTED DOSAGES	COMMENTS
Astragalus (Herb)	
Fluid extract (1:1), ¼–½ tsp (1–2 ml) 3 times daily. or Freeze-dried herb in capsules, 500–1,000 mg 3 times daily. or Powdered solid extract (4:1), 250–500 mg 3 times daily. or Tea, 1 c 3 times daily. or Tincture (1:5), 1–1½ tsp (4–6 ml), 3 times daily. Place in a cup, add 2 tbsp water, and take in a single sip. For dosages used with chemotherapy, *see* **Chemotherapy Side Effects.**	Stops the spread of cancers known to respond to gene p53. Contains compounds that increase the ability of immune-system cells called lymphokine-activated killer (LAK) cells to attack cancers.[7] *Caution:* Do not use when fever or skin infection is present.
Garlic (Herb)	
Enterically coated tablets, as directed on label (usually at least 900 mg daily).	Contains a compound, SAMC, that stops the proliferation of estrogen-dependent breast cancer cells,[8] thus complementing the action of tamoxifen. Another compound, ajoene, counteracts the carcinogenic effect of toxic chemicals.[9] Garlic also increases the effectiveness of selenium supplements in preventing cancer growth and spread.[10] Only enterically coated tablets are effective. *Caution:* Do not use with the blood-thinner warfarin sodium (Coumadin). Garlic will counteract the effects of *Bifidus* and *Lactobacillus* cultures taken as digestive aids.
Ginkgo (Modern Herbal Preparation)	
Ginkgolide extract, 1 40-mg tablet 4 times daily or 1 60-mg tablet 3 times daily. or Quercetin extract, 1–2 125-mg capsules 3 times daily between meals.	Contains quercetin, which accelerates cell death especially in cases of multidrug-resistant breast cancer.[11] Quercetin also increases the effectiveness of doxorubicin hydrochloride (Adriamycin).[12] For best results, take quercetin with bromelain, which increases absorption. *Caution:* Do not take ginkgo or quercetin with the prescription drugs Procardia or Seldane.

SUGGESTED DOSAGES	COMMENTS
Green Tea (Herb)	
Catechin extract, 1 240-mg tablet 3 times daily. or Tea, 1 c 2–5 times daily.	Contains polyphenols, which lock estrogen out of its receptors on cells of estrogen-dependent tumors.[13] This enhances the activity of tamoxifen. Caffeinated green tea also increases the effectiveness of cyclophosphamide. To avoid dilution problems, do not take tea within 1 hour of taking other teas or patent medicines. *Caution:* Avoid if taking thiotepa or Ukrain.
Kelp (Herb)	
Kelp as food, any quantity desired.	May be responsible for low rates of breast cancer in Japan, where it is a dietary staple. Use of kelp increases the rate at which stool passes through the intestines. This lowers the risk that estrogens in the stool can be reabsorbed back into the bloodstream.[14] *Caution:* Limit consumption to once a week.
Kudzu (Herb)	
Dried extract, 1 10-mg tablet 3 times daily. or Tea, 1 c 3 times daily. or Use soy isoflavone extract (see **Soy Isoflavones** in this list).	Contains compounds called isoflavones that are clearly associated with reduced rates of breast and other cancers.[15,16] Daidzein stops cancer cells from growing and blocks estrogen cell receptor sites,[17] which increases the effectiveness of tamoxifen. Genistein reduces bloodstream estrogen levels[18] and activates gene p21, a "molecular patrolman" similar to gene p53.[19] Both isoflavones complement the effects of curcumin (see **Turmeric** in this list).
Lentinan (Modern Herbal Preparation)	
Intramuscular injection (usual form), 0.5–50 mg effective daily dose, depending on patient's condition and circumstances. Smaller, more frequent doses more effective than larger, less frequent doses. Given under professional supervision. or Powder, dosage to be determined by provider. Much greater dosages required than in injectable form.	Activates the immune system's LAK and natural killer (NK) cells against cancer,[20,21] and encourages the maturation of T cells. Prevents immune-system damage when given *before* treatment with mitomycin-C, 5-fluorouracil, or tegafur. When used with immune-system component interleukin-2, can prevent spread of breast cancer to the lung.[22] Can increase survival time after such spread.[23]
Loranthus (Herb)	
Use only under professional supervision (see Appendix A).	Has been shown in at least one study among breast cancer patients to increase the rate at which breast cells were able to repair their DNA, preventing the mutations that can cause cancerous cells to form.[24] Always use as part of an overall cancer treatment program.

Maitake (Modern Herbal Preparation)	
Large dosages are required when used in cancer treatment: Fresh or dried maitake in food, ½–1 oz (15–30 g) daily. or Maitake D-fraction, 4 500-mg capsules 3 times daily before meals. or Tea, 1 c 8–16 times daily. Lower dosages can be used if the cancer is in remission. See listing on page 144.	General immune stimulant that increases the activity of various immune-system cells and reduces tumor formation.[25] When given with mitomycin, inhibits growth of breast cancer cells, even after the tumors are well-formed, and prevents spread to the liver.[26] Tests in the United States with maitake D-fraction have had positive results.[27]

Rhubarb Root (Herb)	
Injectable forms, given under professional supervision. or Non-Kampo Essiac or Hoxie tea, as directed on label.	Contains rhein, which reduces the ability of cancer cells to create protein and glucose.[28] Also contains emodin, which stimulates the production of white blood cells. This makes emodin useful for the treatment of white cell deficiency during chemotherapy.[29] Essiac and Hoxie teas are North American rhubarb formulations recommended because they are readily available and easy to use. *Caution:* Oral forms have laxative effects in dosages larger than those recommended. Do not use if menstruating or if rectal bleeding is present, or if taking any kind of diuretic.

Soy Isoflavones (Modern Herbal Preparation)	
Extract, about 3,000 mg once daily. or Soy germ, 2 tsp (10 g) twice daily, preferably added to cereals or smoothies.	Contains daidzein and genistein (see **Kudzu** in this list). If concentrated isoflavones cause upset stomach, use kudzu.

Turmeric (Herb)	
Curcumin, the yellow pigment found in turmeric, 250–500 mg twice daily between meals.	Curcumin activates gene p53,[30] which complements the action of tamoxifen. May also suppress genes necessary for breast cancer growth. Prevents lung damage caused by the chemotherapy drug cyclophosphamide[31] and reduces lung damage after exposure to whole-body radiation.[32]

HERBS TO AVOID

Individuals who have breast cancer should avoid the following herbs: cordyceps, dan shen, fennel, licorice, and peony. For more information regarding these herbs, see Chapter 3.

KAMPO FORMULAS

See Chapter 4 for dosage information and discussions of individual formulas.

Augmented Rambling Powder
Lowers estrogen levels.[33] Traditionally, this formula is used to treat "hot" symptoms, including dry mouth, red eyes, blurry vision, lower abdominal pressure, red eyes, difficult and painful urination, increased menstrual flow, and uterine bleeding. *Caution:* Should not be used by women who are trying to become pregnant.

Cinnamon Twig and Poria Pill
Reduces the amount of estrogen in the bloodstream by acting on the ovaries.[34] This action reduces the growth of estrogen-dependent breast cancer and augments the effectiveness of tamoxifen. Is not helpful for women who have had their ovaries removed. Traditionally given to women who are experiencing "cold" symptoms, such as weakness, lack of appetite, and fatigue.

Tang-Kuei and Peony Powder
In modern Japanese medicine, is applied to a wide range of conditions that benefit from reduced estrogen production.[35] That includes increasing the effectiveness of tamoxifen in the treatment of breast cancer. Unlike some treatments, does not have a masculinizing effect; decreases ovarian estrogen production[36] without reducing the ratio of estrogen to testosterone in circulation.[37] Traditionally, symptoms for which this formula is appropriate include easy fatigue, soft muscles, and coldness or poor circulation to the bottom half of the body.

Two-Cured Decoction
Reduces estrogen levels in women with breast cancer or fibrocystic breast disease.[38] Traditionally, the symptoms for which this formula was prescribed included coughing large amounts of easily expectorated phlegm, and/or vomiting and nausea. *Caution:* Use with caution if fever is present, and discontinue if preexisting fevers worsen.

FORMULAS TO AVOID

Individuals who have breast cancer should avoid the following formulas: Peony and Licorice Decoction, and Six-Ingredient Pill With Rehmannia (Rehmannia-Six Combination). For more information regarding these formulas, see Chapter 4.

CONSIDERATIONS

❑ The hormone melatonin produces a hundredfold increase in the effectiveness of tamoxifen.[39] In turn, astragalus makes melatonin more effective. Astragalus also increases treatment effectiveness when melatonin is combined with an immune-system component called interleukin-2.

❑ To reduce side effects and increase effectiveness when using chemotherapy, *see* **Chemotherapy Side Effects**; when using radiation therapy, *see* **Radiation Therapy Side Effects.** To learn about herbal treatments that can prevent a cancer from developing its own blood supply, *see* **Cancer.**

BRONCHITIS AND PNEUMONIA

Bronchitis is an infection or irritation of the bronchi, the passageways from the windpipe to the lungs. Pneumonia is an infection or irritation of the lungs themselves. Both of these conditions are much more common in the winter. These disorders are discussed in one entry because Kampo uses the same remedies to treat both of them.

Acute bronchitis usually follows a weakening of the immune system by a viral infection, such as common cold, or exposure to noxious fumes or other irritants, or a combination of both factors. Fever usually occurs first, followed by a dry cough. The cough then becomes raspy, with much sputum production. Repeated airway inflammation may lead to *chronic bronchitis.* In this disorder, the airway walls enlarge, which narrows the passageway. Symptoms range from persistent cough to difficulty in breathing, depending on the illness's severity. If inflammation persists, the damage may become permanent. Smoking, allergies, and asthma can all lead to chronic bronchitis.

Like bronchitis, pneumonia usually follows a viral infection or exposure to respiratory irritants. Pneumonia can also be caused by fluids or objects entering the lungs, as in cases of near-drowning, or by bacterial or fungal infections. Chills and fever are usually the first symptoms, followed by cough with sputum production, chest pain and shortness of breath. Fatigue and muscle aches may be present.

The risk of bronchitis or pneumonia is higher after hospitalization, since a hospital stay often exposes the patient to a variety of germs. Bronchitis and pneumonia are especially common among the elderly, and pneumonia also tends to affect young children. Persons who have alcohol or drug abuse problems are at higher risk for these illnesses, as are persons with AIDS, heart disease, or lung disorders.

Most cases of bronchitis and pneumonia are not helped by antibiotics, since these drugs have no effect on viral infections. Medical researchers have confirmed this fact in carefully controlled clinical studies.[1] Nonetheless, 70 percent of doctors still give bronchitis patients antibiotics for acute bronchitis,[2] based on misconceptions[3] doctors share with the general public. These include the common beliefs that a change in phlegm color from yellow to green is a sign of bacterial infection, or that antibiotic treatment for bronchitis will prevent the disease from progressing to pneumonia. Actually, both disorders can exist at the same time.

There is evidence that taking antibiotics for bronchitis and pneumonia does more harm than good. The person taking the drug gains no resistance against the virus, but loses the beneficial intestinal bacteria that aid digestion. Antibiotic use can also allow drug-resistant strains of bacteria to develop.

Bronchitis was one of the first conditions for which Kampo developed a formula. Kampo regards bronchitis as a manifestation of chronic problems in the body's water usage. Weak lungs and weak digestion are unable to circulate water normally. When the body is invaded by cold, particularly by cold carried on the wind, or wind-cold, the body's water and the pathogenic invader become locked in battle. Their conflict generates heat but also closes the pores, so the result is fever unrelieved by sweating. When the lungs' energy is constrained by cold, they cannot circulate fluids. These fluids accumulate in the epigastric region, or the pit of the stomach, and attack the lungs from below. This process leads to coughing and wheezing with copious, white, stringy sputum that is difficult to expectorate, and a generalized feeling of heaviness, especially in the chest.

The natural approach to treating bronchitis and pneumonia avoids creating new disease problems. It involves two goals: stimulating the normal processes that expel mucus, and stimulating the immune system to deal with viral infection. The expectorant herbs used in Kampo increase the fluidity and volume of phlegm, and stimulate cough. They are *not* cough suppressants, since cough suppression traps mucus in the bronchi and lungs. Use Kampo treatments after receiving a definitive diagnosis, especially if there is a preexisting condition.

INDIVIDUAL KAMPO TREATMENTS

See Chapter 3 for discussions of individual herbs, traditional healing substances, and modern herbal preparations, including directions for making tea.

SUGGESTED DOSAGES	COMMENTS
Coltsfoot (Herb)	
Tea, 1 c no more than twice daily. Do not use for more than 6 weeks.	Small doses open bronchial passages, although large doses close them.[4] Contains mucilages that coat the linings of the throat and relieve irritation. *Caution:* Avoid coltsfoot tinctures, which have a greater toxic potential and less mucilage than teas.
Plantain (Herb)	
Tea, 1 c up to 3 times daily. For this condition, brew using a muslin cloth (see Chapter 3).	Stops cough and expels phlegm. Particularly appropriate for coughs with fever and copious phlegm. Be sure to use the species *Plantago asiatica*, available from Chinese herb shops as *Che Qian Zi.* To avoid absorption problems, take other oral medications 1 hour before using plantain.
Reishi (Modern Herbal Preparation)	
Dried extract, 3 1-g tablets 3 times daily. or Syrup, as directed on label. or Tincture (1:5), 1 tbsp (10 ml) 3 times daily. Place in a cup, add 2 tbsp water, and take in a single sip.	Stimulates the maturation of immune-system cells called macrophages into forms that can "eat" infectious bacteria. This prevents secondary infection in chronic bronchitis.
Snow Fungus (Modern Herbal Preparation)	
Patent medicine *Yin Mi Pian*, 6–12 tablets daily for at least 4 weeks. or Prepared fungus (see Chapter 3) in food, 1 tbsp daily for at least 4 weeks.	Contains compounds that increase the production of or activity of various immune-system components, including interferon,[5] interleukin-2,[6] macrophages,[7,8] and natural killer (NK) cells. They also enhance the effectiveness of antibodies.[9]

White Mustard Seed (Herb)	
Plaster, applied daily (see Chapter 3 for directions).	Rapidly penetrates to the deeper layers of the skin and brings about redness and inflammation. This stimulates the secretion of fluids into the lungs, making expectoration easier. The effect lasts 24–48 hours. Both white and black mustard seeds make effective plasters, but the essential oils in white mustard seed do not evaporate in a hot plaster. *Caution:* When applied too long, can cause skin ulcers. Do not place on varicose veins, and do not use if circulatory problems are present.

KAMPO FORMULAS

See Chapter 4 for dosage information and discussions of individual formulas.

Ephedra Decoction (Four Emperors Combination)

Used to treat persons who are otherwise in good health. Body aches and headache are prominent in the symptom pattern for this formula. A variation, Ephedra, Apricot Kernel, Coix, and Licorice Decoction, is designed to lower fever, in addition to treating other symptoms. Use either formula in patent-medicine form.

Caution: Avoid if nausea or vomiting is present.

Kudzu Decoction

Gentle formula used when neck stiffness and muscle pain are prominent symptoms.

Minor Bluegreen Dragon Decoction

Treats bronchitis marked by fever and chills, with chills predominating. More effective when taken hot as a tea than as a patent medicine.

Caution: Use with caution if fever is present, and discontinue if preexisting fevers worsen.

Minor Bupleurum Decoction

Treats lingering cough. More useful when it is combined with Ephedra, Apricot Kernel, Coicis, and Licorice Decoction or Minor Bluegreen Dragon Decoction.

Caution: Do not use if fever or skin infection is present. Taken long term in patent medicine form, can cause headache, dizziness, and bleeding gums. Side effects can be avoided if the formula is taken as a tea.

Ophiopogonis Decoction

Treats spasmodic cough, dry and irritated throat, scanty and firmly lodged sputum, and laryngitis.

Caution: Use with caution if fever is present, and discontinue if preexisting fevers worsen.

CONSIDERATIONS

❑ The nutritional supplement bromelain both liquefies and decreases bronchial secretions. It also can be used to prevent the progression of sinusitis to bronchitis by breaking up sinus secretions before they can carry the virus to the bronchi.[10]

❑ Mustard seed plasters are more effective when combined with postural draining. After removing the plaster, lie face down on the edge of the bed, forearms on the floor for support. Maintain this position from five to fifteen minutes while expectorating into a basin or newspaper.

❑ *See also* **AIDS; Allergies, Respiratory; Asthma; Colds; Influenza;** and **Sinusitis.**

Burns

Burns are wounds to the skin caused by chemical or thermal injury. Every year, roughly 120,000 Americans suffer burns that are severe enough to require medical assistance.

Burns are graded from first degree to third degree. In a *first-degree burn,* the skin is red but unbroken, and there is no danger of infection. In a *second-degree burn,* the skin is reddened and blistered. Often, there is a massive loss of fluid, and the resulting dehydration may deepen the wound. In a *third-degree burn,* the entire thickness of skin is involved. The skin may be charred, but there may be little initial pain because of the loss of nerve endings. Severity is also judged by how extensive the burn is, based on the percentage of body surface involved. Both the degree and the extent of a burn must be considered in deciding the burn's severity.

Burned skin is initially free of microbial contamination. However, as body fluids ooze through the wound, tissues die, and a variety of infectious agents can affect the skin. Bacteria, fungi, and viruses can enter the wound and cause infection. This invasion of microorganisms is accelerated by the body's immune response to burns. All the body's forms of immune resistance are lowered. Macrophages are less likely to engulf and digest germs. B cells fail to secrete substances that destroy germs, and T cells fail to attach to the germs' surfaces in order to disintegrate the invaders. The larger the burn, the more the immune system is disabled.

Interestingly, the ancient theorists of Kampo viewed burns as symptoms of energy imbalance in the body. When disease disturbed the normal flow of energy, the regions of the body along the disrupted energy channels were more prone to accidents, including burns. The heart's energy channel passed over the tongue, for instance, so disturbance of the heart channel made the person more susceptible to scalding the tongue with a hot drink. The liver's energy channel passes over the eyes, so sunburned eyelids could hint of problems in the liver. In this theory, burns could be a signal of a more systemic disease, particularly if there were more than one burn along a single energy channel.

Use Kampo for first- and second-degree burns that are no larger than 3 inches square (approximately 50 square centimeters). Apply herbs to *dressings* (not to the burn itself) or take herbal teas to stimulate immune response and protect the skin from infection as it regenerates itself. More severe burns require *immediate* medical attention.

INDIVIDUAL KAMPO TREATMENTS

See Chapter 3 for discussions of individual herbs, traditional healing substances, and modern herbal preparations, including directions for making tea.

SUGGESTED DOSAGES	COMMENTS
Aloe (Herb)	
Gel, either commercial or taken from houseplants, used liberally on dressings. Do not use bitters or juice.	Contains complex carbohydrates that activates macrophages,[1] and signal these cells to go into a defensive mode by stimulating the production of nitric oxide.[2] They also stimulate blood circulation on the body's surface and accelerate wound healing.
Astragalus (Herb)	
Fluid extract (1:1), ¼–½ tsp (1–2 ml) 3 times daily. or Freeze-dried herb in capsules, 500–1,000 mg 3 times daily. or Powdered solid extract (4:1), 250–500 mg 3 times daily. or Tea, 1 c. 3 times daily. or Tincture (1:5), 1–1½ tsp (4–6 ml), 3 times daily. Place in a cup, add 2 tbsp water, and take in a single sip.	Increases the body's production of interleukin-2,[3] which reduces stress on the immune system. Starts an immune reaction that produces antigens, which dissolve germs, without stimulating immune-system cells that could cause inflammation at the burn site.[4] *Caution:* Do not use when fever or skin infection is present.
Coptis (Herb)	
Ointment, applied liberally to affected skin. and Tincture (1:5), 15–30 drops 3 times daily. Place in a cup, add 2 tbsp water, and take in a single sip. A clean cloth can also be soaked in the diluted tincture and placed lightly over the burn.	Ointments reduce the incidence of infections in first- and second-degree burns.[5] Tinctures help prevent staph and strep infections. *Caution:* Do not use internally during pregnancy or on a daily basis for more than 2 weeks at a time. Do not use internally with supplements that contain vitamin B_6 or the amino acid histidine.

Cancer

Cancer is a group of diseases in which genetically damaged cells multiply wildly, depriving healthy tissues of nutrients and oxygen. Scientists estimate that there may be as many as 300 types of cancer, and that at any given time, about 40 to 50 percent of the human population has cancer. However, between 95 and 99 percent of all cancers end in spontaneous remission, with the individual totally unaware of the potential disease. These would-be tumors are eliminated by the body's multiple defenses against cancer cells.

Cancer develops through a long series of steps that have to overcome these defenses. It begins when a cell's master code, its DNA, is injured by viruses, toxins, or radiation. This damage may cause the cell to become cancerous. However, cells have other genes that recognize DNA errors, and override the cancer cell's drive to multiply. The "watchdog" genes only fail to "turn off" cancer cells when the watchdogs themselves are damaged. In addition, most cells have an "address," specified by adhesion proteins that "glue" cells into their proper position in the tissues. For a cancer cell to spread, it must have DNA instructions that allow it to break the bonds of that glue, and to make new adhesion proteins before entering other tissues.

Cancer cells also need to requisition their own blood supply. They accomplish this through the process of angiogenesis, which creates new blood vessels to carry nutrients and oxygen. Once a tumor has its own blood supply, it can grow and release cancerous cells into the bloodstream. (These cells, however, are exposed to attack by the immune system.)

Kampo has had a concept of cancer for over 2,000 years. The traditional understanding of the mechanism of cancer was as a depletion of vital energy in the course of personal suffering in life. Shocks and losses—such as the deaths of family or loved ones, war, plagues, famine, storms, or financial ruin—injected a pathogenic "cold" into the body. The body could not redirect this pathogenic energy on its own. The longer destructive energies were left unprocessed, the "harder" they became, first fluid, then phlegm, and finally rocklike, constraining the normal flow of blood and water.

Fortunately, the course of cancer was not unalterable. Correcting energy imbalances early kept them from disturbing the flow of blood and water. Treating "soft" tumors offered a greater chance of success than treating "fixed" tumors. Even advanced tumors occasionally could be treated with herbal medicine.

The ancient formulas to restore the flow of blood and water are the basis of modern Kampo treatments for cancer. However, Kampo physicians use both ancient remedies and modern medicine. The modern use of Kampo relies on the results of painstaking research into every potential cancer cure. For example, scientists have identified compounds in herbs that protect the "watchdog" genes from damage in the first place. There are also Kampo medicines that stimulate the immune system against cancer in the bloodstream and keep cancer cells from establishing themselves in new tissues. (Since cancer treatment differs for each kind of cancer, this book lists the most common cancers separately and makes separate treatment recommendations.)

Kampo is best used as part of a medically directed overall cancer treatment plan, which generally involves some combination of surgery, chemotherapy, and radiation therapy. Despite the fact that most conventional cancer therapies damage at least much healthy tissue as cancer tissue, the blunt force of chemotherapy or radiation therapy can be very effective when applied at the right time. Some Kampo remedies make taking harsh but necessary chemotherapy or radiation therapy easier. Many of the herbs and formulas within the individual cancer sections are suited for this purpose. In addition, treatments that can be used with conventional therapy for a number of different cancers are listed separately in their own sections.

To overcome cancer, use every option conventional medicine and Kampo have to offer. Do not hesitate to discuss any of the suggestions in this book with an oncologist, and be make sure to understand the diagnosis and know precisely what forms of treatment are to be used. Combining the doctor's expertise with natural medicine will provide the greatest opportunity for remission, recovery, and future health.

The therapies listed below *prevent* the process of angiogenesis. Some have other anticancer effects, and are listed under entries for individual cancers.

INDIVIDUAL KAMPO TREATMENTS

See Chapter 3 for discussions of individual herbs, traditional healing substances, and modern herbal preparations, including directions for making tea.

SUGGESTED DOSAGES	COMMENTS
Ginkgo (Herb)	
Ginkgolide extract, 160 to 240 mg daily in 2 or 3 doses.	Deactivates platelet activating factor (PAF), which is necessary for new blood-vessel growth.
Ginseng (Herb)	
Fluid extract or tincture, as directed on label. or Tea, made with Korean or red ginseng, 1 c daily.	In studies with melanoma patients, has been shown to keep tumors from developing blood supplies.[1] If using ginseng extracts or tinctures (which are not as therapeutically active as teas), be sure the product contains *Panax ginseng.* Note that strength may vary by manufacturer.
Kelp (Herb)	
Kelp as food, any quantity desired.	Prevents blood-vessel formation by deactivating the clotting factor thrombin. *Caution:* Limit consumption to once a week.
Kudzu (Herb)	
Dried extract, 1 10-mg tablet 3 times daily. or Tea, 1 c 3 times daily. or Use soy isoflavone extract (see next entry).	Contains genistein, which blocks new blood-vessel formation. *Caution:* Limit consumption to once a week.
Soy Isoflavones (Herb)	
Extract, about 3,000 mg once daily. or Soy germ, 2 tsp (10 g) twice daily, preferably added to cereals or smoothies.	Contains genistein. If concentrated isoflavones cause upset stomach, use **Kudzu** (see previous entry).

KAMPO FORMULAS

See Chapter 4 for dosage information and discussions of individual formulas.

Ten Significant Tonic Decoction (All-Inclusive Great Tonifying Decoction)

Ancient formula to "build up the blood." Found in clinical tests to slow or stop progress of wide variety of cancers.

CONSIDERATIONS

❑ To reduce side effects and increase effectiveness when using chemotherapy, *see* **Chemotherapy Side Effects**; when using radiation therapy, *see* **Radiation Therapy Side Effects.**

❑ *See also* **Bladder Cancer, Bone Cancer, Breast Cancer, Cervical Cancer, Colorectal Cancer, Endometrial Cancer, Hodgkin's Disease, Kidney Cancer, Leukemia, Liver Cancer, Lung Cancer, Melanoma, Ovarian Cancer, Prostate Cancer, Skin Cancer (Basal Cell Carcinoma),** and **Stomach Cancer.**

CATARACTS

Cataracts are white, cloudy blemishes on the normally transparent lens of the eye. They progressively blur vision, and are the leading cause of loss of sight in the United States. At any given time, approximately four million Americans are experiencing some degree of cataract. Most of these people have *senile cataracts,* or those associated with aging, although babies can be born with *congenital cataracts.*

Cataracts can be caused by a number of factors. Exposure to radiation, including that found in sunlight, and to environmental toxins both play a role. Some eye disorders can cause this problem, as can the use of some drugs. Cataracts can also form as a complication of certain diseases, most notably diabetes and atherosclerosis. In turn, cataracts may lead to glaucoma, in which pressure increases within the eye, by causing the lens to swell.

Cataracts result from free-radical damage to the proteins found in the lens, similar to the change that occurs in egg white when the egg is boiled. Free radicals, unstable molecules that can damage cells, are created both as the body uses oxygen and as the result of toxin accumulations. Cataracts form when the normal protective mechanisms of the lens cannot keep up with free-radical damage.

Advanced cases of cataracts are generally treated with lens-replacement surgery. Use of Kampo treatments can prolong the period before surgery becomes necessary.

Modern treatment of cataracts with Japanese medicinal herbs is based on practical experience as well as Kampo theory. Ancient theory explained cataracts as an imbalance of energies in the kidney and the liver. The kidneys stored "essence," roughly corresponding to the modern idea of the instructions stored in DNA, the body's genetic code. All of the organs contributed essence to the eyes. When the kidneys could not send essence upward to the eyes, the eyes formed abnormal tissues. Liver deficiency also contributed to cataracts. The liver stored blood. When the liver could not send blood to nourish the eyes, blurred vision resulted.

INDIVIDUAL KAMPO TREATMENTS

See Chapter 3 for discussions of individual herbs, traditional healing substances, and modern herbal preparations, including directions for making tea.

SUGGESTED DOSAGES	COMMENTS
Ginkgo (Modern Herbal Preparation)	
Ginkgolide extract, 1 40-mg tablet 3 times daily or 1 60-mg tablet twice daily. Increasing dosage to 160 mg (4 40-mg tablets) or 180 mg (3 60-mg tablets) may give increased relief.	Contains quercetin, which helps stop cataract-forming processes seen in diabetic cataracts.[1,2] Quercetin also reinforces the effects of selenium and vitamin E in preventing cataracts associated with the formation of hydrogen peroxide, a free-radical source, within the eye.[3] Other compounds increase circulation within the eye, which also helps prevent free-radical damage.[4]
Turmeric (Herb)	
Curcumin, the yellow pigment found in turmeric, 250–500 mg twice daily between meals.	Curcumin stimulates the production of an enzyme that prevents free-radical damage to cell membranes within the lens.[5]

KAMPO FORMULAS

See Chapter 4 for dosage information and discussions of individual formulas.

Eight-Ingredient Pill With Rehmannia (Rehmannia-Eight Combination)

Balances mineral content of the lens, preventing the formation of cataracts. Tests show it may delay cataract development by 10 to 15 years.[6] Especially useful when cataracts are caused by diabetes, as it provides tighter control of blood-sugar levels[7] and inhibits an enzyme called aldose reductase that allows the formation of diabetic cataracts.[8] Use of this formula should be continued for six months. In the context of cataract treatment, more practitioners are familiar with this formula by the Japanese name *hachimi-jio-gan.*

CONSIDERATIONS

❑ Supplementation with vitamins C and E, the amino acid glutathione, and the trace mineral selenium is associated with a lower incidence of cataracts.[9] Vitamin C has been shown to reduce the need for cataract surgery when used at a daily dose of 1,000 milligrams.[10] Glutathione (100 mg daily) plays a role in maintaining a healthy lens and preventing cataract formation.[11] Glutathione levels are almost always diminished in lenses that develop cataracts.[12] Vitamin E (400 IU daily) and selenium (200 mcg daily) work together to prevent hydrogen peroxide, a major source of free radicals, from forming in the fluid portion of the eye. One study has shown that selenium levels are only 15 percent of normal in lenses affected by cataracts.[13]

❑ Sunglasses can help protect the eyes from the sun's ultraviolet (UV) rays. It is important, though, to buy sunglasses specifically designed to block UV light.

❑ *See also* **Atherosclerosis, Diabetes,** and **Glaucoma.**

CERVICAL CANCER

Cancer of the cervix is one of the most common cancers affecting women. The cervical-cancer rate has dropped over time, though, as more and more women receive annual Pap smears. In this procedure, cells are taken from the surface of the cervix and examined for abnormalities. Pap smears are important because the early stages of cervical cancer usually produce no symptoms.

Cervical cancer has well-defined precancerous stages. It begins as *cervical dysplasia,* the appearance of abnormal cells on the surface of the cervix. Most cervical dysplasias form in response to infection with human papillomavirus (HPV), a sexually transmitted virus that causes genital warts.[1] Two strains, HPV16 and HPV18,[2] have been particularly implicated, and HPV16 infection poses a higher cancer risk if the woman smokes.[3] While women who have had multiple sex partners have the highest rates of cervical cancer (as do those who begin sexual relations early in life), even women who are in lifetime, monogamous relationships can develop the disease.

Another factor that increases the rate at which cervical dysplasia develops into cancer is use of the Pill. Oral contraceptives contain progesterone as well as varying amounts of estrogen. These hormones activate two genes in HPV that enable the virus to cause cancers.[4] In addition, one of the genes creates a protein that poisons the human gene p53, a gene which ordinarily ensures that genetically defective or cancerous cells do not multiply.[5] While HPV-associated cancers may be started by estrogen, the hormone does not stimulate their growth once established.[6] However, cervical cancer not caused by HPV infection *is* stimulated by estrogen. In these cases, reducing estrogen levels allows gene p53 to keep up with cell growth.[7]

In all cases, once cervical cancer has overcome gene p53, it can acquire its own blood supply so that it can grow and spread. When this happens, the disease produces noticeable symptoms, including abnormal vaginal bleeding, foul-smelling discharge, and lower back or pelvic pain. At this point treatment is essential.

Depending on its spread, cervical cancer is classified into stages 0 and I through IV. The extent of spread also determines which type of surgical procedures may be used. Such procedures range from removal of only a part of the cervix to removal of the entire uterus and its supporting structures. Lymph nodes in the groin may also be removed.

When biopsy shows that the cancer has penetrated beyond the first few cell layers, doctors often prescribe chemotherapy with cisplatin and either doxorubicin or mitomycin and possibly additional drugs. Radiation therapy may also be used after surgery. (Doctors usually try avoid radiation in treating younger women, since it can damage the ovaries and induce menopause.) If the cancer has spread, doctors sometimes try combining chemotherapy and radiation, an approach that usually does not alleviate symptoms or extend life.[8] In these cases, immunotherapy is another option.

The Kampo explanation of various forms of cervical irritation was that "damp heat" invading the lymph channels sank down to the cervix, where it could cause infection and atrophy.

Always use Kampo as part of a medically directed over-

Nutrition as a Weapon Against Cervical Cancer

Proper nutrition is helpful both in preventing cervical dysplasia from developing into cancer and in keeping cervical cancer itself from spreading. Women on the Pill who have cervical dysplasia are much less likely to develop more severe dysplasia or cancer if they take folic acid supplements. In one study of such women, 16 percent of those who did not take folic acid had more severe dysplasia after four months, while none of the those taking folic acid (10 milligrams per day) saw their conditions worsen.[1] Vitamin C deficiency also seems to be a risk factor for developing cervical adenocarcinoma, a form of cervical cancer, although it is not certain whether the disease depletes vitamin C or vitamin C stops the disease.[2]

Women who have developed cervical cancer are much less likely to see their cancers spread when their diets are rich in natural antioxidants. A four-year study of 2,189 women with cervical cancer found that those who frequently consumed dark green or yellow vegetables and fruit juices had a lower risk of developing invasive cancer. Compounds in these vegetables that are similar to vitamin A deactivate one of HPV's cancer-causing genes, although they are more effective at the disease's earliest stages.[3] Taking vitamin E (200 to 400 IU per day) provided a threefold decrease in the rate of invasive cancer.[4] Another study found that lower levels of vitamin E were found at every successive stage of cervical cancer, that is, the worse the cancer, the lower the tissue amounts of vitamin E.[5] Similarly, scientists have found lower levels of the amino acid glutathione (and higher levels of the enzyme that destroys it) at every successive stage of the disease.[6] Glutathione (50 milligrams per day) is an important antioxidant building block.

all treatment plan for cervical cancer (see considerations below). Kampo can make chemotherapy or radiation treatment more bearable and effective, and increase the likelihood of achieving remission. Kampo can also slow the development of cervical cancer in cases of cervical dysplasia.

INDIVIDUAL KAMPO TREATMENTS

See Chapter 3 for discussions of individual herbs, traditional healing substances, and modern herbal preparations, including directions for making tea.

SUGGESTED DOSAGES	COMMENTS
Aloe (Herb)	
Juice, 1/3 cup (80 ml) 3 times daily for 2 weeks.	Contains compounds that seem to keep the liver from processing toxins into cancer-causing forms.[9] Can increase effectiveness of cyclophosphamide and 5-fluorouracil treatment.[10]
Astragalus (Herb)	
Fluid extract (1:1), 1/4–1/2 tsp (1–2 ml) 3 times daily. or Freeze-dried herb in capsules, 500–1,000 mg 3 times daily. or Powdered solid extract (4:1), 250–500 mg 3 times daily. or Tea, 1 c 3 times daily. or Tincture (1:5), 1–1 1/2 tsp (4–6 ml), 3 times daily. Place in a cup, add 2 tbsp water, and take in a single sip. For dosages used with chemotherapy, *see* **Chemotherapy Side**	**Effects.** Stops spread of cancers known to respond to gene p53. Contains compounds that stimulate immune-system cells called T cells and that increase the ability of lymphokine-activated killer (LAK) cells to attack cancers.[11] *Caution:* Do not use when fever or skin infection is present.
Green Tea (Herb)	
Catechin extract, 1 240-mg tablet 3 times daily. or Tea, 1 c 2–5 times daily.	Contains compounds that deactivate plasmin, a substance that breaks up tissues and makes a pathway for invading tumors. Other compounds called catechins help prevent both thyroid cancer caused by radiation treatment and deficiencies in white blood cells caused by mitomycin.[12] Caffeine accelerates cell death and increases effectiveness of radiation therapy. To avoid dilution problems, do not take tea within 1 hour of taking other teas or patent medicines.
Lentinan (Modern Herbal Preparation)	
Intramuscular injection (usual form), 0.5–50 mg effective daily dose, depending on patient's condition and circumstances. Smaller, more frequent doses more effective than larger, less frequent doses. Given under professional supervision. or Powder, dosage to be determined by provider. Much greater dosages required than in injectable form.	Activates the immune system's LAK and natural killer (NK) cells against cancer,[13] and encourages the maturation of T cells. Prevents immune-system damage when given *before* treatment with mitomycin-C, 5-fluorouracil, or tegafur.[14]
PSK (Modern Herbal Preparation)	
Dried extract, 6 1,000-mg tablets daily.	Stops tumor spread by disabling the enzymes that allow cancer cells to escape their tissue of origin. Has been found useful in increasing the effectiveness of radiation therapy for cervical cancer. In Japan, this has led to increases in 5-year survival rate.[15]

Scutellaria (Herb)	
Fluid extract (1:1), ¼–½ tsp (1–2 ml) 3 times daily. or Powdered solid extract (4:1), 250–500 mg 3 times daily.	Prevents side effects of immunotherapy treatment with recombinant human tumor necrosis factor (rhTNF).[16] In laboratory studies, stops immune-system damage from cyclophosphamide and 5-fluorouracil.[17,18] *Caution:* Do not use scutellaria tea, which can cause stomach upset during 5-fluorouracil treatment.

Turmeric (Herb)	
Curcumin, the yellow pigment found in turmeric, 250–500 mg twice daily between meals.	Curcumin activates gene p53.[19] Prevents lung damage caused by the chemotherapy drug cyclophosphamide[20] and reduces lung damage after exposure to whole-body radiation.[21]

KAMPO FORMULAS

See Chapter 4 for dosage information and discussions of individual formulas.

Two-Cured Decoction

Contains pinellia, which directly inhibits cervical carcinoma, along with other herbs that enhance pinellia's effectiveness. Also reduces estrogen levels, which may indirectly slow the rate of growth of some cervical cancers.[22]

Caution: Use with caution if fever is present, and discontinue if preexisting fevers worsen.

CONSIDERATIONS

❑ In China, the standard treatment for cervical cancer is a combination of Kampo and electrotherapy, or application of electric current through acupuncture needles.[23] One Chinese study found that the response rate for other forms of cancer treated with Kampo and electrotherapy alone is 69 percent if the cancer is diagnosed before it spreads and 53 percent if diagnosed after it spreads.[24] These figures indicate that Kampo alone is not an acceptable substitute for conventional treatment of cervical cancer. On the other hand, they indicate that Kampo will be helpful in a majority of cases in which it is applied.

❑ Good nutrition is very important in fighting cervical cancer (see "Nutrition as a Weapon Against Cervical Cancer" on page 177).

❑ To reduce side effects and increase effectiveness when using chemotherapy, *see* **Chemotherapy Side Effects**; when using radiation therapy, *see* **Radiation Therapy Side Effects.** To learn about herbal treatments that can prevent a cancer from developing its own blood supply, *see* **Cancer.**

CHEMOTHERAPY SIDE EFFECTS

Chemotherapy is, as its name suggests, the chemical treatment of cancer and other conditions. The drugs used in chemotherapy are very powerful, and can greatly help some people. However, the use of chemotherapy requires a careful consideration of whether its potential effects on the disease outweigh its potential disruption to health. Chemotherapy must be given at precisely the right time in the course of a disease to maximize benefits and minimize side effects.

Where and how chemotherapy is given varies, depending on what drugs are used and the patient's condition. It can be given in a hospital, outpatient clinic, doctor's office, or even at home. The drugs may be given as a single dose each day, continuously over several days, once a week, or once a month. A course of treatment can last from several weeks to several years, and may be repeated if necessary.

Many Kampo herbs and formulas can either make chemotherapy more effective or reduce its side effects. Although chemotherapy is a modern medical invention, the ancient theories of Kampo hint that formulas which stimulate blood circulation, eliminate "blood stasis" (lack of movement), soften hardness, or dissolve masses should help treat cancer.[1] Medical researchers around the world have systematically searched Kampo for treatments that counteract chemotherapy's side effects. Similarly, some of the symptom patterns treated by Kampo match the side effects induced by chemotherapy for cancer, autoimmune diseases, and viral infections.

This section lists, by drug, Kampo recommendations for several of the more commonly used chemotherapy treatments. These recommendations are additions to, rather than replacements for, standard chemotherapy drugs. No herbal treatment from Kampo or any other herbal healing tradition can replace chemotherapy when it is medically required. Always use Kampo in close cooperation with a physician. Except for lentinan, which should be taken before treatment starts, these drugs should be taken at the same time as chemotherapy.

ADRIAMYCIN.

See **Doxorubicin Hydrochloride (Adriamycin).**

CISPLATIN AND CARBOPLATIN

These drugs are used to treat the following cancers: bladder, bone, cervix, endometrium, and lung. Although these drugs can affect cancer cells and healthy cells alike, they are only absorbed by cells that are preparing to make multiple copies of themselves. Since most healthy cells only produce a single replacement, the drugs do more damage to cancer cells than to healthy cells. Once the drug is absorbed, it "glues" strands of DNA together, so that cells cannot make the proteins they need to function and reproduce. Possible side effects include appetite loss, nausea and vomiting, kidney damage, hearing loss, and suppression of red and white blood cell production.

KAMPO FORMULAS

See Chapter 4 for dosage information and discussions of individual formulas.

Ten-Significant Tonic Decoction (All-Inclusive Great Tonifying Decoction)

Increases the drug's effectiveness by stopping anorexia, nausea, and vomiting; reducing kidney damage; and stimulating the bone marrow to produce red blood cells. It also stimulates the immune system, especially useful for helping the body maintain production of interleukins and natural killer (NK) cells.[1]

CYCLOPHOSPHAMIDE

This drug is used for the following cancers: chronic lymphocytic leukemia, Hodgkin's disease, multiple myeloma, sarcoma, and cancers of the breast, cervix, lung, and ovary. It is also used to treat lupus. It keeps tumor cells from multiplying, and works best when given with other chemotherapy drugs. Cyclophosphamide has no effect on cancer until it is activated by the liver, which means a healthy liver is necessary for one to benefit from the drug. The liver changes this drug into a chemical that is harmless in normal cells but destructive in tumor cells. Possible side effects include nausea and vomiting, suppression of red and white blood cell production, bladder and lung damage, infertility, and the development of secondary cancers.

INDIVIDUAL KAMPO TREATMENTS

See Chapter 3 for discussions of individual herbs, traditional healing substances, and modern herbal preparations, including directions for making tea.

SUGGESTED DOSAGES	COMMENTS
Astragalus (Herb)	
Fluid extract (1:1), 1–4 tsp (4–16 ml) 3 times daily. or Freeze-dried herb in capsule form, 1,000–5,000 mg 3 times daily. or Powdered solid extract (4:1), 1,250–2,500 mg 3 times daily. or Tea, 1 c 3 times daily. or Tincture (1:5), 5–8 tsp (20–30 ml) 3 times daily. Place in a cup, add 2 tbsp water, and take in a single sip.	Reverses immune suppression.[1] Begin with the lowest dosage. If fever does not occur, move up to the highest dosage over 4 days.
Cordyceps (Traditional Healing Substance)	
Dried extract, 4 250-mg tablets daily. or Prepared tea, as directed on label.	Restores the body's ability to create red blood cells.[2] *Caution:* Discuss usage with the doctor if a hormone-sensitive cancer, such as breast or prostate cancer, is present.
Galangal (Herb)	
Tea, 1 c 4 times daily.	Stops swelling, inflammation, and pain, particularly in allergic reactions to chemotherapy agents.[3]
Reishi (Modern Herbal Preparation)	
Dried extract, 3 1-g tablets 3 times daily. or Dried mushroom in food, approx. ¼–approx. ½ oz (5–10 g) daily. or Syrup, as directed on label. or Tea, 1 c 3 times daily. or Tincture (1:5), 1 tsp (4 ml) 3 times daily. Place in a cup, add 2 tbsp water, and take in a single sip.	Stimulates protein creation in bone marrow, which increases production of red and white blood cells.[4]
Scutellaria (Herb)	
Dried herb, 1–2 1,000-mg capsules 3 times daily. or Fluid extract (1:1), ¼–½ tsp (0.5 –2 ml) 3 times daily. or Powdered solid extract (4:1), 250–500 mg 3 times daily. or Tea, 1 c 3 times daily. or Tincture (1:5), 1–1½ tsp (4–6 ml) 3 times daily. Place in a cup, add 2 tbsp water, and take in a single sip.	Stops immune-system damage.[5,6]
Turmeric (Herb)	
Curcumin, the yellow pigment found in turmeric, 250–500 mg twice daily between meals.	Curcumin prevents damage to lung tissue.[7]

KAMPO FORMULAS

See Chapter 4 for dosage information and discussions of individual formulas.

Ginseng Decoction to Nourish the Nutritive Qi

Frequently prescribed in Japan to treat cancer patients who have anemia, forgetfulness, hair loss, jaundice, shortness of breath, and tired limbs.

Pinellia Decoction to Drain the Epigastrium

Relieves symptoms frequently experienced by chemotherapy patients: anorexia, feeling of obstruction below the heart, vomiting. Also stops "rumbling" in the stomach and intestines. Most useful for early stages of cancer or at the beginning of a chemotherapy course.

Caution: Use with caution if fever is present, and discontinue if preexisting fevers worsen.

Ten-Significant Tonic Decoction (All-Inclusive Great Tonifying Decoction)

In clinical tests, has been found to prolong survival time. Minimizes side effects. Prevents kidney damage, stimulates production of both red and white blood cells, and reduces the severity of anorexia, nausea, and weight loss.[8] Also prevents the spread of colon cancer to the liver.[9] Is a rich source of the plant chemical daidzein, which stops the growth of leukemia[10] and melanoma.[11]

DOXORUBICIN HYDROCHLORIDE (ADRIAMYCIN)

This drug is used to treat the following cancers: Hodgkin's disease, acute leukemia, and cancers of bone, breast, cervix, endometrium, lung, ovary, and prostate. Doxorubicin tears apart strands of DNA in cells that are preparing to multiply. It affects both cancer cells and healthy cells that frequently reproduce, such as the bone cells that create blood cells. Possible side effects include nausea and vomiting, toxic effects on the heart, infertility, low white blood cell counts, and colon damage.

INDIVIDUAL KAMPO TREATMENTS

See Chapter 3 for discussions of individual herbs, traditional healing substances, and modern herbal preparations, including directions for making tea.

SUGGESTED DOSAGES	COMMENTS
Rhubarb Root (Herb)	
Non-Kampo Essiac or Hoxie tea, as directed on label.	In animal studies, prevents liver damage during treatment.[1] Essiac and Hoxie teas are North American rhubarb formulations recommended because they are readily available and easy to use.
Schisandra (Herb)	
Freeze-dried herb, 100 mg 3 times daily. Available as Hoelen & Schisandra. or Tea, 1 c 3 times daily.	Protects heart muscle,[2,3] but does not interfere with doxorubicin's action on cancer cells.[4]

KAMPO FORMULAS

See Chapter 4 for dosage information and discussions of individual formulas.

Six-Ingredient Pill with Rehmannia (Rehmannia-Six Combination)

In animal studies, shown to protect bone marrow, heart, kidney, and liver function during treatment.[5]

Caution: Avoid if an estrogen-sensitive disorder is present, such as bladder cancer, melanoma, or disorders of the female reproductive system.

Tonify the Middle and Augment the Qi Decoction

Used in Japan to prevent male infertility caused by treatment. Preserves sperm-producing cells in the testes.[6]

5-FLUOROURACIL (5-FU)

This drug is used to treat the following forms of cancer: bladder, breast, colorectal, endometrium, ovary, and stomach. It is also used to treat psoriasis. This drug keeps cancer cells from dividing by making it impossible for their DNA, which is a spiral-shaped double helix, to unwind before cell reproduction. Possible side effects of the topical cream include pain, itching, rash, and ulceration. Possible side effects of the injectable drug include loss of appetite, nausea and vomiting, diarrhea, and low white blood cell counts.

INDIVIDUAL KAMPO TREATMENTS

See Chapter 3 for discussions of individual herbs, traditional healing substances, and modern herbal preparations, including directions for making tea.

SUGGESTED DOSAGES	COMMENTS
Coptis (Herb)	
Compress (see Chapter 3 for directions).	Increases the skin's permeability to topical 5-FU.
Lentinan (Modern Herbal Preparation)	
Intramuscular injection (usual form), less than 10 mg, exact dosage based on patient's condition and circumstances. Given under professional supervision. or Powder, dosage to be determined by provider. Much greater dosages required than in injectible form.	Prevents immune-system damage when given *before* chemotherapy.[1] Prolongs life, induces regression of tumors or lesions, improves immune function, restores appetite, and reduces pain.

MITOMYCIN (MITOCYCIN-C)

This drug is used to treat the following kinds of cancer: bladder, breast, cervix, colorectal, and stomach. It cross-links strands of DNA so that they cannot open. This keeps cancer cells from making copies of themselves, and makes them much more susceptible to radiation treatment. Mitomycin works best in tissues that are oxygen-deprived, such as tumors that have not yet developed their own blood supply. Possible side effects include fever, hair loss, loss of appetite, nausea and vomiting, lung and kidney damage, and suppression of white and red blood cell production.

INDIVIDUAL KAMPO TREATMENTS

See Chapter 3 for discussions of individual herbs, traditional healing substances, and modern herbal preparations, including directions for making tea.

SUGGESTED DOSAGES	COMMENTS
Lentinan (Modern Herbal Preparation)	
Intramuscular injection (usual form), less than 10 mg, exact dosage based on patient's condition and circumstances. Given under professional supervision. or Powder, dosage to be determined by provider. Much greater dosages required than in injectible form.	Prevents immune-system damage when given *before* chemotherapy.[1] Prolongs life, induces regression of tumors or lesions, improves immune function, restores appetite, and reduces pain.
Maitake (Modern Herbal Preparation)	
Fresh or dried maitake in food, ½–1 oz (15–30 g) daily. or Maitake D-fraction, 4 500-mg capsules 3 times daily before meals.	Maitake-D has shown positive results in breast and colorectal cancer patients.[2] When given with mitomycin, inhibits the growth of breast cancer cells, even after the tumors are well-formed, and prevents cells from spreading to the liver.[3,4]

STEROID DRUGS

This family of drugs includes cortisone, dexamethasone, hydrocortisone, methylprednisone, prednisone, and prednisolone. These drugs control inflammation caused by various forms of cancer as well as that caused by a number of other disorders, including allergy, asthma, arthritis, eczema, eye inflammation, psoriasis, and kidney disease. They boost cell metabolism by making cells more receptive to hormones such as adrenalin and cortisol. Possible side effects include weight gain, high blood pressure, acne, osteoporosis, growth of facial hair in women, cataracts, glaucoma, menstrual irregularity, irritability, insomnia, increased vulnerability to infection, and psychosis.

INDIVIDUAL KAMPO TREATMENTS

See Chapter 3 for discussions of individual herbs, traditional healing substances, and modern herbal preparations, including directions for making tea.

SUGGESTED DOSAGES	COMMENTS
Licorice (Herb)	
Glycyrrhizin extract, 200–800 mg daily, depending on severity of symptoms for up to 6 weeks. Resume after a 2-week break. or Tea, 1 c 1–5 times daily for up to 6 weeks. Resume after a 2-week break.	Contains compounds that increase the half-life of cortisol.[1] Avoid deglycyrrhizinated licorice (DGL).

KAMPO FORMULAS

See Chapter 4 for dosage information and discussions of individual formulas.

Ginseng Decoction to Nourish the Nutritive Qi

Increases the effectiveness of prednisolone.

CHRONIC FATIGUE SYNDROME

Chronic fatigue syndrome (CFS) is a state of overwhelming fatigue accompanied by a wide variety of physical and psychological complaints. More than 1 million Americans have CFS, about two-thirds of them young, middle-class women.

The primary symptom is an overwhelming tiredness that does not go away, even with bed rest. There are a number of secondary symptoms that may or may not affect any given patient. These include confusion, depression, difficulty in thinking, excessive irritability, fever and chills, headache, inability to concentrate, pain that seems to move from joint to joint, lymph node pain, muscle weakness, and disturbed sleep. Many CFS patients also have yeast infections, which can themselves produce a variety of symptoms.

The fact that CFS symptoms mimic those of other conditions, such as depression, makes diagnosis difficult, as does the lack of a definitive test for CFS. Diagnosis is based on the elimination of other disorders, and on the length and severity of the fatigue.

Virtually all cases of CFS arise suddenly in active people. It usually starts as a flulike illness the person vividly remembers as the onset of the disease. CFS has been connected to infection with human herpesvirus-6,[1] as well as to cytomegalovirus and Epstein-Barr virus (EBV).[2] It is likely that CFS results from a combination of factors, including viral infection, poor nutrition, exposure to toxins, and long-term stress.

The causes and mechanisms of CFS are still being debated by doctors, and different explanations have emerged. Many doctors see CFS as a disorder in which the brain and the immune system are uncoordinated. Neurologist Jay Lombard and nutritionist Carl Germano describe it as a condition in which "the brain's master conductor misses a beat."[3] According to this explanation, CFS seems to be caused, in large part, by a failure of the brain to stimulate production of cortisol, the hormone that allows the body to handle stress. The lack of cortisol leads to blood-pressure problems. More than 95 percent of CFS patients have a condition in which blood pressure is not properly regulated, which causes pressure to drop. This drop in pressure causes the blood vessels serving the brain to dilate,[4] which aggravates the problem. The end result is that the brain does not get enough blood.[5]

The mechanism behind the blood-pressure drop is a mineral imbalance. The hormonal deficiency causes sodium to leave the body through the urine. Less sodium means less fluid in the blood, so blood volume and pressure fall. Increasing cortisol levels in the bloodstream forces the kidneys to retain more sodium, which leads to an increase in blood pressure.[6]

Another common characteristic of CFS patients is an imbalance of immune-system components called T cells.[7] In CFS, T cells are activated to fight a disease but are unable to "lock on" to their targets. Chinese and Japanese researchers think this imbalance is related to a lack of available zinc compounds. Zinc is necessary for a healthy immune response.

The Kampo view of CFS is that while fatigue is the common denominator of every case of CFS, effective treatment requires distinctions based on the accompanying symptoms. Different individuals will need different treatments to overcome CFS. This view is reflected in the large number of formulas applied to treating the disease. The advantage of Kampo is that formulas can be chosen to meet the combination of symptoms most nearly like those experienced by the individual. Although the exact ways in which Kampo formulas affect CFS are not known, it is likely that they increase the efficiency of the body's hormonal responses to stress. Individual herbs provide a variety of health benefits.

INDIVIDUAL KAMPO TREATMENTS

See Chapter 3 for discussions of individual herbs, traditional healing substances, and modern herbal preparations, including directions for making tea.

SUGGESTED DOSAGES	COMMENTS
Bitter Melon (Herb)	
Juice, 1–2 oz (30–60 ml) 3 times daily. Take with up to 1 tsp of natural sweetener. or Whole fruit, ½–2 fruits (9–15 g) in cooking daily.	More effective than acyclovir in killing the herpesvirus. *Caution:* Bitter melon should be avoided by persons who have cirrhosis or have had hepatitis, or are HIV-positive and have had liver infections. Otherwise, use for 4 weeks, then discontinue for 4 weeks.
Cloves (Herb)	
Oil, 10–15 drops in ¼ c (60 ml) warm water, 3 times daily.	Increases the effectiveness of acyclovir, a prescription drug used to treat CFS.[8]
Dan Shen (Herb)	
Tea, 1 c 3 times daily.	Contains compounds that bind with copper, which increases the body's ability to use zinc. Sedates the nerves that carry pain messages to the brain. Contains a compound, tanshinone IIA,[9] that increases the heart's output, thus increasing the brain's oxygen supply. Do *not* use tincture. *Caution:* Avoid if an estrogen-sensitive disorder is present, such as bladder cancer, melanoma, or disorders of the female reproductive system.
Ginseng (Herb)	
Fluid extract or tincture, as directed on label. or Tea, made with Korean or red ginseng, 1 c daily.	Controls emotional disturbances symptomatic of CFS.[10] If using ginseng extracts or tinctures (which are not as therapeutically active as teas), be sure the product contains *Panax ginseng.* Note that strength may vary by manufacturer.
Lentinan (Modern Herbal Preparation)	
Intramuscular injection (usual form), less than 10 mg, exact dosage based on patient's condition and circumstances. Given under professional supervision. or Powder, dosage to be determined by provider. Much greater dosages required than in injectable form.	Is used in Japan to treat low natural killer cell syndrome (LNKS), which appears to be identical to the Western diagnosis of CFS. Has reversed remittent fever and persistent fatigue. Activates and stimulates production of various immune-system components, particularly helper T cells.[11]
Licorice (Herb)	
Glycyrrhizin extract, 200–800 mg daily, depending on severity of symptoms, for up to 6 weeks. Resume after a 2-week break. or Tea, 1 c 1–5 times daily for up to 6 weeks. Resume after a 2-week break.	Contains glycyrrhizinic acid, which blocks the activity of an enzyme that otherwise would destroy cortisol. Avoid deglycyrrhizinated licorice (DGL). *Caution:* Avoid if high blood pressure is present. Also avoid if an estrogen-sensitive disorder is present, such as bladder cancer, melanoma, or disorders of the female reproductive system.
Maitake (Modern Herbal Preparation)	
Fresh or dried maitake in food, 1–2 tbsp (3–7 g) daily. or Maitake D-fraction in capsule or tablet form, 500 mg 3 times daily. This form will provide the quickest response. or Tea, 1 c 2–4 times daily.	Extracts stimulate the immune system in CFS.[12] Other forms are likely to have the same effect.
Scutellaria (Herb)	
Dried herb, 1–2 1,000-mg capsules 3 times daily. or Fluid extract (1:1), ¼–½ tsp (1–2 ml) 3 times daily. or Powdered solid extract (4:1), 250–500 mg 3 times daily. or Tea, 1 c 3 times daily. or Tincture (1:5), 1–1½ tsp (4–6 ml) 3 times daily. Place in a cup, add 2 tbsp water, and take in a single sip.	Has a high zinc content.[13] Acts against a wide range of bacterial and viral infections without involving the immune system. *Caution:* Avoid in cases of diarrhea caused by foodborne infection or excessive consumption of cold drinks.

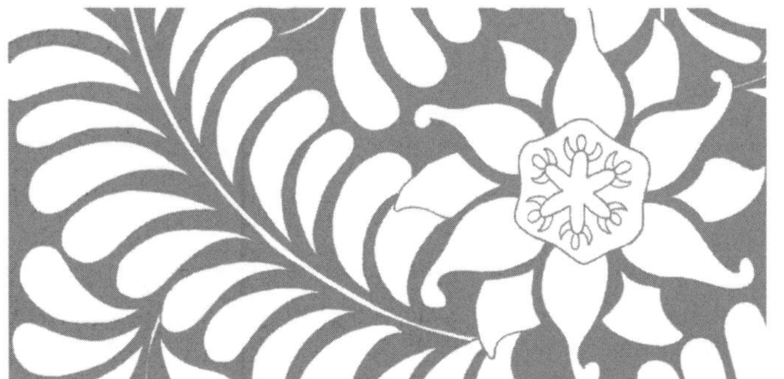

KAMPO FORMULAS

See Chapter 4 for dosage information and discussions of individual formulas.

Calm the Stomach Powder

Relieves a tendency toward easy fatigue with a sense of fullness throughout the digestive tract, loss of taste, heavy sensation in the arms and legs, loose stools or diarrhea, nausea and vomiting, belching, and/or acid regurgitation.

Ginseng Decoction to Nourish the Nutritive Qi

Treats chronic fatigue with weakness of the hands and feet. In the traditional symptom pattern for the formula, there may be pallid or sallow complexion, palpitations with anxiety that may be continuous, reduced appetite, shortness of breath, laconic speech, easy fatigue in the extremities, light-headedness, vertigo, and/or weak pulse. Also used for sores that do not heal.

Honey-Fried Licorice Decoction

Relieves chronic fatigue with "dry" symptoms, that is, dry skin and fever without perspiration. Lubricates the intestines to relieve constipation and sluggish digestion. Traditionally, taken with half a shot glass (at least 10 ml) of sake or clear wine.

Caution: Most manufacturers include the traditional marijuana seed. Will not produce a "high," but will cause a positive urine test for THC, although sophisticated testing methods can distinguish medicinal from illicit use.

Oyster Shell Powder

Treats chronic fatigue with excessive sweating that is worse at night. The patient may be easily startled and suffer palpitations.

Ten-Significant Tonic Decoction (All-Inclusive Great Tonifying Decoction)

Stimulates production of interleukins and natural killer (NK) cells.[14] General immune stimulant traditionally given to persons with abdominal tension, hot flashes in the hands and feet, and lethargy. Traditional Kampo considers it also appropriate when there is anemia or immune disturbances that cause sores which do not heal, conditions frequently confused with CFS.

True Man's Decoction to Nourish the Organs

Treats extreme fatigue after diarrhea. Accompanying symptoms include mild, persistent abdominal pain that responds favorably to local pressure or warmth; lethargy; pale complexion; reduced appetite; soreness of the lower back; and lack of strength in the legs. Not available as a patent medicine, but widely available from TCM practitioners as *zhen ren yang rang tang.*

Caution: Avoid alcohol, wheat, cold or raw foods, fish, and greasy foods. Should not be used by persons with gallbladder problems, obstruction of the bile duct, or a tendency to retain urine, or by pregnant women.

White Tiger Decoction

Strengthens acyclovir's ability to stop a strain of the herpesvirus from replicating.

Caution: Avoid if nausea or vomiting is present.

Yellow Dragon Decoction

Treats extreme fatigue that occurs after diarrhea. Unlike True Man's Decoction to Nourish the Organs, this formula is used when abdominal pain is increased by pressure.

CONSIDERATIONS

❑ A study at the Harvard School of Public Health found that high doses of minerals, vitamins, and antioxidants seldom help CFS.[15] Some scientists go so far as to theorize that CFS may be caused by an excess of free-radical scavengers that compete with superoxide dismutase, the body's own weapon against free radicals.[16] On the other hand, moderate doses of cysteine supplements increase the activity and effectiveness of NK cells.[17] For this reason, it is important to avoid excessive use of antioxidant supplements, but to eat enough protein, especially the amino acid cysteine.

❑ Ginseng may be taken with the non-Kampo herb echinacea to increase the activity of NK cells in CFS.[18] The key is using the right varieties of echinacea and ginseng in the right forms. Take *Echinacea purpurea* as an alcohol tincture, not as a tea. Follow label directions for dosage. Take *Panax ginseng,* also known as Korean or red ginseng, as a tea, not a tincture. Take 1 cup of ginseng tea 2 or 3 times a day.

❑ *See also* **Depression, Herpes,** and **Yeast Infection.**

CIRRHOSIS, ALCOHOLIC

Cirrhosis of the liver is a condition in which the organ's outer layers develop nodules and fibrous scar tissue in response to repeated toxic damage. These nodules and fibers disrupt the blood supply to remaining healthy tissues in the liver. Eventually, cirrhosis leads to a loss of the liver's normal function.

Early cirrhosis may produce no symptoms. It may be discovered during a routine physical or a blood test given for some other reason. Symptoms that may appear as the disease progresses include weight loss, nausea and vomiting, jaundice, weakness, stomach pain, and varicose veins. Some people develop ascites, or abdominal swelling caused by fluid accumulation. If untreated, cirrhosis can lead to a decline in brain function caused by toxins that would normally be disposed of by the liver. It could also cause kidney failure or hepatic coma, and cirrhosis often leads to liver cancer.

While cirrhosis can be caused by several factors, the most common cause in North America is long-term overconsumption of alcohol. The amount and duration of alcohol abuse, rather than the type of alcoholic beverage consumed or the pattern of drinking (binge versus nonbinge) determines the onset of cirrhosis. Women are more susceptible to this disease than men, probably because of differences in body weight and size.

Alcohol causes cirrhosis by activating a liver enzyme called p450. That leads to increased damage from free radicals, toxic substances that can attack liver cells. This enzyme prevents liver tissue from efficiently using oxygen and increases the production of collagen, a substance that becomes fibrous scar tissue.[1] It also increases the rate at which the liver converts alcohol into acetaldehyde, a chemical that damages proteins.[2]

Conventional treatment is more supportive than curative. The idea is to reduce the liver's workload as much as possible so that this resilient organ can repair itself, as long as too much tissue has not been destroyed. Standard treatment also addresses the symptoms and complications seen in cirrhosis. The secret to successful treatment of cirrhosis, though, is activating protective factors in the liver without activating enzyme p450. Kampo herbs can accomplish this goal, and can be used with conventional treatments.

For more than 1,500 years, Kampo has described a symptom pattern corresponding to cirrhosis as "static blood of the liver." When blood cannot leave the liver, it cannot energize the gallbladder, which in turn cannot secrete bile and help the intestines digest food. For more than 600 years, Kampo has recognized another symptom pattern in which the stomach is "cold," and thus fails to energize the circulation of water and nutrients through the body. This causes ascites and loss of appetite. Although Kampo can help treat and even reverse alcoholic cirrhosis, it is important to stop alcohol consumption when undergoing treatment for this disease. Be aware that some herbs may have a negative impact on the liver and/or interact negatively with conventional medicines. Always work with a qualified health care practitioner.

INDIVIDUAL KAMPO TREATMENTS

See Chapter 3 for discussions of individual herbs, traditional healing substances, and modern herbal preparations, including directions for making tea.

SUGGESTED DOSAGES	COMMENTS
Green Tea (Herb)	
Catechin extract, 1 240-mg tablet 3 times daily. or Tea, 1 c 2–5 times daily.	Contains catechins, which deactivate free radicals.[3] Catechins also treat a wide variety of liver conditions that can cause or aggravate cirrhosis, including several forms of hepatitis.[4,5] To avoid dilution problems, do not take tea within 1 hour of taking other teas or patent medicines.
Soy Lecithin (Modern Herbal Preparation)	
Soy phospholipids, 1,500–3,000 mg daily. Identified individually on the label as 3-sn-phospatidylcholine, phosphatidylethanolamine, and phospatidylinositic acid, or as "total phospholipids."	Protects the liver from damage by alcohol and many toxic chemicals. Defends against fatty deposits and buildup of fibrous tissue. Works by stopping free-radical activity and healing cell membranes. *Caution:* Mild diarrhea may occur when soy lecithin is first used.
Turmeric (Herb)	
Curcumin, the yellow pigment found in turmeric, 250–500 mg twice daily between meals.	Curcumin keeps alcohol and other toxins from being converted to a harmful form within the liver, and increases the detoxification rate for any alcohol that is converted.[6]

CONSIDERATIONS

❑ Make sure to visit the doctor for regular blood tests. These will show if the liver is healing.

❑ Eating properly is an important part of cirrhosis treatment. A balanced, low-fat diet will provide the needed nutritional support while reducing stress on the liver. This diet should include grapefruit juice, which contains a substance that can decrease enzyme p450 activity by 30 percent.[7,8] Red chili peppers also contain an enzyme-blocking compound.

❑ The non-Kampo herb milk thistle contains compounds that stop inflammatory processes in the liver,[9] especially in people with cirrhosis who also have diabetes.[10]

❑ *See also* **Alcoholism, Hepatitis,** and **Liver Cancer.** To learn how to use schisandra for protection against liver cancer, see "Schisandra—Kampo's Supreme Liver Herb" on page 251.

COLDS

The common cold is a viral infection characterized by familiar symptoms: dry, sore throat and watery eyes accompanied by nasal discomfort with watery discharge and sneezing. As the cold progresses, the discharge becomes thicker. Throughout the course of a cold, the membranes lining the nasal passages are swollen, and there may be swollen lymph nodes in the neck. Headache, low-grade fever, and muscle aches may also be present.

Colds can be caused by a wide variety of rhinoviruses

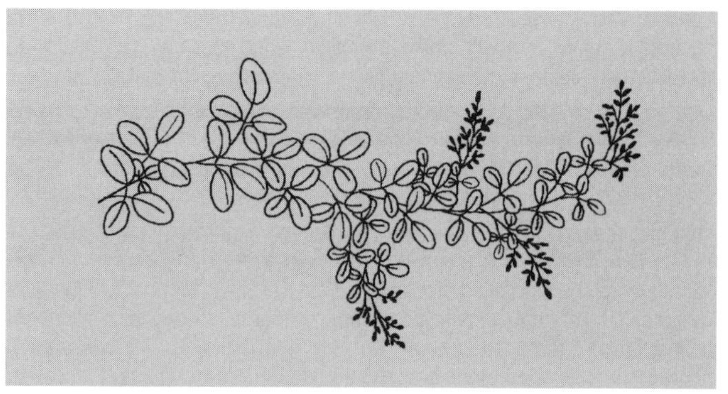

that are capable of infecting the upper respiratory tract. Once a person has been infected with a particular strain of rhinovirus, he or she usually develops an immune defense to it. There are enough strains of rhinovirus, however, that the average adult is exposed to one or two new strains every year. Young children, with their developing, uncoordinated immune systems, can have as many as seven colds a year. Exposure to new strains, combined with a general lack of immune resistance, sets the stage for a cold.

The cure for the common cold continues to evade the best efforts of modern medical science. That is because the rhinovirus is extraordinarily well-adapted to its human host. Rhinoviruses plant themselves on the adhesion molecules that keep human immune-system cells in place on the lining of the respiratory tract. When the virus is attacked by cells called lymphocytes, the body creates more lymphocytes that have to be held in place by more adhesion molecules. This gives more cold viruses places to grow. Eventually, the body defeats the virus by sloughing off the entire virus-lymphocyte mix into the nasal discharge we associate with colds.

Kampo's answer to the question, "Why can't they cure the common cold?" is that what we call the symptoms of a cold are actually its cure. For almost 2,000 years, Kampo has used this condition as the best example of what Kampo calls diseases of the Greater Yang (see Chapter 1). The body's defensive energy in the Greater Yang stage matches the force of the invading pernicious influence, or pathogen. During this time the person is able to resist the pathogen's attack. The body stops the invading disease at its "borders," its skin, muscles, and joints. The fight between the body's defensive energy and the pathogen heats the surface of the body, which causes fever. If the body is strong enough, the invading pathogen is routed and "sweated out." In this process, the pores are opened and heat is allowed to escape, causing chills. The slight fever, the nasal discharge and tearing eyes all work together to expel the invading pathogen from the body and bring the body back into balance.

Kampo treatments for colds accelerate this process. Herbs act against specific infections that can accompany colds, and the aggravation of asthma by colds. Formulas address combinations of symptoms that an individual may experience. If it seems likely that exposure to a secondary infection has occurred, choose from among the herbs. If there are remaining symptoms of a cold that will not go away, choose from among the formulas.

INDIVIDUAL KAMPO TREATMENTS

See Chapter 3 for discussions of individual herbs, traditional healing substances, and modern herbal preparations, including directions for making tea.

SUGGESTED DOSAGES	COMMENTS
Cloves (Herb)	
Oil, 10–15 drops in ¼ c (60 ml) warm water used as mouthwash 2–3 times daily. Or inhale the vapors of 3–4 drops in ½ c hot water.	Oil is 60–95% eugenol, which is thought to give the oil its painkilling properties.[1] Opens nasal passages and prevents secondary infections, although it has no direct effect on rhinoviruses. *Caution:* Do not apply undiluted oil of cloves directly to the nose or throat.
Coltsfoot (Herb)	
Tea, 1 c no more than twice daily.	Relieves acute congestion and dry cough. *Caution:* Avoid coltsfoot tinctures, which have a greater toxic potential and less mucilage than teas.
Fritillaria, Cirrhosa (Herb)	
Fritillaria and Pinellia Syrup, 2–3 tsp (8–12 ml) 3 times daily.	Useful for sticky phlegm, snoring, or chronic sore throat. Available as *Qing Chi Hua Tan Tang.* *Caution:* Avoid if weakness from a chronic health problem is present.
Garlic (Herb)	
Tablets (including deodorized) as directed on label, at least 900 mg daily. Recommended over fresh garlic for this disorder.	Especially useful for treating colds contracted at high altitude.[2] Activates "germ-eating" macrophages.[3] This does not directly affect the rhinovirus, but inhibits other viruses that may also cause upper respiratory infection. *Caution:* Do not use with the blood-thinner warfarin sodium (Coumadin). Garlic will counteract the effects of *Bifidus* and *Lactobacillus* cultures taken as digestive aids.
Lentinan (Modern Herbal Preparation)	
Powder, dosage to be determined by provider. Much greater dosages required than in injectable form.	Stimulates production of interferon, an immune-system chemical, which keeps the rhinovirus from creating proteins. Activates and stimulates production of various other immune-system components, particularly helper T cells.[4] This can counteract bacterial infections that can take hold after serious colds. Lentinan is the "heavy artillery" of herbal cold medication. Use only for colds that persist for weeks and resist all other treatment.

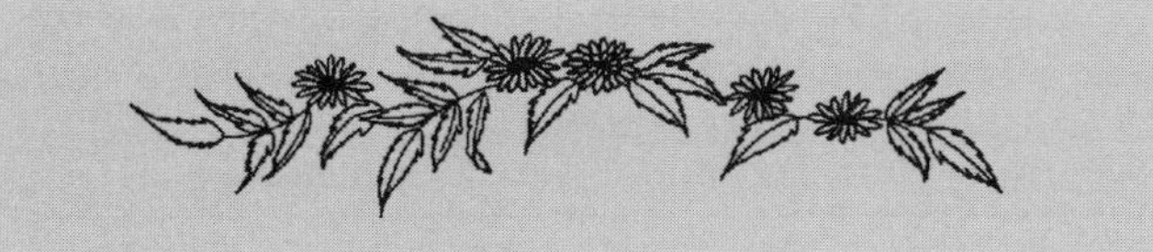

SUGGESTED DOSAGES	COMMENTS
Maitake (Modern Herbal Preparation)	
Fresh or dried maitake in food, 1–2 tbsp (3–7 g) daily. or Maitake D-fraction in capsule or tablet form, 500 mg 3 times daily before meals. or Tea, 1 c 2–4 times daily.	Contains a carbohydrate-based substance known to kill viruses. Effective for treating persistent colds.
Reishi (Modern Herbal Preparation)	
Dried extract, 3 1-g tablets 3 times daily. or Dried mushroom in food, approx. ¼–approx. ½ oz (5–10 g) daily. or Syrup, as directed on label. or Tea, 1 c 3 times daily. or Tincture (1:5), 1 tsp (4 ml) 3 times daily. Place in a cup, add 2 tbsp water, and take in a single sip.	Keeps colds from aggravating asthma. Contains antihistamines,[5] as well as compounds that stop platelet activating factor, a hormone that causes the bronchial passages to constrict.[6]
Scutellaria (Herb)	
Dried herb, 1–2 1,000-mg capsules 3 times daily. or Fluid extract (1:1), ¼–½ tsp (1–2 ml) 3 times daily. or Powdered solid extract (4:1), 250–500 mg 3 times daily. or Tea, 1 c 3 times daily. or Tincture (1:5), 1–1½ tsp (4–6 ml) 3 times daily. Place in a cup, add 2 tbsp water, and take in a single sip.	Keeps colds from progressing to secondary infection with influenza.[7] *Caution:* Avoid in cases of diarrhea caused by foodborne infection or excessive consumption of cold drinks.
Siberian Ginseng (Modern Herbal Preparation)	
Tea, 1 c 3 times daily. Recommended form for this disorder.	Prevents colds after exposure to allergens, cold drafts, and environmental stress. Probably stimulates interferon production. *Caution:* Should be avoided by persons with myasthenia gravis; rheumatoid arthritis and diseases related to it, such as lupus, psoriatric arthritis, and Sjögren's syndrome; or prostate cancer.
Viola (Herb)	
Tea, 1 c 3 times daily. Especially suitable for children (see inset on page 142).	Keeps rhinovirus from leaving infected cells.

KAMPO FORMULAS

See Chapter 4 for dosage information and discussions of individual formulas.

Bupleurum and Cinnamon Twig Decoction

Relieves muscle and joint pain caused by cold and flu.

Caution: Use with caution if fever is present, and discontinue if preexisting fevers worsen.

Cinnamon and Peony Decoction

Treats colds accompanied by conditions that have caused chest congestion. Also relieves headache, stomach pain, and fever and chills.

Cinnamon Twig and Poria Pill

Treats what traditional Japanese doctors call "blood effusive chills." This condition is marked by a symptom pattern that includes "flushing up," that is, feeling of blood rushing to the head, red face, and cough with copious phlegm. Symptoms occur in persons in generally good health.

Cinnamon Twig Decoction

Stops nasal congestion that may be accompanied by headache, stomach pain, or fever and chills. A variation on this formula, Cinnamon Twig and Ginseng Decoction, can prevent allergy symptoms as well as cold symptoms.

Ephedra Decoction

Used by Chinese and Japanese physicians to relieve colds in infants with acute nasal congestion. Seek the advice of the dispensing herbalist on a suitable child's dosage. A variation, Ephedra, Apricot Kernel, Coix, and Licorice Decoction, is designed to lower fever, in addition to treating other symptoms. Use either formula in patent-medicine form.

Kudzu Decoction

Especially relieves nasal congestion accompanied by stiffness or pain in the neck or back.

Minor Bluegreen Dragon Decoction

Treats colds in infants and young children with coughs, phlegm, and profuse, watery nasal discharge. Seek the advice of the dispensing herbalist on a suitable child's dosage.

Caution: Use with caution if fever is present, and discontinue if preexisting fevers worsen.

Tang-Kuei and Peony Powder

Treats summer colds causing nasal congestion and chills throughout the body. Also appropriate for "air conditioning stress," or nasal congestion caused by too many changes from natural to air-conditioned environments in the summer.

Warm the Menses Decoction

Despite its name, this formula is useful to both men and women for relief of colds. Relieves extreme fatigue caused by colds that will not go away.

Caution: Use with caution if fever is present, and discontinue if preexisting fevers worsen.

CONSIDERATIONS

❑ Especially severe symptoms may indicate presence of the flu; *see* **Influenza.** Symptoms that are persistent or that occur at the same time each year may indicate an allergy; *see* **Allergies, Respiratory.**

COLORECTAL CANCER

Cancer of the colon, or large intestine, and rectum is the most common digestive-tract cancer, striking more than 150,000 people a year in the United States. It generally affects older people, and there is a genetic link in some families. Colorectal tumors can grow quite large without obstructing the bowel. Thus, they often remain undetected until they have spread.

The symptoms of colorectal cancer include changes in bowel habits, vague abdominal pain, acid stomach, muscular tension and twitching in the abdomen, and, most notably, blood in the stool. Sometimes rectal bleeding cannot be seen, but can be detected by a home test kit available in drugstores. Blood in the stool can be caused by several conditions, including diverticulitis, hemorrhoids,

Using Kampo With Other Herbal Treatments for Colorectal and Liver Cancer

Doctors have found that the non-Kampo herbs echinacea and arnica can be used to treat colorectal and liver cancer. German researchers have combined an injectable form of echinacea, better known as a cold and flu fighter, with the drugs cyclophosphamide and thymostimulin to extended life expectancies in patients with advanced colorectal cancer by several months.[1] Similar results were found in the research team's experience with patients who had advanced liver cancer.[2]

Arnica, which is generally used as a wound salve, enhances the immune-stimulant power of echinacea. It also has its own anticancer effects. One of its constituent chemicals, helenalin, killed roughly 30 to 40 percent as many cancer cells as the standard chemotherapy drug cyclophosphamide in preliminary studies.[3] German studies have found that arnica stimulates immune-system cells called macrophages to secrete tumor necrosis factor, which dissolves tumors.[4] In addition, the Kampo herb eupatorium also greatly increases the immunostimulant power of echinacea.[5]

Take ½ ounce of echinacea juice (not tincture) or four 500-milligram capsules of dried echinacea powder four times a day. Be sure to use *Echinacea angustifolia.* Take 3 cups of tea made with *dried* eupatorium (never use it fresh) three times a day (see Chapter 3 for tea-making instructions). To make an arnica infusion, steep 4 teaspoons (2 grams) of the chopped herb in 1 cup (250 milliliters) of water for forty-five minutes. Strain and drink *once* a day. Use arnica for no more than two weeks at a time.

inflamed colon, and ulcers. A doctor should always be consulted in cases of rectal bleeding. Polyps, small, stalklike growths, can also cause bleeding. Polyps should be treated promptly, even if benign, because they can become cancerous as they enlarge. In fact, colorectal cancers often start as polyps.

Colorectal cancer is associated with a high-fat, low-fiber diet. Animal fat reduces the amount of oxygen available to the friendly digestive bacteria that normally live in a healthy colon. Without oxygen, these bacteria produce toxins that can cause colorectal cancer. A lack of fiber compounds this problem, since fiber is needed to increase the rate at which these toxins, along with the rest of the stool, pass out of the body. In societies in which people normally eat a high-fiber diet, colorectal cancer is essentially unknown.

The body does have certain defenses against colorectal cancer. One is gene p53, a "molecular patrolman" that stops defective cells from multiplying. Other genes and protective factors also slow or stop colorectal cancer. Some genes protect cells from the "bystander effect," or genetic damage that occurs when bacteria in the colon turn nitrites from food into harmful substances.

Several different staging systems are used to classify colorectal cancer based on how far the cancer has spread, usually to the liver, lungs, or bones. Surgery is the main treatment. When cancer occurs in the rectum, doctors use surgical techniques designed to preserve normal bowel evacuation whenever possible. The standard chemotherapy drug for colorectal cancer is fluorouracil, although other drugs may be employed. Radiation therapy is also used, as is immunotherapy, in which concentrated amounts of the body's own immune-system chemicals are given.

Modern Japanese doctors avail themselves of all scientific diagnostic tools in testing for colorectal cancer, but also use the simple diagnostic techniques of Kampo to confirm test findings. Colorectal cancer is very often accompanied by discoloration of the lower lip. A pale color in the lip is a hint that the colon is not properly processing fatty foods, and the person is at a high risk for this cancer. A dark red lip indicates a high-fat diet, and a greenish tinge to the lower lip is a sign that colorectal cancer has already developed. As the cancer progresses, the lower lip tends to get smaller, receding into the mouth. The color diagnosis is confirmed by looking at the fleshy part of the hand between the thumb and index finger. If this area also has a greenish tint, colorectal cancer is a distinct possibility.

Modern Kampo physicians describe colorectal cancer in terms of overwhelming the yin of the intestines. Within the colon live yin bacteria that break down complex chemicals in food, sharing them with their human host. There are also yang bacteria that reassemble excreted hormones, recycling them for their human host. When the yin bacteria are overwhelmed by high-energy foods such as fats and sugars, or by emotional stress, the foodstuffs they would break down are left to putrefy and form cancer-causing chemicals. At the same time, the yang bacteria are supercharged to recycle carcinogenic hormones. Kampo treatments can help restore the balance of yin and yang in the colon's bacteria. They have also been shown to work within the context of conventional therapy (see considerations below). In addition, there are two non-Kampo herbs that have proven quite helpful in fighting this disease (see "Other Herbal Treatments for Colorectal Cancer" on page 186).

INDIVIDUAL KAMPO TREATMENTS

See Chapter 3 for discussions of individual herbs, traditional healing substances, and modern herbal preparations, including directions for making tea.

SUGGESTED DOSAGES	COMMENTS
Astragalus (Herb)	
Fluid extract (1:1), 1/4–1/2 tsp (1–2 ml) 3 times daily. or Freeze-dried herb in capsules, 500–1,000 mg 3 times daily. or Powdered solid extract (4:1), 250–500 mg 3 times daily. or Tea, 1 c 3 times daily. or Tincture (1:5), 1–1 1/2 tsp (4–6 ml), 3 times daily. Place in a cup, add 2 tbsp water, and take in a single sip. For dosages used with chemotherapy, *see* **Chemotherapy Side Effects.**	Stops spread of cancers known to respond to gene p53. Contains compounds that stimulate immune-system cells called T cells and that increase the ability of lymphokine-activated killer (LAK) cells to attack cancers.[1] Prevents depletion of white blood cells during chemotherapy.[2] Enhances effectiveness of immunotherapy treatment with a combination of melatonin and interleukin-2 (IL-2), which allows a lower dosage of the toxic IL-2 to be used. *Caution:* Do not use when fever or skin infection is present.
Coptis (Herb)	
Tincture (1:5), 15–30 drops 3 times daily. Place in a cup, add 2 tbsp water, and take in a single sip. Recommended form for this disease.	Contains berberine, which stops the multiplication of cancer cells in colorectal and other cancers.[3,4] *Caution:* Do not use during pregnancy or on a daily basis for more than 2 weeks at a time.
Garlic (Herb)	
Enterically coated tablets, as directed on label (usually at least 900 mg daily).	Garlic has been known for many years to reduce the risk of colorectal and other cancers.[5] Contains compounds that stop the bystander effect.[6] Other compounds prevent the spread of tumors once they have started.[7] Reduces production of toxic free radicals in the liver and lungs that may reach the colon.[8] *Caution:* Do not use with the blood-thinner warfarin sodium (Coumadin). Garlic will counteract the effects of *Bifidus* and *Lactobacillus* cultures taken as digestive aids.

Ginkgo (Modern Herbal Preparation)	
Quercetin extract, 1–2 125-mg capsules 3 times daily between meals. Recommended form for this disorder.	Quercetin stops spread of cancer cells by deactivating enzymes that trigger their growth.[9] Plays a special role in preventing colon cancer, since foods containing quercetin or quercetin extracts are in direct contact with the cells lining the colon.[10] For best results, take quercetin with bromelain, which increases absorption. *Caution:* Do not take quercetin with the prescription drugs Procardia or Seldane.

Green Tea (Herb)	
Catechin extract, 1 240-mg tablet 3 times daily. or Tea, 1 c 2–5 times daily.	Stops the bystander effect. Contains compounds called catechins that prevent the growth of nitrite-converting *Clostridium* bacteria. Catechins also prevent tumor growth in animals[11] and help prevent both thyroid cancer caused by radiation treatment and deficiencies in white blood cells caused by mitomycin.[12] Caffeine increases effectiveness of radiation therapy and accelerates cell death. Other compounds deactivate plasmin, preventing tumor invasion. To avoid dilution problems, do not take tea within 1 hour of taking other teas or patent medicines.

Kelp (Herb)	
Kelp as food, any quantity desired.	May be responsible for low rates of colon cancer in Japan, where it is a dietary staple. Use of kelp increases the rate at which stool passes through the intestines. This lowers the risk that cancer-causing estrogens in the stool can be reabsorbed through the colon wall.[13] *Caution:* Limit consumption to once a week.

Maitake (Modern Herbal Preparation)	
Maitake D-fraction, 4 500-mg capsules 3 times daily before meals. Recommended form for this disorder.	General immune stimulant that increases the activity of various immune-system cells and reduces tumor formation.[14] Tests in the United States with maitake D-fraction have had positive results.[15]

PSK (Modern Herbal Preparation)	
Dried extract, 6 1,000-mg tablets daily.	Extensively researched in Japan and the United States. Found to reduce spread of cancer to the lymph nodes, peritoneum and lungs,[16] and liver.[17] Has increased survival rates when given with mitomycin.[18] In laboratory tests, increases the effectiveness of 5-fluorouracil.[19] Also makes T cells more effective.[20]

Reishi (Modern Herbal Preparation)	
Dried extract, 3 1-g tablets 3 times daily. or Syrup, as directed on label. or Tincture (1:5), 1 tbsp (10 ml) 3 times daily. Place in a cup, add 2 tbsp water, and take in a single sip.	Stimulates the body's production of interleukin-2, which fights colorectal and other cancers.[21,22]

Soy Isoflavones (Modern Herbal Preparation)	
Extract, about 3,000 mg once daily. or Soy germ, 2 tsp (10 g) twice daily, preferably added to cereals or smoothies.	Numerous studies show that populations which eat soy products have lower rates of colorectal and other cancers.[23,24] Concentrated source of daidzein, which is known to inhibit human colon cancer.[25]

Turmeric (Herb)	
Curcumin, the yellow pigment found in turmeric, 250–500 mg twice daily between meals.	Curcumin is extraordinarily useful in fighting colorectal cancer. Activates gene p53 and deactivates two genes needed for this cancer to spread.[26] Helps kill cancer cells in the colon and other organs.[27] Stops the bystander effect and prevents cancer caused by aflatoxin, a poison produced during improper storage of grains and peanuts.[28] Reduces lung damage after exposure to whole-body radiation.[29]

HERBS TO AVOID

Individuals who have colorectal cancer should avoid aloe. For more information regarding this herb, including the belief among some scientists that aloe-based laxatives might cause colorectal cancer, see Chapter 3.

KAMPO FORMULAS

See Chapter 4 for dosage information and discussions of individual formulas.

Minor Bupleurum Decoction
Widely used in Japan to treat colorectal cancer. Laboratory studies have found that it acts by stopping creation of DNA, the cell's genetic code, in colon cancer cells.[30] Traditionally used to relieve bitter taste in the mouth, heartburn, nausea and vomiting, and stop fevers and chills. *Caution:* Do not use if fever or skin infection is present. Taken long term in patent medicine form, can cause headache, dizziness, and bleeding gums. Side effects can be avoided if the formula is taken as a tea.

CONSIDERATIONS

❑ Essential fatty acids are an important dietary factor in colorectal cancer. These substances exist in two classes, omega-3s and omega-6s, and omega-3s are lacking in the modern Western diet. This imbalance leads to the overproduction of arachidonic acid, an omega-6, found in relatively large amounts within aggressive tumors. In addition, omega-3s activate gene p53.[31] Increased omega-3 consumption can not only reduce the risk that cancer will develop and spread, it can also make colorectal cancer more responsive to treatment with cisplatin (Platinol), doxorubicin (Adriamycin), or vincristine (Oncovin). These acids are found in cold-water fish and in oils from borage seed, evening primrose, flaxseed (linseed), and hemp. Aspirin also slows the conversion of arachidonic acid into inflammatory substances called prostaglandins. However, aspirin use can cause stomach bleeding, so a doctor should *always* be consulted before using aspirin therapy during treatment for cancer.

❑ Calcium consumption, either in food or in supplements, reduces the risk of colorectal cancer. Calcium combines with toxins to form insoluble soaps. These soaps are repelled from the lining of the digestive tract, and are eliminated through the stool. Always take calcium supplements with magnesium, to avoid creating an imbalance between the two minerals. Take twice as much magnesium as calcium, measured as "elemental magnesium" and "elemental calcium" on the label.

❑ To reduce side effects and increase effectiveness when using chemotherapy, *see* **Chemotherapy Side Effects**; when using radiation therapy, *see* **Radiation Therapy Side Effects.** To learn about herbal treatments that can prevent a cancer from developing its own blood supply, *see* **Cancer.**

❑ Melanoma, a cancer that originates in the skin, may occur in the rectum; *see* **Melanoma.**

Congestive Heart Failure

Congestive heart failure is a condition in which the heart muscle is unable to pump blood fast enough to supply all the nutrients and oxygen needed by the body. About 400,000 new cases are diagnosed every year in the United States. Symptoms include fatigue and weakness, especially on exertion, and swelling associated with fluid retention. Fluid retention in the lungs can also cause shortness of breath. Since congestive heart failure, arrhythmia, and heart attack are all related, all three conditions are discussed in this entry.

The underlying causes of congestive heart failure may be acute or chronic. Acute failure is brought on by *myocardial infarction,* more commonly known as heart attack. Heart attacks that are "silent," in which no symptoms are produced, can still produce heart failure. Heart attacks generally occur as the result of *coronary artery disease,* in which one or more of the arteries serving the heart become blocked with cholesterol deposits. Acute heart failure can also occur after various infections of the heart muscle, which are collectively known as *cardiomyopathy.*

Chronic congestive heart failure is usually a long-term effect of high blood pressure, heart-valve problems, or previous heart attacks. Diabetes, hyperthyroidism, and extreme obesity can also cause chronic heart failure. Chronic lung disease, such as emphysema, and anemia are contributing factors.

Arrhythmia, a slow, fast, or irregular heartbeat, is another cause of chronic heart failure. Arrhythmia can be mild and nothing to worry about or a life-threatening health crisis. The most serious type of heartbeat irregularity is *ventricular fibrillation,* in which the heart cannot pass blood into the arteries because the beat is rapid, uncontrolled, and ineffective.

Congestive heart failure is marked by heart enlargement and fluid retention. When the heart has to work too hard, it enlarges, just as other muscles enlarge during weight training. This helps the heart at first, but eventually the heart muscle weakens. The heart's pumping action decreases as a result. To aid a weakening heart, the body will retain both sodium and fluid, which increases the amount of blood in circulation. Over time the excess fluid seeps into the surrounding tissues, which causes swelling (edema).

Conventional therapy for congestive heart failure consists of treating any underlying disorders while also treating the heart failure itself. Treatment focuses on lifestyle changes, including smoking cessation and improved nutrition (see "Nutritional Support for Congestive Heart Failure" on page 190), and on the use of various drugs. Diuretics increase urine flow, which relieves edema. Vasodilators, such as the ACE inhibitors, relax the blood vessels, which allows more blood to reach the heart. Beta-blockers stabilize arrhythmias, and lower both blood pressure and the heart's need for oxygen. Other drugs control arrhythmias or increase the power of the heartbeat. Many of the heart treatments used in Kampo work on these same principles.

Approximately 700 years ago, Kampo developed ways to treat both heart attack and congestive failure. The physicians of the time identified these diseases by a pattern of symptoms that included weak breathing, cold extremities, dizziness, pallor, and sweating. They reasoned that the cause of these symptoms was a collapse of the yang, or propulsive, energies in the body. The body then had an excess of yin, or containing, energies, and blood and energy could not circulate where they were needed.

The Kampo solution to this condition was strong stimulation with formulas containing aconite, which "jolted" the heart back into activity. Today, standard medical care is always preferable to herbal care for acute heart attack.

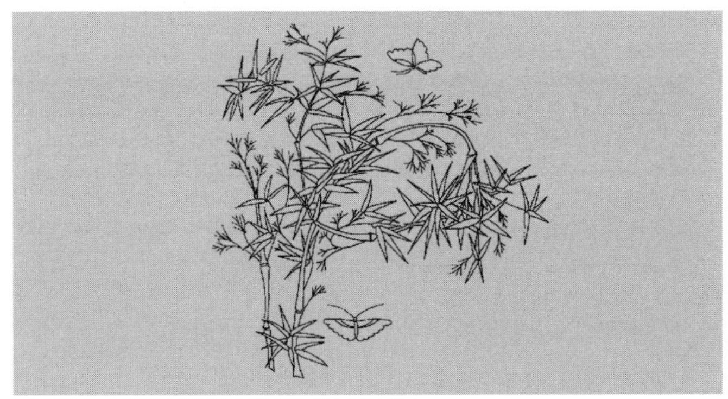

Nutritional Support for Congestive Heart Failure

Nutritional support is an important aspect of congestive heart failure therapy. Not only can the proper supplements help the heart directly, they can also help reduce the side effects of treatment. Prescription medications and their herbal counterparts balance the functions of the heart in terms of their effects on the rest of the body. Nutritional supplements regulate and supply energy to heart muscle at the cellular level.

Furosemide (Lasix), a diuretic widely prescribed for congestive heart failure, can produce muscle spasms, nausea, or vomiting, and increase the severity of ear infections. These side effects can be corrected if patients take the B vitamin thiamin. A daily dosage of 200 milligrams improves functioning of the left ventricle—the chamber that pumps blood throughout the body—in patients with congestive heart disease.[1]

Magnesium is also a potentially useful supplement, but not for every heart patient. Various studies seeking to debunk the use of magnesium supplements have found that taking these supplements does not necessarily cause an increase of magnesium levels in the bloodstream.[2] One study even found that higher blood magnesium levels were associated with a greater risk of death from congestive heart failure.[3] However, this study focused on acutely ill patients over age seventy, and did not determine whether healthier patients got sicker after taking the mineral or sicker patients were taking magnesium in an attempt to get well.

Magnesium supplements are most useful for patients who are taking an ACE inhibitor and/or the heart rhythm stabilizer digitalis (Digoxin). ACE inhibitors, while generally safe, can start hormonal changes that keep heart cells from absorbing magnesium.[4] Digoxin stabilizes heart rhythms but destabilizes magnesium balance. Supplemental magnesium can be used with both drugs.[5] Magnesium supplements also seem to help persons whose heart failure is caused by a heart-valve problem called mitral valve prolapse. Several clinical studies have found that magnesium itself relieves this condition.[6,7] A typical daily dosage is four tablets, each providing 100 milligrams of elemental magnesium.

The two other nutritional supplements widely used to treat congestive heart disease are carnitine and CoQ_{10}. Carnitine is a vitaminlike compound that enables muscle cells to burn fats. It increases the energy available to the heart muscle. Patients with *mild* congestive heart failure who take 500 milligrams of carnitine three times daily have stronger heartbeats and a greater tolerance for physical exertion. The longer the patient uses carnitine, the more dramatic the improvement.[8] Laboratory tests find that carnitine may also be helpful in reversing heart damage that can be caused by the chemotherapy agent doxorubicin hydrochloride (Adriamycin).[9]

CoQ_{10}, also known by its chemical name ubiquinone, improves the heart's energy efficiency. One study tracked 2,664 Italian patients with mild to moderate congestive heart failure. The researchers found that an average dosage of 100 milligrams per day reduced fluid retention, stopped palpitations, and relieved venous congestion in more than 70 percent of the people who took it for three months, and relieved shortness of breath, insomnia, nighttime urination, and vertigo in more than 50 percent of the patients.[10]

After a heart attack occurs, multiple-herb formulas are too potent and could interfere with prescription medication. For continuing care of congestive heart failure, choose, in consultation with the doctor, from among the herbs that reduce fluid retention and those that stimulate the heart. If acute symptoms occur, *immediately* seek professional help.

INDIVIDUAL KAMPO TREATMENTS

See Chapter 3 for discussions of individual herbs, traditional healing substances, and modern herbal preparations, including directions for making tea.

Treatments That Reduce Fluid Retention

SUGGESTED DOSAGES	COMMENTS
Asparagus Root (Herb)	
Tea, 1 cup, 3 times daily between meals.	Stimulates urine production, although both sodium and potassium are eliminated. Is appropriate when diuretics are discontinued. Maintain an adequate potassium supply by taking time-release potassium supplements or by eating fruits and vegetables, especially bananas, oranges, and tomatoes.
Dandelion (Herb)	
Dried extract, up to 3 500-mg tablets daily. or Tea, 1 c 3 times daily on an empty stomach. or Tincture (1:1), 10–15 drops 3 times daily on an empty stomach. Place in a cup, add 2 tbsp water, and take in a single sip.	Relieves fluid retention after excessive salt consumption. Eliminates sodium while sparing potassium, and increased potassium levels reduce muscle spasms and nighttime leg cramps. Also stimulates bile production, which eliminates cholesterol through the stool.

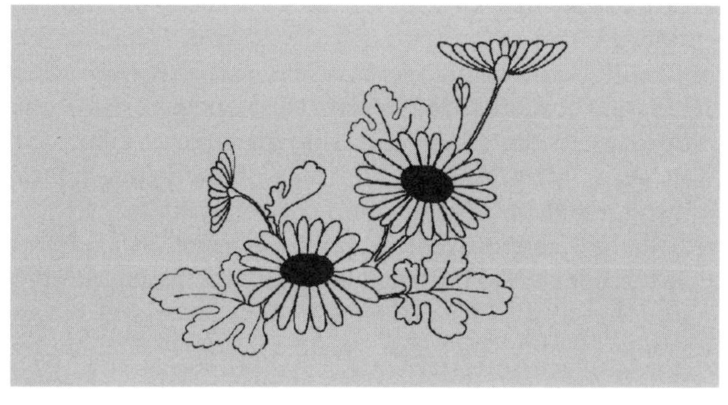

Treatments That Strengthen the Heart

SUGGESTED DOSAGES	COMMENTS
Aconite (Herb)	
Use only under professional supervision.	Carefully regulated doses increase heart output, and relieve shortness of breath and edema.[1] Proper doses stimulate the vagus nerve, which reduces heart rate and dilates the coronary blood vessels. *Caution:* Always use Asian (*Aconitum carmichaeli*), not European (*A. napellus*), aconite. Large doses overstimulate the heart and even cause ventricular fibrillation. Calcium can reverse this effect.
Hawthorn (Herb)	
Dried herb in capsules, 3–5 g daily. or Fluid extract (1:1), ¼–½ tsp (1–2 ml) 3 times daily. or Solid extract, 100–250 mg 3 times daily. Should be standardized to contain 10% proanthocyanidins. or Tea, ⅔ c 3–4 times daily. or Tincture (1:5), 1–1½ tsp (4–6 ml) 3 times daily. Place in a cup, add 2 tbsp water, and take in a single sip.	Best-studied and most effective herbal treatment for this disorder. Dilates the coronary blood vessels by relaxing the smooth muscle surrounding them. Interacts with key enzymes in the heart to change the way in which heart muscle tissue contracts,[2] counteracting the heart muscle's energy-limiting enzyme.[3]
Kudzu (Herb)	
Dried extract, 1 10-mg tablet 3 times daily. or Tea, 1 c 3 times daily.	Improves coronary circulation and lowers the heart's need for oxygen. Contains glycosides, which lower the heart rate and relax the muscles lining the left coronary vessel, and peurarin, a beta-blocker. The most nontoxic herbal treatment for this disorder, and so is most appropriate for very ill patients.
Motherwort (Herb)	
Tea, 1 c 3 times daily.	Strengthens heartbeat but does not increase pulse rate. Instead, it sedates and relaxes the coronary artery for increased circulation to the heart. Recommended for heart irregularities caused by adrenal overstimulation and hyperthyroidism.

HERBS TO AVOID

Individuals who have congestive heart failure should avoid turmeric and curcumin, a compound derived from turmeric. For more information, see Chapter 3.

KAMPO FORMULAS

See Chapter 4 for dosage information and discussions of individual formulas.

Frigid Extremities Decoction

One of Kampo's emergency medicines for acute heart failure. Used only under professional supervision when other treatments are unavailable. May cause a loss of sensation in the mouth and tongue.

Caution: Discontinue the formula if fever occurs.

CONSIDERATIONS

❑ Should circumstances warrant it, consider learning cardiopulmonary resuscitation (CPR).

❑ Lowering sodium intake is one of the best ways to overcome congestive heart failure. Many mild cases of heart failure improve very significantly just by eliminating all salted foods, such as pickles, soy sauce, table salt, and most smoked fish and meats. In more severe cases, there may also be a need to eliminate all commercially prepared breads, canned vegetables and soups, cheese, beets, celery, and spinach.

❑ *See also* **Anemia, Angina, Atherosclerosis, Diabetes, High Blood Pressure, Hyperthyroidism,** and **Obesity.**

CONJUNCTIVITIS

Conjunctivitis, also known as pinkeye, is an inflammation of the membrane that lines the eyelid and wraps around to cover most of the white of the eye. Conjunctivitis may cause the eye to appear swollen and bloodshot, and to feel itchy and irritated. Pus exuding from the inflammation site can cause "sticky eyes" after the eyes are closed for an extended period, such as during sleep.

Most cases of conjunctivitis are caused by viruses, although in rare instances a bacterial infection may be responsible. Bacterial conjunctivitis usually causes a heavier, stickier discharge. Allergies can also cause conjunctivitis.

Conventional treatment for infectious conjunctivitis consists of warm compresses and, if bacterial infection is present, antibiotics. For allergic conjunctivitis, cold compresses and antihistamines are used.

Kampo sees conjunctivitis as a condition in which a pathogen is trying to escape the body through the eyes. The body's reaction to the pathogen can be too strong, or yang, which traps the pathogen inside, or too weak, or yin, which is insufficient to push the pathogen out. Conjunctivitis with yang excess, often producing fever, is treated with profoundly cooling combinations of herbs. Yin or deficient-conformation patients with conjunctivitis, who have chills but not fever, are given warming combinations.

INDIVIDUAL KAMPO TREATMENTS

See Chapter 3 for discussions of individual herbs, traditional healing substances, and modern herbal preparations, including directions for making tea.

SUGGESTED DOSAGES	COMMENTS
Coptis (Herb)	
Tincture (1:5), 1–1½ tsp (4–6 ml) daily. Place in a cup, add 2 tbsp water, and take in a single sip. A clean cloth can also be soaked in the diluted tincture and placed lightly over the eyes. or Use **Coptis Decoction to Relieve Toxicity** (see formulas list).	Fights bacterial conjunctivitis. *Caution:* Do not use during pregnancy or on a daily basis for more than 2 weeks at a time. Do not use with supplements that contain vitamin B_6 or the amino acid histidine.

KAMPO FORMULAS

See Chapter 4 for dosage information and discussions of individual formulas.

Coptis Decoction to Relieve Toxicity

Especially appropriate for treating infectious conjunctivitis accompanied by "hot" symptoms, including bleeding gums, fever, facial flushing caused by embarrassment or emotional tension, headaches, nervousness, or sinusitis. Used when there is fever with sweating, and the discharge from the eye is thin.

Caution: Should not be used by women who are trying to become pregnant.

Gentiana Longdancao Decoction to Drain the Liver

Treats inflamed eyes when there is also ear infection. In China, is also used to treat corneal ulcers.

Caution: Should not be used by women who are trying to become pregnant.

Minor Bluegreen Dragon Decoction

Used when there is fever without sweating, and the discharge from the eye is thin.

Caution: Use with caution if fever is present, and discontinue if preexisting fevers worsen.

Ophiopogonis Decoction

Used to treat conjunctivitis when there is no fever, and the discharge from the eye is thin. Also stops sneezing.

Caution: Use with caution if fever is present, and discontinue if preexisting fevers worsen.

Tang-Kuei, Gentiana Longdancao, and Aloe Pill

Relieves severe "toxicity," or systemic illness, caused by eye infections. Especially appropriate when additional symptoms include a bitter taste in the mouth, dizziness, headache, irritability, and short temper. In women, symptoms may include a shortened menstrual period in which the menstrual blood is reddish-purple.

Caution: Should not be used by women who are trying to become pregnant.

CONSIDERATIONS

❑ *See also* **Allergies, Respiratory.**

CONSTIPATION

Constipation is the infrequent and difficult passage of stools. Although the frequency of elimination varies from individual to individual, constipation is medically defined as fewer than three bowel movements per week. Stomachache may also be present. Constipation is caused by the inability of the cells lining the intestinal walls to balance absorption and secretion of water and minerals.

There are several types of constipation. *Acute constipation* involves short-term bloating, discomfort, and inability to evacuate the bowels. Acute constipation in very rare cases may be caused by bowel obstruction, but is usually caused by failure to consume enough fiber or fluid, or to get adequate exercise.

Chronic constipation is the inability of the person voluntarily to evacuate the bowels for a period of months or years. In chronic constipation, the nerve endings in the rectum that trigger defecation can become desensitized either by the constipation itself or by long-term use of stimulant laxatives. Chronic constipation may also be accompanied by anal fissures, or microscopic tears, caused by straining at stool. *Atonic constipation,* also called colonic inertia, is a form of chronic constipation that afflicts persons who cannot move about freely, generally the elderly or persons confined to bed. This condition can be made worse by prescription medicines for other complaints. Sometimes, atonic constipation can happen if a person, deeply involved in work or other activities, ignores the urge to defecate.

Constipation may cause other digestive problems, including indigestion, diverticulitis, hemorrhoids, and flatulence. Chronic and atonic constipation can cause or play a role in many other health problems, ranging from bad breath and body odor to insomnia and varicose veins. There may also be a link between long-term constipation and several forms of cancer.

There are Kampo equivalents for two of the several types of conventional laxatives used. Bulking agents, as the name implies, add bulk to the stool, which makes it softer and easier to pass. They need to be taken with plenty of fluids. Stimulant laxatives cause the stool-retaining muscles in the intestines to relax and the stool-expelling muscles to contract. Long-term use of stimulant laxatives may result in dependence on the laxative for normal bowel movements.

In Kampo, there are two forms of constipation, "strong" and "weak," known as "convulsing" and "laxing" in TCM. In cases of strong constipation, one must strain to pass tough stools. In cases of weak constipation, one passes small quantities of loose stools. The herbs listed here are most effective for strong constipation. Use herbs only until the constipation eases, and never use any stimulant laxative for more than two weeks. Formulas are used for either strong or weak constipation plus the combination of other symptoms most closely matching those experienced by the individual. (If treating an infant or toddler, see "Easing Children's Constipation.")

Any laxative, herbal or otherwise, affects the rate at which other oral medications are absorbed into the bloodstream. If taking both a prescription medication and a laxative, take them at different times of the day. Be especially careful when taking antibiotics, which harm the friendly bacteria that normally inhabit the colon. These bacteria work on compounds found in herbal stimulant laxatives that otherwise have no laxative effects. Without the bacteria, such laxatives will not work.[1] If constipation occurs while taking antibiotics, use a bulking agent.

INDIVIDUAL KAMPO TREATMENTS

See Chapter 3 for discussions of individual herbs, traditional healing substances, and modern herbal preparations, including directions for making tea.

SUGGESTED DOSAGES	COMMENTS
Aloe (Herb)	
Bitters, standardized to deliver 20–30 mg hydroxyanthracene derivatives daily, calculated as anhydrous aloin. Use up to 2 weeks at the smallest effective dosage.	A stimulant laxative used around the world to relieve constipation. In comparison to other herbal stimulant laxatives, it draws less fluid into the large intestine and thus is less likely to cause dehydration or mineral imbalances.[2] *Caution:* Do not use more than 2 weeks to avoid mineral imbalances as well as possible colon-cell damage (see Chapter 3). Do not use if menstruating or if rectal bleeding is present. Avoid aloe and all stimulant herbal laxatives if taking any kind of diuretic.
Dandelion (Herb)	
Tea, 1 c 3 times daily on an empty stomach. or Tincture (1:5), 10–15 drops 3 times daily on an empty stomach. Place in a cup, add 2 tbsp water, and take in a single sip.	Increases bile flow into the large intestine. Bile contains cholesterol, which disperses in water and lubricates the stool. Dandelion is noted for its ability to relieve constipation without causing diarrhea.
Dioscorea (Herb)	
Tincture (1:5), 20 drops 3 times daily after meals. Place in a cup, add 2 tbsp water, and take in a single sip.	Relieves intestinal spasms and stomach cramps accompanying constipation. Be sure to use an herbal product not mixed with synthetic progesterone.
Ginger (Herb)	
Tea, 1 c 3 times daily.	Helps relieve muscle spasms accompanying constipation.
Kelp (Herb)	
As food; as little as 2 oz (50 g) in a single serving usually reverses constipation.	Up to 45% of kelp's weight consists of algin, a complex carbohydrate that swells in water.[3] Bulk-building algin forms a coating, soothing gel that softens the stool and relieves stress on the blood vessels lining the rectum and anus. *Caution:* Limit consumption to once a week.
Plantain (Herb)	
Cold decoction made with ground seeds, ½ c after morning and evening meals, or ½ c at night. or Tea made with whole seeds, 1 c, up to 3 times daily.	Plantain, or psyllium seed, is a bulking agent[4] and the world's best-known remedy for constipation. Soothes hemorrhoids and does not cause cramps. To avoid absorption problems, take other oral medications 1 hour before using plantain.

Easing Children's Constipation

Infants and toddlers can experience constipation just like older children and adults, but need different treatments. Among newborns, breastfed babies have fewer bowel movements than formula-fed babies, sometimes only one movement every two or three days. If the baby is comfortable and has a good appetite, there is no need to worry about constipation. By the age of twelve months, most children have one comfortable bowel movement every day. If a child goes two or more days without a bowel movement, and then has pain or difficulty passing a large stool, he or she is constipated. Another symptom of constipation is stomachache in which the stomach is firm to the touch.

Avoid harsh stimulant laxatives when treating children. Instead, help the child overcome constipation first by making changes in diet and then by providing gentle, herbal support.

Dehydration can lead to constipation. Increase the child's supply of water, juices, and soup. Do not allow the children to drink too much cow's milk. Cow's milk contains compounds that desensitize the colon walls to stool-moving nerve impulses. Foods high in magnesium, such as spinach and Swiss chard, counteract the constipating effect of cow's milk. Also, increase the amount of fiber in the child's diet. Simply eating a piece of fruit often relieves constipation.

In addition, there are several herbal treatments for constipation. Food-grade aloe vera juice is a safe stimulant laxative. Combine 1½ teaspoons (6 milliliters) of aloe vera juice with applesauce or cereal and use once a day. Flaxseed is a source of lignans, fibers that absorb water and increase stool volume. Mix 1 teaspoon (2.5 grams) of flaxseed in 1 quart (1 liter) of water and simmer for fifteen minutes. Strain and use as the cooking water for cooked cereal. Licorice tea relieves intestinal inflammation caused by stimulant laxatives such as Dulcolax or phenolphthalein, although it has no laxative properties by itself. Make licorice tea by placing 1 teaspoon (3 grams) of the herb in 1 cup of boiling water. Steep for fifteen minutes off the heat, then strain. Give an infant one teaspoon (4 milliliters) of the tea once or twice a day. Give a toddler 2 teaspoons once or twice a day. Do not use for more than three or four days.

Rhubarb Root (Herb)

Tea, 1 c daily. Can be flavored with cinnamon or peppermint.	Stimulant laxative that stops gastrointestinal spasms. Also stimulates the release of bile, adding to its laxative effect and indirectly lowering cholesterol levels.[5] Use only root that has been aged for 1 to 2 years. Fresh root is ineffective. *Caution:* Do not use if menstruating or if rectal bleeding is present. Avoid rhubarb and all stimulant herbal laxatives if taking any kind of diuretic.

KAMPO FORMULAS

See Chapter 4 for dosage information and discussions of individual formulas.

Cinnamon and Peony Decoction

Treats weak constipation in people of poor health who suffer stomach pain. There may also be nosebleeds, chronic fatigue, or varicose veins.

Hemp Seed Pill

Relieves constipation with hard stools that are difficult to expel accompanied by frequent urination. Use this formula in patent-medicine form.

Caution: Most manufacturers include the traditional marijuana seed. Will not produce a "high," but will cause a positive urine test for THC, although sophisticated testing methods can distinguish medicinal from illicit use.

Major Order the Qi Decoction

Relieves strong constipation with flatulence, focal distention and abdominal fullness, abdominal pain that increases upon pressure, and a tense and firm abdomen. Also relieves accompanying symptoms that may include recurring fevers, delirious speech, and profuse sweating from the palms and soles.

Regulate the Stomach and Order the Qi Decoction

Relieves weak constipation in which there is no feeling of fullness in the abdomen. Also relieves mild irritability.

Rhubarb and Licorice Decoction

Relieves strong constipation accompanied by vomiting, as well as weak constipation without vomiting.

CONSIDERATIONS

❑ If constipation is a frequent problem, add more fiber to the diet, but do so gradually to avoid gas and bloating. Drink at least 8 to 10 glasses of water a day, and exercise more frequently.

❑ If constipation recurs at irregular intervals, the problem may be irritable bowel syndrome; *see* **Irritable Bowel Syndrome.** *See also* **Hemorrhoids** and **Indigestion.**

Crohn's Disease

See **Irritable Bowel Syndrome.**

Depression

Almost everyone feels sad or blue from time to time. Such passing moods, though, are not clinical depression. Depression, one of the most common psychological disorders, sometimes goes unrecognized for months or years because it can produce so many different symptoms. These symptoms include: depressed mood on a consistent basis, or in younger people, irritability; the loss of interest or pleasure in all or nearly all activities; either sleeplessness or the desire to sleep all the time; persistent feelings of guilt or worthlessness; decreased energy and fatigue; difficulty in concentration; either decreased or increased appetite; agitation or retardation of motor reflexes; and suicidal thoughts.[1]

Depression is thought to be caused by low brain levels of a chemical called serotonin. Serotonin acts as a neurotransmitter, or a substance that carries impulses from one nerve cell to another. The brain and many other tissues in the body make serotonin from the amino acid tryptophan. The body's tryptophan supplies can run short for various reasons. These include stress-related hormonal changes,[2,3] difficulty in getting tryptophan to cross from the bloodstream into the brain, and, in rare cases, dietary deficiency.[4]

There are several classes of drugs used to treat depression. Fluoxetine (Prozac), paroxetine (Paxil), and sertraline (Zoloft) belong to a class called the selective serotonin reuptake inhibitors (SSRIs). They keep nerve cells from absorbing serotonin, which keeps more serotonin in the clefts between nerve cells. SSRIs have fewer side effects than other drug classes, but those they do have can be serious. SSRI use can cause wild dreams, hallucinations, and aggressive behavior, as well as sexual dysfunction, nausea, headaches, either insomnia or drowsiness, and diarrhea.

Another drug class, the tricyclic antidepressants, stop the reabsorption of other neurotransmitters called dopamine and norepinephrine. Side effects frequently include constipation, dry mouth, and orthostatic hypotension, or a sudden drop in blood pressure when rising from a seated position. A third drug class, known as monoamine oxidase inhibitors (MAOIs), block the action of enzymes that break down norepinephrine, dopamine, and serotonin. Unfortunately, inhibiting these enzymes in the intestines and liver starts a chain reaction that can result in high blood pressure, which, in turn, can lead to stroke. MAOIs also come with a fairly lengthy list of dietary restrictions.

Not just Kampo but most traditions of herbal healing share the view with modern psychiatry that depression is a physical condition that expresses itself in emotional symptoms. Depression is often compared to a "broken heart," and Kampo's ancient theorists developed an elaborate theory of how disorders of the heart caused depression.

One type of depression was thought to result from too little nutritive energy reaching the heart. This condition produced insomnia, nervous unrest, and night sweats. A second type of depression was thought to result from too much nutritive energy reaching the heart. "Blazing heart fire" caused acute mental illness, a condition in which depression alternated with mania, nightmares, palpitations, redness in the face, restlessness, and ulcers of the mouth and tongue. This type of depression was the most dangerous to the patient, and the formulas used to treat it had to be used with the greatest care. Restrained anger could result in a third form of depression known as "liver oppression." This set of symptoms could include acid regurgitation or heartburn, anxiety, bloating, a feeling of fullness in the chest, and pain in the side.

The most effective Kampo treatments for depression are herbal formulas rather than single herbs, since formulas offer a more comprehensive balancing of energies in various parts of the body. Avoid taking more than one Kampo formula for depression. Instead, use the one formula that best fits the symptom pattern. Choosing a formula requires the help of a Kampo or TCM practitioner.

Single herbs are useful for long-term use in cases of mild to moderate depression. However, they do not necessarily substitute for prescribed antidepressant therapy. Rather, they augment antidepressant therapy by acting on the brain in ways different from those of the various drugs.

SSRIs exert effects for between four and six weeks after one stops taking them. During this period they can produce dangerous drug interactions with either MAOIs or certain herbal medications, such as ginkgo-leaf tea and St. John's wort, a non-Kampo herb that may be used with Kampo (see "Kampo and St. John's Wort"). No one should substitute herbal therapies for prescribed antidepressants without first seeking guidance from both a doctor and an Oriental medicine specialist.

INDIVIDUAL KAMPO TREATMENTS

See Chapter 3 for discussions of individual herbs, traditional healing substances, and modern herbal preparations, including directions for making tea.

SUGGESTED DOSAGES	COMMENTS
Barley Sprouts (Herb)	
Powder, 1–3 tbsp (6–15 g) dissolved in 1 c water once daily.	Relieves sadness and mild depression in adults who have both diabetes and attention deficit disorder.[5] If barley sprouts are unavailable, substitute juices or teas of young rice or wheat seedlings. *Caution:* Will inhibit lactation.
Biota (Herb)	
Tea, 1 c 3 times daily before meals. or **Biota Seed Pill to Nourish the Heart** (see formulas list). This is the recommended form.	Used for the treatment of age-related memory loss and accompanying symptoms of depression. Exactly how it works has not been scientifically established. *Caution:* Do not use over the long term, since dizziness, nausea, or vomiting could result. For long-term depression, use the formula.

Kampo and St. John's Wort

St. John's wort, a non-Kampo herb, is quickly becoming one of the most popular herbal antidepressant agents. Traditional Kampo had no knowledge of St. John's wort, which has been known to European herbalists since the time of the ancient Greeks. The modern understanding of St. John's wort and the herbs of Kampo, however, suggests that the two kinds of treatments may be used together.

While the exact way in which St. John's wort works is not yet known, this herb is often described as a natural Prozac. Hypericin, the best-known chemical found in the herb, prevents the reuptake of serotonin by brain tissue[1] in the same manner as Prozac and other SSRIs. St. John's wort has also been described as an MAOI.[2] Repeated laboratory tests on this effect, however, have not yielded consistent results. Yet another explanation of how St. John's wort defeats depression involves hypericin's effects on the immune system. This chemical stops the production of cytokines, hormonal messengers of pain and irritation.[3] Small changes in cytokine balance can make huge differences in brain function, which affects depression.[4] It is important to remember, though, that hypericin is not the only active ingredient in St. John's wort. This herb contains dozens of chemicals, all of which are being extensively researched.

How can St. John's wort and Kampo be used together? When using herbs for depression, it is important to choose those that have complementary effects. None of the investigations of St. John's wort suggests that it increases oxygen circulation to the brain. Therefore, herbs that increase circulation, such as ginkgo, have a complementary effect. St. John's wort has no effect on depression stemming from the body's inability to produce the hormone cortisol. Chronic fatigue syndrome patients do not produce enough cortisol, and these people often suffer from depression. They can often benefit from a combination of St. John's wort and licorice.

What about using St. John's wort with Kampo formulas? Generally speaking, formulas are chosen to have positive "side effects" that reestablish normal function throughout the body. Although the risk of drug interactions between the traditional formulas made of many herbs and St. John's wort is almost nonexistent, the Kampo principle of treating disease with the least possible medication dictates that formulas should be used by themselves.

To use St. John's wort, take capsules as directed by the manufacturer, or use tincture (1:5), 50 to 75 drops four times daily. This herb is useful when depression, tension, and exhaustion are combined. Although some people see an immediate improvement in mood after taking St. John's wort, it is usually necessary to take the herb for several weeks before results are noticeable. It is then necessary to continue taking it for between four and six months.

Ginkgo (Modern Herbal Preparation)

Ginkgolide extract, 1 40-mg tablet 3 times daily or 1 60-mg tablet twice daily. Increasing dosage to 160 mg (4 40-mg tablets) or 180 mg (3 60-mg tablets) may give increased relief. Recommended form for this disorder.

Reverses depression,[6] particularly when used with prescription drugs in elderly patients, by increasing the flow of oxygen to the brain.[7]

Caution: Do not use ginkgo-leaf *tea.*

Licorice (Herb)

Glycyrrhizin extract, 200–800 mg daily, depending on severity of symptoms for up to 6 weeks. Resume after a 2-week break.

or

Tea, 1 c 1–5 times daily for up to 6 weeks. Resume after a 2-week break.

Useful for depression that accompanies chronic fatigue syndrome (CFS). Stimulates the production of cortisol. In most CFS patients, this action can increase blood pressure, which in turn increases the brain's oxygen supply, lifting mood.[8] Avoid deglycyrrhizinated licorice (DGL).

Caution: Avoid if high blood pressure is present. Also avoid if an estrogen-sensitive disorder is present, such as bladder cancer, melanoma, or disorders of the female reproductive system.

Morinda (Herb)

Freeze-dried extract, 2–5 1,000-mg capsules 3 times daily.

or

Tea, 1 c 3 times daily.

An antidepressant herb with the unique property of increasing, rather than diminishing, male sexual function. Increases the rate at which tryptophan is supplied to the brain, but does not affect the rate at which serotonin and other neurotransmitters are made or broken down. Also lowers high blood pressure.[9]

Caution: Avoid in cases of dribbling or difficult urination.

KAMPO FORMULAS

See Chapter 4 for dosage information and discussions of individual formulas.

Biota Seed Pill to Nourish the Heart

Relieves depression in a symptom pattern of low energy, chills, cold limbs, palpitations, insomnia, headache, dizziness, poor memory, agitation, or nightmares.

Bupleurum Plus Dragon Bone and Oyster Shell Decoction

Treats depression that occurs with a combination of symptoms which includes delirious speech, irritability, and palpitations that are frequently accompanied by urinary difficulty, a feeling of fullness in the chest, and difficulty in turning the body sideways and forward. Particularly useful for treating depression accompanied by migraine headaches in men.

Caution: Be sure the formula does *not* include the traditional ingredient minium (lead oxide). Use with caution if fever is present, and discontinue if preexisting fevers worsen.

Coptis Decoction to Relieve Toxicity

Treats depression alternating with episodes of "hot" symptoms, including bleeding gums, fever, facial flushing caused by embarrassment or emotional tension, headaches, nervousness, or sinusitis.

Caution: Should not be used by women who are trying to become pregnant.

Drive Out Stasis from the Mansion of Blood Decoction

Treats depression accompanied by extreme "psychosomatic symptoms," including chest pain, chronic headache with a piercing quality, choking sensation when drinking, dry heaves, insomnia, extreme mood swings, or fever. Particularly useful for depression accompanied by migraine headaches in women.

Frigid Extremities Decoction

Traditional Kampo treatment for depression that is accompanied by a queasy stomach. May cause a loss of sensation in the mouth and tongue.

Caution: Discontinue the formula if fever occurs.

Ginseng Decoction to Nourish the Nutritive Qi

Prescribed in Japan for depression complicated by anemia, forgetfulness, hair loss, jaundice, or tired limbs. It contains small amounts of ginseng, which softens the effects of stress and also stimulates the immune system.

Licorice, Wheat, and Jujube Decoction

Has calming actions similar to those of opium,[10] acts by occupying brain receptor sites that receive sedative drugs such as opium without causing addiction. In Japan, is given to women and children experiencing frequent sobbing and loss of emotional control, and displaying a detached demeanor.[11] Seek the advice of the dispensing herbalist on a suitable child's dosage. Can be made at home in tea form (see Chapter 4).

Pinellia and Magnolia Bark Decoction

Treats a condition TCM labels "plum-pit qi," in which the energy of the body seems to lump in the throat, described by herbalists Bensky and Gamble as "a situation that literally cannot be swallowed."[12]

Caution: Use with caution if fever is present, and discontinue if preexisting fevers worsen.

Restore the Spleen Decoction

The "spleen" is the body's digestive function. This formula regulates digestion to treat depression that manifests itself as anxiety, difficulty in maintaining concentration, fatigue of mind and body, and/or poor memory.

CONSIDERATIONS

❑ Naturopathic medicine links depression to a shortage of a vitaminlike compound called tetrahydrobiopterin (BH_4). This compound is needed for the creation of several neurotransmitters.[13] Although BH_4 is not available as a nutritional supplement, ascorbic acid, folic acid,[14] and vitamin B_{12} stimulate the body's production of BH_4, and are available as supplements.[15] B vitamins are also known to increase the effectiveness of tricyclic antidepressants.[16]

❑ Severe depression can cause overwhelming feelings of guilt, hopelessness, and despair, and even thoughts of suicide. Anyone who experiences suicidal thoughts should *immediately* contact a suicide hotline or local emergency number.

❑ *See also* **Anxiety, Chronic Fatigue Syndrome, Insomnia,** and **Memory Problems.**

DIABETES

Diabetes mellitus affects more than 10 million Americans. It is a chronic disorder in which the body is unable to regulate glucose, the fuel used by cells, and insulin, a hormone that helps glucose enter cells. This causes glucose to accumulate in the bloodstream. Symptoms include fatigue and increases in both thirst and frequency of urination.

There are two types of diabetes mellitus. In *type 1 diabetes,* also known as insulin-dependent or juvenile-onset diabetes, the body cannot produce enough insulin. This usually occurs when the body's own immune defenses destroy the insulin-secreting portions of the pancreas. Type 1 diabetes usually appears in childhood, although it can develop in adults. Treatment consists of insulin injections. *Type 2 diabetes,* also known as non-insulin-dependent or adult-onset diabetes, involves insulin resistance, a condition in which insulin does not reach the cells that need it. This usually happens despite *increased* insulin production, so that the blood contains too much insulin *and* too much glucose. Treatment consists of weight loss, exercise, and drugs.

Insulin can be rendered ineffective for a number of reasons. Obesity or high blood pressure can restrict the flow of insulin to the skeletal muscles. (Since these disorders are more common among older people, the chances of developing type 2 diabetes increase with age.) And since fat cells may compete with other cells for insulin, type 2 diabetes accelerates the accumulation of body fat, which in turn worsens the diabetes. Insulin's effectiveness can be reduced by other factors as well. These include hormonal reactions to emotional stress, antibody reactions to insulin receptors (the cellular "doors" that admit glucose) on red blood cells, and the production of a misshapen form of insulin that is unable to bind with insulin receptors.

Diabetes can have several long-term complications. The brain, nerve tissues, and the lens of the eye—all of which absorb glucose without insulin's help—become saturated with glucose, which is turned into a toxin called sorbitol. This can result in diabetic neuropathy, a nerve disorder that can cause numbness, sensitivity, or pain; difficulty in swallowing or in controlling the bladder; and digestive problems. Vision problems can result from cataracts or a disorder known as diabetic retinopathy, in which blood vessels in the retina break.

Diabetes contributes to atherosclerosis, in which cholesterol plaques develop in the blood vessels. This may cause heart attack, stroke, or intermittent claudication, a painful condition in which blood cannot circulate to the extremities. Poor circulation leaves the skin vulnerable to infections and sores. Diabetes can also cause impotence through both poor circulation and reduced production of an erection-enabling substance called nitrous oxide. In addition, diabetes causes the kidneys to become clogged with excess sugar, which starts a process that leads to kidney damage. The insulin-secreting parts of the pancreas can also become clogged, leading to pancreas damage.

At one time, Kampo and Western medicine alike only diagnosed diabetes when sugar appeared in the urine. By the time this occurs, the disease is usually so far advanced that the body has to break down its own tissues to provide energy. Japanese and Chinese physicians labeled this symptom pattern "wasting and thirsting disorder." They saw this condition as a depletion of the yin, or containing, energies of the kidneys. The kidneys could no longer hold water, causing copious urination. Neither could they "steam" water upward in the body to help the body keep its normal form. The kidneys give information to the liver. When the containing energies of kidneys run out, the liver also becomes deficient. It then sends fiery energy upward to the eyes, causing blurred vision.

When carefully chosen by a Kampo practitioner, herbal formulas are an effective emergency measure to stop the process that leads to ketoacidosis, a life-threatening complication that causes the body to become too acidic. Kampo formulas can dramatically lower blood-sugar levels and stop the process that leads to nerve damage. Once the more severe symptoms of diabetes are controlled, the next step is to help the body maintain a steady flow of energy from the kidneys. The formulas Kampo uses for this purpose help the body use insulin more effectively and evenly. In rare cases, they have even reversed type 1 diabetes—but it is still essential to test blood-sugar levels at least weekly, even in remission.

If taking both antidiabetic medication and a Kampo herb, monitor blood sugar regularly and consult the doctor about any needed medication changes. If discontinuing a medication after starting to use an herb, it may be necessary to resume medication if the herb is then discontinued. Like herbs, formulas may require adjustments in dosages of insulin or prescription antidiabetic drugs. Unlike herbs, formulas do not require such adjustments after the formula is discontinued, provided the appropriate formula is chosen in consultation with a Kampo or TCM practitioner.

INDIVIDUAL KAMPO TREATMENTS

See Chapter 3 for discussions of individual herbs, traditional healing substances, and modern herbal preparations, including directions for making tea.

SUGGESTED DOSAGES	COMMENTS
Aloe (Herb)	
Juice, as directed on label. Typical dosage is 1 fluid oz (30 ml) daily.	Useful in managing levels of blood sugar, cholesterol, and triglycerides in type 2 diabetes. Stimulates the pancreas to produce insulin, but without inducing weight gain.[1,2]
Angelica Dahurica (Herb)	
Freeze-dried root, 1–3 gel caps 3 times daily. or Tea, 1 c 3 times daily.	Contains compounds that stop weight gain caused by oral diabetes medications.[3] Be sure to use *Angelica dahurica,* which may be labeled Radix Angelicae Dahuricae, and not *Angelica sinensis,* or tang-kuei. *Caution:* Do not use during pregnancy.

Astragalus (Herb)	
Fluid extract (1:1), ¼–½ tsp (1–2 ml) 3 times daily. or Freeze-dried herb in capsules, 500–1,000 mg 3 times daily. or Powdered solid extract (4:1), 250–500 mg 3 times daily. or Tea, 1 c 3 times daily. or Tincture (1:5), 1–1½ tsp (4–6 ml), 3 times daily. Place in a cup, add 2 tbsp water, and take in a single sip.	Heals skin ulcers associated with diabetes. Treats peripheral neuropathy, or loss of sensation in hands and feet.[4] *Caution:* Do not use when fever or skin infection is present.

Astragalus, Rehmannia (Herbs)	
Tea, 1 c 3 times daily. Place 1 tsp (3 g) of a 50-50 mixture of ground astragalus and rehmannia in 1 c boiling water. Steep 15 mins and strain before using.	Treats vascular complications of type 2 diabetes.[5] This mixture is available from Oriental herb dealers. *Caution:* Do not use astragalus when fever or skin infection is present.

Atractylodis, Red (Herb)	
Tea, 1 c 3 times daily.	Kampo herb for visual problems. Produces dramatic drops in blood-sugar levels in animal studies of diabetes.[6] Be sure to take *Atractylodis lancea* or *A. chinensis* (*Cang Zhu* in Chinese herb shops), and not *A. macrocephala* (white atractylodis, or *Bai Zhu*). *Caution:* Avoid if diarrhea and excessive sweating are present.

Benincasa (Herb)	
Tea, 1 c up to 3 times daily.	Lowers blood-sugar levels in type 2 diabetes.[7] *Caution:* Use with caution if diarrhea is present.

Bitter Melon (Herb)	
Juice, 1–2 oz (30–60 ml) 3 times daily. or Whole fruit, ½–2 fruits (9–15 g) in cooking daily.	Most widely used herbal remedy for diabetes in the world; effects confirmed in dozens of studies. Increases availability of glucose to muscles, stimulates insulin secretion, and keeps glucose from being absorbed through the intestinal wall.[8] More effective when combined with non-Kampo herb gurmar. *Caution:* Bitter melon should be avoided by persons who have cirrhosis or have had hepatitis, or are HIV-positive and have had liver infections. Otherwise, use for 4 weeks, then discontinue for 4 weeks.

Caltrop (Herb)	
Tea, 1 c up to twice daily.	Lowers blood pressure, stimulates urination, and improves visual acuity, particularly when diabetes causes problems with fluid circulation in the lens.[9]

Corydalis (Herb)	
Powdered herb with food, 2 g twice daily. Must be weighed by an herbalist.	Prevents cataracts caused by diabetes.[10]

Dan Shen (Herb)	
Tablets or tinctures. Use only under professional supervision.	Prevents blood vessel disease caused by diabetes.[11] *Caution:* Avoid if an estrogen-sensitive disorder is present, such as bladder cancer, melanoma, or disorders of the female reproductive system.

Dioscorea (Herb)	
Tincture (1:5), 20 drops 3 times daily after meals. Place in a cup, add 2 tbsp water, and take in a single sip.	Reduces blood-sugar levels in type 1 diabetes.[12] Be sure to use an herbal product not mixed with synthetic progesterone.

Garlic (Herb)	
Cloves in food, preferably raw, 2–3 daily. Recommended form for this disorder.	Lowers blood-sugar levels by stimulating insulin secretion and by preventing insulin deactivation. Does so without stimulating fat accumulation, a common side effect of many diabetes medications.[13] Dried garlic and garlic tablets are not effective in diabetes treatment.[14] *Caution:* Do not use with the blood-thinner warfarin sodium (Coumadin). Garlic will counteract the effects of *Bifidus* and *Lactobacillus* cultures taken as digestive aids.

Ginkgo (Modern Herbal Preparation)	
Ginkgolide extract, 1 40-mg tablet 3 times daily or 1 60-mg tablet twice daily. Increasing dosage to 160 mg (4 40-mg tablets) or 180 mg (3 60-mg tablets) may give increased relief.	Prevents vascular damage in diabetes and reduces risk for diabetic retinopathy. Relieves pain of intermittent claudication, although improvement takes at least 6 weeks. For maximum effectiveness, should be used with conventional medicines or other herbs, or with vigorous exercise.

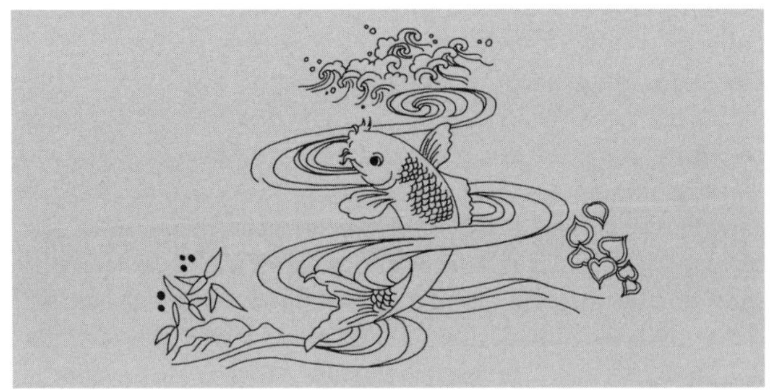

Ginseng (Herb)	
Fluid extract or tincture, as directed on label. or Tea, made with Korean or red ginseng, 1 c daily.	Prolongs the effect of insulin and reduces the amount of insulin required in type 1 diabetes.[15] Also stimulates the pancreas to secrete insulin in type 2 diabetes. Lowers blood-sugar levels.[16] If using ginseng extracts or tinctures (which are not as therapeutically active as teas), be sure the product contains *Panax ginseng.* Note that strength may vary by manufacturer.

Green Tea (Herb)	
Catechin extract, 1 240-mg tablet 3 times daily. or Tea, 2–3 cups daily.	Suppresses the formation of "sticky," vessel-clogging blood proteins,[17] which helps prevent the vascular problems common in later stages of diabetes. Contains tannins, which inhibit enzymes in the mouth and intestines from releasing sugars found in food.[18] Also contains theophylline, which lowers blood-sugar levels through various means.[19] To avoid dilution problems, do not take tea within 1 hour of taking other teas or patent medicines.

Licorice (Herb)	
Glycyrrhizin extract, 200–800 mg daily, depending on severity of symptoms for up to 6 weeks. Resume after a 2-week break. or Tea, 1 c 1–5 times daily for up to 6 weeks. Resume after a 2-week break.	Keeps sorbitol from accumulating in the lens of the eye.[20] Avoid deglycyrrhizinated licorice (DGL). *Caution:* Avoid if high blood pressure is present. Also avoid if an estrogen-sensitive disorder is present, such as bladder cancer, melanoma, or disorders of the female reproductive system.

Maitake (Modern Herbal Preparation)	
Fresh or dried maitake in food, 1/4–1/3 oz (6–9 g) daily. or Maitake D-fraction in capsule or tablet form, 1,000 mg 3 times daily before meals. or Tea, 1 c 4–8 times daily.	Stimulates immune system to fight yeast infections common in diabetes.[21] Should be used for at least 1–2 months to control mild infections and for at least 6–9 months for serious infections.

Reishi (Modern Herbal Preparation)	
Dried extract, 3 1-g tablets 3 times daily. or Fresh or dried reishi in food, 1/4–1/3 oz (6–9 g) daily. or Syrup, as directed on label. or Tincture (1:5), 1 tbsp (10 ml) 3 times daily. Place in a cup, add 2 tbsp water, and take in a single sip.	Stimulates immune system to fight yeast infections common in diabetes.[22] Should be used for at least 1–2 months to control mild infections and for at least 6–9 months for serious infections.

Scutellaria (Herb)	
Dried herb, 1–2 1,000-mg capsules 3 times daily. or Fluid extract (1:1), 1/4–1/2 tsp (1–2 ml) 3 times daily. or Powdered solid extract (4:1), 250–500 mg 3 times daily. or Tea, 1 c 4 times daily. or Tincture (1:5), 1–1 1/2 tsp (4–6 ml) 3 times daily. Place in a cup, add 2 tbsp water, and take in a single sip.	Has a high zinc content.[23] Zinc activates the free-radical fighter superoxide dismutase, which prevents atherosclerosis and is deficient in diabetics.[24] *Caution:* Avoid in cases of diarrhea caused by foodborne infection or excessive consumption of cold drinks.

Shiitake (Modern Herbal Preparation)	
Fresh or dried shiitake in food, 1/4–1/3 oz (6–9 g) daily. or 3 1-g tablets 3 times daily. or Syrup, 1/2 tbsp (4–6 ml) 3 times daily. or Tincture (1:5), 1 tbsp (10 ml) 3 times daily. Place in a cup, add 2 tbsp water, and take in a single sip.	Stimulates immune system to fight yeast infections common in diabetes.[25] Should be used for at least 1–2 months to control mild infections and for at least 6–9 months for serious infections.

Soy Lecithin (Modern Herbal Preparation)	
Soy phospholipids, 1,500–3,000 mg daily. Identified individually on the label as 3-sn-phospatidylcholine, phosphatidylethanolamine, and phospatidylinositic acid, or as "total phospholipids."	Contains genistein, which deactivates an enzyme necessary for the growth of cells associated with atherosclerosis.[26] *Caution:* Mild diarrhea may occur when soy lecithin is first used.

KAMPO FORMULAS

See Chapter 4 for dosage information and discussions of individual formulas.

Coptis Decoction to Relieve Toxicity

Treats yeast infections aggravated by diabetes, especially thrush and esophageal yeast infections causing heartburn.[27]

Caution: Should not be used by women who are trying to become pregnant.

Eight-Ingredient Pill With Rehmannia (Rehmannia-Eight Combination)

Most popular herbal treatment for both type 1 diabetes and type 2 diabetes in Japan. Lowers blood sugar, aids insulin regulation, and treats diabetic neuropathy in type 1 diabetes. Smoothes out insulin's effects, providing tighter control of blood-sugar levels, although it will not reduce the amount of insulin needed. This prevents eye and circulation problems.[28] Has long been recognized to prevent cataract formation.[29]

Major Bupleurum Decoction

Reduces the rate at which glucose enters the bloodstream after meals. Increases the efficiency of insulin.[30] Especially useful for persons who have diabetes and long-term gastrointestinal disorders, with symptoms that include alternating fever and chills, bitter taste in the mouth, nausea, continuous vomiting, burning diarrhea or no bowel movements, despondency, fullness in the chest and upper abdomen on the sides with or without pain, and irritability.

Caution: Use with caution if fever is present, and discontinue if preexisting fevers worsen.

Minor Bupleurum Decoction

Reduces the rate at which glucose enters the bloodstream after meals.[31] Particularly useful for persons who have both diabetes and infection with either HIV or hepatitis.

Caution: Do not use if fever or skin infection is present. Taken long term in patent medicine form, can cause headache, dizziness, and bleeding gums. Side effects can be avoided if the formula is taken as a tea.

Six-Ingredient Pill With Rehmannia (Rehmannia-Six Combination)

Treats the following symptoms that may accompany diabetes: soreness and weakness in the lower back, vertigo, lightheadedness, tinnitus, diminished hearing, night sweats, toothache, hot palms or soles, chronic dry or sore throat, or wasting.

Caution: Avoid if an estrogen-sensitive disorder is present, such as bladder cancer, melanoma, or disorders of the female reproductive system.

White Tiger Plus Atractylodis Decoction

Contains anemarrhena, which lowers blood-sugar levels by increasing the amount of sugar stored in the liver.[32] Many diabetics have found this herb to work when conventional medications have failed.[33] The formula relieves feelings of cold in the lower part of the body, general feeling of heaviness, joint pain, and sweating accompanying diabetes.

Caution: Avoid if nausea or vomiting is present.

White Tiger Plus Ginseng Decoction

Contains anemarrhena, which lowers blood-sugar levels by increasing the amount of sugar stored in the liver.[34] Many diabetics have found this herb to work when conventional medications have failed.[35] The formula increases production of glucagon, a hormone that enables the liver to break down its stored sugar into glucose, but without raising blood-sugar levels.[36] Relieves fever, thirst, profuse sweating, and generalized weakness.

Caution: Avoid if nausea or vomiting is present.

CONSIDERATIONS

❑ Regular eye examinations are important, in addition to periodic blood and urine tests. Daily inspection of the feet is also vital, and infections should be brought to a doctor's attention promptly.

❑ For persons with type 2 diabetes, daily aerobic exercise is important. Exercise stimulates the flow of blood to the skeletal muscles, supplying both glucose and the insulin needed to absorb glucose. This lowers blood-sugar levels and keeps fat cells from depositing fat. Taking medication for type 2 diabetes without exercising aggravates the disease and leads to weight gain. For best results, an exercise program should be combined with a diet that is carefully balanced in terms of fats, carbohydrates, and proteins. This diet should include smaller, more frequent meals to keep blood-sugar levels constant.

❑ In diabetes, it is difficult to maintain constant glucose levels. Therefore, blood-sugar levels can drop too much, causing hypoglycemia. This condition is marked by dizziness, lethargy, sweatiness, and headache. Counteract mild episodes by consuming a quick-acting sugar source, such as orange juice or raisins.

❑ In Japan, type 2 diabetes treatment plans include vanadium[37] and CoQ_{10}.[38] Vanadium, a trace mineral, helps cells use energy properly and inhibits cholesterol creation. CoQ_{10}, a vitaminlike substance, acts as an antioxidant and circulatory aid.

❑ *See also* **Atherosclerosis, Cataracts, Diabetic Retinopathy, High Cholesterol, Kidney Disease, Obesity,** and **Yeast Infections.**

DIABETIC RETINOPATHY

Diabetic retinopathy is an eye disorder that affects the retina, the projection screen on which light that passes through the eye is thrown. In this disorder, the capillaries that nourish the retina leak fluid or blood. This leakage can damage the cells that respond to light and relay visual impulses to the optic nerve, which carries these impulses to the brain. It is a common cause of blindness in persons with severe diabetes.

The risk factors for diabetic retinopathy include age, duration of the diabetes, and the presence of a "sticky" protein in the blood called glycosylated hemoglobin. Another risk factor for diabetic retinopathy is the presence of insulin-like growth factor I, a hormone produced in excess during diabetes.[1] This hormone encourages the growth of fragile capillaries in the eye that easily break and leak fluid. Conventional treatment consists of laser surgery, which seals the leaking blood vessels.

Traditional Japanese physicians saw diabetes as a depletion of the yin, or containing, energies of the kidneys. The kidneys could no longer hold water, causing copious urination. Neither could they "steam" water upward in the body to help the body keep its normal form. In addition, the kidneys control or give information to the liver. When the containing energies of kidneys run out, the liver also becomes deficient. It sends fiery energy upward to the eyes and crown of the head, causing blurred vision.

INDIVIDUAL KAMPO TREATMENTS

See Chapter 3 for discussions of individual herbs, traditional healing substances, and modern herbal preparations, including directions for making tea.

SUGGESTED DOSAGES	COMMENTS
Astragalus, Rehmannia (Herbs)	
Tea, 1 c 3 times daily. Simmer 1 tsp (3 g) of a 50-50 mixture of ground astragalus and rehmannia in 1 c water for 15 mins and strain before using.	Treats eye disease caused by non-insulin-dependent diabetes. Studies with this mixture have noted improvements in blood flow through the eye.[2] This mixture is available from Oriental herb dealers. *Caution:* Do not use astragalus when fever or skin infection is present.

Ginkgo (Modern Herbal Preparation)	
Quercetin extract, 1–2 125-mg capsules 3 times daily between meals.	Contains quercetin, which slows the formation of insulin-like growth factor I. Also counteracts platelet-activating factor, which causes blood clots in the capillaries. For best results, take quercetin with bromelain, which increases absorption. *Caution:* Do not take quercetin with the prescription drugs Procardia or Seldane.

Hawthorn (Herb)	
Fluid extract (1:1), ¼–½ tsp (1–2 ml) 3 times daily. or Solid extract, 100–250 mg 3 times daily. Should be standardized to contain 10% proanthocyanidins. or Tea, ⅔ c 3–4 times daily. or Tincture (1:5), 1–1½ tsp (4–6 ml) 3 times daily. Place in a cup, add 2 tbsp water, and take in a single sip.	Helps maintain integrity of the blood vessels supplying the eye's surface. Also reduces blood-vessel response to emotional tension.

Soy Isoflavones (Modern Herbal Preparation)	
Extract, about 3,000 mg once daily. or Soy germ, 2 tsp (10 g) twice daily, preferably added to cereals or smoothies.	Contains genistein, which slows the formation of insulin-like growth factor I.

CONSIDERATIONS

❑ Formulas can stop the toxic and destructive processes of long-term diabetes. They can dramatically lower blood sugars, and even reverse the process of damage to the retina, eliminating the need for surgery. *See* **Diabetes.**

DIARRHEA

Diarrhea is an increase in the fluidity, frequency, and volume of bowel movements. It may be accompanied by cramping, nausea, and/or vomiting. Diarrhea is a common symptom that usually signifies a mild and temporary condition. However, diarrhea that occurs in a child under age six, is bloody, lasts more than three days, or is accompanied by cramping with weakness between attacks requires medical attention. Diarrhea is also a concern if a person must maintain constant medication levels in the bloodstream, such as levels of lithium, antiseizure drugs, or diabetes medications.

Most cases of diarrhea are caused by various types of food- and waterborne infections, or the toxins produced by such infections. Some of the more common diarrhea-causing microorganisms include *Escherichia coli* (pathogenic *E. coli*), *Campylobacter jejuni, Salmonella, Shigella, Yersinia etereocolitica, Cryptosporidium, Clostridium difficele, Staphylococcus, Giardia lamblia,* and *Vibrio cholerae,* the bacterium that causes cholera.

Diarrhea can be caused by a number of other conditions and disorders. These include food allergies and intolerances; bowel surgery and some drugs; too much vitamin C or artificial sweetener; withdrawal from addictive drugs; gallbladder disease; some forms of cancer; and use of laxatives that contain magnesium, phosphate, or sulfate.

Kampo generally does not treat acute diarrhea, that is, diarrhea occurring suddenly and lasting a short time. Acute diarrhea is the body's defensive mechanism for ridding itself of an "external pernicious influence," what Western medicine would call an infectious microorganism. Kampo understands chronic diarrhea as an imbalance of energy in the digestive system. This form of diarrhea is accompanied by other symptoms, such as muscular weakness, coldness in the hands and feet, irritability, and pain in the chest or side.

Modern investigation has revealed that several Kampo herbs have an antibiotic effect on specific microorganisms that cause diarrhea. Although Kampo traditionally did not treat acute diarrhea, herbal treatments are appropriate for acute diarrhea when it is known that the problem is caused by a specific germ (for example, *Salmonella*) for which an herb is known to be effective. The numerous Kampo formulas that treat diarrhea were designed to correct specific patterns of symptoms. Formulas are intended for long-term use, as they correct the underlying imbalances that produce multiple symptoms, including diarrhea.

It is important to know the cause of diarrhea in each case and match the cause to its treatment. Chronic diarrhea should always be brought to the attention of a health care provider. Kampo is best used as part of an overall home-care plan (see "Home Care for Diarrhea" on page 202).

INDIVIDUAL KAMPO TREATMENTS

See Chapter 3 for discussions of individual herbs, traditional healing substances, and modern herbal preparations, including directions for making tea.

SUGGESTED DOSAGES	COMMENTS
Agrimony (Herb)	
Tea, 1 c 2–3 times daily until symptoms subside. Can be given to children (see inset on page 142).	Acts as an astringent by "tanning" cells in the intestines, which makes them less permeable. *Caution:* Do not use for more than 2 weeks.
Angelica Dahurica (Herb)	
Tea, 1 c, up to 4 times daily.	Stops the growth of *E. coli,* and the bacteria that cause dysentery and typhoid fever,[1] as well as *Salmonella* and *Shigella.*[2] Be sure to use *Angelica dahurica,* which may be labeled Radix Angelicae Dahuricae, and not *Angelica sinensis,* or tang-kuei.

Home Care for Diarrhea

In addition to using specific antidiarrheal agents, home care during an episode of diarrhea requires observing a few simple rules:

• *Avoid solid foods.* It is more important to replace fluids than foodstuffs.

• *Replace water and electrolytes.* Diarrhea causes a person to lose both water and electrolytes, such as chloride, potassium, and sodium. These minerals can be replaced by electrolyte-replacement drinks such as Gatorade and Pedialyte, or by fruit juices, herbal teas, and vegetable broths, but not by water alone.

• *Avoid dairy products.* Acute diarrhea damages the cells lining the walls of the intestine. This creates a temporary lactose intolerance, which will correct itself when the diarrhea is over.

• *Bind diarrhea with carob, kaolin, or pectin.* Carob, often used as a chocolate substitute, is especially rich in dietary fiber. Fiber absorbs water from the intestinal contents, making the stool more solid. Kaolin, a medicinal clay used as a healing substance in Kampo, is the basic ingredient of the antidiarrheal medicines Donangel and Kaodene. Some over-the-counter remedies, such as Kaopectate, combine kaolin with another source of fiber, pectin. Pectin, like carob, absorbs water from the intestinal contents, stopping diarrhea.

Bitter Orange Peel (Herb)	
Tea, 1 c cold or lukewarm 3 times daily 30 mins before meals.	Relaxes the body's smooth muscles, including those in the digestive tract.[3] *Caution:* Kampo urges caution in using this herb if "red" symptoms exist: red tongue, redness in the face with fever and cough, and blood in the stool.

Blue Citrus (Herb)	
Tea, 1 c 3 times daily 30 mins before meals.	Increases gastric secretion. Stimulates movement of food through the digestive tract, stops vomiting, arrests hiccups, and dispels abdominal distention.[4] Only useful after the acute symptoms of diarrhea have passed.

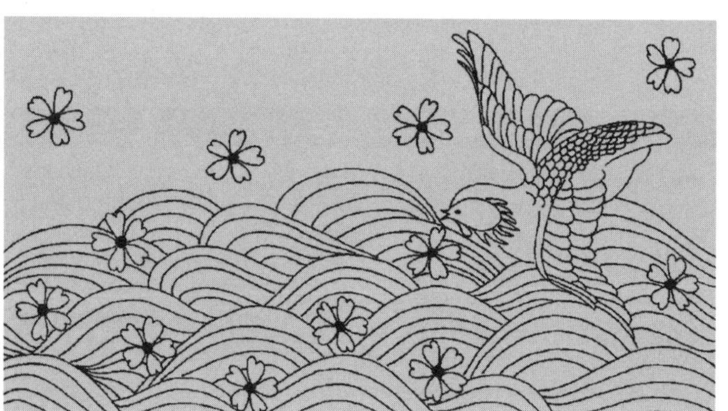

Coptis (Herb)	
Tincture (1:5), 15–30 drops 3 times daily. Place in a cup, add 2 tbsp water, and take in a single sip.	Contains berberine, which is especially useful in treating diarrhea caused by cholera, or by food-poisoning organisms amebiasis, klebsiella, or *Salmonella.* Controls symptoms of giardiasis, but not as effective as metronidazole (Flagyl) in killing the *Giardia* parasite.[5] Should be used with antibiotics for treating bacterial diarrhea, as berberine slows the body's ability to expel pathogens. If coptis is unavailable, substitute tinctures of the non-Kampo herbs barberry, goldenseal, or Oregon grape root (same cautions apply). *Caution:* Only use the herb while taking antibiotics. Do not use with supplements that contain vitamin B_6 or the amino acid histidine.

Forsythia (Herb)	
Tablets, 1 3 times daily. or Tea, 1 c 3 times daily.	Stops the growth of *E. coli* and *Salmonella.*[6] Available in Chinese herb shops as *Wian Qiao.*

Green Tea (Herb)	
Catechin extract, 1 240-mg tablet 3 times daily. or Tea, 1 c 3–5 times daily as desired.	Stops the growth of the following microorganisms: *Campylobacter jejuni, Plesiomonas shigelloides, Staphylococcus aureus, Vibrio cholerae O1* and *non-O1,* and *Vibrio parahaemolyticus.*[7] To avoid dilution problems, do not take tea within 1 hour of taking other teas or patent medicines.

Lonicera (Herb)	
Dried herb, 1 1,000-mg capsule 3 times daily.	Treats diarrhea due to "digestive deficiency," or incomplete digestion. Available as honeysuckle flower or *Jin Yin Hua.* *Caution:* Do not use on a long-term basis.

Plantain (Herb)	
Cold decoction made with ground seeds, ½ c after morning and evening meals, or ½ c at night.	Studies have confirmed that plantain, or psyllium seed, the world's best-known constipation remedy, also treats diarrhea.[8] Ground seeds absorb water from the stool, solidifying it. They also contain soothing mucilages that ease irritation. To avoid absorption problems, take other oral medications 1 hour before using plantain.

Snake Gourd (Trichosanth) Fruit (Herb)	
Fruit, as desired.	Inhibits the growth of *E. coli, Pseudomonas,* and *Shigella sonnei.* *Caution:* Avoid if indigestion is present.

KAMPO FORMULAS

See Chapter 4 for dosage information and discussions of individual formulas.

Five-Accumulation Powder

Treats diarrhea with abdominal pain, borborygmus (gurgling noises), and/or vomiting.

Caution: Use with caution if fever is present, and discontinue if preexisting fevers worsen.

Five-Ingredient Powder with Poria

Treats diarrhea with vomiting and difficulty in urination. Acts by stimulating urination[9] and thus reducing the amount of fluid to be eliminated through the intestines.

Frigid Extremities Decoction

Treats diarrhea with undigested food particles in the stool. Additional symptoms may include abdominal pain, a constant desire to sleep, aversion to cold, and a lack of thirst. May cause a loss of sensation in the mouth and tongue.

Caution: Discontinue the formula if fever occurs.

Kudzu Decoction

Treats diarrhea in children and diarrhea caused by food allergies. Kudzu Decoction is extremely nontoxic. However, seek the advice of the dispensing herbalist on a suitable child's dosage.

Major Ledebouriella Decoction

Reduces diarrhea during drug withdrawal. Acts by inhibiting the secretion of Substance P, a substance that increases the intensity of propulsive motions in the intestinal wall, from the nervous system.[10] Originally prescribed for "crane's-knee wind," in which one or both knees become swollen, enlarged, painful, and immobile, after long-term dysentery. May cause a loss of sensation in the mouth and tongue.

Caution: Discontinue the formula if fever occurs. Do not use for more than 6 weeks.

Pinellia Decoction to Drain the Epigastrium

Traditional remedy for overdoses of formulas used to treat constipation. Prevents gastrointestinal inflammation by inhibiting cAMP, a chemical that causes inflammation.[11] Stops diarrhea without affecting movement of the intestinal muscles,[12] so does not produce constipation if too much is taken. Prevents diarrhea caused by radiation treatment.[13] Particularly useful in controlling diarrhea caused by the chemotherapy drug irinotecan, which is often severe enough that patients must discontinue therapy.[14]

Caution: Use with caution if fever is present, and discontinue if preexisting fevers worsen.

Tonify the Middle and Augment the Qi Decoction

Treats diarrhea occurring at the beginning of menstrual flow.

True Man's Decoction to Nourish the Organs

Treats unremitting diarrhea to the point of incontinence. In severe cases, there may be prolapsed rectum, and the stool may contain pus and blood. Accompanying symptoms include mild, persistent abdominal pain that responds favorably to local pressure or warmth, lethargy, pale complexion, reduced appetite, soreness of the lower back, and lack of strength in the legs. Not available as a patent medicine, but widely available from TCM practitioners as *zhen ren yang rang tang.*

Caution: Patients taking this formula should avoid alcohol, wheat, cold or raw foods, fish, and greasy foods. Should not be used by persons with gallbladder problems, obstruction of the bile duct, or a tendency to retain urine, or by pregnant women.

White Tiger Decoction

Contains the herb anemarrhena, which kills *Salmonella.*[15] Especially appropriate when symptoms include feelings of cold in the lower part of the body, joint pain, and/or sweating.

Caution: Avoid if nausea or vomiting is present.

CONSIDERATIONS

❑ While antidiarrheal medicines, whether herbal or conventional, are very useful in *treating* diarrhea, using them to *prevent* diarrhea may actually cause the disorder. Diarrhea is the body's natural defense against intestinal infection. Taking herbs or drugs to prevent diarrhea while traveling may "lock in" the infection, giving it a chance to multiply and become strong enough to be uncontrollable by the herbs or drugs. Instead, take care to find safe food and drink while traveling, and use medications only if the need arises.

❑ If diarrhea alternates with constipation, irritable bowel syndrome may be the problem; *see* **Irritable Bowel Syndrome.** *See also* **Allergies, Food.**

EAR INFECTIONS

Thirty million times a year in the United States alone, parents take their young children to the pediatrician for middle ear infections. The middle ear—three small bones behind the eardrum—transmits sound vibrations to the inner ear, which passes them on to nerve endings that carry them to the brain. (The inner ear can also become infected, as can the outer ear.)

Otitis media, or middle ear infection, affects one out of three children in the first three years of their lives,[1] although it can strike older children and adults. Acute otitis media causes earache, chills, fever, and redness and bulging of the eardrum. Chronic infections can cause hearing loss, and complications that include fluid accumulations and acute mastoiditis, an infection of the bone behind the ear.

Upper respiratory infections can cause middle ear infections, as can allergies. Allergies can inflame the eustachian tube, which connects the middle ear and the throat, or they can cause nasal passages to swell, which traps air and secretions in the middle ear. Sensitivity to allergens is increased by low humidity, and exposure to secondhand tobacco smoke and smoke from wood-burning stoves. In the United States, where relatively more babies are bottle-fed, ear infections are very frequently associated with food allergies. Cow's milk stresses a baby's developing immune system. Children who develop recurrent ear infections after infancy are more sensitive to cow's milk than children who do not.[2]

The problem in treating middle ear infections is that the exact cause of the infection is often not identified. As a result, the most commonly prescribed antibiotic, amoxicillin, is no more effective than a placebo in actual use.[3] And some strains of the germs that cause ear infections, such as *Haemophilus influenzae,* do not readily respond to medication.[4] Other bacteria are becoming resistant to

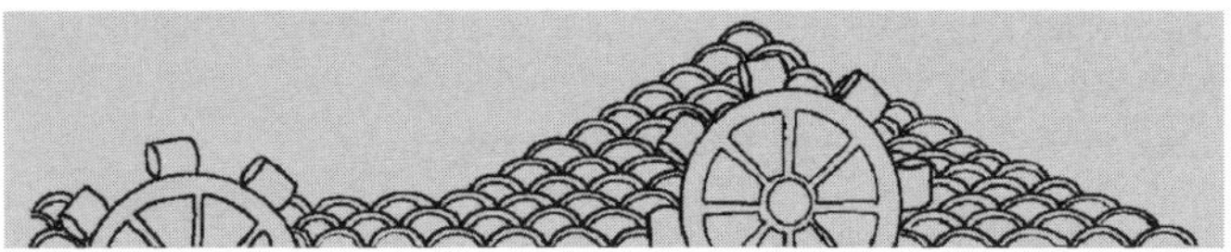

antibiotics, which are often misprescribed. These drug-resistant bacteria affect not only the child in whom they have developed but also any other children who are infected. Viral infections are not affected by antibiotics at all.

Increasingly harsh antibiotics have to be given to control infection. Infections that do not respond to antibiotics are treated with surgery, in which a plastic tube is placed in the ear to help drain fluid. Studies critical of this procedure find that no more than 42 percent of the children who undergo it benefit.[5] Allergy control and herbal medicine together provide a safer, more effective alternative.

The ancient sages of Kampo saw middle ear infection as the invasion of the body by a "seasonal" pathogen. This disease-causing entity caused disease only in certain months of the year. It attacked the body's yang, or outwardly directed, energies, meeting the yang energy in the head. The battle between the body and the infection generated "heat," or fever, and the channeling of defensive energy to the head also caused inflammation of the throat and nose. Over centuries, Kampo refined its understanding of the herbs that treat attacks on yang energies to the herbs that are now known scientifically to stop middle ear infection.

Several Kampo herbs act against the germs that cause ear infections, as does the non-Kampo herb echinacea (see "Understanding Echinacea").

Understanding Echinacea

The non-Kampo herb echinacea is extremely useful for treating ear infections, and is a popular herbal treatment. Echinacea stimulates the production of macrophages, immune-system cells that consume infectious bacteria. However, using echinacea is complicated by the fact that different parts of different species have to be prepared in different ways to maximize their effects on the immune system. The concentrations of active chemicals among species can vary as much as 4,000 percent, depending on what part of each plant is tested.

The easiest way to use echinacea is to use the species *Echinacea angustifolia* for bacterial infections and *E. pallida* for infections of an unknown nature. (A third species, *E. purpurea,* is good for viral infections, but is only effective in the form of alcohol-based tincture, which should not be given to children.) Use flowers, leaves, and stems of *E. angustifolia* to make tea, ¼ to ½ teaspoon (0.5 to 1.0 gram) in ½ cup boiling water. Steep for fifteen to twenty minutes and strain; use three times daily. Use the root of *E. pallida* in either tea form (same directions as *E. angustifolia*) or alcohol-free extract form (follow label directions). Children who are allergic to echinacea can benefit from Kampo.

INDIVIDUAL KAMPO TREATMENTS

See Chapter 3 for discussions of individual herbs, traditional healing substances, and modern herbal preparations, including directions for making tea.

SUGGESTED DOSAGES	COMMENTS
Epimedium (Herb)	
Use as directed by the herbalist.	Used in many Chinese antibacterial formulas. Stimulates the immune system's macrophages, or "germ-eaters," to kill *Streptococcus.*
Garlic (Herb)	
Oil, 1–2 drops in affected ear once daily for up to a week.	Kills *Staphylococcus* and *Streptococcus pneumoniae* infections in the ears, nose, and throat. Can kill some strains that are antibiotic-resistant.[6] Garlic oil can be made at home (see Chapter 3).
Green Tea (Herb)	
Catechin extract, 1 250-mg tablet once daily (child's dosage). or Tea, ½ c once daily (child's dosage). Do not give to a child less than 12 months old.	Helps children with viral middle-ear infections. Also protects against influenza A and B,[7] and helps children with asthma. To avoid dilution problems, do not take tea within 1 hour of taking other teas or patent medicines.
Scutellaria (Herb)	
Fluid extract (1:1), ⅛ tsp (0.5 ml) once daily (child's dosage). Place in a cup and add ¼ c water or juice. or Tea, ¼ c daily (child's dosage). Store in the refrigerator.	Prevents viruses from adhering to cells they would otherwise infect.[8,9] Acts against many strains of *Streptococcus* without stimulating, and potentially exhausting, the immune system. Use herb when viral infections are "going around." *Caution:* Avoid in cases of diarrhea caused by foodborne infection or excessive consumption of cold drinks.

KAMPO FORMULAS

See Chapter 4 for dosage information and discussions of individual formulas.

Gentiana Longdancao Decoction to Drain the Liver

Treats middle ear infections in adults, particularly when accompanied by bitter taste in the mouth, dizziness, headache, hearing loss, irritability, and/or red and sore eyes.

Caution: Should not be used by women who are trying to become pregnant.

Kudzu Decoction

Treats middle ear infections in children and adults. Activates the immune system to fight viral infection. Treats symptoms that include fevers and chills, and stiffness in the neck and upper back.[10] Stops inner ear inflammation caused by food allergies. Seek the advice of the dispensing herbalist on a suitable child's dosage.

CONSIDERATIONS

❑ The process of controlling allergies, and thus reducing the risk of ear infections, begins at a child's birth. The longer a child is breastfed, the less likely ear infections are to be a problem. If a child cannot be or was not breastfed, it is important at least to vary his or her diet as much as possible and avoid giving the same food item every day, especially cow's milk, eggs, and wheat. Some conditions that disrupt digestion are also associated with allergies.[11,12] For more information, *see* **Allergies, Food.**

❑ *See also* **Allergies, Respiratory** and **Asthma.**

Eczema

Eczema is a general term for a pattern of painful skin outbreaks. It causes some areas of skin to become dry, flaky, and red, and other areas to become inflamed, moist, and oozing. In chronic eczema, the cells of the skin may change color, and become thick and scaly. Itching is often quite severe. Eczema leaves the skin open to infection with either *Staphylococcus* (staph) or *Streptococcus* (strep), or to infection with the viruses that cause herpes and warts.

Eczema can stem from an astonishingly broad range of causes, but it is usually the result of either atopic dermatitis or contact dermatitis. *Atopic dermatitis* is a persistent skin condition associated with allergy. Seventy percent of the people who have it also suffer asthma, hay fever, or hives. It can occur anywhere on the body, but is most common on the face, neck, wrists, hands, and eyelids; behind the ears, and in the creases of the groin, knees, and elbows. Atopic dermatitis often starts in childhood, and children with this condition tend to have it over a wider area than adults who develop the disease later in life.

Another chronic form of eczema is *contact dermatitis.* This is a painful, weeping skin reaction caused by contact with an external agent. In North America, the most familiar agents are poison ivy and oak. It can also be caused by other types of plants, as well as perfumes, industrial chemicals, and a variety of other substances.

Both atopic and contact dermatitis cause changes in how the repair mechanism of the skin works. The repair process in the skin is permanently activated, but never completed. Persons with eczema regenerate skin faster than persons without eczema, but the skin never acquires normal immune function.[1]

Standard treatment for eczema consists of use of moisturizers; avoidance of further irritation, such as that caused by drying soaps and hot water; and drug therapy with steroid agents such as hydrocortisone. In short-term use, steroids often stop eczema outbreaks. In long-term use, these drugs can leave the skin fragile and thin, relieving the eczema but increasing the risk of skin breaks and infection. If infection develops, overuse of antibiotics can lead to the development of drug-resistant germs.

The great Kampo theorist Zhang Zhongjing explained eczema as the result of an imbalance between the protective and nutritive energies of the body. When the body was invaded by an outside pernicious influence, or pathogen—in this case, "cold"—the protective energy of the body rushed to the skin to open the pores and purge the infection. In eczema, the protective energies of the body were slightly too weak, so that they opened the pores, but failed to purge the pathogen. At the same time, the nutritive energies of the body were slightly too strong, so that they spilled fluids through the skin. These fluids did not have the energy of protective qi behind them, so they never purged the pernicious influence, or pathogen, causing the disease. Unless herbs were used to reestablish energy balance, eczema became a permanent condition. For best results, herbal medicine should be used with dietary management (see "Managing Eczema Through Diet").

Managing Eczema Through Diet

Dietary eczema control consists of eliminating foods that cause allergies, limiting simple carbohydrates and sugars (including alcohol), and ensuring adequate supplies of the right essential fatty acids. About 75 percent of children's food allergies that contribute to eczema are caused by artificial colors and preservatives, eggs, milk products, peanuts, and tomatoes.[1] Eliminating all these foods, and then resuming them one at a time to see which food aggravates the condition, is the simplest and least disruptive way to manage a child's diet. The sooner allergenic foods are eliminated, the more likely it is that the child will not develop new allergies.[2] (For more information, *see* **Allergies, Food.**)

Adults with eczema are most likely to have food allergies to eggs, milk, peanuts, soy, and/or wheat. Avoiding these food products for an entire year is likely to result in becoming insensitive not only to them but to other food allergens as well.[3] Adults with eczema are also likely to be extremely allergic to the pathogenic yeast *Candida albicans.* Treating yeast infections (*see* **Yeast Infections**) and reducing sugar intake will reduce the body's allergic load and reduce the immune system's hypersensitivity.[4] Reducing sugar consumption has the side benefit of making the intestines less "leaky," and thus less permeable to allergy-causing foods.[5]

Consuming less sugar also leads the body to produce less of an inflammatory hormone called PGE_2. Another way to lower PGE_2 production is by getting enough essential fatty acids (EFAs). There are two classes of these acids, omega-3s and omega-6s, and people with eczema have lower ratios of omega-3s to omega-6s than other people.[6] To provide the needed omega-3 essential fatty acids, take flaxseed oil or fish oil.

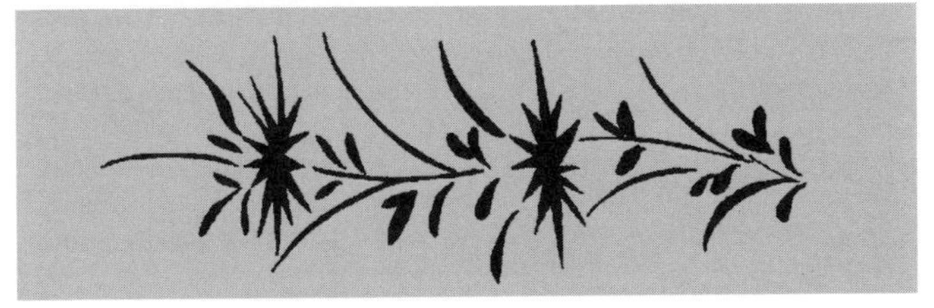

INDIVIDUAL KAMPO TREATMENTS

See Chapter 3 for discussions of individual herbs, traditional healing substances, and modern herbal preparations, including directions for making tea.

SUGGESTED DOSAGES	COMMENTS
Aloe (Herb)	
Gel, either commercial or taken from houseplants, used liberally on the skin.	Contains an anti-inflammatory chemical that is as effective as hydrocortisone without hydrocortisone's detrimental immune-system effects.[2] Can be used *with* hydrocortisone to increase the drug's effectiveness.[3]
Burdock (Herb)	
Cereal from seeds, 1–3 tbsp (3–9 g) once daily. Available in Japanese groceries as *gobi* or *goboshi.* and Dried root, 1–2 tbsp (3–6 g) 3 times daily. or Fluid extract from root (1:1), ½–1 tsp (2–4 ml), 3 times daily. or Powdered solid extract from root (4:1), 2–3 250-mg capsules or tablets 3 times daily. or Tea from root, 1 c up to 6 times daily.	Long used in America, Europe, and Japan for chronic skin diseases, especially eczema. Burdock root contains inulin, which diminishes destruction of skin cells by the immune system.[4] Burdock seed extracts have components that kill both strep and many infectious fungi.[5] *Caution:* Avoid if diarrhea is present.
Dandelion (Herb)	
Fluid extract (1:1), 1–2 tsp (4–8 ml) 3 times daily, preferably on an empty stomach. or Tea, 1 c 3 times daily on an empty stomach.	Detoxifying herb that stimulates the production of bile, which carries cholesterol—the raw material for many inflammatory hormones—into the stool. Do *not* use tincture for this condition.
Forsythia (Herb)	
Tea, 1 c 3 times daily until infection subsides. or Tincture (1:5), 10 drops 3 times daily until infection subsides. Place in a cup, add 2 tbsp water, and take in a single sip.	Acts against staph and many other kinds of bacteria.[6] Also treats inflammation, so is used to treat bacterial infections that enter through cracks in the skin. If there is no improvement in 1 week, see a health care provider.
Ginkgo (Herb)	
Ginkgolide extract, 1 40-mg tablet 4 times daily or 1 60-mg tablet 3 times daily.	Deactivates platelet activating factor (PAF), the chemical messenger that starts allergic reactions.
Green Tea (Herb)	
Catechin extract, 1 240-mg tablet 3 times daily. or Tea, 1 c 3–5 times daily.	Contains flavonoids, which stop allergic reactions, and polyphenols, which act against a wide range of microorganisms. To avoid dilution problems, do not take tea within 1 hour of taking other teas or patent medicines.
Licorice (Herb)	
Topical cream, as needed, no time limit. Simicort is the most widely available brand.	One study found that more eczema sufferers responded to licorice-based creams than to cortisone.[7] Creams are especially useful in treating contact dermatitis caused by poison ivy, oak, or sumac.
PSK (Modern Herbal Preparation)	
Dried extract, 6 1,000-mg tablets daily.	Increases resistance to viral infections that can enter through eczema lesions, especially herpes.[8]
Tang-Kuei (Herb)	
Dried root, 1–2 tsp (1–3 g) daily. or Fluid extract (1:1), ¼–½ tsp (1–2 ml) daily. or Freeze-dried root, 1–2 500-mg capsules daily. or Powdered solid extract (4:1), 250–500 mg daily. or Tea, 1 c daily 2–3 times daily. or Tincture (1:5), 1–1½ tsp (4–6 ml) daily. Place in a cup, add 2 tbsp water, and take in a single sip.	Traditional Chinese herbal treatment for eczema, psoriasis, and vitiligo.[9] Keeps the immune system from attacking the skin at the very beginning of the inflammation process.[10] Also blocks production of inflammation-generating substances called prostaglandins.[11] Long-term use of the herb maintains good skin circulation. Also known as dong quai. *Caution:* Do not exceed recommended dosages; may kill healthy skin cells in overdose.[12] Alcohol tincture inhibits uterine activity and menstrual flow, while other forms have the opposite effect.
Turmeric (Herb)	
Poultice, applied 3 times daily (see Chapter 3 for directions).	Volatile oil has painkilling properties equal to those of steroid preparations such as hydrocortisone and phenylbutazone,[13,14] but without side effects. Do *not* use the turmeric compound curcumin for this disorder. Curcumin does not contain turmeric's volatile oils.

KAMPO FORMULAS

See Chapter 4 for dosage information and discussions of individual formulas.

Kudzu Decoction

Protects eczema-damaged skin from the effects of herpes infection. Especially useful for persons who are HIV-positive, since it blocks tissue-damaging effects of herpes[15] without activating the immune system.

Ledebouriella Powder That Sagely Unblocks

Very helpful in treating eczema; works by preventing allergic hypersensitivity.[16] British studies show that it soothes itching and makes sleeping easier. Relieves eczema in children.[17] Acts "sagely" by not inducing sweating from healthy skin, which could harbor bacteria. Seek the advice of the dispensing herbalist on a suitable child's dosage. Since the formula contains licorice, there are statements in the medical literature that oral preparations of licorice are equivalent to the formula. They are not. In this formula, licorice is a secondary herb used to prevent stomach upset.

Caution: Should not be used by women who are trying to become pregnant, or if nausea or vomiting is present.

CONSIDERATIONS

❑ Eczema is less frequent throughout childhood in children who have been breastfed.[18] A child who cannot be breastfed should be fed as varied a diet as possible instead of being fed the same foods every day. This is especially true of cow's milk, eggs, and wheat, foods that increase the risk of food allergies (see page 146).

❑ If there are silvery, scaly bumps and raised patches of skin, psoriasis may be the problem; *see* **Psoriasis.**

ENDOMETRIAL CANCER

The most common form of uterine cancer affects the lining of the uterus, the endometrium. Endometrial cancer usually strikes after menopause, and its primary warning sign is bleeding (before menopause, bleeding not related to the menstrual period). It can also cause pelvic pain and pain during intercourse.

The growth of endometrial cancer is stimulated by estrogen. Throughout a woman's reproductive life, the lining of the uterus grows and shrinks in response to rising and falling estrogen levels during the menstrual cycle. After menopause, most of the estrogen produced in a woman's body is produced by fat tissue. High-fat diets encourage the development of fat tissue and the production of excess estrogen. (To learn how to reduce estrogen levels through changes in diet, see "Lowering Estrogen Levels Through Diet.")

Endometrial cancer is diagnosed by examining a piece of endometrium, which is usually removed via a biopsy. This cancer is classified into stages 0 and I through IV based on how far it has spread. It generally spreads to other pelvic organs.

The first line of conventional treatment is surgery, usually to remove the uterus, fallopian tubes, and ovaries. If the cancer has spread, chemotherapy or radiation therapy may be used. The doctor may also use hormonal therapy, in which a form of progesterone, another female hormone, is used to counteract the effects of estrogen.

In *Women's Diseases According to Fu Qing-Zhu,* the nineteenth-century Kampo theorist explained endometrial tumors as "cold" taking advantage of the reduced levels of nutrients and energy in the uterus after childbirth. This cold stopped the circulation of blood. The static blood stayed in the womb until, after a period of years, it was eventually transformed into tissue. Endometrial cancer interferes with the circulation of blood and energy in a way that affects other organs, especially the liver and the lungs. Unlike other kinds of cancer that occur in women, this cancer has a highly yin character, or a cancer that contains fat deposits. This reflects the importance of fat to the disease's development.

Several Kampo therapies, including green tea and soy products, lower estrogen levels by providing phytoestrogens, or compounds that act like estrogen within the body without stimulating cancer growth. Other therapies support the immune system and supplement conventional treatments (see considerations below). Always use Kampo as part of a medically directed overall treatment plan for endometrial cancer.

INDIVIDUAL KAMPO TREATMENTS

See Chapter 3 for discussions of individual herbs, traditional healing substances, and modern herbal preparations, including directions for making tea.

Lowering Estrogen Levels Through Diet

A proper diet can reduce lifetime exposure to estrogen, which can reduce the risk of a variety of disorders, including breast cancer, endometriosis, and fibrocystic breast disease. And both proper nutrition and reduced estrogen exposure are important considerations for someone who has or has had an estrogen-influenced disorder. Making the following dietary changes will help reduce estrogen exposure:

• *Reduce calorie intake.* Reducing calorie consumption increases levels of a hormone called SHBG that keeps estrogen from stimulating growth of both healthy and cancerous cells in the breast.[1] And scientists think that calorie reduction has the same effect on other estrogen-influenced disorders. Dieting is not recommended, however, during chemotherapy or radiation treatment.

• *Eat more whole grains, legumes, and berries.* Fiber and lignin from these foods increase the rate at which estrogen is excreted from the body.[2]

• *Cut fat consumption.* Diets that are low in fat do not decrease estrogen production, but do increase estrogen excretion through the urine.[3] Low-fat diets also tend to include a lot of fruits and vegetables, many of which contain compounds, called phytonutrients, that help protect the body against cancer.

• *If overweight, lose weight.* Gradual weight loss after menopause reverses the effects of estrogen overexposure.[4]

• *Use acidophilus supplements.* While the liver breaks down estrogen before sending it to the digestive tract for elimination from the body, bacteria in the intestines can turn these breakdown products back into estrogen. The hormone can then be reabsorbed through the intestinal wall. Using *Lactobacillus acidophilus* supplements can provide the "friendly" microbes that compete with the estrogen-forming bacteria.

SUGGESTED DOSAGES	COMMENTS
Astragalus (Herb)	
Fluid extract (1:1), ¼–½ tsp (1–2 ml) 3 times daily. or Freeze-dried herb in capsules, 500–1,000 mg 3 times daily. or Powdered solid extract (4:1), 250–500 mg 3 times daily. or Tea, 1 c 3 times daily. or Tincture (1:5), 1–1½ tsp (4–6 ml), 3 times daily. Place in a cup, add 2 tbsp water, and take in a single sip. For dosages used with chemotherapy, *see* **Chemotherapy**	**Side Effects.** Slows cancer spread. Increases the ability of immune-system cells called lymphokine-activated killer (LAK) cells to attack cancer tumors, and stimulates other immune-system cells called T cells, which are depleted by the spread of endometrial cancer.
Garlic (Herb)	
Enterically coated tablets, as directed on label (usually at least 900 mg daily). or Raw garlic, 2–3 cloves daily, thoroughly chewed. Recommended form.	Contains compounds that prevent cancer from developing its own blood supply and spreading. Associated with lower rates of estrogen-stimulated cancer.[1] *Caution:* Do not use with the blood-thinner warfarin sodium (Coumadin). Garlic will counteract the effects of *Bifidus* and *Lactobacillus* cultures taken as digestive aids.
Green Tea (Herb)	
Catechin extract, 1 240-mg tablet 3 times daily. or Tea, 1 c 2–3 times daily.	Contains polyphenols, which keep estrogen away from cells of estrogen-dependent tumors.[2] Contains compounds that deactivate plasmin, a substance that breaks up tissues and makes a pathway for invading tumors. Other compounds called catechins help prevent both thyroid cancer caused by radiation treatment and deficiencies in white blood cells caused by mitomycin.[3] Caffeine accelerates cell death and increases effectiveness of radiation therapy. To avoid dilution problems, do not take tea within 1 hour of taking other teas or patent medicines.
PSK (Modern Herbal Preparation)	
Dried extract, 6 1,000-mg tablets daily.	In Japan, has been shown to increase three- and five-year survival rates among women with uterine cancer.[4]
Soy Isoflavones (Modern Herbal Preparation)	
Extract, about 3,000 mg once daily. or Soy germ, 2 tsp (10 g) twice daily, preferably added to cereals or smoothies.	Contains genistein, which inhibits growth of estrogen-dependent cancers.

HERBS TO AVOID

Individuals who have endometrial cancer should avoid the following herbs: cordyceps, dan shen, fennel seed, licorice, peony. For more information regarding these herbs, see Chapter 3.

KAMPO FORMULAS

See Chapter 4 for dosage information and discussions of individual formulas.

Augmented Rambling Powder

Lowers estrogen levels.[5] Traditionally, this formula is used to treat "hot" symptoms, including dry mouth, red eyes, blurry vision, lower abdominal pressure, red eyes, difficult and painful urination, increased menstrual flow, and uterine bleeding.

Cinnamon Twig and Poria Pill

Reduces the amount of estrogen in the bloodstream.[6] Traditionally given to women who are experiencing "cold" symptoms, such as weakness, lack of appetite, and fatigue. Since this formula acts on the ovaries, it will not help women who have had their ovaries removed.

Tang-Kuei and Peony Powder

Decreases estrogen production by the ovaries.[7] Traditionally, symptoms for which this formula is appropriate include easy fatigue, soft muscles, and coldness or poor circulation to the bottom half of the body. Since the formula acts on the ovaries, it will not be helpful for women who have had their ovaries removed.

Two-Cured Decoction

Reduces estrogen levels in women.[8] Traditionally, the symptoms for which this formula was prescribed included coughing large amounts of easily expectorated phlegm, and/or vomiting and nausea.

Caution: Use with caution if fever is present, and discontinue if preexisting fevers worsen.

FORMULAS TO AVOID

Individuals who have endometrial cancer should avoid the following formulas: Peony and Licorice Decoction, and Six-Ingredient Pill With Rehmannia (Rehmannia-Six Combination). For more information regarding these formulas, see Chapter 4.

CONSIDERATIONS

❑ Diets rich in soy products are associated with lower rates of various types of cancer.[9,10] Soy foods include miso and tofu.

❑ To reduce side effects and increase effectiveness when using chemotherapy, *see* **Chemotherapy Side Effects**; when using radiation therapy, *see* **Radiation Therapy Side Effects.** To learn about herbal treatments that can prevent a cancer from developing its own blood supply, *see* **Cancer.**

ENDOMETRIOSIS

Endometriosis is a chronic disease in which tissues that ordinarily develop in the inner layer of the uterine wall are deposited outside the uterus. These tissues form cysts, which may be found in the ovaries, uterine ligaments, fallopian tubes, colon, urethra, bladder, or vagina, and, in rare cases, in the lungs and limbs. More than 12 million American women have endometriosis, which often runs in families.

The main symptom of endometriosis is pain: painful periods, pelvic and lower back pain, ovulatory pain, pain during intercourse. The pain may be barely noticeable, but more often is severe and debilitating. Endometriosis also causes inability to urinate, intestinal discomfort, and infertility. As many as one-third of cases of infertility among menstruating women are caused by endometrial deformities. Because these symptoms are seen in a number of other disorders, an accurate diagnosis is very important.

Like the uterus, endometrial tissue responds to ovarian hormones by building up, breaking down, and bleeding. Endometrial tissues are more receptive to the hormone estrogen, but less receptive to the hormone progesterone.[1] This makes them in effect permanently stuck in the first half of the menstrual cycle, constantly being stimulated to grow and divide by estrogen and never being instructed to stop by progesterone. Endometrial cells also contain an active form of an enzyme known as aromatase.[2] This enzyme converts other hormones into the estrogen that makes endometrial tissues grow.

There are a number of theories as to why endometriosis occurs. They range from the reflux menstruation theory, in which menstrual tissue flows back through the fallopian tubes and into the pelvic cavity, to the fetal defect theory, in which endometrial tissue attaches itself to the wrong body tissues before birth. In addition, there appears to be a link between environmental toxins and endometriosis, since women whose livers are able to effectively detoxify poisons rarely suffer endometriosis.

One way of making estrogen unavailable to endometrial tissue is to surgically remove the tissue. Unfortunately, this usually provides only temporary benefits since the underlying hormonal problems are still there. Surgery can also create painful abdominal adhesions. Laproscopy, in which the doctor removes tissue through a tube passed through a small incision, is often used for diagnostic purposes.

Hormonal therapies are used to stop ovulation and its accompanying hormone production. However, such therapies can produce a wide array of side effects, from stimulating masculinizing changes (such as abnormal hair growth) to nausea, vomiting, vaginal dryness, and mood swings. Production of other hormones can also be affected.

In *Women's Diseases According to Fu Qing-Zhu,* this nineteenth-century Kampo theorist explained endometriosis as "cold" taking advantage of the reduced levels of nutrients and energy in the uterus after childbirth. This cold stopped the circulation of blood. The static blood stayed in the womb until, after a period of years, it was eventually transformed into tissue.

Formulas that stimulate blood circulation became Kampo's mainstay for treating endometriosis. Herbs are used to support liver function and influence hormonal activity. All of these preparations have to be used for at least three months before improvements become noticeable.

INDIVIDUAL KAMPO TREATMENTS

See Chapter 3 for discussions of individual herbs, traditional healing substances, and modern herbal preparations, including directions for making tea.

SUGGESTED DOSAGES	COMMENTS
Dioscorea (Herb)	
Tincture (1:5), 20 drops 3 times daily after meals. Place in a cup, add 2 tbsp water, and take in a single sip.	Treats cramping caused by ovarian cysts.[3] Especially useful for relieving pain that is worsened by doubling over or lying down, but is eased with motion, when stretching out, or bending backwards.[4] Be sure to use an herbal product not mixed with synthetic progesterone.
Green Tea (Herb)	
Catechin extract, 1 240-mg tablet 3 times daily. or Tea, 1 c 2–3 times daily.	Contains compounds that keep inflammatory chemicals called leukotrienes from entering cells.[5] These compounds also stop the production of new fibrous tissue and collagen in endometrial cysts. To avoid dilution problems, do not take tea within 1 hour of taking other teas or patent medicines.
Turmeric (Herb)	
Curcumin, the yellow pigment found in turmeric, 250–500 mg twice daily between meals.	Curcumin stimulates production of an enzyme that both helps the liver deactivate toxins and keeps the liver from activating otherwise harmless chemicals.[6]
Vitex (Herb)	
Tincture (1:5), 1½ tsp (6 ml) 3 times daily. Place in a cup, add 2 tbsp water, and take in a single sip.	Useful when the most prominent symptom is an unusually short period.[7] Increases progesterone secretion, which increases the chance that the endometrial growth cycle will be stopped.

HERBS TO AVOID

Individuals who have endometriosis should avoid the following herbs: cordyceps, dan shen, fennel seed, licorice, and peony. For more information regarding these herbs, see Chapter 3.

KAMPO FORMULAS

See Chapter 4 for dosage information and discussions of individual formulas.

Four-Substance Decoction

Used to treat both fibroids and endometriosis in women who are affected by poor diet or overwork.

Tang-Kuei and Peony Powder

Designed to promote the circulation of blood to its normal channels and release the energies of pent-up emotions from the "liver." Also encourages urination. In modern Japanese medicine, this formula is used for a wide range of conditions that benefit from reduced estrogen production.[8] Reduces the formation of inflammatory compounds in endometrial tissue.[9] Unlike some treatments, this formula does not have a masculinizing effect.[10,11]

FORMULAS TO AVOID

Individuals who have endometriosis should avoid the following formulas: Peony and Licorice Decoction, Ten-Significant Tonic Decoction (All-Inclusive Great Tonifying Decoction). For more information regarding these formulas, see Chapter 4.

CONSIDERATIONS

❑ Since fat produces estrogen, weight loss can reduce estrogen levels. A healthy diet can promote lowered estrogen levels in other ways—see "Lowering Estrogen Levels Through Diet" on page 207.

EPILEPSY

See **Seizure Disorders.**

EYE DISORDERS

Everyone experiences eye trouble at one time or another. Eyes that are bloodshot, blurry, dry, infected, irritated, itchy, sensitive to light, or ulcerated are among the most common health complaints. Chronic eye problems, such as farsightedness, nearsightedness, cataracts, and glaucoma, are usually caused by disorders in the eye itself. Some of these disorders, such as cataracts and glaucoma, are in many cases linked to underlying diseases, such as diabetes or high blood pressure.

The eyeball's tough outer layer is called the sclera, or the "white" of the eye. Beneath the sclera is the middle layer of eye, the choroid, which contains the blood vessels that serve the eye. In the center of the sclera is the highly pigmented iris, and in the center of the iris is the pupil. Behind the iris is the lens. The front of the eye is covered by a transparent membrane called the cornea. At the back of the eye is the retina, a light-sensitive membrane that is connected to the brain by the optic nerve.

The eye contains two important fluids. The aqueous humor, which fills the space between the cornea and the lens, contains all the components of blood except red blood cells. The vitreous humor is a jellylike substance that fills the back of the eyeball, in the space between the lens and the retina.

Some of the more common eye complaints are covered in this section. In addition, a proper diet, especially one that includes natural antioxidants such as beta-carotene and vitamins C and E, can ease or prevent many eye problems. Eat yellow, orange, or dark-green vegetables daily to ensure an adequate supply of these nutrients.

Considerations

❑ *See also* **Cataracts, Conjunctivitis, Diabetic Retinopathy, Glaucoma,** and **Macular Degeneration.**

BAGS BENEATH THE EYES

In the course of aging, the skin and the muscles underlying it can lose tone and sag. When fluids accumulate beneath the flaccid skin, bags beneath the eyes become noticeable. Excessive salt consumption and allergies can also cause bags to form.

Traditional Japanese herbalists regard bags beneath the eyes as an accumulation of blood. The circulation of this blood is energized by the liver, which in turn is weakened by pent-up emotions. Kampo deals with bags under the eyes simply by stimulating blood flow. The underlying imbalance of which they are a symptom may require further treatment.

INDIVIDUAL KAMPO TREATMENTS

See Chapter 3 for discussions of individual herbs, traditional healing substances, and modern herbal preparations, including directions for making tea.

SUGGESTED DOSAGES	COMMENTS
Siberian Ginseng (Modern Herbal Preparation)	
Eleuthero extract, as directed by manufacturer, in 1/4 c water. Be sure to use pure extract, *not* sugar-sweetened ginseng drinks. or Tea, 1 c up to 3 times daily. The recommended form for this disorder.	Relieves puffiness associated with prolonged fatigue. *Caution:* Should be avoided by persons with myasthenia gravis; rheumatoid arthritis and diseases related to it, such as lupus, psoriatic arthritis, and Sjögren's syndrome; or prostate cancer.

KAMPO FORMULAS

See Chapter 4 for dosage information and discussions of individual formulas.

Unblock the Orifices and Invigorate the Blood Decoction

Treats "accumulation of blood" causing swelling or dark circles below the eyes. Also treats dark purple complexion, dizziness, headache, and ringing in the ears.

BLOODSHOT EYES

Bloodshot eyes occur when small blood vessels on the surface of the eye become inflamed. Inflammation of the capillaries on the surface of the eye can be caused by allergies or by exposure to airborne irritant chemicals. Bloodshot eyes can also result from disorders that impair circulation, including diabetes, high blood pressure, and high cholesterol.

Bloodshot eyes are a symptom in literally dozens of the symptom patterns treated with Kampo formulas. In traditional Japanese medicine, red, sore, and bloodshot eyes were thought to be caused by constraints on the flow of blood and energy to the eyes. The flows of nutrients and qi to the eyes was powered by the liver, which could be weakened by constrained anger, excessive consumption of fatty foods and alcohol, or overwork.

Use hawthorn for short-term relief of bloodshot eyes as a single symptom. Use formulas for long-term relief of bloodshot eyes in conjunction with other symptoms.

INDIVIDUAL KAMPO TREATMENTS

See Chapter 3 for discussions of individual herbs, traditional healing substances, and modern herbal preparations, including directions for making tea.

SUGGESTED DOSAGES	COMMENTS
Hawthorn (Herb)	
Dried herb in capsules, 3–5 g daily. or Fluid extract (1:1), ¼–½ tsp (1–2 ml) 3 times daily. or Solid extract, 100–250 mg 3 times daily. Should be standardized to contain 10% proanthocyanidins. or Tea, ⅔ c 3–4 times daily. or Tincture (1:5), 1–1½ tsp (4–6 ml) 3 times daily. Place in a cup, add 2 tbsp water, and take in a single sip.	Contains natural antihistamines called histadine decarboxylase blockers.[1] Helps strengthen the blood vessels supplying the surface of eye. Reduces vascular response to emotional tension.

KAMPO FORMULAS

See Chapter 4 for dosage information and discussions of individual formulas.

Augmented Rambling Powder

Relieves bloodshot eyes during premenstrual syndrome by reducing the body's production of estrogen.[2] Used to treat "hot" symptoms, including bloodshot eyes, blurry vision, difficult or painful urination, increased menstrual flow, and uterine bleeding.

Caution: Should not be used by women who are trying to become pregnant.

Cimicifuga and Kudzu Decoction

Relieves bloodshot eyes caused by allergies. Especially appropriate when additional symptoms include coughing, general body aches, rash, sneezing, and/or tearing.

Considerations

❑ *See also* **Allergies, Respiratory; Diabetes; Hangover; High Blood Pressure;** and **High Cholesterol.**

BLURRED VISION

Vision can become blurred for any number of reasons. Chronically blurred vision is usually caused by common eye defects such as farsightedness, nearsightedness, or astigmatism. Disturbances of the fluid balance in the eye can also cause blurred vision. These disturbances may be limited to the eye itself, as in eyestrain and excessive tearing, or they may reflect disturbances in fluid balance throughout the body, as in diabetes, high blood pressure, and premenstrual syndrome.

Kampo explains blurred vision as resulting from either too much energy flowing to the eyes or too little energy flowing out of the eyes. The eyes lie on the energy channels controlled by the liver. When the liver is disabled by pent-up emotion, excessive consumption of alcohol, or overwork, it cannot supply the eyes with the energy they need. These kinds of disruptions to the liver cause long-term blurred vision. In conditions requiring circulation of an unusually large amount of blood, such as during the menstrual period, the liver may be temporarily unable to supply the eyes with energy. If this is the root disturbance, blurred vision will be periodic rather than permanent.

INDIVIDUAL KAMPO TREATMENTS

See Chapter 3 for discussions of individual herbs, traditional healing substances, and modern herbal preparations, including directions for making tea.

SUGGESTED DOSAGES	COMMENTS
Black Cohosh (Herb)	
Dried root, 2–6 500-mg capsules daily. or Fluid extract (1:1), ¼–½ tsp (1–2 ml) daily. or Freeze-dried root, 1–2 500-mg capsules daily. or Powdered solid extract (4:1), standardized for 27-deoxyacteine, 1–2 250-mg tablets daily. or Tincture (1:5), 1–1½ tsp (4–6 ml) once daily. Place in a cup, add 2 tbsp water, and take in a single sip.	Relieves blurred vision caused by fluid imbalance during premenstrual syndrome.[1] May be necessary to take the herb for 2–3 months before results are obvious.

KAMPO FORMULAS

See Chapter 4 for dosage information and discussions of individual formulas.

Augmented Four-Substance Decoction

Treats blurred vision that occurs with high blood pressure, migraine, or premenstrual syndrome.

Four-Substance Decoction

Treats blurred vision that occurs during emotional tension or premenstrual syndrome. May be necessary to take the formula for 2 to 3 months to notice results.

Gastrodia and Uncaria Decoction

Treats blurred vision caused by high blood pressure.

Caution: Should not be used by women who are trying to become pregnant.

Considerations

❑ *See also* **Diabetes, High Blood Pressure,** and **Premenstrual Syndrome.**

FLOATERS

Floaters are clear flecks that move slowly through the visual field. They are caused by the accumulation of debris in the vitreous humor of the eye, and increase with age.

Kampo explains floaters as concretions of energy that did not pass through normal channels out of the eye. As a relatively minor symptom, floaters go away when circulation is restored.

INDIVIDUAL KAMPO TREATMENTS

See Chapter 3 for discussions of individual herbs, traditional healing substances, and modern herbal preparations, including directions for making tea.

SUGGESTED DOSAGES	COMMENTS
Bupleurum (Herb)	
Saikosaponin extract, 1 300-mg tablet daily. or Tea, 1 c 3 times daily.	Contains compounds that reduce "leakage" from blood vessels into the vitreous humor. *Caution:* Do not use if fever is present. Occasionally causes mild stomach upset. If this happens, reduce the dose. Do not take bupleurum when taking antibiotics.
Ginkgo (Modern Herbal Preparation)	
Ginkgolide extract, 1 40-mg tablet 3 times daily or 1 60-mg tablet twice daily. Increasing dosage to 160 mg (4 40-mg tablets) or 180 mg (3 60-mg tablets) may give increased relief.	Increases microcirculation in the eye, which increases oxygen supply to the retina.
Ligustrum (Herb)	
Tea, 1 c daily.	Contains compounds that reduce "leakage" from blood vessels into the vitreous humor. *Caution:* Avoid if there is diarrhea marked by undigested food in the stool.
Tang-Kuei (Herb)	
Dried root, 1–2 tsp (1–3 g) daily. or Fluid extract (1:1), ¼–½ tsp (1–2 ml) daily. or Freeze-dried root, 1–2 500-mg capsules daily. or Powdered solid extract (4:1), 250–500 mg daily. or Tea, 1 c 2–3 times daily. or Tincture (1:5), 1–1½ tsp (4–6 ml) daily. Place in a cup, add 2 tbsp water, and take in a single sip.	Strengthens the capillaries that supply the eye. Useful in relieving floaters and other symptoms of premenstrual syndrome. Also known as dong quai.

Considerations

❑ Flashing lights and flying sparks are not floaters. When they are accompanied by severe headache and/or a sensation of a curtain falling over the field of vision, they are a symptom of migraine headache. When they occur after an injury to the eye or a blow to the head, they may be symptoms of detached retina. A detached retina requires *immediate* medical attention.

FIBROCYSTIC BREAST DISEASE

Fibrocystic breast disease is marked by the presence of round or oval lumps and/or cysts in the breast. Cysts are soft to firm in texture. Fibrous lumps are rubbery and move freely beneath the skin. These growths are frequently painful, usually in the week or so before menstruation begins. Of the women who have premenstrual syndrome, 20 to 40 percent also have lumpy breasts.

Up to 80 percent of all women have some degree of fibrocystic breast disease, which often goes undetected.[1] While the condition has been associated with a somewhat increased risk for breast cancer, most breast lumps are *not* cancerous. Any breast abnormality, though, should be examined by a doctor.

Fibrocystic breast disease is a progressive condition. A woman in her late teens might start out with a few lumps that become tender before her period begins. As she ages, the breasts become lumpier and more painful. Finally, as she reaches menopause, the discomfort becomes erratic.

Fibrocystic breast disease occurs when the body produces either too much estrogen or too little progesterone, the two main hormones that control the menstrual cycle. Estrogen stimulates tissue growth in the first half of the cycle. Progesterone regulates such growth in the second half. When a woman's body produces more estrogen than progesterone, stimulation exceeds regulation, and breast tissue grows. If a woman's breast cells are also genetically coded to have more estrogen receptors than usual, fibrocystic disease develops.

Fibrocystic breast cells are also affected by other hormones. These include aromatase, which converts testosterone into estrogen, and PGE_2, which makes aromatase more active.[2] Emotional stress and a diet that is high in simple sugar and undesirable fats stimulates this hormonal overactivity, which includes increased estrogen production.

Conventional treatment consists of surgery to either drain or remove cysts. Unfortunately, this usually provides only temporary benefits since the underlying hormonal problems still exist. Hormonal therapy is designed to turn off the growth cycle initiated by estrogen. This often works, although some hormonal treatments may have masculinizing side effects, such as the growth of facial and body hair.

Kampo's traditional explanation of fibrocystic breast disease was that it was caused by an imbalance in the liver. The condition arose when the energy of the liver was constrained and the blood was deficient. When the liver was constrained, usually as a result of emotional tension or bad diet, it could not send its energy upward through the body. Neither could the liver release blood to circulate energy in the rest of the body. Energy gradually built up along the energy channels the liver controls, both of which pass directly over the breast. This energy could be transformed into clumps. The liver could also be constrained by the effects of a rich diet.

Modern science has confirmed that Kampo herbs and formulas treat this condition by reducing estrogen production or by making cells less receptive to estrogen. Kampo practitioners have traditionally prescribed a simple diet for women who have fibrocystic breast disease. Indeed, diet is an important factor in controlling the discomfort this disorder produces (see "Diet Items to Avoid, Supplements to Take for Fibrocystic Breast Disease").

Diet Items to Avoid, Supplements to Take for Fibrocystic Breast Disease

Chocolate, coffee, caffeinated medications (such as certain antifatigue pills), cola drinks, and tea all contain methylxanthines, chemicals that are closely related to caffeine. These chemicals stimulate the production of new fibrous tissue and increase the amount of fluid within cysts. Clinical studies find that virtually all women with fibrocystic breast disease who give up foods and beverages containing methylxanthines improve. Even just reducing consumption helps. The benefits of eliminating these compounds from the diet are greatest in women who are under emotional stress, since the stress hormone cortisol increases the hormonal activity induced by caffeine in fibrocystic breast tissue.[1] Avoiding caffeine may further reduce the already-low risk of breast cysts becoming cancerous. Cysts that become cancerous are highly receptive to adrenal hormones, the production of which is stimulated by caffeine.[2]

Scientists have long known that women with fibrocystic breast disease tend to have low blood concentrations of vitamins A, C, and E.[3] Scientists believe that vitamin A causes fibrocystic breast cells to become less responsive to estrogen.[4] Taking enough vitamin A to affect this disorder can cause headache, and can cause serious birth defects if taken during pregnancy. Fortunately, supplements of beta-carotene, vitamin A's precursor, provide the benefits without the side effects at a dosage of 50,000 IU daily.[5] Vitamin E protects breast tissue against toxins called free radicals. There are studies that both support and contradict the use of vitamin E for fibrocystic breast disease. However, the studies that support its use have used a fairly large dosage of 600 IU a day. Vitamin C is primary useful for chemically recharging vitamin E. A balanced, healthy diet provides enough to recharge E.

INDIVIDUAL KAMPO TREATMENTS

See Chapter 3 for discussions of individual herbs, traditional healing substances, and modern herbal preparations, including directions for making tea.

SUGGESTED DOSAGES	COMMENTS
Ginger (Herb)	
Compresses, applied every 2–6 hours until pain subsides (see Chapter 3 for directions).	Traditional Japanese remedy for breast pain. Works by counteracting chemicals called interleukins,[3] which speed the conversion of other hormones to estrogen within the breast.
Green Tea (Herb)	
Catechin extract, 1 240-mg tablet 3 times daily. or *Decaffeinated* tea, 1 c up to 4 times daily.	Contains polyphenols, which block estrogen from attachment points on cysts.[4] Also contains catechins, which counteract collagenase, a cyst secretion that allows the cyst to break through surrounding tissues.[5] To avoid dilution problems, do not take tea within 1 hour of taking other teas or patent medicines.
Kelp (Herb)	
Kelp as food, any quantity desired.	May be responsible for low rates of fibrocystic breast disease in Japan, where it is a dietary staple. Use of kelp increases the rate at which stool passes through the intestines. This lowers the risk that estrogens in the stool can be reabsorbed back into the bloodstream. Is also a rich source of iodine. Women who are deficient in iodine (a rare occurrence) have breast tissue that is very sensitive to estrogen. *Caution:* Limit consumption to once a week. Persons who are iodine deficient should consult a Kampo or TCM practitioner for dosage advice.
Kudzu (Herb)	
Dried extract, 1 10-mg tablet 3 times daily. or Tea, 1 c 3 times daily. or Use soy isoflavone extract (see **Soy Isoflavones**).	Contains compounds called isoflavones. Daidzen blocks estrogen from attachment points on cysts.[6] Genistein reduces bloodstream estrogen levels.[7]
Soy Isoflavones (Modern Herbal Preparation)	
Extract, about 3,000 mg once daily. or Soy germ, 2 tsp (10 g) twice daily, preferably added to cereals or smoothies.	Contains daidzein and genistein (see **Kudzu**). If concentrated isoflavones cause upset stomach, use kudzu.

HERBS TO AVOID

Individuals who have fibrocystic breast disease should avoid the following herbs: cordyceps, dan shen, fennel seed, licorice, and peony. For more information regarding these herbs, see Chapter 3.

KAMPO FORMULAS

See Chapter 4 for dosage information and discussions of individual formulas.

Augmented Rambling Powder

Lowers estrogen levels in the bloodstream.[8] Traditionally, this formula is used to treat "hot" symptoms, including dry mouth, red eyes, blurry vision, lower abdominal pressure, difficult and painful urination, increased menstrual flow, and uterine bleeding.

Caution: Should not be used by women who are trying to become pregnant.

Tang-Kuei and Peony Powder

Designed to promote the circulation of blood to its normal channels and release the energies of pent-up emotions from the "liver." Also encourages urination. In modern Japanese medicine, this formula is used for a wide range of conditions that benefit from reduced estrogen production.[9] In fibrocystic breast disease, used to stop cyclical growth of tissues. Unlike some treatments, this formula does not have a masculinizing effect.[10,11]

Two-Cured Decoction

Reduces estrogen levels in women with fibrocystic breast disease.[12] Traditionally, the symptoms for which this formula was prescribed included coughing large amounts of easily expectorated phlegm, and/or vomiting and nausea.

Caution: Use with caution if fever is present, and discontinue if preexisting fevers worsen.

FORMULAS TO AVOID

Individuals who have fibrocystic breast disease should avoid the following formulas: Peony and Licorice Decoction, Six-Ingredient Pill With Rhemannia (Rhemannia-Six Combination). For more information regarding these formulas, see Chapter 4.

CONSIDERATIONS

❑ Taking birth control pills that contain a high percentage of estrogen can aggravate fibrocystic breast disease.

❑ Since fat produces estrogen, weight loss can reduce estrogen levels. A healthy diet can promote lowered estrogen levels in other ways—see "Lowering Estrogen Levels Through Diet" on page 207.

❑ *See also* **Premenstrual Syndrome.**

FIBROIDS (UTERINE MYOMAS)

Up to a third of all women over age thirty-five have benign uterine growths known as fibroids or myomas.[1] A fibroid is a well-defined, solid growth in the myometrium, or smooth muscle, supporting the uterus. Fibroids vary in size, from that of the period at the end of this sentence to that of a cantaloupe. Multiple fibroids may occur.

In many of the women who have them, fibroids produce no symptoms. The first symptom may be either pain at the beginning of the period or increased menstrual flow. A fibroid may be forced partially through the cervix, lose its blood supply, and die, resulting in a foul odor. Fibroids usually do not interrupt the menstrual cycle, but as they grow they may cause increased frequency of urination, bladder displacement, urinary retention, and constipation.[2] They can also cause infertility or miscarriage.

Fluctuations in levels of estrogen and progesterone, the two main female hormones, influence fibroids. Fibroid growth, like that of all uterine tissue, is stimulated by estrogen. Estrogen replacement therapy for menopause or the estrogen production that occurs in pregnancy causes the fibroid growth rate to increase. After menopause, when a woman's body produces as much as 80 percent less estrogen, fibroids shrink. And while all uterine tissue responds to estrogen, fibroid tissue is extra-sensitive to progesterone.[3]

In addition to estrogen and progesterone, a third factor, basic fibroblast growth factor (bFGF), determines whether fibroids will grow large enough to cause infertility or other significant symptoms. bFGF is a hormonelike compound that enables fibroids to grow. It interacts with estrogen and progesterone to become especially active just after ovulation, in the middle of the menstrual cycle.[4]

Uterine bleeding is a symptom of a number of different disorders, including cervical and uterine cancer, and so must always be brought to a doctor's attention. Small fibroids may not need treatment, although they should be checked on a regular basis. Doctors are more likely to treat large and actively growing fibroids that are causing extensive bleeding.

Conventional treatment options include drugs and surgery. Drugs are used to reduce estrogen levels. Such drugs can cause a number of side effects, including nausea and masculinizing changes, such as abnormal hair growth. Surgery has traditionally meant hysterectomy, or removal of the entire uterus. Fibroids that are removed without hysterectomy tend to come back. Surgical alternatives to total hysterectomy are relatively new, and are not always successful in the long term.

In *Women's Diseases According to Fu Qing-Zhu,* the nineteenth-century Kampo theorist explained uterine fibroids as "cold" taking advantage of the reduced levels of nutrients and energy in the uterus after childbirth. This cold stopped the circulation of blood. The static blood stayed in the womb until, after a period of years, it was eventually transformed into tissue.

Kampo herbs are used to control bleeding, and to control both estrogen and bFGF levels. While treatments used to control bleeding can work quite quickly, those that control hormone levels usually bring noticeable results in approximately three months. Formulas relieve fibroids by balancing the body's production of estrogen, and relieve combinations of symptoms in three to six months of use. Herbal treatment also stimulates the liver to change estrogen from a more active to less active form. Consult a health care provider before using Kampo with prescription medications. In addition, see "Lowering Estrogen Levels Through Diet" on page 207.

INDIVIDUAL KAMPO TREATMENTS

See Chapter 3 for discussions of individual herbs, traditional healing substances, and modern herbal preparations, including directions for making tea.

SUGGESTED DOSAGES	COMMENTS
Black Cohosh (Herb)	
Dried root, 2–6 500-mg capsules daily. or Fluid extract (1:1), ¼–½ tsp (1–2 ml) daily. or Freeze-dried root, 1–2 500-mg capsules daily. or Powdered solid extract (4:1), standardized for 27-deoxyacteine, 1–2 250-mg tablets daily. or Tincture (1:5), 1–1½ tsp (4–6 ml) once daily. Place in a cup, add 2 tbsp water, and take in a single sip.	Regulates estrogen levels by reducing estrogen activity when levels are high and stimulating production when levels are low. Has been used by American physicians to treat uterine bleeding for over 200 years.[5] Treats uterine pain with a feeling of fullness and weight, and also relieves leg pain.[6]
Cinnamon (Herb)	
Oil, 5–10 drops every 15 mins, up to 4 hours or until bleeding subsides. Place in a cup, add 2 tbsp water, and take in a single sip.	Stops uterine bleeding. Long used in American medicine for this purpose.
Dan Shen (Herb)	
Tincture. Use only under professional supervision.	Treats congealed or stuck blood, dark red clots during menses, and pelvic congestion.[7] *Caution:* Will stop fibroid bleeding, but does increase bloodstream estrogen levels.[8] Therefore, do *not* use on an ongoing basis.
Reishi (Modern Herbal Preparation)	
Dried extract, 3 1-g tablets 3 times daily. or Syrup, as directed on label. or Tincture (1:5), 1 tbsp (10 ml) 3 times daily. Place in a cup, add 2 tbsp water, and take in a single sip.	Keeps the uterine lining from making bFGF and inflammation-causing histamine.[9] Has been shown in laboratory studies to be especially beneficial for patients who do not have severe loss of function in the liver, which processes estrogen into less active forms.[10] In Oriental medicine, reishi is most useful in persons whose "liver" symptoms are compounded by emotional stress or ongoing tension.

HERBS TO AVOID

Individuals who have fibroids should avoid the following herbs: cordyceps, fennel seed, licorice, and peony. For more information regarding these herbs, see Chapter 3.

KAMPO FORMULAS

See Chapter 4 for dosage information and discussions of individual formulas.

Augmented Rambling Powder

Lowers estrogen levels,[11] reducing fibroid growth rate. Traditionally, this formula is used to treat "hot" symptoms, including dry mouth, red eyes, blurry vision, lower abdominal pressure, red eyes, difficult and painful urination, increased menstrual flow, and uterine bleeding.

Caution: Should not be used by women who are trying to become pregnant.

Cinnamon Twig and Poria Pill

Reduces growth of abnormal uterine tissue by reducing the amount of estrogen in the bloodstream.[12] Has been found in laboratory studies not to interfere with the menstrual cycle or to encourage weight gain.[13] Not effective on fibroids that have created a secondary blood supply by attaching to adhesions.

Four-Substance Decoction

Used to treat both fibroids and endometriosis in women who are affected by poor diet or overwork.

Tang-Kuei and Peony Powder

Reduces bloodstream estrogen levels. In modern Japanese medicine, this formula is used for a wide range of conditions that benefit from reduced estrogen production. Unlike some treatments, does not have a "masculinizing" effect.[14,15] Also reduces the formation of inflammatory compounds in the uterus.[16]

FORMULAS TO AVOID

Individuals who have fibroids should avoid the following formulas: Peony and Licorice Decoction, and Six-Ingredient Pill With Rhemannia (Rehmannia-Six Combination). For more information regarding these formulas, see Chapter 4.

CONSIDERATIONS

❑ Progesterone-based drugs, such as the Pill, aggravate uterine fibroids.

❑ Products made with dioscorea, or wild yam, are used by many women to treat menopausal symptoms. Such creams have no detrimental effects on uterine fibroids, and may actually stop bleeding and pain. However, many "dioscorea" creams on the market contain progesterone that is not identified on the label, and which stimulates fibroid growth. Either use dioscorea by itself (see **Dioscorea** in Chapter 3), or use creams that are certified not to contain added progesterone.

❑ Alcohol and caffeine consumption can interfere with liver function, preventing the liver from acting on estrogen. Using vitamin B supplements can help support liver function.

❑ Since fat produces estrogen, weight loss can reduce estrogen levels. A healthy diet can promote lowered estrogen levels in other ways—see "Lowering Estrogen Levels Through Diet" on page 207.

FLATULENCE

See **Indigestion.**

FOOD ALLERGIES

See **Allergies, Food.**

GALLSTONES

The gallbladder is a small, pear-shaped organ located beneath the liver on the right side of the abdomen. It stores bile, a yellow-brown fluid produced by the liver, and secretes bile into the small intestine to help digest fats. The gallbladder is connected to the liver and the small intestine by a series of tubes known as the bile ducts. In roughly 10 percent of the North American population, or 30 million people, these tubes are blocked by hard, crystal-like structures called gallstones. People are more likely to develop gallstones as they age, and women are more prone to them than men.

About 80 percent of all gallstones are made primarily of cholesterol. They form when the bile contains too much cholesterol and not enough bile salts. Cholesterol stones may also form when the gallbladder fails to empty frequently enough, or when the liver fails to secrete certain proteins into the bile.

Other factors play a role in gallstone formation, but the exact cause is not clear. Obesity is a risk factor, probably because of excess cholesterol and because the pressure that fat tissue places on the gallbladder interferes with normal emptying. Very rapid, low-calorie diets also are frequently associated with gallstone formation. Additionally, increased levels of estrogen, such as those seen during pregnancy, or from hormone replacement therapy or hormonal contraceptives, are related to an increased risk of stones.

Gallstone attacks frequently follow a large, fatty meal after a period of fasting. The pain associated with gallstones, steady and severe, is located in the upper abdomen. The pain may last from one to four hours, and then be followed by a residual mild ache or soreness that may persist for a day or so. Nausea and vomiting frequently accompany gallstone attacks, and blood tests will show elevated amounts of the liver pigment bilirubin. Most people, though, have "silent stones," or stones that cause no symptoms.

Fever or chills with a gallstone attack indicate an underlying problem that requires medical attention. Fewer than 2 percent of all persons who have gallstones, however, will require surgery in any given year, and 95 percent of them will be treated with gallstone lithotripsy, in which sound waves are used to break up the stone. People with silent stones detected during routine physicals are usually given cholesterol-lowering medications.

For centuries Kampo medicine has regarded gallstones as "clumps" of heat, generated by the liver, that lodge in the gallbladder, much in the same way that bile acids can "clump" to form stones. In Kampo, however, gallstones are only one aspect of heat in the symptom pattern. Other "heat" generated by the liver is forced to flow upward in the body, producing nausea, headache, blurred vision, and skin discoloration. Gallstone treatments first break up the concentrations of pathological energy that block the bile duct, and then cause the liver's energy to flow in its normal, downward course.

Herbs used in gallstone treatment relieve the symptoms of *cholecystitis,* or gallbladder irritation, which include muscle spasms, pain, and general tension. Generally, herbs should *not* be used when there are actual stones. Kampo formulas relieve the underlying causes of gallstone formation.[1]

INDIVIDUAL KAMPO TREATMENTS

See Chapter 3 for discussions of individual herbs, traditional healing substances, and modern herbal preparations, including directions for making tea.

SUGGESTED DOSAGES	COMMENTS
Gentian (Herb)	
Capsules, as directed on label. Use to avoid bitter taste of other forms.	Treats fiery inflammation of the gallbladder causing intense discomfort. Stimulates bile flow, and also triggers a nerve reflex that promotes the secretion of gastric juice and saliva.[2] *Caution:* Avoid if there is diarrhea with undigested food in the stool.
Peppermint (Herb)	
Oil, enterically coated capsules, 200 mg 3 times daily. or Tea, 1 c 3 times daily between or after meals.	Relieves *mild* spasms of the bile ducts by relaxing the smooth muscles lining them.[3] *Caution:* Should not be used during *acute* gallbladder attacks in which the bile duct may be blocked.
Zanthoxylum (Herb)	
Use as a plaster directly over the painful area (see Chapter 3).	Temporarily relieves pain and spasms of the bile ducts without stimulating bile production. *Caution:* Do not take internally for gallbladder inflammation.

HERBS TO AVOID

Individuals who have gallstones should avoid gardenia and schisandra. For more information regarding these herbs, see Chapter 3.

KAMPO FORMULAS

See Chapter 4 for dosage information and discussions of individual formulas.

Frigid Extremities Powder

Used in Japan to treat gallbladder inflammation and gallstones when symptoms include coldness in the fingers and toes, abdominal pain, diarrhea, and a sensation of fullness in the chest.

Gentiana Longdancao Decoction to Drain the Liver

Traditional remedy for inflammation of the gallbladder and liver. Prescribed in Japan and China for the treatment of cholecystitis, gallstones, and symptoms that may include bitter taste in the mouth, dizziness, hearing loss, irritability, pain in the area of the gallbladder, red and sore eyes, and short temper.

Caution: Should not be used by women who are trying to become pregnant.

Major Bupleurum Decoction

Reduces concentration of cholesterol in the bile, inhibiting the formation of gallstones.[4] Controls symptoms of gallbladder disease, including alternating fever and chills, bitter taste in the mouth, nausea, continuous vomiting, burning diarrhea or no bowel movements, despondency, fullness in the chest and upper sides of the abdomen with or without pain, and irritability.

Caution: Use with caution if fever is present. Discontinue if preexisting fevers worsen.

CONSIDERATIONS

❑ Eat a low-fat diet. Fat digestion places stress on the gallbladder.

GASTRITIS

Gastritis is a group of diseases that causes acid inflammation of the stomach lining. Gastritis differs from peptic ulcer in that it does not usually result in a wound in the stomach wall, and seldom causes much bleeding. Like peptic ulcer, however, gastritis generates nausea, vomiting, and pain in the pit of the stomach or the upper abdomen.

For purposes of treatment, it is useful to think of gastritis as acute or chronic. Acute gastritis occurs immediately when an irritating chemical enters the stomach. The most common culprits are aspirin and nonsteroidal anti-inflammatory drugs (NSAIDs), such as ibuprofen. (These drugs can also cause chronic gastritis.) Such drugs are toxic to the stomach lining. Sometimes the irritating chemical is histamine, which is produced by the body itself. Severe burns, major surgery, respiratory failure, and trauma induce the body to produce huge amounts of stress hormones, which overwhelm the normal functioning of the stomach lining. In addition, radiation therapy can damage the lining.

Fortunately, most cases of acute gastritis respond to antacids and antihistamines, usually given around the clock until symptoms subside. In as little as forty-eight hours the stomach lining begins to regenerate itself, and the crisis usually passes.

Chronic gastritis is more difficult to treat. Sometimes gastritis is the body's response to an infection with *Helicobacter pylori.* In the early stages of infection, the body attempts to flush the infection out of the stomach by increasing production of gastric acids. The bacterium is highly acid resistant, however, and burrows into the stomach wall. Once the infection is established, it actually reduces acid production in the stomach for up to a year, which can create the low-acid conditions in which other viral or fungal infections can flourish. When the stomach regains its ability to produce acid, the gastritis becomes worse instead of better.

The basic medical treatment for chronic gastritis is bismuth, better known as Pepto-Bismol. Doctors usually prescribe a combination of both bismuth and antibiotics, such as amoxicillin, for up to two months.

Kampo's basic understanding of gastritis is that it is a disturbance of the "liver," not the stomach. The liver stores the physical energy generated by emotions. When this energy is not expressed freely, the liver over-controls the digestive process, stimulating the production of digestive juices when they are not needed. Concurrent symptoms, such as breast pain and blurred vision, may also appear along the liver's energy channels, which pass over the breasts and eyes.

Kampo also recognizes gastritis as a symptom of infection. The "invading cold" that causes gastritis simultaneously causes both excess and deficiency. The invading infection produces "heat," which "solidifies" with masses of undigested food in the stomach. The heat also disrupts the stomach's ability to produce its own energy, which powers the movement of food and water downward in the digestive tract. This disruption causes vomiting. The simultaneous presence of deficiency and excess causes gurgling, and excess in the stomach leads to pain.

Modern scientific research has revealed that some herbs act against *H. pylori.* These herbs augment the effects of bismuth, and can be used to replace amoxicillin in cases of amoxicillin allergy. Formulas address the underlying imbalances that predispose the body to gastritis. Chinese studies have found that using Kampo and conventional medicine together increases the cure rate for chronic gastritis from 23 to 84 percent.[1] Treating both the infection and the energy imbalances underlying it offers the greatest chance of success.

INDIVIDUAL KAMPO TREATMENTS

See Chapter 3 for discussions of individual herbs, traditional healing substances, and modern herbal preparations, including directions for making tea.

SUGGESTED DOSAGES	COMMENTS
Coptis (Herb)	
Dried herb, 1 500-mg capsule 3 times daily. or Tincture (1:5), 20 drops 3 times daily. Place in a cup, add 2 tbsp water, and take in a single sip.	Contains berberine, which kills *Helicobacter pylori.*[2] *Caution:* Do not use during pregnancy or on a daily basis for more than 2 weeks at a time. Do not use with supplements that contain vitamin B_6 or the amino acid histidine.
Ginseng (Herb)	
Fluid extract or tincture, as directed on label. or Tea, made with Korean or red ginseng, 1 c daily.	Only effective when there are "cold" symptoms, such as fatigue, listlessness, and pale skin. Stimulates stomach-acid production. If using ginseng extracts or tinctures (which are not as therapeutically active as teas), be sure the product contains *Panax ginseng.* Note that strength may vary by manufacturer. *Caution:* Will make gastritis with "hot" symptoms, such as agitation and sweating, worse.

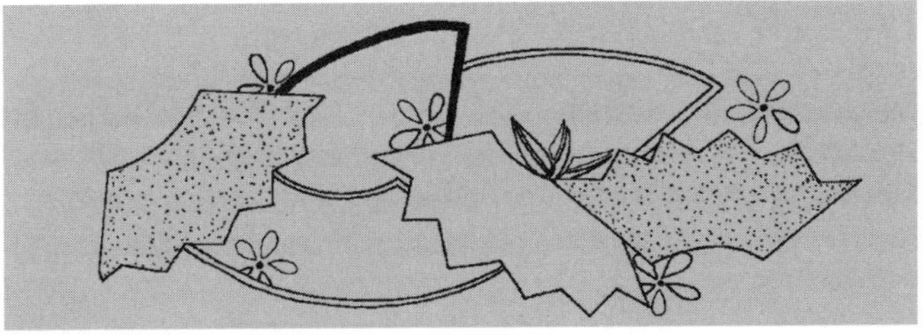

Licorice (Herb)	
Glycyrrhizin extract, 200–600 mg daily, depending on severity of symptoms for up to 6 weeks. Resume after a 2-week break. or Tea, 1 c 1–5 times daily for up to 6 weeks. Resume after a 2-week break.	Stops the production of inflammatory hormones. Avoid deglycyrrhizinated licorice (DGL). *Caution:* Avoid if high blood pressure is present. Also avoid if an estrogen-sensitive disorder is present, such as bladder cancer, melanoma, or disorders of the female reproductive system.

KAMPO FORMULAS

See Chapter 4 for dosage information and discussions of individual formulas.

Augmented Rambling Powder

Treats gastritis with "liver" symptoms caused by emotional stress, such as migraine, eye pain, skin outbreaks on the cheeks, and pain or tenderness in the breasts.

Caution: Should not be used by women who are trying to become pregnant.

Bupleurum Plus Dragon Bone and Oyster Shell Decoction

Treats gastritis with "liver" symptoms caused by emotional stress in cases in which constipation or swelling exists, and there is a sense of heaviness elsewhere in the body.

Caution: Be sure the formula does *not* include the traditional ingredient minium (lead oxide). Use with caution if fever is present, and discontinue if preexisting fevers worsen.

Evodia Decoction

Treats recurrent gastritis with severe pain. Symptom pattern includes diarrhea and vomiting with cold hands and feet, dry heaves or spitting of clear fluids with headache at the crown of the head, and vomiting immediately after eating with acid regurgitation.

Five-Accumulation Powder

Stops belching and reflux in mild gastritis. Sometimes given first so the patient can take another formula more specific to the symptom pattern.

Caution: Use with caution if fever is present, and discontinue if preexisting fevers worsen.

Four-Gentleman Decoction

Treats chronic gastritis induced by major surgery.

Minor Bupleurum Decoction

Treats gastritis when there is also gallbladder disease or hepatitis. Japanese research shows that the formula both protects the stomach lining (like the prescription drug sucralfate) and stops harmful gastric secretions (like the drugs atropine and cimetidine).[3]

Caution: Do not use if fever or skin infection is present. Taken long term in patent medicine form, can cause headache, dizziness, and bleeding gums. Side effects can be avoided if the formula is taken as a tea.

Minor Construct the Middle Decoction

Treats gastritis when there is also anemia. Contains zanthoxylum, which prevents blood loss.[4] Appropriate when there is belching of gastric acid, dull pain below the heart, and sloshing sounds in the stomach.

Warm the Gallbladder Decoction (Bamboo and Hoelen Decoction)

Generally used to treat gastritis when chronic depression is present. Also used when there is gallbladder disease.

Caution: Use with caution if fever is present, and discontinue if preexisting fevers worsen.

CONSIDERATIONS

❑ *See also* **Peptic Ulcer** and **Radiation Therapy Side Effects.**

GLAUCOMA

Glaucoma is a condition in which increased pressure within the eye causes tissue damage. While normal pressure is between 10 and 21 millimeters of mercury, glaucoma can raise this pressure to as high as 40 millimeters. Glaucoma usually affects people over forty, and persons at increased risk for this disorder include African-Americans; those with diabetes, high blood pressure, or hypothyroidism; those with extreme nearsightedness or a family history of glaucoma; and those taking corticosteroid medications.

The eye produces a fluid called aqueous humor, which fills the eye's interior. In glaucoma, aqueous humor is produced faster than it can drain into the capillaries within the eye. The resulting increase in pressure damages both the capillaries and the nerve endings that carry vision impulses to the optic nerve, resulting in blindness. Glaucoma can occur because of tissue abnormalities or because the eye's drainage mechanism is clogged with excess collagen, a protein that forms the eye's supportive structures.

There are two types of glaucoma. In chronic, or *open-angle,* glaucoma there is a persistent, moderate elevation of pressure. This form of glaucoma almost never causes symptoms until tissue destruction is advanced. The most pronounced symptoms are the loss of peripheral vision (the ability to see out of the corner of the eye) and difficulty adjusting to darkness. Other important symptoms are ongoing, low-grade headaches; seeing haloes around lights; and the need for frequent changes in eyeglass prescriptions.

Acute, or *closed-angle,* glaucoma is a medical emergency. This disorder produces severe, throbbing pain with markedly blurred vision. The pupil dilates and becomes fixed, and nausea and vomiting are common. These symptoms call for immediate medical treatment, as irreversible blindness can result in less than forty-eight hours.

Physicians usually treat glaucoma with pilocarpine or a class of drugs known as beta-blockers, such as timolol (Timoptic). Pilocarpine and related drugs act by increasing the resistance of blood-vessel walls to fluids that might swell the eye. The beta-blockers lower blood pressure throughout the body, which relieves stress on the eye. If these drugs do not control glaucoma, physicians then add drugs called systemic carbonic anhydrase inhibitors, such as acetazolamide (Diamox), to stimulate urination. If none of the drug treatments work, the next step is usually laser surgery. A procedure called laser trabeculoplasty burns new channels that allow the fluid to drain.

Kampo conceived of glaucoma as a condition in which overwork, nervous tension, or poor diet created an excess of "heat" in the liver. The liver then pumped its excess energies into its energy channels, which pass directly over the eyes. This energy excess could be cleared as long as the gallbladder was able to supply downward-moving qi. When the gallbladder became inflamed and sent its energy upwards, the liver energy sent to the eyes became trapped there in another channel circling the eyes.

The herbs and formulas listed here do not take the place of pilocarpine or any other prescription medication for glaucoma, but, when used over a period of three to four months, help lower eye pressure and prevent progression of the disease. Using herbs and prescription drugs together, under the guidance of a health care provider, is likely to provide the best control over the disease.

INDIVIDUAL KAMPO TREATMENTS

See Chapter 3 for discussions of individual herbs, traditional healing substances, and modern herbal preparations, including directions for making tea.

SUGGESTED DOSAGES	COMMENTS
Ginkgo (Modern Herbal Preparation)	
Ginkgolide extract, 1–2 40-mg tablets 3 times daily.	Acts by stopping platelet activating factor, a chemical that causes blood clots. This increases blood circulation through the eye, which helps maintain a steady oxygen supply. Has been shown to help patients with severe glaucoma, lowering pressure and widening the field of vision.[1]
Hawthorn (Herb)	
Dried herb in capsules, 3–5 g daily. or Fluid extract (1:1), ¼–½ tsp (1–2 ml) 3 times daily. or Solid extract, 100–250 mg 3 times daily. Should be standardized to contain 10% proanthocyanidins. or Tea, ⅔ c 3–4 times daily. or Tincture (1:5), 1–1½ tsp (4–6 ml) 3 times daily. Place in a cup, add 2 tbsp water, and take in a single sip.	Contains compounds called proanthocyanidins, which help the body use vitamin C to strengthen the collagen in capillary walls.[2–5] Best used as an adjunct treatment when glaucoma does not respond to prescription medications alone. If hawthorn is unavailable, substitute tea or tincture of the non-Kampo herb bilberry. Do not use bilberry-leaf tea if kidney problems exist.
Kudzu (Herb)	
Dried extract, 1 10-mg tablet 3 times daily. or Tea, 1 c 3 times daily.	Contains a natural beta-blocker, peurarin. A Chinese study found peurarin to be useful when pilocarpine does not work, and to sometimes help when timolol (Timoptic) fails.[6] Peurarin increases the effectiveness of timolol, and of beta-1 selective betaxolol (Bepoptic), levobunolol (Betagan), and metipranolol (Optipranolol). Use kudzu *in addition to* these drugs if they cannot keep eye pressure normal.

KAMPO FORMULAS

See Chapter 4 for dosage information and discussions of individual formulas.

Five-Ingredient Powder with Poria

Traditionally used to encourage urination, a usage that has been confirmed by research.[7] In a Chinese study, lowered pressure in 63% of the patients within the first month of use.[8]

CONSIDERATIONS

❑ All sources of caffeine should be avoided, including coffee, green and black tea, cola, and antifatigue pills. Coffee and tea have both been shown to raise eye pressure.[9] Although one cup of either coffee or tea a day is not likely to have any significant effect on glaucoma, constant drinking of either beverage can make controlling eye pressure difficult, especially since caffeine interferes with the beta-blocker drugs and with kudzu.

❑ Insulin stimulates collagen production, which puts persons with type 2 diabetes at risk for glaucoma. This is also true of persons who are overweight, since being overweight in many cases leads to excess insulin production. Vitamin B_3 counteracts insulin's effects on collagen. It is found in any complete B-vitamin tablet yielding at least the Recommended Daily Allowance (RDA) of the vitamin daily. The mineral chromium (200 micrograms per day) complements the B vitamins by allowing the eye's focusing muscles to use glucose more efficiently.

❑ *See also* **Diabetes, High Blood Pressure,** and **Hypothyroidism.**

GLOMERULONEPHRITIS

See **Kidney Disease.**

GRAVES' DISEASE

See **Hyperthyroidism.**

HAIR LOSS

Everyone loses individual hairs—up to fifty scalp hairs a day—constantly. Hair loss only becomes noticeable when fewer hairs are produced after the old ones are shed, or if the new hair is weak and brittle. When hair falls out in patches, it is referred to as *alopecia areata. Alopecia totalis* means the loss of all the hair on the scalp, and *alopecia universalis* means the loss of all the hair on the body.

The most prevalent form of hair loss is androgenetic alopecia (AGA), more commonly called male pattern baldness. AGA occurs in response to the body's production of androgens, or male sex hormones, although the exact mechanism is not completely understood. It generally occurs in men who have a genetic tendency for baldness. Women can also have AGA, since their bodies also produce androgens, but are less likely to lose their hair completely.

Hair loss can occur for other reasons. Severe fungal or bacterial infections can cause hair follicles to be replaced by scar tissue, as can injuries, burns, radiation therapy, and a number of diseases. Various drugs can accelerate hair loss, including chemotherapy agents, birth control pills, anticoagulants, some blood-pressure and anti-inflammatory medications, and the gout medication allopurinol (Zyloprim). Severe illness, usually when accompanied by a high fever, can cause temporary hair loss. Or hair follicles may simply waste away.

Alopecia areata, totalis, and universalis may be caused by overactivity of the immune system. Helper T cells signal other cells to dissolve dead hair follicles, while chemicals called cytokines regulate T-cell activity. When cytokines are not produced properly and the action of the T cells is not checked, hair loss occurs.[1]

A number of conventional drugs are used to fight hair loss, including minoxidil (Rogaine). The steroid drug prednisolone has shown some usefulness in reversing hair loss caused by immune-system factors.[2]

Ancient Kampo medicine developed an explanation of hair loss in terms of bottling up emotional energies in the liver. When the energies of the liver could not rise in the body through their usual channels, the hair became lifeless and dull. If the upward-moving energies of the kidneys were also impaired, by sexual excess or by a condition roughly corresponding to diabetes, the hair fell out. To correct baldness, the first line of treatment is to rejuvenate the kidneys. Then to encourage the growth of healthy hair, the next line of treatment is emotional balancing and general healing of the liver.

Male pattern baldness is relatively rare in Japan. A large proportion of the cases that do occur there fit a symptom pattern known as *satoyoshi.* This disorder results in the destruction of hair follicles by the immune system. It usually also causes diarrhea, dizziness, leg cramps, and sexual problems. The closer the symptoms match this pattern, the more likely a Kampo formula is to work. Japanese doctors fortify Kampo with prednisone or prednisolone therapy to stop the autoimmune destructive process.

Kampo treatments for hair restoration should be undertaken in the context of comprehensive health care under the supervision of a Kampo or TCM practitioner, who should be consulted to see which formula is advisable in each individual case. Complete restoration of hair using Kampo is rare, but is not unknown. Complete restoration will usually not happen if the loss covers over 40 percent of the scalp, and the hair has been gone for more than five years. More often, Kampo formulas restore hair on the side of the head, or in areas of the scalp that have most recently lost hair. Formulas may stimulate the growth of fine hair, which has a subtle cosmetic effect and reduces the risk of sunburn. In addition, Kampo treatments help overcome immune-system factors, and some formulas increase the effectiveness of prescribed steroid drugs.

INDIVIDUAL KAMPO TREATMENTS

See Chapter 3 for discussions of individual herbs, traditional healing substances, and modern herbal preparations, including directions for making tea.

SUGGESTED DOSAGES	COMMENTS
Drynaria Root (Herb)	
Tincture, applied to the scalp as directed on label.	Stimulates hair growth on portions of scalp affected by AGA.[3]

KAMPO FORMULAS

See Chapter 4 for dosage information and discussions of individual formulas.

Cinnamon Twig Decoction Plus Dragon Bone and Oyster Shell

Treats hair loss in men. Most appropriate when the symptom pattern includes diarrhea, dizziness, frequent urination, and impotence or reduced sexual responsiveness.

Cinnamon Twig, Licorice, Dragon Bone, and Oyster Shell Decoction

Treats hair loss in men and women. Especially appropriate when the symptom pattern includes dizziness, insomnia, and/or palpitations. Not available as a patent medicine, but widely available as a prescription from practitioners of Kampo and TCM. The Chinese name is *gui zhi gan cao long gu mu li.*

Seven-Treasure Pill for Beautiful Whiskers

Treats hair loss and premature graying in both sexes. Not available as a patent medicine, but widely available as a prescription from practitioners of Kampo and TCM. The Chinese name is *qi bao mei ran dan.*

Caution: Avoid if either constipation or dark, scanty urine is present.

Unblock the Orifices and Invigorate the Blood Decoction

Treats hair loss in persons who also experience purpura, or the appearance of dark-blue or purple patches on the skin, especially on the face and chest.

CONSIDERATIONS

❑ To combat hair loss resulting from nervous tension, renowned herbalist James Duke recommends making a shampoo using 2 tablespoons of dried carthamus in $^{2}/_{3}$ cup olive oil. Apply and allow to remain for fifteen to thirty minutes before rinsing.

HANGOVER

Alcohol intoxication is the condition of discomfort, impaired judgment, poor coordination, and pain following acute overconsumption of alcoholic beverages. (Intoxication should not be confused with alcoholism, in which the individual depends on regular alcohol consumption to prevent withdrawal symptoms.) Intoxication is often, but not always, followed by hangover, which is marked by nausea, headache, and general malaise. These symptoms are produced by acetaldehyde, a chemical created when the body processes alcohol, that causes headache, nausea, and redness in the face.[1] The body attempts to dilute acetaldehyde in the bloodstream by drawing fluids out of cells, dehydrating them and causing pain.

Hangover severity is related, at least in part, to genetics. Members of certain ethnic groups, especially Japanese and Koreans, feel alcohol's effects to a greater degree because they do not have a gene that breaks down acetaldehyde. Members of other ethnic groups are genetically able to break down acetaldehyde very efficiently, and thus feel alcohol's effects less. Unfortunately, being able to process acetaldehyde efficiently leaves an individual more prone to alcoholism.

Since hangover is not the result of a "pernicious influence" (pathogen) or a stable symptom pattern, Kampo did not develop a theory of the condition. Instead, Kampo remedies for hangover developed from years of experience in finding what works. Most Kampo treatments should be taken immediately after drinking to prevent or reduce hangover, instead of the next morning, and should be discontinued when the hangover subsides. The exception is Chinese senega root, which should be taken *before* alcohol is consumed. Because of alcohol's effects on driving ability, *never* drive after drinking, even if using Kampo.

INDIVIDUAL KAMPO TREATMENTS

See Chapter 3 for discussions of individual herbs, traditional healing substances, and modern herbal preparations, including directions for making tea.

SUGGESTED DOSAGES	COMMENTS
Aloe (Herb)	
Juice, as directed on label. Typical dosage is 1 fluid oz (30 ml) daily.	Prevents the passage of alcohol from the intestines into the bloodstream.[2] Accelerates the rate at which the body recovers from alcohol intoxication by 40–50%.[3] Does not reduce blood alcohol levels as registered by breathalyzers or blood tests.
Chinese Senega Root (Herb)	
Tincture (1:5), maximum of 20 drops. Place in a cup, add 2 tbsp water, and take in a single sip.	Contains compounds that block as much as 90% of the ethanol that otherwise would be absorbed into the body. Only effective if used *before* alcohol consumption. Since alcohol can remain in the mouth, this herb does not necessarily reduce blood alcohol levels as registered by breathalyzers, but lowers alcohol levels as measured by blood tests. *Caution:* Do not use if gastritis or ulcers are present.
Ginseng (Herb)	
Tea, made with Korean or red ginseng, 1 c every 2 hours until intoxication symptoms subside.	Ginseng enhances the breakdown of beverage alcohol in the body. Lowers blood-alcohol concentrations approximately 35% faster than when no treatment is given.[4] Do not use ginseng tincture.
Schisandra (Herb)	
Freeze-dried herb, 100 mg 3 times daily. Available as Hoelen & Schisandra. or Tea, 1 c 3 times daily.	In animal studies, prevents memory loss following excessive alcohol consumption when used in combination with biota (see Chapter 3) and ginseng (see above). Does not accelerate recovery from intoxication.[5] Can be used with ginseng only. *Caution:* Avoid if gallstones or blockages of the bile ducts exist.
Soy Lecithin (Modern Herbal Preparation)	
Soy phospholipids, 1,500–3,000 mg daily. Identified individually on the label as 3-sn-phospatidylcholine, phosphatidylethanolamine, and phospatidylinositic acid, or as "total phospholipids."	Protects liver tissue from effects of alcohol by speeding regeneration and stabilization of cell membrane. Relieves fatigue and hypoglycemia, or low blood sugar, by stopping free-radical activity that would desensitize liver cells to low blood-sugar levels. Ensure that liver releases glucose to cover skipped meals. *Caution:* Mild diarrhea may occur when soy lecithin is first used.

CONSIDERATIONS

❑ Since hangover discomfort partially arises from dehydration, be sure to drink plenty of liquids. Grapefruit and orange juices are the beverages of choice because they contain quercetin, a chemical that stops pain and inflammation.[6]

❑ *See also* **Alcoholism.**

HEADACHES

Headaches are among the most common medical complaints. They can arise from numerous causes, including stress, underlying infections or illnesses, or blood-vessel disturbances in the head.

The most common headaches are those caused by muscle tension in the head, neck, or shoulders, usually due to fatigue or stress. A tension headache is often accompanied by a feeling of tightness around the head, along with weakness or fatigue, and may worsen with sudden movement. Mild painkillers, such as aspirin, acetaminophen, or ibuprofen, are effective against occasional tension headaches.

Intensely painful headaches can precede serious illness, particularly illness involving impaired circulation to the brain. Migraine headaches can bring excruciating pain, distortions in sensory perception, and episodes of complete debility lasting hours or days. Other causes of headache include infections of the ears, sinuses, or mouth; high blood pressure; glaucoma; allergies; brain tumors or abscesses; some drugs; and various foods, especially those containing the additive monosodium glutamate (MSG).

Traditional Japanese medicine created a category of headaches known as *jitsuyo kanpo kyoho,* or "diseases that are not quite diseases," headaches that cause discomfort but do not seriously disrupt normal activities.

As is the case in all Kampo treatments, formulas address combinations of symptoms, which include headache. Choosing the formula that matches the symptom pattern should permanently stop "headaches that are not quite headaches" within four weeks of use.

INDIVIDUAL KAMPO TREATMENTS

See Chapter 3 for discussions of individual herbs, traditional healing substances, and modern herbal preparations, including directions for making tea.

SUGGESTED DOSAGES	COMMENTS
Peppermint (Herb)	
Oil, applied topically (see Chapter 3 for directions).	Eases headache pain.

KAMPO FORMULAS

See Chapter 4 for dosage information and discussions of individual formulas.

Cinnamon Twig Decoction

Stops headache accompanied by nasal allergy or congestion, fever, or chills.

Cinnamon Twig Decoction Plus Kudzu

Stops headache with same symptom pattern as Cinnamon Twig Decoction, along with the additional symptom of stiffness in the neck or back.

Ligusticum Chuanxiong Powder to be Taken With Green Tea

Stops headache in any part of the head, especially when accompanied by dizziness, fever and chills, or nasal congestion.

Unblock the Orifices and Invigorate the Blood Decoction

Relieves headache with "blood effusive" symptoms, such as bags beneath the eyes, purplish complexion, or facial flushing caused by embarrassment or emotional tension.

White Tiger Decoction

Relieves headache with "red" symptoms, including anger, bleeding gums or nose, fever, or irritability.

Caution: Avoid if nausea or vomiting is present.

CONSIDERATIONS

❑ *See also* **Migraine.**

HEART ATTACK, AFTERCARE

See **Congestive Heart Failure.**

HEMORRHOIDS

Hemorrhoids are swollen blood vessels in and around the anus. These blood vessels stretch under pressure in a manner similar to varicose veins in the legs. They are very common and can occur in anyone, but appear more often in older people. Symptoms include blood on the surface of the stool or on the toilet paper, itching, and sometimes pain, although hemorrhoids are often symptomless. While hemorrhoids cause most cases of rectal bleeding, such bleeding can result from a number of conditions, and should always be brought to a doctor's attention.

Internal hemorrhoids are located within the anal canal. *External hemorrhoids* are those that protrude outside the anus. Internal hemorrhoids that grow large enough to protrude from the anus are called prolapsed hemorrhoids, and can be extremely painful.

Hemorrhoids of both types result from increased pressure in the veins, such as that caused by pregnancy, cirrhosis of the liver, or straining to pass hard stool. Hemorrhoids are essentially unknown in cultures in which people eat high-fiber diets and are physically active. Dietary fiber absorbs water, making the stools larger and easier to pass, and exercise stimulates defecation. The low-fiber, highly refined North American diet lacks fiber, which makes stools smaller and more difficult to pass.

Conventional care of hemorrhoids includes the use of stool softeners, and, in stubborn cases, surgery.

As early as the time of the great herbalist Zhang Zhongjing in the second century A.D., Kampo recognized conditions in which the stool could become dry and difficult to pass. Kampo formulas redirected water from the kidneys, where it caused frequent urination, to the intestines, where it softened the stool. The formulas also relieved conditions of "heat" or fever, which also depleted water needed by the intestines.

INDIVIDUAL KAMPO TREATMENTS

See Chapter 3 for discussions of individual herbs, traditional healing substances, and modern herbal preparations, including directions for making tea.

SUGGESTED DOSAGES	COMMENTS
Plantain (Herb)	
Tea, made with whole seeds, 1 c 3 times daily.	Also known as psyllium; gentler alternative to psyllium powder. Softens the stool. Also contains mucilage, which coats and protects the bowel lining. Unlike stimulant laxatives, does not cause cramping. To avoid absorption problems, take other oral medications 1 hour before using plantain. *Caution:* Used in numerous over-the-counter laxatives; avoid those that contain both psyllium and cellulose, since cellulose can cause rectal itching.

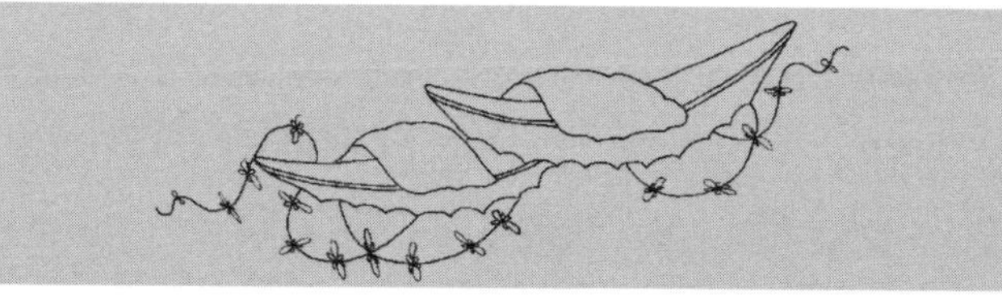

Rhubarb Root (Herb)

Tea, 1 c up to 3 times daily. Can be flavored with cinnamon or peppermint.	Used after surgery for hemorrhoids to ensure soft stools. Use only root that has been aged for 1 to 2 years. *Caution:* Do not use if menstruating or if rectal bleeding is present. Avoid rhubarb and all stimulant laxatives if taking any kind of diuretic.

KAMPO FORMULAS

See Chapter 4 for dosage information and discussions of individual formulas.

Cinnamon Twig and Poria Pill

Used in Japan especially to treat bleeding hemorrhoids in men who also have prostate problems. Most effective when used with hemorrhoidal ointments or suppositories.[1]

Hemp Seed Pill

Softens the stool by stimulating the release of fluids into the intestines. Particularly useful for hemorrhoids aggravated by postpartum or postsurgical constipation. Use this formula in patent-medicine form.

Caution: Most manufacturers include the traditional marijuana seed. Will not produce a "high," but will cause a positive urine test for THC, although sophisticated testing methods can distinguish medicinal from illicit use.

Peach Blossom Decoction

Treats hemorrhoids with blood in the stool or with bleeding noticed after defecation. Also relieves syndromes that include pus or blood in the stool and abdominal pain.

CONSIDERATIONS

❑ There are two supplements that act against hemorrhoids by strengthening the rectal blood vessels. A plant-based supplement called hydroxyethylrutoside (HER, or HER flavonoids), taken in dosages of from 1,000 to 2,000 milligrams per day, heals both hemorrhoids and varicose veins.[2] If HER flavonoids are unavailable, citrus bioflavonoids (rutin and hesperidin) can be taken in dosages of from 3,000 to 6,000 milligrams per day. An animal-based supplement called glycosaminoglycan (GAG, or aortic GAGs), taken in dosages of 100 milligrams per day, provides the protein building blocks for healthy veins and helps control pain.[3]

❑ Bathing external hemorrhoids in a warm-water sitz bath relieves irritation and pain. To take a sitz bath, fill a basin or bathtub with enough water to cover up to the middle of the abdomen. Use water that is about 110°F, and no hotter than 120°F. (If the water is uncomfortably hot, try using a cold forehead compress.) Stay in the bath for between twenty and forty minutes, and finish by splashing the area with cool water or taking a quick cold shower.

❑ *See also* **Constipation.**

HEPATITIS

Hepatitis is an inflammation of the liver. This disease results from chronic overconsumption of alcohol, exposure to toxic chemicals, allergic reactions, or overdoses of some prescription drugs, but it is most commonly caused by viral infection. Most cases of viral hepatitis tend to be acute, that is, they generally last for a few weeks. Chronic hepatitis is an inflammation that lasts more than six months.

At least seven different hepatitis viruses cause liver infection (see "The ABCs of Hepatitis" on page 224), so blood tests are needed for an accurate diagnosis. Hepatitis symptoms vary widely. Initially they may include flulike complaints, such as malaise and loss of appetite. Later symptoms may include fever, nausea, sensitivity to light, vomiting, headache, swollen joints, and dark urine. Symptoms vary because the liver is an extremely robust organ, able to function even when large portions are destroyed.

In chronic hepatitis, the nutrients ordinarily distributed by the liver become unavailable. Low blood-sugar levels and fatigue result. Chronic hepatitis also keeps the liver from breaking down toxins it normally removes from the body. The buildup of toxins in the bloodstream can result in depression, delirium, or loss of short-term memory. Toxic buildup can also cause jaundice, a condition in which the skin and eyes turn any color from faint yellow to bright tangerine. Frequently, however, there is no change in skin color at all.

The destructive agent in viral hepatitis is not the virus, but rather the immune system itself. As long as the virus lies dormant in the liver cell, it is undetectable to the immune system. When the virus begins to multiply, however, immune-system cells engulf and destroy the cell. Thus, the immune response destroys liver tissue and causes hepatitis's most serious symptoms. Asymptomatic viral hepatitis may wait for months or years for a "trigger"—such as a drinking binge, or exposure to a poisonous chemical or certain prescription drugs—to manifest itself. This trigger stresses the liver and activates the infection. When this happens, symptoms appear.

Mild cases of hepatitis often clear up by themselves. Steroids are sometimes used in more serious cases to suppress the immune system, and thus reduce tissue damage. Interferon, one of the body's own chemical defenders, is used for hepatitis B and C, and severe cases of A. Unfortunately, interferon causes flulike symptoms and depression, and is effective only 20 percent of the time.

Kampo's understanding of hepatitis predates the scientific explanation by almost 2,000 years. Kampo recognizes hepatitis as a disease of the Lesser Yang (see Chapter 1). In this stage of disease, the body and the invading infection reach a stalemate that can last for years at a time. During this stalemate, the disease is half "exterior" and half "interior." As an external condition, it can produce chills and fever, and a sense of fullness in the abdomen and chest. As an internal condition, it can redirect energies normally cycled downward through the liver upward to the mouth and throat, causing thirst and a bitter taste in the mouth. By debilitating the liver, it can also interfere with the function of the gallbladder, producing anorexia, heartburn, nausea, or vomiting. Most of the time, however, the forces of the body and the pathogen are equally matched.

A basic principle of Kampo treatment is "never oppose force with like force." Kampo treatments for hepatitis redirect rather than attack the pathogens causing the disease. This drains the heat of infection, redirects "rebellious" digestive energies in order to stop nausea and vomiting, and restores the stalemate between body and pathogen. Kampo does not offer an immediate cure for difficult cases of hepatitis (and neither does modern medicine), but controls the disease with a minimum of tissue damage. Be aware that some herbs may have a negative impact on the liver and/or interact negatively with conventional medicines. Always work with a qualified health care practitioner.

INDIVIDUAL KAMPO TREATMENTS

See Chapter 3 for discussions of individual herbs, traditional healing substances, and modern herbal preparations, including directions for making tea.

SUGGESTED DOSAGES	COMMENTS
Hoelen (Herb)	
Dried or fresh hoelen in food, ⅛–¼ oz (3–6 g) daily. or Tea, 1 c 3 times daily. or Tincture, as directed on label. Place in a cup, add 2 tbsp water, and take in a single sip.	Greatly increases the effectiveness of metronidazole, used to treat liver inflammation caused by hepatitis.[1] Hoelen by itself sometimes brings about relief of symptoms. A chemically treated extract has been reported to produce an immediate cure in nearly half of all viral hepatitis patients.[2] The natural extract, pachymaran, is less readily absorbed but still readily available to the body, especially when the whole mushroom is used. *Caution:* Do not use in cases of long-term illness that cause excessive urination.
Licorice (Herb)	
Glycyrrhizin extract, 200–800 mg daily, depending on severity of symptoms for up to 6 weeks. or Tea, 1 c 3 times daily for up to 6 weeks.	In Japan, used extensively against hepatitis B. Contains glycyrrhizin, which "locks" the virus into cells to keep the infection from spreading. Glycyrrhizin consistently improves liver function and occasionally brings about total recovery from hepatitis B.[3,4] Makes interferon more effective against hepatitis C and severe cases of hepatitis A.[5,6] Avoid deglycyrrhizinated licorice (DGL). *Caution:* Avoid if high blood pressure is present. Also avoid if an estrogen-sensitive disorder is present, such as bladder cancer, melanoma, or disorders of the female reproductive system.
Peppermint (Herb)	
Oil, enterically coated capsules, 200 mg 3 times daily. or Tea, 1 c 3 times daily between or after meals.	Calms upset stomach and cramping. Has no direct effect on the disease. *Caution:* Should not be used if the bile duct may be blocked.
Schisandra (Herb)	
Freeze-dried herb, 100 mg 3 times daily. Available as Hoelen & Schisandra. or Tea, 1 c 3 times daily.	Protects the liver against hepatitis viruses[7] and toxic chemicals,[8] and helps the liver regenerate after surgery or infection.[9] *Caution:* Avoid during pregnancy, or if gallstones or blockages of the bile ducts exist.

The ABCs of Hepatitis

Some viruses that can cause hepatitis, such as Epstein-Barr virus and cytomegalovirus, can cause other illnesses as well. In addition, there are at least seven viruses that exclusively infect the liver. They are identified as hepatitis A, B, C, D, E, F, and G.

The most common form of viral hepatitis, hepatitis A, is almost always a short-term, self-limiting illness. It is spread by person-to-person contact, or by contaminated food or water. Before symptoms arise, the infection can be halted with gamma-globulin injections.

Hepatitis B is a much more serious infection. Formerly known as serum hepatitis, it is spread by blood-to-blood contact or sexual contact with an infected person. Infected mothers can also pass the virus to their babies during birth. In some parts of the developing world, hepatitis B is also spread by food and water contamination because of poor sanitation. While the virus sometimes persists for many years, most people recover within a year, compared with a usual recovery time of six weeks for hepatitis A. Hepatitis B can cause cirrhosis and an increased susceptibility to liver cancer. Fortunately, there is a highly successful vaccination for hepatitis B.

Hepatitis C (formerly called non-A, non-B hepatitis) is carried by nearly 4 million people in the United States alone. It is usually spread through transfusions or shared needles. Hepatitis C is a potentially deadly infection that is extremely difficult to detect because repeated blood tests may be necessary to identify the disease. It has many of the same long-term consequences as hepatitis B.

About 20 percent of all cases of hepatitis are caused by four other viruses, hepatitis D, E, F, and G. Hepatitis D (formerly called delta hepatitis) and E (formerly called enteric hepatitis) are seldom encountered in North America, but are often epidemic in other parts of the world. The hepatitis D virus only multiplies in the presence of the B virus,[1] and makes hepatitis B symptoms worse. Hepatitis E is sometimes epidemic in tropical areas after widespread flooding. It produces symptoms similar to hepatitis A, except that it is much more dangerous to pregnant women. Hepatitis F is an extremely rare strain of the virus that is transmitted from primates to humans. Hepatitis G, on the other hand, is a relatively common infection, accounting for as many as 9 percent of all hepatitis infections.[2] A mild form of the disease, hepatitis G does not seem to cause ongoing liver damage.[3]

KAMPO FORMULAS

See Chapter 4 for dosage information and discussions of individual formulas.

Minor Bupleurum Decoction

Usefulness in hepatitis treatment has been confirmed by dozens of studies; in Japan, over 90% of chronic hepatitis patients take this formula. Traditionally used to stop fever and chills, dry throat, bitter or sour taste in the mouth, dizziness, irritability, heartburn, nausea, and vomiting—some of the symptoms of viral hepatitis. Also effective against hepatitis caused by drug exposure. Especially useful in treating children. In early stages of infection, stimulates gamma interferon production, which interferes with the virus's ability to reproduce.[10] In chronic hepatitis, stimulates immune-system cells to destroy precancerous lesions,[11] and causes immune-system cells to "clump" over sites of infection.[12] Prevents progression of hepatitis C.[13] Seek the advice of the dispensing herbalist on a suitable child's dosage.

Caution: Modern Kampo practitioners caution that this formula is not helpful in cases of "yin deficiency," which expresses itself as night sweats, low-grade fevers, irritability, and thirst.[14] Do not use if fever or skin infection is present. Taken long term in patent medicine form, can cause headache, dizziness, and bleeding gums. Side effects can be avoided if the formula is taken as a tea.

CONSIDERATIONS

❑ An individual who is being treated for *amebic* hepatitis with a drug such as metronidazole (Flagyl) should consult with an herbalist about taking a tea that combines hoelen, peony, and tang-kuei (see Chapter 3) along with the prescription medication. This herbal combination can double the effectiveness of the antiamebic drugs.[15]

❑ *See also* **Alcoholism** and **Liver Cancer.** To learn how to use schisandra for protection against liver cancer, see "Schisandra—Kampo's Supreme Liver Herb" on page 251.

HERPES

There are a number of disease-causing herpesviruses. Herpes simplex virus 1 (HSV-1) causes mild skin outbreaks, generally in the form of cold sores (fever blisters) of the mouth, though sometimes the genitals are affected. Herpes simplex virus 2 (HSV-2) causes more severe outbreaks, generally in the form of genital herpes, though sometimes the mouth is affected. HSV-1 can also cause a painful eye disease called ocular keratitis, although Japanese doctors have seen cases in which this disorder is caused by HSV-2.[1] Herpes varicella-zoster (herpes zoster) causes shingles and chickenpox, and it too can damage the eye. Herpesvirus infections are extremely common.

All three herpes infections can cause painful blisters. Herpes blisters are highly infectious until they are completely healed, which may take two to four weeks. Although herpes infections can be contagious even after healing, the rate of transmission drops dramatically at that point. In some cases, there are no symptoms.

HSV-1 initially produces burning or tingling around the lips and nose. In a few hours, this is followed by small red pimples, and then by the blisters. There may be a mild fever and enlarged lymph nodes in the neck. Recurrences often happen after sunburn or exposure to intense sunlight. Outbreaks can also occur after other infections weaken the immune system.

The first symptoms of HSV-2 usually occur four to eight days after exposure. They include a burning or itching in the genital area, followed by the blisters that turn into red, painful sores which are easily infected. There may be pain upon urination, and fever, flulike symptoms, and headache may also occur. Symptoms tend to be more severe in women. Outbreaks may be triggered by nerve damage, especially to the trigeminal nerve underlying the cheekbones, where HSV-2 frequently settles. (Dental procedures that disturb this nerve cause outbreaks in up to 40 percent of infected patients.) HSV-2 can cause serious complications, including liver damage. An infected mother can pass the disease to her baby during birth, creating a risk of blindness or brain damage.

The first symptoms of shingles may include malaise, chills, fever, and intestinal or urinary difficulties. Three or four days later, the blisters develop, generally along the path of a nerve on one side of the trunk. Shingles often occur decades after a person has the chickenpox, although recurrences of the shingles themselves are rare. Possible complications include skin infections and lasting pain along the affected nerve.

The herpesvirus operates in two distinct modes. During acute infection, the virus reproduces and disperses to adjoining tissues. After acute infection, it implants itself in the nerve tissue, where it does not attempt to reproduce. Only when the security of its "home" is threatened will the virus reactivate into a disease-causing form.

The key to managing herpes infections is making sure they do not implant themselves. A strong antibody response can keep the virus from entering cells.[2] Herbs and drugs that stimulate antibody production, such as aloe, offer a first line of defense against the disease. After implantation, the standard medical therapy for chronic herpes infection is a group of drugs that includes acyclovir. Acyclovir destroys the virus, and is relatively safe. However, it cannot reach every herpesvirus in every cell, so reinfection is always possible unless, and sometimes even if, the medication is continued.

Kampo's approach to treating herpes is very different. Kampo medicines do not attack the virus directly and do not stimulate any part of the immune system to attack the virus.[3] Instead, they prevent the inflammation that would signal the virus that its cellular "home" was about to be attacked and it should become active. The Kampo theory behind this kinder and gentler treatment of the virus was that virus was a pathogen seeking a route of escape. Formulas that "opened the pores" of the skin, which relieved tension and relaxed muscles, made such escape easier. While we now know that the herpesvirus does not "escape" after Kampo treatment, its destructive potential is reduced.

Since mainstream medicine and Kampo act through different mechanisms, the best way to control recurrences is to combine the two approaches. A wide variety of herbs work with acyclovir to offer better protection against implantation than either herbs or acyclovir alone.[4] One herb, licorice, can be used as a "morning-after" treatment if herpes exposure is suspected.[5] In addition, scutellaria helps stop skin infections that can complicate shingles.

INDIVIDUAL KAMPO TREATMENTS

See Chapter 3 for discussions of individual herbs, traditional healing substances, and modern herbal preparations, including directions for making tea.

SUGGESTED DOSAGES	COMMENTS
Aloe (Herb)	
Gel, either commercial or taken from houseplants, used liberally on dressings.	Encourages formation of antibodies against herpes.[6] Creams or lotions made with the non-Kampo herb St. John's wort can also be used for this purpose.[7]
Bitter Melon (Herb)	
Juice, 1–2 oz (30–60 ml) 3 times daily. Take with up to 1 tsp of natural sweetener. or Whole fruit, ½–2 fruits (9–15 g) in cooking daily.	In laboratory studies, two to three times more effective than acyclovir in killing the herpesvirus; 100 to 1,000 times more effective in killing acyclovir-resistant strains.[8] *Caution:* Bitter melon should be avoided by persons who have cirrhosis or have had hepatitis, or are HIV-positive and have had liver infections. Otherwise, use for 4 weeks, then discontinue for 4 weeks.
Cloves (Herb)	
Oil, 10 drops in ¼ c (60 ml) warm water, 3 times daily.	Increases effectiveness of acyclovir without side effects.[9]
Dendrobium (Herb)	
Tea or tincture, as directed by herbalist.	Traditional remedy for mouth sores activated by exposure to the sun.
Green Tea (Herb)	
Tea, applied lukewarm as a compress.	Contains caffeine, which increases effectiveness of topical interferon treatment.[10] Also helps prevent secondary infections.
Licorice (Herb)	
Glycyrrhizin extract, 200–800 mg daily, depending on severity of symptoms for up to 6 weeks. or Tea, 1 c 3 times daily for up to 6 weeks.	Kills herpes simplex and herpes zoster viruses. Avoid deglycyrrhizinated licorice (DGL). *Caution:* Avoid if high blood pressure is present. Also avoid if an estrogen-sensitive disorder is present, such as bladder cancer, melanoma, or disorders of the female reproductive system.
Scutellaria (Herb)	
Dried herb, 1–2 1,000-mg capsules 3 times daily. or Fluid extract (1:1), ¼–½ tsp (1–2 ml) 3 times daily. or Powdered solid extract (4:1), 250–500 mg 3 times daily. or Tea, 1 c 3 times daily. or Tincture (1:5), 1–1½ tsp (4–6 ml) 3 times daily. Place in a cup, add 2 tbsp water, and take in a single sip.	Kills a number of viruses and bacteria that commonly affect persons with shingles, including *E. coli, Proteus, Pseudomonas, Salmonella, Shigella, Staphylococcus,* and *Streptococcus.* Also prevents infection by influenza A and B. Should be used at first sign of skin rash for best effect. *Caution:* Avoid in cases of diarrhea caused by foodborne infection or excessive consumption of cold drinks.

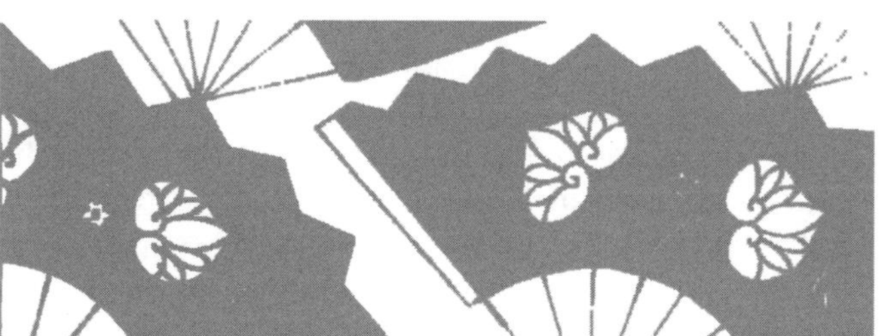

HERBS TO AVOID

Individuals who have herpes infections should avoid pinellia and tang-kuei. For more information regarding these herbs, see Chapter 3.

KAMPO FORMULAS

See Chapter 4 for dosage information and discussions of individual formulas.

Gentiana Longdancao Decoction to Drain the Liver

Relieves symptoms of both herpes simplex and herpes zoster outbreaks. Traditionally used to "draw fire" from the skin. Especially appropriate when symptoms include eye irritation, fatigue, irritability, whitish vaginal discharge, painful urination, and swelling or inflammation in the ears.

Caution: Should not be used by women who are trying to become pregnant.

Kudzu Decoction

Scientifically demonstrated to prevent recurrences of HSV-1 and ocular keratitis. Works by stopping inflammatory reaction to the virus rather than by stimulating the immune system to act against the virus. Thus, the virus is given fewer opportunities to mutate into an untreatable form.[11]

White Tiger Decoction

The anemarrhena in this formula contains mangiferin,[12] which strengthens acyclovir's ability to stop HSV-1 from replicating. In laboratory tests, mangiferin is more effective than acyclovir in stopping replication.[13]

Caution: Avoid if nausea or vomiting is present.

HIGH BLOOD PRESSURE (HYPERTENSION)

Blood pressure—the force circulating blood exerts against the walls of arteries—that is too high can cause arteries to narrow, which can lead to arteriosclerosis, heart attack, kidney disease, memory loss, and stroke. It is estimated that more than 50 million Americans have high blood pressure, which is often symptomless. More than 90 percent of these people have primary, or essential, high blood pressure, that which is not due to a single known cause. High blood pressure is more common among African-Americans than among members of other ethnic groups, and affects more men than women.

Doctors are not sure exactly what causes primary high blood pressure. There may be a genetic component, since it seems to run in families. But there may also be a lifestyle component, as high blood pressure has been linked to diet, smoking, alcohol use, excessive caffeine and salt intake, and lack of exercise. Certain medications, such as birth control pills, can elevate blood pressure, as can pregnancy.

Blood pressure is measured as a pair of numbers. The first number is the systolic pressure, exerted when the heart beats, and represents blood pressure at its highest. The second number is the diastolic pressure, exerted when the heart rests between beats, and represents pressure at its lowest. Pressure varies throughout the day in response to stress, activity level, and other factors. Normal readings for adults range from 110/70 to 140/90, with 120/80 generally considered to be the norm. Elevation of the diastolic pressure is of greater concern than that of the systolic pressure, with a sustained diastolic blood pressure over 140 almost always considered to be a medical emergency.

Two factors contribute to many cases of primary high blood pressure. First, excessive blood levels of the hormone insulin stimulate the arterial walls to contract and cause the kidneys to retain sodium. Both actions increase pressure. Second, sodium is found in salt, and how strongly the kidneys react to sodium is determined by a person's salt sensitivity. In about 60 percent of the people who have primary high blood pressure, an increase in blood-sodium levels leads to kidney production of angiotensin II, a substance that also stimulates the arteries to contract.

Doctors urge patients with high blood pressure to lose weight, exercise, and cut salt consumption. If these measures don't work, doctors prescribe various drugs. Diuretics promote urination, reducing the amount of fluid in the bloodstream. Beta-blockers cause the heart to slow down and lower its blood output, which reduces pressure. Other drugs inhibit angiotensin II production, and are called angiotensin-converting enzyme (ACE) inhibitors. The various drugs have different side effects, including fatigue, depression, fainting when rising from a seated position (orthostatic hypotension), unfavorable blood-fat and -sugar changes, and impaired male sexual function. Often drugs are combined, or a patient must switch from one drug to another.

In Kampo, any of a large number of related disorders of the liver, kidneys, and blood can result in high blood pressure. The liver can be overheated by bad diet, emotional tension, or overwork so that it sends "fire" upward through the body. Liver fire manifests itself as dizziness, dry mouth, splitting headaches, irritability, nightmares, and a flushed face. Too little liver energy can also result in high blood pressure, as blood and energy tend to become congested in the head because the liver does not supply the energy to move them. Symptoms include all of those found when there is liver fire, with the addition of back pain, forgetfulness, and blurry vision.

When the kidneys are unable to hold fluids and instead "steam" them upward through the body, the result can be high blood pressure. Kampo treatments for this class of high blood pressure increase the kidneys' yin, or containing, energies.

Finally, high blood pressure can result from the "solidifying" of stagnant energy into "phlegm" that obstructs blood flow through the head. This produces a sensation of tightness in the head, palpitations, poor appetite, and vomiting. It also produces blue or purple streaks and enlarged veins in the tongue, the signs traditional Japanese medicine uses to diagnose high blood pressure.

Clinical researchers have found that Kampo lowers blood pressure within a few days' use just as prescription drugs do, but the amount of the change may be slightly less. For this reason, the gentler Kampo products are best for "borderline" cases.[1] Kampo is also useful for people who know they are sensitive to salt or who suffer depression. Although all of Kampo's traditional treatments for high blood pressure are formulas, many single herbs also help lower blood pressure. Use single herbs first, checking blood pressure regularly. High blood pressure often occurs at the same time as high cholesterol levels, and a number of these herbs fight both problems. If the herbs do not help—although they probably will—then see a Kampo or TCM practitioner about choosing an appropriate formula.

Never discontinue a blood-pressure medication abruptly, especially if it is a beta-blocker. Gradually lowering the dose over a period of weeks prevents rebound hypertension, blood pressure that goes higher when a medication is stopped than it was before treatment. Perform weekly pressure checks, and consult a physician before discontinuing medication.

INDIVIDUAL KAMPO TREATMENTS

See Chapter 3 for discussions of individual herbs, traditional healing substances, and modern herbal preparations, including directions for making tea.

SUGGESTED DOSAGES	COMMENTS
Amaranth (Herb)	
Tea, 1 c 3 times daily.	Causes blood vessels near the surface of the body to dilate, which reduces blood pressure. Contains ecdysterone, which strengthens heartbeat and prevents high blood-sugar levels in laboratory tests.[2] Listed in Chinese herb shops as achyranthis; may also be labeled as *Niu Xi* or *Tu Niu Xi*. *Caution:* Avoid during pregnancy.
Caltrop (Herb)	
Tea, 1 c up to twice daily.	Prevents blurred vision associated with high blood pressure and/or diabetes due to fluid-balance changes in the lens of the eye.[3]

Epimedium (Herb)	
Use as directed by the herbalist.	Lowers blood pressure by dilating coronary arteries, which reduces both stress on the heart and the risk of atherosclerosis. Unlike many drug treatments, stimulates rather than lessens sexual desire and capacity in men. *Caution:* Avoid if a prostate disorder is present.

Ginseng (Herb)	
Fluid extract or tincture, as directed on label. or Tea, made with Korean or red ginseng, 1 c daily.	Contains chemicals that relax the blood-vessel linings.[4] Also acts as a sexual stimulant. If using ginseng extracts or tinctures (which are not as therapeutically active as teas), be sure the product contains *Panax ginseng.* Note that strength may vary by manufacturer. *Caution:* Avoid using a form of ginseng called *Tienqi* (*Panax notoginseng*).

Green Tea (Herb)	
Catechin extract, 1 240-mg tablet 3 times daily. or *Decaffeinated* tea, 1 c 2–3 times daily.	Contains compounds called catechins, which lower blood pressure by inhibiting the action of ACE.[5] To avoid dilution problems, do not take tea within 1 hour of taking other teas or patent medicines.

Hawthorn (Herb)	
Dried herb in capsules, 3–5 g daily. or Fluid extract (1:1), $\frac{1}{4}$–$\frac{1}{2}$ tsp (1–2 ml) 3 times daily. or Solid extract, 100–250 mg 3 times daily. Should be standardized to contain 10% proanthocyanidins. or Tea, $\frac{2}{3}$ c 3–4 times daily. or Tincture (1:5), 1–1$\frac{1}{2}$ tsp (4–6 ml) 3 times daily. Place in a cup, add 2 tbsp water, and take in a single sip.	Dilates the blood vessels, lowers blood pressure, and dissolves cholesterol deposits.[6] Increases circulation within and around the heart, and compensates for mild cases of cardiac deficiency.[7]

Lycium (Herb)	
Concentrate, 1 1,000-mg tablet 3 times daily. Available as Longevity Tonic (recommended) or *Gou Qi Zi.* or Tea, 1 c 3 times daily.	Lowers blood pressure, and reduces blood-cholesterol and -sugar levels.[8] Corrects blurred vision and male sexual dysfunction caused by long-term high blood pressure. Unlike some prescription drugs, lycium does not cause orthostatic hypotension. *Caution:* Do not use if diarrhea is present.

Scutellaria (Herb)	
Dried herb, 1–2 1,000-mg capsules 3 times daily. or Fluid extract (1:1), $\frac{1}{4}$–$\frac{1}{2}$ tsp (1–2 ml) 3 times daily. or Powdered solid extract (4:1), 250–500 mg 3 times daily. or Tea, 1 c 4 times daily. or Tincture (1:5), 1–1$\frac{1}{2}$ tsp (4–6 ml) 3 times daily. Place in a cup, add 2 tbsp water, and take in a single sip.	Acts by dilating blood vessels and stimulating urination. In animal studies, also lowers cholesterol levels.[9] *Caution:* Avoid in cases of diarrhea caused by foodborne infection or excessive consumption of cold drinks.

Tang-Kuei (Herb)	
Dried root, 1–2 tsp (1–3 g) daily. or Fluid extract (1:1), $\frac{1}{4}$–$\frac{1}{2}$ tsp (1–2 ml) daily. or Freeze-dried root, 1–2 500-mg capsules daily. or Powdered solid extract (4:1), 250–500 mg daily. or Tea, 1 c 2–3 times daily. or Tincture (1:5), 1–1$\frac{1}{2}$ tsp (4–6 ml) daily. Place in a cup, add 2 tbsp water, and take in a single sip.	Particularly useful for lowering high blood pressure during premenstrual syndrome. Prolongs resting period between heartbeats and increases coronary blood flow. Prevents formation of atherosclerotic plaques. Also known as dong quai.

HERBS TO AVOID

Individuals who have high blood pressure should avoid the following herbs: barley sprouts, coltsfoot, dan shen, ephedra, and licorice. For more information regarding these herbs, see Chapter 3.

KAMPO FORMULAS

See Chapter 4 for dosage information and discussions of individual formulas.

Bupleurum Plus Dragon Bone and Oyster Shell Decoction
Treats high blood pressure caused by "liver fire." Counteracts the action of stress hormones, especially norepinephrine, in increasing blood pressure.[10] *Caution:* Be sure the formula does *not* include the traditional ingredient minium (lead oxide). Use with caution if fever is present, and discontinue if preexisting fevers worsen.

Coptis Decoction to Relieve Toxicity
Lowers blood pressure and reduces the likelihood of blood clot formation. Increases blood flow to the brain.[11] Traditionally used to treat "hot" symptoms, including acne, bleeding gums, fever, facial flushing caused by embarrassment or emotional tension, headaches, nervousness, or sinusitis. *Caution:* Should not be used by women who are trying to become pregnant.

Eight-Ingredient Pill With Rehmannia (Rehmannia-Eight Combination)

Traditionally prescribed when symptoms include dizziness, light-headedness, night sweats, ringing in the ears or diminished hearing, and soreness and weakness in the lower back. In laboratory studies, reduces blood pressure caused by sensitivity to salt, and protects kidney tissue against damage.[12]

Four-Substance Decoction

Treats high blood pressure caused by too little liver energy. Has been found to be useful in controlling high blood pressure caused by salt sensitivity.[13]

Gentiana Longdancao Decoction to Drain the Liver

Treats high blood pressure caused by liver fire.

Caution: Should be used with caution by persons who take insulin and are on a low-carbohydrate diet. Should not be used at all by women who are trying to become pregnant.

Pinellia, Atractylodis Macrocephala, and Gastrodia Decoction

Treats high blood pressure caused by the solidifying of stagnant energy. This type is aggravated by overwork and emotional stress. Secondary symptoms may include dizziness, headache, sensation of fullness in the chest, and copious amounts of sputum with deep cough.

Caution: Use with caution if fever is present, and discontinue if preexisting fevers worsen.

Prepared Aconite Decoction

Treats high blood pressure accompanied by edema and cold sensations in the body. May cause a loss of sensation in the mouth and tongue.

Caution: Discontinue the formula if fever occurs.

True Warrior Decoction

Treats high blood pressure accompanied by diarrhea or difficulty in urination. May cause a loss of sensation in the mouth and tongue.

Caution: Discontinue the formula if fever occurs.

CONSIDERATIONS

❑ Kudzu is the most appropriate herbal treatment for nerve damage in persons with a long history of high blood pressure. Any herb or herbal formula taken for degenerative diseases affecting hearing or sight should not be used on a long-term basis. Instead, take kudzu three to six months, three times daily (1 ten-milligram tablet or 1 cup tea; tea-making directions in Chapter 3), then replace it with another herb that has similar effects. See a doctor for regular checkups, and consult with a Kampo or TCM practitioner as needed.

❑ Cutting salt intake may or may not lower pressure. The effort only helps about fifty percent of people with high blood pressure, and too *little* salt can cause adrenalin surges, rapid heartbeat, and disturbed sleep.[14] Another approach is to increase potassium in the diet, since potassium counteracts sodium's pressure-raising effects. Eating fruits and vegetables daily—and even eating dairy products and moderate quantities of lean beef, chicken, or pork three or more times a week—provides enough potassium to lower blood pressure.[15]

❑ *See also* **High Cholesterol** and **Obesity.**

HIGH CHOLESTEROL

Cholesterol is a fatty, waxy substance that occurs naturally in the body. Although cholesterol is often misunderstood as a toxic substance, the body needs it for everything from cell membrane creation to hormone production to nerve function. In fact, cholesterol is so important to health that 85 percent of the body's supply is made in the liver. Disturbances in the body's use of cholesterol can result in "high cholesterol," or levels above those doctors consider normal and safe. "High cholesterol" can lead to atherosclerosis, in which cholesterol gathers into artery-clogging plaques that can eventually plug arteries. This process can lead, often after many years, to heart attack or stroke. About 60 million Americans have cholesterol levels high enough to warrant treatment.

Cholesterol, being fatty, cannot travel through the watery bloodstream by itself. Therefore, it is attached to a protein, forming a lipoprotein, for delivery to cells throughout the body. There are several different types of lipoproteins, but the two most important are low-density lipoprotein (LDL) and high-density lipoprotein (HDL). While LDL is thought of as "bad" cholesterol, and HDL as "good" cholesterol, they are actually two stages in the body's use of the same substance, with LDL particles being much larger than HDL particles. The problem with cholesterol arises when LDL becomes "stuck" in the linings of arteries injured by high blood pressure or infection. This LDL attracts macrophages, immune cells that get their cholesterol supplies from LDL, which attach to the trapped LDL particles and themselves become part of the growing plaque. The area of injury can grow larger and even calcify.

Doctors recognize that total cholesterol is not as important a measure of disease risk as the *ratio* of HDL to LDL. Doctors look for an LDL level under 130 milligrams per deciliter of blood (mg/dl) and a HDL level over 30 mg/dl. This corresponds to a LDL/HDL ratio of 4.3 to 1 or lower. Disease risk is increased by untreated high blood pressure, and by factors that make the blood "sticky," including smoking and high blood-sugar levels.

Diet is the first weapon in fighting a high cholesterol level (see "Cholesterol and Diet—The Whole Picture" on page 230). When cholesterol levels cannot be lowered through diet, doctors will prescribe various types of cholesterol-controlling drugs. All have possible side effects, ranging from digestive upsets to liver disturbances.

There is no concept in Kampo that directly corresponds to a laboratory finding of high cholesterol. However, Kampo has described many of the herbs that are useful for treating high cholesterol as treatments for toxins. A true "antitoxin" for high cholesterol would have to lower both cholesterol and blood sugar levels. This is precisely what garlic does. Kampo described the soybean, source of soy lecithin, as an agent which—when combined with scallion to make a simple miso soup—"arrested inner strife" in the arteries and the lungs. And Kampo described Minor Bupleurum Decoction,

Cholesterol and Diet—The Whole Picture

Most people believe that eating larger amounts of fatty foods causes cholesterol levels to go up, and eating smaller amounts of fatty foods causes cholesterol levels to go down. The reality, however, is not quite that straightforward. Doctors have observed that some high-fat diets—such as the traditional diet of Arctic peoples, which is based on whale blubber—do not automatically cause high cholesterol levels. There are also studies casting doubt on the relationship between elevated total cholesterol levels and heart disease. The National Health Examination Follow-Up Survey, for example, found no direct links between total cholesterol levels and heart attack or stroke.[1]

The reason some high-fat diets do not raise cholesterol is that, while they provide a high proportion of fat, the total available calories are severely limited. (In the case of the traditional Arctic diet, even whale blubber was scarce.) It is important to remember that the body's first priority is to obtain enough glucose for fuel, especially for the brain. Carbohydrate, protein, and fat can all be turned into glucose. Only when this need is met can the body turn to making cholesterol and storing fat. Moreover, most of the body's cholesterol is made by the liver itself, and not taken from the diet.

When reducing cholesterol levels, the proportion of fat in the diet is not as important as the total amount of fat that the diet provides. "Sensible" reductions in the amount of fat eaten will not necessarily lower cholesterol levels. Moreover, the way one lowers fat intake also has an effect on cholesterol. Most "fat-free" foods are loaded with sugar. The glucose absorbed from them can build up in the bloodstream faster than the body can use it. This excess sugar glycosylates, or "sugar-coats," red blood cells, making red blood cells "stickier." This creates the single greatest risk factor for heart disease. It also indirectly increases levels of LDL. In addition, high blood-sugar levels lead to high levels of insulin, the hormone that moves sugar into both muscle cells and fat cells. In fact, insulin moves glucose into fat cells much more efficiently, so that high insulin levels spur weight gain. This explains why a large-scale French study found that insulin levels, rather than cholesterol levels, provided the single best measure of predicting cardiovascular disease risk.[2]

The secret of dieting to lower cholesterol, then, is to reduce consumption of both saturated fat and excess calories. This makes exercise an essential companion to proper diet. Exercise burns excess calories, takes sugar out of circulation, reduces glycosylation, and increases the liver's ability to process LDL into HDL. It also reduces the need for insulin and decreases the deposit of fat. Consult a physician before beginning any exercise program.

---

which prevents cholesterol from being attacked by free radicals, as a means of clearing "turbidity" in the center of the body. These treatments work best when combined with a program of diet and exercise.

INDIVIDUAL KAMPO TREATMENTS

See Chapter 3 for discussions of individual herbs, traditional healing substances, and modern herbal preparations, including directions for making tea.

SUGGESTED DOSAGES	COMMENTS
Cordyceps (Traditional Healing Substance)	
Dried extract, 4 250-mg tablets daily. or Prepared tea, as directed on label.	Lowers LDL and total cholesterol while raising HDL.[1] *Caution:* Avoid if a hormone-sensitive disorder is present, such as bladder cancer, melanoma, prostate disorders, or disorders of the female reproductive system.
Garlic (Herb)	
Cloves in food, preferably raw, 2–3 daily. The recommended form. or Tablets (including deodorized) as directed on label, at least 900 mg daily.	Lowers LDL and total cholesterol while raising HDL.[2] Lowers blood-sugar levels without increasing insulin production, another heart disease factor.[3] *Caution:* Do not use with the blood-thinner warfarin sodium (Coumadin). Garlic will counteract the effects of *Bifidus* and *Lactobacillus* cultures taken as digestive aids.
Shiitake (Modern Herbal Preparation)	
Fresh or dried shiitake in food, ¼–½ oz (6–16 g) daily. or 3 1-g tablets 3 times daily. or Syrup, ½ tbsp (4–6 ml) 3 times daily. or Tincture (1:5), 1 tbsp (10 ml) 3 times daily. Place in a cup, add 2 tbsp water, and take in a single sip.	Lowers both LDL and total cholesterol by concentrating fats in the liver, where they are broken down.[4]
Soy Lecithin (Modern Herbal Preparation)	
Soy phospholipids, 1,500–3,000 mg daily. Identified individually on the label as 3-sn-phospatidylcholine, phosphatidylethanolamine, and phospatidylinositic acid, or as "total phospholipids." or Tofu, 2–4 oz (50–100 g) daily.	Lowers *total* cholesterol levels without side effects, and protects the liver against toxins. *Caution:* Mild diarrhea may occur when soy lecithin is first used.

KAMPO FORMULAS

See Chapter 4 for dosage information and discussions of individual formulas.

Bupleurum Plus Dragon Bone and Oyster Shell Decoction

Increases the ratio of HDL to LDL.[5] Reduces nervous tension that may contribute to high blood pressure.

Caution: Be sure the formula does *not* include the traditional ingredient minium (lead oxide). Use with caution if fever is present, and discontinue if preexisting fevers worsen.

Minor Bupleurum Decoction

Reduces atherosclerotic plaque formation by destroying free radicals.[6] This disables macrophages' ability to "dock" in artery linings. Increases the ratio of HDL to LDL.

Caution: Do not use if fever or skin infection is present. Taken long term in patent medicine form, can cause headache, dizziness, and bleeding gums. Side effects can be avoided if the formula is taken as a tea.

CONSIDERATIONS

❑ Low cholesterol levels can also cause health problems. For instance, people with low cholesterol levels have higher-than-average rates of cancer, and respiratory and digestive illnesses,[7] and low levels are associated with, among other things, depression, schizophrenia,[8] and the progression of HIV to AIDS.[9]

❑ *See also* **Atherosclerosis** and **High Blood Pressure.**

HIV INFECTION

HIV is the human immunodeficiency virus, the virus that causes AIDS. Millions of people worldwide now carry the virus, which is usually passed through sexual contact or blood-to-blood contact. Infected mothers can also pass the virus to their children, either during birth or through breast-feeding. It is *not* passed through coughing or sneezing, nor through everyday contact, such as shaking hands.

Most people who are infected with HIV are not aware at first that they have it. While the virus can sometimes cause a flulike illness two to four weeks after infection, it usually takes two to five years for symptoms to appear. Antigen tests can detect HIV infection before symptoms appear, but even frequent HIV testing usually cannot detect the virus in the first six months of infection. In many cases, HIV is discovered only when the infected person develops one or more of the opportunistic infections or cancers associated with AIDS.

HIV affects immune-system cells called T cells. There are two types. Helper T cells help the immune system respond against bacteria, viruses, and cancerous cells. Suppresser T cells suppress the immune system's response against these invaders, a process meant to keep the system from becoming overactive. The decrease in helper T cells and the increase in suppresser T cells results in an increased susceptibility to infections and cancer.

The key to understanding HIV infection is understanding that helper T cells are destroyed not only by HIV, but also by the immune system itself.[1] HIV changes the surface of helper T cells so that they are recognized as foreign matter

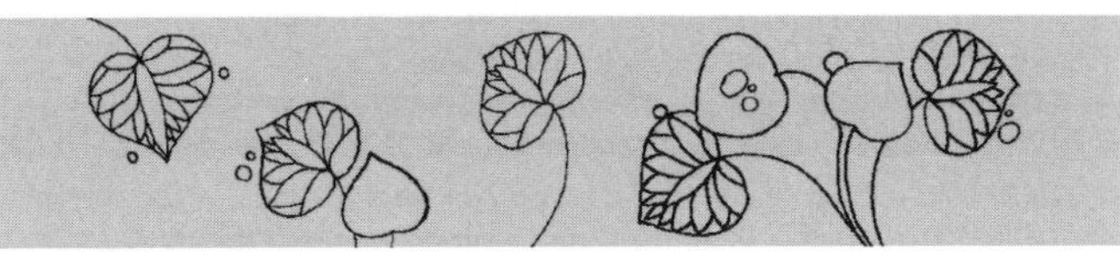

and eliminated by suppresser T cells.[2] As long as the immune system's response to the infected helper T cells is not too strong, there is relatively little damage to the immune system as a whole. In this steady state, the symptoms of AIDS do not appear. Stimulating the immune system *without* regard to which components of the system will be activated, however, makes HIV worse, not better.

The precise relationship between HIV and the immune system was discovered when doctors gave tetanus booster, which acts as an immune-system stimulant, to volunteers with HIV. The doctors' expectation was that boosting the immune system would lower the amount of HIV in the volunteers' bloodstream. Instead, the amount of the virus present in the volunteers' blood increased 200 to 400 percent.[3] Even worse, their remaining virus-free blood cells became more susceptible to HIV infection. On the other hand, medical attempts to *depress* the immune system in order to *treat* HIV have also failed.[4]

At this point, the most effective approach to healing is to deal, not with the immune system, but with the virus itself. This is the approach used in "AIDS cocktails," in which drugs are combined to disable the virus in as many different ways as possible. These potent drug combinations extend life, but also cause serious complications, including blood abnormalities and damage to the liver or pancreas.

HIV was unknown before 1981, so traditional Japanese medicine did not have a concept of either viruses in general or HIV. However, Kampo medicine did have a concept of diseases of the Lesser Yang (see Chapter 1). This is a condition of stalemate between the destructive energies of infection, which are trying to involve more and more of the body, and the body's defensive energies, that are trying to drive the infection out. Scientists in the United States and Japan noted that HIV infection sometimes matches these symptoms. Some people who contract HIV develop a skin rash in the early stages of their infection. The virus then lies dormant for months or years until some other factor limits immune resistance. Then HIV infection overcomes the body's inner organs.

Kampo offers ways to fill in the gaps of traditional treatment. Minor Bupleurum Decoction, the formula most often used for diseases of the Lesser Yang, has a profound effect on HIV, particularly in cases in which AIDS symptoms have not yet appeared. This includes an ability to complement AIDS cocktails.[5] Systematic testing has revealed many other traditional herbs that are extremely helpful in treating AIDS. Before using any of these herbs, however, be sure to discuss them with a physician, who can determine if a specific herb's effect is appropriate for any specific stage of the disease.

INDIVIDUAL KAMPO TREATMENTS

See Chapter 3 for discussions of individual herbs, traditional healing substances, and modern herbal preparations, including directions for making tea.

SUGGESTED DOSAGES	COMMENTS
Astragalus (Herb)	
Fluid extract (1:1), ¼–½ tsp (1–2 ml) 3 times daily. or Freeze-dried herb in capsules, 500–1,000 mg 3 times daily. or Powdered solid extract (4:1), 250–500 mg 3 times daily. or Tea, 1 c 3 times daily. or Tincture (1:5), 1–1½ tsp (4–6 ml), 3 times daily. Place in a cup, add 2 tbsp water, and take in a single sip.	Stops infections that can accelerate the progress of HIV to AIDS, including hepatitis B[6] and *Streptococcus,* without stimulating the immune system overall. Prevents cell-to-cell transmission of some viruses. *Caution:* Do not use when fever or skin infection is present.
LEM (Modern Herbal Preparation)	
Powder, as directed on label.	Prevents progression of HIV to AIDS by stopping cell-to-cell transmission of the virus.[7] *Caution:* Can occasionally cause mild diarrhea or skin rashes. Should these symptoms occur, consult a health care provider.
Maitake (Modern Herbal Preparation)	
Fresh or dried maitake in food, 1–2 tbsp (3–7 g) daily. or Maitake D-fraction in capsule or tablet form, 500 mg 3 times daily before meals. or Tea, 1 c 2–4 times daily.	Contains a carbohydrate-based substance known to kill HIV and to keep HIV from killing T cells.[8]
Prunella (Herb)	
Tea, 1 c 3 times daily between meals.	Blocks cell-to-cell transmission of HIV and interferes with the virus's ability to bind with T cells.[9] *Caution:* Do not use if diarrhea, nausea, stomachache, or vomiting is present.
Scutellaria (Herb)	
Dried herb, 1–2 1,000-mg capsules 3 times daily. or Fluid extract (1:1), ¼–½ tsp (1–2 ml) 3 times daily. or Powdered solid extract (4:1), 250–500 mg 3 times daily. or Tea, 1 c 3 times daily. or Tincture (1:5), 1–1½ tsp (4–6 ml) 3 times daily. Place in a cup, add 2 tbsp water, and take in a single sip.	Contains baicalin, which deactivates reverse transcriptase, an enzyme HIV needs to insert itself into human DNA, without affecting the T cells' ability to replicate.[10] Also prevents many other kinds of infections without stimulating the immune system. *Caution:* Avoid in cases of diarrhea caused by foodborne infection or excessive consumption of cold drinks.
Turmeric (Herb)	
Curcumin, the yellow pigment found in turmeric, 250–500 mg twice daily between meals.	Curcumin stops HIV replication by deactivating the virus's long terminal repeat gene.[11] Also inhibits the activity of HIV integrase, an enzyme that allows the virus to use a human cell for its own replication.[12] Inhibits other factors necessary for HIV replication.[13]
Viola (Herb)	
Use under professional supervision.	Reported to keep HIV from "erupting" from infected cells.[14,15] Use *Viola yedoensis* instead of *Viola tricolor.* Sold in bulk in Chinese herb shops as *Zi Hua Di Ding.*

HERBS TO AVOID

Individuals who have HIV infection should avoid the following immune-stimulant herbs: aloe, American ginseng, asparagus root, bamboo, chrysanthemum, coix, ginseng, ligustrum, psoralea, and Solomon's seal. For more information regarding these herbs, see Chapter 3. In addition, avoid the following popular non-Kampo herbs: chamomile, echinacea, saw palmetto, and wheat grass.

KAMPO FORMULAS

See Chapter 4 for dosage information and discussions of individual formulas.

Minor Bupleurum Decoction

Can prevent the progression of HIV to AIDS.[16,17] Stops 90% of the activity of the enzyme reverse transcriptase.[18] Does not interfere with T-cell reproduction.[19] Especially useful for people with AIDS who also have hepatitis.

Caution: Do not use if fever or skin infection is present. Taken long term in patent medicine form, can cause headache, dizziness, and bleeding gums. Side effects can be avoided if the formula is taken as a tea.

Ten-Significant Tonic Decoction (All-Inclusive Great Tonifying Decoction)

Useful as a general tonic for persons with HIV. Stimulates production of interleukins and NK cells.[20] Kampo physicians traditionally give this formula to persons with abdominal tension, hot flashes in the hands and feet, and lethargy.

CONSIDERATIONS

❑ While immune suppression through the use of powerful drugs is harmful to people with HIV, immune suppression through strenuous exercise seems to help. Such exercise reduces numbers of both helper T and suppresser T cells. People with HIV who exercise tend to have fewer complications and to progress much more slowly to AIDS. Ask at a local health club about designing an appropriate exercise regimen.

❑ Persons who are HIV-positive should avoid recreational drug use. Some drugs, notably cocaine[21] and marijuana,[22] may not affect HIV infection itself but disable T-cell response to other kinds of infections.

❑ *See also* **AIDS** and **Hepatitis.**

HODGKIN'S DISEASE

Hodgkin's disease is a little-understood cancer of lymph tissue, the tissue that houses much of the body's immune function. This tissue is organized into lymph nodes found in various parts of the body. In North America, Hodgkin's disease usually strikes either young boys or elderly men.

Often the only symptoms of Hodgkin's disease at first are night sweats with low-grade fever. In approximately 10 percent of cases, there may be a skin itch in the early stages. As the disease progresses, it causes increasing inflammation. The lymph nodes become swollen, and there may be coughing, chest pain, and bone pain. Because the initial symptoms resemble those of many other disorders, a positive diagnosis for Hodgkin's disease can only be made by examining an enlarged lymph node.

Hodgkin's disease seems to be caused by a virus that has not yet been identified. The longer the infection lasts, which may be years or decades, the greater the chance that this disorder will develop. The body is more susceptible to the virus that appears to cause Hodgkin's after infection with Epstein-Barr virus or mononucleosis, and after tonsillectomy or appendectomy.

Although Hodgkin's disease is a cancer of the immune system, it usually affects only one group of white blood cells. This cancer attacks T cells and specifically helper T cells, the cells that stimulate the immune response against infectious organisms. Also, it usually affects only a part of the lymphatic system, rather than spreading throughout it. The net effect of the disease on the immune system is that it does not greatly increase vulnerability to infection, except to herpes and viral warts.

Hodgkin's disease is classified into stages I through IV based on the number of lymph node regions involved. Medical treatment is set by stage. Early stages are usually treated with radiation therapy. Later stages of the disease are usually treated with "MOPP" chemotherapy, named after the chemicals used in treatment.

Before the twentieth century, Japanese doctors, like doctors elsewhere, lacked the scientific tools needed to diagnose Hodgkin's disease. As early as 1119, however, they recognized a symptom pattern in which the kidneys were unable to help the bones generate marrow (where white blood cells are created). If the debility to the kidneys continued, they eventually lost their store of "essence," or guiding information for the body. Essence roughly corresponds to the modern idea of DNA, except it is localized in the kidneys. This lack of guiding essence would cause night sweats and fevers. Although the loss of essence affected the entire body, pain was localized to the area near the kidneys, particularly the lower back, and the channels for transporting lymph. Modern Japanese medicine has found that formulas that treat this symptom pattern, such as Six-Ingredient Pill with Rehmannia, also treat Hodgkin's disease.

Always use Kampo as part of a medically directed overall treatment plan for Hodgkin's disease (see considerations below). Especially in treating childhood Hodgkin's disease, always work with a Kampo or TCM practitioner along with the physician; the dosages provided in this entry are meant for adults.

INDIVIDUAL KAMPO TREATMENTS

See Chapter 3 for discussions of individual herbs, traditional healing substances, and modern herbal preparations, including directions for making tea.

SUGGESTED DOSAGES	COMMENTS
Astragalus (Herb)	
Fluid extract (1:1), ¼–½ tsp (1–2 ml) 3 times daily. or Freeze-dried herb in capsules, 500–1,000 mg 3 times daily. or Powdered solid extract (4:1), 250–500 mg 3 times daily. or Tea, 1 c 3 times daily. or Tincture (1:5), 1–1½ tsp (4–6 ml), 3 times daily. Place in a cup, add 2 tbsp water, and take in a single sip. For dosages used with chemotherapy, *see* **Chemotherapy Side Effects.**	Stimulates the activity of T cells.[1] *Caution:* Do not use when fever or skin infection is present.
Siberian Ginseng (Modern Herbal Preparation)	
Eleuthero extract, as directed by manufacturer, in ¼ c water. Be sure to use pure extract, not sugar-sweetened ginseng drinks. or Tea, 1 c 3 times daily.	Contains compounds that both increase interferon production and stimulate the immune-protection activity of T cells.[2] *Caution:* Should be avoided by persons with myasthenia gravis; rheumatoid arthritis and diseases related to it, such as lupus, psoriatic arthritis, and Sjögren's syndrome; or prostate cancer.

KAMPO FORMULAS

See Chapter 4 for dosage information and discussions of individual formulas.

Capital Qi Pill

Relieves night sweats. Also effective for shortness of breath that may be accompanied by soreness and weakness in the lower back, lightheadedness, vertigo, tinnitus, or diminished hearing.

Six-Ingredient Pill with Rehmannia (Rehmannia-Six Combination)

Relieves bone pain in the lower half of the body and spine.

CONSIDERATIONS

❑ To reduce side effects and increase effectiveness when using chemotherapy, *see* **Chemotherapy Side Effects**; when using radiation therapy, *see* **Radiation Therapy Side Effects.**

HYPERACTIVITY

See **Attention Deficit Disorder/Attention Deficit Hyperactivity Disorder (ADD/ADHD).**

HYPERTHYROIDISM

Over 2.5 million Americans suffer from hyperthyroidism, a condition in which the thyroid gland at the base of the neck becomes overactive. When this happens, the gland produces too much of the hormone thyroxine, which speeds up the body's functions. It occurs most often in women between the ages of twenty and forty, and often arises following physical or emotional stress. A blood test is used for diagnosis.

The overwhelming majority of persons with hyperactive thyroids suffer from a condition known as *Graves' disease.* This is an autoimmune disease in which the thyroid, mistakenly responding to immune-system signals, pumps more and more thyroxine into circulation.

In Graves' disease the appetite is disturbed, and there is weight loss, no matter how much food is consumed, because nutrients are poorly absorbed. Other symptoms include nervousness, irritability, insomnia, fatigue, and a constant feeling of being hot, with increased perspiration. Graves' disease increases the frequency of bowel movements, decreases menstrual flow, and causes hair loss, and induces rapid heartbeat, separation of the nails from the nail beds, hand tremors, and, sometimes, protruding eyeballs and vision disturbances. The thyroid gland may swell as the disease progresses, forming a goiter.

Japanese researchers have linked Graves' disease to bouts of severe allergies, specifically to cedar pollen.[1] Graves' disease may also be linked to a class of respiratory viruses known as the spumaretroviruses[2] and a virus known as HTLV-1.[3]

There are other forms of hyperthyroidism: *Plummer's disease* and a potentially dangerous form called *thyroid storm,* which appears suddenly and causes mood swings, fever, extreme agitation, and weakness. Neither form is related to the immune system. If left untreated, all forms of hyperthyroidism can lead to bone and heart disorders.

Conventional medicine treats hyperthyroidism with drugs that lower thyroxine output. Sometimes in cases of Graves' disease, steroid drugs are used. If drugs do not work, radiation is used to destroy overactive thyroid tissue. This may result in underactive thyroid, and the lifelong need for thyroid supplements.

Kampo developed a number of formulas to treat symptom patterns corresponding to hyperthyroidism. Most of these formulas were designed to correct excess heat in the liver and gallbladder. When the liver is "heated" by overwork, bad diet, or toxins from infection, it sends its energy out along an energy channel extending from the external genitalia to the breasts and eyes. If the gallbladder is similarly heated, it sends its energy upward to meet the liver energy, blocking both energies' normal flow through the body. Energy became trapped in the external genitalia, breasts, and eyes. A similar pattern can result from heat in the kidneys.

Kampo formulas relieve heat and stop the symptoms of hyperthyroidism, and some also increase the effectiveness of steroids (see considerations below).

INDIVIDUAL KAMPO TREATMENTS

See Chapter 3 for discussions of individual herbs, traditional healing substances, and modern herbal preparations, including directions for making tea.

SUGGESTED DOSAGES	COMMENTS
Scutellaria (Herb)	
Dried herb, 1–2 1,000-mg capsules 3 times daily. or Fluid extract (1:1), ¼–½ tsp (1–2 ml) 3 times daily. or Powdered solid extract (4:1), 250–500 mg 3 times daily. or Tea, 1 c 3 times daily. or Tincture (1:5), 1–1½ tsp (4–6 ml) 3 times daily. Place in a cup, add 2 tbsp water, and take in a single sip.	Useful for prevention of common infections, such as colds, flu, and other upper respiratory infections, in place of immune-stimulant herbs. A compound in the herb shuts down the reproduction process in influenza viruses A and B provided it is administered 18 to 54 hours *before* infection.[4,5] *Caution:* Avoid in cases of diarrhea caused by foodborne infection or excessive consumption of cold drinks.

HERBS TO AVOID

Individuals who have Graves' disease should avoid the following herbs: aloe, American ginseng, astragalus, bamboo, burdock, chrysanthemum, ginger, ginseng, and Siberian ginseng. For more information regarding these herbs, see Chapter 3. In addition, avoid the following popular non-Kampo herbs: echinacea, lemon balm (melissa), and wheat grass. There is no need to avoid these herbs if the hyperthyroidism is *not* caused by Graves' disease.

KAMPO FORMULAS

See Chapter 4 for dosage information and discussions of individual formulas.

Bupleurum Plus Dragon Bone and Oyster Shell Decoction

Treats hyperthyroidism when the primary symptoms are difficulties in concentration and speech, irritability, nervousness, and rapid pulse.

Caution: Be sure the formula does *not* include the traditional ingredient minium (lead oxide). Use with caution if fever is present, and discontinue if preexisting fevers worsen.

Eight-Ingredient Pill With Rehmannia (Rehmannia-Eight Combination)

Stops continuous sweating.

Gentiana Longdancao Decoction to Drain the Liver

Useful when the primary symptoms of hyperthyroidism are irritability, headache, and short temper. It is particularly useful for women who experience a shortened period.

Caution: Should not be used by women who are trying to become pregnant.

Honey-Fried Licorice Decoction

Treats anxiety, irritability, and insomnia with weight loss.

Minor Bupleurum Decoction

Increases the effectiveness of the steroid drug prednisone. Relieves secondary symptoms, including asthma, chills alternating with hot flashes, and nausea or acid stomach.

Caution: Do not use if fever or skin infection is present. Taken long term in patent medicine form, can cause headache, dizziness, and bleeding gums. Side effects can be avoided if the formula is taken as a tea.

Ophiopogonis Decoction

Increases effectiveness of the steroid drug methylprednisolone. Sometimes used to treat bulging eyes.

Caution: Use with caution if fever is present, and discontinue if preexisting fevers worsen.

CONSIDERATIONS

❑ Ironically, it possible to have both Graves' disease and Hashimoto's thyroiditis, which causes underactivity of the thyroid, at the same time. Both conditions can occur with still other autoimmune diseases, including rheumatoid arthritis, lupus, chronic hepatitis, diabetes, pernicious anemia, and Sjögren's syndrome.[6] Persons who have any of these diseases need periodic monitoring of thyroid function.

❑ To reduce side effects and increase effectiveness when using steroid drugs, *see* **Chemotherapy Side Effects.**

❑ *See also* **Hypothyroidism.**

HYPOTHYROIDISM

Hypothyroidism is caused by low activity of the thyroid gland. This gland, which lies at the base of the neck, produces the hormone thyroxine, which regulates virtually all bodily functions. A lack of this hormone can cause these functions to slow down. Thyroxine deficiencies range from barely detectable (subclinical hypothyroidism) to severe (myxedema). From 1 to 4 percent of all adults have severe hypothyroidism, and up to 10 percent of all adults have some form of thyroid deficiency. The percentages go up with age. Many cases of hypothyroidism are not detected, since the blood test used for diagnosis is not part of a standard physical examination.

Hypothyroidism can cause depression, weight gain or difficulty in losing weight, numbness and tingling in the feet and hands, constipation, fatigue, headache, menstrual problems, recurrent infections, swelling, or sensitivity to the cold. The tongue may thicken, and the voice may change in quality. There may be dry skin, dull or thinning hair, thinning of eyebrows, and brittle nails. Women with hypothyroidism may be infertile.

Almost all cases of hypothyroidism occur as a sequel to an immune-system malfunction known as *Hashimoto's thyroiditis.* This is an autoimmune disease in which the thyroid, mistakenly responding to immune-system signals, becomes inactive. Fibrous tissue forms, and swelling and inflammation set in. This causes goiter, or an enlarged thyroid gland. The thyroid continues to function for a long time before the body suffers a thyroxine shortage. As a result the disease can come on so gradually that the person is at first aware of only vague, low-grade symptoms.

Hypothyroidism can have other causes. Treatment of hyperthyroidism can destroy the thyroid gland. Problems in the pituitary gland can disrupt the supply of thyroid-stimulating hormone. In some parts of the world, iodine deficiency is a common cause of hypothyroidism.

Almost all cases of hypothyroidism require thyroid hormone replacement therapy. The replacement may be a mixture of several thyroid hormones, or just thyroxine, the main hormone. In most cases, therapy must be continued for life.

Kampo views the symptoms modern medicine identifies as hypothyroidism as a manifestation of internal "cold." This is cold that has attacked the kidneys, the organs that warm the entire body. Cold congests, congeals, and contracts, stopping the normal flow of energy and causing weight gain. It contracts the pores of the skin, causing the skin to dry out and locking pathogens under the skin, resulting in recurrent infections. It overcomes the yang, or outwardly directed, energies of the kidneys. Water that is not circulated properly by the kidneys may flood or spill over into the flesh and skin, where it causes aching, swelling, and puffiness. It can also "veil the sensory orifices" and create a dull, stuffy feeling in the head.

Kampo formulas relieve symptoms and can treat established cases of hypothyroidism.[1] They can be used along with thyroid hormone replacement therapy.

INDIVIDUAL KAMPO TREATMENTS

See Chapter 3 for discussions of individual herbs, traditional healing substances, and modern herbal preparations, including directions for making tea.

SUGGESTED DOSAGES	COMMENTS
Scutellaria (Herb)	
Dried herb, 1–2 1,000-mg capsules 3 times daily. or Fluid extract (1:1), ¼–½ tsp (1–2 ml) 3 times daily. or Powdered solid extract (4:1), 250–500 mg 3 times daily. or Tea, 1 c 3 times daily. or Tincture (1:5), 1–1½ tsp (4–6 ml) 3 times daily. Place in a cup, add 2 tbsp water, and take in a single sip.	Helps prevent recurrent infections in place of immune-stimulant herbs. A compound in the herb shuts down the reproduction process in influenza viruses A and B provided it is administered 18 to 54 hours *before* infection.[2,3] *Caution:* Avoid in cases of diarrhea caused by foodborne infection or excessive consumption of cold drinks.

HERBS TO AVOID

Individuals who are in the early stages of hypothyroidism may avoid losing remaining thyroid function by avoiding the following immune-stimulant herbs: aloe, American ginseng, astragalus, bamboo, burdock, chrysanthemum, ginger, ginseng, kelp, motherwort, and Siberian ginseng. For more information regarding these herbs, see Chapter 3. In addition, avoid the following popular non-Kampo herbs: echinacea, lemon balm (melissa), and wheat grass.

KAMPO FORMULAS

See Chapter 4 for dosage information and discussions of individual formulas.

Frigid Extremities Decoction

Yang-stimulating formula designed for a symptom pattern that includes extremely cold hands and feet; abdominal pain; aversion to cold; constant desire to sleep, and to sleep with the knees drawn up; diarrhea with undigested food particles; and a lack of thirst. May cause a loss of sensation in the mouth and tongue.

Caution: Discontinue the formula if fever occurs.

Kidney Qi Pill From *The Golden Cabinet*

Especially affects circulation of water. Treats copious urination or urinary incontinence in hypothyroidism. May cause a loss of sensation in the mouth and tongue.

Caution: Discontinue the formula if fever occurs.

Prepared Aconite Decoction

Yang-stimulating formula, like **Frigid Extremities Decoction** (see this list), but for more advanced cases of the disease. May cause a loss of sensation in the mouth and tongue.

Caution: Discontinue the formula if fever occurs.

True Warrior Decoction

Primary treatment in modern Japanese herbal medicine for hypothyroidism. Especially useful for treating abdominal pain and diarrhea. May cause a loss of sensation in the mouth and tongue.

Caution: Discontinue the formula if fever occurs.

CONSIDERATIONS

❑ Persons who are taking the prescription drug thyroxine may benefit from also taking desiccated thyroid tablets, available over the counter in health food stores. These tablets provide all thyroid hormones except thyroxine, which is present only in trace amounts. Since these tablets do not contain thyroxine, they cannot be used in place of medically prescribed therapy.

❑ Subclinical hypothyroidism, or that which produces no symptoms, may exist even if blood tests are normal. Test for this condition by taking a body-temperature reading three mornings in a row. Before getting out of bed, hold a thermometer in either armpit for fifteen minutes, keeping as still as possible. Add the temperatures, and divide by three. If the average temperature is below 97.5°F, see the doctor. Women should avoid taking their temperatures while ovulating or during the first week of the period.

❑ Ironically, it is possible to have both Hashimoto's thyroiditis and Graves' disease, which causes overactivity of the thyroid, at the same time. Both conditions can occur with still other autoimmune diseases, including rheumatoid arthritis, lupus, chronic hepatitis, diabetes, pernicious anemia, and Sjögren's syndrome.[4] Persons who have any of these diseases need periodic monitoring of thyroid function.

❑ Avoid consuming large amounts of soy foods, such as tofu or miso. These foods contain a chemical that interferes with the body's use of thyroid hormone.

IMPOTENCE

Impotence is a condition in which a man does not have the ability to achieve or maintain an erection adequate for normal sexual intercourse. Impotence may be chronic or recurrent, or it may happen as a single isolated incident. This condition often has both psychological and physical factors.

Erections are made possible by a complex combination of blood vessel and nerve functions that are affected by hormones, especially the main male hormone, testosterone. Anything that interferes with these interactions can interfere with erections. Diabetes, which leads to atherosclerosis and impaired circulation, is the most frequent cause of impotence, but impotence can also be caused by high blood pressure and the medications given for it (and other drugs as well), insufficient testosterone production, hypothyroidism or hyperthyroidism, repeated infections of sexually transmitted diseases, excessive alcohol consumption, and smoking. Fatigue, overwork, and poor nutrition can compound the problem.

Many of the factors associated with impotence become more common with age. This explains why most men who suffer from at least occasional impotence are older, the condition affecting one out of three men over age sixty (although it can affect younger men as well). While it often takes longer for older men to achieve erections, impotence is *not* a normal consequence of aging.

Conventional medicine treats impotence with medications, including Viagra, that can adversely affect the cardiovascular system. Penile injections or implants and external vacuum-type devices may also be used.

Kampo understands that impotence sometimes results from, ironically, too much of the yang, or "masculine," principle. The sex organ expands so much that its tissues become loose. Excessive consumption of foods with a yang principle, such as dairy products, fats, and meat, aggravate the energy imbalance. Treatment for this form of impotence is dietary rather than herbal. Impotence may also result from a deficiency of yang energies in the kidneys, such as that associated with diabetes. Treatment for this form of impotence consists of activating the "kidneys" to produce testosterone, enabling erection.

Both an excess of yang energy from food and deficiency of yang energy from the kidneys can exist at the same time. Combining dietary restraint with herbal treatment helps both causes of impotence. Any of the preparations listed here should be effective within three to four weeks of use.

INDIVIDUAL KAMPO TREATMENTS

See Chapter 3 for discussions of individual herbs, traditional healing substances, and modern herbal preparations, including directions for making tea.

SUGGESTED DOSAGES	COMMENTS
Cistanche (Herb)	
Dried herb, 1 1-gm capsule 3 times daily.	The primary herb in many combinations marketed as "herbal Viagra." Can increase erectile strength in most men who take it, but is especially useful for impotence caused by diabetes. Available as *Rou Cong Rong.*
Epimedium (Herb)	
Use as directed by the herbalist.	Has testosteronelike effects, stimulates sexual activity and desire. Increases sperm production. *Caution:* Avoid if a prostate disorder is present.
Ginseng (Herb)	
Fluid extract or tincture, as directed on label. or Tea, made with Korean or red ginseng, 1 c daily.	A traditional aphrodisiac. Stimulates secretion of gonadotrophins, which stimulate cell growth and healing in the sex organs.[1] Relaxes the penis's erectile tissue, allowing inward blood flow.[2] If using ginseng extracts or tinctures (which are not as therapeutically active as teas), be sure the product contains *Panax ginseng.* Note that strength may vary by manufacturer. *Caution:* Not used in men with a strong physique and a symptom pattern of strong pulse with tension in the abdomen, resistance and pain when pressed over the heart and below the ribs, tendency toward constipation, and bad breath. In such men, ginseng will cause impotence to worsen.[3]
Siberian Ginseng (Modern Herbal Preparation)	
Eleuthero extract, as directed by manufacturer, in ¼ c water. Be sure to use pure extract, *not* sugar-sweetened ginseng drinks. or Tea, 1 c up to 3 times daily.	Stimulates production of testosterone.[4] *Caution:* Should be avoided by persons with myasthenia gravis; rheumatoid arthritis and diseases related to it, such as lupus, psoriatic arthritis, and Sjögren's syndrome; or prostate cancer. Same symptom-pattern restriction as **Ginseng.**

KAMPO FORMULAS

See Chapter 4 for dosage information and discussions of individual formulas.

Restore the Right Kidney Pill

Treats impotence occurring after long or debilitating disease. Additional symptoms in the pattern may include aversion to cold, coolness of the hands and feet, and pain in the lower back and knees. May cause a loss of sensation in the mouth and tongue.

Caution: Discontinue the formula if fever occurs. Avoid if there is constipation or dark, scanty urine.

CONSIDERATIONS

❑ Anxiety, depression, stress, guilt, and fear of intimacy can all contribute to impotence. Seek counseling if necessary.

❑ Some well-known non-Kampo herbal remedies for impotence, including damiana and yohimbine, act by stimulating blood circulation into and blocking circulation out of the penis. When taken in overdose, use of these herbs may result in a painful and potentially damaging condition called priapism, the opposite of impotence, in which blood becomes trapped in the erect penis.

❑ *See also* **Alcoholism, Atherosclerosis, Diabetes, High Blood Pressure, Hyperthyroidism,** and **Hypothyroidism.**

INCONTINENCE

Incontinence is the inability to control the bowels or bladder in a person old enough to do so. Older people are more likely to suffer incontinence, especially urinary incontinence, because they are more likely to have the disorders that often interfere with bowel or bladder control.

Both urination and defecation depend on a complex series of nerve and muscle reactions. These reactions may be disrupted at any step, resulting in incontinence. Urinary incontinence can be caused by bladder infection (the most common cause) or medication side effects. Prostate disorders may be the cause of incontinence in men, while a lack of estrogen may pose a problem in postmenopausal women. Women are particularly susceptible to *stress incontinence,* in which urine is released during laughing, coughing, or sneezing. Bowel incontinence may accompany diarrhea. Both types of incontinence can result from surgery, spinal cord injuries, stroke, dementia, or damage to nerves associated with either the bladder or the rectum.

Conventional medicine deals with incontinence after first diagnosing any underlying disorder. The patient may be trained to void at regular intervals for urinary incontinence, or to make changes in diet for bowel incontinence. Drugs and surgery may also be used.

By Kampo definition, incontinence is a failure of yin, or containing, energies. These energies are essential to the action of what Chinese Kampo calls the "middle burner," an energy organ that keeps energy flowing upward in the center of the body. When the digestive system fails to supply energy to the middle burner, either bowel or urinary incontinence may result.

The first step in controlling incontinence, therefore, is to ensure a healthful diet and good digestion. In addition, any underlying disorders should be treated. If incontinence persists, Kampo provides formulas to treat individual symptom patterns.

INDIVIDUAL KAMPO TREATMENTS

See Chapter 3 for discussions of individual herbs, traditional healing substances, and modern herbal preparations, including directions for making tea.

SUGGESTED DOSAGES	COMMENTS
Cardamom (Herb)	
Tincture (1:5), 10 drops in ¼ c hot water 3 times daily for 21 days.	Stops urinary incontinence in both men and women. Treats urinary tract infection caused by *E. coli*.[1]

KAMPO FORMULAS

See Chapter 4 for dosage information and discussions of individual formulas.

Gentiana Longdancao Decoction to Drain the Liver

Reduces incontinence caused by prostate enlargement or irritation. Treats "vague" symptoms not directly related to prostate disease, which may include headache, dizziness, red and sore eyes, swelling in the ears, hearing loss, bitter taste in the mouth, or short temper.

Kidney Qi Pill From *The Golden Cabinet*

Relieves lower back pain and weakness of the lower extremities. Symptoms may also include a cold sensation in the lower half of the body, tension in the lower abdomen, and irritability to the point of having difficulty in lying down. There is often either urinary difficulty with edema, or excessive urination, sometimes to the point of incontinence. In extreme cases, the patient has difficulty breathing, and breathes more easily when leaning against a support. May cause a loss of sensation in the mouth and tongue.

Caution: Discontinue the formula if fever occurs.

True Man's Decoction to Nourish the Organs

Treats unremitting diarrhea to the point of incontinence. Accompanying symptoms include mild, persistent abdominal pain that responds favorably to local pressure or warmth, lethargy, pale complexion, reduced appetite, soreness of the lower back, and lack of strength in the legs. Not available as a patent medicine, but widely available from TCM practitioners as *zhen ren yang rang tang.*

Caution: Patients taking this formula should avoid alcohol, wheat, cold or raw foods, fish, and greasy foods. Should not be used by persons with gallbladder problems, obstruction of the bile duct, or a tendency to retain urine, or by pregnant women.

CONSIDERATIONS

❑ If urinary incontinence is present, try eliminating or cutting alcohol and caffeine intake. If bowel incontinence is present, try adding small amounts of fiber to the diet, keeping in mind that too much fiber can make matters worse.

❑ If urinary incontinence is caused by weak pelvic muscles, try strengthening them with Kegel exercises. A physical therapist can provide guidance on how to do these exercises correctly. For bowel incontinence, it may be possible to strengthen the anal sphincters through biofeedback-guided exercises. Again, a physical therapist can help.

❑ *See also* **Bladder Infection** and **Diarrhea.**

INDIGESTION

Indigestion, medically known as *dyspepsia,* is a term used to describe a variety of abdominal discomforts associated with eating. Some people experience indigestion as abdominal pain, pressure, or heartburn. Other people experience indigestion as belching, a feeling of excessive gas, or flatulence. Still others use the term to describe a vague feeling that digestion has not proceeded naturally or that they react badly to specific foods. Indigestion is one of the most common medical complaints in North America, with sales of over-the-counter digestive aids running into the billions of dollars.

Indigestion can arise from a number of causes. Among the most common are poor diet, rushed meals, stress, and lack of exercise. A number of drugs, especially painkillers such as aspirin and ibuprofen, can affect the stomach. In addition, a number of serious illnesses can produce the same symptoms, including colitis, colorectal or stomach cancer, extremely high blood-sugar levels, gallstones, gastritis, heart attack, hepatitis, intestinal obstruction, irritable bowel syndrome, and pancreatitis.

Chronic indigestion should always be brought to a doctor's attention. However, it is possible to distinguish simple indigestion from symptoms caused by other conditions. Indigestion occurs only after eating, and the pain it causes is dull rather than sharp. It spreads symmetrically to both the left and right of the abdomen, and, when gas is not a problem, is felt above the navel. Pain below the navel is more likely to originate in the appendix or colon, while pain around the navel is usually associated with disorders of the small intestine. Pain caused by serious disease of the gallbladder, liver, or pancreas usually begins as an intense pain in a single spot that then spreads upward in the body.

Pain under the breastbone is especially significant. This pain may be caused by a malfunction of the esophagus, or by failures of circulation in and to the heart. Seek *immediate* medical attention if chest pain radiates to the jaw or arm; is vicelike or squeezing in nature; or is accompanied by heartburn, dizziness, nausea, or cold sweats.

Some of the more common indigestion symptoms are covered in this section. In addition, a proper diet, especially when combined with a program of exercise and stress relief, can ease or prevent simple indigestion. Use herbs as needed after eating, but take formulas on a long-term basis.

Considerations

❑ *See also* **Allergies, Food; Constipation;** and **Diarrhea.**

BELCHING

A belch is a regurgitation of swallowed air. When excess air is swallowed, belching is the body's way of reestablishing normal pressure in the stomach. If the air cannot be expelled, it accumulates in the stomach and causes sharp pain. Predispositions to belching include chronic anxiety, poorly fitting dentures, and postnasal drip, as well as drinking carbonated beverages or drinking through a straw, eating rapidly, smoking cigarettes, or sucking on hard candy.

Kampo explains belching in terms of "entangled energy," which escapes from traps in the digestive tract explosively and unpredictably. Warming the cold that traps digestive energy releases gas and normalizes the flow of energy.

INDIVIDUAL KAMPO TREATMENTS

See Chapter 3 for discussions of individual herbs, traditional healing substances, and modern herbal preparations, including directions for making tea.

SUGGESTED DOSAGES	COMMENTS
Fennel Seed (Herb)	
Tea, 1–3 tsp.	Relieves belching and gas in infants. *Caution:* Do not give infants essential oil.[1]
Peppermint (Herb)	
Oil, 10–15 drops. Place in a cup, add 2 tbsp water, and take in a single sip. or Tea, 1 c.	The quickest herbal relief for belching in adults. Relaxes the lower esophagus and equalizes pressures between the throat and stomach.[2] *Caution:* Should not be used if the bile duct may be blocked.

KAMPO FORMULAS

See Chapter 4 for dosage information and discussions of individual formulas.

Calm the Stomach Powder

Treats recurrent belching, especially when there is acid regurgitation.

BLOATING AND FLATULENCE

"Gas" causes a feeling of dull abdominal pain and bloating. The physiological process that produces feelings of bloating actually does not create more gas than is usually present in the lower digestive tract. Instead, it is a super-sensitivity to gas that is only present in normal amounts. One is more sensitive to the presence of gas when blood-sugar levels are elevated, such as after eating a large dessert.[1]

Flatulence, on the other hand, results from excess gas production. The gases involved include the odorless carbon dioxide and hydrogen, and the odor-producing hydrogen sulfide. Hydrogen sulfide is toxic, and failure to release it can cause tissue damage.[2]

Kampo explains bloating and flatulence as the simultaneous presence of deficiency (bloating) and excess (flatulence) in the intestines. Treatments for bloating and flatulence encourage downward motion through the intestines, passing the imbalance out of the body.

INDIVIDUAL KAMPO TREATMENTS

See Chapter 3 for discussions of individual herbs, traditional healing substances, and modern herbal preparations, including directions for making tea.

SUGGESTED DOSAGES	COMMENTS
Cinnamon (Herb)	
Oil, 15–30 drops. Place in a cup, add 2 tbsp warm water, and take in a single sip. or Tea, 1 c.	Relieves bloating and flatulence as well as cramps.
Fennel Seed (Herb)	
Tea, 1–3 tsp.	Relieves bloating and flatulence in infants. *Caution:* Do not give infants essential oil.

KAMPO FORMULAS

See Chapter 4 for dosage information and discussions of individual formulas.

Major Order the Qi Decoction

Treats severe constipation with flatulence.

Considerations

❑ If prone to flatulence, avoid (in addition to beans) dates, figs, and prunes. Asparagus, onions, and wheat may also pose problems for some people.

HEARTBURN

Heartburn is a sensation of warmth or burning beneath the breastbone or in the stomach above the navel. Heartburn pain can radiate to the neck and arms, mimicking heart pain caused by angina. Heartburn most often occurs after the person has eaten a large meal, and then bends, stoops, or lies down. The change in position weakens the sphincter at the bottom of the esophagus, allowing acidic material from the stomach to back up into the esophagus. Aspirin, alcohol, spicy food and citrus fruit juices can also induce heartburn, as can excess weight, overeating, stress, smoking, and pregnancy.

Kampo describes heartburn in terms of heat and cold. "Heat" generated from the emotional energy of inordinate anger, anxiety, or joy can disrupt the flow of energy between the liver and stomach and cause acid reflux, belching, bitter taste in the mouth, nausea, and vomiting. Cold foods or "cold" in the form of infection can weaken the energies of the stomach and cause food to stagnate. When the mass of food in the stomach keeps it from passing "turbid" fluids downward, they rise and cause nausea and heartburn.

INDIVIDUAL KAMPO TREATMENTS

See Chapter 3 for discussions of individual herbs, traditional healing substances, and modern herbal preparations, including directions for making tea.

SUGGESTED DOSAGES	COMMENTS
Coptis (Herb)	
Tincture (1:5), 20 drops. Place in a cup, add 2 tbsp water, and take in a single sip.	Drains fluids from the stomach, stopping heartburn associated with emotional tension. If coptis is unavailable, substitute tincture of the non-Kampo herb goldenseal (same caution applies). *Caution:* Do not use during pregnancy or on a daily basis for more than 2 weeks at a time.

Turmeric (Herb)	
Powder, 1 tsp in 1 c of water. or Tea, 1 c.	Clears "energy debris" resulting from cold in the digestive tract, and stops irritation. Do *not* use the turmeric compound curcumin.

KAMPO FORMULAS

See Chapter 4 for dosage information and discussions of individual formulas.

Calm the Stomach Powder

Especially useful when heartburn is accompanied by physical or mental fatigue.

Evodia Decoction

Useful when heartburn is accompanied by severe vomiting. Use under supervision of an herbalist for this purpose.

HICCUPS

Hiccups are sudden, involuntary contractions of the diaphragm. They can occur in persons of any age, but are more common in infants and small children than in adults. The most frequent causes of hiccups are indigestion and swallowing air while eating. When air is swallowed with food or drink, it has no place to go except back through the esophagus in a hiccup.

Kampo describes hiccups in terms of either emotional or physical causes. Unrelieved emotional tension can build up energy in the liver, which spreads laterally and causes tightness across the stomach. The lungs' energy then escapes in spasmodic bursts, or hiccups. Alternatively, hiccups result from either abnormal "heat" (infection and irritation) or abnormal "cold" (undigested food) in the stomach. The stomach is no longer able to contain its energy, which "rebels" by escaping upward.

INDIVIDUAL KAMPO TREATMENTS

See Chapter 3 for discussions of individual herbs, traditional healing substances, and modern herbal preparations, including directions for making tea.

SUGGESTED DOSAGES	COMMENTS
Galangal (Herb)	
Tea, 1 c.	Galangal contains chemicals that stop hiccup-causing inflammation. Also stops stomach upset caused by incomplete digestion.

INFERTILITY, FEMALE

As many as one out of every four American couples experiences infertility, defined as the failure to conceive after at least one year of unprotected intercourse. Infertility in women can have many causes, including ovarian cysts and blockages of the fallopian tubes, endometriosis, hypothyroidism, and uterine fibroids. This entry concerns female infertility caused by ovulatory failure, or the failure of the ovary to release an egg.

In a woman of childbearing age, the ovaries normally release one egg per menstrual cycle. The pituitary gland secretes follicle stimulating hormone (FSH), which allows the egg to "mature" in the ovary. The pituitary also secretes luteinizing hormone (LH), which triggers ovulation. In addition, a form of estrogen called estradiol causes the uterine lining to thicken, which gives a fertilized egg a nutrient-rich attachment point in the womb. If an egg is not fertilized, the lining is broken down, both the egg and the lining are eliminated through menstruation, and a new cycle begins.

Anything that upsets this complex hormonal balance can interfere with ovulation. Stress, whether physical or psychological in origin, can disrupt the system. So can age, especially as a woman reaches her midthirties. Ovulatory failure can also occur for no detectable reason.

Conventional medicine first treats ovulatory failure with fertility drugs. The drugs can not only have a number of different side effects, but can also increase a woman's risk of developing ovarian cancer if used over too long a period of time. If this does not work, a woman can opt for in vitro fertilization. In this procedure, the ovaries are hormonally stimulated to release multiple eggs, which are then extracted, fertilized in a laboratory, and returned to her body. In vitro fertilization is expensive and often not successful.

Japanese physicians often find the cause of female infertility through yin-yang diagnosis, or evaluation of the body's two main types of energy. Yang energies project outward, while yin energies curve inward. Straight eyelashes indicate an excess of yang energy, corresponding to the excessive production of testosterone, a male hormone that can "turn off" LH production. Curved eyelashes indicate an excess of yin energy, such as the failure to produce LH. Women who are infertile due to the presence of ovarian cysts tend to manifest yang energies in the center of the cheeks in the form of skin outbreaks, rashes, or pimples. Ovarian cysts are also related to the presence of spots in the whites of the eyes. Fibroid tumors tend to show themselves as a yellowish coloration in the whites of the eyes. Japanese physicians often interpret white vaginal discharges as potential for tumors, yellow discharges as active formation of tumors, and green discharges as growth of existing tumors. Other menstrual irregularities are indicated by the presence of a horizontal line between the lips and the nose when the woman smiles.

Diagnosing the energy imbalance underlying infertility is critical to successful treatment. Obviously, the first step is to treat any reproductive-tract disorders that may be present. Since energy imbalance in infertility caused by ovulatory failure is influenced by many factors, treatment usually requires the use of formulas rather than of single herbs. Consult a Kampo or TCM practitioner to determine the formula most likely to help, or consult a gynecologist regarding the type of hormonal rebalancing needed. Kampo formulas for fertility should be effective within three months of consistent daily use.

INDIVIDUAL KAMPO TREATMENTS

See Chapter 3 for discussions of individual herbs, traditional healing substances, and modern herbal preparations, including directions for making tea.

SUGGESTED DOSAGES	COMMENTS
Artemisia (Herb)	
Use under professional supervision.	Increases chances of conception. Also used to treat threatened miscarriage when there is vaginal bleeding.

HERBS TO AVOID

Individuals who have an infertility-causing disorder should avoid the following herbs: amaranth (achyranthus), barley sprouts, gardenia, snake gourd root, and tang-kuei. For more information regarding these herbs, see Chapter 3.

KAMPO FORMULAS

See Chapter 4 for dosage information and discussions of individual formulas.

Cinnamon Twig and Poria Pill

Stimulates ovulation. Increases blood levels of estradiol, FSH, and LH, and increases the weight of the uterus.[1]

Peony and Licorice Decoction

Increases chances of pregnancy, particularly in women with ovarian cysts. Acts by increasing the ratio of estradiol to testosterone and FSH to LH.[2] Not a traditional use of the formula.

Warm the Menses Decoction

Treats infertility in a symptom pattern of bleeding between periods, continuous or extended menstrual flow, irregular menstruation (either early or late), or persistent uterine bleeding, and cold in the lower abdomen, dry lips and mouth, low-grade fever in the late afternoon, or warm palms and soles.

Caution: Discontinue if preexisting fevers worsen.

CONSIDERATIONS

❑ *See also* **Endometriosis, Fibroids, Hypothyroidism,** and **Ovarian Cysts.**

INFERTILITY, MALE

As many as one out of every four American couples experiences infertility, defined as the failure to conceive after at least one year of unprotected intercourse. Male infertility can be caused by a variety of injuries to and disorders of the sperm-producing organs, the testes. These include damage caused by the mumps and certain other viruses; radiation damage, whether through industrial accident or in the course of cancer treatment; exposure to environmental toxins; heat damage caused by snug-fitting briefs or pants; the use of medications or recreational drugs, including alcohol, marijuana, heroin, or methadone; smoking; and the cancer treatments cyclophosphamide and doxorubicin hydrochloride (Adriamycin). In addition, systemic illnesses, including cirrhosis of the liver, Hodgkin's disease, sickle-cell anemia, and acute fevers, can also lead to infertility.

Male infertility can also be caused by physical abnormalities. One is a vascular condition known as *varicocele,* in which blood accumulates in the testicles, a condition similar to varicose veins. Varicocele accounts for 20 to 40 percent of cases of male infertility, and usually can be surgically corrected. Infertility can also result from blockage of the spermatic ducts, the tubes that carry sperm away from the testes. This also can be corrected through surgery.

Infertility occurs when blood levels of testosterone, the main male hormone, are reduced, generally because illness or injury reduces blood flow to the testes. Lower levels of testosterone result in lowered sperm production. Even if a man produces enough sperm for conception (about 100 million per milliliter of semen), he may still be infertile if his sperm is not mobile, or in biological terms, motile. Sperm cells that are not motile cannot swim up into the woman's fallopian tubes, where conception generally occurs.

Despite the identification of various causes of male infertility, almost half of all cases have *no* cause that can be pinpointed through examination. Consequently, these cases cannot be medically treated. Injections of testosterone or other hormones do not increase male fertility. Such injections may even have feminizing side effects if the body converts the extra testosterone into female hormones. Other techniques that may be tried are in vitro fertilization (see page 240) or artificial insemination, in which either the man's or a donor's sperm is introduced directly into the woman's reproductive tract.

Traditional Japanese medicine's understanding of infertility associated the condition with imbalances in the liver and kidneys. The body's generative energy, or *jing,* is seen by Oriental medicine to reside in the kidneys. In this view, excessive ejaculation depletes the *jing* and drains both the kidney and the penis of vital energy, or qi.

Male sexual dysfunction is also associated with "liver" imbalance. The energy channel controlled by the liver encircles the penis, and the liver controls the blood which supplies the erect penis. Symptoms of liver imbalance include impaired libido with chest congestion, depression, irritability, red eyes, and sore neck and shoulders.

Herbal treatments of infertility emphasize astringing, or conserving, *jing,* and preventing the loss of sperm from the body. (Almost all Kampo and TCM practitioners also suggest that male sexual vigor requires sexual intercourse with the avoidance of ejaculation, limiting ejaculation to once every ten days for men in their twenties to no ejaculation at all preferably, and no more than once a month for men over sixty.)

INDIVIDUAL KAMPO TREATMENTS

See Chapter 3 for discussions of individual herbs, traditional healing substances, and modern herbal preparations, including directions for making tea.

SUGGESTED DOSAGES	COMMENTS
Astragalus (Herb)	
Fluid extract (1:1), 1/4–1/2 tsp (1–2 ml) 3 times daily. or Freeze-dried herb in capsules, 500–1,000 mg 3 times daily. or Powdered solid extract (4:1), 250–500 mg 3 times daily. or Tea, 1 c 3 times daily. or Tincture (1:5), 1–1 1/2 tsp (4–6 ml), 3 times daily. Place in a cup, add 2 tbsp water, and take in a single sip.	Enhances male fertility by increasing sperm motility.[1] *Caution:* Do not use when fever or skin infection is present.
Epimedium (Herb)	
Use as directed by the herbalist.	Stimulates semen formation and nerve activity in the male sex organs. Do not use more than 3 months. There are no side effects, but the herb becomes less effective with continued use. *Caution:* Avoid entirely if a prostate disorder is present.

HERBS TO AVOID

Men who have fertility problems should avoid vitex. For more information regarding this herb, see Chapter 3.

KAMPO FORMULAS

See Chapter 4 for dosage information and discussions of individual formulas.

Cinnamon Twig and Poria Pill

Treats male infertility due to variocele, increases sperm count and sperm motility.[2] Improves circulation in the lower abdominal region and reduces blood retention. Traditionally is given to men who are "warm-natured," preferring cold temperatures to warm temperatures, and who have a tendency to muscle strain.

Tonify the Middle and Augment the Qi Decoction

Helps developing sperm cells receive the amino acids they need to reach the egg in the uterus. Has been clinically proven to raise both testosterone levels and sperm counts. Widely used in Japan for treating male infertility for which there is no readily discernible cause. Also effective in alleviating infertility caused by the cancer treatment Adriamycin.[3] Traditionally given to men who are "cold natured," preferring warm temperatures to cold temperatures.

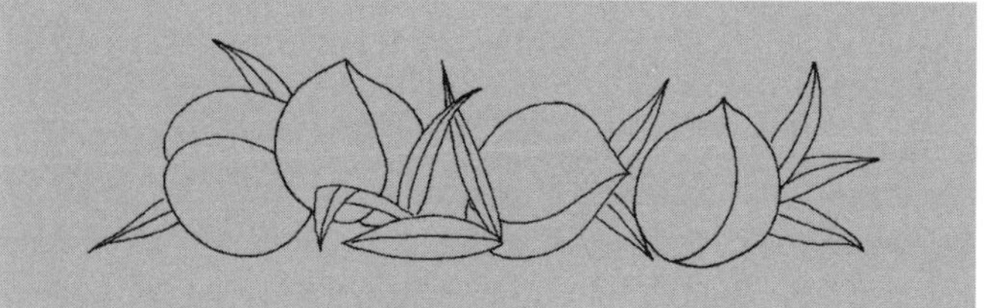

CONSIDERATIONS

❑ Purified ferulic acid, a male fertility aid derived from the herb tang-kuei (see Chapter 3), is available in health food stores. Follow the package directions.

INFLUENZA

Influenza, commonly called the flu, is a viral respiratory infection. The symptoms include chills, fever, headache, muscle aches, fatigue, weakness, nasal discharge, and cough. These are similar to the symptoms of a cold, except that flu symptoms tend to come on more suddenly and be more severe. The fatigue and weakness associated with the flu can last for several weeks after the initial infection.

The human body can build immunity to the influenza virus, which comes in two main strains, A and B. However, the virus can reproduce and mutate inside the bodies of domestic animals, and these mutations cause worldwide epidemics every one to three years. Flu epidemics generally occur during the winter.

Flu is transmitted through extremely small particles generated by coughs and sneezes. The virus begins to replicate within four to six hours of its arrival in the body, but the spread of infection sufficient to produce symptoms requires an incubation period of from two to three days. The worse the case of the flu, the more likely it is to be contagious.

Medical treatment for flu consists mostly of pain relief. (It is important never to give children under the age of fifteen aspirin, as the use of aspirin during viral infections can result in Reye's syndrome, an extremely serious complication.) The A strain of flu can be treated with the prescription drug amantadine hydrocholoride (Symmetrel), if taken within the first forty-eight hours of infection. This drug reduces the flu's duration by about 50 percent, although it can cause nervousness. Another prescription drug, ribavirin (Virazole), is effective against both A and B.

Kampo sees influenza the same way it sees the common cold, as the initial assault of an invading outside pernicious influence, or "cold." The body stops the invading disease at its "borders," its skin, muscles, and joints. The fight between the body's defensive energy and the pathogen heats the surface of the body, causing fever in the process. If the body is strong enough, the invading pathogen is routed and "sweated out" of the body. This process opens the pores and allows heat to escape the body, causing chills. Fever, nasal discharge, and tearing eyes all work together to expel the invading pathogen from the body and bring it back to balance. Kampo treatments help the body's natural defense mechanisms vanquish the flu without causing damage to tissues.

Some single herbs can be used to prevent the flu. Note that these herbs have to be taken up to two days *before* infection.

INDIVIDUAL KAMPO TREATMENTS

See Chapter 3 for discussions of individual herbs, traditional healing substances, and modern herbal preparations, including directions for making tea.

SUGGESTED DOSAGES	COMMENTS
Fritillaria, Cirrhosa (Herb)	
Fritillaria and Pinellia Syrup, 2–3 tsp (8–12 ml) 3 times daily.	Useful for sticky phlegm, snoring, or chronic sore throat. Available as *Qing Chi Hua Tan Tang.* *Caution:* Avoid if weakness from a chronic health problem is present.
Green Tea (Herb)	
Catechin extract, 1 240-mg tablet 3 times daily. or Tea, 1 c 2–3 times daily.	Helps prevent infection by either influenza A or influenza B.[1] To avoid dilution problems, do not take tea within 1 hour of taking other teas or patent medicines.
Scutellaria (Herb)	
Dried herb, 1–2 1,000-mg capsules 3 times daily. or Fluid extract (1:1), ¼–½ tsp (1–2 ml) 3 times daily. or Powdered solid extract (4:1), 250–500 mg 3 times daily. or Tea, 1 c 4 times daily. or Tincture (1:5), 1–1½ tsp (4–6 ml) 3 times daily. Place in a cup, add 2 tbsp water, and take in a single sip.	Contains a compound that shuts down the reproduction process in influenza viruses A and B.[2,3] *Caution:* Avoid in cases of diarrhea caused by foodborne infection or excessive consumption of cold drinks.

KAMPO FORMULAS

See Chapter 4 for dosage information and discussions of individual formulas.

Bupleurum and Cinnamon Twig Decoction

Relieves joint pain from flu.

Caution: Use with caution if fever is present, and discontinue if preexisting fevers worsen.

Warm the Gallbladder Decoction (Bamboo and Hoelen Decoction)

Relieves insomnia in persons who have not completely recovered from the flu and are troubled by coughing and sputum production.

Caution: Use with caution if fever is present, and discontinue if preexisting fevers worsen.

CONSIDERATIONS

❑ *See also* **Colds.**

INSOMNIA

Insomnia is a state of inadequate sleep. It may take the form of an inability to fall asleep, or of a tendency to wake up in the night and be unable to go back to sleep.

Insomnia may be transient, lasting from one to several nights. This is caused by short-term stress, changes in schedule or surroundings, or jet lag. Insomnia may be short-term, persisting for between a few days and three weeks. This is caused by protracted stress, such as surgery or short-term illness. Chronic insomnia can persist for months or years, caused by a fundamental imbalance in the body or the emotions. Depression, chronic pain, and breathing difficulties can all contribute to chronic insomnia.

If there is no obvious underlying physical cause of insomnia, doctors treat this condition with a variety of mild tranquilizers and antidepressants. In addition to other side effects, some of these drugs can be habit-forming, and some can cause daytime sleepiness.

Kampo sees insomnia as a collection of related symptom patterns that compromise the yin, or containing, energies of the liver and heart. In some forms of insomnia, the liver, agitated by emotional stress, poor diet, or overwork, discharges its energy as "fire" flowing upward in the body. Liver fire creates bloodshot or tired eyes, blurred vision, headache, and thirst. In Kampo theory, the organs, or energy centers of the body, "take turns" being the most active, and the liver and gallbladder are at their most active between 11 P.M. and 3 A.M. The inability to sleep during this time, particularly if accompanied by stiff neck or shoulders, or irritability or bursts of anger, or headache, is attributed to a liver disturbance.

Other kinds of insomnia result when the heart cannot contain the emotions. This form of insomnia causes vivid dreams, nightmares, palpitations, and memory problems. Insomnia also can result from deficiencies of blood or energy that cause lack of self-confidence, constant worrying, easy fright, and frequent urination.

INDIVIDUAL KAMPO TREATMENTS

See Chapter 3 for discussions of individual herbs, traditional healing substances, and modern herbal preparations, including directions for making tea.

SUGGESTED DOSAGES	COMMENTS
Schisandra (Herb)	
Freeze-dried herb, 100 mg 3 times daily. Available as Hoelen & Schisandra. or Tea, 1 c 3 times daily.	Relieves insomnia accompanied by nightmares. *Caution:* Avoid if gallstones or blockages of the bile ducts exist.

KAMPO FORMULAS

See Chapter 4 for dosage information and discussions of individual formulas.

Bupleurum and Kudzu Decoction to Release the Muscle Layer From *Medical Revelations*

Relieves insomnia when secondary symptoms include fever and chills, with fever becoming worse and chills lessening; dry nasal passages; pain in the eye or eye socket; headache; irritability; and stiffness in the extremities.

Caution: Avoid if nausea or vomiting is present.

Bupleurum Decoction to Clear the Liver

Treats insomnia generated by constant emotional stress, particularly when secondary symptoms include hearing loss, bad breath, flushed cheeks, severe headaches, or ringing in the ears.

Caution: Avoid during pregnancy.

Cinnamon Twig Decoction Plus Dragon Bone and Oyster Shell

Treats persons of strong constitution who have insomnia accompanied by depression, dream-filled sleep, feelings of frustration, and palpitations.

Coptis Decoction to Relieve Toxicity

Treats insomnia in persons with "blood effusive" symptoms: redness in the face, a feeling of blood rushing to head, high blood pressure, and possibly chronic constipation.

Caution: Should not be used by women who are trying to become pregnant.

Emperor of Heaven's Special Pill to Tonify the Heart

Treats insomnia with "dry" symptoms, such as constipation or scratchy throat.

Caution: Do not use this formula if there is loss of appetite or diarrhea, or if there are aches and pains from influenza.

Licorice, Wheat, and Jujube Decoction

Treats insomnia in children who are awake all night crying. Seek the advice of the dispensing herbalist on a suitable child's dosage. Can be made at home in tea form (see Chapter 4).

Peony and Licorice Decoction

Treats insomnia in children and infants. Traditionally given when a green vein appears on the stomach. Seek the advice of the dispensing herbalist on a suitable child's dosage.

Pill for Deafness That is Kind to the Left Kidney

Relieves insomnia caused by tinnitus, described in ancient sources as "the sound of swarms of insects in the ear all night."

Polyporus Decoction

Treats insomnia accompanied by nausea or vomiting.

Warm the Gallbladder Decoction (Bamboo and Hoelen Decoction)

Relieves insomnia in persons who have not completely recovered from a cold or lung infection and are troubled by coughing and sputum production.

Caution: Use with caution if fever is present, and discontinue if preexisting fevers worsen.

CONSIDERATIONS

❑ Polygonum, usually sold as *Ho She Wou,* is useful in cases of repeated nightmares (see Chapter 3).

❑ Avoid over-the-counter sleep aids.

IRRITABLE BOWEL SYNDROME

A number of disorders can cause intestinal pain and discomfort, among them irritable bowel syndrome (IBS) and Crohn's disease. IBS is a condition in which the rhythmic muscular contractions of the digestive tract become irregular and uncoordinated, and the normal movement of food and waste material is impaired. Crohn's disease is a condition in which severe inflammation causes ulceration of part or all of the digestive tract. These disorders produce similar symptoms, and Kampo views them in a similar light. For that reason, they are both discussed in this entry.

In IBS, trapped gas and stools cause bloating, distention, and constipation and/or diarrhea, often alternating. Eating may result in intense pain that is relieved by moving the bowels or by vomiting. Crohn's disease also causes diarrhea and pain. In addition, there are fever, headache, steatorrhea (fatty stools that float), fatigue, loss of appetite, and loss of weight. Nutrients are not properly absorbed, which leads to malnutrition. While complications stemming from IBS are rare, chronic bleeding from Crohn's disease may cause iron-deficiency anemia, and the presence of open sores increases the risk of infection. Crohn's disease may become chronic, which can result in bowel obstruction.

IBS is a fairly common disorder, affecting an estimated one out of every five Americans, most of them women. Crohn's disease, once rare, is becoming more common, with as many as 500,000 cases diagnosed each year. It occurs more often among Jews than among members of other ethnic groups.

Although the physical cause of IBS is not known, some studies suggest that this disorder can be caused by an unusual reaction to opiates, which can cause diarrhea in hypersensitive persons.[1] Opiates exist in medications, such as codeine and morphine, and in foods, including beef, milk, and wheat. Stress is another likely factor. Like IBS, Crohn's disease has no known cause, but is linked to food allergies. IBS and Crohn's disease also share a common link in that depression occurs frequently in people with either disorder.

Crohn's disease is diagnosed through the use of either a barium enema, in which barium highlights the digestive tract on an x-ray, or an endoscope, in which a tube is used to view the intestinal wall. Crohn's disease and other digestive disorders must be ruled out before the doctor can make a firm diagnosis of IBS, which does not involve an observable physical illness. Both disorders are treated with drugs that relieve symptoms. In the case of Crohn's disease, this includes steroid drugs such as prednisolone. Surgery is another option in Crohn's disease.

In Kampo theory, both IBS and Crohn's disease result from an overcontrolling liver. The liver can be so charged by the emotions it stores that it overdirects the small intestine, which in turn overdirects the digestive organ, the spleen. The spleen tries to circulate energies upward in the body, but these nutritive energies collide with the liver energy and create "turbidity," a liquid of variable composition. The turbidity descends by fits and starts to the intestines, where it alternately causes and relieves abdominal cramping. Because the disease processes in both IBS and Crohn's disease are complex, Kampo generally uses formulas rather than single herbs.

INDIVIDUAL KAMPO TREATMENTS

See Chapter 3 for discussions of individual herbs, traditional healing substances, and modern herbal preparations, including directions for making tea.

SUGGESTED DOSAGES	COMMENTS
Peppermint (Herb)	
Oil, enterically coated capsules, 200 mg once or twice daily between meals.	Stops colon spasms by relaxing intestinal muscles. *Caution:* Should not be used if the bile duct may be blocked.

KAMPO FORMULAS

See Chapter 4 for dosage information and discussions of individual formulas.

Formulas That Treat IBS

Calm the Middle Powder

Relieves spastic abdominal pain.

Four-Gentlemen Decoction

Treats a pattern of symptoms that includes loose stools, low and soft voice, pallid complexion, and weakness in the limbs, without pain in the digestive tract.

Minor Construct the Middle Decoction

Treats a pattern of symptoms that includes intermittent, spasmodic abdominal pain and reduced appetite. There may also be cold hands and feet, dry mouth and throat, irritability, low-grade fever, or palpitations.

Pinellia Decoction to Drain the Epigastrium

Treats a pattern of symptoms that includes diarrhea with rumbling in the lower digestive tract, fullness and tightness over the stomach with little pain, and reduced appetite.

Caution: Use with caution if fever is present, and discontinue if preexisting fevers worsen.

Formulas That Treat Crohn's Disease

Ginseng Decoction to Nourish the Nutritive Qi

Relieves abdominal discomfort without causing sedation. Use allows reduction in prednisolone dosage.[2]

Minor Bupleurum Decoction

Increases the effectiveness of prednisone. Relieves sensation of fullness in the chest with bitter taste in the mouth, nausea, and fever and chills.

Caution: Do not use if fever or skin infection is present. Taken long term in patent medicine form, can cause headache, dizziness, and bleeding gums. Side effects can be avoided if the formula is taken as a tea.

Ophiopogonis Decoction

Increases the effectiveness of a wide range of steroid drugs. Also effective against asthmatic symptoms, including coughing, wheezing, and involuntary spitting of saliva.

Caution: Use with caution if fever is present, and discontinue if preexisting fevers worsen.

True Man's Decoction to Nourish the Organs

This formula treats diarrhea or dysenteric disorders with unremitting diarrhea to the point of incontinence. In severe cases, there may be prolapsed rectum, and the stool may contain pus and blood. Accompanying symptoms include mild, persistent abdominal pain that responds favorably to local pressure or warmth, lethargy, pale complexion, reduced appetite, soreness of the lower back, and lack of strength in the legs. Not available as a patent medicine, but widely available from TCM practitioners as *zhen ren yang rang tang.*

Caution: Avoid alcohol, wheat, cold or raw foods, fish, and greasy foods. Should not be used by persons with gallbladder problems, obstruction of the bile duct, or a tendency to retain urine, or by pregnant women.

True Warrior Decoction

This formula is appropriate to advanced stages of the disease, with coldness in the hands and feet, and such a severe state of weakness that cramping has disappeared. May cause a loss of sensation in the mouth and tongue.

Caution: Discontinue the formula if fever occurs.

CONSIDERATIONS

❑ Treatment for IBS requires a high-fiber diet, and avoidance of foods that cause mucus secretion from the bowel membranes—animal fats, butter, carbonated beverages, chocolate, coffee, the food additives mannitol and sorbitol, ice cream, margarine, nuts, orange juice, and wheat bran among them—and foods that contain natural opiates, such as beef, milk, and wheat products. On the other hand, too much fiber can worsen Crohn's disease. This disorder requires a diet that is low in fat and high in both protein (from chicken or fish) and vegetables, especially garlic, carrots, turnips, and cole vegetables, such as broccoli and cabbage.

❑ *See also* **Allergies, Food.**

Kidney Cancer (Renal Cell Carcinoma)

There are several types of cancer that affect the kidney, but the most common type is called renal cell carcinoma. It appears twice as often in men as in women and generally strikes people in their late fifties. The causes of kidney cancer are not exactly known, although increased risk is associated with smoking and high-fat diets.

Blood in the urine, flank pain, and a palpable abdominal mass are the three main symptoms of kidney cancer, although all three symptoms seldom occur together. While blood in the urine is the only symptom in 60 percent of all cases, it is by no means a sure sign of kidney cancer. Kidney stones; infections of the kidney, bladder, and urethra; yeast infections; and urinary-tract injuries can also cause bleeding. A cancer diagnosis must be confirmed by a biopsy.

Kidney cancer is classified according to systems that measure tumor size and extent of spread. This form of cancer tends to spread early in its development, especially to the lungs. It also disables the immune system, which makes treatment more difficult. In early stages, the kidney and adjacent lymph nodes may be removed. In later stages, surgery may be combined with radiation therapy. Chemotherapy is sometimes used, although kidney cancer is resistant to most drugs.

Newer treatments for kidney cancer include immunotherapy, or the use of agents that stimulate the immune system. Interferon-alpha slows the growth of cancer cells, and alters their surfaces so that immune-system cells called macrophages can recognize and destroy them. Interleukin-2 (IL-2) activates two kinds of immune-system cells—tumor-infiltrating lymphocytes (TIL) and lymphokine-activated killer (LAK) cells—that attack cancer cells, and other parts of the immune system to fight infection. Sometimes the hormone melatonin is used with IL-2 for increased effectiveness. While these therapies do help some patients,[1,2] they have side effects that may be severe enough to stop treatment. These effects include swelling caused by IL-2, and loss of appetite, fatigue, fever and chills, and nausea caused by interferon-alpha. Using the two therapies together has shown positive results,[3] but also combines the side effects.

Kampo medicine identifies kidney cancer through symptoms that are subtler than those recognized by conventional medicine. In Kampo diagnosis, bags under the eyes, bedwetting, getting up at night to go to the bathroom, getting up late in the morning, groaning, lower back pain, and snoring are all signs of kidney cancer. These symptoms tend to occur together. They also tend appear at an earlier stage of cancer, when it is usually easier to treat. Kampo associates this disorder with "extreme yang" foods, such as eggs, meat, and unleavened baked goods, and with an "extreme yang" environment of unremitting emotional tension.[4]

Bags under the eyes are especially indicative of kidney health. Fluid, puffy bags under the eyes reflect the kidneys' inability to move water. Hard, rigid bags reflect the accumulation of fats and toxins in the kidneys that may turn into tumors.

Kampo should always be used as part of a medically directed overall treatment program for kidney cancer, especially since making immunotherapy bearable is the principal use of Kampo in this disease (see considerations on the next page).

INDIVIDUAL KAMPO TREATMENTS

See Chapter 3 for discussions of individual herbs, traditional healing substances, and modern herbal preparations, including directions for making tea.

SUGGESTED DOSAGES	COMMENTS
Astragalus (Herb)	
Fluid extract (1:1), ¼–½ tsp (1–2 ml) 3 times daily. or Freeze-dried herb in capsules, 500–1,000 mg 3 times daily. or Powdered solid extract (4:1), 250–500 mg 3 times daily. or Tea, 1 c 3 times daily. or Tincture (1:5), 1–1½ tsp (4–6 ml), 3 times daily. Place in a cup, add 2 tbsp water, and take in a single sip. For dosages used with chemotherapy, *see* **Chemotherapy Side Effects.**	Contains compounds that slow the spread of kidney cancer. These compounds also stimulate activity of T cells and increase the ability of LAK cells to attack cancerous tumors.[5] Increases the effectiveness of therapy with melatonin and/or IL-2.[6] Stops opportunistic infection by *Streptococcus.* *Caution:* Do not use when fever or skin infection is present.
Cordyceps (Traditional Healing Substance)	
Dried extract, 4 250-mg tablets daily. or Prepared tea, as directed on label.	Contains compounds that stimulate NK cells.[7] *Caution:* Avoid if a hormone-sensitive disorder is present, such as bladder cancer, melanoma, prostate disorders, or disorders of the female reproductive system.
Lentinan (Modern Herbal Preparation)	
Intramuscular injection (usual form), 0.5–50 mg effective daily dose, depending on patient's condition and circumstances. Smaller, more frequent doses more effective than larger, less frequent doses. Given under professional supervision. or Powder, dosage to be determined by provider. Much greater dosages required than in injectable form.	Lentinan activates LAK and NK cells to attack carcinoma,[8] including that of the kidney.
Licorice (Herb)	
Glycyrrhizin extract. Use only under professional supervision for this disorder.	Has eliminated kidney tumors in test animals.[9] Reduces inflammation secondary to kidney cancer.
Reishi (Modern Herbal Preparation)	
Dried extract, 3 1-g tablets 3 times daily. or Dried mushroom in food, approx. ¼–approx. ½ oz (5–10 g) daily. or Syrup, as directed on label. or Tincture (1:5), 1 tsp (4 ml) 3 times daily. Place in a cup, add 2 tbsp water, and take in a single sip.	Contains compounds that stimulate the body's production of IL-2[10,11] and increase the effectiveness of melatonin. Also deactivates mast cells, which cause swelling and promote delayed allergic reactions.
Siberian Ginseng (Modern Herbal Preparation)	
Eleuthero extract, as directed on label, in ¼ c water. Be sure to use pure extract, *not* sugar-sweetened ginseng drinks. or Tea, 1 c up to 3 times daily.	Effective against cancer cells that respond to immunotherapy, including kidney cancer. Contains compounds that stimulate various immune-system components, including natural production of interferon.[12] *Caution:* Should be avoided by persons with prostate cancer.

KAMPO FORMULAS

See Chapter 4 for dosage information and discussions of individual formulas.

Guide Out the Red Powder

Used in treatment of diseases in which blood in the urine is a symptom. It relieves a sensation of heat, particularly in the chest, with cravings for cold beverages. It also stops nightmares and calms nervous unrest.

Ten-Significant Tonic Decoction (All-Inclusive Great Tonifying Decoction)

Stimulates production of interleukins and NK cells.[13] Prolongs survival time and minimizes side effects of cancer treatment, including treatment with fluorouracil.

FORMULAS TO AVOID

Individuals who have kidney cancer should avoid Tonify the Middle and Augment the Qi Decoction. For more information regarding this formula, see Chapter 4.

CONSIDERATIONS

❑ Since kidney cancer is a yang condition, supplying the body with yin, macrobiotic foods should slow or reverse the progress of disease. For more information on this subject, see *The Macrobiotic Way* by Michio Kushi.
❑ Supplemental L-carnitine, an amino acid, can reduce (but not eliminate) the swelling associated with IL-2 therapy. Use 500 milligrams three times daily.
❑ To reduce side effects and increase effectiveness when using chemotherapy, *see* **Chemotherapy Side Effects**; when using radiation therapy, *see* **Radiation Therapy Side Effects.** To learn about herbal treatments that can prevent a cancer from developing its own blood supply, *see* **Cancer.**

KIDNEY DISEASE

The main function of the kidneys is to eliminate wastes and to regulate fluid balance in the body. A number of disorders can cause the kidneys to malfunction.

The basic functional unit of the kidney is the nephron. It contains structures that filter out wastes from the blood, retain essential nutrients, and concentrate the remaining fluid into urine, which passes into the ureters and then the bladder.

The most easily recognized symptom of nephritis, or kidney inflammation, is blood in the urine. Bloody urine should always be brought to a doctor's attention, as it appears in a number of urinary-tract disorders. Kidney damage is sometimes signaled by swelling, as the kidneys cannot move fluids out of the body. When advanced nephritis cripples the kidneys' ability to retain protein, the urine can actually take on a gel-like appearance.

Kidney disorders can be roughly divided into two categories, acute and chronic. The acute disorders are caused by infection, last for relatively short periods of time, and cause relatively few side effects. Chronic disorders, though, have more long-lasting consequences. *Idiopathic rapidly progressive glomerulonephritis* (IRPG) is a collection of diseases that cause the kidneys to leak massive quantities of protein into the urine. It may be caused by an autoimmune disease, such as lupus or rheumatoid arthritis, or by an allergic reaction to drugs or chemotherapy. It may also be a complication of the body's immune response to infections or cancer. *Nephrotic syndrome* also causes the kidneys to lose protein. In addition, it causes high cholesterol levels, mineral deficiencies, and swelling. It can arise from many of the same conditions that cause IRPG. It can also be caused by diabetes, HIV infection, overuse of NSAID painkillers, or allergic reactions to bee stings.

Standard medical treatment for chronic kidney disease includes steroid drugs such as prednisone, which deactivate the immune system, and/or cyclophosphamide, which inhibits capillary formation and thus reduces bleeding. Treatment with these drugs increases the risk of infection with chicken pox, measles, tuberculosis, and yeast. Other treatments include dialysis, in which a machine takes over the blood-cleansing function, or kidney transplantation.

The herbal combinations useful in treating nephritis were first formulated on the principle of counteracting "cold," or infection, that reached the body' interior. These formulas treated what we now call acute, infectious glomerulonephritis. Kampo physicians devised other formulas to "guide out the red" in treating bloody urine. These formulas encouraged urination to relieve swelling.

The herbs and formulas most commonly used today, however, have been chosen on the basis of scientific, clinical studies rather than traditional symptom patterns, and are generally used for chronic kidney disease. Kampo should always be used as part of a medically directed overall treatment plan that includes conventional treatment (see considerations below).

INDIVIDUAL KAMPO TREATMENTS

See Chapter 3 for discussions of individual herbs, traditional healing substances, and modern herbal preparations, including directions for making tea.

SUGGESTED DOSAGES	COMMENTS
Bupleurum (Herb)	
Saikosaponin extract, 1 300-mg tablet daily. or Tea, 1 c 3 times daily. or Use combination formula *sairei-to* (see formulas list). Recommended form.	Stimulates the body's production of its own steroids.[1] Prevents protein loss and tissue damage to the kidney. Use the herb alone if the formula is not available.[2] *Caution:* Do not use if fever is present. Occasionally causes mild stomach upset. If this happens, reduce the dose. Do not take antibiotics when taking bupleurum.
Hoelen (Herb)	
Dried or fresh hoelen in food, ⅛–¼ oz (3–6 g) daily. or Tea, 1 c 3 times daily. or Tincture, as directed on label. Place in a cup, add 2 tbsp water, and take in a single sip.	Immune suppressant that prevents lesions in kidney tissue.[3] *Caution:* Do not use in cases of long-term illness that cause excessive urination. In such cases, use Five-Ingredient Powder With Poria (see *Sairei-to* on formulas list).

KAMPO FORMULAS

See Chapter 4 for dosage information and discussions of individual formulas.

Sairei-to

This is a combination of two commonly available formulas: Five-Ingredient Powder with Poria and Minor Bupleurum Decoction. Japanese study has found this combination to be especially useful in preventing kidney damage in children.[4] Five-Ingredient Powder with Poria helps promote the flow of fluids in the kidney, and increases the effectiveness of prednisone.[5] Minor Bupleurum Decoction prevents loss of protein and tissue damage to the kidney,[6] enhances immunotherapy for nephritis,[7] and reduces cholesterol in kidney tissue, which is especially helpful in diabetic nephritis.[8] Seek the advice of the dispensing herbalist on a suitable child's dosage.

CONSIDERATIONS

❑ To reduce side effects and increase effectiveness when using steroid drugs, *see* **Chemotherapy Side Effects.**

Kidney Stones

Kidney stones are crystals that form in the kidneys or the bladder. These crystals are composed of calcium salts, uric acid, or struvite, a kind of crystal that contains magnesium. Since Japanese cuisine uses almost no dairy products, the main source of dietary calcium, Kampo physicians did not develop treatments that target calcium-based stones. Therefore, this entry will focus on uric acid and struvite stones.

A passed stone's appearance is a clue to its composition. Struvite stones are the color of maple syrup and are faceted. Uric acid stones are shaped like footballs and are reddish-brown or tan. (Calcium stones may be mulberry-shaped.)

Kidney stones usually cause no symptoms until they are dislodged. A dislodged kidney stone can cause excruciating, radiating pain originating in the flank or kidney area, along with chills, fever, nausea, and vomiting. Struvite and uric acid stones may form "staghorns" that imbed the stone into the kidney. Imbedded stones can also cause extreme pain.

Kidney stones can form when there is an increase in stone-causing minerals or a decrease in the factors that protect against stone formation. Among the metabolic problems that cause kidney stones are Cushing's syndrome, or overactive adrenal glands; cystinuria, or elevated levels of the amino acid cystine in the urine; and sarcoidosis, an immune-cell disease. Diet is another important factor in stone formation (see "Using Diet to Prevent Kidney Stones"). In addition, stones can form in response to hepatitis, yeast infections, and especially bacterial urinary tract infections (which can affect the stones themselves).

The diagnosis of kidney stones is made by noting the passage of the stone or by ultrasound, in which sound waves are used to produce a "picture" of the urinary tract. Small stones may be simply monitored to see that they do not grow. Large stones may be treated with lithotripsy, in which high-frequency sound waves are used to crush the stone. If lithotripsy does not work, surgery may be necessary.

While scientific explanations of kidney stones are based on the understanding of the chemicals that make up the stones, Kampo's explanation is based on its understanding of the injuries that predispose the kidneys to make stones. The problem arises from a disorder in the Yang Brightness or Lesser Yin, the third and fourth stages of disease progression in Kampo theory (see Chapter 1). In these stages, the body has battled an infectious agent, such as bacteria or yeast, for a long time. The infection creates its own energy in the form of "heat." This is not the desirable form of heat that warms the body, but a destructive form that disturbs the body's energy and water channels. The energy of the water in the kidneys has nowhere to go, and eventually solidifies into a stone. Kampo treatment "cools" pathogenic heat, which breaks up the stone.

Using Diet to Prevent Kidney Stones

The best way to avoid the pain of a kidney stone attack is to avoid developing a stone in the first place, and this means paying careful attention to diet. Dietary factors associated with a high risk of kidney stones include consuming large amounts of alcohol,[1] animal protein,[2] and fat,[3] and low amounts of fiber.[4] Even vegetarians are at risk for developing kidney stones,[5] but among meat-eaters the more vegetables are eaten, the fewer the attacks.[6]

In addition to restrictions on meat and alcohol, each type of stone also carries its own dietary restrictions. Uric acid stones are formed from proteins in foods that are rich in purines, such as anchovies, herring, mackerel, sardines, shellfish, and yeast. Struvite or cystine stones form when the diet is rich in foods that contain the amino acid methionine, such as dairy products (except whole milk), fish, garbanzo beans (chickpeas), lima beans, mushrooms, and all nuts except hazelnuts and sunflower seeds.

INDIVIDUAL KAMPO TREATMENTS

See Chapter 3 for discussions of individual herbs, traditional healing substances, and modern herbal preparations, including directions for making tea.

SUGGESTED DOSAGES	COMMENTS
Aloe (Herb)	
Bitters, standardized to deliver 5–10 mg hydroxyanthracene derivatives daily, calculated as anhydrous aloin. Use up to 2 weeks during acute attacks.	Contains compounds called anthroquinones, which reduce crystal growth.[1,2] *Caution:* Has laxative effects if taken in dosages larger than those recommended. Do not use more than 2 weeks. Do not use if menstruating or if rectal bleeding is present, or if taking any kind of diuretic.
Eupatorium (Herb)	
Tincture (1:5), 15 drops in ¼ c hot water every 2–3 hours until symptoms abate.	Prevents acute attacks of kidney stones. Use at the first sign of flank pain and if urine is scanty or contains fine stones.

Rhubarb Root (Herb)	
Non-Kampo Essiac or Hoxie tea, as directed on label. Use up to 2 weeks during acute attacks.	Contains anthroquinones, which stimulate the muscles underlying the urinary canal to propel stones out of the body.[3,4] Essiac and Hoxie teas are North American rhubarb formulations recommended because they are readily available and easy to use. *Caution:* Has laxative effects in dosages larger than those recommended. Do not use if menstruating or if rectal bleeding is present, or if taking any kind of diuretic. Avoid if there have been prior attacks of calcium-based stones.

KAMPO FORMULAS

See Chapter 4 for dosage information and discussions of individual formulas.

Polyporus Decoction
Relieves nausea and vomiting accompanying acute attacks of kidney stones. Prevents urinary tract infection. Provides relief from what Japanese doctors call "urethral syndrome," which is marked by painful urination and a sensation of retained urine. Unlike many prescription treatments, does not force the body to excrete vitamin C. Modern Chinese formulas employ 2 to 3 times the amount of herbs that are traditionally used. Kidney-stone treatment requires "Japanese" dosages, since "Chinese" formulas have no effect on kidney stones.[5]

CONSIDERATIONS

❑ The Japanese beverage lisymachia or *kinsenso* tea, available from Japanese grocery stores, increases urination and helps the kidneys flush out stones while they are still small.[6] Take 1 to 2 cups daily for three to four months.

❑ High-protein and "crash" diets greatly increase the acidity of the urine, which can promote the development of some types of stones. A person with a family or personal history of kidney stones should avoid these diets.

❑ Calcium-based stones can be treated with varuna, an herb used in Ayurvedic, or traditional Indian, healing. See an herbalist for assistance. To prevent calcium stones from forming, avoid dairy products, meats, beet greens, black tea, cocoa, cranberries, nuts, parsley, pepper, spinach, Swiss chard, and especially rhubarb. Also, consider taking magnesium (600 milligrams per day) and vitamin B_6 (25 milligrams per day) as a preventative.

❑ *See also* **Bladder Infection, Hepatitis,** and **Yeast Infections.**

LEUKEMIA

Leukemia is an overall name for a group of cancers that originate in the blood-producing cells of the bone marrow. Most leukemias are classified by two major criteria: cell of origin (lymphoid or myeloid) and the course of the disease (acute or chronic). Acute leukemia tends to affect children more often than adults, while the opposite is true of chronic leukemia. Acute leukemias develop more rapidly than chronic forms.

The two main acute leukemias are acute lymphocytic or lymphoblastic leukemia (ALL) and acute myelocytic leukemia (AML). Symptoms include fatigue; weight loss; shortness of breath; blood in the stool, urine, or sputum; and easy bruising. Acute leukemia tends to spread to the liver, lymph nodes, and spleen. The two main chronic leukemias are chronic myelocytic (or granulocytic) leukemia (CML) and chronic lymphocytic leukemia (CLL). The symptoms tend to be more subtle than those of acute leukemia, and include abdominal fullness, a "run down" feeling, sweating, and easy bruising. The spleen, where chronic leukemia concentrates its effects, may be enlarged, causing a feeling of fullness in the left side of the abdomen. Diagnosis of the precise form of leukemia in each case is made by taking a bone marrow biopsy.

Different types of leukemia have different risk factors. In adults, smoking is associated with all forms.[1] Some types are associated with environmental hazards, such as exposure to industrial solvents or radiation (including radiation treatment for other forms of cancer). Others are linked to genetic disorders. Still others are linked to viruses, including the Epstein-Barr virus and the human T-cell leukemia virus type I.

All forms of leukemia increase the number of white blood cells and decrease the number of red blood cells. White blood cells are essential for fighting infection. While the total number of white cells rises dramatically in leukemia, the bone marrow fails to produce all the different kinds of white cells the body needs to fight infection. At the same time, the body's resources for producing red blood cells are consumed by the production of the cancerous white blood cells. In particular, the bone cannot produce platelets, which stop bleeding.

Chemotherapy is the main conventional treatment for leukemia, with different types of drugs and administration methods being used for different specific diseases. Chemotherapy-resistant leukemias may be treated with interferon, a naturally occurring immune component. Doctors sometimes treat cases that do not respond to either chemotherapy or interferon with bone marrow transplantation.

Kampo medicine has recognized a symptom pattern corresponding to acute leukemia since the seventh century. Traditionally, Kampo explained acute leukemia as an invasion of "heat" reaching the deepest, yin levels of the blood. Heat expands the blood, and causes it to move recklessly and leave its normal pathways. In recent years, Japanese scientists have found that some of the formulas originally designed to "shrink the blood" actually work by stopping leukemia cells from producing inflammatory hormones.[2]

Kampo therapies fight leukemia by supporting the immune system, helping toxic-substance fighters called free radical scavengers, and causing leukemia cells to enter the normal processes of cell death and replacement. Kampo should be part of a medically directed overall leukemia treatment program (see considerations below). Especially in treating childhood leukemia, always work with a Kampo or TCM practitioner along with the physician.

INDIVIDUAL KAMPO TREATMENTS

See Chapter 3 for discussions of individual herbs, traditional healing substances, and modern herbal preparations, including directions for making tea.

SUGGESTED DOSAGES	COMMENTS
Garlic (Herb)	
Allicin tablets, as directed on label.	Allicin stops leukemia cells from reproducing so that they die naturally.[3] Do *not* use fresh garlic or garlic oil. The allicin in fresh garlic is highly unstable at room temperature. Garlic oil does not contain allicin, and contains concentrated amounts of ajoene, a chemical that can increase bleeding.
Green Tea (Herb)	
Catechin extract, 1 240-mg tablet 3 times daily. or Tea, 1 c 2–5 times daily.	Catechins increase the effectiveness of free-radical scavengers, substances that act against leukemia cells. Green tea stops proliferation of cancer cells.[4] Also stops cancer-causing chemicals from damaging chromosomes,[5] which guide cell reproduction, and keeps chromosomes in cancerous cells from dividing.[6] Increases the effectiveness of standard chemotherapy.[7] Most helpful in AML in Japanese clinical studies.[8] To avoid dilution problems, do not take tea within 1 hour of taking other teas or patent medicines.
Hawthorn (Herb)	
Dried herb in capsules, 3–5 g daily. or Fluid extract (1:1), $\frac{1}{4}$–$\frac{1}{2}$ tsp (1–2 ml) 3 times daily. or Solid extract, 100–250 mg 3 times daily. Should be standardized to contain 10% proanthocyanidins. or Tea, $\frac{2}{3}$ c 3–4 times daily. or Tincture (1:5), 1–1$\frac{1}{2}$ tsp (4–6 ml) 3 times daily. Place in a cup, add 2 tbsp water, and take in a single sip.	Contains rutin, which accelerates the death of leukemia cells. Especially useful for persons who have both leukemia and high blood pressure, since it also lowers blood pressure.
Kudzu (Herb)	
Dried extract, 1 10-mg tablet 3 times daily. or Tea, 1 c 3 times daily. or **Kudzu Decoction** (see formulas list).	Contains daidzein, which stops the growth of certain strains of leukemia cells.[9]
PSK (Modern Herbal Preparation)	
Dried extract, 6 1,000-mg tablets daily.	Increases the effectiveness of free-radical scavengers.[10] Stops invasion of normal tissues by leukemia cells.[11] Reduces likelihood of relapse in childhood ALL after chemotherapy is discontinued.[12]
Turmeric (Herb)	
Curcumin, the yellow pigment found in turmeric, 250–500 mg twice daily between meals.	Curcumin increases differentiation in leukemia cells (which keeps them from multiplying indefinitely) when combined with vitamin D and beta-caratones from daily servings of green leafy, yellow, or orange vegetables.[13] Do not take vitamin D supplements. The body's own supply is sufficient.

KAMPO FORMULAS

See Chapter 4 for dosage information and discussions of individual formulas.

Kudzu Decoction

The kudzu in this formula contains daidzein (see **Kudzu** on treatments list).

Minor Bupleurum Decoction

Especially appropriate for persons with leukemia who also have either HIV infection or hepatitis. Reduces by 80 percent the rate at which some leukemia-causing viruses can reproduce[14] without interfering with reproduction of the body's own T cells.[15]

Caution: Do not use if fever or skin infection is present. Taken long term in patent medicine form, can cause headache, dizziness, and bleeding gums. Side effects can be avoided if the formula is taken as a tea.

Polyporus Decoction

Contains polypusterones, which stop reproduction of some kinds of leukemia cells.[16] Relieves a symptom pattern of urinary difficulty accompanied by fever and thirst, sometimes with diarrhea, nausea, cough, insomnia, or irritation.

CONSIDERATIONS

❑ Eat 3 to 4 ounces of soy foods, such as tofu or miso, daily. Leukemia cells require large amounts of the amino acid asparagine, and soy foods contain asparaginase, an enzyme that breaks down asparagine. For reasons that are not completely understood, the asparaginase from soy is more stable in the body than the enzyme used in chemotherapy. However, discontinue using large amounts of soy foods once remission is achieved, as asparaginase can interfere with the body's use of thyroid hormone.

❑ Modern Kampo recognizes all of the conventional risk factors for leukemia, plus abnormalities of diet. White blood cells are larger and more flexible than red blood cells, and are therefore relatively more "yin." Foods and beverages that expand yin increase the number of white blood cells and contribute to leukemia. Yin foods include chocolate, honey, and sugar; cottage cheese, ice cream, milkshakes, and yogurt; and breads, rolls, and pretzels.

❑ Japanese clinical tests have found that Ten-Significant Tonic Decoction (All-Inclusive Great Tonifying Decoction)

Schisandra—Kampo's Supreme Liver Herb

The main Kampo herb for liver problems is schisandra. This herb is an important ingredient in formulas used to treat complications of liver cancer involving the digestive tract and lungs. However, it is notable when used by itself for its ability to help protect the liver against the kinds of damage that can lead to cancer. Schisandra protects the liver against the effects of carcinogens, particularly carbon tetrachloride,[1] and also air pollution, alcohol, dioxin, exhaust and paint fumes, pesticides, and steroid drugs. These chemicals have to become activated by enzymes within the liver before they can become poisonous, and schisandra short-circuits this process.[2] In laboratory studies, schisandra increases the liver's ability to protect itself from toxic substances called free radicals, which are byproducts of the body's normal oxygen usage.[3] A schisandra extract called gomisin A stimulates production of an enzyme called glutathione peroxidase, which helps offset liver damage caused by chronic viral hepatitis and HIV. This reduces the likelihood that chronic hepatitis will progress to liver cancer.[4] Gomisin A also blocks inflammation[5] and tissue destruction. This stimulates liver regeneration, which helps the liver recover after surgery.[6]

To use schisandra, take the tea three times daily (see Chapter 3 for tea-making instructions). Or use the freeze-dried herb in capsules, available as Hoelen and Schisandra, 100 milligrams three times daily. Avoid if gallstones or blockages of the bile ducts exist.

prevents leukemia caused by chemotherapy for other forms of cancer (see Chapter 4).[17]

❑ To reduce side effects and increase effectiveness when using chemotherapy, *see* **Chemotherapy Side Effects.**

LIVER CANCER

The liver is a common site of cancers that have spread from other parts of the body. Cancer that arises in the liver itself is less common, at least in North America. In Asia, however, this type of liver cancer occurs more frequently. That is because hepatitis and poisoning with aflatoxin, a mold that affects improperly stored grains, are more common in Asia, and these disorders increase the risk of developing liver tumors. As a result, liver cancer is the type of malignancy most helped by Kampo.

In North America, the most common cause of liver cancer is cirrhosis of the liver. Other contributing factors are use of oral contraceptives, alcohol consumption, exposure to chemical carcinogens, and use of anabolic steroids.[1]

The symptoms of liver cancer include abdominal pain, a severe form of abdominal swelling known as ascites, jaundice, weakness, and loss of both appetite and weight, although symptoms only appear when the disease is advanced. The liver may be enlarged, and hard masses may be present. Diagnosis is confirmed by biopsy.

Surgery may be used for localized growths, although liver cancer often occurs as multiple tumors. A number of different chemotherapy drugs may be used. In addition, doctors may employ interferon, a chemical produced by the immune system.

Kampo conceived of liver cancer and other chronic liver diseases as a disease of the Lesser Yang stage of illness (see Chapter 1). This is a condition of stalemate between the destructive energies of a pathogen, which is trying to involve more and more of the body, and the body's defensive energies, which are trying to drive the pathogen out. The principal formula to correct symptoms of the Lesser Yang was Minor Bupleurum Decoction, which modern medicine has revealed to be exceptionally useful in treating liver cancer. Other treatments support the immune system, slow the cancer's growth, increase the effectiveness of conventional medical therapies, and reduce the side effects of chemotherapy.

Modern Japanese medicine treats most cases of liver cancer with a combination of herbs and conventional drugs (see considerations below). Also see "Using Kampo With Other Herbal Treatments for Colorectal and Liver Cancer" on page 186. In cases of secondary liver cancer, see the primary-cancer entry, such as breast cancer, for additional information and treatments. Be aware that some herbs may have a negative impact on the liver and/or interact negatively with conventional medicines. Always work with a qualified health care practitioner.

INDIVIDUAL KAMPO TREATMENTS

See Chapter 3 for discussions of individual herbs, traditional healing substances, and modern herbal preparations, including directions for making tea.

SUGGESTED DOSAGES	COMMENTS
Astragalus (Herb)	
Fluid extract (1:1), ¼–½ tsp (1–2 ml) 3 times daily. or Freeze-dried herb in capsules, 500–1,000 mg 3 times daily. or Powdered solid extract (4:1), 250–500 mg 3 times daily. or Tea, 1 c 3 times daily. or Tincture (1:5), 1–1½ tsp (4–6 ml), 3 times daily. Place in a cup, add 2 tbsp water, and take in a single sip. For dosages used with chemotherapy, *see* **Chemotherapy Side Effects.**	Contains compounds that increase the ability of lymphokine-activated killer (LAK) cells to attack tumors.[2] Also prevents progression of hepatitis B to liver cancer.[3] *Caution:* Do not use when fever or skin infection is present.

Cinnamon (Herb)	
Freshly grated cinnamon in food, at least 1 tsp daily. or Oil, 15–30 drops, up to 3 times daily. Place in a cup, add 2 tbsp warm water, and take in a single sip. or Tea, 1 c up to 3 times daily. Use freshly ground cinnamon.	Contains camphornin and cinnamonin, which stop the growth of human liver cancer cells under laboratory conditions.[4] Contains compounds known to deactivate plasmin, a substance that allows cancer cells to invade healthy tissue. Stimulates the body's production of, and increases the effectiveness of, tumor necrosis factor, which destroys cancer cells.

Coptis (Herb)	
Dried herb, 1 500-mg capsule 3 times daily. or Tincture (1:5), 15–30 drops 3 times daily. Place in a cup, add 2 tbsp water, and take in a single sip.	Contains berberine, which stops the multiplication of human liver cancer cells.[5] If coptis is unavailable, substitute capsules or tinctures of the non-Kampo herbs goldenseal or Oregon grape root (same caution applies). *Caution:* Do not use during pregnancy or on a daily basis for more than 2 weeks at a time.

LEM (Modern Herbal Preparation)	
Powder, as directed on label.	In animal studies, injections of LEM slowed the growth of cancerous liver tumors.[6] Clinical studies have shown that LEM has the ability to help the liver to produce antibodies to hepatitis B,[7] which reduces future risk of liver cancer. *Caution:* Can occasionally cause mild diarrhea or skin rashes. Should these symptoms occur, consult a health care provider.

Reishi (Modern Herbal Preparation)	
Dried extract, 3 1-g tablets 3 times daily. or Dried mushroom in food, approx. ¼–approx. ½ oz (5–10 g) daily. or Syrup, as directed on label. or Tea, 1 c 3 times daily. or Tincture (1:5), 1 tsp (4 ml) 3 times daily. Place in a cup, add 2 tbsp water, and take in a single sip.	Contains compounds called ganoderic acids, which act against liver cancer.[8]

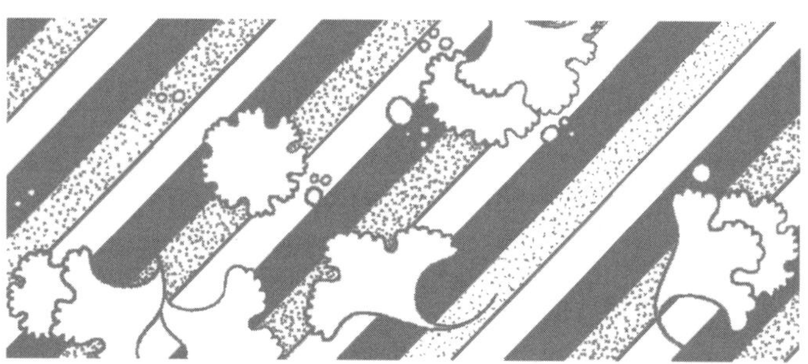

Rhubarb Root (Herb)	
Injectable forms, given under professional supervision. Or Non-Kampo Essiac or Hoxie tea, as directed on label.	Contains compounds called rhein and emodin. These stop a cancer from developing its own blood supply, a step that allows it to spread. Rhein reduces the ability of cancer cells to create protein and glucose.[9] Emodin stimulates the production of white blood cells. This makes it useful for the treatment of white blood cell deficiency during chemotherapy.[10] Essiac and Hoxie teas are North American rhubarb formulations recommended because they are readily available and easy to use.

Scutellaria (Herb)	
Dried herb, 1–2 1,000-mg capsules 3 times daily. or Fluid extract (1:1), ¼–½ tsp (1–2 ml) 3 times daily. or Powdered solid extract (4:1), 250–500 mg 3 times daily. or Tea, 1 c 3 times daily. or Tincture (1:5), 1–1½ tsp (4–6 ml) 3 times daily. Place in a cup, add 2 tbsp water, and take in a single sip.	Contains compounds that induce both cell death in liver cancer cells and stop immune-system damage from chemotherapy with 5-fluorouracil.[11,12] *Caution:* Avoid in cases of diarrhea caused by foodborne infection or excessive consumption of cold drinks.

KAMPO FORMULAS

See Chapter 4 for dosage information and discussions of individual formulas.

Major Bupleurum Decoction

Controls *symptoms* of liver cancer, including alternating fever and chills, bitter taste in the mouth, nausea, continuous vomiting, burning diarrhea or no bowel movements, despondency, fullness in the chest with or without pain, and irritability.

Caution: Use with caution if fever is present, and discontinue if preexisting fevers worsen.

Minor Bupleurum Decoction

Controls *progression* of liver cancer. Contains compounds that "turn off" liver cancer cells and keep them from multiplying.[13,14] Acts without reducing the body's production of white or red blood cells,[15] a common side effect of other treatments. Also sensitizes the liver to, and increases the effectiveness of, dexamethasone, a drug sometimes used to treat liver inflammation caused by cancer.[16] The formula also prevents the progression of chronic hepatitis to liver cancer, and prevents liver cancer caused by aflatoxin exposure.[17]

Caution: Do not use if fever or skin infection is present, or if receiving interferon therapy.[18] Taken long term in patent medicine form, can cause headache, dizziness, and bleeding gums. Side effects can be avoided if the formula is taken as a tea.

CONSIDERATIONS

❑ Persons who have fevers or are receiving interferon cannot take Minor Bupleurum Decoction, but they can take the non-

Kampo herb milk thistle. Silybinin, a chemical in milk thistle, protects the liver's Kuppfer cells from inflammation. These specialized immune cells engulf foreign matter in the liver, and also play a role in destroying cancer cells that have entered the bloodstream. Silybinin acts without interfering with tumor necrosis factor, an immune-system chemical that accelerates the destruction of cancer cells.[19] This herb is available in a standardized form that delivers 120 milligrams of silymarin in a 500-milligram capsule. It is also possible to use 500-milligram capsules of milk thistle seeds themselves. Take either form three times daily. Or make milk thistle tea by placing $^{1}/_{3}$ to $^{1}/_{2}$ ounce (12 to 15 grams) of seed in 2 cups (500 milliliters) of boiling water, and allowing it to steep for forty-five minutes. Strain and drink one-third of the tea in three doses per day. Since milk thistle tinctures are made with alcohol, they must be avoided by persons with liver cancer.

❑ For information on the herb Kampo uses most often in liver disease, see "Schisandra—Kampo's Supreme Liver Herb" on page 251.

❑ To reduce side effects and increase effectiveness when using chemotherapy, *see* **Chemotherapy Side Effects.** To learn about herbal treatments that can prevent a cancer from developing its own blood supply, *see* **Cancer.** *See also* **Cirrhosis, Alcoholic** and **Hepatitis.**

LUNG CANCER

Lung cancer is one the most common forms of cancer; every year it is diagnosed in approximately 100,000 men and 50,000 women in the United States. The most significant risk factor is smoking. Smoking two packs a day for twenty years increases the risk for lung cancer to between sixty and seventy times the risk of a nonsmoker who is not exposed to secondhand smoke.[1] Passive exposure to secondhand smoke increases one's risk approximately 50 percent. Exposure to asbestos, pollution, or industrial metals also increases the risk of developing this disease.

Symptoms of lung cancer include cough, bloody or rusty sputum, hoarseness, and wheezing. There may be pain radiating from the shoulder to the arm. These symptoms often appear late in the course of the disease. Most lung cancers take one of several main forms: adenocarcinoma, large cell, small cell (also called oat cell), and squamous cell. In addition, cancers that originate elsewhere in the body may spread to the lung.

Many lung cancers can be detected by chest x-ray. It some cases, a CAT scan, which is more sensitive, is needed to find small tumors. The diagnosis must then be confirmed via a biopsy. At that point the cancer is classified according to tumor size and how extensively it has spread.

Conventional treatment includes surgery for small, localized tumors. However, since lung cancers usually spread before they are detected, the main treatments are chemotherapy using a wide variety of drugs and radiation therapy.

Kampo medicine describes lung cancer in terms of an imbalance between yang, or outward-directed energy, and yin, or inward-directed energy. Tobacco is an extremely yang substance, and heating tobacco adds to its yang energies. Smokers are usually thinner (more yang) than nonsmokers, and most smokers put on weight (become more yin) when they stop.

Kampo medicine diagnoses the condition of the lungs by observing their corresponding area on the face, the cheeks. Deficient lung energy produces a pale complexion with puffiness in the cheeks. Deficient energy in general leads to both anemia and overweight, labored breathing, weak chest muscles and rounded shoulders, and tendency to stoop. Lung cancer will also produce blemishes and discoloration along the lung meridian, which runs along the arm down to the seam between the first finger and the thumb, and then extends down the thumb. One of the most common signs of lung cancer is tension or weakness in the thumb, which is the end of the lung channel.

While Kampo offers no cure for lung cancer, several Kampo therapies can greatly extend life. In one Chinese test, not duplicated in Western studies, some persons with advanced lung cancer who received Six-Ingredient Pill with Rehmannia along with chemotherapy and radiation have lived as long as seven years. Other preparations reduce side effects of conventional medical treatments of the disease (see considerations below), and increase resistance to infection during chemotherapy. Still other treatments slow lung cancer's growth and spread.

In cases of secondary lung cancer, see the primary-cancer entry, such as breast cancer, for additional information and treatments.

INDIVIDUAL KAMPO TREATMENTS

See Chapter 3 for discussions of individual herbs, traditional healing substances, and modern herbal preparations, including directions for making tea.

SUGGESTED DOSAGES	COMMENTS
Astragalus (Herb)	
Fluid extract (1:1), ¼–½ tsp (1–2 ml) 3 times daily. or Freeze-dried herb in capsules, 500–1,000 mg 3 times daily. or Powdered solid extract (4:1), 250–500 mg 3 times daily. or Tea, 1 c 3 times daily. or Tincture (1:5), 1–1½ tsp (4–6 ml), 3 times daily. Place in a cup, add 2 tbsp water, and take in a single sip. For dosages used with chemotherapy, *see* **Chemotherapy Side Effects.**	Contains compounds that both stimulate T cells and increase the ability of immune-system cells called lymphokine-activated killer (LAK) cells to attack cancerous tumors.[2] Supports the immune system during therapy with cyclophosphamide.[3] *Caution:* Do not use when fever or skin infection is present.

Lentinan (Modern Herbal Preparation)	
Intramuscular injection (usual form), 0.5–50 mg effective daily dose, depending on patient's condition and circumstances. Smaller, more frequent doses more effective than larger, less frequent doses. Given under professional supervision. or Powder, dosage to be determined by provider. Much greater dosages required than in injectable form.	Lentinan activates LAK and natural killer (NK) cells to attack carcinoma, including that of the lung. Can improve survival time in cases of advanced secondary lung cancer.[4] Prevents immune-system damage when given *before* treatment with mitomycin-C, 5-fluorouracil, or tegafur.[5]

PSK (Modern Herbal Preparation)	
Dried extract, 6 1,000-mg tablets daily.	Has extended longevity in advanced non-small cell lung cancer when used with radiation therapy[6] or chemotherapy.[7] Also stops the spread of cancer from other parts of the body to the lungs.[8]

Psoralea (Herb)	
Freeze-dried herb, 1 1,000-mg capsule 3 times daily. Use only under supervision of an herbalist.	Contains compounds that inhibit lung cancer.[9] Sold as Psoralea Seed capsule, Scruffy Pea, or *Bu Gu Zhi.* *Caution:* Use sunscreen or avoid exposure to sunlight.

Scutellaria (Herb)	
Dried herb, 1–2 1,000-mg capsules 3 times daily. or Fluid extract (1:1), ¼–½ tsp (1–2 ml) 3 times daily. or Powdered solid extract (4:1), 250–500 mg 3 times daily. or Tea, 1 c 3 times daily. or Tincture (1:5), 1–1½ tsp (4–6 ml) 3 times daily. Place in a cup, add 2 tbsp water, and take in a single sip.	Stops inflammatory processes in lung cancer. Relieves cough.[10] Laboratory studies show that it can thwart immune-system damage caused by cyclophosphamide and 5-fluorouracil.[11,12] *Caution:* Avoid in cases of diarrhea caused by foodborne infection or excessive consumption of cold drinks.

KAMPO FORMULAS

See Chapter 4 for dosage information and discussions of individual formulas.

Ginseng Decoction to Nourish the Nutritive Qi

Frequently prescribed in Japan to treat cancer patients who experience anemia, forgetfulness, hair loss, jaundice, shortness of breath, and tired limbs. Relieves symptoms, but does not affect the disease itself.

Pinellia Decoction to Drain the Epigastrium

Useful for relieving the following symptoms frequently experienced by cancer patients: anorexia, feeling of obstruction below the heart, vomiting. Also stops "rumbling" in the stomach and intestines. This formula is most useful for persons in the early stages of cancer or who are beginning chemotherapy. Particularly useful in controlling diarrhea caused by the chemotherapy drug irinotecan, which is often severe enough that patients must discontinue therapy.[13]

Caution: Use with caution if fever is present, and discontinue if preexisting fevers worsen.

Six-Ingredient Pill with Rehmannia (Rehmannia-Six Combination)

Chinese physicians have found this formula to increase survival time for patients with small cell lung cancer when used with either chemotherapy or radiation therapy.[14] The symptom pattern for which this formula was designed includes soreness or weakness in the lower back, diminished hearing or ringing in the ears, light-headedness, chronically dry or sore throat, night sweats, and toothache or inflamed gums. This symptom pattern is seen in patients who undergo radiation therapy or chemotherapy with vinblastine or cyclophosphamide.

Caution: Patients whose lung cancer is secondary to cancer of the breast, cervix, or uterus should not use this formula.

CONSIDERATIONS

❑ To reduce side effects and increase effectiveness when using chemotherapy, *see* **Chemotherapy Side Effects**; when using radiation therapy, *see* **Radiation Therapy Side Effects.** To learn about herbal treatments that can prevent a cancer from developing its own blood supply, *see* **Cancer.**

LUPUS

Lupus (systemic lupus erythematous, or SLE) is a chronic inflammatory condition that affects connective tissue. The first sign of the disease in a number of patients is a butterfly-shaped rash over the nose and cheeks that looks like the facial markings of a wolf. For this reason the disease is termed *lupus,* which in Latin means "wolf." Another form of lupus, discoid lupus erythematous (DLE), affects primarily the hair follicles and skin on the scalp, and two other forms, subacute cutaneous lupus erythematous (SCLE) and acute cutaneous lupus erythematous (ACLE), affect only the skin.

About 90 percent of all lupus patients are women, generally young adults. Genetic factors play a strong role in lupus. But there are other risk factors associated with this disorder, including stress, infections, severe drug reactions, and hormonal imbalances.

Because lupus affects many parts of the body, it produces a number of symptoms. These include scaling skin lesions, nausea, headaches, diarrhea and/or constipation, malaise, fatigue, and weight loss. Mental symptoms include confusion, irritability, and depression. Attacks of lupus can induce arthritis, with both swollen joints and fever, and can destroy tissues in the lungs, spleen, heart, and brain, and especially the kidneys. Not all patients experience all these symptoms, however, and the range and variability of symptoms can make lupus a difficult disease to diagnose.

Lupus is caused by a misdirected attack by the body's white blood cells on its own organs. This occurs when the immune system produces substances called antibodies, which normally attack infection-causing organisms, that "lock on" to and attack DNA in the patient's skin cells. In some lupus patients, another immune-system component called the T cell becomes involved. When this happens, the immune response is even stronger than normal, and greatly increases the severity of symptoms.[1]

Because DNA is normally contained within the cells, the antibodies are only activated when skin cells are damaged by some other event, such as sunburn or the natural aging process. For this reason, lupus is characterized by periodic attacks followed by remissions. Without treatment, however, each subsequent attack produces worse symptoms than the episode preceding it.

Mild cases of lupus are treated with painkillers such as aspirin or ibuprofen. Advanced cases are usually treated with large doses of steroid drugs, which inhibit immune-system activity. This drug group includes methylprednisolone, dexamethasone, prednisone, and prednisolone. Although these drugs are useful in preventing lupus attacks, they have so many side effects that they are usually taken only every other day.

Kampo distinguished a symptom pattern corresponding to kidney damage by lupus in the time of master herbalist Zhang Zhongjing in the third century A.D. However, before the twentieth century Kampo practitioners did not recognize a symptom pattern for the earlier stages of the disease. Kampo practitioners in Japan and China today discuss lupus in terms of damaged yin, or containing energy, in the kidneys and liver, but they choose herbs and formulas to treat lupus on the basis of laboratory and clinical research.

Japanese and Chinese physicians use Kampo to augment rather than replace prescription medicines. In fact, Kampo's ability to make steroid drugs more effective is one of its most helpful modern applications in treating lupus. Almost a dozen clinical studies confirm that several Kampo treatments allow lupus control with smaller doses of steroid drugs. This minimizes the side effects of the drugs and extends lupus control over days when steroids are not taken.

INDIVIDUAL KAMPO TREATMENTS

See Chapter 3 for discussions of individual herbs, traditional healing substances, and modern herbal preparations, including directions for making tea.

SUGGESTED DOSAGES	COMMENTS
Astragalus (Herb)	
Fluid extract (1:1), 1/4–1/2 tsp (1–2 ml) 3 times daily. or Freeze-dried herb in capsules, 500–1,000 mg 3 times daily. or Powdered solid extract (4:1), 250–500 mg 3 times daily. or Tea, 1 c 3 times daily. or Tincture (1:5), 1–1 1/2 tsp (4–6 ml), 3 times daily. Place in a cup, add 2 tbsp water, and take in a single sip. For this disorder, use only under professional supervision, and only for up two weeks at a time.	Increases activity of natural killer (NK) cells, which fight infection.[2] For patients who are responding well to steroid drugs, taking astragalus reduces the risk of infection, especially when infections are "going around." *Caution:* Since this herb increases the body's response to steroids, inform the doctor when using it. Do not take astragalus for more than two out of every four weeks. Avoid this herb if *not* taking steroids.
Codonopsis (Herb)	
Tablets, 1 g 3 times daily. Available as *Dang Shen.* or Tea, 1 c 3 times daily. or Tincture (1:5), 1/2–1 tsp (2–4 ml) 3 times daily. Place in a cup, add 2 tbsp water, and take in a single sip.	Decreases the formation of antibodies that target DNA.[3]
Gentian (Herb)	
Capsules, as directed on label. Use to avoid bitter taste of other forms.	In Chinese clinical studies, use of gentian with a minimal dose of prednisone more than doubles the chances of going into remission, compared with use of prednisone alone.[4] *Caution:* Avoid if there is diarrhea with undigested food in the stool.
Hoelen (Herb)	
Dried or fresh hoelen in food, 1/8–1/4 oz (3–6 g) daily. or Tea, 1 c 3 times daily. or Tincture, as directed on label. Place in a cup, add 2 tbsp water, and take in a single sip.	Immune suppressant that stops symptoms. *Caution:* Do not use in cases of long-term illness that cause excessive urination.
Licorice (Herb)	
Glycyrrhizin extract, 200–800 mg daily, depending on severity of symptoms for up to 6 weeks. Resume after a 2-week break. or Tea, 1 c 1–5 times daily for up to 6 weeks. Resume after a 2-week break.	Relieves pain and inflammation, and increases effectiveness of steroid drugs, especially prednisolone. Avoid deglycyrrhizinated licorice (DGL). *Caution:* Avoid if high blood pressure is present. Also avoid if an estrogen-sensitive disorder is present, such as bladder cancer, melanoma, or disorders of the female reproductive system.
Scutellaria (Herb)	
Dried herb, 1–2 1,000-mg capsules 3 times daily. or Fluid extract (1:1), 1/4–1/2 tsp (1–2 ml) 3 times daily. or Powdered solid extract (4:1), 250–500 mg 3 times daily. or Tea, 1 c 3 times daily. or Tincture (1:5), 1–1 1/2 tsp (4–6 ml) 3 times daily. Place in a cup, add 2 tbsp water, and take in a single sip.	Prevents infections without stimulating the immune system. Prevents flu (provided it is used 18 to 54 hours *before* exposure).[5,6] Inhibits several types of bacterial infections, including staph and strep. *Caution:* Avoid in cases of diarrhea caused by foodborne infection or excessive consumption of cold drinks.

HERBS TO AVOID

Individuals who have lupus should avoid the following herbs: American ginseng, bamboo, burdock, chrysanthemum, Siberian ginseng, and wheat grass. For more information regarding these herbs, see Chapter 3. Also avoid the non-Kampo herb echinacea. All these herbs stimulate the immune system. In addition, these individuals should avoid ginseng unless under the care of a Kampo or TCM practitioner who is familiar with lupus treatment. Ginseng can either stimulate or suppress the immune system, depending on the dosage.

KAMPO FORMULAS

See Chapter 4 for dosage information and discussions of individual formulas.

Ginseng Decoction to Nourish the Nutritive Qi

Increases the effectiveness of prednisolone.[7] There are over-the-counter variations of this formula that substitute codonopsis for the much more expensive red ginseng. This "imitation" formula is probably better for treating lupus.

Sairei-to

This is a combination of two commonly available formulas: Five-Ingredient Powder with Poria and Minor Bupleurum Decoction. This combination reduces the number of antibodies that destroy skin DNA,[8] and relieves pain and swelling.[9]

CONSIDERATIONS

❑ *See also* **Kidney Disease.**

MACULAR DEGENERATION

Macular degeneration is the progressive destruction of the macula, the part of the retina responsible for fine vision. It is the leading cause of vision loss among people over age fifty-five in North America. About 20,000 new cases are diagnosed each year.[1]

There are two forms of macular degeneration: dry (atrophic) or wet (exudative). In the dry form, which is more common, cells in the macula accumulate sacs of debris called drusens. These drusens swell and block off circulation to the microscopic blood vessels that serve the macula. In the wet form, blood vessels themselves swell, and unnecessary vessels form beneath the retina. These vessels leak fluid and may bleed, which causes scarring.

Aging, atherosclerosis, high blood pressure, and smoking all contribute to blood-vessel damage in the eye. As blood vessels are damaged, less oxygen reaches the retina, and the blood vessels constrict to preserve the available oxygen. When normal blood flow is restored from time to time, the vessels don't relax right away, and oxygen-rich blood gathers in the retina. As a result, oxygen-based toxins called free radicals accumulate.

Historically, macular degeneration was relatively rare in Japan, although the number of cases has increased recently.[2] Japanese researchers have extensively studied the value of combining herbal and nutritional treatment with technology-based treatments, such as hyperbaric oxygen treatment, surgery, and radiation. Japanese researchers are also exploring the use of interferon to reverse the overgrowth of blood vessels.[3]

Despite the fact that macular degeneration was uncommon in ancient Japan, Kampo has provided an explanation for it. Shortly after the time of Kampo master Zhang Zhongjing in the third century A.D., Kampo scholars developed a theory of visual impairment in terms of energy blockages. When the organs in the lower part of the body lacked yin, or containing, energy, they could release energy to travel to the head but could not reabsorb it when it was circulated back to them. Energy accumulated in the eyes and caused visual distortion.

When ginkgo is used to treat macular degeneration, it must be taken with the non-Kampo herbs bilberry and grape seed extract. A person who has a bad reaction to ginkgo should use either of the formulas listed below.

INDIVIDUAL KAMPO TREATMENTS

See Chapter 3 for discussions of individual herbs, traditional healing substances, and modern herbal preparations, including directions for making tea.

SUGGESTED DOSAGES	COMMENTS
Ginkgo (Modern Herbal Preparation), Bilberry, Grape Seed Extract	
Ginkgolide extract, 1–2 40-mg tablets 3 times daily. and Bilberry extract, standardized to contain at least 25% anthocyanidins, 40–80 mg 3 times daily. and Grape seed extract, standardized to contain 95% procyanidins, 150–300 mg once daily.	These three treatments complement one another. Ginkgo increases microcirculation in the eye, which allows for a steadier supply of oxygen to the retina. Deactivates platelet activating factor (PAF), which is needed to form new blood vessels.[4] Contains quercetin, which protects retina from effects of low oxygen levels.[5] Bilberry slows down atherosclerosis, deactives PAF,[6] and prevents free-radical damage. Grape seed extract also prevents free-radical damage.
Shiitake (Modern Herbal Preparation)	
Fresh or dried shiitake in food, ¼–⅓ oz (6–9 g) daily. or 3 1-g tablets 3 times daily. or Syrup, ½ tbsp (4–6 ml) 3 times daily. or Tincture (1:5), 1 tbsp (10 ml) 3 times daily. Place in a cup, add 2 tbsp water, and take in a single sip.	General immune stimulant that increases interferon production.

KAMPO FORMULAS

See Chapter 4 for dosage information and discussions of individual formulas.

Augmented Rambling Powder

Treats both macular degeneration and optic nerve atrophy caused by "toxin accumulation," the underlying cause of which is energy blockage in the liver caused by repressed emotion. Traditionally given to persons with vigorous constitutions and "hot" symptoms, including bloodshot eyes, blurry vision, and difficult or painful urination, and in women, increased menstrual flow and uterine bleeding.

Caution: Should not be used by women who are trying to become pregnant.

Six-Ingredient Pill With Rehmannia (Rehmannia-Six Combination)

Treats both macular degeneration and optic nerve atrophy caused by yin deficiencies in the kidneys. Traditionally given to persons with weak constitutions and symptoms that include back pain, dizziness, hearing problems or ringing in the ears, and a weak, rapid pulse.

Caution: Avoid if an estrogen-sensitive disorder is present, such as bladder cancer, melanoma, or disorders of the female reproductive system.

CONSIDERATIONS

❑ The key findings of Japanese research are that nutrition can slow the development of macular degeneration and good circulation can enhance surgical treatment of it. To slow the course of the disease, be sure to get enough vitamins and minerals, especially zinc and vitamin E.[7] To get the best results from surgery, try to maintain circulatory health.[8] This means keeping high blood pressure, if present, under control, and keeping cholesterol and triglyceride levels down (*see* **High Blood Pressure** and **High Cholesterol**).

MASTITIS

Nursing mothers can develop mastitis, an infection of the milk ducts. Diabetes increases the risk of developing all types of infections, including mastitis. As a result, diabetic women are approximately thirteen times more likely to be affected by mastitis than women who do not have diabetes.

Mastitis can be caused by either *Staphylococcus* (staph) or by an infectious yeast called *Candida.* The first symptom of staph mastitis is fatigue. This is followed about twenty-four hours later by breast swelling and inflammation, and by fever. The infection usually occurs when the baby picks up the germ in a shared hospital nursery and then passes it to the mother through cracks in the mother's nipples. Sometimes staph toxins are passed to the mother by milk from cows that had mastitis,[1] and cause an allergic reaction. Staph mastitis usually clears up in three to four weeks.

Mastitis can also be caused by yeast infection, which causes a burning pain that radiates outward from the nipple to the rest of the breast. The pain can be severe enough to prevent breastfeeding. Yeast mastitis usually takes several months to resolve.

Doctors usually recommend that mothers with either type of mastitis continue nursing. The exception is when an abscess, or a localized collection of pus, forms. When this happens the concentration of infection may harm the baby, causing pneumonia and even lung abscesses.

Sterile hot packs are used to ease the pain of mastitis. Women with yeast mastitis may need prescription pain relievers, since it is often unaffected by over-the-counter pain relievers.[2] Both kinds of mastitis are frequently treated with penicillin or streptomycin. In many cases, these antibiotics are very effective, although their overuse in veterinary medicine, especially in animals used for food, has created some strains of both staph and yeast mastitis that do not respond to antibiotics. Also, on rare occasions penicillin and streptomycin can provoke dangerous allergic reactions.

Kampo choose herbs for mastitis treatment on the basis of their ability to reestablish energy circulation to the body's surface, including the breasts. Kampo thought of mastitis as a collapse of "heat" into the body's center. The invading pathogen, or germ, caused fever that overcame the body's yang, or outwardly directed, energies. Reviving the yang restored circulation to the surface of the body and healed the breasts.

In the case of breast abscess, herbal treatments are inappropriate. Swift antibiotic action is needed for the health of both mother and baby. For staph mastitis without abscess, Kampo treatments reduce breast inflammation and pain, allowing the body to heal itself, without any harmful chemicals that can be passed on to the child. Yeast infections require herbs with stronger antimicrobial properties, so nursing must be suspended until after treatment.

INDIVIDUAL KAMPO TREATMENTS

See Chapter 3 for discussions of individual herbs, traditional healing substances, and modern herbal preparations, including directions for making tea.

Treatments for Use by Nursing Mothers

SUGGESTED DOSAGES	COMMENTS
Coix (Herb)	
Cereal, 1 oz (30 g) daily. Available in Japanese groceries as *hatomugi.*	Standard remedy in Japan for mastitis. Draws fluids away from the skin, reduces pain and swelling, and increases lactation. *Caution:* Promotes urination, so should not be used during pregnancy.
Viola (Herb)	
Tea, 1 c 3 times daily.	Treats enlarged, painful breasts, especially when accompanied by constipation and headache.

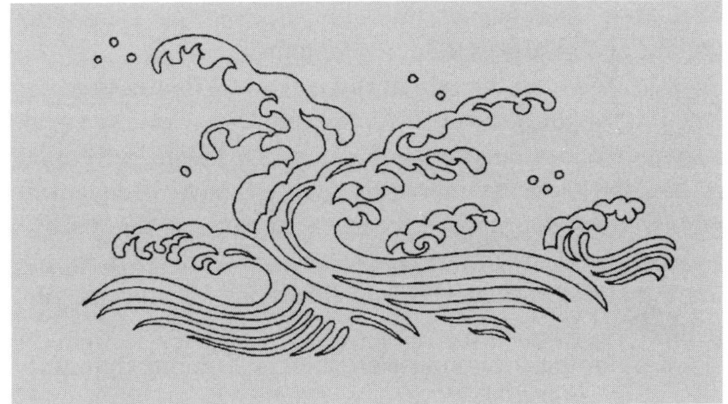

Treatments for Use by Mothers Who Are Not Nursing

Coptis (Herb)	
Dried herb, 1 500-mg capsule 3 times daily. or Tincture (1:5), 20 drops 3 times daily. Place in a cup, add 2 tbsp water, and take in a single sip.	Kills *Candida.*[3] This herb also kills not only staph but a wide range of other bacteria that occasionally cause mastitis.[4] If coptis is unavailable, substitute capsules or tinctures of the non-Kampo herbs barberry, goldenseal, or Oregon grape root (same cautions apply). *Caution:* Do not use while nursing (or pregnant), and do not nurse for 1 week afterwards. Do not use on a daily basis for more than 2 weeks at a time. Do not use with supplements that contain vitamin B_6 or the amino acid histidine.

KAMPO FORMULAS

See Chapter 4 for dosage information and discussions of individual formulas.

Frigid Extremities Powder

Treats mastitis with cold fingers and toes, a feeling of fullness in the lungs, irritability, and body warmth.

Caution: Should not be used by nursing mothers.

CONSIDERATIONS

❑ Diabetic men can also develop mastitis, since in diabetes extra sugar is present in all the body's tissues.[5] Men respond better to antibiotic treatment for mastitis than women.

MEASLES

Measles (rubeola) is a highly contagious viral infection that produces a characteristic splotchy rash. The rash appears about four days after the initial symptoms, which include fatigue, fever, irritability, cough, and runny nose. The rash erupts on the forehead and spreads downward over the face, neck, trunk, limbs, and feet. Fevers can run as high as 105°F (40.6°C). The disease runs its course in about ten days. People with measles become infectious five days after they have been exposed to the disease (more than a week before symptoms appear) until five days after the rash breaks out. German measles (rubella) is a similar illness that is less contagious and produces milder symptoms.

Measles, long thought of as a childhood illness, is prevalent among children in developing countries. However, since vaccination has been available, a much larger percentage of measles patients in North America have been adults who were never exposed to, or vaccinated for, the disease. Measles causes more severe symptoms in adults than in children, and the vaccine can sometimes cause fever and joint pain.

Recovering from measles confers lifetime immunity from future infection. The disease also causes immune-system changes that may have some beneficial effects, notably a reduced risk of developing asthma[1] and hay fever.[2] In rare cases, however, recovery from measles can be complicated when the immune system overreacts and fails to "turn off" after it has contained the virus. This can cause damage to the lungs, eyes, heart, liver, kidneys, or brain. Conventional treatment for measles consists of using aspirin or other painkillers to ease pain and reduce fever. (It is important never to give children under the age fifteen aspirin, as the use of aspirin during viral infections can result in Reye's syndrome, an extremely serious complication.)

Kampo teaches that the symptoms of measles arise only after a struggle between the body and a pathogen in which the body has almost won, sending the pathogen to the surface of the body to be expelled. Immediately after infection, Kampo treatments bolster immune defenses by taking on some of the antiviral activity. This results in less severe symptoms, reduces the risk of complications, and shortens the course of the disease. After the pathogen has "escaped," Kampo treatments relieve irritation and heal the rash. In addition, Kampo can ease post-vaccination symptoms. These treatments also apply to German measles.

INDIVIDUAL KAMPO TREATMENTS

See Chapter 3 for discussions of individual herbs, traditional healing substances, and modern herbal preparations, including directions for making tea.

SUGGESTED DOSAGES	COMMENTS
Licorice (Herb)	
For post-vaccination symptoms: Glycyrrhizin extract, 200–800 mg daily, depending on severity of symptoms for up to 1 week. or Tea, 1 c 1–5 times daily for 1 week. *After rash appears:* Topical cream, as needed until rash disappears. Simicort is the most widely available brand.	Oral forms ease joint pain and fever after vaccination. Cream relieves external inflammation without affecting internal immune processes. Oral dosages are for adults only. Avoid deglycyrrhizinated licorice (DGL). *Caution:* Do not use licorice products for more than 2 weeks.

KAMPO FORMULAS

See Chapter 4 for dosage information and discussions of individual formulas.

Kudzu Decoction

To be used after possible infection, but before symptoms appear. Can moderate symptoms by supplementing the antiviral activity of the immune system. Traditionally used to "open the pores" of the face and neck so that pathogens could escape.

CONSIDERATIONS

❑ Although many parents are concerned about vaccinating their children, the side effects of measles shots for kids are usually at most mild and temporary. However, that is not true of all adults. Women who are pregnant or could become pregnant within three months should not be vaccinated. The same is true for men and women who have uncontrolled tuberculosis or are receiving chemotherapy. Otherwise, persons who were born after 1957 and have never had measles should consult a physician about vaccination. This is particularly true for those who travel to areas of the world where measles is still common.

❑ If measles does strike, taking vitamin A supplements in doses of 400,000 IU per day for two days can reduce the risk of complications. (Pregnant women should not take vitamin A, since high dosages of this vitamin can harm the baby.) Take it only when symptoms appear after known exposure to measles, since it can interfere with the immune response if taken too early. Vitamin A is only effective in the presence of zinc, so take 30 to 60 milligrams of zinc at the same time.[3]

MELANOMA

Melanoma is an increasingly common form of skin cancer, particularly in the United States, Israel, and Australia. Most patients are between the ages of forty and sixty-five, and are fair-skinned. It affects men and women in equal numbers.

This form of cancer can lie latent for as long as fifty years after the sunburn that usually triggers it. Scientists believe that repeated exposure to sunlight itself weakens the immune system's ability to search for and destroy melanoma cells. Any other drain on the immune system, such as a long-term infection or extensive burn, can also contribute to the development of melanoma.

Melanoma can begin as a new growth. Often, though, it appears as a change to an existing mole. Melanomas are asymmetric, and have irregular borders, multiple colors, and a diameter greater than that of a pencil eraser (6 millimeters). A smaller, more circular skin lesion may be basal cell carcinoma, a much more common and less aggressive form of cancer. All suspicious growths should be brought to a doctor's attention.

Melanoma is diagnosed by removing and examining the growth. This disease is classified in stages, from I to IV, depending on how thick the growth is and whether it has spread. Melanoma can spread to almost anywhere in the body, but usually spreads to the liver, lungs, bones, or brain.

Some forms of melanoma are stimulated by the hormone insulin. Insulin production is increased by stress and the consumption of sugar or saccharin. Other forms of melanoma are stimulated by the hormone estrogen. Excess estrogen production can occur for a number of reasons, including dietary ones (see "Lowering Estrogen Levels Through Diet" on page 207; these dietary changes can also help reduce insulin production.)

Surgery is the primary conventional treatment for melanoma, especially for small, early tumors. Chemotherapy is used, although it is not as helpful in this disease as it is in some other cancers. Immunotherapy, in which concentrated amounts of the body's own immune-system chemicals are given, is also used. The agents most often employed are interleukin-2 (IL-2) and lymphokine-activated killer (LAK) cells. Sometimes the hormone melatonin is added to the treatment program.

Kampo explains melanoma as a disturbance of the energy channels underlying the skin by "heat," such as the heat of the sun. Heat blocks the normal flow of energy, which is transformed into small, hard lumps. If the body does not receive more heat once the lumps form, they do not spread. If the body later experiences an energy disturbance that heats the skin, melanoma results.

The Kampo herbs included in this entry are those verified as effective by both ancient Kampo theory and recent scientific investigation. Kampo treatments for melanoma either reduce its spread in the very earliest stages of the disease or increase the effectiveness of immunotherapy. Other therapies lower estrogen levels. Kampo should always be used as part of a medically directed overall treatment plan for melanoma (see considerations below).

INDIVIDUAL KAMPO TREATMENTS

See Chapter 3 for discussions of individual herbs, traditional healing substances, and modern herbal preparations, including directions for making tea.

SUGGESTED DOSAGES	COMMENTS
Aloe (Herb)	
Gel, either commercial or taken from houseplants, used liberally on the skin.	Contains antihistamines that prevent the production of basic fibroblast growth factor (bFGF), which is needed for melanoma growth.[1] Apply to damaged skin, including unusual growths, but if melanoma is suspected, *seek medical attention.*
Astragalus (Herb)	
Fluid extract (1:1), ¼–½ tsp (1–2 ml) 3 times daily. or Freeze-dried herb in capsules, 500–1,000 mg 3 times daily. or Powdered solid extract (4:1), 250–500 mg 3 times daily. or Tea, 1 c 3 times daily. or Tincture (1:5), 1–1½ tsp (4–6 ml), 3 times daily. Place in a cup, add 2 tbsp water, and take in a single sip. For dosages used with chemotherapy, *see* **Chemotherapy Side Effects.**	Contains compounds that increase the effectiveness of both IL-2 alone (in laboratory tests) and melatonin and IL-2 used together. These compounds also increase the ability of LAK cells to attack cancerous tumors,[2] and reverse immune suppression caused by cyclophosphamide treatment.[3] *Caution:* Do not use when fever or skin infection is present.
Kudzu (Herb)	
Dried extract, 1 10-mg tablet 3 times daily. or Tea, 1 c 3 times daily. or Use soy isoflavone extract (see **Soy Isoflavones** in this list).	Contains daidzein, which stops the growth of certain strains of melanoma.[4]

Lentinan (Modern Herbal Preparation)	
Intramuscular injection (usual form), 0.5–50 mg effective daily dose, depending on patient's condition and circumstances. Smaller, more frequent doses more effective than larger, less frequent doses. Given under professional supervision. or Powder, dosage to be determined by provider. Much greater dosages required than in injectable form.	Reduces rate at which melanoma cells can invade tissues outside the skin.[5]

PSK (Modern Herbal Preparation)	
Dried extract, 6 1,000-mg tablets daily.	Reduces the rate at which melanoma spreads to the lungs.[6] Increases the effectiveness of treatment with cyclophosphamide and IL-2.[7]

Reishi (Modern Herbal Preparation)	
Dried extract, 3 1-g tablets 3 times daily. or Dried mushroom in food, approx. ¼–approx. ½ oz (5–10 g) daily. or Syrup, as directed on label. or Tea, 1 c 3 times daily. or Tincture (1:5), 1 tbsp (10 ml) 3 times daily. Place in a cup, add 2 tbsp water, and take in a single sip.	Contains compounds that stimulate the body's production of IL-2.[8,9]

Siberian Ginseng (Modern Herbal Preparation)	
Eleuthero extract, as directed on label, in ¼ c water. Be sure to use pure extract, *not* sugar-sweetened ginseng drinks. or Tea, 1 c up to 3 times daily.	Useful in forms of cancer that respond to immunotherapy, including melanoma. Contains compounds that stimulate various immune-system components.[10] *Caution:* Should be avoided by persons with myasthenia gravis; rheumatoid arthritis and diseases related to it, such as lupus, psoriatric arthritis, and Sjögren's syndrome; or prostate cancer.

Soy Isoflavones (Modern Herbal Preparation)	
Extract, about 3,000 mg once daily. or Soy germ, 2 tsp (10 g) twice daily, preferably added to cereals or smoothies.	Contains daidzein (see **Kudzu** in this list). If concentrated isoflavones cause upset stomach, use kudzu.

HERBS TO AVOID

Individuals who have melanoma should avoid the following herbs: cordyceps, dan shen, fennel, licorice, and peony (estrogen stimulators), and also garlic (insulin stimulator). For more information regarding these herbs, see Chapter 3.

KAMPO FORMULAS

See Chapter 4 for dosage information and discussions of individual formulas.

Augmented Rambling Powder
Lowers estrogen levels.[11] Traditionally used to treat "hot" or "red" symptoms, in which the melanoma lesion appears as a bright red nodule with an elevated border. *Caution:* Should not be used by women who are trying to become pregnant.

Cinnamon Twig and Poria Pill
Reduces the amount of estrogen in the bloodstream.[12]

Tang-Kuei and Peony Powder
Decreases estrogen production by the ovaries.[13] Like **Augmented Rambling Powder** (see this list), treats "hot" or "red" symptoms, in which the melanoma lesions appear as a bright red nodule with an elevated border, but is more focused on correcting toxin accumulations in the liver.

FORMULAS TO AVOID

Individuals who have melanoma should avoid the following estrogen-stimulating formulas: Peony and Licorice Decoction and Six-Ingredient Pill With Rehmannia (Rehmannia-Six Combination). For more information regarding these formulas, see Chapter 4.

CONSIDERATIONS

❑ To reduce side effects and increase effectiveness when using chemotherapy, *see* **Chemotherapy Side Effects.** To learn about herbal treatments that can prevent a cancer from developing its own blood supply, *see* **Cancer.**
❑ *See also* **Skin Cancer (Basal Cell Carcinoma).**

MEMORY PROBLEMS

Occasional lapses of memory are an almost universal condition among persons of all ages. Chronic memory problems, however, most often occur among older people, and can cause considerable anxiety and concern.

While memory loss is most commonly associated with Alzheimer's disease and stroke, this problem can be caused by other disorders as well. Brain tissue can be damaged by free radicals, toxins produced by normal body processes. Impaired circulation (*see* **Atherosclerosis**) can reduce the flow of oxygen and nutrients to the brain. Thyroid disease and low blood-sugar levels can also affect memory.

The ability to remember can be affected by a variety of other factors. Some of these are short-term situations, such as fever, dehydration, chemical byproducts of bacterial infection, and disturbances in body chemistry. Anxiety and depression (and the drugs used to treat them) can cause memory problems, as can drug and alcohol use. Certain prescription drugs can affect memory, including blood-pressure medications, painkillers, antihistamines, and muscle relaxants. Toxic metals, such as aluminum, lead, and arsenic, can impair memory if they accumulate in the body. Stress can also affect memory, both through its physical effects and because it makes a person less likely to concentrate on the matter at hand. The first step in dealing with memory loss involves a full examination, so that obvious physical causes can be ruled out.

Although modern thinking is that memory problems are a disorder primarily of the brain and secondarily of the circulatory system, Kampo teaches that memory problems are a disorder primarily of the spirit and secondarily of the soul. Normally the heart is the organ that gives the individual control over the spirit while awake. Memory is part of the spirit's authority over will and emotional control. If the heart is weak, it cannot contain the spirit. When this happens, the energy of memory "drifts upward." This is the kind of disorder that creates false memories when the spirit seeks a truth and apprehends a falsehood. Herbs that bolster yang energy are needed to force the spirit down.

On the other hand, Kampo teaches that the soul retreats from the top of the body to the liver during sleep. This is the collection of life experiences. Memory problems result when the liver cannot "contain" the soul. This is the kind of disturbance that results in words or facts lingering "on the tip of the tongue." False memories do not interfere, but true memories are not available. To correct this condition, herbs that bolster yin energy are needed to bring the soul up to the top of the body.

In both kinds of memory problems, deficiencies of blood keep the soul and spirit from rising and falling normally day and night. Herbs that act on the heart and liver to move energy in the proper directions are the same herbs that have been found through research to help memory. Use formulas when memory problems occur as part of an overall symptom pattern.

INDIVIDUAL KAMPO TREATMENTS

See Chapter 3 for discussions of individual herbs, traditional healing substances, and modern herbal preparations, including directions for making tea.

SUGGESTED DOSAGES	COMMENTS
Biota (Herb)	
Tea, 1 c 3 times daily until memory improves, or for 3 months. or Use **Biota Seed Pill to Nourish the Heart** (see formulas list).	Prevents loss of memory, especially short-term memory. If biota is unavailable, substitute the non-Kampo herb yellow cedar.[1] Same caution applies. *Caution:* Long-term use can result in nausea and vomiting.
Ginkgo (Modern Herbal Preparation)	
Ginkgolide extract, up to 500 mg daily in a single dose.	Widely used memory herb. Affects the brain's use of acetylcholine (see inset on page 149). Corrects impaired mental function, dementia, fear, dizziness, and visual problems associated with memory loss.
Hawthorn (Herb)	
Dried herb in capsules, 3–5 g daily. or Fluid extract (1:1), ¼–½ tsp (1–2 ml) 3 times daily. or Solid extract, 100–250 mg 3 times daily. Should be standardized to contain 10% proanthocyanidins. or Tea, ⅔ c 3–4 times daily. or Tincture (1:5), 1–1½ tsp (4–6 ml) 3 times daily. Place in a cup, add 2 tbsp water, and take in a single sip.	Helps maintain the integrity of blood vessels in the brain by reducing artery-clogging plaques.
Jujube Fruit (Herb)	
Pitted fruits, 10 daily.	Reported to restore memory.[2]
Rose Hips (Herb)	
Natural rose-hip vitamin C, 1,000 mg. Rose-hip vitamins have a shelf life of 6 mos. or Tea, 1 cup as desired.	Traditional remedy for "restraining essence"; protects the function of memory against genetic disease. Contains both vitamin C and the vitamin C cofactors needed to increase capillary circulation in brain tissue. *Caution:* Should not be used when there is danger of increasing aluminum absorption.
Soy Lecithin (Modern Herbal Preparation)	
Very high doses of soy phospholipids, 15–25 g (15,000–25,000 mg, or 30–50 500-mg capsules). Identified individually on the label as 3-sn-phospatidylcholine, phosphatidylethanolamine, and phospatidylinositic acid, or as "total phospholipids." or Tofu, 2–4 oz (50–100 g) daily.	Source of brain chemical phosphatidylcholine. Prevents destruction of brain tissue under conditions of oxygen deprivation. *Caution:* If there is no noticeable improvement within 2 weeks, supplements should be stopped, since soy lecithin at this dosage is expensive and can cause mild diarrhea.

KAMPO FORMULAS

See Chapter 4 for dosage information and discussions of individual formulas.

Biota Seed Pill to Nourish the Heart

Relieves poor memory with low energy, chills, cold limbs, palpitations, insomnia, headache, dizziness, poor memory, agitation, or nightmares.

Bupleurum Plus Dragon Bone and Oyster Shell Decoction

Treats anxiety, insomnia, palpitations, and other manifestations of nervous tension in persons suffering memory loss who are physically strong.

Caution: Be sure the formula does *not* include the traditional ingredient minium (lead oxide). Use with caution if fever is present, and discontinue if preexisting fevers worsen.

Coptis Decoction to Relieve Toxicity

Potent free-radical scavenger. Protects brain tissue from the effects of inadequate oxygen supply.[3] Its historical use was in treating delirious speech.

Caution: Should not be used by women who are trying to become pregnant.

Emperor of Heaven's Special Pill to Tonify the Heart

Relieves mild, transient memory loss with "dry" symptoms, such as constipation or scratchy throat.

Caution: Do not use this formula if there is loss of appetite or diarrhea, or if there are aches and pains from influenza.

Gastrodia and Uncaria Decoction

These herbs increase the brain's production of a chemical, superoxide dismutase, that fights toxins called free radicals. They also prevent free radicals from starting a process that destroys brain cell walls.[4]

Caution: Should not be used by women who are trying to become pregnant.

Eight-Ingredient Pill With Rehmannia (Rehmannia-Eight Combination)

Regulates blood sugar and prevents diabetic nerve damage, which helps preserve mental function. Traditionally used to treat a symptom pattern that includes weakness in the lower half of the body, including poor circulation to the legs and feet, and impotence in men. There may also be back and knee weakness, increased urination, cold hands and feet, lumbago, reduced resistance to infection, and fatigue.

Settle the Emotions Pill

Combines four herbs—acorus, ginseng, hoelen, and Chinese senega root—widely prescribed in China and Japan for age-related loss of mental function. Treats poor memory compounded by insomnia, dizziness, hot flashes, or dry mouth.

CONSIDERATIONS

❑ Individuals who suspect that they may have been exposed to toxic metals should consider having their hair analyzed. Such metals are incorporated into the hair, and an analysis would indicate any toxin buildup.

❑ Eat green or yellow vegetables and fruit daily. If this is not possible, take a multivitamin tablet every day, and supplement it with vitamin E, 800 IU a day.

❑ *See also* **Alzheimer's Disease** and **Stroke.**

MÉNIÈRE'S DISEASE

Ménière's disease is an inner-ear disorder that causes attacks of vertigo, or dizziness and loss of balance. The vertigo may be accompanied by nausea and vomiting, and there may be a sense of fullness in the ear. Milder forms of the disease cause only slight difficulty in concentration, discomfort in the head, and momentary dizzy spells. Severe forms of the disease cause profound dizziness, ringing in the ears, and eventually deafness. Once deafness occurs, attacks of dizziness cease. In most people, Ménière's disease affects only one ear, although it is possible to have it in both ears.

In Ménière's disease there is a swelling of the channels that carry lymph away from the inner ear, an organ important to both hearing and balance. The swelling damages the delicate hairs with which the ear detects sound. They also

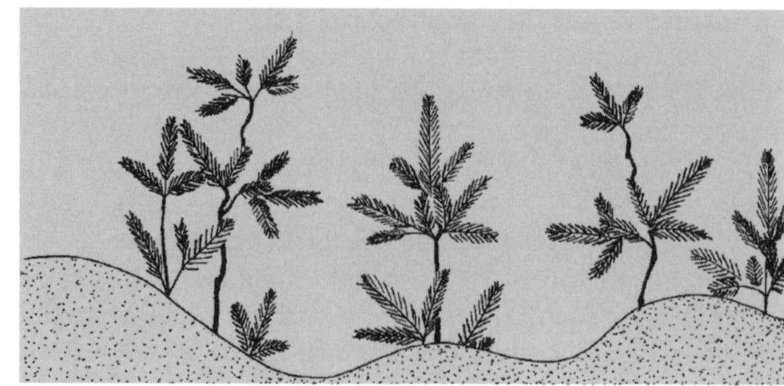

change the flow of fluid in the ear so that it cannot adjust to rapid changes in body position, such as getting out of bed or rising from a chair. Changes in spinal-fluid pressure aggravate the condition.[1]

Ménière's disease usually follows a blow to the head or a middle ear infection. In recent years, scientists have recognized that either of these conditions can trigger an autoimmune reaction, or one in which the immune system causes a disruption in normal bodily functioning. White blood cells do not recognize that collagen, a gelatinous protein, is building up within the inner ear.[2] The collagen clogs the inner ear, and, combined with changes in spinal-fluid pressure, causes the ear's balance mechanism to malfunction. Over a period of months or years, the pressure also destroys the cilia, or microscopic hairs, by which the ear detects sound.

Conventional medical treatment of the condition has used drugs combined with a low-salt diet to reduce both inflammation and the amount of fluid circulating in the body. Unfortunately, these measures do nothing to help people who have already lost their hearing.[3] More recently, doctors have used antibiotic therapy to alter the mineral balance of the fluid within the inner ear, which alleviates swelling. Overdoses, however, can cause hearing loss.

Kampo theorists who wrote the *Imperial Grace Formulary of the Tai Ping Era* (written in the eleventh century A.D.) conceived of this disease as a disorder of the body's immune organ, or what was called the "middle burner." First the body experienced dampness, clogging not only physical channels but also energy channels. Congested energy became "phlegm," in both a physical sense and a metaphorical sense, and accumulated in the middle burner. This obstruction blocked the flow of yang, or outward-directed, energies upward, especially to the ears.

To correct the symptoms of what we would call Ménière's disease, Kampo first cleared the middle burner, or immune system, and then treated dizziness and hearing loss. Kampo herbs help move lymph and prevent autoimmune damage to the inner ear. Kampo formulas relieve Ménière's disease as a part of different symptom patterns. As with conventional medicine, early treatment is essential. Once deafness occurs, attacks of dizziness cease, but the damage cannot be corrected.

INDIVIDUAL KAMPO TREATMENTS

See Chapter 3 for discussions of individual herbs, traditional healing substances, and modern herbal preparations, including directions for making tea.

SUGGESTED DOSAGES	COMMENTS
Coptis (Herb), Scutellaria (Herb)	
Coptis tincture (1:5), 1–1½ tsp (4–6 ml) 3 times daily. Place in a cup, add 2 tbsp water, and take in a single sip. and Scutellaria tincture (1:5), 1–1½ tsp (4–6 ml) 3 times daily. Place in a cup, add 2 tbsp water, and take in a single sip.	Together these herbs help control infection and circulate lymph away from the inner ear. Other forms of these herbs may be used if tinctures are not available. *Caution:* Do not use coptis during pregnancy or on a daily basis for more than 2 weeks at a time. Avoid scutellaria in cases of diarrhea caused by foodborne infection or excessive consumption of cold drinks.
Siberian Ginseng (Modern Herbal Preparation)	
Eleuthero extract, as directed by manufacturer, in ¼ c water. Be sure to use pure extract, *not* sugar-sweetened ginseng drinks. or Tea, 1 c 3 times daily.	Deactivates mast cells, which produce chemicals that cause inflammation and tissue destruction. Useful in early stages of the disease.[4] *Caution:* Should be avoided by persons with myasthenia gravis; rheumatoid arthritis and diseases related to it, such as lupus, psoriatric arthritis, and Sjögren's syndrome; or prostate cancer.

HERBS TO AVOID

Individuals who have Ménière's disease should avoid licorice. For more information regarding this herb, see Chapter 3.

KAMPO FORMULAS

See Chapter 4 for dosage information and discussions of individual formulas.

Bupleurum Plus Dragon Bone and Oyster Shell Decoction

Treats Ménière's disease when secondary symptoms include constipation, delirious speech, inability to turn the torso, rapid pulse, and/or a sensation of heaviness throughout the entire body.

Caution: Be sure the formula does *not* include the traditional ingredient minium (lead oxide). Use with caution if fever is present, and discontinue if preexisting fevers worsen.

Five-Ingredient Powder with Poria

Treats Ménière's disease caused by trauma or accompanying fever; other symptoms include headache, irritability, strong thirst but with vomiting after drinking, and/or urinary difficulty.

Prepared Aconite Decoction

Treats Ménière's disease accompanied by body aches. May cause a loss of sensation in the mouth and tongue.

Caution: Discontinue the formula if fever occurs.

True Warrior Decoction

Treats Ménière's disease accompanied by cold sensations in the body, swelling, and urinary difficulty, but no pain. May cause a loss of sensation in the mouth and tongue.

Caution: Discontinue the formula if fever occurs.

CONSIDERATIONS

❑ The hormone melatonin activates the white blood cells in the inner ear to recognize and dispose of collagen. Take 3 milligrams a day for up to a month when symptoms first appear.

Menopause-Related Problems

Menopause is when menstruation ends. It occurs after a period of several years in which production of the main female hormone, estrogen, diminishes, a period known as the climacteric. Unless brought about by injury, surgery, or chemotherapy, the climacteric, also called perimenopause, usually begins in the midforties. Menopause is usually complete by age fifty to fifty-five.

During the climacteric, the ovaries greatly reduce their estrogen production (although small amounts are produced by other bodily tissues), while the production of other hormones greatly increases. As a result the woman's menstrual cycle starts to shorten. Eventually, the period becomes irregular—sometimes longer, sometimes much shorter. The vagina and fallopian tubes shrink, vaginal lubrication decreases, and the ligaments supporting the uterus and vagina lose their strength.

It is important to remember that menopause is not a disorder, but a natural part of life. Nevertheless, it can produce symptoms that range from mildly uncomfortable to extremely distracting, and that affect each woman differently. Most women experience hot flashes, which generally occur in the first two years. Other symptoms include spontaneous sweating, heart palpitations, urinary urgency, head and body aches, fatigue, mood swings, nervousness, depressed feelings, deficiencies in concentration and memory, and insomnia. Backache and a tendency to back sprain are common. The skin becomes drier. Sex drive may either increase or decrease.

The decline in estrogen production has other important effects. The bones no longer retain as much calcium and phosphorous. A condition called osteoporosis can result, in which the bones become soft, and even minor stresses can result in fractures. Decreased estrogen production is also associated with an increased risk of heart disease. The ovaries form estrogen from low-density lipoprotein (LDL), the "bad," artery-clogging kind. This action decreases the ratio of LDL to "good," artery-clearing high-density lipoprotein (HDL).

The most common conventional treatment for menopausal symptoms is estrogen replacement therapy, in which estrogen and another female hormone, progesterone, are taken in a carefully balanced monthly cycle. This therapy may lower the risk of death from heart disease after several years' use, and greatly reduces the loss of bone due to osteoporosis. On the other hand, oral estrogen replacement therapies frequently result in nausea, and because the replacement hormone is processed in the liver, liver damage can result. Estrogen replacement given via vaginal suppositories may cause breast discomfort and bloating. Worst of all, estrogen replacement therapy is associated with an increased risk of breast cancer.

Kampo explains the problems of menopause as a combination of blood deficiency and energy constraints. When a woman's body does not produce enough blood to supply the liver, which houses emotional energy, the liver seeks to force the digestive system to process more food that can be "transformed" into blood. The energy normally circulated by the liver fails to reach the organs along its energy channel, producing tensions or swellings in the breasts, vision abnormalities, and headache. More complicated imbalances involve the kidneys and the lungs, which keep fluids from circulating properly, especially to the skin and mucous membranes. These imbalances result in tension in the bloodstream (high blood pressure) and dryness of the skin and vagina.

Many women with menopausal symptoms find relief using Kampo alone. However, Kampo can be used to supplement estrogen replacement therapy, or estrogen replacement therapy can be used to supplement Kampo; see a health care provider. Either kind of treatment usually takes several months to work.

INDIVIDUAL KAMPO TREATMENTS

See Chapter 3 for discussions of individual herbs, traditional healing substances, and modern herbal preparations, including directions for making tea.

SUGGESTED DOSAGES	COMMENTS
Black Cohosh (Herb)	
Dried root, 2–6 500-mg capsules daily. or Fluid extract (1:1), ¼–½ tsp (1–2 ml) daily. or Freeze-dried root, 1–2 500-mg capsules daily. or Powdered solid extract (4:1), standardized for 27-deoxyacteine, 1–2 250-mg tablets daily. or Tincture (1:5), 1–1½ tsp (4–6 ml) once daily. Place in a cup, add 2 tbsp water, and take in a single sip.	About 80 percent effective in relieving symptoms of menopause when taken 4 weeks or longer.[1] Increases vaginal lubrication as effectively as estrogen replacement therapy.[2] Relieves headaches and muscle pain. Stops irregular bleeding.
Tang-Kuei (Herb)	
Dried root, 1–2 tsp (1–3 g) daily. or Fluid extract (1:1), ¼–½ tsp (1–2 ml) daily. or Freeze-dried root, 1–2 500-mg capsules daily. or Powdered solid extract (4:1), 250–500 mg daily. or Tea, 1 c 2–3 times daily. or Tincture (1:5), 1–1½ tsp (4–6 ml) daily. Place in a cup, add 2 tbsp water, and take in a single sip.	Increases circulation, protects the heart, and increases the effectiveness of other herbal or prescription treatments. Contrary to some published reports, has not been confirmed to relieve hot flashes or vaginal dryness when used by itself.[3] Also known as dong quai.
Vitex (Herb)	
Fluid extract (1:1), 1 tsp (4 ml) 3 times daily. or Solid extract (4:1), 250–500 mg 3 times daily.	Stops hot flashes with sensation of movement in the skin, dizziness, and depression. This herb must be used for 3–6 months to have a noticeable effect on symptoms.

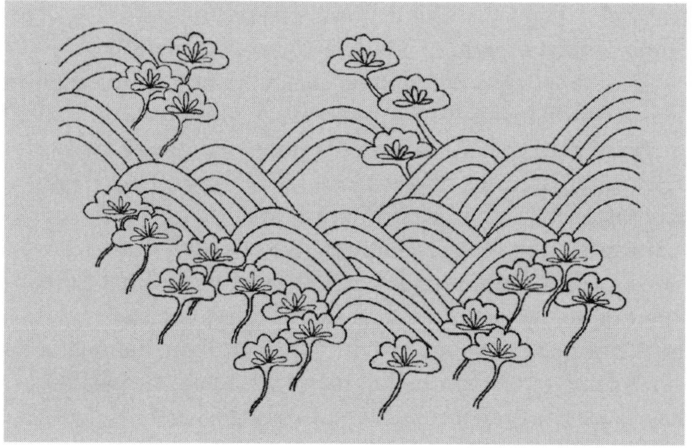

KAMPO FORMULAS

See Chapter 4 for dosage information and discussions of individual formulas.

Augmented Rambling Powder

Most commonly used formula for menopause in Japan. Treats hot flashes, especially when they are triggered by emotional distress.

Bupleurum and Cinnamon Twig Decoction

Treats eye problems (myopia spuria), headache, hot flashes, and spontaneous sweating, especially with stiff neck and shoulders. Also useful for tension headaches and migraines. Not appropriate for women who are either unusually active (more than 1 hour exercise per day) or completely sedentary (no exercise at all).

Caution: Use with caution if fever is present, and discontinue if preexisting fevers worsen.

Bupleurum Plus Dragon Bone and Oyster Shell Decoction

Treats hot flashes, ringing in the ears, and overreaction to stimuli, especially being startled out of sleep. Also treats difficulty concentrating and short-term memory problems. Not appropriate for physically active women.

Caution: Be sure the formula does *not* include the traditional ingredient minium (lead oxide). Use with caution if fever is present, and discontinue if preexisting fevers worsen.

Cinnamon Twig and Poria Pill

Treats hot flashes when they are accompanied by "static blood," that is, abnormal genital bleeding or pelvic congestion. Treats osteoporosis in women not receiving estrogen replacement therapy.

Cinnamon Twig, Licorice, Dragon Bone, and Oyster Shell Decoction

Used to treat anxiety in physically robust women. Symptoms include hot flashes, palpitations, sweating.

Coptis Decoction to Relieve Toxicity

Treats "hot" symptoms, especially hot flashes, outbreaks on the skin, thirst, and bad breath.

Caution: Should not be used by women who are trying to become pregnant.

Eight-Ingredient Pill With Rehmannia (Rehmannia-Eight Combination)

Used when there is sensitivity to cold weather in the hands and feet, dry and itchy skin, impaired vision and hearing, and/or abnormalities in urination. Used to treat osteoporosis, especially when symptoms of bone weakness are more severe in the lower half of the body.

Kudzu Decoction

Used when there is severe tightness of the muscles in the neck and/or back.

Ledebouriella Powder That Sagely Unblocks

Used when symptoms include weight gain, constipation, high blood pressure, and/or sudden outbursts of emotion.

Caution: Should not be used if nausea or vomiting is present.

Licorice, Wheat, and Jujube Decoction

Treats disorientation, frequent attacks of melancholy and crying spells, inability to control oneself, restless sleep, night sweats, and frequent bouts of yawning. Can be made at home in tea form (see Chapter 4).

Tang-Kuei and Peony Powder

Treats hot flashes when they are accompanied by muscle tremor and/or fluid retention.

Tonify the Middle and Augment the Qi Decoction

Especially appropriate when dominant symptom is fatigue and/or loss of muscle tone. Useful for incontinence and prolapse of the uterus. In formulas for menopause, sometimes identified as Center-Supplementing Qi-Boosting Decoction.

Warm the Menses Decoction

Stops mild, persistent uterine bleeding, irregular menstruation (either early or late), extended or continuous menstrual flow, bleeding between periods that may be accompanied by cold in the lower abdomen, dry lips and mouth, low-grade fever in the late afternoon, or warm palms and soles.

Caution: Discontinue if preexisting fevers worsen.

MENSTRUAL PROBLEMS

Every month, as part of the menstrual cycle, a woman's body sheds the tissues that line the uterus. This occurs because the body must prepare every month for a possible pregnancy, and does so by growing a thicker, spongier uterine lining meant to nourish a growing fetus. If no pregnancy occurs, this lining is not needed and breaks down.

Two problems associated with menstruation are pain before or during the beginning of the period (*dysmenorrhea*) and unusually heavy bleeding (*menorrhagia*). Menstrual pain is an extremely common condition. It can be accompanied by nausea, vomiting, diarrhea, headache, dizziness, and blurred vision. The pain, sometimes intense, often spreads to the legs and lower back. Primary dysmenorrhea is the medical term for pain for which no physical cause can be identified. Secondary dysmenorrhea is pain associated with a clear physical condition, such as endometriosis, ovarian cysts and tumors, pelvic inflammatory disease, uterine polyps, and fibroid adenomyosis, a nonmalignant condition in which the uterine lining invades the muscles of the uterine wall.

A heavy period involves the loss of more than two ounces (eighty milliliters) of blood. This loss occurs during regular menstrual cycles (cycles of normal length) unless caused by another disorder, such as endometriosis or uterine fibroids.

Primary menstrual pain and heavy bleeding are usually related to the production of inflammatory substances called series-2 prostaglandins. These hormonelike compounds produce pain by causing uterine contractions to increase, and heavy bleeding by promoting inflammation and clotting in the uterine lining. Blood clots, oddly enough, can actually cause bleeding by blocking the normal flow of blood through the uterus.

Conventional treatment of primary dysmenorrhea consists of painkillers and, if needed, bed rest. If a narrow cervix is discovered, it may be dilated. Treatment of primary menorrhagia consists of using female hormones, such as those used in birth control pills, to correct the hormonal imbalance linked to prostaglandin production.

Using Shepherd's Purse With Kampo to Stop Bleeding

The non-Kampo herb shepherd's purse stops bleeding through the action of a plant protein that acts like the hormone oxytocin.[1] Oxytocin stimulates the constriction of the smooth muscles that surround blood vessels, especially those in the uterus, which prevents too much blood from entering the uterine lining. It complements Kampo therapies used to stop the bleeding of heavy periods or nosebleed.

The most effective way to take shepherd's purse is as a tea two to three times a day. Pour ⅔ cup (150 milliliters) of boiling water over 3 to 4 teaspoons (4.5 to 6 grams) of finely chopped herb. Allow the mixture to stand for fifteen minutes, then strain and drink. Shepherd's purse should be taken on an empty stomach, or at least between meals. It is possible to make a large quantity of shepherd's purse tea ahead of time and store it under refrigeration for up to three months. The tea's medicinal potency increases as it is stored. Shepherd's purse is also available as a fluid extract or tincture. Take ¼ to ½ teaspoon (1 to 2 milliliters) of fluid extract or 1½ to 2 teaspoons (4 to 6 milliliters) three times a day. Although this herb stops uterine bleeding, it does not cause contractions, and thus can be used for nosebleeds during pregnancy. However, if the bleeding persists more than three days or becomes greater during treatment, consult a physician.

Modern Oriental medicine sees menstrual pain as being caused by one of three main factors. One is the intrusion of "cold" and "damp" into the womb. This can occur if a woman swims or becomes chilled in the rain, sits or sleeps in damp places, or drinks unusually large amounts of cold drinks. A second factor is a deficiency of the body's energy and blood, caused by physical thinness or weakness that results from dieting. In this situation, the body's energy channels do not have enough energy to maintain smooth menstrual blood flow. In the third factor, excessive emotion, such as joy, anger, worry, thought, sadness, fear, or shock, can affect the flows of blood and energy. Blood circulation in the womb is disrupted as a result, and the relationship between energy and blood goes out of balance.

Kampo theorists believed that a normal menstrual cycle depended on the liver's ability to provide and restrain the flow of blood at appropriate times. When the liver lost its yin, or holding, energies, it released too much blood into the menstrual flow. Restoring the liver's yin energies prevented heavy periods. Heavy periods could also result from "heated" blood. This is blood that leaves its natural course after it is energized too strongly by the liver, which has to release the energy of strong emotions it is unable to store.

Both herbs and formulas may have to be used for three to four months before results are apparent. Use of the menstrual-pain herbs is tied to a regular monthly cycle; if periods are irregular, see a doctor. These treatments should only be used after secondary causes, such as endometriosis, are ruled out. A non-Kampo herb, shepherd's purse, may be used to make Kampo treatment for heavy periods more effective (see page 265).

INDIVIDUAL KAMPO TREATMENTS

See Chapter 3 for discussions of individual herbs, traditional healing substances, and modern herbal preparations, including directions for making tea.

Treatments That Reduce Menstrual Pain

SUGGESTED DOSAGES	COMMENTS
Amaranth (Herb)	
Tea, 1 c 3 times daily.	Relieves menstrual pain. Listed in Chinese herb shops as achyranthis; may also be labeled as *Niu Xi* or *Tu Niu Xi*.
Lindera (Herb)	
Fluid extract (1:1), $\frac{1}{4}$–$\frac{1}{2}$ tsp (1–2 ml) 3 times daily.	Used for a symptom pattern that includes painful menstruation, tightness in the chest, pain in the flanks, and frequent urination. Available as *Wu Yao*.

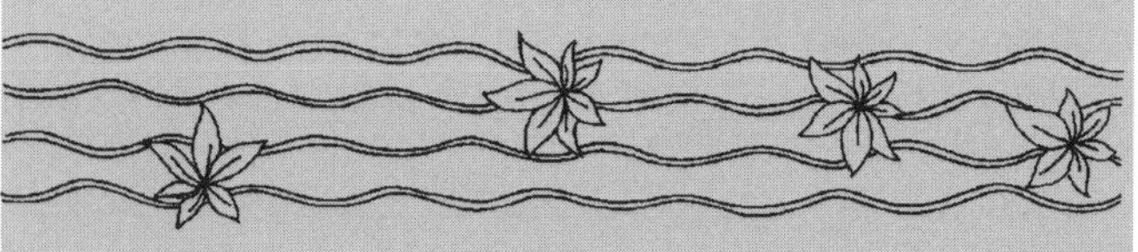

Tang-Kuei (Herb)	
Dried root, 1–2 tsp (1–3 g) daily. or Fluid extract (1:1), $\frac{1}{4}$–$\frac{1}{2}$ tsp (1–2 ml) daily. or Freeze-dried root, 1–2 500-mg capsules daily. or Powdered solid extract (4:1), 250–500 mg daily. or Tea, 1 c daily 2–3 times daily. or Tincture (1:5), 1–1$\frac{1}{2}$ tsp (4–6 ml) daily. Place in a cup, add 2 tbsp water, and take in a single sip.	Regulates menstrual function. Use during first fourteen days of the cycle (before ovulation) for 3 to 4 months. Also known as dong quai.
Vitex (Herb)	
Tincture (1:5), $\frac{3}{4}$–1 tbsp (9–12 ml) 3 times daily. Place in a cup, add 2 tbsp water, and take in a single sip.	Regulates menstrual function. Use during the last fourteen days of the cycle (after ovulation) for 3–4 months.

Treatments That Reduce Heavy Menstrual Bleeding

Agrimony (Herb)	
Tea, 1 c 2–3 times daily.	Kampo has used agrimony for thousands of years to stop bleeding of all kinds. *Caution:* Do not use for more than 2 weeks.
Cinnamon (Herb)	
Oil, 15–30 drops, up to 3 times daily. Place in a cup, add 2 tbsp warm water, and take in a single sip. or Tea, 1 c up to 3 times daily.	Alleviates both heavy periods and other types of abnormal uterine bleeding by stimulating the flow of blood out of the uterus. The standard remedy for this condition before the twentieth century.

KAMPO FORMULAS

See Chapter 4 for dosage information and discussions of individual formulas.

Formulas That Reduce Menstrual Pain

Augmented Rambling Powder

Treats menstrual pain with tenderness in the breasts and lower abdomen, irritability, edema, headache, and digestive disturbance at the beginning of the period.

Caution: Should not be used by women who are trying to become pregnant.

Cinnamon Twig and Poria Pill

Stops sharp, severe pain with discharge of clotted blood. Also stops excessive menstrual flow in 90 percent of women who use it for at least 3 months.[1]

Formulas That Reduce Heavy Menstrual Bleeding

Four-Substance Decoction

Regulates blood flow to relieve either heavy periods or lack of periods. Most useful when other symptoms indicate a general lack of energy: blurred vision, dizziness, lusterless nails, lower abdominal pain.

CONSIDERATIONS

❑ The prostaglandin imbalances that cause both menstrual pain and heavy periods result from an imbalance in the types of fats in the diet. In the modern Western diet, there is a deficiency of omega-3 essential fatty acids, substances that promote healing and calm inflammation. These fatty acids are highly concentrated in flaxseed and flaxseed oil, and are more available when the diet contains less animal fat. They should be taken daily for a period of three to four months. In addition, vitamin C, taken in doses of 500 to 1,000 milligrams three times a day, helps stabilize fragile capillaries that may break and bleed, causing heavy menstrual bleeding.

❑ *See also* **Endometriosis, Fibroids (Uterine Myomas), Pelvic Inflammatory Disease,** and **Premenstrual Syndrome (PMS).**

MIGRAINE

Migraine is commonly thought of as the ultimate headache. Attacks are excruciatingly painful and recurrent, but can occur without pain. Symptoms include temporary slurring or loss of speech; distortion of sight, with "shooting stars" and kaleidoscopic color patterns; temporary paralysis; and short-term memory loss. Migraine may be heralded by an aura or prodrome, which may be experienced as a "curtain falling" over the field of vision or as a wave of inexplicable depression and emotional pain. Migraines may last for a few hours or a few days, and may occur a few times a year or every day. The first attack usually occurs between the ages of ten and thirty, but many people "outlast" migraines by the age of fifty. Since the blood-vessel changes that occur in the brain during migraine are influenced by estrogen, more women are affected than men.

Noise and other forms of environmental disturbance aggravate migraine. Water retention associated with the menstrual cycle also seems to increase the likelihood of an attack, as do stress, long-term eyestrain, and holding the same position for long periods of time, such as during a long phone call or when behind the wheel of a car.

Until recently, migraines were thought to be caused by spasms of the blood vessels supplying the brain. However, brain-scan studies have not detected this problem in those parts of the brain where migraine starts. Migraine is now frequently described as "spreading depression," a kind of seizure disorder in which pain fibers in the brain, blood vessels supplying the brain, and chemical balances all go awry at the same time. Migraine has also been linked to toxic-chemical exposure, allergies, drug use, and other factors.

The problem in treating migraines is that no single drug is enough to bring relief. Conventional treatment of migraine uses painkillers (if the headache is mild enough) and drugs meant to redirect blood flow. Many migraine sufferers are successfully treated with antiseizure medication, although these drugs must be used very carefully.

Even Kampo had multiple, conflicting explanations of migraine. One theory was that migraine was set off by the wind. Pathogenic atmospheric changes invaded the body and followed the energy channels to the head and eyes, obstructing the flow of "clear qi." Another theory was that the migraine resulted from the accumulated energies of emotional or premenstrual tension stored in the liver. Migraines ceased when the liver and gallbladder were "drained" of heat. Still another theory was that migraines were a symptom of an infection that was between two of the "yang," or outermost, layers of the body's natural defenses. In the Kampo multistage model of disease (see Chapter 1), migraine created fever and chills and vomiting like an early disease stage, but physical weakness and racing pulse like a later stage. Treatment required a careful balance of herbs to strengthen the body in general and herbs to weaken the pathogen.

Since Kampo also has many theories of migraine, it offers many treatments. The advantage of using herbs is their ability to complement standard treatments and to complement each other. Keep a small supply of the herbs listed below for use when migraines strike. When using formulas, matching the formula to the overall symptom pattern is essential; see a Kampo or TCM practitioner.

INDIVIDUAL KAMPO TREATMENTS

See Chapter 3 for discussions of individual herbs, traditional healing substances, and modern herbal preparations, including directions for making tea.

SUGGESTED DOSAGES	COMMENTS
Ginger (Herb)	
Tea, 1 c 2–3 times daily.	Prevents the formation of enzymes[1] necessary for a set of hormonal reactions that cause inflammation and pain.
Vitex (Herb)	
Fluid extract (1:1), 25 drops every 30 mins until pain subsides. Place in a cup, add 2 tbsp water, and take in a single sip.	Relieves migraines that occur with premenstrual syndrome.

KAMPO FORMULAS

See Chapter 4 for dosage information and discussions of individual formulas.

Bupleurum Plus Dragon Bone and Oyster Shell Decoction

Used in Japan to treat migraines caused by environmental stresses, such as weather changes, noise, allergens, and drafts. Clinical tests show that this formula helps to prevent formation of $5HT_1$, a substance that causes blood-vessel constriction.[2]

Caution: Be sure the formula does *not* include the traditional ingredient minium (lead oxide). Use with caution if fever is present, and discontinue if preexisting fevers worsen.

Evodia Decoction

Used to relieve migraines with any of the following digestive disturbances: vomiting immediately after eating, indeterminate gnawing hunger, or acid reflux; dry heaves or spitting of fluids with worst pain at the top of the head; and vomiting and diarrhea with cold hands and feet.

Four-Substance Decoction

Relieves migraine with a symptom pattern generally seen in women: dizziness, blurred vision, lusterless complexion and nails, general muscle tension, lower abdominal pain, and irregular menstruation with little flow or amenorrhea.

Ligusticum Chuanxiong Powder to be Taken With Green Tea

Relieves migraine accompanied by fever and chills, dizziness, and nasal congestion. As the name suggests, it is taken with a cup of green tea.

Major Bupleurum Decoction

Relieves migraine with alternating fevers and chills, bitter taste in the mouth, nausea, and either burning diarrhea or severe constipation. Usually emotional symptoms are not severe when they occur with the symptoms that call for this formula.

Caution: Use with caution if fever is present, and discontinue if preexisting fevers worsen.

Rhubarb and Moutan Decoction

Prevents disturbances of numbness, paralysis, blurred vision, or slurred speech due to migraine.

Caution: If these symptoms appear in someone who has not been diagnosed as having migraine by a physician, *immediately* seek professional help.

Tang-Kuei, Gentiana Longdancao, and Aloe Pill

Stops migraine that occurs with a shortened menstrual period, and red and sore eyes, hearing loss, or swelling in the ears.

Caution: Should not be used by women who are trying to become pregnant.

CONSIDERATIONS

❑ Women who suffer from migraines should not use high-estrogen birth control pills. This increases the risk of stroke.[3]

❑ Not to be overlooked in treating migraine is the reliable standby, aspirin. Taking aspirin at the beginning of an attack can keep a one-sided migraine from spreading to the other eye. Taking a single aspirin two or more times a week can minimize the severity of future attacks.[4]

❑ Many migraine sufferers report that monosodium glutamate (MSG), nitrates in cured meats, caffeine, and alcohol can all trigger attacks, and should thus be avoided by persons who are prone to migraine.

MULTIPLE MYELOMA

See **Bone Cancer.**

MULTIPLE SCLEROSIS

Multiple sclerosis (MS) is a disease of the central nervous system. Nerve cells are sheathed in a substance called myelin. In MS, there is chronic inflammation and destruction of these sheaths. This leaves the underlying nerves vulnerable to damage, which can result in scarred areas called plaques. MS affects more than 350,000 persons in the United States alone, and is the most frequent cause of neurologic disability in early to middle adulthood.

The symptoms of MS may be dramatic or mild, and those experienced by each individual depend on which nerve fibers in the brain or spinal cord are damaged. Common problems include weakness of the limbs, which causes difficulty in climbing stairs; loss of dexterity; and the recurrent stubbing of the big toe due to a "foot drop." There may also be blurred vision or partial blindness, facial pain, dizziness, tingling, numbness, and spasms. Urinary or bowel urgency or incontinence may occur, and men may experience impotence. Mental symptoms, such as mood swings, may occur. Almost all cases of MS are marked by heat sensitivity, that is, the appearance or worsening of symptoms after exposure to heat (such as a hot shower) and fatigue.

MS may occur as *relapsing* MS, in which acute attacks lasting from days to weeks are followed by some degree of recovery; *chronic progressive* MS, in which symptoms become gradually worse without periods of stability; or *inactive* MS, with fixed areas of damage that do not worsen with time. The varied nature of this illness means that there is no one test that can detect it. Diagnosis depends on observation of the disease and testing to rule out other causes.

While the exact cause of MS is unknown, scientists currently believe that MS requires a combination of genetic predisposition and a triggering factor, usually a viral infection in late childhood. In MS, the infection causes the body to create misdirected immune-system cells called T cells, which secrete tumor necrosis factor (TNF). TNF, in turn, signals other immune-system cells called macrophages to attack the nerve cells. MS patients also have an abnormal blood-brain barrier that is "opened" by extremely small blood clots, which allows toxic chemicals to enter the brain.[1,2]

There is no one conventional treatment for MS. Steroid drugs, such as prednisone, are used to reduce symptoms during relapses, but can also cause a number of side effects. Other drugs are used to reduce the frequency of relapses, or to protect myelin from destruction.

MS is much more common in temperate climates than in tropical ones, and marked differences in the prevalence of MS exist between different ethnic groups. It occurs more frequently in Scandinavia and northern Europe, while it is virtually unknown in sub-Saharan Africa and almost completely unknown in Japan.

Because MS is not seen in Japan, Kampo has not developed a symptom pattern corresponding to that seen in MS. The *sho,* or symptom pattern, however, has been adapted to allow a Kampo understanding of MS. At this point, Kampo therapies are being used *experimentally* in treatment. Always speak to a doctor before taking these therapies, and use them under the guidance of a Kampo or TCM practitioner.

INDIVIDUAL KAMPO TREATMENTS

See Chapter 3 for discussions of individual herbs, traditional healing substances, and modern herbal preparations, including directions for making tea.

SUGGESTED DOSAGES	COMMENTS
Ginkgo (Modern Herbal Preparation)	
Ginkgolide extract, 4 40-mg tablets once daily.	Contains factors that prevent clots from forming in the blood-brain barrier. Ginkgo also improves blood flow to the brain and helps brain cells function more efficiently. Laboratory studies indicate it is more helpful in preventing relapses than in treating acute symptoms.[3–5]
Soy Lecithin (Modern Herbal Preparation)	
Phosphatidylserine extract, 300 mg daily. Leci-PS is a good preparation, but any soy lecithin tablet labeled for phosphatidylserine content is useful.	Contains phosphatidylserine, a chemical that reduces TNF production. Persons with MS have low levels of this substance in their bloodstreams.[6] *Caution:* Mild diarrhea may occur when soy lecithin is first used.

HERBS TO AVOID

Individuals who have multiple sclerosis should avoid maitake. For more information regarding this herb, see Chapter 3.

KAMPO FORMULAS

See Chapter 4 for dosage information and discussions of individual formulas.

Augmented Four-Substance Decoction

Provides symptomatic relief of blurred vision and dizziness.

Ginseng Decoction to Nourish the Nutritive Qi

Increases the effectiveness of prednisolone. Prescribed in Japan to treat any medical condition complicated by forgetfulness or tired limbs.

Ophiopogonis Decoction

Relieves respiratory distress (coughing, wheezing) accompanying MS. Increases the effectiveness of steroid drugs.

Caution: Use with caution if fever is present, and discontinue if preexisting fevers worsen.

Sairei-to

This is a combination of two commonly available formulas: Five-Ingredient Powder with Poria and Minor Bupleurum Decoction. It increases the effectiveness of prednisone.[7]

Caution: Avoid if taking alpha interferon.

FORMULAS TO AVOID

Individuals who have multiple sclerosis and are receiving alpha-interferon therapy should avoid Minor Bupleurum Decoction. For more information regarding this formula, see Chapter 4.

CONSIDERATIONS

❑ Modern scientists point out that one of the reasons MS is very rare in Japan may be that the traditional diet contains generous supplies of substances called omega-3 fatty acids. Omega-3 fatty acids form chains of fat that elongate to cover nerve cells and protect them from damage.[8] While it is also possible that there is a genetic difference that allows people in Japan to use fatty acids more effectively, following a Japanese-style diet, including seafood, seeds, and soyfoods, may help prevent relapses.

MUMPS

Mumps is a viral disease causing acute and painful inflammation of the salivary glands and sometimes other glands in the body. The virus is passed through infected saliva. First symptoms can include headache, chills, loss of appetite, malaise, and, if the body's immune resistance is especially low, a fever of from 103°F to 106°F (39.4°C to 41.1°C). For many patients, however, the first symptom is the swelling of the salivary glands, the mumps, which generally starts about a day after any initial symptoms.

Once in the body, the virus incubates for between twelve to twenty-five days before the swelling appears. A person is infectious for approximately five days before the mumps appear until approximately nine days afterwards. This disease appears most often in children, but can occur in adults as well. Adults with the mumps tend to experience greater discomfort and suffer more complications.

From 20 to 30 percent of males past puberty who get mumps experience swelling of the testicles. Shaking chills and high fevers are frequent, and may be accompanied by headache, nausea, and vomiting. Usually testicular swelling eases after seven to nine days. Even if the testicles atrophy after the infection runs its course, complete infertility is rare even when both testicles are inflamed. Other, rarer complications include inflammation of the brain, pancreas, or other organs, or a particularly fatiguing form of low blood sugar.

The current scientific understanding of mumps is that the immune system both defends against the virus by producing interferon,[1] and causes the pain and swelling characteristic of the disease[2] by needlessly activating other immune-system components called T cells. Conventional treatment consists of using aspirin or other painkillers to ease pain and reduce fever. (It is important never to give children under the age fifteen aspirin, as the use of aspirin during viral infections can result in Reye's syndrome, an extremely serious complication.) Bed rest cannot prevent testicular swelling, contrary to popular belief, but can ease testicular pain.

Kampo describes mumps as a condition that is half "interior" and half "exterior." The pathogen, or virus, struggles to go deeper and lower into the body, even as the immune system tries to force it upward and out. The result is a "fullness" of energies causing swelling at whatever depth and height the body can stop the disease. Formulas to treat mumps are chosen for the ability to "vent" the pathogen while restoring the flow of protective energies downward through the body. All Kampo therapies should only be used until the swelling subsides.

INDIVIDUAL KAMPO TREATMENTS

See Chapter 3 for discussions of individual herbs, traditional healing substances, and modern herbal preparations, including directions for making tea.

SUGGESTED DOSAGES	COMMENTS
Siberian Ginseng (Modern Herbal Preparation)	
Eleuthero extract, as directed by manufacturer, in 1/4 c water. Be sure to use pure extract, *not* sugar-sweetened ginseng drinks. or Tea, 1 c 3 times daily. Can be given to children (see inset on page 142).	Increases interferon production.[3] Use as soon as possible after exposure to the mumps. *Caution:* Should be avoided by persons with myasthenia gravis; rheumatoid arthritis and diseases related to it, such as lupus, psoriatric arthritis, and Sjögren's syndrome; or prostate cancer.

HERBS TO AVOID

Individuals who have the mumps should avoid the non-Kampo herb echinacea, which activates the T cells.

KAMPO FORMULAS

See Chapter 4 for dosage information and discussions of individual formulas.

Kudzu Decoction

Can moderate symptoms by supplementing the antiviral activity of the immune system. Traditionally used to "open the pores" of the face and neck so that pathogens could escape.

Minor Bupleurum Decoction

Relieves pain and swelling, prevents progression of viral diseases.

Caution: Avoid this formula if mumps is accompanied by bleeding or painful gums, nosebleed, peptic ulcer, or unusual emotional agitation not related to concerns about the disease. Do not use if fever or skin infection is present.

NEPHRITIS

See **Kidney Disease.**

NOSEBLEED

Nosebleeds occur when the delicate capillaries in the nasal linings rupture. This can arise from a number of causes, most commonly through injury, such as a fall or by a child placing a foreign object in the nose. Other nosebleeds are caused by irritation of the mucus membranes lining the nasal passages and sinuses.

Often injury-related nosebleeds produce what looks like a lot of blood, although the amount of blood usually lost is slight. Irritation nosebleeds involve chronic, light bleeding.

Traditional Japanese medicine associated chronic nosebleed with emotional tension and with "inverted bleeding," a tendency to develop nosebleeds and bleeding gums during the menstrual period. Kampo saw nosebleed and other forms of bleeding as blood that became heated, so that it lost its course and spilled out of the body. Kampo's strategy for treating bleeding is to remove the pathogen that "heats" or causes irritation while also stanching the flow of blood.

The preparations listed here are appropriate for chronic, light nosebleeds associated with irritation, or with emotional or hormonal factors. Use any of these therapies until nosebleeds no longer recur. These preparations can be used with the non-Kampo herb shepherd's purse (see "Using Shepherd's Purse With Kampo to Stop Bleeding" on page 265.) Since chronic nosebleed can be associated with an underlying illness, such as high blood pressure, see a doctor if nosebleeds recur.

INDIVIDUAL KAMPO TREATMENTS

See Chapter 3 for discussions of individual herbs, traditional healing substances, and modern herbal preparations, including directions for making tea.

SUGGESTED DOSAGES	COMMENTS
Agrimony (Herb)	
Tea, 1 c 2–3 times daily. Can be given to children (see inset on page 142).	Kampo has used agrimony for thousands of years to stop bleeding of all kinds. Especially useful for treating children's nosebleeds. *Caution:* Do not use for more than 2 weeks.

KAMPO FORMULAS

See Chapter 4 for dosage information and discussions of individual formulas.

Frigid Extremities Decoction

Stops recurrent nosebleed in a "cold" symptom pattern that includes abdominal pain, aversion to cold, cold hands or feet, constant desire to sleep, diarrhea with undigested food particles, cold extremities, lack of thirst, and/or sleeping with the knees drawn up. May cause a loss of sensation in the mouth and tongue.

Caution: Discontinue the formula if fever occurs.

Regulate the Stomach and Order the Qi Decoction

Stops nosebleeds caused by long-standing infection.

White Tiger Decoction

Stops nosebleed caused by high blood pressure or that occurs with emotional stress.

Caution: Avoid if nausea or vomiting is present.

OBESITY

Obesity is the presence of excessive body fat. It can be measured in several ways, but a simple way is to consider a person obese if he or she weighs 20 percent or more over the normal weight for his or her height, build, age, and sex. Obesity is a health problem, and not just a cosmetic concern, because it can lead to a number of serious disorders. These include heart disease, diabetes, stroke, high blood pressure, and certain kinds of cancer.

Weight loss is the most easily understood principle of health. All that is necessary to lose weight is to make sure that the calories consumed in food are fewer than the calories spent on exercise and daily activities. That is because excess calories, no matter what their source, are turned into fat before being stored. There are several ideas as to why this happens, including genetic predisposition, the existence of excess fat cells, and a malfunction in the brain's appetite control center. It is likely that several different factors play a role in this disorder.

The most popular approach to weight loss is through any one of various diet plans. Some involve calorie restrictions with no food-choice restrictions, some exclude all fat, some contain 30 percent fat. While most participants in any diet program will fail to lose weight and keep it off, every plan produces a few success stories. This implies that different people need different approaches to weight control.

Kampo offers an entirely different perspective on the problems of obesity and overweight. The many different Western explanations of excess weight all point to the excess nutrient consumption. The Kampo explanation involves misplaced energy.

Kampo divides obesity into two categories, "strong" and "weak." Strong obesity occurs in people who have a strong constitution. These are robust, muscular individuals who are active in their daily life. Their excessive weight is a physical manifestation of blockages that keep energy from circulating downward in their bodies. These energy "dams" force qi, or energy, upward, where it causes headache, high blood pressure, irritability, and redness in the face. In addition, if body energies cannot circulate fluids downward, constipation results.

Weak obesity is a deficiency of the body's yin, or containing, energies. Persons who have weak obesity are flabby, and suffer water retention and puffiness. They fatigue easily, and may be depressed. They have disorders associated in Kampo with failures of the kidneys, such as lack of sexual vigor, lower back pain, and skin disorders. Yin energies can be depleted by repeated dieting.

Individual herbs are generally used to address specific issues, such as water retention. Formulas are used to address differences in the type of obesity involved. Formulas for strong obesity redirect the body's energies into a normal pattern. Not only do functional manifestations of the energy blockage, such as constipation and headache, disappear, but so do the physical manifestations, namely excess weight. Formulas for weak obesity restore yin energies, which causes both obesity and its associated symptoms to abate. Either type of formula should produce weight loss within three months.

INDIVIDUAL KAMPO TREATMENTS

See Chapter 3 for discussions of individual herbs, traditional healing substances, and modern herbal preparations, including directions for making tea.

SUGGESTED DOSAGES	COMMENTS
Angelica Dahurica (Herb)	
Freeze-dried root, 1–3 gel caps 3 times daily. or Tea, 1 c up to 4 times daily before meals.	Contains compounds that stop insulin from promoting the deposit of fat into body tissues. This action prevents weight gain caused by drugs for diabetes.[1] Be sure to use *Angelica dahurica*, which may be labeled Radix Angelicae Dahuricae, and not *Angelica sinensis*, or tang-kuei. *Caution:* Do not use during pregnancy.
Dandelion (Herb)	
Tea, 1 c 3 times daily on an empty stomach. or Tincture (1:5), 10–15 drops 3 times daily on an empty stomach. Place in a cup, add 2 tbsp water, and take in a single sip.	Gentle diuretic, stops short-term weight gain caused by consumption of salty foods.[2]
Ephedra (Herb)	
Tea, 1 c 1–3 times daily. or Tincture (1:5), 15 drops 3 times daily. Place in a cup, add 2 tbsp water, and take in a single sip. and **Green Tea** (tea form only) for up to 3 months.	Contains ephedrine, which when combined with a low-calorie diet, has been shown to promote loss of fat without loss of muscle.[3,4] *Caution:* Do not use ephedra if taking an MAO inhibitor, or if high blood pressure, anxiety, glaucoma, or a prostate disorder is present. To avoid possible kidney stone development, drink 8 glasses of water daily.
Green Tea (Herb)	
Catechin extract, 1 240-mg tablet 3 times daily. or Tea, 1 c 2–3 times daily.	Stops short-term weight gain caused by consumption of salty foods.[5] To avoid dilution problems, do not take tea within 1 hour of taking other teas or patent medicines.

KAMPO FORMULAS

See Chapter 4 for dosage information and discussions of individual formulas.

Ledebouriella Powder That Sagely Unblocks

Used for strong obesity. Treats "beer barrel" pattern of fat deposits. Particularly useful if any of the following symptoms occurs frequently: difficulty in swallowing; nasal congestion with thick, sticky discharge; strong fever and chills; red eyes; bitter taste in the mouth; dry mouth; constipation; dark urine. Research has confirmed that this formula activates the brown fat cells, which burn fat to produce body heat. Reduces both percentage of body fat and total body weight without changes in the number of calories consumed.[6]

Caution: Should not be used by women who are trying to become pregnant, or if nausea or vomiting is present.

Major Bupleurum Decoction

Used for strong obesity. Treats a constant feeling of fullness. Lowers total cholesterol levels while raising levels of high-density lipoprotein (HDL), the "good," artery-clearing kind.

Caution: Use with caution if fever is present, and discontinue if preexisting fevers worsen.

Peach Pit Decoction to Order the Qi

Used for weak obesity. Also promotes weight loss by stimulating the body to burn fat. Relieves weight the body had built up after an assault by a "pathogenic influence," such as weight gain after prolonged illness or after many attempts at dieting. Used to treat overweight in women who also experience chronic menstrual irregularities.

Stephania and Astragalus Decoction

Used for weak obesity. Designed for weight loss in persons whose excess weight is caused by fluid retention. In Japan, this formula is particularly prescribed for weight loss in persons who suffer pain in the knees or lower back.

OSTEOARTHRITIS

Osteoarthritis is the most common disorder in the world—nearly everyone has some degree of it by age sixty. It results from wear and tear on joints. The hands and the weight-bearing joints—the knees, hips, and spine—are the areas most often affected.

Arthritic joints are painful and stiff, and lose their flexibility. The pain of osteoarthritis can range from mild to excruciating. The bones can also become deformed, often quite badly, even if the person experiences no pain.[1] If the deformity is bad enough, the affected joint's range of motion can be severely limited.

Osteoarthritis primarily affects the synovial pads that line the bones within the joint. Cumulative stress breaks down collagen, a protein found in the pads. With age, the ability to produce new collagen decreases. As the pads wear away, the bones rub together, causing pain and inflammation. Osteoarthritis can also occur when there is traumatic stress on a joint, such as fracture or surgery.

Conventional treatment for osteoarthritis depends on a variety of painkillers, both prescription and over-the-counter. Long-term use of these drugs can cause a variety of side effects, including intestinal bleeding.

Kampo considers osteoarthritis to be a local obstruction of the body's normal flow of energy. It results when an "outside pernicious influence," either a pathogen or mechanical wear and tear, settles into a joint. When there is lower back pain, the local obstruction of energy causing arthritic inflammation also interferes with the normal function of the kidneys, which must be "tonified," or rebalanced, to control the disease. This tonic process to balance a pattern of symptoms requires formulas, although individual herbs can control individual symptoms.

Complementing Kampo With Other Therapies in Osteoarthritis

The Kampo herb hawthorn (see treatments list) is best used with the nutritional supplements glucosamine sulfate and chondroitin, along with one or all of the herbs devil's claw, salia guggul, and yucca. Glucosamine sulfate and chondroitin provide a protein "net" along which collagen can gather, while hawthorn helps the joint produce the needed collagen. Devil's claw stops pain. Salia guggul, like glucosamine, helps stabilize collagen fibers.[1] Yucca reduces intestinal absorption of bacterial toxins that can break down cartilage.[2]

Take glucosamine sulfate and chondroitin in dosages of from 1,000 to 1,500 milligrams per day. Take salia guggul in the form of tincture of myrrh. The dosage is between fifteen to thirty drops in a small amount of water daily. (Do not use the standardized myrrh extract gugulipid, which is used for high cholesterol.) Use saponin extract of yucca leaf as directed by manufacturer, or eat about ½ ounce (12 to 16 grams) of yucca leaf daily. The analgesics in devil's claw break down in the stomach, so take it in enterically coated capsule form, 400 milligrams three times a day.[3]

INDIVIDUAL KAMPO TREATMENTS

See Chapter 3 for discussions of individual herbs, traditional healing substances, and modern herbal preparations, including directions for making tea.

SUGGESTED DOSAGES	COMMENTS
Asiasarum (Herb)	
Topical massage oil, as needed.	Relieves pain. May also be labeled as "wild ginger" oil. *Caution:* Do *not* take internally.
Hawthorn (Herb)	
Dried herb in capsules, 3–5 g daily. or Fluid extract (1:1), ¼–½ tsp (1–2 ml) 3 times daily. or Solid extract, 100–250 mg 3 times daily. Should be standardized to contain 10% proanthocyanidins. or Tea, ⅔ c 3–4 times daily. or Tincture (1:5), 1–1½ tsp (4–6 ml) 3 times daily. Place in a cup, add 2 tbsp water, and take in a single sip.	Contains compounds that help stabilize collagen in cartilage.[2] Also protects cartilage from the effects of steroid drugs.[3] See "Complementing Kampo with Other Therapies in Osteoarthritis" for treatments that should be used with hawthorn.
Turmeric (Herb)	
Poultice, applied 3 times daily (see Chapter 3 for directions).	Valuable painkiller. Do *not* use the turmeric compound curcumin for this disorder.

KAMPO FORMULAS

See Chapter 4 for dosage information and discussions of individual formulas.

Kidney Qi Pill From *The Golden Cabinet*

Relieves lower back pain and weakness of the lower extremities. May cause a loss of sensation in the mouth and tongue.

Caution: Discontinue the formula if fever occurs.

Prepared Aconite Decoction

Designed to treat persons with a weak constitution with aching bones and joints, aversion to cold, and cold extremities. Given when primary symptom is pain. May cause a loss of sensation in the mouth and tongue.

Caution: Discontinue the formula if fever occurs.

True Warrior Decoction

Designed to treat persons with a weak constitution with aching bones and joints, aversion to cold, and cold extremities. Given when primary symptom is swelling. May cause a loss of sensation in the mouth and tongue.

Caution: Discontinue the formula if fever occurs.

CONSIDERATIONS

❑ *See also* **Rheumatoid Arthritis.**

OSTEOSARCOMA

See **Bone Cancer.**

OVARIAN CANCER

Approximately one of every seventy women in the United States will contract ovarian cancer at some point in her life. Risk for this form of cancer increases with early age at first menstruation, late menopause, and no pregnancies. All of these conditions increase the chances that estrogen, the primary female hormone, will stimulate the development of ovarian cancer. High-fat diets and the use of talcum powder in the underwear have also been associated with an increased risk for ovarian cancer.[1] (To learn how to reduce estrogen levels through dietary means, see "Lowering Estrogen Levels Through Diet" on page 207.)

The symptoms of ovarian cancer are abdominal swelling, masses in the abdomen, bleeding, lower back pain, and urinary difficulties. These symptoms can also be caused by benign ovarian cysts. (Sudden, sharp, and severe pain is usually caused by an ovarian cyst.) Because the symptoms of ovarian cancer overlap several other conditions, this cancer is frequently diagnosed only at an advanced stage.

A firm diagnosis is made by biopsy, although a number of other tests may be performed. Ovarian cancer is classified into stages I through IV by the extent of spread and by the type of cell from which it originated. It most often spreads to nearby organs within the abdomen, and then to the liver, lungs, or bones.

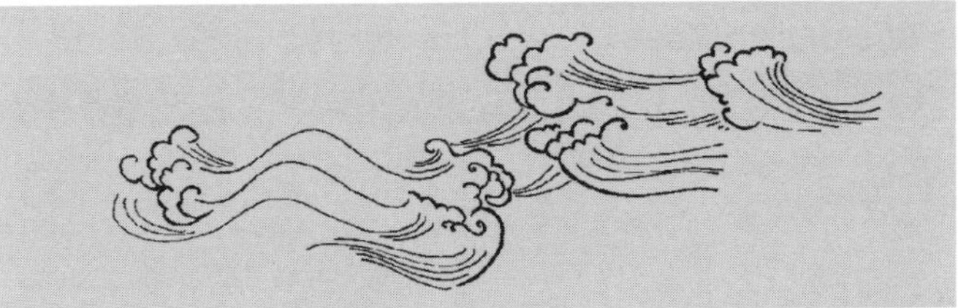

Surgery is the first treatment for ovarian cancer. In addition to the ovary, the uterus and fallopian tubes may also be removed, as may the membrane that lines the abdomen. After surgery, physicians give combinations of chemotherapy, immunotherapy, and radiation. In recent years, the trend has been to use multiple chemotherapy drugs, including cisplatin, cyclophosphamide, doxorubicin hydrochloride (Adriamycin), and 5-fluorouracil in various combinations over a longer period of time.[2,3] The use of extended chemotherapy often harms the immune system and the bone marrow.

The authoritative scholars of Kampo medicine place ovarian cancer into four groups of symptoms. They are, in decreasing order of seriousness: accumulation of "damp heat," or infection, sinking to the lower reaches of the body; loss of yin, or containing, energies of the liver and kidney; inadequate digestion; and misdirection of emotional energies through the liver. The value of these categories is that they give external clues to the development of this frequently hidden disease.

The accumulation of damp heat is characteristic of stages III and IV of ovarian cancer. There may be a bloody, foul-smelling vaginal discharge and lower back pain. There is usually constipation, dark urine, and a bitter taste in the mouth.

Loss of yin in the liver and kidney is characteristic of stages II and III of ovarian cancer. In this stage there may be a bitter taste in the mouth, blurred vision, constipation, dark urine, dry throat, pain in the lower abdomen, and vaginal bleeding.

Inadequate digestion (known in TCM as "spleen and kidney vacuity") is also associated with stages II and III. It is a combination of aversion to cold, a blood-tinged vaginal discharge, loose stools, pain in the lower back and around the waist, and chronic fatigue.

The symptom of "binding depression" in the liver gives the earliest warning of cancer, at stages I and II. Its symptoms are abdominal swelling and pain, depression, dreaming, a feeling of fullness in the chest, headache, irritability, loss of appetite, and vaginal discharge with blood.

Any of these symptom patterns should be brought to a physician's attention immediately. The doctor can do a preliminary test for ovarian cancer, using either ultrasound or a cancer marker test called CA-125, without resorting to surgery. Kampo formulas can be extremely helpful for individuals who are receiving conventional treatment (see considerations below).

INDIVIDUAL KAMPO TREATMENTS

See Chapter 3 for discussions of individual herbs, traditional healing substances, and modern herbal preparations, including directions for making tea.

SUGGESTED DOSAGES	COMMENTS
Green Tea (Herb)	
Catechin extract, 1 240-mg tablet 3 times daily. or Tea, 1 c 2–5 times daily.	Contains compounds that deactivate plasmin, a substance that breaks up tissues and makes a pathway for invading tumors. Other compounds called catechins help prevent both thyroid cancer caused by radiation treatment and deficiencies in white blood cells caused by mitomycin.[4] Caffeine accelerates cell death and increases effectiveness of radiation therapy. Decreases the availability of estrogen.[5] To avoid dilution problems, do not take tea within 1 hour of taking other teas or patent medicines.
PSK (Modern Herbal Preparation)	
Dried extract, 6 1,000-mg tablets daily.	Helps maintain the body's production of interleukin-2, an immune-system chemical, during chemotherapy.[6]
Siberian Ginseng (Modern Herbal Preparation)	
Eleuthero extract, as directed on label, in 1/4 c water. Be sure to use pure extract, *not* sugar-sweetened ginseng drinks. or Tea, 1 c up to 3 times daily.	Useful in forms of cancer that respond to immunotherapy, including ovarian cancer. Contains compounds that stimulate various immune-system components.[7] *Caution:* Should be avoided by persons with myasthenia gravis; rheumatoid arthritis and diseases related to it, such as lupus, psoriatric arthritis, and Sjögren's syndrome; or prostate cancer.
Turmeric (Herb)	
Curcumin, the yellow pigment found in turmeric, 250–500 mg twice daily between meals.	Prevents fibrin formation, a step by which cancerous tumors acquire their own blood supply.[8]

HERBS TO AVOID

Individuals who have ovarian cancer should avoid the following herbs: cordyceps, dan shen, fennel, licorice, and peony. For more information regarding these herbs, see Chapter 3.

KAMPO FORMULAS

See Chapter 4 for dosage information and discussions of individual formulas.

Coptis Decoction to Relieve Toxicity

Contains coptis, which stops multiplication of many types of ovarian cancer cells,[9,10] and scutellaria, which prevents damage to the immune system from chemotherapy. This formula can be used during chemotherapy to reduce side effects.

FORMULAS TO AVOID

Individuals who have ovarian cancer should avoid the following formulas: Peony and Licorice Decoction, and Six-Ingredient Pill With Rehmannia (Rehmannia-Six Combination). For more information regarding these formulas, see Chapter 4.

CONSIDERATIONS

❑ To reduce side effects and increase effectiveness when using chemotherapy, *see* **Chemotherapy Side Effects**; when using radiation therapy, *see* **Radiation Therapy Side Effects.** To learn about herbal treatments that can prevent a cancer from developing its own blood supply, *see* **Cancer.**

OVARIAN CYSTS

The ovaries are made up of follicles, each of which contains an egg. Once a month, a follicle ruptures and releases an egg. Ovarian cysts are enlarged follicles that have failed to rupture. Often an ovarian cyst will cause few symptoms. Some women, however, experience generalized aching, heaviness, disruption of the menstrual cycle, back pain, abdominal pain, and pain during sexual intercourse.

When discomfort is slight, and the size of the cyst is less than four centimeters, physicians typically wait two or three periods before deciding how to treat the cyst. *Functional* cysts are small and usually disappear within several menstrual cycles. *Pathological* cysts, which are caused by disease, require medical intervention. This includes cysts that result from a disorder called polycystic ovarian disease, in which the ovaries contain many cysts and high levels of male hormones are present. Twisting of an ovary by a cyst can cause sudden, extreme pain and necessitate surgery.

In most cases of ovarian cysts, the woman's body produces enough or even too much estrogen, but produces it at the wrong time in her menstrual cycle. Therefore, the first step in treatment is to reduce estrogen overproduction. Fatty tissues make estrogen, so the patient is usually advised to lose weight. She is also usually told to stop any *daily* use of estrogen-based contraceptive pills or estrogen replacement therapy. Since completely eliminating estrogen supplements can cause another problem, excess testosterone, doctors often prescribe short-term doses of estrogen-based birth control pills for those days in the menstrual cycle when extra estrogen is needed. In addition, drugs are used that help regulate the balance between two other sex hormones, luteinizing hormone (LH) and follicle stimulating hormone (FSH), which together control the release of eggs from the ovaries.

As early as the third century A.D., Kampo physicians recognized a pattern of symptoms corresponding to ovarian cysts. They reasoned that ovarian cysts were caused by "static blood" in the womb. The blood supply of the ovaries could remain constricted and prevent normal periods, or it could spill out and cause pain, persistent bleeding, and abdominal spasms.

Modern science has learned that the blood-circulating herbs Kampo practitioners chose for this symptom pattern also lower estrogen levels (in addition, see "Lowering

Estrogen Levels Through Diet" on page 207). Some formulas also lower testosterone levels, preventing the appearance of masculine secondary sex characteristics. All of these preparations have to be used on a long-term basis, at least three months, before changes in symptoms can be expected. They can be used with short-term birth control pills and hormone-regulating drugs as well; discuss such usage with a doctor.

INDIVIDUAL KAMPO TREATMENTS

See Chapter 3 for discussions of individual herbs, traditional healing substances, and modern herbal preparations, including directions for making tea.

SUGGESTED DOSAGES	COMMENTS
Dioscorea (Herb)	
Tincture (1:5), 15–20 drops 3 times daily after meals. Place in a cup, add 2 tbsp water, and take in a single sip.	Treats cramping caused by ovarian cysts.[1] Especially useful for relieving pain that is worsened by doubling over or lying down, but eases with motion, or when stretching out or bending backwards.[2] Be sure to use an herb product not mixed with synthetic progesterone.
Tang-Kuei (Herb)	
Dried root, 1–2 tsp (1–3 g) daily. or Fluid extract (1:1), ¼–½ tsp (1–2 ml) daily. or Freeze-dried root, 1–2 500-mg capsules daily. or Powdered solid extract (4:1), 250–500 mg daily. or Tea, 1 c daily 2–3 times daily. or Tincture (1:5), 1–1½ tsp (4–6 ml) daily. Place in a cup, add 2 tbsp water, and take in a single sip.	Relieves pain caused by ovarian cysts. Take during the two weeks after menstruation, then discontinue until the next period. Tincture inhibits uterine activity and menstrual flow, while other forms have the opposite effect. Also known as dong quai.
Vitex (Herb)	
Tincture (1:5), ¾–1 tbsp (9–12 ml) 3 times daily.	Reduces amount of estrogen in the bloodstream.[3]

HERBS TO AVOID

Individuals who have ovarian cysts should avoid the following herbs: cordyceps, dan shen, fennel seed, licorice, and peony. For more information regarding these herbs, see Chapter 3.

KAMPO FORMULAS

See Chapter 4 for dosage information and discussions of individual formulas.

Augmented Rambling Powder

Lowers estrogen levels.[4] Traditionally, this formula is used to treat "hot" symptoms, including dry mouth, red eyes, blurry vision, lower abdominal pressure, difficult and painful urination, increased menstrual flow, and uterine bleeding.

Caution: Should not be used by women who are trying to become pregnant.

Cinnamon Twig and Poria Pill

Original Kampo treatment for ovarian cysts. Reduces the growth of ovarian tissues by reducing estrogen levels in the bloodstream.[5] Traditionally given to women who are experiencing "cold" symptoms, such as weakness, lack of appetite, and fatigue.

Peony and Licorice Decoction

Corrects abnormal hair growth (hirsutism) in women with long-term polycystic ovarian disease.[6]

Caution: Should be used with caution, since it acts by converting testosterone, which causes hirsutism, into estrogen, which may aggravate ovarian cysts.[7] Use under the supervision of a Kampo practitioner, and only until symptoms are reversed or up to 6 months. Do *not* use for ovarian cysts not associated with polycystic ovarian disease.

Tang-Kuei and Peony Powder

Reduces amount of estrogen in circulation, thereby reducing cyclical growth of cysts. Unlike some treatments, does not have a "masculinizing" effect, since the formula decreases estrogen production by the ovaries[8] without reducing the ratio of estrogen to testosterone in circulation.[9] Also reduces the formation of inflammatory compounds in endometrial tissue, or the tissue lining the uterus.[10]

Two-Cured Decoction

Reduces estrogen levels.[11] Traditionally prescribed for ovarian cysts in women coughing up large amounts of easily expectorated phlegm, and/or experiencing vomiting and nausea.

Caution: Use with caution if fever is present, and discontinue if preexisting fevers worsen.

FORMULAS TO AVOID

Individuals who have ovarian cysts should avoid Six-Ingredient Pill With Rehmannia (Rehmannia-Six Combination). For more information regarding this formula, see Chapter 4.

PELVIC INFLAMMATORY DISEASE

Pelvic inflammatory disease (PID) is an infection of the female reproductive tract. Most cases of PID result from infection with a sexually transmitted disease, such as chlamydia or gonorrhea. PID can also develop after surgical injury to the uterus or insertion of an intrauterine device (IUD) for contraception. Experts estimate that PID affects more than a million women each year in the United States.[1]

Vaginal discharge is the first symptom of PID, and may be followed by tension in the anal area, fever, nausea, pain along the midline of the abdomen, and vaginal bleeding once the infection has entered the uterus. Women infected with chlamydia or gonorrhea often experience pain when leaning the trunk to the left or right. PID infections are often so mild that they go undetected until they are discovered as the cause of infertility, which occurs when scar tissue forms in the fallopian tubes.

PID is conventionally treated with antibiotics after the infectious agent is identified. Surgery may be needed to remove abscesses.

About 20 percent of women treated with standard antibiotics do not respond to treatment.[2] These are the women who can most benefit from treatment with Kampo. Kampo viewed PID as a manifestation of "damp heat," or infection with inflammation, flowing downward into the reproductive tract. Kampo treatments restore the upward circulation of energy in the body as they cool and soothe. More severe cases of PID include "blood stasis," in which misplaced energy "gels" into pain and swelling. Kampo treatments for PID increase general circulation to break up this kind of energy.

INDIVIDUAL KAMPO TREATMENTS

See Chapter 3 for discussions of individual herbs, traditional healing substances, and modern herbal preparations, including directions for making tea.

SUGGESTED DOSAGES	COMMENTS
Coptis (Herb)	
Dried herb, 1 500-mg capsule 3 times daily. or Tincture (1:5), 20 drops 3 times daily. Place in a cup, add 2 tbsp water, and take in a single sip.	Fights gonorrhea, as well as giardiasis and trichomonas infections that can be misidentified as PID.[3] If coptis is unavailable, substitute capsules or tinctures of the non-Kampo herbs goldenseal or Oregon grape root (same cautions apply). *Caution:* Do not use during pregnancy or on a daily basis for more than 2 weeks at a time. Do not use with supplements that contain vitamin B_6 or the amino acid histidine.
Scutellaria (Herb)	
Dried herb, 1–2 1,000-mg capsules 3 times daily. or Fluid extract (1:1), ¼–½ tsp (1–2 ml) 3 times daily. or Powdered solid extract (4:1), 250–500 mg 3 times daily. or Tea, 1 c 3 times daily. or Tincture (1:5), 1–1½ tsp (4–6 ml) 3 times daily. Place in a cup, add 2 tbsp water, and take in a single sip.	Multipurpose infection fighter that may treat antibiotic-resistant strains of gonorrhea. *Caution:* Avoid in cases of diarrhea caused by foodborne infection or excessive consumption of cold drinks.

KAMPO FORMULAS

See Chapter 4 for dosage information and discussions of individual formulas.

Eight-Ingredient Pill with Rehmannia (Rehmannia-Eight Combination)

Relaxes the walls of the bladder and increases urination,[4] effectively flushing PID organisms (which have a very short life span) out of the genitourinary tract before they can cause damage.

Gentiana Longdancao Decoction to Drain the Liver

Treats PID with fever, especially when there is a shortened menstrual period with unusually dark blood.

Peony and Licorice Decoction

Treats PID compounded by abdominal or perianal pain and cramping. Increases estrogen production, and can increase probability of pregnancy.[5]

Caution: Avoid in cases of breast or bladder cancer, melanoma, or fibrocystic breast disease.

Tang-Kuei and Peony Powder

Used in Japan to prevent miscarriage in women who have had PID.

Tang-Kuei, Gentiana Longdancao, and Aloe Pill

Treats PID in women who also have herpes.

FORMULAS TO AVOID

Individuals who have PID should not use formulas that contain snake gourd root. See Chapter 3 for more information regarding this herb, and see Chapter 4 for listings of formula ingredients.

CONSIDERATIONS

❑ Kampo experts in both Japan and the United States have noted that PID which does not respond to antibiotics sometimes dramatically improves after the removal of dental amalgams containing mercury. Dr. Yoshiaki Omura of the Heart Disease Research Foundation has also noted that "purging" the body of mercury compounds—by taking 100 milligrams of dried Chinese parsley (cilantro) four times a day—has a similar, positive effect.[6] Although the science behind these findings is still being examined, these methods pose no risk and may help when other treatments do not.

❑ Epimedium reduces infection in male sexual partners of women with PID by stimulating urination. It also prevents the buildup of scar tissue in the testes, a condition that can reduce male fertility. Use as directed by the herbalist. Do not use more than directed, since high dosages decrease, rather than increase, frequency of urination, leading to retention of disease-causing microorganisms.

PEPTIC ULCER

Peptic ulcers are inflamed lesions in the lining of the upper digestive tract. They occur when the lining is exposed to stomach, or gastric, juices. The major forms of peptic ulcer are duodenal ulcer (intestinal ulcer) and gastric ulcer (stomach ulcer). Men experience ulcers more often than women, by a ratio of two to one.

Normally, the stomach and duodenum (the upper segment of the small intestine) are protected from stomach acid by a layer of mucus. If too much acid is produced, or too little mucus, the acid then starts to break down the body's own tissues. The lining can also be irritated by aspirin, alcohol, and a group of pain relievers known as nonsteroidal anti-inflammatory drugs (NSAIDs). In addition, *Helicobacter pylori*, a bacterium often found in the stomach, is strongly associated with ulcer formation.

The main symptom of peptic ulcer is a burning pain that occurs either before a meal, about an hour after a meal, or during the night. There may be discomfort in the chest or back. Some people find that they eat more when ulcer pain strikes, while others become queasy and lose appetite.

Conventional treatment of peptic ulcers focuses on neutralizing stomach acid and reducing its production, along with eliminating *H. pylori* infection. Some over-the-counter antacids use aluminum, which can be toxic if it builds up in the body, and all antacids can produce a rebound effect, in which acid production increases when one stops taking them.

Kampo offers three main theories of the origin of peptic ulcers. In one theory, emotional disturbance causes the liver's energy to overact on the stomach, since in Oriental medicine the liver stores emotional energy. Signs and symptoms of the liver "oppressing" the stomach include "belly" pain, headache, gas, irritability, anger, and fatigue. In the second theory, cold can shut down the "furnace" of the stomach. This condition is thought to be brought on by actual weather conditions, or by overeating raw or cold foods. It is marked by fatigue, diarrhea, anorexia, and a pale complexion. In the third theory, dietary irregularities are thought to affect the flow of energy and blood to the stomach. Alcohol and spicy foods, as well as mental strain, weaken the ability of the spleen to transform and transport food. Symptoms of this irregularity are focused on the left side of the stomach area, and include loss of appetite, vomiting, nausea, diarrhea, and pain.

Kampo treatments are designed to avoid both overstimulation of acid production and understimulation of blood and energy circulation to the stomach. Formulas should be used for ulcers that occur as part of overall symptom patterns.

INDIVIDUAL KAMPO TREATMENTS

See Chapter 3 for discussions of individual herbs, traditional healing substances, and modern herbal preparations, including directions for making tea.

SUGGESTED DOSAGES	COMMENTS
Licorice (Herb)	
Deglycyrrhizinated licorice (DGL): *When ulcers are active:* 2–4 380-mg chewable tablets between or 20 mins before meals. *For maintenance:* 1–2 380-mg chewable tablets 20 mins before meals.	Stimulates the stomach to secrete a protective lining of mucus.[1] DGL must be taken before meals; taking it after meals cancels its effect. Do not take capsules; DGL must be chewed to be effective in ulcer treatment. Therapeutic results may take 2–4 months, but DGL can be used indefinitely.

HERBS TO AVOID

Individuals who have peptic ulcer should avoid gentian. For more information regarding this herb, see Chapter 3.

KAMPO FORMULAS

See Chapter 4 for dosage information and discussions of individual formulas.

Astragalus Decoction to Construct the Middle

Especially useful when pain is spasmodic rather than continuous. Relieves respiratory problems, such as allergies or asthma, that occur at the same time as ulcer attacks.

Calm the Stomach Powder

Relieves peptic ulcers accompanied by distention and fullness throughout the digestive tract, loss of taste and appetite, heavy sensation in the arms and legs, loose stool or diarrhea, easy fatigue, increased desire for sleep, nausea and vomiting, belching, and/or acid regurgitation.

Coptis Decoction to Relieve Toxicity

Traditionally used to treat peptic ulcers accompanied by signs of stress, such as redness in the face, headaches, and mood swings. Japanese research has found that different herbs in this formula defend the mucous lining, stop changes in the stomach lining caused by alcohol, and act against *H. pylori*.[2]

Caution: Should not be used by women who are trying to become pregnant.

Four-Gentlemen Decoction

Treats peptic ulcers caused by improper eating habits, excessive consumption of alcohol, excessive deliberation, or overwork.

Ophiopogonis Decoction

Treats peptic ulcers accompanied by symptoms of allergy or asthma, such as coughing and spitting of saliva, dry and uncomfortable sensation in the throat, dry mouth, rapid pulse, shortness of breath, and/or wheezing.

Caution: Use with caution if fever is present, and discontinue if preexisting fevers worsen.

Six-Gentlemen Decoction

Treats peptic ulcers accompanied by loss of appetite, nausea, stifling sensation in the chest and over the stomach, and/or vomiting.

Caution: Use with caution if fever is present and discontinue if preexisting fevers worsen.

Warm the Gallbladder Decoction

Treats peptic ulcers accompanied by anxiety, bitter taste in the mouth, dizziness or vertigo, insomnia, nausea or vomiting, palpitations, and slight thirst.

Caution: Use with caution if fever is present, and discontinue if preexisting fevers worsen.

CONSIDERATIONS

❑ *See also* **Gastritis.**

PNEUMONIA

See **Bronchitis and Pneumonia.**

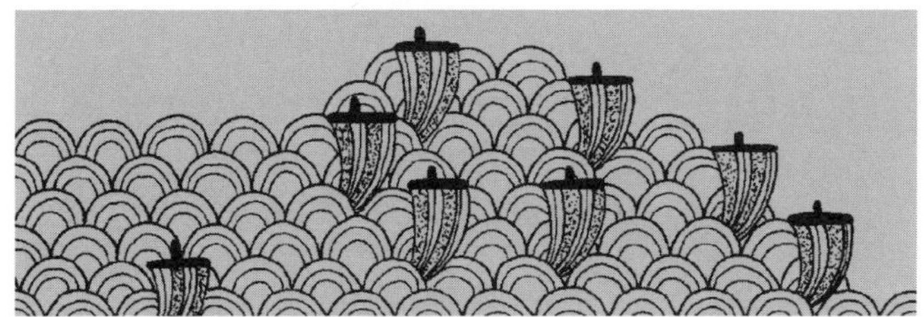

PREMENSTRUAL SYNDROME (PMS)

Premenstrual syndrome (PMS) covers a variety of symptoms, both emotional and physical, experienced by many women a week or two before the start of menstruation. Emotional symptoms include depression, apprehension, irritability, mood swings, and changes in sex drive. Physical symptoms include swollen limbs and fingers, acne, backache, breast tenderness, food cravings, and water retention. Most women find that one symptom, such as depression, predominates, but that there is a great deal of overlap. Many women will have months in which they have no symptoms.

One of the causes of PMS is hormonal imbalance in the form of excessive estrogen, the primary female hormone. Hormonal fluctuations lead to fluid retention. This affects circulation, which reduces the amount of oxygen reaching the brain, ovaries, and uterus. PMS is also related to a monthly depletion of the chemical serotonin, which both maintains mood and regulates bodily rhythms.

Conventional treatment for PMS seeks to correct symptoms rather than correct the underlying process. Different types of drugs are used, including antidepressants, antianxiety agents, diuretics, and oral contraceptives.

Oriental medicine sees PMS as a stagnation of liver energy; that is, the free flow of the body's energy is impeded by the liver. The breasts and the external sex organs lie on the liver's energy meridians, or channels, so stagnation of liver energy creates breast tenderness, headache, and anger and irritability. Kampo therapies not only relieve symptoms, but several of them also reduce estrogen production to bring about long-term relief (see also "Lowering Estrogen Levels Through Diet" on page 208).

INDIVIDUAL KAMPO TREATMENTS

See Chapter 3 for discussions of individual herbs, traditional healing substances, and modern herbal preparations, including directions for making tea.

SUGGESTED DOSAGES	COMMENTS
Asiasarum (Herb)	
Topical massage oil, as needed.	Treats premenstrual pain in the small of the back that worsens when taking a deep breath.[1] May also be labeled as "wild ginger" oil. *Caution:* Do *not* take internally.
Black Cohosh (Herb)	
Dried root, 2–6 500-mg capsules daily. or Fluid extract (1:1), ¼–½ tsp (1–2 ml) daily. or Freeze-dried root, 1–2 500-mg capsules daily. or Powdered solid extract (4:1), standardized for 27-deoxyacteine, 1–2 250-mg tablets daily. or Tincture (1:5), 1–1½ tsp (4–6 ml) once daily. Place in a cup, add 2 tbsp water, and take in a single sip.	Contains compounds that act like a very mild dose of estrogen, which blocks the more potent natural estrogen from acting on cells throughout the body.[2] Relieves depression and muscular pain. Especially useful to women who have both PMS and uterine fibroids. This herb must be used for 2–3 months to obtain relief of symptoms.
Dandelion (Herb)	
Tea, 1 c 3 times daily. or Tincture (1:5), 1 tsp–1 tbsp (4–12 ml) 3 times daily on an empty stomach. Place in a cup, add 2 tbsp water, and take in a single sip.	Relieves water weight and breast swelling.[3] Also reduces food cravings.
Dioscorea (Herb)	
Tincture (1:5), 10 drops twice daily after meals. Place in a cup, add 2 tbsp water, and take in a single sip.	Relieves cramps. Be sure to use an herbal product not mixed with synthetic progesterone.
Motherwort (Herb)	
Tea, 1 c 3 times daily.	Relieves headache and dizziness, and reduces appetite. Especially helpful for women who also have overactive thyroid.[4]
Tang-Kuei (Herb)	
Fluid extract (1:1), ¼–½ tsp (1–2 ml) 3 times daily. or Tincture (1:5), 1 tsp (4 ml) daily. Place in a cup, add 2 tbsp water, and take in a single sip.	Especially useful for cramps. Initially contracts, and then releases the uterus.[5] Start taking on day 14 of menstrual cycle and continue until menstruation begins. Also known as dong quai.
Vitex (Herb)	
Fluid extract (1:1), ½ tsp (2 ml) daily. or Solid extract capsules, 175–225 mg daily. or Tincture (1:5), 1½ tsp (6 ml) 3 times daily. Place in a cup, add 2 tbsp water, and take in a single sip.	Reduces the body's production of estrogen, and thereby relieves depression, cramps, migraines, mood swings, water retention, and weight gain. For long-term relief, this herb must be used for 3–6 months after symptoms dissappear.[6] *Caution:* Has been known to stimulate the release of multiple eggs from the ovary, potentially resulting in multiple births.[7]

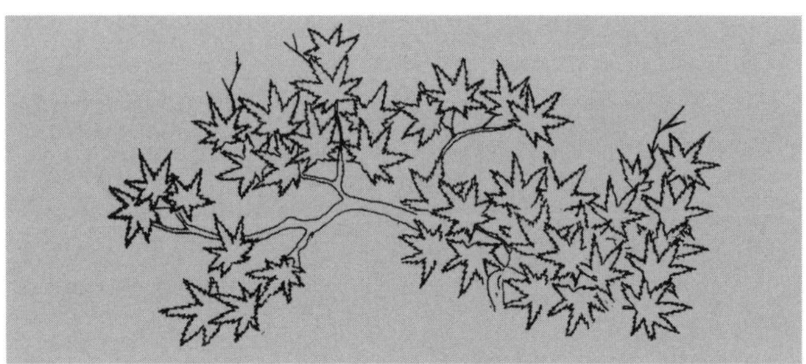

HERBS TO AVOID

Individuals who have PMS should avoid the following

herbs: cordyceps, dan shen, fennel, licorice, and peony. For more information regarding these herbs, see Chapter 3.

KAMPO FORMULAS

See Chapter 4 for dosage information and discussions of individual formulas.

Augmented Rambling Powder

Treats PMS by lowering estrogen levels.[8] Traditionally, this formula is used to treat "hot" symptoms, including dry mouth, red eyes, blurry vision, lower abdominal pressure, difficult and painful urination, increased menstrual flow, and uterine bleeding.

Caution: Should not be used by women who are trying to become pregnant.

Bupleurum and Cinnamon Twig Decoction

Treats joint pain and swelling during PMS.

Caution: Use with caution if fever is present, and discontinue if preexisting fevers worsen.

Bupleurum, Cinnamon Twig, and Ginger Decoction

Treats sweating, swelling, thirst, and urinary difficulty during PMS.

Caution: Avoid during pregnancy. Avoid if there is any kind of bleeding, and use with caution if fever is present. Discontinue if preexisting fevers worsen.

FORMULAS TO AVOID

Individuals who have PMS should avoid the following formulas: Peony and Licorice Decoction, and Six-Ingredient Pill With Rhemannia (Rehmannia-Six Combination). For more information regarding these formulas, see Chapter 4.

CONSIDERATIONS

❑ If depression is a problem, especially when accompanied by tension and exhaustion, try the non-Kampo herb St. John's wort (see "Kampo and St. John's Wort" on page 195).

PROSTATE CANCER

Prostate cancer is the most common type of cancer in men. One in every eight men in the United States will develop the disease. About 80 percent of all cases occur after age sixty-five, and about 80 percent of all men have some degree of prostate cancer by age eighty. Rates are higher among African-Americans than among members of other ethnic groups.

The prostate is a walnut-sized gland that encircles the urethra, the tube through which urine is voided. This gland produces the seminal fluid, which forms the bulk of the ejaculate. Both prostate cancer and benign prostate enlargement have the same symptoms: difficulty in passing urine, frequent urination and getting up at night to urinate, pain or burning sensation during urination, blood in the urine, and pain in the lower back or pelvis. Such symptoms should always be brought to a doctor's attention.

More prostate cancers are now detected at earlier stages because of the prostate-specific antigen (PSA) test. This test measures levels of a chemical produced by all prostate cells, but in larger amounts by cancer cells (see consideration below).

The exact cause of prostate cancer is unknown, although there is evidence that a high-fat diet may play a role in promoting its development. It is known that testosterone, a male sex hormone, stimulates the growth of both the prostate itself and any cancer cells it may contain.

Once prostate cancer is diagnosed, it is classified into stages, using one of several staging systems, based on how aggressive it is and how far it has spread. Prostate cancer spreads first to the lymph glands, and then to the bones, lungs, liver, or bladder.

Conventional medicine uses a variety of treatments in prostate cancer. In some elderly men with localized, slow-growing tumors, treatment consists of simply watching the cancer carefully, and treating it if it spreads. For other patients, various types of surgery may be appropriate, ranging from complete removal of the prostate to removal of tissue through a tube passed up the urethra. While chemotherapy is not often employed, radiation therapy is used to slow the cancer's spread. Impotence and incontinence are potential side effects of these therapies.

Prostate cancer is often treated with hormonal therapy, which attempts to reduce the effect testosterone has on the prostate. Drugs called LHRH stimulants reduce the concentration of testosterone in the bloodstream to very low levels. However, they also can cause breast pain, impotence, loss of sex drive, and hot flashes.

Since prostate cancer almost always strikes after age fifty and for hundreds of years few men lived to age fifty, Kampo historically did not have a theory of the disease. However, modern Kampo practitioners have linked symptom patterns to various stages of the disease. The first stage of prostate cancer is kidney "deficiency," or an inability of the kidneys to contain fluids. There is frequent urination with reduced flow, weakness in the legs and knees, lower back pain, and dry mouth without thirst. As the tumor grows, there is accumulation of "dampness" and "heat." Urination becomes still more difficult, and there may be a feeling of fullness in the abdomen. The next step is "blood stasis," or lack of blood circulation, and retention of toxins. There is fever and irregularity in defecation as well as urination. The final stage of prostate cancer corresponds to what the classic Kampo writers called "evil overcoming the right." There is anemia and pallor, anorexia, fever, wasting of the muscles, and shortness of breath with even the mildest physical exertion.[1]

Saw Palmetto and the Prostate

A non-Kampo herb, saw palmetto, is well known for its effects on the prostate. It blocks testosterone from reaching prostate cells, but without affecting the amount of testosterone in circulation. This action proves useful for preserving sexual function in both prostate cancer and benign prostate enlargement.[1] Researchers have found that saw palmetto also has a mild toxic effect on prostate cancer cells.[2] Take 300 milligrams of this herb three times a day.

Kampo herbs act in the same way as conventional hormonal therapy, but on a gentler scale. This reduces side effects. Kampo should always be used as part of a medically directed comprehensive treatment plan (see the considerations).

INDIVIDUAL KAMPO TREATMENTS

See Chapter 3 for discussions of individual herbs, traditional healing substances, and modern herbal preparations, including directions for making tea.

SUGGESTED DOSAGES	COMMENTS
Lithospermum (Herb)	
Tincture (1:5), 15 drops 3 times daily. Place in a cup, add 2 tbsp water, and take in a single sip. Use for 6 mos.	Reduces formation of testosterone and other sex hormones.[2] May be labeled "Stone Seed."
PSK (Modern Herbal Preparation)	
Dried extract, 6 1,000-mg tablets daily.	Reduces rate of spread in those types of prostate cancer that can spread to the lungs.[3]
Soy Isoflavones (Modern Herbal Preparation)	
Extract, about 3,000 mg once daily. or Soy germ, 2 tsp (10 g) twice daily, preferably added to cereals or smoothies.	Soy contains genistein, which inhibits the spread of prostate cancer.[4]
Turmeric (Herb)	
Curcumin, the yellow pigment found in turmeric, 300 mg twice daily between meals for 6 mos.	Reduces the spread of prostate cancer.
Vitex (Herb)	
Tincture (1:5), 15 drops 3 times daily. Place in a cup, add 2 tbsp water, and take in a single sip.	Reduces testosterone production.[5]

HERBS TO AVOID

Individuals who have prostate cancer should avoid the following herbs: American ginseng, cinnamon, cordyceps, ephedra, epimedium, ginseng, and Siberian ginseng. For more information regarding these herbs, see Chapter 3.

KAMPO FORMULAS

See Chapter 4 for dosage information and discussions of individual formulas.

Gentiana Longdancao Decoction to Drain the Liver

Reduces incontinence caused by prostate enlargement or irritation. Treats symptoms not directly related to prostate cancer, which may include headache, dizziness, red and sore eyes, swelling in the ears, hearing loss, bitter taste in the mouth, or short temper.

Peony and Licorice Decoction

Adjusts sex hormone levels to reduce spread of prostate cancer.[6,7]

FORMULAS TO AVOID

Individuals who have prostate cancer should avoid Eight-Ingredient Pill With Rhemannia (Rhemannia-Eight Combination). For more information regarding this formula, see Chapter 4.

CONSIDERATIONS

❑ The introduction of the prostate-specific antigen (PSA) test has led to a jump in prostate cancer diagnoses.[8] This test provides an early-warning system for the potential development of cancerous growths in the prostate. However, since many conditions cause prostate irritation, and PSA is a measurement of the irritation rather than a count of cancer cells, PSA readings can produce false positive results.[9] Simply taking the blood sample for the PSA test a few minutes after a digital exam of the prostate can raise PSA levels. If the doctor is performing both a rectal exam and a PSA screening, it is important to have the blood drawn for the PSA test *before* the rectal exam. It is also important that the doctor forms a diagnosis from more information than just the PSA test. Most physicians make a decision to treat prostate cancer on the basis of PSA, digital examination, and ultrasound.[10]

❑ Diets rich in soy products are associated with lower rates of prostate and other cancers.[11,12] Soy foods include miso and tofu.

❑ Many men use the non-Kampo herb saw palmetto for prostate problems (see "Saw Palmetto and the Prostate" on page 279).

❑ To reduce side effects and increase effectiveness when using radiation therapy, *see* **Radiation Therapy Side Effects.** To learn about herbal treatments that can prevent a cancer from developing its own blood supply, *see* **Cancer.**

❑ *See also* **Prostate Enlargement, Benign.**

PROSTATE ENLARGEMENT, BENIGN

Prostate enlargement—also known as benign prostatic hyperplasia (BPH)—is a noncancerous enlargement of the prostate gland. This walnut-sized gland encircles the urethra, the tube through which urine passes. This gland produces the seminal fluid, which forms the bulk of the ejaculate. The condition ordinarily will not arise until a man has reached middle age, usually at least age fifty.

In the beginning stages, there may be no symptoms. As the prostate grows, however, symptoms can develop, most notably difficulty in passing urine, frequent urination, and getting up at night to urinate. These symptoms can be aggravated by immobility, exposure to cold, or alcohol consumption. It can become difficult to achieve orgasm. As the prostate continues to swell, there can be pain or burning sensation during urination, blood in the urine, and pain in the lower back or pelvis. Bladder infections and kidney disorders may develop. Since the symptoms of BPH are also seen in prostate cancer, they should always be brought to a doctor's attention.

BPH is linked to changes in hormonal levels that occur as a man ages. These changes causes the glandular tissue of the prostate to grow in the presence of testosterone, the primary male hormone.

If there is severe obstruction of the urethra, surgery may be used to widen the opening. In addition, drugs are used to reduce prostate swelling. These drugs, however, can have a number of side effects, including a decrease in libido, and may not always be effective.[1]

Kampo formulas offer yet another approach to treating prostate enlargement. The formula most commonly used in Japan, Eight-Ingredient Pill with Rehmannia, has no effect on sex hormones, but keeps cells in the prostate, and only in the prostate, from using the amino acid thymidine, effectively shutting down their capacity to grow and multiply.[2] At the same time, it stimulates the use of testosterone, thus increasing rather than decreasing sex drive,[3] without encouraging the growth of prostate cancer.[4]

The Kampo sage Fu-Qing Zhu, who invented this formula, explained its effect in terms of restoring vital masculine energy. With advancing age, a man's yang, or masculine, energies could become depleted. The kidney qi, or energy, could no longer force "turbidity" and "dampness" out through the urine, so these energy coagulations could accumulate in the prostate. The formula reinvigorated the kidneys and allowed them to disperse congestion. Modern Japanese medicine uses several other formulas to treat BPH, but doctors note that the formulas which work do not exactly match the traditional *sho,* or symptom pattern, for the condition.[5]

Use Kampo formulas for prostate problems. Choose formulas in consultation with an experienced practitioner.

HERBS TO AVOID

Individuals who have prostate enlargement should avoid the following herbs: American ginseng, cinnamon, cordyceps, ephedra, epimedium, and Siberian ginseng. Korean or red ginseng should be used with caution. For more information regarding these herbs, see Chapter 3.

KAMPO FORMULAS

See Chapter 4 for dosage information and discussions of individual formulas.

Eight-Ingredient Pill With Rehmannia (Rehmannia-Eight Combination)

Found in clinical tests to restore ease of urination in men with prostate inflammation. Traditionally given to men with "cold" symptoms, including coldness and numbness of the legs and lower back, and frequent urination at night. If the lower abdomen is flaccid and the upper abdomen is taut, this formula is appropriate. This formula is thought to help the body convert yang (ability to move) into yin (ability to hold, in this case, urine) at "Bladder Time," that is 3 to 7 P.M.

Caution: This formula should only be used when a definitive diagnosis of BPH has been made. It should *not* be used for prostate cancer.

Gentiana Longdancao Decoction to Drain the Liver

Reduces incontinence caused by prostate enlargement or irritation. Treats symptoms not directly related to prostate enlargement, which may include headache, dizziness, red and sore eyes, swelling in the ears, hearing loss, bitter taste in the mouth, or short temper.

Kidney Qi Pill From *The Golden Cabinet*

Treats excessive urinary frequency. May cause a loss of sensation in the mouth and tongue.

Caution: Discontinue the formula if fever occurs.

Sairei-to

This is a combination of two commonly available formulas: Five-Ingredient Powder with Poria and Minor Bupleurum Decoction. It helps reestablish normal urination after prostate surgery.[6]

CONSIDERATIONS

❑ Many men use the non-Kampo herb saw palmetto for prostate problems (see "Saw Palmetto and the Prostate" on page 279).

❑ Besides saw palmetto, there are other non-Kampo natural treatments for BPH. Micronized pollen stops the process of inflammation and swelling in the prostate without affecting sex hormones.[7] Another herb commonly used for prostate problems, pygeum, both lowers the amount of testosterone in circulation[8] and stops prostate inflammation.[9] This allows it to be used in dosages that do not cause sexual dysfunction.

❑ *See also* **Prostate Cancer.**

PSORIASIS

Psoriasis is a skin disorder marked by well-defined reddish, scaling, elevated lesions. The area of the skin affected by psoriasis can range from a few spots of dandruff-like scaling to widespread lesions over the elbows, knees, torso, and scalp. The disorder follows a pattern of acute flareups followed by periods of remission. It most often affects people in their teens or early twenties.

Psoriasis results when skin cells reproduce too rapidly, roughly at a rate 1,000 times greater than in normal skin. New skin cells appear so rapidly that dead skin cells cannot be shed, and the accumulated pileup of cells forms the characteristic silvery scales. The speeded-up reproduction results from an imbalance between two chemicals, one that accelerates cell division and one that decelerates it.

About fifty percent of people who have psoriasis come from families in which the disease runs. This indicates that a strong genetic factor is at work in this disorder. There is also a strong link between psoriasis and toxins that reach the skin from the digestive tract. These toxins, which form when the bowels are sluggish, help accelerate cell division.[1] In addition, psoriasis is linked to toxins produced during periods of emotional stress. These toxins both affect nerve cells that carry pain messages in the skin[2] and prolong the imbalances that lead to psoriasis.[3] This explains why about 40 percent of psoriasis patients develop the disease shortly after a specific, stressful event.[4]

Medical treatment of psoriasis does not cure but can bring a measure of relief. Ultraviolet light, from either natural sunlight or an artificial source, has a healing effect.

Smaller outbreaks of the disease are treated with a combination of drugs, including steroids, that together dissolve scales and prevent inflammation. Discontinuing the steroids, unfortunately, can bring on a severe flareup.

Modern Kampo theorists characterize psoriasis as a condition of "blood stasis," "blood dryness," and "blood heat."[5] This concept is a variation of the idea ancient Kampo theorists had about the disease. The sages of Kampo reasoned that psoriasis resulted when two different invading pathogens met in the body and fought each other. The weaker pathogen sought to leave the body through the skin, but its escape route was blocked by the other pathogen, which was attempting to enter the body through the skin. The blood was heated as it battled the pathogen trying to enter the body. The heat of the blood then transformed the original pathogen, which was trapped under the skin, into a toxin.

The individual herbs in this entry have been scientifically validated, and are used to promote specific healing actions. Kampo's ancient formulas for psoriasis, which have more general actions, have also been scientifically proven.

INDIVIDUAL KAMPO TREATMENTS

See Chapter 3 for discussions of individual herbs, traditional healing substances, and modern herbal preparations, including directions for making tea.

SUGGESTED DOSAGES	COMMENTS
Coptis (Herb), Milk Thistle	
Coptis tincture (1:5), 15–30 drops 3 times daily. Place in a cup, add 2 tbsp water, and take in a single sip. and Milk thistle, silymarin extract in tablets, 70–120 mg 3 times daily.	Combination prevents new outbreaks. Coptis stops the production of intestinal toxins, while the non-Kampo herb milk thistle activates the liver to detoxify the poisonous bacterial byproducts. Milk thistle improves liver function, inhibits inflammation, and reduces the rate at which skin cells multiply.[6] If coptis is unavailable, substitute tincture of the non-Kampo herb goldenseal (same caution applies). *Caution:* Do not use coptis during pregnancy or on a daily basis for more than 2 weeks at a time. Milk thistle can be used indefinitely.
Licorice (Herb)	
Topical cream, as needed, no time limit. Simicort is the most widely available brand.	Acts in the same manner as steroid creams. Was found to be more effective than steroids in one study.[7]
Psoralea (Herb)	
Freeze-dried herb, 1 1,000-mg capsule 3 times daily.	Contains psoralens, which increases the effectiveness of light therapy. Sold as Psoralea Seed capsule, Scruffy Pea, or *Bu Gu Zhi.* Must be activated by UV light to be effective. *Caution:* Do not use when taking prescription psoralens.
Soy Isoflavones (Modern Herbal Preparation)	
Extract, about 3,000 mg once daily. or Soy germ, 2 tsp (10 g) twice daily, preferably added to cereals or smoothies.	Contains genistein, which reduces the formation of keratin, a skin protein associated with psoriasis.[8]

KAMPO FORMULAS

See Chapter 4 for dosage information and discussions of individual formulas.

Four-Substance Decoction

Used in China to treat children's psoriasis.[9] Seek the advice of the dispensing herbalist on a suitable child's dosage.

Warming and Clearing Decoction

Traditionally prescribed for chronic skin diseases. Found in laboratory studies to neutralize the action of leukocytes, immune-system cells involved in tissue destruction in psoriasis.[10]

Caution: Should not be used by women who are trying to become pregnant.

CONSIDERATIONS

❑ Add fiber to the diet. It encourages bowel movements and reduces the production of intestinal toxins.[11] In addition, avoid alcohol. It makes psoriasis worse.[12]

❑ Avoid excessive skin dryness. In particular, it is important to avoid detergents and soaps, since detergents activate a chemical that promotes cell reproduction in psoriasis-affected skin.[13] Lubricating the skin with petrolatum or vegetable oils brings relief without side effects.

❑ If emotional stress is a problem, try hypnosis. In some cases, this has been enough to cure psoriasis.[14]

❑ If blisters and oozing are present, or there is scabby and scaling skin, eczema may be the problem; *see* **Eczema.**

RADIATION THERAPY SIDE EFFECTS

Radiation therapy is part of conventional medicine's standard arsenal against cancer. It kills cells by inducing the formation of free radicals, toxic byproducts of oxygen usage. Its effects are most pronounced on cells that are rapidly reproducing, such as cancer cells. The idea is that more cancer cells than healthy cells will be killed by the radiation.

Doctors try to aim radiation precisely at the cancer itself. However, it is impossible to not affect healthy cells. This causes a number of side effects, including fatigue, nausea, diarrhea, hair loss, and dry mouth or eyes. Different individuals experience different effects, depending on what part of the body is involved and how much radiation is received.

While radiation therapy is a purely modern medical technique, Japanese Kampo experts describe radiation injury in terms of simultaneous excesses of both yin and yang. Too much yin, or containing, energy keeps the powerful pulses of energy received during radiation therapy locked in the body's energy channels, which leads to increased damage. Too much yang, or combative, energy keeps the body from healing once the radiation has been discharged.

Although these explanations link modern treatment to ancient theory, the remedies modern Kampo physicians use to treat radiation-related problems are chosen on a systematic, scientific basis. The herbs that are helpful are those that sensitize target organs to the effects of radiation without affecting other organs, or that protect healthy organs easily damaged by radiation, such as the thyroid. Many Kampo formulas that protect tissues from radiation's effects protect both cancerous and healthy tissues. That is why the formulas listed here have clinically proven, specific applications in protecting healthy tissues during radiation therapy. Except as directed by a physician, start Kampo therapies after the last radiation treatment, so as to avoid counteracting the radiation's effects.

INDIVIDUAL KAMPO TREATMENTS

See Chapter 3 for discussions of individual herbs, traditional healing substances, and modern herbal preparations, including directions for making tea.

SUGGESTED DOSAGES	COMMENTS
Green Tea (Herb)	
Catechin extract, 1 240-mg tablet 3 times daily. or Tea, 1 c 2–5 times daily.	Catechin compounds protect the body from the effects of repeated exposure to gamma radiation, preventing thyroid cancer.[1] Caffeine increases effectiveness of radiation therapy. Use caffeinated tea only. To avoid dilution problems, do not take tea within 1 hour of taking other teas or patent medicines.
Loranthus (Herb)	
Use only under professional supervision (see Appendix A).	Prolongs survival time. Reduces risk of low white blood cell count (leukopenia).[2] Always use as part of an overall cancer treatment program.
PSK (Modern Herbal Preparation)	
Dried extract, 6 1,000-mg tablets daily.	Relieves pain, poor appetite, fatigue, weakness, and dryness of the mouth and throat. Has been shown to increase two- and five-year survival rates when used with radiation.[3] Sensitizes cervical and uterine tumors to radiation therapy.
Snow Fungus (Modern Herbal Preparation)	
Patent medicine *Yin Mi Pian*, 6–12 tablets daily. or Prepared fungus (see Chapter 3) in food, 1 tbsp daily.	Increases resistance to side effects.[4]

KAMPO FORMULAS

See Chapter 4 for dosage information and discussions of individual formulas.

Pinellia Decoction to Drain the Epigastrium

Helps inhibit inflammation.[5] In animal studies, effective in preventing damage from radiation burns when taken after radiation exposure.[6] Also treats anorexia, feeling of obstruction below the heart, and vomiting.

Caution: Use with caution if fever is present, and discontinue if preexisting fevers worsen.

Ten-Significant Tonic Decoction (All-Inclusive Great Tonic Decoction)

Prevents damage to the bone marrow, thymus, and spleen.[7] Traditionally given to persons with abdominal tension, hot flashes in the hands and feet, and lethargy.

Tonify the Middle and Augment the Qi Decoction

Prevents deficiencies in white blood cells after treatment. Also activates immune-system cells called macrophages to fight bacterial infection.[8] Traditionally given to persons weakened by long bouts with disease.

True Warrior Decoction

Treats diarrhea without cramps, but with coldness in the hands and feet. May cause a loss of sensation in the mouth and tongue.

Caution: Discontinue the formula if fever occurs.

CONSIDERATIONS

❑ Since radiation therapy depletes the body's stores of beta-carotene, and vitamins C and E,[9] it would seem natural to take supplements during radiation treatment. However, there is some evidence that the greater the body's stores of these free-radical scavenging vitamins (and of the mineral selenium) during treatment, the larger the tumor will be after treatment.[10] Do not take vitamin or mineral supplements during radiation treatment except on an oncologist's advice.

RHEUMATOID ARTHRITIS

Rheumatoid arthritis (RA) is a joint inflammation that causes pain, stiffness, swelling, and deformity, and often limits the joint's range of motion. RA most frequently strikes women between the ages of twenty and forty. The disease usually follows a pattern of flareups followed by remissions.

RA usually starts with an infection by any one or more of a variety of infectious microorganisms.[1,2] At first there is loss of appetite, fatigue, and vague pain in the muscles and bones. During this stage of the disease, the body produces large numbers of immune-system cells called T cells to fight the infection. Over the course of several weeks, some of these T cells find their way to the lining of a joint called the synovial membrane. The T cells attack cells in the membrane as if they were germs, and the membrane swells until it no longer fits in the joint. The immune system produces chemicals to clean up the dead cells, and the resulting inflammation causes acute pain, and swelling, thickening, and distortion of the joint lining. As the disease progresses, it dissolves a protein called collagen in cartilage, and eventually attacks the bone itself. RA is, in effect, a disease in which the body can turn on the immune system but cannot turn it off.

RA can be a complication of many other autoimmune diseases, such as lupus, psoriasis, Reiter's syndrome (an inflammation of the joints and mucous membranes), or Sjögren's syndrome (an inflammation that dries the mucous membranes). It also can be aggravated by a condition known as "leaky gut," in which the intestines admit semidigested food particles into the bloodstream. These particles cause a delayed allergic reaction that can compound the symptoms of RA.[3]

Ironically, the very agents most commonly used to treat RA pain, aspirin and other nonsteroidal anti-inflammatory drugs (NSAIDs), increase the "leakiness" of the intestinal lining and accelerate the faulty immune response.[4] When these agents no longer stop pain, most RA patients are then given steroid drugs such as cortisone. Steroids can be very effective in relieving pain and preventing new attacks. On the other hand, they increase the risk of infection and have a host of other side effects.

Kampo attempts to treat the sources of RA without disrupting the body's ability to fight other diseases. As early as 1481, the Kampo teacher Zhu Dan-xi noted that joint pain and swelling follow "damp heat," or infection, "lodged in the lower burner," or immune system. In this condition, the immune system does not know that it has defeated the invading pathogen and continues to fight it. In time the fight depletes the body's energy and heat becomes cold, obstructing the kidney-driven flow of water and warmth, especially to the joints.

In the early stages of the disease, Kampo's strategy is simply to "tell" the lower burner that the infection is over. Bitter herbs remove toxins, and the immune system is no longer compelled to respond to them. In later stages of the disease, Kampo fights cold. Strongly warming herbs stimulate circulation and move water out of joints. Formulas are generally used to treat overall symptom patterns.

INDIVIDUAL KAMPO TREATMENTS

See Chapter 3 for discussions of individual herbs, traditional healing substances, and modern herbal preparations, including directions for making tea.

SUGGESTED DOSAGES	COMMENTS
Asiasarum (Herb)	
Topical massage oil, as needed.	Relieves pain. May also be labeled as "wild ginger" oil. *Caution:* Do *not* take internally.
Clematis (Herb)	
Dried herb, 1 1,000-mg capsule 3 times daily. or Tea, 1 c daily.	Cools and soothes arthritic pain and swelling,[5] raises the threshold of pain.[6] Available as *Wei Ling Xian.*
Ginger (Herb)	
Dried ginger, 2 1,000-mg capsules twice daily. or Ginger in food, fresh or pickled, about 2/3 oz (20 g) or 1/2-inch slice daily. or Tea, 1 c 2–3 times daily.	Stops the formation of chemicals that cause inflammation and pain.[7–9] Improves circulation to, and accelerates fluid flow out of, joints. Often helps when conventional drugs do not.[10]
Hoelen (Herb)	
Dried or fresh hoelen in food, 1/8–1/4 oz (3–6 g) daily. or Tea, 1 c 3 times daily. or Tincture, as directed on label. Place in a cup, add 2 tbsp water, and take in a single sip.	Especially helpful in RA secondary to lupus. Contains poriatin, which suppresses immune processes that cause both RA and lupus.[11,12] *Caution:* Do not use in cases of long-term illness that cause excessive urination.
Turmeric (Herb)	
Curcumin, the yellow pigment found in turmeric, 400 mg 3 times daily between meals.	Stops production of inflammatory chemicals.[13] Also "primes" cells to receive the hormones released during steroid treatment and keeps these hormones from being broken down, making the steroids more effective. Unlike NSAID medications, does not cause toxic reactions even in overdose.[14] Pain relief comparable to steroids.[15] For best results, take curcumin with bromelain, which increases absorption.

HERBS TO AVOID

Individuals who have RA should avoid the following herbs: agrimony and Siberian ginseng. For more information regarding these herbs, see Chapter 3.

KAMPO FORMULAS

See Chapter 4 for dosage information and discussions of individual formulas.

Cinnamon Twig and Prepared Aconite Decoction

Relieves acute pain, especially in older persons. Variation of Cinnamon Twig Decoction (see Chapter 4) that is available in patent-medicine form.

Ephedra Decoction (Four Emperors Combination)

Used in the early stages of RA to relieve swelling and pain. Appropriate when symptoms are worse in cold weather. A variation, Ephedra, Apricot Kernel, Coix, and Licorice Decoction, is designed to lower fever, in addition to treating other symptoms. Use either formula in patent-medicine form.

Caution: Avoid if nausea or vomiting is present.

Kidney Qi Pill From *The Golden Cabinet*

Relieves lower back pain and weakness of the lower extremities. Symptoms may also include a cold sensation in the lower half of the body, tension in the lower abdomen, and irritability to the point of having difficulty lying down. There is often either urinary difficulty with swelling, or excessive urination, sometimes to the point of incontinence. In extreme cases, the patient will have difficulty breathing, and breathe more easily when leaning against a support. Particularly appropriate for persons suffering from both arthritis and diabetes. May cause a loss of sensation in the mouth and tongue.

Caution: Discontinue the formula if fever occurs.

Ledebouriella Decoction That Sagely Unblocks

Historically prescribed for "crane's-knee wind," in which one or both knees become swollen, enlarged, and painful and cannot be moved. Symptoms may also include aversion to cold, attraction to warmth, or shortness of breath.

Ophiopogonis Decoction

Especially helpful for RA secondary to Sjögren's syndrome; increases salivary secretions 40% in clinical tests.[16] Traditionally given to treat dry mouth and dry throat.

Caution: Use with caution if fever is present, and discontinue if preexisting fevers worsen.

Prepared Aconite Decoction

Designed to treat persons with a weak constitution who have aching bones and joints, aversion to cold, and cold extremities. Given to persons whose primary symptom is pain. Especially effective against collagen-induced RA, in which swelling does not allow fluids to circulate freely.[17] May cause a loss of sensation in the mouth and tongue.

Caution: Discontinue the formula if fever occurs.

Prolong Life Decoction

Useful when the individual cannot turn to the side. Also improves memory and responsiveness.

Caution: To avoid ill effects from eating apricot seeds (see Chapter 3), it is best to use this formula in patent-medicine form. Do not use this formula at all if nausea or vomiting is present.

Sairei-to

In this combination formula, Five-Ingredient Powder with Poria stimulates fluid circulation and relieves swelling,[18] and Minor Bupleurum Decoction regulates the immune system. Combination stimulates the natural production of steroids that can prolong the effects of cortisone and related drugs.[19] Also prevents kidney damage in advanced RA.[20]

True Warrior Decoction

Designed to treat persons with a weak constitution who have aching bones and joints, aversion to cold, and cold extremities. Given to persons whose primary symptom is swelling. May cause a loss of sensation in the mouth and tongue.

Caution: Discontinue the formula if fever occurs.

FORMULAS TO AVOID

Individuals who have RA should avoid Ten-Significant Tonic Decoction (All-Inclusive Great Tonifying Decoction). For more information regarding this formula, see Chapter 4.

CONSIDERATIONS

❑ *See also* **Lupus, Osteoarthritis,** and **Psoriasis.**

SEIZURE DISORDERS

A seizure is a temporary change in behavior caused by the abnormal firing of neurons (nerve cells) in the brain. This abnormal activity disrupts cell-to-cell communication in the brain. Seizures can result in loss of consciousness, tingling or numbness, inattention, loss of speech, unexplained emotions, and/or staring. Seizures that involve intense, uncontrolled muscle movements are called *convulsions.*

Seizures can occur for many reasons, including high fever, electric shock, poisoning, drug reactions, head injury, and fluctuations in blood-sugar levels. Often the seizure is an isolated incident. When seizures reoccur because of a problem within the brain itself, the condition is called *epilepsy.* Epilepsy is usually first diagnosed in childhood or adolescence. However, anyone who has had a seizure needs a medical evaluation, which may involve brain scans and brainwave tests.

Scientists believe that epileptic seizures originate in the portion of the brain associated with thinking, the cerebral cortex. The extent to which the electrical disturbance in the cortex spreads throughout the brain determines the severity of the seizure. Partial seizures begin and remain at a single site in the cortex. Generalized seizures begin in the cortex but rapidly involve other parts of the brain, and cause loss of consciousness. One type of generalized seizure, the absence seizure, causes a brief (30 second) period of staring with no unusual muscle movements.

If seizures occur chronically, a wide variety of antiseizure medications may be used, either singly or in combination. For the most part, these drugs do not reliably control seizures.[1] Such drugs need to be used with great care, not only because of side effects but also because the range between an ineffective blood level of medication and a toxic one is narrow. Avoiding drastic changes in fluid volume within the body is critical.

Changes in fluid volume is the key to Kampo's understanding of seizure disorders. While neurology usually explains seizure disorders in terms of physical lesions in the brain, Kampo explains seizure disorders in terms of the energy-flow blockages by "phlegm." This phlegm—which, unlike the Western idea of phlegm, is not detectable on conventional physical examination—results from a disruption of the body's ability to circulate fluid. This disruption occurs over such a long period of time that fluid "solidifies," and stops the free flow of energy and information. Underlying the creation of phlegm is the body's failure to utilize nutritive energy. Restoring normal fluid flow stops the creation of phlegm and energizes the heart, the seat of emotion, to once again contain emotions.

Kampo is helpful in the treatment of partial epileptic seizures, and especially beneficial in borderline cases in which the physician does not prescribe any other anticonvulsant. *Never* discontinue any conventional medication without a physician's advice. Except as otherwise noted, only use the herbs and formulas listed here with guidance from both a Kampo practitioner and a neurologist.

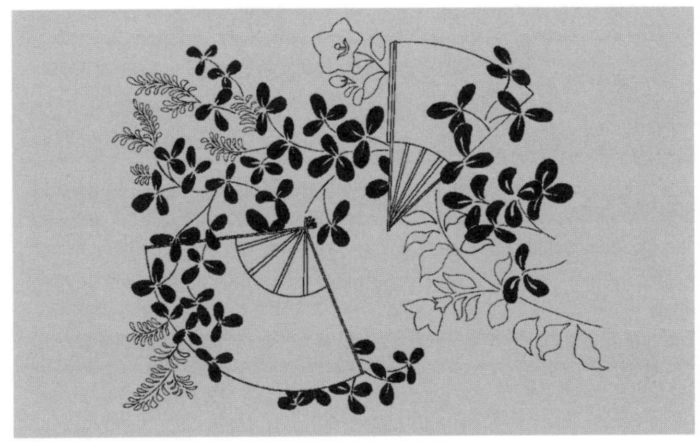

INDIVIDUAL KAMPO TREATMENTS

See Chapter 3 for discussions of individual herbs, traditional healing substances, and modern herbal preparations, including directions for making tea.

SUGGESTED DOSAGES	COMMENTS
Acorus (Herb)	
Use only under professional supervision.	Used to treat absence seizures.
Chinese Senega Root (Herb)	
Use only under professional supervision.	Removes phlegm obstructing the "orifices of the heart," which shows itself as seizures, and as emotional and mental disorientation. Considered most effective in treating seizures that seem to be related to pent-up emotions or brooding. *Caution:* Do not use during pregnancy, or if gastritis or ulcers are present.
Ginger (Herb)	
Dried ginger, 2 1,000-mg capsules twice daily. or Ginger in food, fresh or pickled, about 2/3 oz (20 g) or 1/2-inch slice daily. or Tea, 1 c 2–3 times daily.	Has no direct effect on seizures, but protects the liver from damage by treatment with valproic acid (Depakene, Depakote).[2] No professional supervision is needed.

HERBS TO AVOID

Individuals who are taking medication for a seizure disorder should avoid the following herbs: akebia, alisma, aloe, Cornelian cherry, ephedra, green tea, hawthorn, hoelen, Japanese watermelon, lophatherum, mulberry bark, polyporus, and rhubarb root. They promote fluid loss through increased urination or regularity, and when used in excess can cause antiseizure drugs to become overly concentrated in the bloodstream. For more information regarding these herbs, see Chapter 3.

KAMPO FORMULAS

See Chapter 4 for dosage information and discussions of individual formulas.

Bupleurum Plus Dragon Bone and Oyster Shell Decoction

Especially useful for controlling partial seizures that result in slurred speech.

Caution: Be sure the formula does *not* include the traditional ingredient minium (lead oxide). Use with caution if fever is present, and discontinue if preexisting fevers worsen.

Cinnamon Twig, Licorice, Dragon Bone, and Oyster Shell Decoction

Used to treat seizure disorders in men who also display what Kampo calls "kidney symptoms," such as frequent urination, erection difficulties, loss of sensation in the penis, hair loss, or disturbed sleep.

Gastrodia and Uncaria Decoction

Combination of gambir and gastrodia, the two most effective herbs for treating seizures. Japanese research shows that they act by destroying free radicals, toxins found in the body's tissues, and by increasing the brain's own defenses against free radicals. These herbs also keep free radicals from activating compounds that destroy cell walls.[3] Kampo uses this formula for the treatment of childhood epilepsy. Seek the advice of the dispensing herbalist on a suitable child's dosage.

Caution: Should not be used by women who are trying to become pregnant.

Warm the Gallbladder Decoction

Used for seizure disorders that occur with frothing at the mouth and/or ongoing digestive problems.

Caution: Use with caution if fever is present, and discontinue if preexisting fevers worsen.

FORMULAS TO AVOID

Individuals who have seizure disorders should avoid Kidney Qi Pill From *The Golden Cabinet.* For more information regarding this formula, see Chapter 4.

SHINGLES

See **Herpes.**

SINUSITIS

Sinusitis is an inflammation or infection of the sinuses, the open spaces found within the facial bones. Like the nose, the sinuses are lined with membranes that can become irritated. The membranes then swell, blocking the free passage of air and secretions. Sinus infections are triggered by events that alter mucous production, such as allergic attacks, and by changes in body temperature favorable to the growth of infectious bacteria. Airborne irritants, such as air pollution, cigarette smoke, disinfectants, household cleaners, and pesticides, can also injure the sinus linings and give bacteria a foothold.

The main symptom of sinusitis is a discharge of mucus. Other symptoms include headache, earache, facial pain or pressure, and bad breath. Sinusitis can, in rare cases, lead to more serious conditions, such as pneumonia. Conventional treatment consists of antibiotics, decongestants, and painkillers.

Kampo's concept of sinusitis is one of an invasion of "cold," carried by the wind. Cold interferes with the normal circulation of qi, or energy, through the energy channels. Since the energy channels meet in the head, this cold causes headache. It also disables the lungs, which control the nose. The nose then becomes stuffy and congested.

Subtle differences in the total pattern of symptoms are accommodated by different formulas, while herbs are used for specific problems. Treatment of sinusitis usually requires at least three weeks of consistent use of the chosen herb or formula.

INDIVIDUAL KAMPO TREATMENTS

See Chapter 3 for discussions of individual herbs, traditional healing substances, and modern herbal preparations, including directions for making tea.

SUGGESTED DOSAGES	COMMENTS
Coptis (Herb)	
Tincture (1:5), 20 drops 3 times daily. Place in a cup, add 2 tbsp water, and take in a single sip.	Potent antimicrobial agent; stops bleeding. *Caution:* Do not use during pregnancy or on a daily basis for more than 2 weeks at a time. Do not use with supplements that contain vitamin B_6 or the amino acid histidine.
Ligusticum (Herb)	
Fluid extract (1:1), 15–20 drops 4 times daily until nasal secretions stop.	Stops profuse clear or white nasal secretion. If ligusticum is unavailable, substitute the non-Kampo herb osha (same cautions apply). *Caution:* Should not be used by infertile women, or by women who have irregularities of the skin and nails, menstrual irregularities, or pallor.

KAMPO FORMULAS

See Chapter 4 for dosage information and discussions of individual formulas.

Ephedra, Apricot Kernel, Gypsum, and Licorice Decoction

Treats nasal congestion and flaring accompanied by cough, fever with or without sweating, labored breathing, nasal pain, thirst, and/or wheezing.

Caution: Avoid if nausea or vomiting is present.

Gentiana Longdancao Decoction to Drain the Liver

Treats severe headache, nasal obstruction (membranes red and swollen), and thick, yellow nasal discharge with a bad odor.

Kudzu Decoction

Treats nasal congestion or sinusitis with stiff upper back.

Ligusticum Chuanxiong Powder to be Taken With Green Tea

Treats nasal congestion with headache. Especially appropriate when there is dizziness.

CONSIDERATIONS

❑ To prevent relapses, avoid irritating chemicals or allergens. Persons who live in a part of the country that has extremely dry air during the winter should use a humidifier to keep the sinus membranes from drying and cracking.

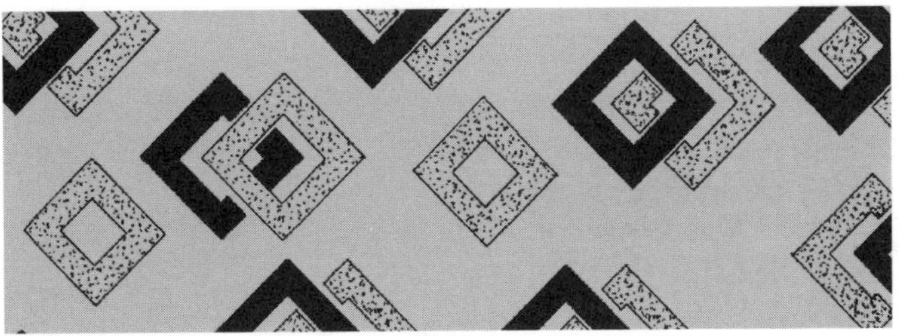

SKIN CANCER (BASAL CELL CARCINOMA)

Basal cell carcinoma is among the most common forms of cancer, with more than half a million new cases reported each year. Fortunately, it is a relatively benign disease with a very high cure rate. It develops on skin that is exposed to the ultraviolet (UV) light of the sun over a period of years. It can also develop after exposure to arsenic. Basal cell carcinoma is most common on the scalp, face, neck, hands, and forearms.

Basal cell carcinoma appears as small patches of white, hard skin, usually smaller in diameter than a pencil eraser. These growths almost never break out of protein capsules that contain them, but may bleed and form scars. Left unattended over a period of years, however, they can eventually invade adjacent soft tissues. (Melanoma is a skin cancer that occurs much less frequently, but is much more aggressive. Therefore, any abnormal skin growths should be brought to a doctor's attention.)

Unless the cancer has spread, conventional treatment consists of surgery. If the cancer has spread, radiation therapy may be recommended (see considerations below).

Kampo explains basal cell carcinoma as a disturbance of the energy channels underlying the skin caused by "heat," such as the heat of the sun. Heat blocks the normal flow of energy, which is transformed into small, hard lumps. If the body does not receive more heat once the lumps form, they do not spread. Herbs that treat the effects of heat also treat basal cell carcinoma.

INDIVIDUAL KAMPO TREATMENTS

See Chapter 3 for discussions of individual herbs, traditional healing substances, and modern herbal preparations, including directions for making tea.

SUGGESTED DOSAGES	COMMENTS
Aloe (Herb), Vitamin E	
Aloe gel, either commercial or taken from houseplants, used liberally on dressings. and Vitamin E cream, as directed on label.	Aloe contains antihistamines, which prevent the production of chemicals needed for the growth of basal cell carcinoma and other skin cancers. Combination has been shown to produce remission in about a third of the people who use it.[1] When added to dressings, accelerates healing after liquid nitrogen treatment.

KAMPO FORMULAS

See Chapter 4 for dosage information and discussions of individual formulas.

Two-Cured Decoction

Contains pinellia, which directly inhibits the growth of basal cell carcinoma. Also reduces estrogen levels, indirectly slowing the rate of growth of some other forms of skin cancer.[2]

Caution: Use with caution if fever is present, and discontinue if preexisting fevers worsen.

CONSIDERATIONS

❑ Actinic keratosis, a precancerous condition caused by excessive exposure to sunlight, may be treated with a skin ointment that contains 5-fluorouracil (Fluoroplex). A coptis compress, applied and removed before applying Fluoroplex, (see Chapter 3) increases the skin's ability to absorb this drug.[3]

❑ Other Kampo herbs can be used by themselves to help prevent skin damage from progressing to skin cancer. Schisandra contains compounds that prevent the skin cancer development after chemical injury,[4] and is especially recommended for persons exposed to arsenic compounds. Take 100 milligrams three times daily of the freeze-dried herb (available as Hoelen & Schisandra) or 1 cup of schisandra tea three times daily (see Chapter 3 for tea-making directions). Do not use this herb if gallstones or bile-duct blockages exist. Turmeric contains curcumin, which prevents development of skin cancer caused by UV light[5] and also prevents chemically-induced skin cancers.[6] Apply a turmeric poultice three times daily (see Chapter 3 for instructions). This poultice can also be used as a natural sunscreen to prevent UV damage.

❑ To reduce side effects and increase effectiveness when using radiation therapy, *see* **Radiation Therapy Side Effects.**

❑ *See also* **Melanoma.**

STOMACH CANCER

In North America, stomach cancer is a disease that mostly affects older people. In Japan, however, it is more common among adults in general owing to a diet that includes pickled vegetables and extremely hot tea (the problem being the heat rather than the tea itself). As a result, Kampo practitioners have long experience in treating stomach cancer.

In North America, the consumption of nitrates in processed or "cured" meats and fish contribute to the development of stomach cancer. Nitrates are converted to cancer-causing nitrites by bacteria in the stomach, and *Helicobacter pylori* is the bacterium most closely linked to this process.[1] Zinc deficiency is also implicated as a cause of stomach cancer,[2] since a lack of zinc reduces the immune system's effectiveness.[3]

The early symptoms of stomach cancer include a feeling of fullness or discomfort after eating. Weakness or weight loss may be present. Low-level bleeding may cause anemia. In rare instances, the person will vomit blood or pass tarry, black stools. As the cancer spreads it can affect the liver, causing jaundice and abdominal fluid accumulations.

Surgery is most successful if the cancer is contained within the stomach itself. If the cancer has spread, radiation therapy or chemotherapy may be used.

Kampo sees stomach cancer as the result of toxic assault from eating too many foods that are either extremely yin or extremely yang. Extremely yin foods, such as alcohol, refined grains, pastries, sugar, and cold drinks (sweetened or unsweetened), reduce the energy level of the stomach. This forces it to produce more acid in order to digest food. Extremely yang foods, such as animal protein, fats, and oils, also require the stomach to produce more acid. In either case, excess acid inflames the lining of the stomach. Inflammation becomes ulceration, and tumors eventually "solidify" from the excess of digestive energy.

Kampo physicians can detect a risk for stomach cancer through external examination, since the skin as a whole shows the condition of the stomach. A splotchy brown skin color, or freckles, especially on the nose, indicates excessive acidity. Skin discoloration along the stomach's energy channel, especially over the knees or on the top of the feet in the area of the second and third toes, also indicates stomach imbalances. A swollen upper lip indicates problems from the overconsumption of alcohol, refined grain products, and sugar. A receded upper lip indicates problems from eating too much meat, eggs, and salt.

Five-year survival rates for stomach cancer in Japan are much higher than those in the United States.[4,5] This is the result of both the widespread practice of early detection through *sho* diagnosis, as described above, and of the widespread use of appropriate Kampo therapies. Kampo should always be used as part of a medically directed overall treatment plan for stomach cancer (see considerations below).

INDIVIDUAL KAMPO TREATMENTS

See Chapter 3 for discussions of individual herbs, traditional healing substances, and modern herbal preparations, including directions for making tea.

SUGGESTED DOSAGES	COMMENTS
Garlic (Herb)	
Enterically coated tablets, as directed on label (usually at least 900 mg daily). or Raw garlic, 2–3 cloves daily, thoroughly chewed. Recommended form.	Contains compounds that prevent spread of cancer to the lymph nodes. Use of garlic is associated with lower rates of stomach and other cancers.[6] Ajone, a cancer-fighting garlic compound, builds up in the bloodstream after 3–4 weeks of constant use. Individuals who cannot tolerate garlic can try **Shiitake** (see consideration below).
Houttynia (Herb)	
Tea, as directed by herbalist.	Slows the development of stomach cancer.[7] Available in Chinese herb shops as *Yu Xing Cao.*
Lentinan (Modern Herbal Preparation)	
Intramuscular injection (usual form), 0.5–50 mg effective daily dose, depending on patient's condition and circumstances. Smaller, more frequent doses more effective than larger, less frequent doses. Given under professional supervision. or Powder, dosage to be determined by provider. Much greater dosages required than in injectable form.	Used successfully to treat stomach cancer.[8,9] Activates the immune system to attack most kinds of solid cancers.[10–13]

PSK (Modern Herbal Preparation)	
Dried extract, 6 1,000-mg tablets daily.	Increases the effectiveness of mitomycin.[14]

KAMPO FORMULAS

See Chapter 4 for dosage information and discussions of individual formulas.

Coptis Decoction to Relieve Toxicity

Kills *Helicobacter pylori.* Contains berberine, which prevents cell multiplication in cancers of the digestive tract.[15,16] Protects the stomach lining.[17] Although this formula is available as a patent medicine, use it only after consultation with a Kampo or TCM practitioner who has experience in treating stomach cancer.

Caution: Should not be used by women who are trying to become pregnant.

CONSIDERATIONS

❑ Shiitake can be used to help prevent stomach cancer in persons who cannot tolerate garlic. It works by blocking the formation of cancer-causing chemicals from dietary nitrates. Use the fresh or dried mushroom in food, $^1/_4$ to $^1/_3$ ounces (6 to 9 grams) daily. Or take one of the following types of shiitake extract three times daily: three 1-gram tablets, $^1/_2$ tablespoon (4 to 6 milliliters) syrup, or 1 tablespoon (10 milliliters) tincture (1:5). Place the tincture in a cup, add 2 tablespoons water, and take in a single sip.

❑ To reduce side effects and increase effectiveness when using chemotherapy, *see* **Chemotherapy Side Effects**; when using radiation therapy, *see* **Radiation Therapy Side Effects.** To learn about herbal treatments that can prevent a cancer from developing its own blood supply, *see* **Cancer.**

STREP THROAT

Most cases of sore throat are caused by viral infections, and disappear in a few days. However, some are caused by infection with *Streptococcus* (strep) bacteria, which can take weeks to go away. Strep throat causes pain on swallowing, redness of the throat, swollen tonsils, and tender lymph nodes in the neck. Strep throat cannot be distinguished from viral sore throat just by looking at the throat and tonsils. Fortunately, physicians now have swabs that can immediately test for the presence of strep.[1]

Strep throat can lead to rheumatic fever, which causes arthritis, fever, and heart inflammation. Therefore, unlike viral infections, strep infections are treated with antibiotics to prevent damage to other organs. Unfortunately, antibiotics usually have little effect on the bacteria in the throat itself,[2] and do not always prevent complications.[3] About 20 percent of the time antibiotics fail to kill off all of the strep bacteria. This occurs when other bacteria secrete a chemical that deactivates penicillin and related drugs.

Kampo treatments for strep throat circumvent this problem, since Kampo therapies are unaffected by the antibiotic-deactivating chemical. Kampo physicians noted over the course of centuries that certain herbs relieved a condition characterized as "damp heat." Damp heat is a fever-producing disease that invades the body. Being damp, it sinks downward, until it reaches the lungs and bottles up their upward-moving energies. The captured energy closes the throat, and is transformed into a form of blocked energy, phlegm. Herbs used to treat damp heat clear the infection and the toxins it produces, and then redirect the energy of the lungs.

Only a doctor can diagnose strep throat. Scientific study has confirmed that some Kampo therapies act directly on strep, and do so without the side effects of many commonly prescribed antibiotics. Other herbs relieve symptoms. Strep throat treated with these preparations should improve within three days and go away within three weeks. If it does not, it is possible that a more serious secondary infection is present. In that case, see a health care professional.

INDIVIDUAL KAMPO TREATMENTS

See Chapter 3 for discussions of individual herbs, traditional healing substances, and modern herbal preparations, including directions for making tea.

SUGGESTED DOSAGES	COMMENTS
Amaranth (Herb)	
Tea, 1 c 3 times daily.	Relieves sore throat pain. Listed in Chinese herb shops as achyranthis; may also be labeled as *Niu Xi* or *Tu niu xi.* *Caution:* Avoid during pregnancy.
Arisaema (Herb)	
Use only under supervision of an herbalist.	Relieves intensely sore throat, bleeding, fullness, and swelling of throat and tongue. Also identified as jack-in-the-pulpit.
Coptis (Herb)	
Tincture (1:5), 15–30 drops 3 times daily for 10 days. Place in a cup, add 2 tbsp water, and take in a single sip.	Keeps strep from attaching to the throat lining.[4] Kills some bacteria that have become resistant to antibiotics.[5] Prevents secondary infection with yeast (thrush).[6] *Caution:* Do not use during pregnancy or on a daily basis for more than 2 weeks at a time. Do not use with supplements that contain vitamin B_6 or the amino acid histidine.
Garlic (Herb)	
Oil, 3–4 drops in $^1/_4$ cup water. Use once daily as a gargle.	Relieves difficulty in swallowing.
Ginger (Herb)	
Ginger tea, 1 c 3 times daily.	Relieves pain.

Myrrh (Traditional Healing Substance)	
Tincture (1:5), 10–30 drops up to 3 times daily as needed. Place in a cup, add 2 tbsp water, and use as a gargle.	Treats ulcerated, enlarged tissues and stops excessive mucous secretion.

Scrophularia (Herb)	
Tea, 1 c 4 times daily.	Draws out "fire," relieves red, dry, inflamed tissue. Sold as *Xuan Shen* in Chinese herb shops.

KAMPO FORMULAS

See Chapter 4 for dosage information and discussions of individual formulas.

Clear Summerheat and Augment the Qi Decoction

Relieves burning sensation, especially when there is profuse sweating.

Caution: This formula should not be used for fevers and upper respiratory infection accompanied by an upset stomach.

Lily Bulb Decoction to Preserve the Metal

Stops coughing with blood-streaked sputum, wheezing, dry sore throat, and feverish hands and feet.

Caution: Always see a doctor if bloody sputum is present.

Lonicera and Forsythia Powder (Honeysuckle and Forsythia Powder)

Shown in laboratory tests to kill strep.[7] Contains platycodon, an immune-stimulant herb that is safe for use by persons with HIV.[8]

STRESS

Stress is a reaction to any life event that upsets the body's balance. Stress can have physical causes, such as pain or cold, or emotional causes, such as worry or frustration. (Even pleasure can cause stress!) Chronic stress is implicated in a plethora of disorders, including addiction, anorexia, anxiety, high blood pressure, and immune deficiency.

The stress response first developed as a way of releasing quick energy in the face of physical danger, or what is known as the "fight or flight" response. The pituitary gland, located at the base of the brain, responds to the perception of stress by releasing adrenocorticotrophic hormone (ACTH). This hormone is circulated to the adrenal glands, which lie on top of the kidneys. The adrenals convert cholesterol into cortisol, which initiates a series of profound changes in body chemistry.

In the liver, cortisol stimulates the release of the body's principal fuel, glucose. Cortisol also short-circuits the immune system's ability to cause inflammation in response to tissue damage. Less inflammation means that muscles can move more freely and there is less pain. In addition, cortisol makes the red blood cells more likely to clot. When loss of blood is causing the stress, the release of cortisol is a lifesaving response.

The problem with stress arises when the body cannot turn off the cycle started by ACTH. This situation can be produced by the chronic stress often found in modern life. Ordinarily, cortisol is broken down during sleep, and is replenished every morning. When stress is unremitting, the body goes out of balance. As the excess glucose is burned, it creates toxins called free radicals. These free radicals disrupt processes throughout the body, including normal immune function. The blood continues to clot easily, and the blood vessels constrict. This raises blood pressure and weakens artery walls.

Eventually the adrenal glands themselves may "burn out." Lengthy periods of high adrenal-hormone levels in the bloodstream signal the immune system to attack the glands themselves. As a result, unhealthy high blood pressure becomes unhealthy low pressure, and fatigue and depression often follow.

The key to using Kampo to prevent stress-related illness is to recognize the stage of the illness. Early stages of stress-related disease produce symptoms of "yang stage" disorders, that is, excesses of outwardly directed energy. Imbalances of yang manifest themselves as excessive energy and also tight (although easily fatigued) muscles, easy bruising, flushing in the face, high blood pressure, high blood-sugar levels, striations on the skin, and, in women, development of masculine features, especially hair growth. Late stages of stress-related diseases produce symptoms of "yin stage" disorders, that is, the inability to contain fluids in their proper paths and appropriate tissues. Imbalances of yin manifest themselves primarily as fatigue, but also in loose muscles, a pale complexion, low blood pressure, low blood-sugar levels, a brownish or copper cast to the entire skin, and, in women, loss of body hair. Recognizing the symptom pattern makes it possible to choose the best therapy. Distinguishing yang and yin is essential to effective Kampo treatment, and should be done by a Kampo or TCM practitioner. In addition, since stress-related symptoms mimic those of various disorders, it would be wise to have such symptoms evaluated by a health care professional.

INDIVIDUAL KAMPO TREATMENTS

See Chapter 3 for discussions of individual herbs, traditional healing substances, and modern herbal preparations, including directions for making tea.

SUGGESTED DOSAGES	COMMENTS
Ginseng (Herb)	
Fluid extract or tincture, as directed on label. or Tea, made with Korean or red ginseng, 1 c daily.	Ancient Kampo remedy for stress. Benefits the central nervous system by preserving memory and reflexes, and the heart, lungs, and kidneys by relaxing blood vessels.[1] If using ginseng extracts or tinctures (which are not as therapeutically active as teas), be sure the product contains *Panax ginseng.* Note that strength may vary by manufacturer. *Caution:* Beware of ginseng anti-stress tonics imported from China in which ginseng may be combined with *Wu Ling Zhi,* or squirrel droppings. This ingredient is effective,[2] but many people may find it objectionable. May be identified on the label as Excrementum Trogopteri seu Peteroni.

Scutellaria (Herb)	
Dried herb, 1–2 1,000-mg capsules 3 times daily. or Fluid extract (1:1), ¼–½ tsp (1–2 ml) 3 times daily. or Powdered solid extract (4:1), 250–500 mg 3 times daily. or Tea, 1 c 3 times daily. or Tincture (1:5), 1–1½ tsp (4–6 ml) 3 times daily. Place in a cup, add 2 tbsp water, and take in a single sip.	Stops the overproduction of ACTH in laboratory studies,[3] supporting this herb's traditional use for this purpose. Useful in preventing viral infections that often follow immune impairment. *Caution:* Avoid in cases of diarrhea caused by foodborne infection or excessive consumption of cold drinks.

Siberian Ginseng (Modern Herbal Preparation)	
Eleuthero extract, as directed by manufacturer, in ¼ c water. Be sure to use pure extract, *not* sugar-sweetened ginseng drinks. or Tea, 1 c 3 times daily.	Treats difficulty in concentrating and sensitivity to environmental stresses, such as noise, drafts, and changes in weather. Also fights depression, supports the immune system, and prevents viral infection.[4,5] *Caution:* Should be avoided by persons with myasthenia gravis; rheumatoid arthritis and diseases related to it, such as lupus, psoriatric arthritis, and Sjögren's syndrome; or prostate cancer.

KAMPO FORMULAS

See Chapter 4 for dosage information and discussions of individual formulas.

Bupleurum Plus Dragon Bone and Oyster Shell Decoction

Reduces the rate at which the body produces cortisol in response to stress. More effective for emotional stress than for immediate, physical stresses caused by accident or disease.[6]

Caution: Be sure the formula does *not* include the traditional ingredient minium (lead oxide). Use with caution if fever is present, and discontinue if preexisting fevers worsen.

Four-Substance Decoction

Treatment for anxiety and depression that helps maintain intellectual sharpness and short-term memory.[7]

Sairei-to

This is a combination of two commonly available formulas: Five-Ingredient Powder with Poria and Minor Bupleurum Decoction. It is especially helpful in preventing burnout from long-term stress. Reduces the cortisol's inhibiting effects on the pituitary and adrenal glands.[8] Minor Bupleurum Decoction itself is effective for "cold chills" caused by fear or awe.[9]

Tang-Kuei and Peony Powder

Prevents free-radical cell damage in the brain caused by aging or prolonged stress.[10]

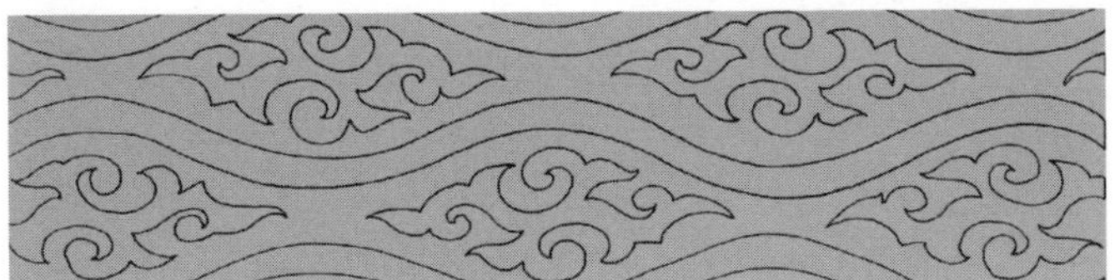

STROKE

Stroke is a neurological injury that occurs when the brain's supply of oxygen is interrupted. Generally, the longer the oxygen supply is cut off, the greater the damage to brain tissue. Most strokes are caused by blood clots blocking the arteries supplying the brain, or by compression of the artery linings. Other strokes are caused by blood-vessel ruptures within the brain. Atherosclerosis, in which fatty deposits build up within artery walls, and high blood pressure are both risk factors for stroke.

The nature and persistence of any disability following a stroke depend on where the stroke occurs and how much of the brain is involved. Possible disabilities include speech or swallowing difficulties, paralysis, blurred vision, loss of bladder or bowel control, or mental difficulties. Very brief "mini-strokes," or *transient ischemic attacks* (TIAs), may produce strokelike effects, or cause a momentary sense of distraction or dizziness.

While strokes cut off circulation within minutes, medical researchers have learned that the resulting damage to brain tissue is often a long-term process. A blood clot can shut down all circulation to a very small part of the brain. Those nerve tissues die, creating an infarct. Surrounding tissues, however, still receive—and adapt to—a minimal amount of oxygen. When natural healing processes reestablish circulation to the surviving brain cells, though, those cells are suddenly overwhelmed with oxygen. This oxygen produces toxins called free radicals, which attack previously undamaged cells and create further damage. As free radical damage spreads farther and farther from the infarct, outward symptoms become more severe, and new disabilities may appear.[1]

Anticipating the scientific explanation of stroke by several centuries, Kampo medicine termed stroke as *oketsu,* or "static blood syndrome." When blood is unable to circulate, energy is unable to circulate. Since the energy channels pass through the head, static blood in the head paralyzes, weakens, or denervates every muscle supplied by any blocked channel. Japanese researchers have found that Kampo formulas heal *oketsu* by stopping the production of free radicals as circulation is reestablished in the brain.

Never use any herbal remedy for the aftereffects of stroke before medical diagnosis or without consulting a physician. Herbal remedies are *only* effective for strokes caused by blocked arteries, and can be harmful if used for those caused by blood-vessel rupture. The doctor will perform the necessary brain scans and other tests to determine the cause of the stroke. Once this has been done, the following treatments accelerate recovery. Always use Kampo as part of a medically directed aftercare program for stroke. If acute stroke symptoms occur—sudden numbness, paralysis, blurred vision, or slurred speech—*immediately* seek professional help.

INDIVIDUAL KAMPO TREATMENTS

See Chapter 3 for discussions of individual herbs, traditional healing substances, and modern herbal preparations, including directions for making tea.

SUGGESTED DOSAGES	COMMENTS
Ginkgo (Herb)	
Ginkgolide extract, 240 mg once daily.	Preserves blood flow in healthy portions of the brain by counteracting the clotting process. Can also increase blood flow to the brain.[2] *Caution:* Since combinations of blood-thinning drugs and gingko can cause risk of bleeding, always consult a physician before using ginkgo.
Hawthorn (Herb)	
Dried herb in capsules, 3–5 g daily. or Fluid extract (1:1), ¼–½ tsp (1–2 ml) 3 times daily. or Solid extract, 100–250 mg 3 times daily. Should be standardized to contain 10% proanthocyanidins. or Tea, ⅔ c 3–4 times daily. or Tincture (1:5), 1–1½ tsp (4–6 ml) 3 times daily. Place in a cup, add 2 tbsp water, and take in a single sip.	Contains antioxidants that help maintain the integrity of tiny blood vessels in brain tissue during stress caused by either high blood pressure or microscopic blood clots.[3]

KAMPO FORMULAS

See Chapter 4 for dosage information and discussions of individual formulas.

Rhubarb and Moutan Decoction

Most potent free-radical scavenger of all the Kampo formulas.[4] Successfully used in Japan to treat *oketsu* syndrome, especially the loss of the ability of self-expression after a stroke.

CONSIDERATIONS

❑ *See also* **Atherosclerosis** and **High Blood Pressure.**

TINNITUS (RINGING IN THE EARS)

Tinnitus is the sensation of sound in the absence of actual sound. The sounds that may be heard include tinkling, ringing, buzzing, hissing, and roaring noises. These noises may come and go, or they may be persistent. There may also be hearing loss.

Tinnitus can result from one-time exposure to an unusually loud noise. These sonic assaults can include the roar of aircraft engines, explosions, gunfire, or loud music. Tinnitus can also result from repeated exposure to loud noises. It may follow sudden changes in air pressure, the toxic effects of certain antibiotics or chemotherapy agents, exposure to carbon monoxide or heavy metals, or even using too much aspirin.

Tinnitus is marked by damage to the inner ear, a fluid-filled structure that contains thousands of hairlike cells. These delicate "hairs" help translate sound impulses into nerve impulses that are sent on to the brain, and are easily damaged by loud noise or toxicity. These conditions cause the release of toxins called free radicals. Once the hair cells are destroyed, they cannot be replaced.

The literature of Kampo is filled with references to an annoying condition of "unending noise like swarms of cicadas" and an even more serious condition likened to "constant hearing of the wind." In Kampo, progressively worsening cases of tinnitus are part of a symptom pattern caused by weak kidneys. Deficient yin, or containing energy, in the kidneys keeps them from circulating fluids and nourishment upward to the ears. The first stage of this disease causes a constant, annoying sensation of sound, but does not greatly interfere with normal hearing. Later, the still-weaker kidneys release too much of their fluids downward into the bladder. The blood supply to the ears becomes deficient as well, and the sufferer experiences the audible sensation of wind. The internal wind becomes all that the person can hear. To prevent this progression, most of the formulas Kampo uses to treat tinnitus are tonic formulas for the kidneys.

It is always necessary to have tinnitus medically evaluated in order to ensure that the right problem is being treated. If no underlying disorder is discovered, using free-radical fighting herbs and formulas over a period of three to four weeks can treat the condition. It is essential, however, to start treatment in the first few days or weeks after any *hearing loss* begins, or treatment is not likely to be effective.

INDIVIDUAL KAMPO TREATMENTS

See Chapter 3 for discussions of individual herbs, traditional healing substances, and modern herbal preparations, including directions for making tea.

SUGGESTED DOSAGES	COMMENTS
Black Cohosh (Herb), Goldenseal	
Black cohosh, dried root, 2–6 500-mg capsules daily. or Black cohosh, fluid extract (1:1), 20–30 drops 4 times daily. and Goldenseal tincture (1:5), 10–15 drops 4 times daily. Place in a cup, add 2 tbsp water, and take in a single sip.	Combination treats ringing in the ears. Black cohosh relieves dizziness, while the non-Kampo herb goldenseal relieves inner ear inflammation.

Cordyceps (Traditional Healing Substance)	
Dried extract, 4 250-mg tablets daily. or Prepared tea, as directed on label.	Relieves ringing in the ears caused by fluid accumulation in the middle ear. Effective if taken in the first 6–8 weeks after the condition is first noticed, but is not useful if hairs within inner ear have been irreversibly damaged.[1] If there is no improvement after 8 weeks, discontinue usage. *Caution:* Avoid if a hormone-sensitive disorder is present, such as bladder cancer, melanoma, prostate disorders, or disorders of the female reproductive system.

Ginkgo (Modern Herbal Preparation)	
Ginkgolide extract, 1 40-mg tablet 3 times daily or 1 60-mg tablet 4 times daily.	Prevents free-radical damage. Effective if taken in the first 6–8 weeks after the condition is first noticed,[2] but is not useful if hairs within inner ear have been irreversibly damaged.[3] If there is no improvement after 8 weeks, discontinue usage.

Ligustrum (Herb)	
Tea, 1 c once daily.	Treats ringing in the ears, as well as spots before the eyes, dizziness, and prematurely gray hair. *Caution:* Avoid if there is diarrhea with undigested food in the stool.

KAMPO FORMULAS

See Chapter 4 for dosage information and discussions of individual formulas.

Gentiana Longdancao Decoction to Drain the Liver

Treats ringing in the ears or hearing loss accompanied by blurred vision, body aches, dizziness, headache, insomnia, irritability, dizziness, headache, palpitations, or sensation of heat in the head.

Caution: Should not be used by women who are trying to become pregnant.

Pill for Deafness That Is Kind to the Left Kidney

Treats ringing in the ears that sounds like swarming insects and is worse at night.

Six-Ingredient Pill With Rehmannia (Rehmannia-Six Combination)

Treats ringing in the ears accompanied by deafness and dizziness, and/or body aches, dry mouth, dry throat, low-grade fever, and spontaneous sweating.

Caution: Avoid if an estrogen-sensitive disorder is present, such as breast or uterine cancer, fibroids, ovarian cysts, or fibrocystic breast disease.

CONSIDERATIONS

❑ *See also* **Ménière's Disease.**

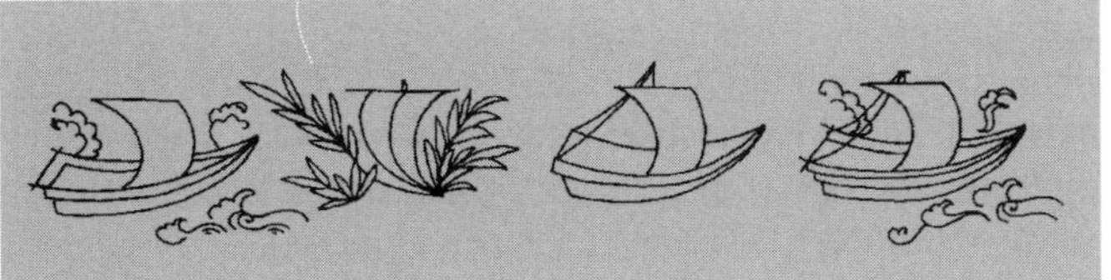

TUBERCULOSIS

Tuberculosis (TB) is a chronic disease caused by the bacterium *Mycobacterium tuberculosis.* Scientists estimate that as many as two billion people worldwide have been infected.[1] Tens of thousands of cases have recently appeared in the United States, generally in people whose immune systems have been weakened by HIV infection.

TB is passed when bacteria are released during coughing, sneezing, and speech. Symptoms include chronic cough with blood-streaked sputum, fatigue, fever and night sweats, and weight loss. In some people, the disease becomes inactive. In others, it takes an active form, and can cause severe lung damage. TB also can start tissue damage in the adrenal glands, bones, chest cavity, kidneys, eyes, sex organs, and throat.

TB bacteria are first met and engulfed by immune-system cells called macrophages. The bacteria can survive this process, but as long as they are confined to the macrophages, no symptoms occur. Once the macrophage dies and the bacterium escapes, though, the rest of the immune system sends out huge numbers of fresh immune-system cells to destroy the TB. In the process nearby healthy tissues are also destroyed.

TB is usually treated with a number of antibiotics at once. In a small number of people—especially in those who start, but do not finish, a course of treatment—the germ becomes resistant to antibiotics. The problem of drug resistance has become so widespread that doctors now often treat TB with chemotherapy, which controls TB without activating immune responses that destroy tissue.[2]

Kampo anticipated the modern explanation of tuberculosis as a process of destruction triggered by the immune system itself. Ancient scholars of Kampo conceived of TB as an insidious progression of invading "heat," or infection. This heat destroys the yin, or containing, energies of the organs it affects. They can no longer contain protective qi, or energy. This energy rises to the surface of the body as fire, where it causes night sweats and fever. This disruption of protective energy affects not just the lungs, but also the "kidneys" (in this case, corresponding to the adrenal glands) and liver. It causes *oketsu,* or "blood stasis," which blocks blood flow out of the lungs, leading to the coughing up of blood, and further disrupting the flow of protective energy. Kampo treatments for TB restore the yin, freeing the blood and allowing the organs to house the protective qi, and stop qi's transformation into fire. In effect, they do the work of the immune system without destroying healthy tissue.

Always take any drugs the doctor prescribes for TB exactly as given for the full course of treatment. Although Kampo treatments can help TB, they are most useful in increasing the effectiveness and diluting the side effects of standard treatment. Always consult a physician before taking any herbal treatment for TB.

INDIVIDUAL KAMPO TREATMENTS

See Chapter 3 for discussions of individual herbs, traditional healing substances, and modern herbal preparations, including directions for making tea.

SUGGESTED DOSAGES	COMMENTS
Bletilla (Herb)	
Use only under professional supervision.	Has helped patients who have not responded to other therapies; can reduce sputum production, coughing, and spitting and coughing of blood.[3]
Cardamom (Herb)	
Tincture (1:5), 10 drops 3 times daily. Place in a cup, add 2 tbsp water, and take in a single sip.	Increases the effectiveness of the antibiotic streptomycin against TB.[4]
Fennel Seed (Herb)	
Tea, 1 c 3 times daily.	Increases the effectiveness of streptomycin.[5] *Caution:* Avoid if an estrogen-sensitive disorder is present, such as bladder cancer, melanoma, or disorders of the female reproductive system.

KAMPO FORMULAS

See Chapter 4 for dosage information and discussions of individual formulas.

Minor Bupleurum Decoction and Tonify the Middle and Augment the Qi Decoction

This combination enables patients to take multiple forms of chemotherapy simultaneously. Minor Bupleurum Decoction increases the effectiveness of 3TC (lamivudine) treatment or 3TC plus AZT for TB patients who also have HIV.[6] Licorice, found in both formulas, reduces hepatitis flareups in patients infected with both hepatitis B and TB.[7]

Ophiopogonis Decoction

Traditional TB remedy for symptoms that include coughing and spitting of saliva, dry and uncomfortable sensation in the throat, dry mouth, red tongue, shortness of breath, and wheezing.

Caution: Use with caution if fever is present, and discontinue if preexisting fevers worsen.

CONSIDERATIONS

❑ *See also* **AIDS** and **HIV Infection.**

ULCERS

See **Peptic Ulcers.**

URINARY TRACT INFECTION

See **Bladder Infection.**

UTERINE CANCER

See **Endometrial Cancer.**

YEAST INFECTIONS

The human body is normally host to a great variety of bacteria and fungi which play neutral or even helpful roles in normal bodily functioning. A yeast infection occurs when one of these organisms, the yeast *Candida albicans,* grows out of control. *C. albicans* only becomes a problem when the "good" bacteria that normally keep it in check, such as *Lactobacillus acidophilus,* become weakened.

C. albicans is normally found in the gastrointestinal and female reproductive tracts. When it overgrows, it may show itself in babies as diaper rash. In adults, it can cause oral thrush—white plaques in the mouth and throat—or skin infections marked by redness, inflammation, and itching. In women, it can cause vulvovaginitis, which produces itching, burning, and a sticky white or yellow discharge.

The growth of *C. albicans* can be spurred by several factors. Broad-spectrum antibiotics can kill off the good bacteria that keep the yeast under control. When antibiotic treatment is over, new bacterial and fungal strains that are capable of resisting the antibiotic take hold. Also, *C. albicans* is a sugar-loving organism. Candidiasis, another term for *C. albicans* infection, can be aggravated by high levels of sugar in the diet, or by the high blood-sugar levels associated with diabetes. (Thrush is a common problem among diabetics.) And yeast can overgrow when the immune system does not function as it should, especially in people with HIV infection. *C. albicans* overgrowth is also associated with chronic fatigue syndrome, and with chronic skin or vaginal irritation.

"Damp heat" is the Oriental description of the body's environment during *C. albicans* infection. In Kampo, yeast infection is considered a parasitic disorder. When the digestive process is weakened by poor diet, stress, or the influence of "heart fire" (traumatic emotions), it can no longer separate pure from impure. This leads to an accumulation of dampness. Dampness, being heavy, sinks in the body. Damp, hot stasis in the "lower burner," or what conventional medicine calls the immune system, can interfere with the circulation of blood and energy, so candidiasis can be accompanied by what Kampo sees as blood circulation disorders, such as lack of periods, painful periods, or endometriosis.

Kampo therapies for yeast infection either act on the yeast directly, soothe inflammation, or correct underlying imbalances. With the exception of coptis, which should not be used for more than two weeks at a time, it may be necessary to take herbs for as long as six months to control yeast overgrowth. This is also true for the formula listed, unless it is taken in patent medicine form.

INDIVIDUAL KAMPO TREATMENTS

See Chapter 3 for discussions of individual herbs, traditional healing substances, and modern herbal preparations, including directions for making tea.

SUGGESTED DOSAGES	COMMENTS
Coptis (Herb)	
Dried herb, 1 500-mg capsule 3 times daily. or Tincture (1:5), 20 drops 3 times daily. Place in a cup, add 2 tbsp water, and take in a single sip.	Very effective against yeast and a number of other infections. *Caution:* Do not use during pregnancy or on a daily basis for more than 2 weeks at a time. Do not use with supplements that contain vitamin B_6 or the amino acid histidine.
Garlic (Herb)	
Cloves in food, preferably raw, 2–3 daily. The recommended form. or Tablets (including deodorized) as directed on label, at least 900 mg daily.	Kills yeasts. *Caution:* Do not use with the blood-thinner warfarin sodium (Coumadin). Garlic will counteract the effects of *Bifidus* and *Lactobacillus* cultures taken as digestive aids.
Lonicera (Herb)	
Dried herb, 1 1,000-mg capsule 3 times daily.	Treats burning urination caused by damp heat.
Plantain (Herb)	
Cold decoction made with ground seeds, ½ c after morning and evening meals, or ½ c at night. or Tea made with whole seeds, 1 c, up to 3 times daily.	Contains mucilages that soothe irritation.[1] To avoid absorption problems, take other oral medications 1 hour before using plantain.
Reishi (Modern Herbal Preparation)	
Dried extract, 3 1-g tablets 3 times daily. or Dried mushroom in food, approx. ¼–approx. ½ oz (5–10 g) daily. or Syrup, as directed on label. or Tea, 1 c 3 times daily. or Tincture (1:5), 1 tsp (4 ml) 3 times daily. Place in a cup, add 2 tbsp water, and take in a single sip.	Stops inflammatory processes.

KAMPO FORMULAS

See Chapter 4 for dosage information and discussions of individual formulas.

Gentiana Longdancao Decoction to Drain the Liver

Traditionally used to "draw fire" from the urinary tract and other parts of the body inflamed by infection. Especially useful when yeast infection is accompanied by emotional stress or overwork. Also appropriate when symptoms include eye irritation, fatigue, irritability, whitish vaginal discharge, painful urination, and swelling or inflammation in the ears. Used when a woman has a generally healthy constitution.

Caution: Should not be used by women who are trying to become pregnant.

CONSIDERATIONS

❑ Women who have recurrent yeast infections usually benefit from the reintroduction of friendly bacteria into the vagina. The best way to do this is by using commercially available *Lactobacillus acidophilus* capsules or tablets, sometimes labeled only as "Acidopholous." Place one or two capsules in the vagina before going to bed every other night for two weeks.

Appendices

Appendix A

Sources of Kampo Services and Products

This appendix provides information on where to find Kampo services and products, including a chart listing the brand-name versions of the formulas used in this book. It also includes a section on finding doctors who use loranthus in cancer treatment and some sources for general herbal information.

WHERE TO FIND KAMPO SERVICES

Over 9,600 professional herbalists throughout the United States prepare Kampo formulas from individual herbs. They can be located through the following associations.

American Association of Acupuncture and Oriental Medicine (AAAOM)

433 Front Street
Catasauqua PA 18032
610-266-1433
Fax: 610-264-2768
Website: www.aaom.org

Members of the AAAOM meet professional standards of training and practice. The group can provide names of local practitioners. The website contains a current list of imported herbal patent formulas that are contaminated with either heavy metals or prescription drugs.

American Association of Naturopathic Physicians

601 Valley Street, Suite 105
Seattle WA 98109
206-298-0126 (main offices)
206-298-0125 (referrals)
Fax: 206-298-0129
Website: www.naturopathic.org

Although naturopathic physicians are not necessarily trained in Kampo, any naturopath will recognize the conditions and formulas described in this book. The association provides referrals to a nationwide network of licensed practitioners.

WHERE TO FIND KAMPO PRODUCTS

All of the herbs and formulas listed in this book are available from Kampo physicians, herbalists, and retailers. As a general rule, it is always best to buy locally from people who provide information about their products. If the local herbalist does not have the herb or patent medicine for the formula fitting a specific diagnosis, contact one of the mail-order sources listed below. A Kampo physician or local herb retailer can also contact any of the wholesale suppliers of herbs and formulas listed.

All Kampo herbs are used in Chinese and Japanese medicine. To serve the Chinese community, some companies sell Kampo herbs and formulas under their Mandarin or Cantonese pinyin names, instead of their English or Japanese names. Formula strength also differs from manufacturer to manufacturer. Be sure to follow the manufacturer's dosage recommendations. See the chart that starts on page 302 for brand-name versions of the formulas mentioned in this book.

Every effort has been made to list all Kampo products and suppliers serving the United States. Product lines change, however, and some products included here may be discontinued, while new products may be added. Retailers can help locate current versions of Kampo products.

United States—Mail Order Marketers

Absolutely Healthy

c/o Intelligent Choice, Inc.
10490 Wilshire Blvd., Suite 402
Los Angeles CA 90024-4647
888–252–7873
310–474–1040 (overseas orders)
Fax (toll-free): 888–686–819
Fax (overseas): 310–474–2060
Website: info@AbsolutelyHealthy.com

LEM.

Blue Light, Inc.

111 South Cayuga Street
Ithaca NY 14850
888–258–3548
Fax: 888–666–9888
Website: www.treasureofeast.com

Freeze-dried herbal concentrates, patent medicines.

Bioherb Inc.
P.O. Box 611
Elk Grove IL 60009
708–364–5679

Maitake, polyporus, reishi, and shiitake mushroom products.

Center for Natural Wellness
334 Central Avenue
Albany NY 12206
518–449–2353
Fax: 518–449–1507
Website: www.chineseherbs.com

Herbs, patent medicines.

Crane Enterprises (sells to licensed practitioners only)
745 Falmouth Road
Mashpee MA 02649
800–227–4118
Fax: 508–329–2369
Website: www.craneherb.com

Herbs, formulas.

East Earth Herbs
P.O. Box 2802
Eugene OR 97402
800–258–6878

Reishi extracts, herbs.

East Earth Trade Winds
P.O. Box 493151
Redding CA 96049-3151
800–258–6878 (orders)
530–223–2346 (information)
Fax: 800–258–1384

Herbs, ready-made formula teas, patent medicines.

Excel
2552 Barrington Court
Hayward CA 94580
800–878–8871 ext. 50
510–278–8008 ext. 50 (outside the United States)
Fax: 510–782–4701
Website: www.excelmass.com

Lentinan, Kasugai, and Sugureta brand shiitake products.

GMHP
P.O. Box 515
Graton CA 95444
800–789–9121
Fax: 707–823–9091
E-mail: admin@health.pon.net

Mushrooms, mushroom products.

Green Kingdom Herbs
1610 Stanton Street
Bay City MI 48708
517–895–1275

Herbs, formulas, custom-made formulas.

Healing Arts Alliance Herbal Pharmacy
Phone / fax: 888–449–8908
Website: www.kshin.com

Herbs in bulk.

Health Concerns
8001 Capwell Drive
Oakland CA 94621-2107
510–639–0280
Fax: 510–639–9410

Reishi mushroom products, patent medicines (Health Concerns, Seven Forests).

Herbal Traditions
67 Santa Maria Drive
Novato CA 94947
415–893–0086
Website: www.herbaltraditions.com

Imported patent medicines, formulas.

JHS Natural Products
P.O. Box 50398
Eugene OR 97405
888–330–4691
Fax: 541–344–3107

PSK.

KPC Products, Inc.
16305–A Vineyard Boulevard
Morgan Hill CA 95037
800–572–8188 (orders)
408–782–1200 (information)
Fax: 408–782–1555
Website: www.kpc.com

KPC herbal formulas for southern California and southwestern states.

Maitake Products
P.O. Box 2354
Paramas NJ 07653
800–747–7418

Organically grown maitake mushroom products.

Maypro Industries
550 Mamaroneck Avenue
Harrison NY 10528
914–381–3808

PSK.

Min Tong Herbs
4175 Lakeside Drive, Suite 120
Richmond CA 94806
800–562–5777

Reishi products, Oriental herbs.

Miracle Exclusives
P.O. Box 349
Locust Valley NY 11560
800–645–6360
Shiitake extract.

Sinoking
116 Nassau Street
New York NY 10038
888–293–3298
Fax: 212–385–8949
Retail supplier of Chinese herbal formulas nationwide. Call for nearest location.

Spring Wind Herbs Company
2325 Fourth Street, #6
Berkeley CA 94710
800–588–4883 (orders)
510–849–1820 (information)
Fax: 510–849–4886
KPC herbal formulas for northern California and northwestern states.

Tong Ren Herbs
1130 North Dixie Highway
Hollywood FL 33020
800–219–5165 (orders)
954–929–9010 (information)
Fax: 954–929–0096
KPC herbal formulas for states east of the Mississippi.

Canada—Mail Order Marketers

Botanicum
492 Main Street
Winnipeg R3B 1B7 Manitoba
204–942–0950
Fax: 204–942–0405
KPC herbal formulas for western Canada.

Lotus Blanc
1127 rue Clark
Montreal H2Z 1K3 Quebec
888–532–5650
Fax: 514–672–4229
KPC herbal formulas for eastern Canada.

North American Reishi Ltd.
Box 1780
Gibson V0N 1V0 British Columbia
604–886–7799
Cordyceps, maitake, reishi, shiitake.

Uptown Health Foods
130-22529 Lougheed Highway
Maple Ridge V2X OL4 British Columbia
604–467–5587
E-mail: uptown@getset.com
Herbs, Zand formulas.

Australia—Information on Kampo Suppliers

Focus on Herbs
P.O. Box 203
Launceston 7250 Tasmania
Phone: +61–3–63301493
Fax: +61–3–63301498
Website: www.focusonherbs.com.au

Europe—Mail Order Marketer

Sinecura
Krijgslaan, 151
9000 Gent
Belgium
Phone: 32–9–244–6868
Fax: 32–9–244–6849
Website: www.sinecura.be
E-mail: sinecura@sinecura.be

Wholesalers and Brands Carried

Products from these suppliers are available to the trade only. No calls from individual product users will be accepted.

Brion Herbs Corporation
6380 East Sheri Lane
Long Beach CA 90815-4741
310–493–5405
Brion, Health Concerns.

East Earth Trade Winds
See retail listing on page 300.
Herbs, mixed raw herbs for teas, patent medicines.

Golden Flower Chinese Herbs
7001 San Antonio Drive NE #K
Albuquerque NM 87109
800–729–8509 (orders)
505–821–8857 (information)
Fax: 505–827–3285
Golden Flower.

Health Concerns
See retail listing on page 300.
Health Concerns, Seven Forests.

Herbal Apothecary
360 Oak Avenue
San Anselmo CA 94960
415–456–1184
Herbal Apothecary.

KPC Products, Inc.

See retail listing on page 300.
Wholesaler of KPC formulas throughout the United States.

Mayway Trading Corporation

1338 Cypress Street
Oakland CA 94607
510–208–3113
Fax: 510–208–3069
Chinese patent medicines.

NF Formulas

9775 S.W. Commerce Circle
Wilsonville OR 97070-9602
503–682–9755
Fax: 503–682–9529
NF.

Nuherbs

3820 Penniman Avenue
Oakland CA 94619-1759
510–534–4372
Fax: 510–534–4384
Chinese patent medicines.

Qualiherb

13340 East Firestone Blvd, Suite N
Santa Fe Springs CA 90670
E-mail: qualiherb@worldnet.att.net
Qualiherb, Sheng Chang.

Zand Chinese Classics

P.O. Box 5312
Santa Monica CA 90405
310–457–5535
Website: www.zand.com
Zand.

PATENT-MEDICINE VERSIONS OF KAMPO FORMULAS

All Kampo formulas used in this book that are available in patent-medicine form are listed below, along with patent-medicine brand names and manufacturers. Since many retailers, direct mail marketers, and wholesalers may not carry all brands, persistence in locating a specific product may be necessary. Formulas that are *not* available in patent-medicine form (see Chapter 4 and Part Two) are available by prescription from practitioners of Oriental medicine.

Formula	Patent-Medicine Brand Name (Manufacturer)
Arrest Wheezing Decoction	Ding Chuan Tang (Blue Light, KPC, Qualiherb) Mahuang & Ginkgo Combination (Blue Light, Brion, Herbal Apothecary, KPC, Ming Tong, Sheng Chang) Mahuang & Ginkgo Formula (Zand)
Astragalus Decoction to Construct the Middle	Astragalus Combination (Blue Light, KPC) Astragalus Formula (Center for Natural Wellness, Golden Flower) Huang Qi Jian Zhong Tang (Blue Light, Center for Natural Wellness, Golden Flower)
Augmented Four-Substance Decoction	Jia Wei Si Wu Tang (Center for Natural Wellness, Golden Flower) Tang Kuei and Salvia Formula (Center for Natural Wellness, Golden Flower)
Augmented Rambling Powder	Bupleurum & Peony Formula (Brion, Herbal Apothecary, KPC, Ming Tong, Sheng Chang, Zand) Free and Easy Wanderer Plus (Center for Natural Wellness, Golden Flower) Free Wanderer Plus (Kanpo) Jia Wei Xiao Yao San (Center for Natural Wellness, Golden Flower, KPC, Qualiherb) Relaxed Wanderer (Jade Pharmacy) Women's Balance (Health Apothecary, Health Concerns)
Biota Seed Pill to Nourish the Heart	Biota & Codonopsis Combination (Blue Light) Biota Sedative Pill (Asian Patents) Bo Zi Yang Xin Wan (Blue Light) Pai Tzu Yang Xin Wan (Asian Patents)
Bupleurum and Cinnamon Twig Decoction	Bupleurum & Cinnamon (Kanpo, NF, Qualiherb) Bupleurum & Cinnamon Combination (Blue Light, Brion, Herbal Apothecary, KPC, Ming Tong, Sheng Chang) Bupleurum & Cinnamon Formula (Zand) Chai Hu Gui Zhi Tang (Blue Light, KPC, Qualiherb) Ease 2 (Health Concerns)
Bupleurum and Kudzu Decoction to Release the Muscle Layer From *Medical Revelations*	Bupleurum & Pueraria Combination (Blue Light, Brion, KPC, Ming Tong, Qualiherb, Sheng Chang) Chai Ge Jie Ji Tang (Blue Light, KPC, Qualiherb)
Bupleurum, Cinnamon Twig, and Ginger Decoction	Bupleurum, Cinnamon & Ginger Combination (KPC) Chai Hu Gui Zhi Gan Jiang Tang (KPC)
Bupleurum Decoction to Clear the Liver	Bupleurum & Rehmannia (Qualiherb) Bupleurum & Rehmannia Combination (Blue Light, Brion, KPC, Sheng Chang) Chai Hu Qing Gan Tang (Blue Light) Chai Hu Qing Gen Tang (KPC, Qualiherb) Forsythia 18 (Seven Forests)
Bupleurum Plus Dragon Bone and Oyster Shell Decoction	Ardisia Sixteen (Seven Forests) Bupleurum & D.B. Combination (Blue Light) Bupleurum & Dragon Bone Combination (Brion, Herbal Apothecary, Ming Tong, Sheng Chang) Bupleurum & Dragon Bone Formula (Zand)

Formula	Patent-Medicine Brand Name (Manufacturer)
Bupleurum Plus Dragon Bone and Oyster Shell Decoction (cont.)	Bupleurum D Formula (Center for Natural Wellness, Golden Flower) Bupleurum with Dragon Bone & Oyster Shell (Kanpo) Calm Dragon Formula (K'an Traditionals) Chai Hu Jia Long Gu Mu Li Tang (Golden Flower) Chai Hu Long Gu Mu Li Tang (Blue Light, Center for Natural Wellness) Ease Plus (Health Concerns) Qing Gan (Probotannix) Zheng Jing (Probotannix)
Calm the Middle Powder	An Zhong San (KPC, Qualiherb) Cardamom & Fennel (Qualiherb) Cardamom and Fennel Formula (Brion, Ming Tong, Sheng Chang, Zand) Fennel & Galanga Formula (KPC) Peaceful Middle (Kanpo)
Calm the Stomach Powder	Magnolia & Ginger (Qualiherb) Magnolia & Ginger Formula (Blue Light) Magnolia & Ginger Powder (Brion, Herbal Apothecary, Ming Tong, Sheng Chang) Peaceful Stomach Tablets (Herbal Traditions) Ping Wei San (Blue Light, Qualiherb) Ping-Wei San (Herbal Traditions) Stomach Tabs (Health Concerns)
Capital Qi Pill	Rehmannia & Schizandra Formula (Brion, Sheng Chang)
Cimicifuga and Kudzu Decoction	Cimicifuga & Pueraria (Qualiherb) Cimicifuga & Pueraria Combination (Brion, KPC, Sheng Chang) Sheng Ma Ge Gen Tang (KPC, Qualiherb)
Cinnamon and Peony Decoction	Cinnamon & Peony (Qualiherb) Cinnamon & Peony Combination (Brion, Herbal Apothecary, Ming Tong, Sheng Chang) Cinnamon and Peony Combination (KPC) Gui Zhi Jia Shao Yao Tang (KPC, Qualiherb)
Cinnamon Twig and Ginseng Decoction	Cinnamon & Ginseng Combination (Brion)
Cinnamon Twig and Poria Pill	Cinnamon & Hoelen (NF, Qualiherb) Cinnamon & Hoelen Formula (Blue Light, Brion, Herbal Apothecary, KPC, Ming Tong, Sheng Chang, Zand) Cinnamon & Poria (Kanpo) Cinnamon & Poria Formula (Center for Natural Wellness) Cinnamon and Poria Formula (Golden Flower) Gui Zhi Fu Ling Wan (Blue Light, Center for Natural Wellness, Golden Flower, KPC, Qualiherb) Women's Palace (Jade Pharmacy)
Cinnamon Twig and Prepared Aconite Decoction	Cinnamon, Aconite & Ginger Combination (Brion)
Cinnamon Twig Decoction	Cinnamon Combination (Blue Light, Brion, KPC, Ming Tong, Qualiherb, Sheng Chang) Gui Zhi Tang (Blue Light, KPC, Qualiherb) Also contained in Children's Herbal Sentinel (Three Treasures)
Cinnamon Twig Decoction Plus Dragon Bone and Oyster Shell	Cinnamon & Dragon Bone Combination (Brion, KPC, Ming Tong, Sheng Chang) Cinnamon Twig Plus (Alembic Herbals) Gui Zhi Jin Long Gu Mu Li Tang (KPC)
Cinnamon Twig Decoction Plus Kudzu	Cinnamon & Pueraria Combination (Brion, Herbal Apothecary)
Clear Summerheat and Augment the Qi Decoction	Astragalus & Atractylodes (Qualiherb) Astragalus & Atractylodis Combination (KPC) Qing Shu (Alembic) Qing Shu Yi Qi Tang (KPC)
Coptis Decoction to Relieve Toxicity	Copticlear (K'an Traditionals) CoptiDetox (K'an Traditionals) Coptis & Scute Combination (Blue Light, Brion, Herbal Apothecary, KPC, Ming Tong, Sheng Chang) Coptis Detox (Kanpo) Coptis Relieve Fire (Qualiherb) Coptis Relieve Toxicity Formula (Center for Natural Wellness, Golden Flower) Huan Lian Jie Du Pian (Golden Flower) Huang Lian Jie Du Tang (Blue Light, Center for Natural Wellness, KPC, Qualiherb)
Drive Out Stasis From the Mansion of Blood Decoction	Blood Mansion (Alembic Herbals) Persica & Carthamus Combination (Blue Light, KPC, Sheng Chang) Red Stirring (Three Treasures) Xue Fu Zu Yu Tang (Alembic Herbals, Blue Light, KPC, Three Treasures)
Eight-Ingredient Pill With Rehmannia (Rehmannia-Eight Combination)	Ba Wei Di Huang Wan (Blue Light, Health Concerns, KPC, Qualiherb) Dynamic Warrior (Jade Pharmacy) Eight Flavors Rehmannia (Kanpo) Golden Book Tea Pills (Chinese patent medicine) Rehmannia 8 (Qualiherb) Rehmannia Eight (Health Concerns) Rehmannia Eight Formula (Blue Light, Brion, Herbal Apothecary, KPC, Ming Tong, Sheng Chang) Rehmannia Eight Plus (NF) Rehmannia Eight Plus Formula (Zand) Sexoton Pills (Chinese patent medicine)
Emperor of Heaven's Special Pill to Tonify the Heart	Celestial Emperor's Blend (K'an Traditionals) Emperor Tea (Asian Patents) Ginseng & Zizyphus (Qualiherb) Ginseng & Zizyphus Formula (Blue Light, KPC) Heavenly Empress (Women's Treasure) Tian Wang Bu Xin Dan (Blue Light, Golden Flower, KPC, Qualiherb, Women's Treasure)
Ephedra Decoction (Four Emperors Combination)	Mahuang (Kanpo) Mahuang Combination (Brion, Herbal Apothecary, KPC, Ming Tong, Qualiherb, Sheng Chang) Mahuang Tang (KPC, Qualiherb)
Ephedra, Apricot Kernel, Coix, and Licorice Decoction	Great White Lung Clearing Formula (K'an Traditionals) Ma Xing Gan Shi Tang (KPC) Ma Xing Shi Gan Tang (Blue Light, K'an Traditionals, Qualiherb) Mahuang & Apricot Seed (Qualiherb)

Formula	Patent-Medicine Brand Name (Manufacturer)
Ephedra, Apricot Kernel, Coix, and Licorice Decoction (cont.)	Mahuang & Apricot Seed Combination (Blue Light, KPC) Mahuang & Coix Combination (Brion, Ming Tong, Sheng Chang)
Ephedra, Apricot Kernel, Gypsum, and Licorice Decoction	Ephedra and Apricot Kernel Stop Cough Tablets (Herbal Traditions) Ma Hsing Chih Ke Pian (Herbal Traditions) Ma Hsing Chih Ke Pien (Chinese patent medicine) Ma Xing Shi Gan Tang (Blue Light) Mahuang & Apricot Seed Combination (Blue Light, Brion, Herbal Apothecary, Ming Tong, Sheng Chang) Mahuang, Apricot Seed, Licorice & Gypsum (Kanpo) Zhi Sou Ding Chuang Wan (Chinese patent medicine)
Ephedra, Asiasarum, and Prepared Aconite Decoction	Ma Huang Fu Zi Xi Xin Tang (KPC) Ma Huang Xi Xin Fu Zi Tang (Blue Light, Qualiherb) Mahuang & Asarum (Qualiherb) Mahuang & Asarum Combination (Blue Light, KPC)
Evodia Decoction	Evodia Combination (Blue Light, Brion, KPC, Ming Tong, Qualiherb, Sheng Chang) Wu Zhu Yu Tang (Blue Light, KPC, Qualiherb)
Five-Accumulation Powder	Dang Gui & Magnolia (Qualiherb) Five-Accumulation (Kanpo) Tangkuei & Magnolia Combination (Brion, Herbal Apothecary, Ming Tong, Sheng Chang) Tangkuei and Magnolia Five Formula (KPC) Wu Ji San (KPC)
Five-Ingredient Powder With Poria	Drain Dampness (Health Concerns) Gardenia & Hoelen Formula (Blue Light) Hoelen Five Formula (Zand) Hoelen Five Herb Formula (Brion, KPC, Ming Tong, Sheng Chang) Hoelen 5-Herb (Qualiherb) Li Shui (Probotannix) Poria Five (Kanpo) Water's Way (K'an Traditionals) Wu Lin San (Blue Light, KPC) Wu Ling San (Health Concerns, K'an Traditionals, Qualiherb)
Four-Gentleman Decoction	Four Gentleman (NF) Four Gentlemen Combo (Herbal Apothecary) Four Gentlemen Formula (Zand) Four Major Herb Combination (Blue Light, Sheng Chang) Major Four-Herbs Combination (Brion, Ming Tong) Si Jun Zi Tang (Blue Light)
Four-Substance Decoction	Angelica Restorative Formula (K'an Traditionals) Bend Bamboo (Three Treasures) Brighten the Eyes (Three Treasures) Dang Gui 4 (Qualiherb) Dang Gui Four Combination (Blue Light) Four Agents (Kanpo) Si Wu Tang (Blue Light, KPC) Tangkuei Four Combination (KPC, Sheng Chang) Tangkuei Four Formula (Brion, Herbal Apothecary, Ming Tong, Sheng Chang, Zand) Women's Essence (Jade Chinese Herbals) Included in Invigorate Blood and Stem Flow (Three Treasures) and Women's Rhythm (Jade Pharmacy)
Frigid Extremities Decoction	Aconite & G.L. Combination (Blue Light) Aconite, Ginger & Licorice Combination (Brion, KPC, Qualiherb, Sheng Chang) Si Ni Tang (Blue Light, KPC)
Frigid Extremities Powder	Bupleurum & Aurantium (Qualiherb) Bupleurum & Aurantium Formula (Blue Light) Bupleurum & Chih-shih Formula (Brion, Sheng Chang) Jin Qi Cao Stone Formula (Health Concerns) Si Ni San (Blue Light, Qualiherb)
Gastrodia and Uncaria Decoction	Gastrodia & Gambir Combination (KPC) Gastrodia & Uncaria Combination (Blue Light) Gastrodia and Uncaria Formula (Center for Natural Wellness, Golden Flower) Gastrodia Relieve Wind (Health Concerns) Jiang Ya (Probotannix) Tian Ma Gou Teng Yin (Blue Light, Center for Natural Wellness, Golden Flower, KPC, Qualiherb) Uncaria & Gastrodia (Qualiherb)
Gentiana Longdancao Decoction to Drain the Liver	Drain Fire (Three Treasures) Gentiana Combination (Blue Light, Brion, Herbal Apothecary, KPC, Ming Tong, Sheng Chang) Gentiana Drain Fire Formula (Center for Natural Wellness, Golden Flower) Gentiana Formula (Zand) Gentiana Liver-Purging (Kanpo) Gentiana 12 (Seven Forests) Long Dan Sie Gan Tang (Golden Flower) Long Dan Xie Gan Tang (Blue Light, Center for Natural Wellness, KPC; do not use for more than 1 week, as prolonged use can cause appetite loss and loose stools) Lung Tan Xie Gan Pill (Chinese patent medicine) Quell Fire (Jade Pharmacy) Yi Jun (Probotannix)
Ginseng Decoction to Nourish the Nutritive Qi	Ganoderma 18 (Seven Forests) Ginseng & Rehmannia Combination (KPC) Ginseng Combination (Brion, Ming Tong) Ginseng Construction Nourishing Pills (Asian Patents) Ginseng Nourishing Formula (Center for Natural Wellness, Golden Flower) Ginseng Nutri Combination (Blue Light) Ginseng Nutritive Combination (Herbal Apothecary, Sheng Chang) Ginseng Nutritive Formula (Zand) Ginseng Tonic Pills (Asian Patents) Lung Tan Xie Gan Pill (Chinese patent medicine, available from East Earth Trade Winds) Ren Shen Yang Rong Tang (Blue Light, Golden Flower) Ren Shen Yang Ying Tang (Golden Flower, KPC) Ren Shen Yang Ying Wan (Asian Patents, Center for Natural Wellness) Yang Ying Wan (Chinese patent medicine, available from Chinese pharmacies)
Guide Out the Red Powder	Dao Chi San (Blue Light, KPC, Qualiherb) Rehmannia Akebia Formula (KPC) Rehmannia & Akebia Formula (Blue Light, Brion, Qualiherb, Sheng Chang) Tao Chih Pien (Chinese patent medicine)

Formula	Patent-Medicine Brand Name (Manufacturer)
Hemp Seed Pill	Apricot Seed & Linum (Qualiherb) Apricot Seed & Linum Formula (Blue Light, Brion, Herbal Apothecary, KPC, Ming Tong, Sheng Chang) Ma Zi Ren Wan (Blue Light, Jade Chinese Herbals, KPC)
Honey-Fried Licorice Decoction	Baked Licorice (Kanpo) Baked Licorice Combination (Blue Light, Brion, Ming Tong, Qualiherb, Sheng Chang) Licorice Combination (KPC) Zhi Gan Cao Tang (Blue Light, KPC, Qualiherb)
Kidney Qi Pill From *The Golden Cabinet*	Dynamic Warrior (Jade Pharmacy) Essential Yang (Golden Flower) Jin Gui Shen Qi Wan (Blue Light)
Kudzu Decoction	Ge Gen Tang (Blue Light, Center for Natural Healing, Golden Flower, KPC) Pueraria (Kanpo) Pueraria Combination (Brion, Herbal Apothecary, KPC, Ming Tong, Qualiherb, Sheng Chang) Pueraria Formula (Blue Light, Center for Natural Healing, Golden Flower) Pueraria Plus Formula (Zand) Shu Jin 1 (Probotannix)
Ledebouriella Powder That Sagely Unblocks	Astragalus 18 Diet Fuel (Health Concerns) Fang Feng Tong Sheng San (Blue Light, KPC) Ledebouriella & Platycodon (Qualiherb) Ledebouriella & Platycodon Formula (Blue Light) Ledebouriella Wondrous Panacea (Kanpo) Siler & Platycodon Formula (Brion, KPC, Ming Tong, Sheng Chang, Zand)
Licorice, Wheat, and Jujube Decoction	Gan Mai Da Zao Tang (Blue Light, KPC) Licorice & Jujube Combination (Blue Light, Brion, KPC, Ming Tong, Sheng Chang)
Ligusticum Chuanxiong Powder to Be Taken With Green Tea	Chuan Xiong Cha Tiao San (Blue Light, KPC) Chuan Xiong Cha Tiao Wan (Herbal Traditions) Cnidium & Tea Formula (Blue Light, Brion, KPC, Ming Tong, Sheng Chang) Febrifugal Pills (Chinese patent medicine) Ligusticum Green Tea Pill (Herbal Traditions)
Lily Bulb Decoction to Preserve the Metal	Bai He Gu Jin Tang (Blue Light, Center for Natural Healing, KPC, Qualiherb) Lily Combination (KPC, Qualiherb) Lily Formula (Blue Light) Lily Preserve Metal Formula (Center for Natural Healing)
Lonicera and Forsythia Powder (Honeysuckle and Forsythia Powder)	Lonicera and Forsythia Heat-Dispelling Tablets (Herbal Traditions) Yin Chiao (Asian Patents, available with and without sugar coating) Yin Chaio Chieh Tu Pien (Herbal Traditions) Yin Chiao Formula (Center for Natural Wellness, Golden Flower)
Major Bupleurum Decoction	Da Chai Hu Tang (Blue Light, KPC, Qualiherb) Major Bupleurum (Kanpo) Major Bupleurum Combination (Blue Light, Brion, KPC, Ming Tong, Qualiherb, Sheng Chang)
Major Construct the Middle Decoction	Da Jian Zhong Tang (Blue Light, KPC) Major Zanthoxylum (Qualiherb) Major Zanthoxylum Combination (Blue Light, Brion, KPC, Ming Tong, Sheng Chang)
Major Ledebouriella Decoction	Clematis 19 (Seven Forests) Da Fang Feng Tang (KPC) Major Siler Combination (Brion, KPC)
Major Order the Qi Decoction	Da Cheng Qi Tang (Blue Light, KPC, Qualiherb) Major Rhubarb Combination (Blue Light, Brion, Herbal Apothecary, KPC, Qualiherb, Sheng Chang)
Minor Bluegreen Dragon Decoction	Blue Green Lung Clearing Formula (K'an Traditionals) Minor Blue Dragon (Health Concerns, Qualiherb) Minor Blue Dragon Combination (Blue Light, Brion, KPC, Ming Tong, Sheng Chang) Minor Blue Dragon Formula (Center for Natural Wellness, Golden Flower, Herbal Apothecary, Zand) Minor Cyan Dragon (Kanpo) Xiao Qing Long Tang (Blue Light, Center for Natural Wellness, Golden Flower, K'an Traditionals, KPC, Qualiherb)
Minor Bupleurum Decoction	Minor Bupleurum (Kanpo, NF) Minor Bupleurum Combination (Blue Light, Brion, KPC, Ming Tong, Sheng Chang) Minor Bupleurum Formula (Center for Natural Wellness, Golden Flower, Qualiherb, Zand) Minor Bupleurum Formulation (K'an Traditionals) Xiao Chai Hu Tang (Blue Light, Center for Natural Wellness, Golden Flower, KPC, also available as an imported Chinese patent medicine from East Earth Trade Winds)
Minor Construct the Middle Decoction	Minor Cinnamon & Peony (Qualiherb) Minor Cinnamon & Peony Combination (Blue Light, Brion, KPC, Ming Tong, Sheng Chang) Xiao Jian Zhong Tang (Blue Light, KPC)
Ophiopogonis Decoction	Juan Tong (Probotannix) Mai Men Dong Tang (Blue Light) Ophiopogon (Kanpo) Ophiopogon Combination (Blue Light, Brion, Herbal Apothecary, KPC, Ming Tong, Qualiherb, Sheng Chang)
Oyster Shell Powder	Mu Li (Qualiherb) Oyster Shell (Qualiherb)
Peach Blossom Decoction	Kaolin & Oryza Combination (Brion)
Peach Pit Decoction to Order the Qi	Persica & Rhubarb Combination (Blue Light, Brion, Herbal Apothecary, Ming Tong, Qualiherb, Sheng Chang) Persica Qi-Supporting (Kanpo) Tao He Cheng Qi Tang (Blue Light, KPC, Qualiherb)
Peony and Licorice Decoction	Corydalis Formula (Golden Flower) Jie Jing (Probotannix) Peony & Licorice (Kanpo, Qualiherb) Peony & Licorice Combination (Blue Light, Brion, KPC, Ming Tong, Sheng Chang) Shao Yao Gan Cao Tang (Blue Light, KPC, Qualiherb) SPZM (Health Concerns)
Pill for Deafness That Is Kind to the Left Kidney	Tso-Tzu Otic Pills (Asian Patents, also available from East Earth Trade Winds)

Formula	Patent-Medicine Brand Name (Manufacturer)
Pinellia and Magnolia Bark Decoction	Ban Xia Hou Po Tang (Blue Light, Center for Natural Healing, Golden Flower, KPC, Qualiherb) Pinellia & Magnolia (Kanpo, Qualiherb) Pinellia & Magnolia Bark Combination (Golden Flower) Pinellia & Magnolia Combination (Blue Light, Brion, Herbal Apothecary, KPC, Ming Tong, Sheng Chang) Pinellia and Magnolia Bark Formula (Center for Natural Healing, Golden Flower)
Pinellia, Atractylodis Macrocephala, and Gastrodia Decoction	Ban Xia Tian Ma Bai Zhu Tang (Blue Light, KPC) Pinellia & Gastrodia Combination (Blue Light, Brion, KPC, Ming Tong, Sheng Chang)
Pinellia Decoction to Drain the Epigastrium	Ban Xia Xie Xin Tang (KPC, Qualiherb) Fu-Shen 16 (Seven Forests) Pinellia Combination (KPC, Qualiherb)
Polyporus Decoction	Polyporus (Kanpo) Polyporus Combination (Blue Light, Brion, Ming Tong, Qualiherb, Sheng Chang) Zhu Ling (Qualiherb) Zhu Ling Tang (Blue Light)
Prepared Aconite Decoction	Aconite Combination (Brion)
Prolong Life Decoction	Mahuang & Ginseng Combination (Brion, KPC, Ming Tong, Sheng Chang) Xu Ming Tang (KPC)
Rambling Powder	Bupleurum and Danggui (Qualiherb) Bupleurum and Tang-kuei Formula (Center for Natural Wellness, Golden Flower) Free Flow (Three Treasures) Freeing the Moon (Three Treasures) Hsiao Yao Wan (Chinese import, available through East Earth Trade Winds) Mind Peak (Jade Chinese Herbals) Relaxed Wanderer (Jade Pharmacy) Tangkuei and Bupleurum Formula (KPC) Tiao Jing (Probotannix) Xiao Yao San (Center for Natural Wellness, Golden Flower, KPC)
Regulate the Stomach and Order the Qi Decoction	Rhubarb & Mirabilitum (Qualiherb) Rhubarb & Mirabilitum Combination (Brion, KPC, Sheng Chang) Stomach-Regulating, Qi-Supporting (Kanpo) Tiao Wei Cheng Qi Tang (KPC, Qualiherb)
Restore the Right Kidney Pill	Ease the Journey Yang (Three Treasures) Eucommia & Rehmannia Formula (KPC) Restore Right Kidney Pill (Blue Light, Three Treasures) Strengthen the Root (Three Treasures) You Gui Wan (Blue Light, KPC)
Restore the Spleen Decoction	Calm the Spirit (Three Treasures) Gather Vitality (Jade Pharmacy) Ginseng & Longan (Qualiherb) Ginseng & Longan Combination (Blue Light, KPC) Gui Pi Tang (Blue Light, Jade Pharmacy, KPC, Qualiherb, Three Treasures) Gui Pi Wan (Chinese import, available through East Earth Trade Winds) Jen Shem (Health Concerns)

Formula	Patent-Medicine Brand Name (Manufacturer)
Rhubarb and Licorice Decoction	Rhubarb & Licorice (Kanpo) Rhubarb & Licorice Combination (Brion)
Rhubarb and Moutan Decoction	Rhubarb & Moutan Combination (Brion, Ming Tong, Sheng Chang)
Settle the Emotions Pill	Ding Xin Wan (Chinese patent medicine)
Shut the Sluice Pill	Firm Vessel (Jade) Sang Piao Xiao (Jade) Suo Quan Wan (Jade) Available to practitioners only from Crane Herb Company
Six-Gentleman Decoction	Liu Jun Zi Tang (Blue Light, Center for Natural Wellness, KPC) Major Six-Herbs Combination (Brion, Ming Tong) Prosperous Farmer (Jade Pharmacy) Six Gentlemen (Kanpo) Six Gentlemen Formula (Center for Natural Wellness, Golden Flower) Six Major Herb (Qualiherb) Six Major Herb Combination (Blue Light, KPC, Sheng Chang)
Six-Ingredient Pill With Rehmannia (Rehmannia-Six Combination)	Liu Wei Di Huang Wan (Blue Light, Golden Flower, KPC, Qualiherb, also available as a Chinese import from East Earth Trade Winds) Nourish Essence Formula (Golden Flower) Quiet Contemplative (Jade Pharmacy) Rehmannia 6 (Qualiherb) Rehmannia Six Formula (Blue Light, Brion, Herbal Apothecary, KPC, Ming Tong, Sheng Chang, Zand) Six Flavor Tea (Asian Patents, also available as import from East Earth Trade Winds) Six Flavors Rehmannia (Kanpo)
Stephania and Astragalus Decoction	Fang Ji Huang Qi Tang (Blue Light, KPC, Qualiherb) Stephania & Astraglus (Qualiherb) Stephania & Astragalus Combination (Blue Light, KPC) Stephania & Hoelen Combination (Brion)
Tang-Kuei and Peony Powder	Dan Gui & Peony (Kanpo) Dang Gui & Peony Formula (Blue Light, KPC) Dang Gui Shao Yao San (Blue Light, Center for Natural Wellness, Golden Flower, Qualiherb) Danggui & Peony (Qualiherb) Tang Kuei and Peony Formula (Center for Natural Wellness, Golden Flower, KPC) Tangkuei & Peony (NF) Tangkuei & Peony Formula (Brion, Herbal Apothecary, Ming Tong, Sheng Chang, Zand)
Tang-Kuei, Gentiana Long-dancao, and Aloe Pill	Dang Gui Long Hui Wan w/o She Xiang (KPC) Tangkuei, Gentiana & Aloe Formula, Minus Musk (KPC)
Ten-Significant Tonic Decoction (All-Inclusive Great Tonifying Decoction)	General Tonic Formula (Center for Natural Wellness, Golden Flower) General Tonic Pills (Chinese patent medicine) Ginseng & Dang Gui Ten Combination (Blue Light) Ginseng & Danggui 10 (Qualiherb) Ginseng & Dongquai Combination (Zand) Ginseng & Tangkuei Ten Combination (Brion, KPC, Ming Tong, Sheng Chang)

Formula	Patent-Medicine Brand Name (Manufacturer)
Ten-Significant Tonic Decoction (cont.)	Qiang Jin 1 (Probotannix) Shi Quan Da Bu Tang (Blue Light, KPC, Qualiherb) Shi Quan Da Bu Wan (Center for Natural Wellness, Golden Flower) Shih Chuan Da Wu Wang (Chinese patent medicine, available from East Earth Trade Winds) Ten Flavor Tea (Chinese patent medicine, available from East Earth Trade Winds)
Tonify the Middle and Augment the Qi Decoction	Arouse Vigor (Jade Pharmacy) Bu Zhong Yi Qi Tang (Blue Light, Center for Natural Wellness, Golden Flower, KPC, Qualiherb) Center-Supplementing, Qi Boosting (Kanpo) Central Chi Pills (Asian Patents) Central Qi Pills (Chinese patent medicine) Ginseng & Astragalus (NF, Qualiherb) Ginseng & Astragalus Combination (Blue Light, Brion, Golden Flower, Herbal Apothecary, KPC, Ming Tong, Sheng Chang) Ginseng & Astragalus Formula (Center for Natural Wellness, Zand) Tonify Qi and Ease the Muscles (Three Treasures) Yi Qi (Probotannix) Also available as herb mixture for making tea from East Earth Trade Winds
Trauma Pill	Die Da Wan (Center for Natural Wellness, Golden Flower) Tieh Ta Formula (Center for Natural Wellness, Golden Flower)
True Warrior Decoction	Ginger, Aconite, Hoelen & Peony Combination (KPC) True Warrior (Kanpo) Vita Combination (Brion, Ming Tong) Vital Energy Combination (Sheng Chang) Vitality Combination (Herbal Apothecary) Zhen Wu Tang (KPC)
Two-Cured Decoction	Citrus & Pinellia (Qualiherb) Citrus & Pinellia Combination (Blue Light, KPC) Er Chen Tang (Blue Light, KPC, Qualiherb, Three Treasures) Limpid Sea (Three Treasures)
Unblock the Orifices and Invigorate the Blood Decoction	Musk & Persica (Qualiherb) Musk & Persica Combination (Kanpo) Tong Qiao Huo Xue Tang (Qualiherb)
Warm the Gallbladder Decoction (Bamboo and Hoelen Decoction)	Bamboo & Hoelen Combination (Herbal Apothecary, Sheng Chang) Clear Phlegm (Health Concerns) Clear the Moon (Women's Treasures) Clear the Soul (Three Treasures) Hoelen & Bamboo Combination (Blue Light, Brion, KPC, Ming Tong) Wen Dan Tang (Blue Light, KPC)
Warm the Menses Decoction	Tangkuei & Evodia Combination (Brion, KPC, Ming Tong, Sheng Chang) Warm the Menses (Women's Treasure) Wen Jing Tang (KPC) Included in Women's Journey (Jade Pharmacy)
Warming and Clearing Decoction	Tangkuei & Gardenia Combination (Brion, KPC, Ming Tong, Sheng Chang) Warming & Clearing (Kanpo) Wen Qing Yin (KPC)
White Tiger Decoction	Bai Hu Tang (KPC) Gypsum Combination (Brion, Sheng Chang, KPC)
White Tiger Plus Ginseng Decoction	Ginseng & Gypsum Combination (Brion, Sheng Chang)
Yellow Dragon Decoction	Coptis Combination (KPC) Huang Lian Tang (KPC)

WHERE TO FIND DOCTORS WHO USE LORANTHUS IN CANCER TREATMENT

While this section does list American sources of information on loranthus, centers specializing in the use of this herb for cancer treatment are concentrated in Europe. It is important to keep in mind that loranthus extracts are used only in conjunction with other, medically approved cancer treatments.

Hufeland Klinik for Holistic Immunotherapy

Bismarckstr. 16
D-6990 Bad Mergentheim
Germany
011–49–7931–7082

Klinik Friedenweiler

Kurhausweg 2
D-7829 Friedenweiler
Germany
Phone: 011–07651–208–0
Fax: 011–07651–208–116

Lukas Klinic

CH-4144 Arlesheim
Switzerland
011–41–61–72–3333

Physicians Association for Anthroposophical Medicine

P.O. Box 269
Kimberton PA 19442

Rudolf Steiner Fellowship Foundation

241 Hungry Hollow Road
Spring Valley NY 10977
914–356–8494
Fax: 914–425–6835

GENERAL HERBAL INFORMATION

American Botanical Council

P.O. Box 144345
Austin TX 78714
512–926–4900
Website: www.herbalgram.org

The Herb Research Foundation

1007 Pearl Street
Suite 200
Boulder CO 80302
303–449–2265
Website: www.herbs.org

Appendix B

Identifying Japanese Medicinal Herbs

This appendix lists the common name(s), botanical name(s), pharmaceutical name, part of plant used, plant family name, and Japanese-, Chinese-, and Korean-language names for each of the herbs and some of the other medicinal substances described in Chapter 3. This appendix also lists common dosages for use of the herb when used as a single preparation—that is, not as part of a formula—and tips for recognizing good quality in the unprocessed herb.

Aconite

Other common names: Blue monkshood, wolfbane
Botanical name: *Aconitum carmichaeli* Debx.; European aconite is *Aconitum mapellus* L.
Pharmaceutical name: Radix Lateralis Aconiti Carmichaeli Praeparata
Part of plant used: Root, only after steaming or boiling
Plant family: Ranunculaceae (Peony Family)
Japanese name: *Bushi*
Chinese name: *Fu Zi*
Korean name: *Puja*
Dosage when used by itself in decoctions: 1.5 –15.0 grams
How to recognize good quality in the unprocessed herb: Large, solid, salty white surface

Acorus

Other common names: Gramineus, sweetflag rhizome
Botanical name: *Acorus gramineus* Soland.
Pharmaceutical name: Rhizoma Acori Graminei
Part of plant used: Rhizome
Plant family: Araceae (Sweet Flag Family)
Japanese name: *Shobu*
Chinese name: *Shi Chang Pu*
Korean name: *Ch'angp'o*
Dosage when used by itself in decoctions: 3.0–9.0 grams
How to recognize good quality in the unprocessed herb: Firm but not fibrous, fragrant, white cross section

Agrimony

Other common names: Cocklebur
Botanical name: *Agrimonia pilosa* Ledeb. var. *japonica (Miq.) Nakai; American and European herbalists usually substitute Agrimonia eupatoria* L.
Pharmaceutical name: Herba Agrimoniae Pilosae
Part of plant used: Above-ground parts
Plant family: Rosaceae (Rose Family)
Japanese name: *Senkakuso*
Chinese name: *Xian He Cao*
Korean name: *Sonhakch'o*
Dosage when used by itself in decoctions: 9.0–30.0 grams
How to recognize good quality in the unprocessed herb: Red-purple stems

Akebia (Mu Tong)

Botanical name: *Akebia trifoliata* (Thunb.) Koidz. var. *australis* (Diels) Rehd., *A. quinata* (Thunb.) Decne. Varieties of wild ginger (Artistolochia) and clematis are also substituted for this herb
Pharmaceutical name: Caulis Mutong
Part of plant used: Stalk and stem; TCM practitioners also use fruit for some conditions
Plant family: Lardizabalaceae (Akebia Family)
Japanese name: *Mokutsu*
Chinese name: *Mu Tong*
Korean name: *Mokt'ong*
Dosage when used by itself in decoctions: 3.0–9.0 grams
How to recognize good quality in the unprocessed herb: Green without dust or roots

Alisma

Other common names: Water plantain
Botanical name: *Alisma plantago-aquatica* L. var. *orientale* Samuels
Pharmaceutical name: Rhizoma Alismatis Orientalitis
Part of plant used: Rhizome
Plant family: Alismataceae (Water Lily Family)
Japanese name: *Takusha*
Chinese name: *Ze Xie, Fu Ze Xie*
Korean name: *T'aeksa*
Dosage when used by itself in decoctions: 6.0–15.0 grams
How to recognize good quality in the unprocessed herb: Lustrous, off-white color, powdery

Aloe

Other common names: Aloe vera
Botanical name: *Aloe vera* N.L. Burm
Pharmaceutical name: Herba Aloes
Part of plant used: Dried concentrate of juice found in the leaf
Plant family: Liliaceae (Lily Family)
Japanese name: *Rokai*
Chinese name: *Lu Hui*
Korean name: *Nohwa*
Dosage when used by itself in decoctions: 0.3–1.5 grams
How to recognize good quality in the unprocessed herb: Dark green, lustrous color, bitter taste

Amaranth (Achyranthis)

Other common names: Tuniuxi root
Botanical name: *Achyranthes aspea* L., *A. longifolia* Mak.
Pharmaceutical name: Radix Achyranthis
Part of plant used: Root
Plant family: Amaranthaceae (Amaranth Family)
Japanese name: *Dogoshitsu*
Chinese name: *Tu Niu Xi*
Korean name: *T'ousul*
Dosage when used by itself in decoctions: 15.0–30.0 grams
How to recognize good quality in the unprocessed herb: White cross section, no root hairs

American Ginseng

Botanical name: *Panax quinquefolium* L.
Pharmaceutical name: Panacis Quinquefolii Radix
Part of plant used: Root
Plant family: Araliaceae (Ginseng Family)
Japanese name: *Seiyojin*
Chinese name: *Xi Yang Shen*
Korean name: *Soyangsam*
Dosage when used by itself in decoctions: 2.0–9.0 grams
How to recognize good quality in the unprocessed herb: Hard, lightweight, dense striations on the surface, aromatic, sweet with bitter aftertaste

Anemarrhena

Other common names: Anemarrhena rhizome
Botanical name: *Anemarrhena asphodeloides* Bge.
Pharmaceutical name: Rhizoma Anemarrhenae Asphodeloidis
Part of plant used: Rhizome
Plant family: Liliaceae (Lily Family)
Japanese name: *Chimo*
Chinese name: *Zhi Mu, Zhi Mu Rou*
Korean name: *Chimo*
Dosage when used by itself in decoctions: 6.0–12.0 grams
How to recognize good quality in the unprocessed herb: Hard, thick root with yellowish white cross section

Angelica Dahurica (Wild Angelica)

Other common names: Chinese angelica root
Botanical name: *Angelica dahurica* (Fisch. Ex Hoffm.) Benth. et Hook.
Pharmaceutical name: Radix Angelicae Dahuricae
Part of plant used: Root
Plant family: Apiaceae (Parsley Family)
Japanese name: *Byakushi*
Chinese name: *Bai Zhi (Chuan bai zhi, Hang bai zhi)*
Korean name: *Paegchi*
Dosage when used by itself in decoctions: 3.0–9.0 grams
How to recognize good quality in the unprocessed herb: Aromatic, dark yellow root bark, no branches on taproot

Apricot Seed

Other common names: Apricot kernel
Botanical name: *Prunus armeniaca* L.
Pharmaceutical name: Semen Pruni Armeniacae
Part of plant used: Shelled kernels of seed
Plant family: Rosaceae (Rose Family)
Japanese name: *Kyonin*
Chinese name: *Xing Ren*
Korean name: *Sain*
Dosage when used by itself in decoctions: 3.0–9.0 grams. *Never eat whole apricot kernels*
How to recognize good quality in the unprocessed herb: Bitter, full, intact, oily

Arisaema

Other common names: Jack-in-the-pulpit rhizome, wild turnip
Botanical name: *Arisaemea consanguineum* Schott, *Arisaema amurense* Maxim.
Pharmaceutical name: Rhizoma Arisaematis
Part of plant used: Rhizome
Plant family: Araceae (Sweet Flag Family)
Japanese name: *Tennansho*
Chinese name: *Tian Nan Xing*
Korean name: *Ch'onnamsong*
Dosage when used by itself in decoctions: 4.5–9.0 grams
How to recognize good quality in the unprocessed herb: Firm yet powdery, white

Artemisia

Other common names: Artemisia yinchenhao, capillaris
Botanical name: *Artemisia capillaris* Thunb.
Pharmaceutical name: Herba Artemisiae Annuae
Part of plant used: Above-ground parts
Plant family: Asteraceae (Composite Family)
Japanese name: *Inchinko*
Chinese name: *Yin Chen Hao*
Korean name: *Kyunchinho*
Dosage when used by itself in decoctions: 3.0–24.0 grams
How to recognize good quality in the unprocessed herb: Fragrant and green

Asiasarum

Other common names: Asarum, Chinese wild ginger
Botanical name: *Asarum sieboldii* Miq.
Pharmaceutical name: Herba cum Radice Asari
Part of plant used: Roots and above-ground parts
Plant family: Aristolochiaceae (Wild Ginger Family)
Japanese name: *Saishin*
Chinese name: *Xi Xin*
Korean name: *Sesin*
Dosage when used by itself in decoctions: 1.0–3.0 grams
How to recognize good quality in the unprocessed herb: Green leaves and gray-yellow root. Should make the tongue numb when tasted

Asparagus Root

Botanical name: *Asparagus cochinchinensis* (Lour.) Merr. The garden asparagus, *Asparagus officinale* L., has the same medicinal properties
Pharmaceutical names: Tuber Asparagi Cochinchinensis
Part of plant used: Root or tuber
Plant family: Liliaceae (Lily Family)
Japanese name: *Tenmondo*
Chinese name: *Tian Men Dong*
Korean name: *Ch'onmundong*
Dosage when used by itself in decoctions: 6.0–15.0 grams
How to recognize good quality in the unprocessed herb: Translucent, yellow-white

Astragalus

Other common names: Locoweed, milk vetch root
Botanical name: *Astragalus membranaceus* (Fisch.) Bge.

Pharmaceutical name: Radix Astragali Membranaceus
Part of plant used: Root
Plant family: Fabaceae (Legume Family)
Japanese name: *Ogi*
Chinese name: *Huang Qi*
Korean name: *Hwanggi*
Dosage when used by itself in decoctions: 9.0–60.0 grams
How to recognize good quality in the unprocessed herb: Firm yet cottonlike, few striations, long, sweet, thick

Atractylodis, Red

Other common names: Black atractylodis, lance-leafed atractylodis
Botanical name: *Atractylodes lancea* Thunb.
Pharmaceutical name: Rhizoma Atractylodis
Part of plant used: Rhizome
Plant family: Astreaceae (Composite Family)
Japanese name: *Sojutsu*
Chinese name: *Cang Zhu*
Korean name: *Ch'angch'ul*
Dosage when used by itself in decoctions: 4.5–9.0 grams
How to recognize good quality in the unprocessed herb: Aromatic, cinnabar-colored cross section, lacking small hairs on surface

Atractylodis, White

Other common names: White atractylodis rhizome
Botanical name: *Atractylodes macrocephala* Koidz.
Pharmaceutical name: Rhizoma Atractylodis Macrocephalae
Part of plant used: Rhizome
Plant family: Asteraceae (Composite Family)
Japanese name: *Byakujutsu*
Chinese name: *Bai Zhu*
Korean name: *Paekch'ul*
Dosage when used by itself in decoctions: 4.5–9.0 grams
How to recognize good quality in the unprocessed herb: Firm, fragrant, long, solid, creamy white color in cross section

Bamboo Shavings

Botanical name: *Phyllostachys nigra* (Lodd.) Munro var. *henonis* (Mitf.) Stapf ex Rendle
Pharmaceutical name: Caulis Bambusae in Taeniis
Part of plant used: Stem
Plant family: Gramineae (Grass Family)
Japanese name: *Chikujo*
Chinese name: *Zhu Ru*
Korean name: *Chukchu*
Dosage when used by itself in decoctions: 4.5–9.0 grams (1 or 2 bundles)
How to recognize good quality in the unprocessed herb: Soft, thin, yellow-green

Barley Sprouts

Other common names: Barley shoots
Botanical name: *Hordeum vulgare* L.
Pharmaceutical name: Fructus Hordei Vulgaris Germinantus
Part of plant used: Sprouts
Plant family: Gramineae (Grass Family)
Japanese name: *Bakuga*
Chinese name: *Mai Ya*
Korean name: *Maek'ga*
Dosage when used by itself in decoctions: 6.0–60.0 grams
How to recognize good quality in the unprocessed herb: Fully sprouted, large, and yellow

Benincasa

Other common names: Petha, winter melon, wax gourd
Botanical name: *Benicasa hispida* (Thunb.)
Pharmaceutical name: Semen Benincasae Hispidae
Part of plant used: Seed
Plant family: Cucurbitaceae (Gourd Family)
Japanese name: *Tokanin*
Chinese name: *Dong Gua Ren*
Korean name: *Tonggwain*
Dosage when used by itself in decoctions: 3.0–12.0 grams
How to recognize good quality in the unprocessed herb: Full, round, white seed

Biota

Other common names: Arborvitae
Botanical name: *Biota orientalis* (L.) Endl.
Pharmaceutical name: Semen Biotae Orientalis
Part of plant used: Seed
Plant family: Cupressaceae (Cypress Family)
Japanese name: *Hakushinin*
Chinese name: *Bai Zi Ren*
Korean name: *Paekchain*
Dosage when used by itself in decoctions: 6.0–18.0 grams
How to recognize good quality in the unprocessed herb: Full, oily, yellowish white

Bitter Melon

Other common names: Balsam pear, bitter gourd, cerasee, momordica
Botanical name: *Momordica charantia* L.
Pharmaceutical name: Fructus Mormordicae Charantiae
Part of plant used: Fruit, whole or juiced
Plant family: Cucurbitaceae (Gourd Family)
Japanese name: *Rahanka*
Chinese name: *Luo Han Guo*
Korean name: *Nahan'gwa*
Dosage when used by itself in decoctions: 25.0–50.0 grams juice
How to recognize good quality in the unprocessed herb: Solid, green fruit covered with bumps

Bitter Orange (Whole Bitter Orange)

Other common names: Chih-shih
Botanical name: *Citrus aurantium* L.
Pharmaceutical name: Fructus Immaturus Citri Aurantii
Part of plant used: Whole fruit
Plant family: Rutaceae (Citrus Family)
Japanese name: *Kijitsu*
Chinese name: *Zhi Shi*
Korean name: *Chisil*
Dosage when used by itself in decoctions: 3.0–9.0 grams
How to recognize good quality in the unprocessed herb: Solid fruit with blue-black rind

Bitter Orange Peel

Botanical name: *Citrus reticulata* Blanco
Pharmaceutical name: Pericarpium Citri Reticulatae
Part of plant used: Rind of the fruit
Plant family: Rutaceae (Citrus Family)
Japanese name: *Chinpi*
Chinese name: *Chen Pi, Ju Pi, Guang Gan Pi, Guang Chen Pi*
Korean name: *Chinp'i*
Dosage when used by itself in decoctions: 3.0–9.0 grams
How to recognize good quality in the unprocessed herb: Oily, aromatic, pliable, thin-skinned pieces of peel in large sections

Black Cardamom

Other common names: Alpinia oxyphylla fruit, bitter-seeded cardamom, intelligence nut
Botanical name: *Alpinia oxyphylla* Miq.
Pharmaceutical name: Fructus Alpiniae Oxyphyllae
Part of plant used: Seed
Plant family: Zingiberaceae (Ginger Family)
Japanese name: *Yakuchinin*
Chinese name: *Yi Zhi Ren*
Korean name: *Ikchiin*
Dosage when used by itself in decoctions: 3.0–9.0 grams
How to recognize good quality in the unprocessed herb: Intensely aromatic

Black Cohosh

Other common names: Black cohosh rhizome, black snakeroot, bugbane rhizome, cimicifuga, squawroot
Botanical name: *Cimicifuga foetida* L., *C. dahurica* (Turcz.), *C. heracleifolia* Kom.
Pharmaceutical name: Rhizoma Cimicifugae
Part of plant used: Rhizome
Plant family: Ranunculaceae (Peony Family)
Japanese name: *Shoma*
Chinese name: *Sheng Ma*
Korean name: *Sungma*
Dosage when used by itself in decoctions: 1.5–9.0 grams
How to recognize good quality in the unprocessed herb: Black root with few rootlets. Cross section of the root may be white or light green *(C. foetida)*, light green *(C. dahurica)*, or gray *(C. heracleifolia)*

Bletilla

Other common names: Bletilla rhizome
Botanical name: *Bletilla striate* (Thunb.) Reichb. F.
Pharmaceutical name: Rhizoma Bletillae Striatae
Part of plant used: Rhizome
Plant family: Orchidaceae (Orchid Family)
Japanese name: *Byakukyu*
Chinese name: *Bai Ji*
Korean name: *Paekkup*
Dosage when used by itself in decoctions: 3.0 –15.0 grams
How to recognize good quality in the unprocessed herb: Solid, thick, white, without odor

Blue Citrus (Qing Pi)

Other common names: Green tangerine peel
Botanical name: *Citrus reticulata* Blanco
Pharmaceutical name: Pericarpium Citri Reticulatae Viride
Part of plant used: Rind of the fruit
Plant family: Rutaceae (Citrus Family)
Japanese name: *Jyohi*
Chinese name: *Qing Pi*
Korean name: *Ch'ongpi*
Dosage when used by itself in decoctions: 3.0–9.0 grams
How to recognize good quality in the unprocessed herb: Aromatic, oily, pliable, thin-skinned pieces of peel in large sections

Brucea

Other common names: Java brucea fruit
Botanical name: *Brucea javanica* (L.) Merr.
Pharmaceutical name: Fructus Brucae Javanicae
Part of plant used: Fruit
Plant family: Simaroubaceae (Quassia or Tree of Heaven Family)
Japanese name: *Atanshi*
Chinese name: *Ya Dan Zi*
Korean name: *Adancha*
Dosage when used by itself in decoctions: 10.0–30.0 grams
How to recognize good quality in the unprocessed herb: Hard, oily, solid, white

Bupleurum

Other common names: Bupleurum root, hare's ear root, throwax root
Botanical name: *Bupleurum chinense* D.C. (northern bupleurum), *Bupleurum scorzoneraefolium* Wild. (southern bupleurum)
Pharmaceutical name: Radix Bupleuri
Part of plant used: Root
Plant family: Apiaceae (Parsley Family)
Japanese name: *Saiko*
Chinese name: *Chai Hu*
Korean name: *Siho*
Dosage when used by itself in decoctions: 3.0 –12.0 grams
How to recognize good quality in the unprocessed herb: Thin root bark and few if any side branches

Burdock (Arctium Lappa)

Other common names: Arctium, great burdock fruit
Botanical name: *Arctium lappa* L.
Pharmaceutical name: Fructus Arctii Lappae
Part of plant used: Seed
Plant family: Asteraceae (Composite Family)
Japanese name: *Goboshi*
Chinese name: *Niu Bang Zi*
Korean name: *Ubangja*
Dosage when used by itself in decoctions: 3.0–9.0 grams
How to recognize good quality in the unprocessed herb: Full seed with a grayish red outer skin

Caltrop

Other common names: Puncture-vine fruit, tribulus
Botanical name: *Tribulus terrestris* L.
Pharmaceutical name: Fructi Tribuli Terrestris
Part of plant used: Fruit
Plant family: Zygophyllaceae (Cloves Family)
Japanese name: *Byakushitsuri*
Chinese name: *Bai Ji Li*
Korean name: *Paekchillyo*
Dosage when used by itself in decoctions: 6.0–12.0 grams
How to recognize good quality in the unprocessed herb: Grayish white, thorny

Cardamom

Other common names: Cardamon, grains-of-paradise
Botanical name: *Amomum villosum* Lour.
Pharmaceutical name: Fructus Amomi
Part of plant used: Whole pods
Plant family: Zingiberaceae (Ginger Family)
Japanese name: *Shukusha*
Chinese name: *Sha Ren*
Korean name: *Sa'in*
Dosage when used by itself in decoctions: 1.5–4.5 grams
How to recognize good quality in the unprocessed herb: Full, thin-skinned, yellow-green

Carthamus

Other common names: Safflower
Botanical name: *Carthamus tinctorius* L.
Pharmaceutical name: Flos Carthami Tinctorii
Part of plant used: Flower
Plant family: Asteraceae (Composite Family)
Japanese name: *Koka*
Chinese name: *Hong Hua*
Korean name: *Honghwa*
Dosage when used by itself in decoctions: 0.9–9.0 grams
How to recognize good quality in the unprocessed herb: Long, soft, petals, picked when changing from yellow to red

Chebula

Other common names: Tribulus
Botanical name: *Terminalia chebula* Retz.
Pharmaceutical name: Fructus Terminaliae Chebulae
Part of plant used: Fruit
Plant family: Zygophyllaceae (Chaparral Family)
Japanese name: *Kashi*
Chinese name: *He Zi*
Korean name: *Hacha*
Dosage when used by itself in decoctions: 3.0–9.0 grams, crushed before decocting
How to recognize good quality in the unprocessed herb: Shiny, hard, yellowish-brown

Chinese Senega Root

Other common names: Polygala, polygala tenuifolia root
Botanical name: *Polygala tenuifolia* Willd.
Pharmaceutical name: Radix Polygalae Tenuifoliae
Part of plant used: Root
Plant family: Polygalaceae (Senga Family)
Japanese name: *Onji*
Chinese name: *Yuan Zhi*
Korean name: *Woji*
Dosage when used by itself in decoctions: 3.0–9.0 grams
How to recognize good quality in the unprocessed herb: White exterior

Chrysanthemum

Botanical name: *Chrysanthemum morifolium* Ramat.
Pharmaceutical name: Flos Chrysanthemi Morifolii
Part of plant used: Flower
Plant family: Asteraceae (Composite Family)
Japanese name: *Kikuka* (cultivated), *Nogikuka* (wild)
Chinese name: *Ju Hua*
Korean name: *Kukhwa*
Dosage when used by itself in decoctions: 4.5–15.0 grams
How to recognize good quality in the unprocessed herb: Fragrant, brightly colored

Cinnamon, bark

Other common names: Cinnamon bark, Saigon cinnamon bark
Botanical name: *Cinnamomum* cassia Presl.
Pharmaceutical name: Cortex Cinnamomi Cassiae
Part of plant used: Bark
Plant family: Lauraceae (Laurel Family)
Japanese name: *Nikkei*
Chinese name: *Rou Gui*
Korean name: *Yukkye*
Dosage when used by itself: 1.5–4.5 grams. Very seldom used in teas; usually taken in pill or tablet form to preserve essential oils
How to recognize good quality in the unprocessed herb: Aromatic; thick, reddish purple cross section, oily

Cinnamon, twig

Other common names: Cassia twig, cinnamon twig, Saigon cinnamon twig
Botanical name: *Cinnamomum cassia* Blume
Pharmaceutical name: Ramulus Cinnamomi Cassiae
Part of plant used: Twig
Plant family: Lauraceae (Laurel Family)
Japanese name: *Keishi*
Chinese name: *Gui Zhi*
Korean name: *Kyechi*
Dosage when used by itself in decoctions: 3.0–15.0 grams
How to recognize good quality in the unprocessed herb: Aromatic, brownish red,

Cistanche

Other common names: Broomrape
Botanical name: *Cistanche deserticola* Y. C. Ma
Pharmaceutical name: Herba Cistanches Deserticolae
Part of plant used: Above-ground parts
Plant family: Orobanchaceae (Broomrape Family)
Japanese name: *Nikujuyo*
Chinese name: *Rou Cong Rong*
Korean name: *Yukch Ongyong*
Dosage when used by itself in decoctions: 9.0–21.0 grams
How to recognize good quality in the unprocessed herb: Soft, brownish red, long, thick, dense scales

Clematis

Other common names: Chinese clematis root
Botanical name: *Clemantis* spp.
Pharmaceutical name: Radix Clematidis
Part of plant used: Root
Plant family: Ranunculaceae (Peony Family)
Japanese name: *Ireisen*
Chinese name: *Wei Ling Xian*
Korean name: *Wojoksum*
Dosage when used by itself in decoctions: 6.0–12.0 grams
How to recognize good quality in the unprocessed herb: Black bark, white center, solid

Cloves

Other common names: Clove flower bud
Botanical name: *Syzygium aromaticum* (L.) Merr. et Perry
Pharmaceutical name: Flos Caryophylli
Part of plant used: Unopened flower buds
Plant family: Myrtaceae (Cloves Family)
Japanese name: *Choko*
Chinese name: *Ding Xiang, Gong Ding Xiang*
Korean name: *Chonghyang*
Dosage when used by itself in decoctions: 1.5–4.5 grams of blossoms; when taken in powder form, 500–1,000 milligrams
How to recognize good quality in the unprocessed herb: Fragrant, full, oily, dark red. Does not float when added to decoction

Codonopsis

Botanical name: *Codonopsis pilosula* (Franch.) Nannf.
Pharmaceutical name: Radix Codonopsitis Pilosulae
Part of plant used: Root
Plant family: Campanulaceae (Bluebell or Lobelia Family)

Japanese name: *Tojin*
Chinese name: *Dang Shen*
Korean name: *Tangsam*
Dosage when used by itself in decoctions: 9.0–30.0 grams
How to recognize good quality in the unprocessed herb: Firm, moist, sweet, thick, many striations on bark

Coix

Other common names: Coicis, *hatomugi*, Job's tears
Botanical name: *Coix lachryma-jobi* L.
Pharmaceutical name: Semen Coicis Lachryma-jobi
Part of plant used: Seed
Plant family: Gramineae (Grass Family)
Japanese name: *Yokuinin*
Chinese name: *Yi Yi Ren*
Korean name: *Uii-in*
Dosage when used by itself in decoctions: 9.0–30.0 grams
How to recognize good quality in the unprocessed herb: Full, large, round, white seed

Coltsfoot

Other common names: Tussilago
Botanical name: *Tussilago farfarae* L.
Pharmaceutical name: Flos Tussilaginis Farfarae
Part of plant used: Flower buds
Plant family: Asteraceae (Composite Family)
Japanese name: *Kantoka*
Chinese name: *Kuan Dong Hua*
Korean name: *Kwandonghwa*
Dosage when used by itself in decoctions: 1.5–9.0 grams. Do *not* use wildcrafted coltsfoot in tincture form
How to recognize good quality in the unprocessed herb: Firm, fresh, purple

Coptis

Other common names: Chinese goldthread, coptidis, coptis rhizome
Botanical name: *Coptis chinensis* Franch.
Pharmaceutical name: Rhizoma Coptidis
Part of plant used: Root
Plant family: Berberidaceae (Barberry Family)
Japanese name: *Oren*
Chinese name: *Huang Lian*
Korean name: *Hwangnyon*
Dosage when used by itself in decoctions: 1.5–9.0 grams
How to recognize good quality in the unprocessed herb: Reddish yellow or yellow cross section, turns tea inky black

Cordyceps

This appears in Chapter 3 under Other Traditional Healing Substances.
Botanical name: *Cordyceps sinensis* (Berk.) Sacc.
Pharmaceutical names: Cordyceps Sinensis
Part of plant used: All
Plant family: Clavicipitaceae (Antler Fungus Family)
Japanese name: *Tochukaso*
Chinese name: *Dong Chong Xia Cao*
Korean name: *Tongch'unghach'o*
Dosage when used by itself in decoctions: 4.5–12.0 grams
How to recognize good quality in the unprocessed herb: Fat, full, round with a bright yellow exterior and a light yellow cross section

Cornelian Cherry

Other common names: Cornelian cherry fruit, cornus, Japanese dogwood fruit
Botanical name: *Cornus officinalis* Sieb. et Zucc.
Pharmaceutical name: Fructus Corni Officinalis
Part of plant used: Fruit
Plant family: Cornaceae (Dogwood Family)
Japanese name: *Sanshuyu*
Chinese name: *Shan Zhu Yu*
Korean name: *Sansuyok*
Dosage when used by itself in decoctions: 3.0–60.0 grams
How to recognize good quality in the unprocessed herb: Fat, seedless, soft, thick, purplish red

Corydalis

Other common names: Corydalis rhizome
Botanical name: *Corydalis yanhusuo* W. T. Wang. Other species of corydalis are also used in Kampo
Pharmaceutical name: Rhizoma Corydalis Yanhusuo
Part of plant used: Rhizome
Plant family: Papaveraceae (Opium Poppy Family)
Japanese name: *Engsoaku*
Chinese name: *Yan Hu Suo*
Korean name: *Yonhosaek*
Dosage when used by itself in decoctions: 4.5–12.0 grams
How to recognize good quality in the unprocessed herb: Hard, large, bright yellow

Cuscuta

Other common names: Chinese dodder seeds
Botanical name: *Cuscuta chinensis* Lam.
Pharmaceutical name: Semen Cuscutae Chinensis
Part of plant used: Seed
Plant family: Convolvulaceae (Dodder or Love-Vine Family)
Japanese name: *Toshishi*
Chinese name: *Tu Si Zi*
Korean name: *T'osacha*
Dosage when used by itself in decoctions: 9.0–15.0 grams
How to recognize good quality in the unprocessed herb: Yellow-gray, full, rounded

Dan Shen

Other common names: Cinnabar root, red sage, salvia miltiorrhiza
Botanical name: *Salvia miltiorrhiza* Bge.
Pharmaceutical name: Radix Salviae Miltiorrhizae
Part of plant used: Root
Plant family: Lamiaceae (Mint Family)
Japanese name: *Tanjin*
Chinese name: *Dan Shen*
Korean name: *Tansam*
Dosage when used by itself in decoctions: 6.0–60.0 grams
How to recognize good quality in the unprocessed herb: Coarse, purple-black inside with small white spots

Dandelion

Other common names: Taraxicum (in TCM)
Botanical name: *Taraxacum mongolicum* Hand.-Mazz. Other species may be substituted
Pharmaceutical name: Herba cum Radice Taraxaci Mongolici
Part of plant used: Whole plant
Plant family: Asteraceae (Composite Family)
Japanese name: *Hokoei*

Chinese name: *Pu Gong Ying*
Korean name: *P'ongongyong*
Dosage when used by itself in decoctions: 9.0–30.0 grams
How to recognize good quality in the unprocessed herb: Intact root with many green leaves

Dendrobium

Botanical name: *Dendrobium nobile* Lindl.
Pharmaceutical name: Herba Dendrobii
Part of plant used: Above-ground parts
Plant family: Orchidaceae (Orchid Family)
Japanese name: *Sekkoku*
Chinese name: *Shi Hu*
Korean name: *Sokkok*
Dosage when used by itself in decoctions: 6.0–15.0 grams
How to recognize good quality in the unprocessed herb: Pliable, golden, shiny

Dioscorea

Other common names: Chinese yam, medicinal yam, Mexican yam, tokoro, wild yam
Botanical name: *Dioscorea opposita* Thunb., although any species of *Dioscorea* may be substituted
Pharmaceutical name: Rhizoma Dioscoreae
Part of plant used: Rhizome
Plant family: Dioscoreaceae (Yam Family)
Japanese name: *Sanyaku*
Chinese name: *Shan Yao*
Korean name: *Sanyak*
Dosage when used by itself in decoctions: 9.0–15.0 grams
How to recognize good quality in the unprocessed herb: Long, thick, firm, powdery, yellowish white cross section

Dracaena Lily

Botanical name: *Dracaena cambodiana* Pierre ex Gagnep.
Pharmaceutical names: Sanguis Draconis
Part of plant used: Resin
Plant family: Liliaceae (Lily Family)
Japanese name: *Kekketsu*
Chinese name: *Xue Jie*
Korean name: *Hyolgal*
Dosage when used by itself in decoctions: 0.3–1.5 grams
How to recognize good quality in the unprocessed herb: Iron-black when gathered, blood-red when powdered

Drynaria Rhizome

Botanical name: *Drynaria fortunei* (Kunze) J. Sm.
Pharmaceutical name: Rhizoma Drynariae
Part of plant used: Rhizome
Plant family: Polypodiaceae (Fern Family)
Japanese name: *Kotsusaiho*
Chinese name: *Gu Sui Bu*
Korean name: *Kolswaebo*
Dosage when used by itself in decoctions: 6.0–18.0 grams
How to recognize good quality in the unprocessed herb: Brown, large, thick

Ephedra

Other common names: Ma huang
Botanical name: *Ephedra sinica* Stapf., *E. equisetina Bunge., E. intermedia* Schrenk et Mey
Pharmaceutical name: Herba Ephedrae
Part of plant used: Above-ground parts
Plant family: Ephedraceae (Ephedra Family)
Japanese name: *Mao*
Chinese name: *Ma Huang*
Korean name: *Mahwang*
Dosage when used by itself in decoctions: 3.0–9.0 grams
How to recognize good quality in the unprocessed herb: Light green, solid center in the stem

Epimedium

Other common names: Goat wort
Botanical name: *Epimedium grandiflorum* Morr.
Pharmaceutical name: Herba Epimedii
Part of plant used: Above-ground parts
Plant family: Berberidaceae (Barberry Family)
Japanese name: *Inyokaku*
Chinese name: *Yin Yang Huo*
Korean name: *Umyanggwak*
Dosage when used by itself in decoctions: 6.0–15.0 grams
How to recognize good quality in the unprocessed herb: Yellow-green, many stems

Eucommia

Other common names: Eucommia bark, gutta percha
Botanical name: *Eucommia ulmoides* Oliv.
Pharmaceutical name: Cortex Eucommiae Ulmoidis
Part of plant used: Bark
Plant family: Eucommiaceae (Eucommia Family)
Japanese name: *Tochu*
Chinese name: *Du Zhong*
Korean name: *Tuch'ung*
Dosage when used by itself in decoctions: 6.0–15.0 grams
How to recognize good quality in the unprocessed herb: Yellowish brown outside and dark purple inside, bark should reveal many white threads when broken

Eupatorium

Other common names: Boneset
Botanical name: *Eupatorium japonicum* Thunb., *Eupatorium fortunei* Turcz.
Pharmaceutical name: Herba Eupatorii Japonicum
Part of plant used: Above-ground parts
Plant family: Asteraceae (Composite Family)
Japanese name: *Hairan*
Chinese name: *Pei Lan*
Korean name: *P'e-nan*
Dosage when used by itself in decoctions: 4.5–9.0 grams
How to recognize good quality in the unprocessed herb: Numerous leaves, strongly aromatic

Evodia

Other common names: Evodia fruit
Botanical name: *Evodia rutaecarpa* (Juss.) Benth.
Pharmaceutical name: Fructus Evodiae Rutaecarpae
Part of plant used: Fruit
Plant family: Rutaceae (Citrus Family)
Japanese name: *Goshuyu*
Chinese name: *Wu Zhu Yu*
Korean name: *Osuyu*
Dosage when used by itself in decoctions: 3.0–9.0 grams
How to recognize good quality in the unprocessed herb: Full, brownish green, round, aromatic

Fennel Seed

Other common names: Fennel fruit
Botanical name: *Foeniculum vulgare* Mill.
Pharmaceutical name: Fructus Foeniculi Vulgaris
Part of plant used: Seed
Plant family: Apiaceae (Parsley Family)
Japanese name: *Shouikyo*
Chinese name: *Xiao Hui Xiang*
Korean name: *Sohoehyang*
Dosage when used by itself in decoctions: 3.0–9.0 grams
How to recognize good quality in the unprocessed herb: Aromatic, green-yellow

Forsythia

Other common names: Forsythia fruit, weeping forsythia fruit
Botanical name: *Forsythia suspensa* (Thunb.) Vahl
Pharmaceutical name: Fructus Forsythiae Suspensae
Part of plant used: Fruit
Plant family: Oleaceae (Olive Family)
Japanese name: *Rengyo*
Chinese name: *Lian Qiao*
Korean name: *Yon'gyo*
Dosage when used by itself in decoctions: 6.0–15.0 grams
How to recognize good quality in the unprocessed herb: Unripe: blue-green, no branches or stems in the package. Ripe: yellow, thick shell, no seeds. Unripe fruit is preferred

Frankincense

This appears in Chapter 3 under Other Traditional Healing Substances.
Other common names: Boswellia, mastic, olibanum
Botanical name: *Boswellia carterii* Birdw.
Pharmaceutical name: Gummi Olibanum
Part of plant used: Resin
Plant family: Burseraceae (Frankincense and Myrrh Family)
Japanese name: *Nyuko*
Chinese name: *Ru Xiang*
Korean name: *Yuhyang*
Dosage when used by itself in decoctions: 3.0–9.0 grams
How to recognize good quality in the unprocessed herb: Aromatic, granular but not containing sand, translucent, light yellow

Fritillaria (Cirrhosa)

Botanical name: *Fritillaria cirrhosa* D. Don.
Pharmaceutical name: Bulbus Fritillariae Cirrhosae
Part of plant used: Bulb
Plant family: Liliaceae (Lily Family)
Japanese name: *Senbaimo*
Chinese name: *Chuan Bei Mu*
Korean name: *Ch'onp'aemo*
Dosage when used by itself in decoctions: 3.0–12.0 grams, 1.0–1.5 grams as a powder *Never take the raw herb internally*
How to recognize good quality in the unprocessed herb: White, powdery

Fritillaria (Thunberg Fritillaria Bulb)

Botanical name: *Fritillaria thunbergii* Miq.
Pharmaceutical name: Bulbus Fritillariae Thunbergii
Part of plant used: Bulb
Plant family: Liliaceae (Lily Family)
Japanese name: *Setsubaimo*
Chinese name: *Zhe Bei Mu*
Korean name: *Cholp'ameo*
Dosage when used by itself in decoctions: 3.0–9.0 grams. *Never take the raw herb internally*
How to recognize good quality in the unprocessed herb: Firm yet powdery, white flesh

Galangal

Other common names: Galanga, lesser galangal rhizome
Botanical name: *Alpinia officinarum* Hance
Pharmaceutical name: Rhizoma Alpiniae Officinari
Part of plant used: Rhizome
Plant family: Zingiberaceae (Ginger Family)
Japanese name: *Koryokyo*
Chinese name: *Gao Liang Jiang*
Korean name: *Koyanggang*
Dosage when used by itself in decoctions: 1.5–9.0 grams
How to recognize good quality in the unprocessed herb: Fragrant, reddish brown, solid

Gambir

Other common names: Hookvine, hutch, pale catechu, uncaria. Most patent medicines use the term "uncaria"
Botanical name: *Uncaria gambir* Roxb. Chinese Kampo physicians also use *Uncaria rhynchophylla* (Miq.) and *Uncaria sinensis* Roxb.
Pharmaceutical name: Ramulus cum Uncis Uncariae
Part of plant used: Stems with "hooks"
Plant family: Rubiaceae (Madder Family)
Japanese name: *Chotoko*
Chinese name: *Gou Teng*
Korean name: *Kuduing*
Dosage when used by itself in decoctions: 6.0–15.0 grams
How to recognize good quality in the unprocessed herb: Glossy, purplish red, many hooks, no dry stems

Gardenia

Other common names: Cape jasmine fruit, gardenia fruit
Botanical name: *Gardenia jasminoides* Ellis
Pharmaceutical name: Fructus Gardenia Jasminoidis
Part of plant used: Fruit
Plant family: Rubiaceae (Madder Family)
Japanese name: *Sanshishi*
Chinese name: *Zhi Zi*
Korean name: *Ch'icha*
Dosage when used by itself in decoctions: 3.0–12.0 grams
How to recognize good quality in the unprocessed herb: Full, round, thin-skinned, reddish yellow

Garlic

Other common names: Garlic bulb, garlic cloves
Botanical name: *Allium sativa* L.
Pharmaceutical name: Bulbus Alli Sativi
Part of plant used: Bulb
Plant family: Alliaceae (Onion Family)
Japanese name: *Taisan*
Chinese name: *Da Suan*
Korean name: *Taesan*
Dosage when used by itself in decoctions: 3–5 cloves (6.0–15.0 grams)
How to recognize good quality in the unprocessed herb: Full, firm cloves with tight skin

Gastrodia

Other common names: Gastrodia rhizome
Botanical name: *Gastrodia elata* Blume
Pharmaceutical name: Rhizoma Gastrodiae Elatae
Part of plant used: Rhizome
Plant family: Orchidaceae (Orchid Family)
Japanese name: *Tenma*
Chinese name: *Tian Ma*
Korean name: *Ch'onma*
Dosage when used by itself in decoctions: 3.0–9.0 grams, or 0.9–1.5 grams in powder form
How to recognize good quality in the unprocessed herb: No hole in the middle, translucent, yellowish white

Gentian

Other common names: Chinese gentian root, gentiana, Gentiana Longdancao
Botanical name: *Gentiana scabra* Bge. The European *Gentiana lutea* L. may be substituted
Pharmaceutical name: Radix Gentianae Longdancao
Part of plant used: Root
Plant family: Gentianaceae (Gentian Family)
Japanese name: *Ryutan*
Chinese name: *Long Dan Cao*
Korean name: *Yongdanch'o*
Dosage when used by itself in decoctions: 3.0–9.0 grams
How to recognize good quality in the unprocessed herb: Intact, yellow or yellow-brown, elongated

Ginger, dried

Other common names: Dried ginger rhizome
Botanical name: *Zingiber officinalis* Roscoe
Pharmaceutical name: Rhizoma Zingiberis Officinalis
Part of plant used: Rhizome (dried)
Plant family: Zingiberaceae (Ginger Family)
Japanese name: *Kankyo*
Chinese name: *Gan Jiang*
Korean name: *Kongang*
Dosage when used by itself in decoctions: 3.0–12.0 grams
How to recognize good quality in the unprocessed herb: Yellow-gray exterior with powdery, white interior

Ginger, fresh

Botanical name: *Zingiber officinale* Roscoe
Pharmaceutical name: Rhizoma Zingiberis Recens
Part of plant used: Rhizome
Plant family: Zingiberaceae (Ginger Family)
Japanese name: *Shokyo*
Chinese name: *Sheng Jiang*
Korean name: *Saenggang*
Dosage when used by itself in decoctions: 3.0–9.0 grams
How to recognize good quality in the unprocessed herb: Full, large, young, no withering, soft skin on root

Ginkgo Nut

Botanical name: *Ginkgo biloba* L.
Pharmaceutical name: Semen Ginkgo Bilobae
Part of plant used: Seed, usually crushed before use
Plant family: Ginkgoaceae (Ginkgo Family)
Japanese name: *Ginkyo*
Chinese name: *Bai Guo*
Korean name: *Unhaeng*
Dosage when used by itself in decoctions: 4.5–9.0 grams
How to recognize good quality in the unprocessed herb: Full, round, white

Ginseng

Other common names: Ginseng root, Korean ginseng, red ginseng
Botanical name: *Panax ginseng* C. A. Meyer
Pharmaceutical name: Radix Ginseng
Part of plant used: Root
Plant family: Araliaceae (Ginseng Family)
Japanese name: *Ninjin*
Chinese name: *Ren Shen*
Korean name: *Insam*
Dosage when used by itself in decoctions: 1.0–9.0 grams
How to recognize good quality in the unprocessed herb: Long taproot with long branches. White ginseng should be a pale yellow. Red ginseng should be a translucent reddish brown

Green Tea

Botanical name: *Camellia sinensis* (L.) O. Kuntze
Pharmaceutical name: Theae Folium
Part of plant used: Leaf
Plant family: Theaceae (Tea Family)
Japanese name: *O'cha*
Chinese name: *Cha*
Korean name: *Cha*
Dosage when used by itself in decoctions: 2.0–3.0 grams
How to recognize good quality in the unprocessed herb: Light green or yellow, fragrant

Hawthorn

Other common names: Crataegus, hawthorn fruit
Botanical name: *Crataegus* spp.
Pharmaceutical name: Fructus Crataegi
Part of plant used: Fruit
Plant family: Rosaceae (Rose Family)
Japanese name: *Sanzashi*
Chinese name: *Shan Zha*
Korean name: *Sanza*
Dosage when used by itself in decoctions: 9.0–15.0 grams
How to recognize good quality in the unprocessed herb: Large and thick, either red or brown skin

Hoelen

Other common names: China-root, poria, tuckahoe
Botanical name: *Poria cocos* (Schw.) Wolf
Pharmaceutical name: Sclerotium Poriae Cocos
Part of plant used: Stem
Plant family: Polyporaceae (Polypore Mushroom Family)
Japanese name: *Bukuryo*
Chinese name: *Fu Ling*
Korean name: *Pongnyong*
Dosage when used by itself in decoctions: 9.0–15.0 grams
How to recognize good quality in the unprocessed herb: Red outer skin with deep wrinkles, white cross section

Houttynia

Botanical name: *Houttuynia cordata* Thunb.
Pharmaceutical name: Herba cum Radice Houttuyniae Cordatae
Part of plant used: Whole plant
Plant family: Saururaceae (Lizard's Tail Family)
Japanese name: *Juyaku*
Chinese name: *Yu Xing Cao*

Korean name: *Osaengch'o*
Dosage when used by itself in decoctions: 15.0–60.0 grams
How to recognize good quality in the unprocessed herb: Fishy smell, well-shaped leaves

Japanese Mint

Other common names: Schizonepeta, tenuifolia
Botanical name: *Schizonepeta tenuifolia* Briq.
Pharmaceutical name: Schizonepetae Folium
Part of plant used: Above-ground parts
Plant family: Lamiaceae (Mint Family)
Japanese name: *Keigai*
Chinese name: *Jing Jie*
Korean name: *Hyongkae*
Dosage when used by itself in decoctions: 9.0–27.0 grams
How to recognize good quality in the unprocessed herb: Light purple, thin stem, numerous spikes

Japanese Watermelon

Other common names: Citrullus
Botanical name: *Citrullus vulgaris* Schrad.
Pharmaceutical name: Fructus Citrulli Vulgaris
Part of plant used: Fruit
Plant family: Curcubitaceae (Curcubit or Gourd Family)
Japanese name: *Suika*
Chinese name: *Xi Gua*
Korean name: *Sogwa*
Dosage when used by itself in decoctions: 15.0–30.0 grams or 1 cup of fresh juice
How to recognize good quality in the unprocessed herb: Juicy, sweet

Jujube Fruit

Other common names: Chinese date
Botanical name: *Ziziphus jujuba* Mill. var. *inermis* (Bge.) Rehd.
Pharmaceutical name: Fructus Zizyphi Jujubae
Part of plant used: Date (pitted)
Plant family: Rhamnaceae (Buckthorn Family)
Japanese name: *Taiso*
Chinese name: *Da Zao*
Korean name: *Taecho*
Dosage when used by itself in decoctions: 3–12 dates (10.0–30.0 grams)
How to recognize good quality in the unprocessed herb: Full, very small seeds, if any

Kelp

Other common names: Bladderwrack (*Fucus vesiculosus*), kelp thallus
Botanical name: various genera—*Fucus, Laminaria, Macrocystis, Nerocystis*
Pharmaceutical name: Algae Thallus
Part of plant used: Entire plant
Plant family: Sargassum (Kelp Family)
Japanese name: *Kaiso*
Chinese name: *Hai Zhao*
Korean name: *Haecho*
Dosage when used by itself in decoctions: 4.5–15.0 grams
How to recognize good quality in the unprocessed herb: No offensive odor

Kudzu

Other common names: Pueraria, pueraria root
Botanical name: *Pueraria lobata* (Willd.) Ohwi.
Pharmaceutical name: Radix Puerariae
Part of plant used: Root
Plant family: Fabaceae (Legume Family)
Japanese name: *Kakkon*
Chinese name: *Ge Gen*
Korean name: *Kalgun*
Dosage when used by itself in decoctions: 6.0–12.0 grams
How to recognize good quality in the unprocessed herb: Powdery, unfragmented, white root. Traditionally roasted for use in treating diarrhea

Ledebouriella

Other common names: Ledebouriella root, siler
Botanical name: *Ledebouriella divaricata* Turcz., *Saposhinikovia divaricata* (Turcz.) Schischk
Pharmaceutical name: Radix Ledebouriella Divaricatae
Part of plant used: Root
Plant family: Apiaceae (Parsley Family)
Japanese name: *Bofu*
Chinese name: *Fang Feng*
Korean name: *Bangp'ung*
Dosage when used by itself in decoctions: 3.0–9.0 grams
How to recognize good quality in the unprocessed herb: Strong roots with a thin skin, cross section should have light yellow center surrounded by brown rings

Licorice

Other common names: Licorice root
Botanical name: *Glycyrrhiza uralensis* Fischer. Other species are equally effective
Pharmaceutical name: Radix Glycyrrhizae Uralensis
Part of plant used: Root
Plant family: Fabaceae (Legume Family)
Japanese name: *Kanzo*
Chinese name: *Gan Cao, Guo Lao*
Korean name: *Kamch'o*
Dosage when used by itself in decoctions: 2.0–12.0 grams
How to recognize good quality in the unprocessed herb: Outer skin should be brown-red, thin, free of wrinkles. Cross section should be yellow-white and powdery

Ligusticum

Other common names: Chinese lovage root, kao-pen, ligusticum root
Botanical name: *Ligusticum sinsense* Olive., *L. jeholense* Nakai et Kigag
Pharmaceutical name: Rhizoma et Radix Ligusticum
Part of plant used: Root
Plant family: Apiaceae (Parsley Family)
Japanese name: *Kohon*
Chinese name: *Gao Ben*
Korean name: *Kobon*
Dosage when used by itself in decoctions: 3.0–9.0 grams
How to recognize good quality in the unprocessed herb: Aromatic

Ligustrum

Other common names: Privet fruit
Botanical name: *Ligustrum lucidum* Ait.
Pharmaceutical name: Fructus Ligustri Lucidi
Part of plant used: Fruit
Plant family: Oleaceae (Olive Family)
Japanese name: *Joteishi*

Chinese name: *Nu Zhen Zi*
Korean name: *Yojungja*
Dosage when used by itself in decoctions: 4.5–15.0 grams
How to recognize good quality in the unprocessed herb: Firm, full, gray-black

Lily Bulb

Botanical name: *Lilium brownii* F.E. Brown var. *colchesteri*, *Lilium pumilum* D.C., or *Lilium longiflorum* Thunb.
Pharmaceutical name: Bulbus Lilii
Part of plant used: Bulb
Plant family: Liliaceae (Lily Family)
Japanese name: *Byakugo*
Chinese name: *Bai He*
Korean name: *Paekhap*
Dosage when used by itself in decoctions: 9.0–30.0 grams
How to recognize good quality in the unprocessed herb: Yellowish white with uniform scales

Lindera

Botanical name: *Lindera strychnifolia* (Sieb. et Zucc.) Villar
Pharmaceutical name: Radix Linderae Strychnifoliae
Part of plant used: Root
Plant family: Lauraceae (Laurel Family)
Japanese name: *Uyaku*
Chinese name: *Wu Yao*
Korean name: *Oyak*
Dosage when used by itself in decoctions: 3.0–9.0 grams
How to recognize good quality in the unprocessed herb: Powdery, brown

Lithospermum

Other common names: Arnebia, groomwell root
Botanical name: *Lithospermum erythrorhizon* Sibe. et Zucc.
Pharmaceutical name: Radix Lithospermi
Part of plant used: Root
Plant family: Boraginaceae (Borage Family)
Japanese name: *Shiso*
Chinese name: *Zi Cao*
Korean name: *Chach'o*
Dosage when used by itself in decoctions: 3.0–9.0 grams. Also used in ointments and pills
How to recognize good quality in the unprocessed herb: Purple

Lobelia

Botanical name: *Lobelia chinensis* Lour.
Pharmaceutical name: Herba et Radix Lobeliae Chinensis
Part of plant used: Entire plant
Plant family: Campanulaceae (Bluebell Family)
Japanese name: *Hanpenren*
Chinese name: *Ban Bian Lian*
Korean name: *Panpyonpyon*
Dosage when used by itself in Kampo decoctions: 15.0–30.0 grams
How to recognize good quality in the unprocessed herb: Green leaves, yellow root

Longan

Other common names: Kan-sui root
Botanical name: *Euphoria kansui* Liou
Pharmaceutical name: Arillus Euphoriae Longanae
Part of plant used: Fruit, flesh only
Plant family: Sapindaceae (Longan Family)
Japanese name: *Ryuganniku*
Chinese name: *Long Yan Rou*
Korean name: *Yonganyuk*
Dosage when used by itself in decoctions: 6.0–30.0 grams in decoction
How to recognize good quality in the unprocessed herb: Soft, thick-fleshed, sweet

Lonicera

Other common names: Japanese honeysuckle
Botanical name: *Lonicera japonica* Thunb.
Pharmaceutical name: Flos Lonicerae Japonicae
Part of plant used: Flower buds
Plant family: Caprifoliaceae (Honeysuckle Family)
Japanese name: *Kinginka*
Chinese name: *Jin Yin Hua*
Korean name: *Kumunhwa*
Dosage when used by itself in decoctions: 9.0–15.0 grams
How to recognize good quality in the unprocessed herb: Aromatic, pale yellow, flowers not yet open

Lophatherum

Botanical name: *Lophatherum gracile* Brongn.
Pharmaceutical name: Herba Lophatheri Gracilis
Part of plant used: Above-ground parts
Plant family: Gramineae (Grass Family)
Japanese name: *Tanchikuyo*
Chinese name: *Dan Zhu Ye, Zhu Ye*
Korean name: *Tamchukyop*
Dosage when used by itself in decoctions: 6.0–9.0 grams
How to recognize good quality in the unprocessed herb: Blue-green, large leaves, few stems, no flower spikes or roots

Loranthus (Mulberry Mistletoe)

Botanical name: *Viscum coloratum* (Kom.) Nakai, *V. album* L. This is *not* the mistletoe found in North America, which is poisonous
Pharmaceutical name: Ramulus Sangjisheng
Part of plant used: Whole plant
Plant family: Loranthaceae (Mistletoe Family)
Japanese name: *Sokisei*
Chinese name: *Sang Ji Sheng*
Korean name: *Sanggisaeng*
Dosage when used by itself in decoctions: 9.0–30.0 grams
How to recognize good quality in the unprocessed herb: Young with many leaves, intact, green

Lotus

Botanical name: *Nelumbo nucifera* Gaertn.
Pharmaceutical name: Folium Nelumbinis Nuciferae (Lotus Leaf), Nodus Nelumbinis Nuciferae Rhizomatis (Lotus Rhizome Node), Semen Nelumbinis Nuciferae (Lotus Seed), Receptaculum Nelumbinis Nuciferae (Lotus Seed Receptacle), Plumula Nelumbinis Nuciferae (Lotus Sprout), Stamen Nelumbinis Nuciferae (Lotus Stamen)
Part of plant used: All
Plant family: Nymphaeceae (Water Lily Family)
Japanese name: *Kayo* (leaf), *Gusetsu* (rhizome node), *Renshi* (seed), *Renbo* (seed receptacle), *Renshin* (sprout), *Renniku* (stamen)
Chinese name: *He Ye; Ou Jie; Lian Zi, Lian Rou, Lian Shi, Lian Ren; Lian Fang, Lian Peng, Lian Peng Guo; Lian Xin; Lian Xu*
Korean name: *Hayop, Ujol, Yoncha, Yonbang, Yonsim, Yonwa*
Dosage when used by itself in decoctions: Leaf—9.0–15.0 grams, up to 30 grams when used alone; rhizome nodes—9.0–15.0

grams fresh, 30.0–60.0 grams dried, juice preferred to tea; seed—6.0–15.0 grams; seed receptacle—3.0–9.0 grams; sprout—1.5–6.0 grams; stamen—1.5–9.0 grams
How to recognize good quality in the unprocessed herb: Leaf—green without spots; rhizome nodes—dark, no rootlets; seed—full, round; seed receptacle—reddish purple, at least 3 inches across; sprout—blue-green, large terminal bud at top; stamen—no dirt, grit, or stem pieces

Lycium, fruit

Other common names: Chinese wolfberry fruit, lycium fruit, matrimony vine fruit
Botanical name: *Lycium barbarum* L.
Pharmaceutical name: Fructus Lycii
Part of plant used: Fruit
Plant family: Solanaceae (Nightshade Family)
Japanese name: *Kukoshi*
Chinese name: *Gou Qi Zi*
Korean name: *Kugicha*
Dosage when used by itself in decoctions: 6.0–18.0 grams
How to recognize good quality in the unprocessed herb: Large, red, soft, sweet

Lycium, root bark

Other common names: Lycium bark, wolfberry bark
Botanical name: *Lycium chinense* Mill., *L. barbarum* L.
Pharmaceutical name: Cortex Lycii Radicis
Part of plant used: Root bark
Plant family: Solanaceae (Nightshade Family)
Japanese name: *Jikoppi*
Chinese name: *Di Gu Pi*
Korean name: *Chigolp'i*
Dosage when used by itself in decoctions: 6.0–15.0 grams
How to recognize good quality in the unprocessed herb: Large, thick, lacking heartwood

Magnolia, bark

Botanical name: *Magnolia officinalis* Rehd. et Wils
Pharmaceutical name: Cortex Magnoliae Officinalis
Part of plant used: Bark
Plant family: Mangoliaceae (Magnolia Family)
Japanese name: *Koboku*
Chinese name: *Hou Po*
Korean name: *Mubak*
Dosage when used by itself in decoctions: 3.0–9.0 grams
How to recognize good quality in the unprocessed herb: Aromatic, thick, finely textured, oily, with a deep purple inner surface

Magnolia, flower

Botanical name: *Magnolia liliflora* Desr. (and three lesser-used species)
Pharmaceutical name: Flos Magnoliae
Part of plant used: Flower. Since the flower has a hairy surface, it should be rubbed with a clean cloth or wrapped in a cheesecloth before use in teas
Plant family: Magnoliaceae (Magnolia Family)
Japanese name: *Shini*
Chinese name: *Xho Yi Hua* (for *Magnolia liliflora), Xho Yi Hua* (for *Magnolia officinalis)*
Korean name: *Sinihwa*
Dosage when used by itself in decoctions: 3.0–9.0 grams
How to recognize good quality in the unprocessed herb: Dry, green, unopened buds, no branches or stems

Malt Sugar

This appears in Chapter 3 under Other Traditional Healing Substances.
Other common names: Barley malt sugar, maltose
Pharmaceutical name: Saccharum Granorum
Japanese name: *Koi*
Chinese name: *Yi Tang*
Korean name: *Idang*
Dosage when used by itself in decoctions: 30.0–60.0 grams
How to recognize good quality in the unprocessed herb: Granular, no clumps or foreign matter, readily dissolves in decoctions

Marijuana Seed

Other common names: Cannabis seed, hemp seed, marijuana
Botanical name: *Cannabis sativa* L.
Pharmaceutical name: Semen Cannabis Sativae
Part of plant used: Seed
Plant family: Cannabaceae (Hemp Family)
Japanese name: *Mashinin*
Chinese name: *Huo Ma Ren*
Korean name: *Hwamain*
Dosage when used by itself in decoctions: 9.0–45.0 grams (weight after grinding)
How to recognize good quality in the unprocessed herb: Only used in patent medicines.
Unprocessed marijuana seed is illegal under federal law; Kampo preparations use heat-treated marijuana seed, which is permitted. More restrictive state and local laws may apply

Morinda

Other common names: Morinda root
Botanical name: *Morinda officinalis* How.
Pharmaceutical name: Radix Morindae Officinalis
Part of plant used: Root
Plant family: Rubiaceae (Madder Family)
Japanese name: *Hagekiten*
Chinese name: *Ba Ji Tian*
Korean name: *P'agukch'on*
Dosage when used by itself in decoctions: 6.0–15.0 grams
How to recognize good quality in the unprocessed herb: Interconnected, large, purple

Motherwort

Other common names: Leonurus
Botanical name: *Leonurus heterophyllus* Sweet
Pharmaceutical name: Herba Leonuri Heterophylli
Part of plant used: Above-ground parts
Plant family: Lamiaceae (Mint Family)
Japanese name: *Yakumoso*
Chinese name: *Yi Mu Cao*
Korean name: *Ikmoch'o*
Dosage when used by itself in decoctions: 9.0–120.0 grams. Extremely large dosages should be taken under professional supervision
How to recognize good quality in the unprocessed herb: Green with thin stems

Moutan (Giant Peony)

Other common names: Tree peony root
Botanical name: *Paeonia suffruticosa* Andr.
Pharmaceutical name: Cortex Moutan Radicis
Part of plant used: Root bark

Plant family: Ranunculaceae (Peony Family)
Japanese name: *Botanpi*
Chinese name: *Mu Dan Pi*
Korean name: *Moktanp'i*
Dosage when used by itself in decoctions: 6.0–12.0 grams
How to recognize good quality in the unprocessed herb: Aromatic, coarse, long, powdery. Outside should be a dusky yellow, pink, or reddish brown. Inside should be pale yellow or brown

Mulberry Root

Other common names: Morus root
Botanical name: *Morus alba* L.
Pharmaceutical name: Cortex Mori Albae Radicis
Part of plant used: Root bark
Plant family: Moraceae (Mulberry Family)
Japanese name: *Sohakuhi*
Chinese name: *Sang Bai Pi*
Korean name: *Sangbaekpi*
Dosage when used by itself in decoctions: 6.0–15.0 grams
How to recognize good quality in the unprocessed herb: Powdery, white

Musk

This appears in Chapter 3 under Other Traditional Healing Substances.
Zoological name: *Moschus moschiferus* L. or *Moschus berezovskii* Flerov
Pharmaceutical name: Secretio Moschus
Part of animal used: Navel gland secretions
Animal family: Cervidae (Deer Family)
Japanese name: *Jako*
Chinese name: *She Xiang*
Korean name: *Sahyang*
Dosage when used by itself: 0.06–0.15 grams (60–150 milligrams). Not used in decoctions; given in pills, plasters, and compresses
How to recognize good quality in unprocessed musk: Soft, oily, granular, intensely aromatic before processing. The original Kampo formulas call for musk collected from wild deer, but because of the animal's endangered status, musk is almost always collected from domesticated deer. All musk is extremely expensive. Look for collected musk rather than synthetic muscone

Myrrh

This appears in Chapter 3 under Other Traditional Healing Substances.
Botanical name: *Commiphora myrrha* Engl.
Pharmaceutical name: Myrrha
Part of plant used: Resin
Plant family: Burseraceae (Frankincense and Myrrh Family)
Japanese name: *Motsuyaku*
Chinese name: *Mo Yao*
Korean name: *Molyak*
Dosage when used by itself in decoctions: 3.0–12.0 grams
How to recognize good quality in the unprocessed herb: Aromatic, reddish brown

Notopterygium

Other common names: Notch-leafed fern
Botanical name: *Notopterygium incisum* Ting. ex H.T. Chang
Pharmaceutical name: Rhizoma et Radix Notopterygii
Part of plant used: Root
Plant family: Apiaceae (Parsley Family)
Japanese name: *Kyokatsu*
Chinese name: *Qiang Huo*
Korean name: *Kanghwal*
Dosage when used by itself in decoctions: 6.0–15.0 grams
How to recognize good quality in the unprocessed herb: Irregular shape, shows many red spots when sliced

Nutmeg

Botanical name: *Myristica fragrans* Houtt.
Pharmaceutical name: Semen Myristicae Fragrantis
Part of plant used: Whole nut
Plant family: Myristicaceae (Nutmeg Family)
Japanese name: *Nikuzuku*
Chinese name: *Rou Dou Kou*
Korean name: *Yuktugu*
Dosage when used by itself in decoctions: 1.5–9.0 grams
How to recognize good quality in the unprocessed herb: Aromatic, hard, glossy

Ophiopogon

Other common names: Japanese lily
Botanical name: *Ophiopogon japonicus* Ker-Gawl.
Pharmaceutical name: Tuber Ophiopogonis Japonici
Part of plant used: Tuber
Plant family: Liliaceae (Lily Family)
Japanese name: *Bakumondo*
Chinese name: *Mai Men Dong*
Korean name: *Maekmundong*
Dosage when used by itself in decoctions: 6.0–15.0 grams
How to recognize good quality in the unprocessed herb: Aromatic, chewy, large, light yellow-white, soft, sweet

Opium Poppy Husk

Botanical name: *Papaver somniferum* L.
Pharmaceutical name: Pericarpium Papaveris Somniferi
Part of plant used: Fruit husk
Plant family: Papaveraceae (Opium Poppy Family)
Japanese name: *Ozokukoku*
Chinese name: *Ying Su Ke*
Korean name: *Aengokkak*
Dosage when used by itself in decoctions: 1.5–6.0 grams
How to recognize good quality in the unprocessed herb: Hard, large, thick, yellowish white

Peach Seed

Other common names: Peach kernel, persica
Botanical name: *Prunus persica* (L.) Batsch.
Pharmaceutical name: Semen Persicae
Part of plant used: Shelled seed
Plant family: Rosaceae (Rose Family)
Japanese name: *Tonin*
Chinese name: *Tao Ren*
Korean name: *Toin*
Dosage when used by itself in decoctions: 4.5–9.0 grams
How to recognize good quality in the unprocessed herb: Whole kernels

Peony

Other common names: White peony root
Botanical name: *Paeonia lactiflora* Pall.
Pharmaceutical name: Radix Paeoniae Lactiflorae
Part of plant used: Root
Plant family: Ranuculaceae (Peony Family)

Japanese name: *Byakushaku*
Chinese name: *Bai Shao*
Korean name: *Paekchak*
Dosage when used by itself in decoctions: 6.0–15.0 grams
How to recognize good quality in the unprocessed herb: Firm, powdery, straight, thick, without cracks

Peppermint

Botanical name: *Mentha haplocalyx* Briq. (mint). Many American Kampo practitioners substitute *Mentha x piperita* L. (peppermint)
Pharmaceutical names: Herba Menthae Hapolcalycis (mint), Herba Menthae Piperitae (peppermint)
Part of plant used: Leaves and stem
Plant family: Lamiaceae (Mint Family)
Japanese name: *Hakka*
Chinese name: *Bo He*
Korean name: *Pakha*
Dosage when used by itself in decoctions: 1.5–6.0 grams
How to recognize good quality in the unprocessed herb: Dry, fragrant, green, contains no roots

Perilla

Botanical name: *Perilla frutescens* (L.) Britt. var. crispa (Thunb.) Hand.-Mazz., or *Perilla frutescens* (L.) Britt. var. acuta (Thunb.) Kudo.
Pharmaceutical names: Folium Perillae Frutescentis (leaf), Fructus Perillae Frutescentis (seed)
Parts of plant used: Leaf, seeds (used separately)
Plant Family: Lamiaceae (Mint Family)
Japanese names: *Shisoyo* (leaf), *Soshi* (seed)
Chinese names: *Zi Su Ye* (leaf), *Su Zi* (seed)
Korean names: *Chasoyop* (leaf), *Soja* (seed)
Dosage when used by itself in decoctions: Leaf—3.0–9.0 grams; Seed—4.5–9.0 grams
How to recognize good quality in the unprocessed herb: Leaf—large, fragrant, purple; Seed—full, round, grayish-brown

Phellodendron

Other common names: Amur cork-tree bark, yellow fir
Botanical name: *Phellodendron amurense* Rupr.
Pharmaceutical name: Cortex Phellodendri
Part of plant used: Bark
Plant family: Rutaceae (Citrus Family)
Japanese name: *Obaku*
Chinese name: *Huang Bai*
Korean name: *Hwangbaek*
Dosage when used by itself in decoctions: 3.0–12.0 grams
How to recognize good quality in the unprocessed herb: Full, bright yellow

Pinellia

Other common names: Pinellia rhizome
Botanical name: *Pinellia ternata* (Thunb.) Breit.
Pharmaceutical name: Rhizoma Pinelliae Ternatae
Part of plant used: Rhizome. Raw pinellia is for external use only. Pinellia for decoctions has been fried with ginger or vinegar
Plant family: Araceae (Sweet-Flag or Calamus Family)
Japanese name: *Hange*
Chinese name: *Ban Xia*
Korean name: *Panha*
Dosage when used by itself in decoctions: 4.5–12.0 grams
How to recognize good quality in the unprocessed herb: Prepared herb should smell of ginger or vinegar. Raw herb is usually not available

Plantain

Other common names: Plantago, psyllium seed
Botanical name: *Plantago asiatica* L.
Pharmaceutical name: Semen Plantaginis
Part of plant used: Seed. Wrap in cheesecloth before using in decoctions
Plant family: Plantaginacae (Plantain Family)
Japanese name: *Shazenshi*
Chinese name: *Che Qian Zi*
Korean name: *Ch'ajonja*
Dosage when used by itself in decoctions: 4.5–9.0 grams
How to recognize good quality in the unprocessed herb: Black, full, round

Platycodon

Other common names: Balloon flower, Japanese bellflower
Botanical name: *Platycodon grandiflorum* (Jacq.) A. DC.
Pharmaceutical name: Radix Platycodi Grandiflori
Part of plant used: Root
Plant family: Campanulaceae (Bluebell Family)
Japanese name: *Kikyo*
Chinese name: *Jie Geng*
Korean name: *Kilgyong*
Dosage when used by itself in decoctions: 3.0–9.0 grams
How to recognize good quality in the unprocessed herb: Large, thick, bitter, firm, white

Polygonum

Other common names: Chinese cornbind, fleeceflower root, ho-shu-wou, polygonum hosuwu
Botanical name: *Polygonum multiflorum* Thunb.
Pharmaceutical name: Radix Polygoni Multiflori
Part of plant used: Root
Plant family: Polygonaceae (Cornbind Family)
Japanese name: *Kashuu*
Chinese name: *He Shou Wu*
Korean name: *Hasuo*
Dosage when used by itself in decoctions: 9.0–30.0 grams
How to recognize good quality in the unprocessed herb: Reddish brown, heavy, powdery, solid

Polyporus

Other common names: Polypore mushroom, umbrella polypore
Botanical name: *Polyporus umbellatus* (Pers.) Fr.
Pharmaceutical name: Sclerotium Polypori Umbellati
Part of plant used: Stem
Plant family: Polyporaceae (Polypore Mushroom Family)
Japanese name: *Chorei*
Chinese name: *Zhu Ling*
Korean name: *Cheyyong*
Dosage when used by itself in decoctions: 6.0–15.0 grams
How to recognize good quality in the unprocessed herb: Dark red, lustrous outer skin, white, powdery cross section

Prunella

Other common names: Self-heal
Botanical name: *Prunella vulgaris* L.
Pharmaceutical name: Spica Prunellae Vulgaris
Part of plant used: Above-ground parts
Plant family: Lamiaceae (Mint Family)

Japanese name: *Kagoso*
Chinese name: *Xia Ku Cao*
Korean name: *Hagoch'o*
Dosage when used by itself in decoctions: 30.0 grams
How to recognize good quality in the unprocessed herb: Dark crimson with large spikes

Psoralea

Other common names: Psoralea fruit
Botanical name: *Psoralea corylifolia* L.
Pharmaceutical name: Fructus Psoralea Corylifoliae
Part of plant used: Seed
Plant family: Fabaceae (Legume Family)
Japanese name: *Hokotsushi*
Chinese name: *Bu Gu Zhi*
Korean name: *Pogolchi*
Dosage when used by itself in decoctions: 3.0–9.0 grams
How to recognize good quality in the unprocessed herb: Black, full, solid

Reed Root

Other common names: Phragmitis
Botanical name: *Phragmites communis* L.
Pharmaceutical name: Rhizoma Phragmitis Communis
Part of plant used: Rhizome
Plant family: Gramineae (Grass Family)
Japanese name: *Rokon*
Chinese name: *Lu Gen*
Korean name: *Nogun*
Dosage when used by itself in decoctions: 15.0–60.0 grams
How to recognize good quality in the unprocessed herb: Coarse, shiny, strong, yellowish white, no small rootlets

Rehmannia, cooked

Other common names: Chinese foxglove root
Botanical name: *Rehmannia glutinosa* (Gaertn.) Libosch.
Pharmaceutical name: Radix Rehmanniae Glutinosae Conquitae
Part of plant used: Root. Should be charred if used to stop bleeding
Plant family: Scophulariaceae (Spinach Family)
Japanese name: *Jukujio*
Chinese name: *Shu Di Huang*
Korean name: *Sukchihwang*
Dosage when used by itself in decoctions: 9.0–30.0 grams
How to recognize good quality in the unprocessed herb: Black

Rehmannia, raw

Other common names: Chinese foxglove root
Botanical name: *Rehmannia glutinosa* (Gaertn.) Libosch.
Pharmaceutical name: Radix Rehmanniae Glutinosae
Part of plant used: Root
Plant family: Scrophulariaceae (Spinach Family)
Japanese name: *Shojio*
Chinese name: *Sheng Di Huang*
Korean name: *Saengjihwang*
Dosage when used by itself in decoctions: 9.0–30.0 grams
How to recognize good quality in the unprocessed herb: Thick, reddish yellow

Rhubarb Root

Other common names: Chinese rhubarb
Botanical name: *Rheum palmatum* L.
Pharmaceutical name: Radix et Rhizoma Rhei
Part of plant used: Root
Plant family: Polygonaceae (Rhubarb Family)
Japanese name: *Daio*
Chinese name: *Da Huang*
Korean name: *Taehwang*
Dosage when used by itself in decoctions: 3.0 –12.0 grams
How to recognize good quality in the unprocessed herb: Golden brown, bitter, hard, heavy, oily, solid

Rose Hips

Other common names: Chinese rose, dog rose
Botanical name: *Rosa rugosa* Thunb., *Rosa cania* L., *Rosa chinensi* Jacq.
Pharmaceutical name: Flos et Pseudofructus Rosae Rugosae, Flos et Pseudofructus Rosae Caninae, Flos et Pseudofructus Rosae Chinensis
Part of plant used: Hips and petals together
Plant family: Rosaceae (Rose Family)
Japanese name: *Gekkika*
Chinese name: *Yue Ji Hua*
Korean name: *Wolgyehwa*
Dosage when used by itself in decoctions: 3.0–6.0 grams
How to recognize good quality in the unprocessed herb: Fragrant, large, purple to red, thick

Saussurea

Other common names: Aucklandia, costus root
Botanical name: *Aucklandia lappa* Decne., also known as *Saussurea lappa* Clask.
Pharmaceutical name: Radix Aucklandiae Lappae
Part of plant used: Root
Plant family: Asteraceae (Composite Family)
Japanese name: *Mokko*
Chinese name: *Mu Xiang*
Korean name: *Mokhyang*
Dosage when used by itself in decoctions: 1.5–9.0 grams
How to recognize good quality in the unprocessed herb: Aromatic, slightly oily, solid

Scallion

Other common names: Spring onion
Botanical name: *Allium pstulosum* L.
Pharmaceutical name: Bulbus Allii Fistulosi
Part of plant used: Bulb, including the root
Plant family: Alliaceae (Onion Family)
Japanese name: *Sohaku*
Chinese name: *Cong Bai*
Korean name: *Ch'ongbaek*
Dosage when used by itself in decoctions: 2–5 scallions
How to recognize good quality in the unprocessed herb: Fresh, white bottoms with bright green tops

Schisandra

Other common names: Schisandra fruit
Botanical name: *Schisandra chinensis* (Turcz.) Baill.
Pharmaceutical name: Fructus Schisandrae Chinensis
Part of plant used: Fruit
Plant family: Schisandraceae (Schisandra Family)
Japanese name: *Gomishi*
Chinese name: *Wu Wei Zi*
Korean name: *Omicha*
Dosage when used by itself in decoctions: 1.5–9.0 grams
How to recognize good quality in the unprocessed herb: Fleshy, large, oily, purplish red, shiny, thick

Scrophularia

Other common names: Ningpo figwort root
Botanical name: *Scrophularia ningpoensis* Hemsl.
Pharmaceutical name: Radix Scrophulariae Ningpoensis
Part of plant used: Root
Plant family: Scrophulariaceae (Spinach Family)
Japanese name: *Genjin*
Chinese name: *Xuan Shen*
Korean name: *Hyonsam*
Dosage when used by itself in decoctions: 9.0–30.0 grams
How to recognize good quality in the unprocessed herb: Black, hard, and thick, with a thin skin

Scutellaria

Other common names: Baical skullcap root, scute, scutellaria root, skullcap
Botanical name: *Scutellaria baicalensis* Georgi
Pharmaceutical name: Radix Scutellariae Baicalensis
Part of plant used: Root
Plant family: Lamiaceae (Mint Family)
Japanese name: *Ogon*
Chinese name: *Huang Qin*
Korean name: *Hwanggum*
Dosage when used by itself in decoctions: 6.0–15.0 grams
How to recognize good quality in the unprocessed herb: Long, solid, thick, yellow, without noticeable root bark

Siberian Ginseng

This appears in Chapter 3 under Modern Japanese Herbal Preparations.
Other common names: Eleuthero, eleutherococcus
Botanical name: *Eleutherococcus senticosus* Ruprecht et Maximovich
Pharmaceutical name: Cortex Acanthopanacis Gracilistyli Radicis
Part of plant used: Root and root bark
Plant family: Araliaceae (Ginseng Family)
Japanese name: *Gokahi*
Chinese name: *Wu Jia Pi*
Korean name: *Ogap'i*
Dosage when used by itself in decoctions: 2.0–3.0 grams
How to recognize good quality in the unprocessed herb: Aromatic, long, thick sections of bark with grayish white cross section, no wood in center

Snake Gourd (Trichosanth) Fruit

Botanical name: *Trichosanthes kirilowii* Maxim.
Pharmaceutical name: Fructus Trichosanthis
Part of plant used: Whole melon
Plant family: Cucurbitaceae (Gourd Family)
Japanese name: *Karo*
Chinese name: *Gua Luo Shi*
Korean name: *Kwalwi*
Dosage when used by itself in decoctions: 9.0–30.0 grams
How to recognize good quality in the unprocessed herb: Intact, orange-yellow, sugary taste

Snake Gourd (Trichosanth) Root

Botanical name: *Trichosanthes kirilowii* Maxim.
Pharmaceutical name: Radix Trichosanthi Kirilowii
Part of plant used: Root
Plant family: Cucurbitaceae (Gourd Family)
Japanese name: *Tenkafun*
Chinese name: *Tian Hua Fen*
Korean name: *Ch'onhwabun*
Dosage when used by itself in decoctions: 9.0–15.0 grams
How to recognize good quality in the unprocessed herb: Firm, powdery, white

Solomon's Seal

Other common names: Jade bamboo, polygonatum
Botanical name: *Polygonatum odoratum* (Mill.) Druce var. *pluriflorum,* also known as *Polygonatum officinale* All.
Pharmaceutical name: Rhizoma Polygonati Odorati
Part of plant used: Rhizome
Plant family: Liliaceae (Lily Family)
Japanese name: *Gyokuchiku*
Chinese name: *Yu Zhu*
Korean name: *Okchuk*
Dosage when used by itself in decoctions: 9.0–15.0 grams
How to recognize good quality in the unprocessed herb: Long, thick, yellowish white

Solomon's Seal, Siberian

Other common names: Polygonati, polygonatum, Siberian Solomon's seal rhizome
Botanical name: *Polygonatum sibiricum* Redoute
Pharmaceutical name: Rhizoma Polygonati
Part of plant used: Rhizome
Plant family: Liliaceae (Lily Family)
Japanese name: *Osei*
Chinese name: *Huang Jing*
Korean name: *Hwangchong*
Dosage when used by itself in decoctions: 6.0–18.0 grams
How to recognize good quality in the unprocessed herb: Moist, yellow with translucent cross section

Stephania

Herbs used equivalently: Moonseed, sinomenium
Botanical name: *Sinomenium acutum* (Thunb.) Rehd. et Wils. (Japanese formulas), *Stephania tetranda* S. Moore (Chinese formulas)
Pharmaceutical name: Radix Stephaniae Tetrandrae
Part of plant used: Root
Plant family: Menispermaceae (Stephania Family)
Japanese name: *Kanboi*
Chinese name: *Han Fang Ji*
Korean name: *Hanbanggi*
Dosage when used by itself in decoctions: 3.0–9.0 grams
How to recognize good quality in the unprocessed herb: Firm, powdery

Tang-Kuei (Chinese Angelica)

Other common names: Chinese angelica root, dong quai, tang-gui
Botanical name: *Angelica sinensis* (Oliv.) Diels
Pharmaceutical name: Radix Angelicae Sinensis
Part of plant used: Root
Plant family: Apiaceae (Parsley Family)
Japanese name: *Toki*
Chinese name: *Dang Gui*
Korean name: *Tanggwi*
Dosage when used by itself in decoctions: 3.0–15.0 grams
How to recognize good quality in the unprocessed herb: Oily, fragrant, long, moist, yellow-brown exterior, yellow-white cross section. Do not use dry roots

Turmeric, rhizome

Botanical name: *Curcuma longa* L., *C. aromatica* Salisb.
Pharmaceutical name: Tuber Curcumae
Part of plant used: Rhizome
Plant Family: Zingiberaceae (Ginger Family)
Japanese name: *Ukon*
Chinese name: *Yu Jin, Guang Yu Jin, Chuan Yu Jin*
Korean name: *Ukkum*
Dosage when used by itself in decoctions: 3.0–5.0 grams
How to recognize good quality in the unprocessed herb: Thin wrinkles on the surface, orange-yellow cross section

Turmeric, root

Botanical name: *Curcuma longa* L.
Pharmaceutical name: Rhizoma Curcumae Longae
Part of plant used: Root
Plant Family: Zingiberaceae (Ginger Family)
Japanese name: *Kyoo*
Chinese name: *Jiang Huang*
Korean name: *Kanghwang*
Dosage when used by itself in decoctions: 3.0–5.0 grams
How to recognize good quality in the unprocessed herb: Solid, brownish yellow, columnlike shape

Viola

Other common names: Yedeon's violet
Botanical name: *Viola yedoensis* Mak. *V. mandshurica* W. Beck may be substituted
Pharmaceutical name: Herba cum Radice Violae Yedoensitis
Part of plant used: Whole plant
Plant family: Violaceae (Pansy Family)
Japanese name: *Shikajicho*
Chinese name: *Zi Hua Di Ding*
Korean name: *Chahwachi*
Dosage when used by itself in decoctions: 9.0–15.0 grams
How to recognize good quality in the unprocessed herb: Yellow-green and intact

Vitex

Other common names: Chaste tree fruit
Botanical name: *Vitex rotundifolia* L.
Pharmaceutical name: Fructus Viticis
Part of plant used: Fruit
Plant family: Verbenaceae (Verbena Family)
Japanese name: *Mankeishi*
Chinese name: *Man Jing Zi*
Korean name: *Manhyongja*
Dosage when used by itself in decoctions: 6.0–12.0 grams
How to recognize good quality in the unprocessed herb: Fragrant, solid, yellow-red

Wheat

Other common names: Green wheat, wheat berries
Botanical name: *Triticum aestivum* L.
Pharmaceutical name: Semen Tritic Aestivi Levis
Part of plant used: Seed
Plant family: Gramineae (Grass Family)
Japanese name: *Fushobaku*
Chinese name: *Fu Xiao Mai*
Korean name: *Pusomaek*
Dosage when used by itself in decoctions: 9.0–15.0 grams
How to recognize good quality in the unprocessed herb: Not quite ripened kernels of wheat of uniform size. Should float when added to decoction or when stewed with jujube and licorice

White Mustard Seed

Other common names: Mustard seed
Botanical name: *Brassica alba* (L.) Boiss.
Pharmaceutical name: Semen Sinapis Albae
Part of plant used: Seed
Plant family: Brassicaceae (Cabbage Family)
Japanese name: *Kakugaishi*
Chinese name: *Bai Jie Zi*
Korean name: *Paekkaecha*
Dosage when used by itself in decoctions: 3.0–9.0 grams
How to recognize good quality in the unprocessed herb: Full, round, white

Zanthoxylum

Other common names: Chinese prickly ash, Szechuan pepper
Botanical name: *Zanthoxylum bungeanum* Maxim.
Pharmaceutical name: Pericarpium Zanthoxyli Bungeani
Part of plant used: Fruit
Plant family: Rutaceae (Citrus Family)
Japanese name: *Shokusho*
Chinese name: *Chuan Jiao*
Korean name: *Ch'onch'o*
Dosage when used by itself in decoctions: 1.5–6.0 grams
How to recognize good quality in the unprocessed herb: Shiny red, thin-skinned

Zizyphus

Other common names: Sour jujube seed
Botanical name: *Ziziphus spinosa* Hu, also known as *Ziziphus jujuba* Mill.
Pharmaceutical name: Semen Zizyphi Spinosae
Part of plant used: Fruit. Crush before use
Plant family: Rhamnaceae (Buckthorn Family)
Japanese name: *Sansonin*
Chinese name: *Suan Zao Ren*
Korean name: *Sanchoin*
Dosage when used by itself in decoctions: 9.0–18.0 grams
How to recognize good quality in the unprocessed herb: Large, full, purplish red

Appendix C

Glossary

ACLE. Acute cutaneous lupus erythematous.

ACTH. Adrenocortitrophic hormone. A hormone that stimulates the secretion of ephinephrine (adrenaline) as part of the body's response to stress.

actinic keratosis. Abnormal skin growth stimulated by ultraviolet radiation from sunlight; may lead to a type of cancer called basal cell carcinoma.

acute illness. An illness that may cause severe symptoms but is of limited duration. Term is also sometimes used to mean "severe."

ADD. Attention Deficit Disorder.

Addison's disease. A disease caused by failure of the adrenal glands, marked by lack of appetite, weakness, digestive problems, and darkening of the skin.

ADHD. Attention Deficit Hyperactivity Disorder.

AIDS. Acquired immune deficiency syndrome.

aldose reductase. An enzyme that converts glucose into a toxin called sorbitol, a step that can lead to the formation of diabetic cataracts.

allergen. A normally harmless substance, such as pollen, that provokes an immune response.

allergy. An overreactive immune response to an allergen, such as hay fever developing in response to grass pollen.

alopecia. Baldness.

amino acid. One of the twenty-two nitrogen-bearing substances that the body uses to create proteins.

analgesic. An agent that reduces pain.

anaphylactic shock. A severe allergic reaction that can occur within seconds of contact with the allergen, marked by very low blood pressure and breathing difficulties.

anemia. A condition in which the bloodstream cannot carry enough oxygen to meet the needs of the body's tissues.

angina. A spasmodic, choking, or suffocative pain caused by a reduction in the heart muscle's supply of oxygen.

angiogenesis. The development of blood vessels that provide oxygen and nutrients to a tissue, healthy or malignant.

antibiotic. An agent derived from a mold or bacterium that acts against bacteria, fungi, and other microorganisms.

antibody. A protein, created by the immune system, designed to react to a specific microorganism or other foreign matter.

antigen. A foreign substance that triggers the body to produce antibodies.

antihistamine. An agent that opposes the action of histamine (*see* histamine).

aromatase. An enzyme involved in regulating sex hormone balances.

arrhythmia. Any deviation from the heartbeat's normal rhythm.

arteriosclerosis. A stiffening and thickening of the walls of arteries caused by calcium deposits.

artery. A blood vessel that carries blood away from the heart and towards the rest of the body's tissues.

ascites. The accumulation of fluid in the abdominal cavity, usually after liver disease.

astringent. In Oriental medicine, an agent that helps the body avoid loss of fluids, particularly blood or semen. Also an agent that causes contraction, especially after being applied to the skin.

atherosclerosis. A common form of arteriosclerosis in which fatty deposits form within the inner linings of arteries.

autoimmune disease. A condition in which the immune system attacks the body's own tissues. Examples include lupus, multiple sclerosis, and rheumatoid arthritis.

B cell. An immune-system cell that creates antibodies (*see* antibody).

bacteria. Single-celled microbes. Some bacteria can cause disease, while others, known as "friendly" bacteria, help the body by aiding digestion and protecting against harmful organisms.

basic fibroblast growth factor (bFGF). A hormone that stimulates the growth of blood vessels.

benign. Pertaining to cells or tumors that are not cancerous.

bile. A yellowish secretion, created in the liver, that is released into the small intestine to aid in fat digestion.

biopsy. Removal of tissue for diagnostic purposes.

blood (*ketsu*). An Oriental medicine term for body fluid that produces the essential energy qi (*see* qi).

blood imbalance (*ketsu sho*). An Oriental medicine term for irregularities in circulation that cause disease.

blood-brain barrier. A protective feature, involving capillary walls and other cells, that permits the entry of only certain substances into the brain.

BPH. Benign prostatic hypertrophy.

candidiasis. Infection with the yeast *Candida,* especially *Candida albicans.*

capillaries. Tiny blood vessels that link arteries with veins, and through which nutrients and wastes pass to and from the body's cells.

carcinoma. A cancer that arises from the cells, called epithelial cells, that line the body inside and out.

cardiac. Pertaining to the heart. Also, pertaining to the stomach area adjacent to the esophagus.

cervical dysplasia. Abnormal cell growth on the cervix that may lead to cervical cancer.

CFS. Chronic fatigue syndrome.

chemotherapy. The use of drugs to treat disease, especially drug therapy for cancer.

cholecystitis. Inflammation of the gallbladder.

cholesterol. A waxy substance used by the body for a number of purposes, including the creation of cell membranes and hormones. Most of the body's cholesterol supply is made in the liver, with the rest being obtained from food.

chronic illness. An illness that recurs or persists for an extended period of time.

cirrhosis. Liver disease marked by the development of scar tissue and nodules, and which eventually leads to loss of liver function.

climacteric. A period of transition from fertility to menopause in which production of estrogen, the main female hormone, diminishes. Also called perimenopause.

cold (*kan*). An Oriental medicine term for sensations of coldness or lack of energy, usually affecting the feet, legs, and lower torso.

collagen. A gelatinous protein found in connective tissue.

complication. A secondary problem that arises as the result of the initial illness, and that tends to make recovery longer and/or more difficult.

compress. A cloth used to apply heat, cold, or drugs to the body's surface.

constipation. A condition in which bowel movements are infrequent or difficult.

constitutional state (*taishitsu*). An Oriental medicine term for a qualitative measure of resistance or susceptibility to illness. One can have either a strong, robust constitution (*jitsu-sho*) or a weak, deficient constitution (*kyo-sho*).

cor pulmonale. Enlargement of the right ventricle of the heart caused by lung disease.

cortisol. A hormone produced in response to stress.

costochondritis. Inflammation of the cartilage attached to a rib.

Crohn's disease. A chronic inflammatory disease that leads to ulceration within the intestines.

cystitis. Inflammation of the bladder.

damp heat. An Oriental medicine concept equivalent to infection with inflammation. Damp heat moves downward in the body.

decoction. Liquid medicine made with boiled extracts of water-soluble substances.

deficiency (*kyo, kyosei taishitsu*). An Oriental medicine term for a frail constitutional state that produces symptoms such as weak reactions to stimuli, loss of muscle tone, lack of fluids, or other signs of energy deficiency. Usually called "vacuity" in TCM (*see* TCM).

dementia. A breakdown of mental function, marked by personality changes and decline in the ability to speak, remember, think, and/or orient oneself to the outside world.

dermatitis. Inflammation of the skin.

DGL. Deglycyrrhizinated licorice.

DHEA. Dehydroepiandrosterone. The most abundant hormone in the bloodstream, converted by the body into sex hormones.

diarrhea. A condition in which bowel movements are more frequent or fluid than normal.

diastolic pressure. The blood pressure exerted between heartbeats.

diuretic. An agent that increases urine output.

DLE. Discoid lupus erythematous.

dopamine. A substance created by the body that serves as a neurotransmitter (*see* neurotransmitter).

duodenal. Pertaining to the first portion of the intestine just after the stomach.

dysenteric wind. An Oriental medicine term for a condition of being unable to stand or walk, or to do so only with great difficulty, after infection with dysentery.

dysentery. Inflammation of the large intestine marked by bloody diarrhea and cramps.

dysmenorrhea. Difficult or painful menstruation.

edema. Swelling caused by fluid retention.

electrolyte. A substance, such as calcium and other minerals, that can conduct electrical impulses when dissolved in body fluids. Usually associated with maintenance of the body's fluid balance.

enzyme p450. A related group of liver enzymes necessary for the activation of many chemicals, including some cancer treatment drugs. Unbalanced p450 activity can lead to the development of toxins that damage liver tissue.

epididymitis. Inflammation of the ducts through which sperm leave the testes.

epinephrine (adrenaline). Stimulant hormone that increases rate and force of the heartbeat, quickens the breathing, and causes the liver to break down its energy stores for immediate use. Also serves as a neurotransmitter (*see* neurotransmitter).

Epstein-Barr virus (EBV). A virus responsible for infectious mononucleosis (a disease marked by fatigue, sore throat, and swollen glands) and linked to a number of other disorders.

essence. *See* jing.

essential fatty acid (EFA). A fatty acid that is required by the body, but which the body cannot create itself. There are two types of EFAs, omega-3s and omega-6s, which must be obtained from food.

essential oil. A volatile substance responsible for the odor or taste of a plant.

estradiol. The most active form of estrogen in the body.

estrogen. The main female hormone, important to both the menstrual cycle and to the development of such secondary sex characteristics as breast growth.

excess (*jitsu, jissei taishitsu*). An Oriental medicine term for an energetic constitutional state that produces symptoms such as excessive reactions to stimuli, muscle tension, excessive blood or fluids, and other signs of energy excess. Usually called "repletion" in TCM (*see* TCM).

expectorant. An agent that promotes the elimination of mucus from the respiratory tract.

exudate. Fluid expelled through the skin.

fibrin. A protein-based substance that forms strands on which new blood vessels may grow.

Five Delays. An Oriental medicine term for delayed development in children, consisting of delays in standing up, in walking, in growth of hair on the head, in the development of teeth, and in the development of speech.

flatulence. The presence of an abnormally large amount of gas in the stomach and intestines.

fluid imbalance (*suisho, suidoku*). An Oriental medicine term for abnormal fluid release (sweating) or retention (edema), which gives an indicator of how advanced a disease is.

follicle stimulating hormone (FSH). A hormone that allows eggs to "mature" within the ovary.

free radical. An unstable molecule produced during the body's use of oxygen. Such a molecule can damage tissues.

free radical scavenger. A substance that eliminates free radicals.

frostbite. Localized tissue destruction resulting from exposure to extreme cold.

gallstone. A hard, crystal-like structure found in the gallbladder or a bile duct, composed chiefly of cholesterol.

gastric. Pertaining to the stomach.

gastritis. Inflammation of the stomach lining.

gene p53. A gene that stops the multiplication of defective cells.

gingivitis. Inflammation of the gums.

glomerulnephritis. Inflammation of that portion of the kidney, the glomerulus, that filters wastes from the blood.

glucose. A simple sugar that is the body's primary source of energy.

***gobi* (also *goboshi*).** Prepared burdock, found in Japanese grocery stores.

Greater Yang. The first stage in the Oriental medicine six-stage model of disease, in which cold or a pathogen invades the outermost defensive layers of the body, and the body vigorously defends itself.

***hatomugi*.** Coix cereal, found in Japanese grocery stores.

HDL. High-density lipoprotein.

heat (*netsu*). An Oriental medicine term for overactivity of any bodily process, such as the reaction to infection that results in fever.

hemorrhage. Abnormal or profuse bleeding.

hepatitis. Inflammation of the liver, usually caused by a virus but sometimes caused by other agents, such as toxins.

herpes. A family of viruses responsible for a number of different disorders, including chickenpox, cold sores, genital herpes, ocular keratitis, and shingles.

histamine. A chemical, produced by the body in response to an allergen, that can cause breathing difficulties and low blood pressure.

HIV. Human immunodeficiency virus.

hormone. A chemical messenger that regulates bodily functions.

hot flushes (*nobose*). An Oriental medicine term for a rush of heat to the head with an uncomfortable sensation of heat, congestion, pressure, or muscular tension.

human papillomavirus (HPV). A virus that causes genital warts and is involved in cervical cancer.

hypertension. High blood pressure.

hypertrophy. A general increase in the bulk of a tissue or organ that is not due to a tumor.

hypoglycemia. Low blood sugar.

hypotension. Low blood pressure.

IBS. Irritable bowel syndrome.

immunity. The ability to resist infection or illness.

immunotherapy. The use of immune-strengthening techniques to fight illness.

incontinence. The inability to hold urine or stool for voluntary excretion.

infection. Invasion of the body by harmful microorganisms, such as bacteria, fungi, or viruses.

inflammation. The body's response to irritation or injury, generally involving redness, swelling, and warmth.

insomnia. The inability to sleep.

insulin. A hormone that enables the transport of sugar or fatty acids into most of the body's cells.

insulin resistance. *See* type 2 diabetes.

insulin-like growth factor I. A hormone that, when produced in excess, encourages the growth of weak, easily broken capillaries.

intercostal. Pertaining to the spaces between the ribs.

interferon. Any of a family of protein compounds that slow the course of viral infection.

interleukin. Any of a family of hormonelike substances that stimulate the immune system to produce B cells and T cells (*see* B cell, T cell).

intermittent claudification. A condition caused by interrupted blood supply to the muscles, chiefly the calf muscles. It is marked by attacks of lameness and pain.

intramuscular. Refers to injections given into muscle tissue.

jaundice. A yellowish staining of the skin, eyes, and mucous membranes, caused by too much bile pigment (bilirubin) in the blood.

***jing* (Chinese term; in Japanese, *sei*).** An Oriental medicine term for the essence that underlies all life, thought of as fluid-like, supportive, nutritive, and essential to reproduction, both physically and in the sense of passing on personal values. In terms of conventional medicine, roughly equivalent to DNA.

jitsuyo kanpo kyoho. An Oriental medicine term that means "diseases that are not diseases," or minor disorders, such as tension headaches, that cause discomfort but do not threaten essential body functions.

keratitis. Inflammation of the cornea.

ketoacidosis. Acidification of the blood, generally caused by diabetes.

laxative. An agent that loosens the bowels.

LDL. Low-density lipoprotein.

leaky gut syndrome. A condition in which the intestinal walls allow relatively large food particles to pass into the bloodstream. This condition can result in allergic reactions.

Lesser Yang. The second stage in the Oriental medicine six-stage model of disease, in which a stalemate exists between an invading pathogen and the body's defensive energies.

leukocyte. *See* white blood cell.

leukopenia. Low white blood cell count.

lipid peroxides. Substances that break down fats.

lipoprotein. A molecule that combines protein and fat, which allows fatty substances to be transported through the watery bloodstream.

lower burner. An Oriental medicine term for an energy organ that circulates defensive or immune energies upward from the portions of the torso below the navel.

luteinizing hormone (LH). A hormone that stimulates the release of eggs from the ovary.

lymph node. One of a number of organs that filter foreign material from lymph, a clear fluid that circulates within the body's tissues. Lymph nodes also create lymphocytes (*see* lymphocyte).

lymphocyte. Any of a group of white blood cells with specialized immune functions, such as B cells and T cells (*see* B cell, T cell).

lymphokine activated killer (LAK) cell. A hormonally activated immune cell that uses chemicals to destroy tumor cells.

macrophage. A "germ-eating" immune-system cell.

malignant. Pertaining to cells that are cancerous.

melatonin. An antioxidant hormone that protects damaged cells; also involved in sleep-wake cycle.

menopause. The termination of menstruation, caused by decreases in the levels of estrogen and progesterone.

menorrhagia. Abnormally heavy menstrual periods.

metastatic. Pertaining to cancer that has spread from the site where it first developed.

middle burner. An Oriental medicine term for an energy organ that circulates defensive or immune energies upward through the middle portion of the torso.

MS. Multiple sclerosis.

mucous membrane. Any of the membranes that line those moist parts of the body in contact with air, such as the anus, mouth, nasal passages, and vagina.

myasthenia gravis. A condition in which the immune system attacks the connection between nerves and muscles, especially the muscles around the eyes and the lungs.

myeloma. A tumor composed of the blood-producing cells in the bone marrow.

myoma. A benign growth composed of muscle tissue.

natural killer (NK) cell. An immune-system cell, activated by antibodies, that secretes chemicals to destroy cancer cells and infectious microbes.

neuralgia. Severe, throbbing, or stabbing pain along the course of a nerve.

neuropathy. Damage to nerve tissue.

neurotransmitter. A substance that relays impulses from one nerve cell to another.

norepinephrine. A stimulant hormone produced in response to low blood pressure and physical stress. Also serves as a neurotransmitter (*see* neurotransmitter).

orchitis. Inflammation of the testes.

orifice. A term for a body opening and, in Oriental medicine, any of the sense organs in the head.

osteomyelitis. Inflammation of the bone.

osteoporosis. A thinning and weakening of the bones, caused by the loss of minerals from bone tissue.

ovarian polycystic disease. A condition in which the ovaries contain many cysts, and high levels of male hormones are present.

Paired Organs. A TCM system in which five organ pairs—spleen/stomach, lung/large intestine, kidney/bladder, liver/gallbladder, and heart/small intestine—are responsible for, among other actions, housing and circulating energy.

parasite. An organism that lives on or in, and obtains nourishment from, another organism.

pathogen. A disease-causing entity.

peritoneum. The membrane lining the abdominal cavity.

pernicious anemia. Anemia caused by vitamin B_{12} deficiency, marked by red blood cells that are very large.

pharyngitis. Inflammation of the pharynx, the upper portion of the digestive tube from the esophagus to the mouth and nasal cavities.

phlegm. A term for mucus and, in Oriental medicine, a congestion of energy that impedes circulation or sensory perception.

PID. Pelvic inflammatory disease.

placebo. An inactive substance used in research to provide a basis for comparison with an active substance.

plaque. A deposit of undesired material on tissue, such as the buildup of plaque in arteries that leads to atherosclerosis.

plasmin. A substance that breaks up tissues, which creates a pathway for tumor invasion.

platelet activating factor (PAF). A substance that causes red blood cells to clump together. This starts a process that leads to allergic and asthmatic reactions.

PMS. Premenstrual syndrome. Term for a variety of symptoms that may be experienced a week or two before the start of menstruation, including acne, backache, breast tenderness, irritability, mood swings, and water retention.

poultice. A soft mush prepared by wetting powders or other absorbent substances with oils or water. The mash is then placed in a cloth and applied to the skin.

progesterone. A female sex hormone that acts in concert with estrogen to control the menstrual cycle.

prolactin. A hormone that starts and maintains milk flow.

prolapse. The sinking or falling of an organ or other body part, especially at its orifice.

prostaglandin. Any of a class of hormonelike substances present in many tissues. These substances regulate bodily processes such as blood pressure, inflammation reaction, and smooth muscle contraction in the windpipe, intestines, and uterus.

pulmonary. Pertaining to the lungs.

purgative. An agent that empties the bowels by encouraging defecation.

purpura. Purple discoloration of the skin, caused by bleeding.

qi. An Oriental medicine term for vital energy that circulates through the body in identifiable channels, connecting various organs.

radiation therapy. The use of radiation to treat disease, especially when used to treat cancer.

receptor site. A site on a cell that accepts a specific substance, such as an estrogen receptor site on a breast cell.

red blood cell. A cell that contains hemoglobin, a substance that carries oxygen through the bloodstream.

reflux. Upward flow of substances that should normally flow downward, such as stomach acid backing up into the esophagus.

remission. The reduction or reversal of symptoms in such chronic diseases as cancer or multiple sclerosis.

renal. Pertaining to the kidneys.

reverse transcriptase. An enzyme that allows HIV and similar viruses to insert their genetic information into the DNA of a human cell, causing the cell to produce more viruses.

Reye's syndrome. A condition that can follow viral infection. It involves brain inflammation and fatty-tissue invasion of the internal organs.

rhinovirus. A family of viruses that cause colds.

sarcoma. A cancer of the connective tissue.

SCLE. Subacute cutaneous lupus erythematous.

sedative. An agent that quiets nervous excitement.

serotonin. A hormone that influences a number of bodily functions, including digestion, respiration, and blood pressure maintenance. Also serves as a neurotransmitter (*see* neurotransmitter).

shingles. An infection with the herpes varicella-zoster virus, marked by painful blisters that follow the course of a nerve.

sho **(also called** ***hosho*** **or** ***yakusho*****).** An Oriental medicine term for a pattern of symptoms calling for treatment with a specific formula.

sign. An indication of disease that is not necessarily noticeable to the patient, but that is noticeable to the examiner.

Sjögren's syndrome. A condition in which the immune system attacks the body's moisture-producing glands. It is marked by dryness of the eyes and mouth.

SLE. Systemic lupus erythematous.

Smöyogi effect. A rebound effect in which blood sugar levels drop after consumption of a sugar-rich snack or meal.

spasm. Involuntary contraction of one or more muscle groups.

sperm motility. A sperm cell's ability to move through the female reproductive tract.

spermatorrhea. Any condition involving the involuntarily release of sperm.

static blood (*oketsu*). An Oriental medicine term for blood that is no longer free-flowing and that has lost its physiological function. Such blood may form clots or tumors.

stomatitis. Inflammation of the mouth.

summerheat. An Oriental medicine term for an external force that enters the body's interior and drives fluid out through the skin.

symptom. An indication of disease that is noticeable to the patient.

systolic pressure. The blood pressure exerted during heartbeats.

T cell. Any of a group of immune-system cells. Helper T cells coordinate the immune response against infectious microbes and cancerous cells, enabling the body to defend itself, while suppresser T cells suppress the immune response, preventing the immune system from attacking the body itself.

tachycardia. Excessively rapid heart rate.

TCM. Traditional Chinese Medicine.

tea. An infusion made by simmering plant material in water.

testosterone. The main male hormone, important to proper sexual function, fertility, and the development of such secondary sex characteristics as beard growth.

thrush. An infection by the fungus *Candida albicans* of the mouth and throat, as shown by white spots on the tongue and insides of the cheeks.

tincture. An alcohol solution prepared from herbal materials.

tinnitus. A ringing or roaring in the ear in the absence of any actual sound.

tonic. An agent designed to restore enfeebled function, and to promote vigor and a sense of well-being.

tonifying. Promoting vigor in an organ system.

topical. Pertaining to the surface of the body.

toxin. A poison that impairs bodily health; in Oriental medicine, pathogenic energy.

transient ischemic attack (TIA). A brief (lasting anywhere from several minutes to two hours) disruption in brain function caused by a temporary interruption in the brain's oxygen supply. It may produce momentary dizziness or any of the symptoms associated with a stroke, such as slurred speech, paralysis, or vision problems.

trigeminal. Pertaining to the nerves that enable facial sensation and movement.

triglycerides. The primary form in which fat is both found in food and stored in the body.

tumor necrosis factor (TNF). An immune-system chemical that causes inflammation and can kill cancer cells.

type 1 diabetes. A form of diabetes in which the body cannot produce enough insulin to meet its needs. Also called insulin-dependent or juvenile-onset diabetes.

type 2 diabetes. A form of diabetes in which the body produces enough insulin, but cannot use that insulin properly (insulin resistance). Also called non-insulin-dependent or adult-onset diabetes.

ulcer. A lesion on the skin or a mucous membrane.

upper burner. An Oriental medicine term for an energy organ that circulates defensive or immune energies from the torso to the head.

uveitis. Inflammation of the uveal tract, the vascular system of the eye.

vacant blood (*kekkyo*). An Oriental medicine term for blood that is inadequate to supply the organs.

vascular. Pertaining to the blood vessels.

vein. A blood vessel that carries blood away from the body's tissues and towards the heart.

vertigo. Faintness, dizziness, or inability to maintain one's balance.

virus. Any of a group of tiny disease-causing entities with very simple structures. They cannot reproduce on their own, and so must take over cells within the host organism to do so.

vitiligo. Appearance of nonpigmented patches on otherwise normal skin.

volatile oils. Easily evaporated taste- and aroma-imparting compounds found in plants.

weak gastrointestinal function (*icho kyojaku*). An Oriental medicine term for a state of poor digestion in which herbs and formulas taken by mouth may be poorly absorbed.

white blood cell (leukocyte). An immune-system cell that destroys invading organisms along with infected or damaged cells.

wind. An Oriental medicine term for any disease-causing entity that has sudden appearance and movement. Also refers to the abnormal movement of energy within the body.

wind-cold. An Oriental medicine term for infectious disease that is literally or figuratively caused by wind.

yang. An Oriental medicine term for any of the three early stages of disease, in which the body's energy is directed toward fighting the pathogen. Also used to described defensive energy directed outward from the body.

yeast. Any of a group of single-celled fungi. Some yeasts, such as *Candida albicans,* can cause infection.

yin. An Oriental medicine term for any of the later stages of disease, in which the body's energy is directed toward containing blood and fluids, and keeping organs within their normal contours. Also used to describe energy used to contain blood or fluid.

References

Chapter 1

What Is Kampo?

1. Soukichi, H., "Legends About the Initial Chou," in *The Great System of Oriental Culture,* unpublished, c. 1930.

2. English translations of this book, known in Chinese as *Huang Di Nei Jing Su Wen,* are widely available. The title is also translated as *The Yellow Emperor's Internal Canon.*

3. Quoted in Dharmananda, S. *Chinese Herbology: A Professional Training Program* (Portland: Institute for Preventative Medicine and Traditional Health Care, 1992), p. 508.

4. Quoted by Otsuka, K. in Hsu, H.Y., Peacher, W.G. (eds). *Shang Han Lun: Wellspring of Chinese Medicine* (Long Beach, California: Oriental Healing Arts Press, 1981), p. 82.

5. Bensky, D., Barolet, R. *Chinese Herbal Medicine: Formulas and Strategies* (Seattle: Eastland Press, 1990), p. 12.

6. Most modern theorists of Chinese medicine use from eighteen to twenty-two categories for classifying formulas, including: tonify and nourish (*bu yang*), disperse the exterior (*fa biao*), induce vomiting (*yong tu*), attack the interior (*gong li*), harmonize and relieve (*he jie*), regulate qi (*li qi*), regulate blood (*li xue*), dispel cold (*qu han*), dispel wind (*qu feng*), resolve dampness (*li shi*), clear summerheat (*qing shu*), moisten dryness (*run zao*), drain fire (*xie huo*), eliminate phlegm (*chu taan*), eliminate stagnation (*xiao dao*), kill parasites (*sha chong*), improve vision (*ming mu*), abscesses and sores (*yong yang*), menstruation and childbirth (*jing chan*), and emergencies (*jiu ji*).

7. In Bensky, D., Barolet, R., p. 5.

8. This section is based on Otsuka Keisetsu's *Kampo I Gaku* (Tokyo: Sogensha Publishing Company, 1945). Assistance provided by Dr. Helmut Bacowsky.

9. Tsumura, A. *Kampo: How the Japanese Updated Traditional Herbal Medicine* (San Francisco: Kodansha, 1991), p. 18.

10. Tsumura, A., pp. 16–17.

11. Shirota, F., Cyong, J.C. *What Is Kampo? The Role of Kampo Medicine in Japanese Health Care* (Tokyo: Tsumura and Company, 1996), pp. 22–24.

12. Shirota, F., Cyong, J.C., p. 16.

13. "Kampo Makes Large Inroads in Japanese Medical Care, Survey Indicates," *Kampo Today: News of Japanese Herbal Medicine,* Vol. 2, No. 1 (February 1997), p. 1.

14. *Kampo Today,* p. 1.

15. Based on Shirota, F., Cyong, J.C., p. 20.

16. *Kokumin Eisei no Doko, Kosei no Sihyo, Rinji Zokan* (Tokyo: Health and Welfare Statistics Association, 1995), p. 42 (9).

17. Varro Tyler, in an article in *HerbalGram* 38, p. 70.

18. Comments of Dr. Rudi Bauer at "Plants for Food and Medicine: Joint Meeting of the Society for Economic Botany and International Society for Ethnopharmacology," meeting held in London, England, 1–6 July 1996.

19. Comments of Dr. Max Wichtl at "Plants for Food and Medicine: Joint Meeting of the Society for Economic Botany and International Society for Ethnopharmacology," meeting held in London, England, 1–6 July 1996.

Chapter 3

The Medicines of Kampo

1. Lin, W.S., Chan, W.C., Hew, C.S., "Superoxide and traditional Chinese medicines," *Journal of Ethnopharmacology,* 48(3), 165–171 (3 November 1995).

Aconite

1. Hikino, H., Takahashi, M., Konno, C., Hashimoto, I., Namiki, T., "Pharmacological study of *Aconitum* roots. XV. Subacute and subchronic toxicity of *Aconitum* extracts and mesaconitine," *Sohyakugaku Zasshi,* 37, 1–9 (1983).

2. Ikeda, Y., Oyama, T., Taki, M., "Effect of processed Aconiti tuber on catecholamine and indoleamine contents in brain in rats," *Acta Anaesthesiologica Belgica,* 45(3), 113–118 (1994).

3. Oyama, T., Isono, T., Suzuki, Y., Hayakawa, Y., "Anti-nociceptive effects of Aconiti tuber and its alkaloids," *American Journal of Chinese Medicine,* 22(2), 175–182 (1994).

4. Hikino, H., Konno, C., Takata, H., Yamada, Y., Chizuko, O., Ohizumi, Y., Sugio, K., Fujimura, H., "Antiinflammatory principles of *Aconitum* roots," *Journal of Pharmacobiodynamics,* 3, 514–515 (1980).

Acorus

1. Nishiyama, N., Zhou, Y., Saito, H., "Beneficial effects of DX-9386, a traditional Chinese prescription, on memory disorder produced by lesioning the amygdala in mice," *Biological & Pharmaceutical Bulletin,* 17(12), 1679–1681 (December 1994).

2. Tang, W., Eisenbrand, G., *Chinese Drugs of Plant Origin: Chemistry, Pharmacology, and Use in Traditional and Modern Medicine* (Berlin: Springer-Verlag, 1992), p. 44.

Agrimony

1. Swanston-Flatt, S.K., Day, C., Bailey, C.J., Flatt, P.R., "Traditional plant treatments for diabetes. Studies in normal and streptozotocin diabetic mice," *Diabetologia,* 33(8), 462–464 (August 1990).

Akebia

1. Yamahra, J., Takagi, Y., Sawada, T., Fujimura, H., Shirakawa, K., Yoshikawa, M., Kitagawa, I., "Effects of crude drugs on congestive edema," *Chemical Pharmacy Bulletin,* 27, 1464–1468 (1979).

2. Tsen, T.T., "Pharmacological studies on the components of *Akebia longeracemosa,* especially on the chemical and pharmacological properties of *Akebia* saponins," *Shikoku Igaku Zasshi,* 29, 65–83 (1973).

Alisma

1. Bensky, D., Barolet, R., Kaptchuk, T., Bensky, L.L. *Chinese Herbal Medicine: Materia Medica,* Revised Edition (Seattle: Eastland Press, 1993), p. 146.

2. Huang, K.C. *The Pharmacology of Chinese Herbs* (Boca Raton, Florida: CRC Press, 1993), p. 105.

3. Shimizu, N., Ohtsu, S., Tomoda, M., Gonda, R., Ohara, N., "A glucan with immunological activities from the tuber of *Alisma orientale," Biological & Pharmaceutical Bulletin,* 17(12), 1666–1668 (December 1994).

Aloe

1. Cole, H.N., Chen, K.K., *"Aloe vera* in Oriental dermatology," *Archives of Dermatology and Syphilology,* 47, 250–257 (1943).

2. Zhang, L., Tizard, I.R., "Activation of a mouse macrophage cell line by acemannan, the major carbohydrate fraction from Aloe vera gel," *Immunopharmacology,* 35(2), 119–128 (November 1996).

3. Karaca, K., Sharma, J.M., Nordgren, R., "Nitric oxide production by chicken macrophages activated by Acemannan, a complex carbohydrate extracted from *Aloe vera," International Journal of Immunopharmacology,* 17(3), 183–188 (March 1995).

4. Visuthikosol, V., Chowchuen, B., Sukwanarat, Y., Sriurairatana, S., Boonpucknavig, V., "Effect of aloe vera gel to healing of burn wound: a clinical and histologic study," *Journal of the Medical Association of Thailand,* 78(8), 403–409 (August 1995).

5. Fulton, J.E., Jr., "The stimulation of postdermabrasion wound healing with stabilized aloe vera gel-polyethylene oxide dressing," *Journal of Dermatologic Surgery & Oncology,* 16(5), 460–467 (May 1990).

6. Danhof, I., "Potential reversal of chronological and photoaging of the skin by topical application of natural substances," *Phytotherapy Research,* 7, S53–S56 (1993).

7. Miller, M.B., Koltai, P.J., "Treatment of experimental frostbite with pentoxifylline and aloe vera cream," *Archives of Otolaryngology—Head & Neck Surgery,* 121(6), 678–680 (June 1995).

8. Hutter, J.A., Salman, M., Stavinoha, W.B., Satsangi, N., Williams, R.F., Streeper, R.T., Weintraub, S.T., "Anti-inflammatory C-glucosyl chromone from *Aloe barbadensis," Journal of Natural Products,* 59(5), 541–543 (May 1996).

9. Davis, R.H., Parker, W.L., Murdoch, D.P., "Aloe vera as a biologically active vehicle for hydrocortisone acetate," *Journal of the American Podiatric Medical Association,* 81(1), 1–9 (January 1991).

10. Syed, T.A., Ahmad, S.A., Holt, A.H., Ahmad, S.A., Ahmad, S.H., Afzal, M., "Management of psoriasis with *Aloe vera* extract in a hydrophilic cream, a placebo-controlled, double-blind study," *Tropical Medicine & International Health,* 1(4), 505–509 (August 1996).

11. Suzuki, I., Saito, H., Inoue, S., Migita, S., Takahashi, T., "Purification and characterization of two lectins from *Aloe arborescens* Mill.," *Journal of Biochemistry,* 85, 163–171 (1979).

12. Imanishi, K., "Aloctin A, an active substance of *Aloe arborescens* Miller, as an immunomodulator," *Phytotherapy Research,* 7, S20–S23 (Spring 1993).

13. Womble, D., Helderman, J.H., "Enhancement of allo-responsiveness of human lymphocytes by acemannan (Carrisyn)," *International Journal of Immunopharmacology,* 10(8), 967–974 (1988).

14. Saito, H., Imanishi, K., Suzuki, I., "Pharmacological studies on a plant lectin, Aloctin A. II. Inhibitory effect of Aloctin A on experimental models of inflammation in rats," *Japanese Journal of Pharmacology,* 32, 139–142 (1982).

15. Imanishi, K., Ishiguro, T., Saito, H., Suzuki, I., "Pharmacological studies on a plant lectin, Aloctin A. I. Growth inhibition of mouse methylcholanthrene-induced fibrosarcoma (Meth A) in ascites form by Aloctin A," *Experientia,* 37, 1186–1187 (1981).

16. Desai, K.N., Wei, H., Lamartiniere, C.A., "The preventive and therapeutic potential of the squalene-containing compound, Roidex, on tumor promotion and regression," *Cancer Letters,* 101(1), 93–96 (19 March 1996).

17. Kim, H.S., Lee, B.M., "Inhibition of benzoapyrene-DNA adduct formation by *Aloe barbadensis* Miller," *Carcinogenesis,* 18(4), 771–776 (April 1997).

18. Gribel, N.V., Pashinskii, V.G., "Antimetastatic properties of aloe juice," *Voprosy Onkologii,* 32(12), 38–40 (1986).

19. Egger, S.F., Brown, G.S., Kelsey, L.S., Yates, K.M., Rosenberg, L.J., Talmadge, J.E., "Hematopoietic augmentation by a beta-(1,4)-linked mannan," *Cancer Immunology, Immunotherapy,* 43(4), 195–205 (December 1996).

20. Roberts, D.B., Travis, E.L., "Acemannan-containing wound dressing gel reduces radiation-induced skin reactions in C3H mice," *International Journal of Radiation Oncology, Biology, Physics,* 32(4), 1047–1052 (15 July 1995).

21. Sakai, R., "Epidemiologic survey on lung cancer with respect to cigarette smoking and plant diet," *Japanese Journal of Cancer Research,* 80(6), 513–520 (June 1989).

22. Fan, Y.J., Li, M., Yang, W.L., Qin, L., Zou, J., "Protective effect of extracts from *Aloe vera* L. var. *chinensis* (Haw.) Berg. on experimental hepatic lesions and a primary clinical study on the injection of aloe in patients with hepatitis," *Chung-Kuo Chung Yao Tsa Chih—China Journal of Chinese Materia Medica,* 14(12), 746–748 (December 1989).

23. Sydiskis, R.J., Owen, D.G., Lohr, J.L., Rosler, K.H., Blomster, R.N., "Inactivation of enveloped viruses by anthraquinones extracted from plants," *Antimicrobial Agents and Chemotherapy,* 35(12), 2463–2466 (December 1991).

24. Agarwal, O.P., "Prevention of atheromatous heart disease," *Angiology,* 36, 485–492 (1985).

25. Ghannam, N., Kingston, M., al-Meshall, I.A., Tariq, M., Parman, N.S., Woodhouse, N., "The antidiabetic activity of Aloes: Preliminary clinical and experimental observations," *Hormone Research,* 24, 288–294 (1986).

26. Ibid.

27. Yagi, T., Yamauchi, K., Kuwano, S., "The synergistic purgative action of aloe-emodin anthrone and rhein anthrone in mice, synergism in large intestinal propulsion and water secretion," *Journal of Pharmacy & Pharmacology,* 49(1), 22–25 (January 1997).

28. Akao, T., Che, Q.M., Kobashi, K., Hattori, M., Namba, T., "A purgative action of barbaloin is induced by *Eubacterium* sp. strain BAR, a human intestinal anaerobe, capable of transforming barbaloin to aloe-emodin anthrone," *Biological & Pharmaceutical Bulletin,* 19(1), 136–138 (January 1996).

29. Saito, H., Imanishi, K., Okabe, S., "Effects of Aloe extract, Aloctin A, on gastric secretion and on experimental gastric lesions in rats," *Yakugaku Zasshi,* 109, 335–339 (1989).

30. Ibid.

31. Chung, J.H., Cheong, J.C., Lee, J.Y., Roh, H.K., Cha, Y.N., "Acceleration of the alcohol oxidation rate in rats with aloin, a quinone derivative of *Aloe,*" *Biochemical Pharmacology,* 52(9), 1461–1468 (8 November 1996).

32. Sakai, K., Saitoh, Y., Ikawa, C., Nishihata, T., "Effect of water extracts of aloe and some herbs in decreasing blood ethanol concentration in rats. II.," *Chemical & Pharmaceutical Bulletin,* 37(1), 155–159 (January 1989).

33. Fahim, M.S., Wang, M., "Zinc acetate and lyophilized *Aloe barbadensis* as vaginal contraceptive," *Contraception,* 53(4), 231–236 (April 1996).

34. Brusick, D., Mengs, U., "Assessment of the genotoxic risk from laxative senna products," *Environmental & Molecular Mutagenesis,* 29(1), 1–9 (1997).

35. Siegers, C.P., von Hertzberg-Lottin, E., Otte, M., Schneider, B., "Anthranoid laxative abuse—a risk for colorectal cancer?" *Gut,* 34(8), 1099–1101 (August 1993).

Amaranth (Achyranthis)

1. Ogawa, S., Nishimoto, N., Matsuda, H., "Pharmacology of ecdysones in vertebrates," in Burdette, W. J. (ed). *Invertebrate Endocrinology and Hormonal Heterophylly* (Berlin: Springer-Verlag, 1974), pp. 341–344.

2. Pakrashi, A., Bhattacharya, N., "Abortifacient principle of *Achyranthis aspera* Linn.," *Indian Journal of Experimental Biology,* 15, 856–858 (1977).

American Ginseng

1. Benishin, C.G., Lee, R., Wang, L.C., Liu, H.J., "Effects of ginsenoside Rb1 on central cholinergic metabolism," *Pharmacology,* 42(4), 223–229 (1991).

2. Chen, X., Yang, S.J., Chen, L., Ma, X.L., Chen, Y.P., Wang, L.L., Sun, C.W., "The effects of *Panax quinquefolium* saponin (PQS) and its monomer ginsenoside on heart," *Chung-Kuo Chung Yao Tsa Chih—China Journal of Chinese Materica Medica,* 19(10), 617–620 (October 1994).

3. Wang, W.K., Chen, H.L., Hsu, T.L., Wang, Y., "Alteration of pulse in human subjects by three Chinese herbs," *American Journal of Chinese Medicine,* 22(2), 197–203 (1994).

4. Huang, K.C. *The Pharmacology of Chinese Herbs* (Boca Raton, Florida: CRC Press, 1993), p. 35.

5. Fujimoto, Y., Satoh, M., Takeuchi, N., Kirisawa, M., "Cytotoxic acetylenes from *Panax quinquefolium,*" *Chemical Pharmacy Bulletin* (Tokyo), 39(2), 521–523 (February 1991).

Anemarrhena

1. Nakashima, N., Kimura, I., Kimura, M., Matsuura, H., "Isolation of pseudoprototimosaponin AIII from rhizomes of *Anemarrhena asphodeloides* and its hypoglycemic activity in streptozotocin-induced diabetic mice," *Journal of Natural Products,* 56(3), 345–350 (March 1993).

2. Bensky, D., Gamble, A., Kaptchuk, T., Bensky, L.L. *Chinese Herbal Medicine: Materia Medica,* Revised Edition (Seattle: Eastland Press, 1993), p. 57.

Angelica Dahurica (Wild Angelica)

1. Kimura, Y., Ohminami, H., Arichi, H., Okuda, H., Baba, K., Kozawa, M., Arichi, S., "Effects of various coumarins from roots *Angelica dahurica* on actions of adrenaline, ACTH, and insulin in fat cells," *Planta Medica,* 45, 183–187 (1982).

2. Huang, K.C. *The Pharmacology of Chinese Herbs* (Boca Raton, Florida: CRC Press, 1993), p. 158.

3. Bensky, D., Gamble, A., Kaptchuk, T., Bensky, L.L. *Chinese Herbal Medicine: Materia Medica,* Revised Edition (Seattle: Eastland Press, 1993), p. 35.

Apricot Seed

1. Huang, K.C. *The Pharmacology of Chinese Herbs* (Boca Raton, Florida: CRC Press, 1993), p. 215.

2. Yamamoto, K., Osaki, Y., Kato, T., Miyazaki, T., "Antimutagenic substances in the Armeniacae semen and Persicae semen," *Yakugaku Zasshi—Journal of the Pharmaceutical Society of Japan,* 112(12), 934–939 (December 1992).

Arisaema

1. Chang, H.M., But, P.P.H. *Pharmacology and Applications of Chinese Materia Medica,* Volume 1 (Singapore: World Scientific Publishing, 1986), p. 156.

2. Bensky, D., Gamble, A., Kaptchuk, T. Bensky, L.L. *Chinese Herbal Medicine: Materia Medica.* Revised Edition (Seattle: Eastland Press, 1993), p. 192.

Inset: Arisaema, the Lost Herb

1. Hu, S.L., "A comment on two medicinal aroids *huzhang* and *tiannanxing,*" *Chung-Kuo Chung Yao Tsa Chih—China Journal of Chinese Materia Medica,* 18(4), 195–196, 239, 253 (April 1993).

Artemisia

1. Zhang, L.H., Wang, J.Z., Zhou, X.B., Wu, B.J., "A comparative study on cholagogic effect of *Artemisia,*" *Chung-Kuo Chung Yao Tsa Chih—China Journal of Chinese Materia Medica,* 18(9), 560–561, 575 (September 1993).

2. Bensky, D., Gamble, A., Kaptchuk, T., Bensky, L.L. *Chinese Herbal Medicine: Materia Medica,* Revised Edition (Seattle: Eastland Press, 1993), p. 147.

3. Huang, K.C. *The Pharmacology of Chinese Herbs* (Boca Raton, Florida: CRC Press, 1993), p. 344.

4. "Differentiations to UTI protocol," *Protocol Journal of Botanical Medicine,* 1(1), 135 (Summer 1995).

Asiasarum

1. Hashimoto, K., Yanagisawa, T., Okui, Y., Ikeya, Y., Maruno,

M., Fujita, T., "Studies on anti-allergic components in the roots of *Asiasarum sieboldi,*" *Planta Medica,* 60(2), 124–127 (April 1994).

2. Bensky, D., Gamble, A., Kaptchuk, T., Bensky, L.L. *Chinese Herbal Medicine: Materia Medica,* Revised Edition (Seattle: Eastland Press, 1993), p. 36.

3. Huang, K.C. *The Pharmacology of Chinese Herbs* (Boca Raton, Florida: CRC Press, 1993), p. 145.

4. Winston, D., "Eclectic specific condition review: premenstrual syndrome," *Protocol Journal of Botanical Medicine,* 1(4), 179 (Spring 1996).

Asparagus Root

1. Bensky, D., Gamble, A., Kaptchuck, T., Bensky, L.L. *Chinese Herbal Medicine: Materia Medica,* Revised Edition (Seattle, Washington: Eastland Press, 1993), pp. 359–360.

Astragalus

1. Lin, L, et al., "A clinical study on treatment of vascular complications of diabetes with the sugar-reducing and pulse-invigorating capsule," *Journal of Traditional Chinese Medicine* (English-language version), 14(1), 3–9 (1994).

2. Chen, L.X., Liao, J.Z., Guo, W.Q., "Effects of *Astragalus membranaceus* on left ventricular function and oxygen free radical in acute myocardial infarction patients and mechanism of its cardiotonic action," *Chung-Kuo Chung Hsi I Chieh Ho Tsa Chih—Chinese Journal of Modern Developments in Traditional Medicine,* 15(3), 141–143 (March 1995).

3. Huang, W.M., Yan, J., Xu, J., "Clinical and experimental study on inhibitory effect of *sanhuang* mixture on platelet aggregation," *Chung-Kuo Chung Hsi I Chieh Ho Tsa Chih—Chinese Journal of Modern Developments in Traditional Medicine,* 15(8), 465–467 (August 1995).

4. Shi, H.M., Dai, R.H., Fan, W.H., "Intervention of lidocaine and *Astragalus membranaceus* on ventricular late potentials," *Chung-Kuo Chung Hsi I Chieh Ho Tsa Chih—Chinese Journal of Modern Developments in Traditional Medicine,* 14(10), 598–600 (October 1994).

5. Deng, C.Q., Ge, J.W., Wang, Q., "Comparison of effect of *Astragalus membranaceus* and *huoxuefang* on thromboxane, prostacyclin and adenosine cyclic monophosphate in cerebral reperfusion injury in rabbits," *Chung-Kuo Chung Hsi I Chieh Ho Tsa Chih—Chinese Journal of Modern Developments in Traditional Medicine,* 15(3), 165–167 (March 1995).

6. Luo, H.M., Dai, R.H., Li, Y., "Nuclear cardiology study on effective ingredients of *Astragalus membranaceus* in treating heart failure," *Chung-Kuo Chung Hsi I Chieh Ho Tsa Chih—Chinese Journal of Modern Developments in Traditional Medicine,* 15(12), 707–709 (December 1995).

7. Li, S.Q., Yuan, R.X., Gao, H., "Clinical observation on the treatment of ischemic heart disease with *Astragalus membranaceus,*" *Chung-Kuo Chung Hsi I Chieh Ho Tsa Chih—Chinese Journal of Modern Developments in Traditional Medicine,* 15(2), 77–80 (February 1995).

8. Liang, H., Wang, Z., Tian, F., Geng, B., "Effects of astragalus polysaccharides and ginsenosides of ginseng stems and leaves on lymphocytes membrane fluidity and lipid peroxidation in traumatized mice," *Chung-Kuo Chung Yao Tsa Chih—China Journal of Chinese Materia Medica,* 20(9), 558–560, inside backcover (September 1995).

9. Yan, H.J., "Clinical and experimental study of the effect of *kang er xin-i* on viral myocarditis," *Chung Hsi I Chieh Ho Tsa Chih—Chinese Journal of Modern Developments in Traditional Medicine,* 11(8), 468–470, 452 (August 1991).

10. Guo, Q., Peng, T.Q., Yang, Y.Z., "Effect of *Astragalus membranaceus* on Ca2+ influx and coxsackie virus B3 RNA replication in cultured neonatal rat heart cells," *Chung-Kuo Chung Hsi I Chieh Ho Tsa Chih—Chinese Journal of Modern Developments in Traditional Medicine,* 15(8), 483–485 (August 1995).

11. Chu, D.T., Lin, J.R., Wong, W., "The in vitro potentiation of LAK cell cytotoxicity in cancer and AIDS patients induced by F3—a fractionated extract of *Astragalus membranaceus,*" *Chung-Hua Chung Liu Tsa Chih—Chinese Journal of Oncology,* 16(3), 167–171 (May 1994).

12. Cha, R.J., Zeng, D.W., Chang, Q.S., "Non-surgical treatment of small cell lung cancer with chemo-radio-immunotherapy and traditional Chinese medicine," *Chung-Hua Nei Ko Tsa Chih—Chinese Journal of Internal Medicine,* 33(7), 462–466 (July 1994).

13. Khoo, K.S., Ang, P.T., "Extract of *Astragalus membranaceus* and *Ligustrum lucidum* does not prevent cyclophosphamide-induced myelosuppression," *Singapore Medical Journal,* 36(4), 387–390 (August 1995).

14. Jin, R., Wan, L.L., Mitsuishi, T., "Effects of *shi-ka-ron* and Chinese herbs in mice treated with anti-tumor agent mitomycin C," *Chung-Kuo Chung Hsi I Chieh Ho Tsa Chih—Chinese Journal of Modern Developments in Traditional Medicine,* 15(2), 101–103 (February 1995).

15. Weng, X.S., "Treatment of leukopenia with pure Astragalus preparation—an analysis of 115 leukopenic cases," *Chung-Kuo Chung Hsi I Chieh Ho Tsa Chih—Chinese Journal of Modern Developments in Traditional Medicine,* 15(8), 462–464 (August 1995).

16. Chang, H.M., But, P.P.H. *Pharmacology and Applications of Chinese Materia Medica,* Volume 2 (Teaneck, New Jersey: World Scientific Publishing, 1987), pp. 1041–1046.

17. Zhang, B.Z., Ding, F., Tan, L.W., "Clinical and experimental study on *yi-gan-ning* granule in treating chronic hepatitis B," *Chung-Kuo Chung Hsi I Chieh Ho Tsa Chih—Chinese Journal of Modern Developments in Traditional Medicine,* 13(10), 597–599, 580 (October 1993).

18. Zhao, X.Z., "Effects of *Astragalus membranaceus* and *Tripterygium hypoglancum* on natural killer cell activity of peripheral blood mononuclear in systemic lupus erythematosus," *Chung-Kuo Chung Hsi I Chieh Ho Tsa Chih—Chinese Journal of Modern Developments in Traditional Medicine,* 12(11), 669–671, 645 (November 1992).

19. Wagner, H., Proksch, A., Riess-Maurer, I., Vollmar, A., Odenthal, S., Stuppner, H., Jurcic, K., Le Turdu, M., Fang, J.N., "Immunostimulatory effects of polysaccharides (heteroglycans) of higher plants," *Arzneimittel-Forschung,* 35, 1069–1075 (1985).

20. Tu, L.H., Huang, D.R., Zhang, R.Q., Shen, Q., Yu, Y.Y., Hong, Y.F., Li, G.H., "Regulatory action of *Astragalus* saponins and *buzhong yiqi* compound on synthesis of nicotinic acetylcholine receptor antibody in vitro for myasthenia gravis," *Chinese Medical Journal,* 107(4), 300–303 (April 1994).

21. Chen, Y.C., "Experimental studies on the effects of *danggui buxue* decoction on IL-2 production of blood-deficient mice," *Chung-Kuo Chung Yao Tsa Chih—China Journal of Chinese Materia Medica,* 19(12), 739–741, 763 (December 1994).

22. Liang, H., Zhang, Y., Geng, B., "The effect of astragalus poly-

saccharides (APS) on cell mediated immunity (CMI) in burned mice," *Chung-Hua Cheng Hsing Shao Shang Wai Ko Tsa Chih—Chinese Journal of Plastic Surgery & Burns,* 10(2), 138–141 (March 1994).

23. Hong, C.Y., Ku, J., Wu, P., "*Astragalus membranaceus* stimulates human sperm motility in vitro," *American Journal of Chinese Medicine,* 20(3–4), 289–294 (1992).

24. Hong, G.X., Qin, W.C., Huang, L.S., "Memory-improving effect of aqueous extract of *Astragalus membranaceus* (Fisch.) Bge.," *Chung-Kuo Chung Yao Tsa Chih—China Journal of Chinese Materia Medica,* 19(11), 687–688, 704 (November 1994).

25. Bensky, D., Gamble, A., Kaptchuk, T., Bensky, L.L. *Chinese Herbal Medicine: Materia Medica,* Revised Edition (Seattle: Eastland Press, 1993), p. 320.

Atractylodis, Red

1. Bensky, D., Gamble, A., Kaptchuk, T., Bensky, L.L. *Chinese Herbal Medicine: Materia Medica,* Revised Edition (Seattle: Eastland Press, 1993), p. 217.

Atractylodis, White

1. Tang, W., Eisenbrand, G. *Chinese Drugs of Plant Origin: Chemistry, Pharmacology, and Use in Traditional and Modern Medicine* (Berlin: Springer-Verlag, 1992), p. 200.

2. Bensky, D., Gamble, A., Kaptchuk, T., Bensky, L.L. *Chinese Herbal Medicine: Materia Medica,* Revised Edition (Seattle: Eastland Press, 1993), p. 322.

Bamboo Shavings

1. Bensky, D., Gamble, A., Kaptchuk, T., Bensky, L.L. *Chinese Herbal Medicine: Materia Medica,* Revised Edition (Seattle: Eastland Press, 1993), p. 183.

2. Sato, T., Matsuhashi, M., Iida, O., "Fungi isolated from diseased medicinal plants," *Eisei Shikenjo Hokoku—Bulletin of National Institute of Hygienic Sciences,* 110, 60–66 (1992).

Barley Sprouts

1. Pollmer, U., personal communication with author, 8 January 1995.

Benincasa

1. Kumazawa, Y., Nakatsuru, Y., Yamada, A., Yadomae, T., Nishimura, C., Otsuka, Y., Nomoto, K., "Immunopotentiator separated from hot water extract of the seed of *Benincasa cerifera* Savi (Tohgashi)," *Cancer Immunology, Immunotherapy,* 19(2), 79–84 (1985).

2. Chandrasekar, B., Mukherjee, B., Mukherjee, S.K., "Blood sugar lowering potentiality of selected Cucurbitaceae plants of Indian origin," *Indian Journal of Medical Research,* 90, 300–305 (August 1989).

Biota

1. Nishiyama, N., Wang, Y.L., Saito, H., "Beneficial effects of S-113m, a novel herbal prescription, on learning impairment model in mice," *Biological & Pharmaceutical Bulletin,* 18(11), 1498–503 (November 1995).

2. Huang, K.C. *The Pharmacology of Chinese Herbs* (Boca Raton, Florida: CRC Press, 1993), p. 263.

3. Bensky, D., Gamble, A., Kaptchuk, T., Bensky, L.L. *Chinese Herbal Medicine: Materia Medica,* Revised Edition (Seattle: Eastland Press, 1993), p. 259.

4. Ibid.

Bitter Melon

1. Bever, B.O., Zahnd, G.R., "Plants with oral hypoglycemic action," *Quarterly Journal of Crude Drug Research,* 17, 139–196 (1979).

2. Welihinda, J., Arvidson, G., Gylfe, E., Hellman, B., Karlsson, E., "The insulin-releasing activity of the tropical plant *Momordica charantia,*" *Acta Biologica et Medica Germanica,* 41(12), 1229–1240 (1982).

3. Bourinbaiar, A.S., Lee-Huang, S., "The activity of plant-derived antiretroviral proteins MAP30 and GAP31 against herpes simplex virus in vitro," *Biochemical & Biophysical Research Communications,* 219(3), 923–929 (February 1996).

4. Lee-Huang, S., Huang, P.L., Huang, P.L., Bourinbaiar, A.S., Chen, H.C., Kung, H.F., "Inhibition of the integrase of human immunodeficiency virus (HIV) type 1 by anti-HIV plant proteins MAP30 and GAP31," *Proceedings of the National Academy of Sciences of the United States of America,* 92(19), 8818–8822 (12 September 1995).

5. Bourinbaiar, A.S., Lee-Huang, S., "Potentiation of anti-HIV activity of anti-inflammatory drugs, dexamethasone and indomethacin, by MAP30, the antiviral agent from bitter melon," *Biochemical & Biophysical Research Communications,* 208(2), 779–785 (17 March 1995).

6. Takemoto, D.J., Dunford, C., McMurray, M.M., "The cytotoxic and cytostatic effects of the bitter melon (*Momordica charantia*) on human lymphocytes," *Toxicon,* 20(3), 593–599 (1982).

7. Cakici, I., Hurmoglu, C., Tunctan, B., Abacioglu, N., Kanzik, I., Sener, B., "Hypoglycaemic effect of *Momordica charantia* extracts in normoglycaemic or cyproheptadine-induced hyperglycaemic mice," *Journal of Ethnopharmacology,* 44(2), 117–121 (October 1994).

8. Tennekoon, K.H., Jeevathayaparan, S., Angunawala, P., Karunanayake, E.H., "Effect of *Momordica charantia* on key hepatic enzymes," *Journal of Ethnopharmacology,* 44(2), 93–97 (October 1994).

Bitter Orange

1. Hosoda, K., Noguchi, M., Chen, Y.P., Hsu, H.Y., "Studies on the preparation and evaluation of *Kijitsu,* the immature citrus fruits. IV. Biological activities of immature fruits of different citrus species," *Yakugaku Zasshi—Journal of the Pharmaceutical Society of Japan,* 111(3), 188–192 (March 1991).

2. Bensky, D., Gamble, A., Kaptchuk, T., Bensky, L.L. *Chinese Herbal Medicine: Materia Medica,* Revised Edition (Seattle: Eastland Press, 1993), p. 235.

Bitter Orange Peel

1. Tang, W., Eisenbrand, G. *Chinese Drugs of Plant Origin: Chemistry, Pharmacology, and Use in Traditional and Modern Medicine* (Berlin: Springer-Verlag, 1992), p. 350.

2. Bruneton, J. *Pharmacognosy, Phytochemistry, Medicinal Plants* (Paris: Lavoisier Publishing, 1995), pp. 280–281.

Black Cardamom

1. Shoji, N., Umeyama, A., Takemoto, T., Ohizumi, Y., "Isolation of a cardiotonic principle from *Alpinia oxyphylla*," *Planta Medica*, 50, 186–187 (1984).

2. Shoji, N., Umeyama, A., Asakawa, Y., Takemoto, T., Nomoto, K., Ohizumi, Y., "Structural determination of nootkato, a new sesquiterpene isolated from *Alpina oxyphylla* Miquel possessing calcium-antagonistic activity," *Journal of Pharmaceutical Science*, 73, 843–844 (1984).

Black Cohosh

1. Bruneton, J. *Pharmacognosy, Phytochemistry, Medicinal Plants* (Paris: Lavoisier Publishing, 1995), pp. 296–297.

2. Einer-Jensen, N., Zhao, J., Andersen, K.P., Kristoffersen, K., "*Cimicifuga* and *Melbrosia* lack oestrogenic effects in mice and rats," *Maturitas*, 25(2), 149–153 (October 1996).

3. Düker, E.M., Kopanski, L., Jarry, H., Wuttke, W., "Effects of extracts from *Cimicifuga racemosa* on gonadotropin release in menopausal women and ovariectomized rats," *Planta Medica*, 57(5), 420–424 (October 1991).

4. Lehmann-Willenbrock, E., Riedel, H.H., "Clinical and endocrinologic studies of the treatment of ovarian insufficiency manifestations following hysterectomy with intact adnexa," *Zentralblatt für Gynakologie*, 110(10), 611–618 (1988).

5. Zheng, R.L., Zhang, H., "Effects of ferulic acid on fertile and asthenozoospermic infertile human sperm motility, viability, lipid peroxidation, and cyclic nucleotides," *Free Radical Biology & Medicine*, 22(4), 581–586 (1997).

Bletilla

1. Huang, K.C. *The Pharmacology of Chinese Herbs* (Boca Raton, Florida: CRC Press, 1993), p. 267.

2. Bensky, D., Gamble, A., Kaptchuk, T., Bensky, L.L. *Chinese Herbal Medicine: Materia Medica*, Revised Edition (Seattle: Eastland Press, 1993), p. 254–255.

3. Bensky, D., Gamble, A., Kaptchuk, T., Bensky, L.L., p. 255.

Blue Citrus (Qing Pi)

1. Huang, K.C. *The Pharmacology of Chinese Herbs* (Boca Raton, Florida: CRC Press, 1993), p. 177.

Brucea

1. Chang, M. *Anticancer Chinese Herbs* (Hunan Changha, China: Hunan Science and Technology Press, 1992).

2. Bensky, D., Gamble, A., Kaptchuk, T., Benksy, L.L. *Chinese Herbal Medicine: Materia Medica*, Revised Edition (Seattle, Washington: Eastland Press, 1993), p. 98.

Bupleurum

1. Yen, M.H., Lin, C.C., Chuang, C.H., Liu, S.Y., "Evaluation of root quality of *Bupleurum* species by TLC scanner and the liver protective effects '*xiao-chai-hu-tang*' prepared using three different *Bupleurum* species," *Journal of Ethnopharmacology*, 34(2–3), 155–165 (September 1991).

2. Huang, K.C. *The Pharmacology of Chinese Herbs* (Boca Raton, Florida: CRC Press, 1993), p. 152.

3. Bensky, D., Gamble, A., Kaptchuk, T., Bensky, L.L. *Chinese Herbal Medicine: Materia Medica*, Revised Edition (Seattle: Eastland Press, 1993), p. 50.

4. Hiai, S., Yokoyama, H., Nagasawa, T., Oura, H., "Stimulation of the pituitary-adrenocortical axis by saikosaponin of Bupleuri radix," *Chemical Pharmaceutical Bulletin*, 29, 495–499 (1981).

5. Yamamoto, M., Kumagai, A., Yokoyama, Y., "Structure and actions of saikosaponins isolated from *Bupleurum falcatum* L.," *Arzneimittel-Forschung*, 25, 1021–1040 (1975).

6. Huang, K.C. , p. 152.

7. Ushio, Y., Abe., H., "Inactivation of measles virus and herpes simplex virus by saikosaponin d," *Planta Medica*, 58(2), 171–173 (April 1992).

8. Sakurai, M.H., Matsumoto, T., Kiyohara, H., Yamada, H., "Detection and tissue distribution of anti-ulcer pectic polysaccharides from *Bupleurum falcatum* by polyclonal antibody," *Planta Medica*, 62(4), 341–346 (August 1996).

9. Sung, C.K., Kang, G.H., Yoon, S.S., Lee, I.K., Kim, D., Sankawa, U., Ebizuka, Y., "Glycosidases that convert natural glycosides to bioactive compounds," in Waller, G., Yamasaki, K. (eds). *Saponins Used in Traditional and Modern Medicine*, Advances in Experimental Medicine and Biology Volume 404 (New York: Plenum Press, 1996), p. 28.

Burdock (Arctium Lappa)

1. Lin, C.C., Lu, J.M., Yang, J.J., Chuang, S.C., Ujiie, T., "Anti-inflammatory and radical scavenge effects of *Arctium lappa*," *American Journal of Chinese Medicine*, 24(2), 127–137 (1996).

2. Umehara, K., Nakamura, M., Miyase, T., Kuroyanagi, M., Ueno, A., "Studies on differentiation inducers. VI. Lignan derivatives from Arctium Fructus. (2)," *Chemical & Pharmaceutical Bulletin*, 44(12), 2300–2304 (December 1996).

3. Morita, K., Kada, T., Namiki, M., "A dismutagenic factor isolated from burdock (*Arctium lappa* Linne)," *Mutation Research*, 129(1), 25–31 (October 1984).

4. Pizzorno, J.E., Murray, M.T. *A Textbook of Natural Medicine* (Seattle: John Bastyr College Publications, 1985), p. IV: Food A1.

5. Bensky, D., Gamble, A., Kaptchuk, T., Bensky, L.L. *Chinese Herbal Medicine: Materia Medica*, Revised Edition (Seattle: Eastland Press, 1993), p. 42.

6. Morita, T., Ebihara, K., Kiriyama, S., "Dietary fiber and fat-derivatives prevent mineral oil toxicity in rats by the same mechanism," *Journal of Nutrition*, 123(9), 1575–1585 (September 1993).

7. Nose, M., Fujimoto, T., Takeda, T., Nishibe, S., Ogihara, Y., "Structural transformation of lignan compounds in rat gastrointestinal tract," *Planta Medica*, 58(6), 520–523 (December 1992).

Caltrop

1. Huang, K.C. *The Pharmacology of Chinese Herbs* (Boca Raton, Florida: CRC Press, 1993), p. 140.

Cardamom

1. Huang, Z.Y., Lin, B.H., Sun, H.X., Wu, Z.P., Wu, Q.D., Huang, Y.C., Gu, C.F., Rao, D.Y., Huang, Z., Lin, Y.Q., Chen, Z.M., "Therapeutic effect of *Alpinia japonica* on peptic ulcers," *Fujian Medical Journal*, 6, 24–25 (1984).

2. Bensky, D., Gamble, A., Kaptchuk, T., Bensky, L.L. *Chinese Herbal Medicine: Materia Medica*, Revised Edition (Seattle: Eastland Press, 1993), p. 218.

3. Huang, K.C. *The Pharmacology of Chinese Herbs* (Boca Raton, Florida: CRC Press, 1993), p. 177.

4. Dharmananda, S. *Chinese Herbology: A Professional Training Program* (Portland: Institute for Traditional Medicine and Preventive Health Care, 1992), p. 177.

Carthamus

1. Duke, J.A. *The Green Pharmacy* (Emmaus, Pennsylvania: Rodale Press, 1997), p. 80.

2. Yasukawa, K., Akihisa, T., Kasahara, Y., Kaminaga, T., Kanno, H., Kumaki, K., Tamura, T., Takido, M., "Inhibitory effect of alkane-6,8-diols, the components of safflower, on tumor promotion by 12-O-tetradecanoylphorbol-13-acetate in two-stage carcinogenesis in mouse skin," *Oncology,* 53(2), 133–136 (March–April 1996).

3. Ibid.

4. Chang, H.M., But, P.P.H. *Pharmacology and Applications of Chinese Materia Medica,* Volume 1 (Singapore: World Scientific Publishing, 1986), p. 535.

5. Shi, M., Chang, L., He, G., "Stimulating action of *Carthamus tinctorius* L., *Angelica sinensis* (Oliv.) Diels and *Leonurus sibiricus* L. on the uterus," *Chung-Kuo Chung Yao Tsa Chih—China Journal of Chinese Materia Medica,* 20(3), 173–175, 192 (March 1995).

Chebula

1. Bensky, D., Gamble, A., Kaptchuk, T., Bensky, L.L. *Chinese Herbal Medicine: Materia Medica,* Revised Edition (Seattle, Washington: Eastland Press, 1993), pp. 380–381.

Chinese Senega Root

1. Huang, K.C. *The Pharmacology of Chinese Herbs* (Boca Raton, Florida: CRC Press, 1993), p. 224.

2. Yoshikawa, M., Yamahara, J., "Inhibitory effect of oleanene-type triterpene oligoglycosides on ethanol absorption: the structure-activity relationships," in Waller, G., Yamasaki, K. *Saponins Used in Traditional and Modern Medicine,* Advances in Experimental Medicine and Biology Volume 404 (New York: Plenum Press, 1996), pp. 207–218.

Chrysanthemum

1. Tang, W., Eisenbrand, G. *Chinese Drugs of Plant Origin: Chemistry, Pharmacology, and Use in Traditional and Modern Medicine* (Berlin: Springer-Verlag, 1992), p. 312.

Cinnamon

1. Yu, S.M., Wu, T.S., Teng, C.M., "Pharmacological characterization of cinnamophilin, a novel dual inhibitor of thromboxane synthase and thromboxane A_2 receptor," *British Journal of Pharmacology,* 111(3), 906–912 (March 1994).

2. Okano, K., Iwai, M., Iga, Y., Yokoyama, K., "Antiulcerogenic compounds isolated from Chinese cinnamon," *Planta Medica,* 55(3), 245–248 (June 1989).

3. Quale, J.M., Landman, D., Zaman, M.M., Burney, S., Sathe, S.S., "In vitro activity of *Cinnamomum zeylanicum* against azole-resistant and sensitive *Candida* species and a pilot study of cinnamon for oral candidiasis," *American Journal of Chinese Medicine,* 24(2), 103–109 (1996).

4. Osawa, K., Matsumoto, T., Yasuda, H., Kato, T., Naito, Y., Okuda, K., "The inhibitory effect of plant extracts on the collagenolytic activity and cytotoxicity of human gingival fibroblasts by *Porphyromonas gingivalis* crude enzyme," *Bulletin of Tokyo Dental College,* 32(1), 1–7 (February 1991).

5. Singh, H.B., Srivastava, M., Singh, A.B., Srivastava, A.K., "Cinnamon bark oil, a potent fungitoxicant against fungi causing respiratory tract mycoses," *Allergy,* 50(12), 995–999 (December 1995).

6. Ling, J., Liu, W.Y., "Cytotoxicity of two new ribosome-inactivating proteins, cinnamomin and camphorin, to carcinoma cells," *Cell Biochemistry & Function,* 14(3), 157–161 (September 1996).

Cistanche

1. Xiong, Q., Kadota, S., Tani, T., Namba, T., "Antioxidative effects of phenylethanoids from *Cistanche deserticola,*" *Biological and Pharmaceutical Bulletin,* 19(12), 1580–1585 (December 1996).

2. Zhao, W.K., Jin, G.Q., "Effect of *guzhen* recipe on glucocorticoid receptor in senile rat thymocyte," *Chung-Kuo Chung Hsi I Chieh Ho Tsa Chih—Chinese Journal of Modern Developments in Traditional Medicine,* 15(2), 92–94 (February 1995).

Clematis

1. Bensky, D., Gamble, A., Kaptchuk, T., Bensky, L.L. *Chinese Herbal Medicine: Materia Medica,* Revised Edition (Seattle: Eastland Press, 1993), p. 159.

2. Tang, W., Eisenbrand, G. *Chinese Drugs of Plant Origin: Chemistry, Pharmacology, and Use in Traditional and Modern Medicine* (Berlin: Springer-Verlag, 1992), p. 351.

3. Bensky, D., Gamble, A., Kaptchuk, T., Bensky, L.L., p. 158.

Cloves

1. Bensky, D., Gamble, A., Kaptchuk, T., Bensky, L.L. *Chinese Herbal Medicine: Materia Medica,* Revised Edition (Seattle: Eastland Press, 1993), p. 306.

2. Kurokawa, M., Nagasaka, K., Hirabayashi, T., Uyama, S., Sato, H., Kageyama, T., Kadota, S., Ohyama, H., Hozumi, T., Namba, T., et al., "Efficacy of traditional herbal medicines in combination with acyclovir against herpes simplex virus type 1 infection in vitro and in vivo," *Antiviral Research,* 27(1–2), 19–37 (May 1995).

Codonopsis

1. Wang, Z.T., Du, Q., Xu, G.J., Wang, R.J., Fu, D.Z., Ng, T.B., "Investigations on the protective action of *Codonopsis pilosula* (*Dangshen*) extract on experimentally-induced gastric ulcer in rats," *General Pharmacology,* 28(3), 469–473 (March 1997).

2. Chang, H.M., But, P.P.H. *Pharmacology and Applications of Chinese Materia Medica,* Volume 2 (Teaneck, New Jersey: World Scientific Publishing, 1987), p. 975.

3. Zeng, X.L., Li, X.A., Zhang, B.Y., "Immunological and hematopoeietic effect of *Codonopsis pilosula* on cancer patients during radiotherapy," *Chung-Kuo Chung Hsi I Chieh Ho Tsa Chih—Chinese Journal of Modern Developments in Traditional Medicine,* 12(10), 607–608 (October 1992).

4. Chen, Y.R., Yen, J.H., Lin, C.C., Tsai, W.J., Liu, W.J., Tsai, J.J., Lin, S.F., Liu, H.W., "The effects of Chinese herbs on improving survival and inhibiting anti-ds DNA antibody production in

lupus mice," *American Journal of Chinese Medicine,* 21(3–4), 257–262 (1993).

Coix

1. Numata, M., Yamamoto, A., Moribayashi, A., Yamada, H., "Antitumor components isolated from the Chinese herbal medicine *Coix lachryma-jobi,*" *Planta Medica,* 60(4), 356–359 (August 1994).

2. Kaneda, T., Hidaka, Y., Kashiwai, T., Tada, H., Takano, T., Nishiyama, S., Amino, N., Miyai, K., "Effect of coix seed on the changes in peripheral lymphocyte subsets," *Rinsho Byori—Journal of Clinical Pathology,* 40(2), 179–181 (February 1992).

3. Hidaka, Y., Kaneda, T., Amino, N., Miyai, K., "Chinese medicine, Coix seeds increase peripheral cytotoxic T and NK cells," *Biotherapy,* 5(3), 201–203 (1992).

4. Check, J.B., K'Ombut, F.O., "The effect on fibrinolytic system of blood plasma of Wistar rats after feeding them with Coix mixed diet," *East African Medical Journal,* 72(1), 51–55 (January 1995).

5. Park, Y., Suzuki, H., Lee, Y.S., Hayakawa, S., Wada, S., "Effect of coix on plasma, liver, and fecal lipid components in the rat fed on lard- or soybean oil-cholesterol diet," *Biochemical Medicine & Metabolic Biology,* 39(1), 11–17 (February 1988).

Coltsfoot

1. Bensky, D., Gamble, A., Kaptchuk, T., Bensky, L.L. *Chinese Herbal Medicine: Materia Medica,* Revised Edition (Seattle: Eastland Press, 1993), p. 201.

2. Huang, K.C. *The Pharmacology of Chinese Herbs* (Boca Raton, Florida: CRC Press, 1993), p. 218.

3. Wiedenfeld, Helmut, personal correspondence with author, 6 April 1996.

Coptis

1. Mitscher, L.A., "Plant-derived antibiotics," in Weinstein, M.J., Wagman, G.H. (eds). *Antibiotics,* Volume 15 (New York: Plenum Press, 1978), pp. 363–477.

2. Kaneda, Y., Tanaka, T., Saw, T., "Effects of berberine, a plant alkaloid, on the growth of anaerobic protozoa in axenic culture," *Tokai Journal of Experimental & Clinical Medicine,* 15(6), 417–423 (November 1990).

3. Bensky, D., Gamble, A., Kaptchuk, T., Bensky, L.L. *Chinese Herbal Medicine: Materia Medica,* Revised Edition (Seattle: Eastland Press, 1993), p. 78.

4. Zhang, L., Yang, L.W., Yang, L.J., "Relation between *Helicobacter pylori* and pathogenesis of chronic atrophic gastritis and the research of its prevention and treatment," *Chung-Kuo Chung Hsi I Chieh Ho Tsa Chih—Chinese Journal of Modern Developments in Traditional Medicine,* 12(9), 515–516 (September 1992).

5. Franzblau, S.G., Cross C., "Comparative in vitro antimicrobial activity of Chinese medicinal herbs," *Journal of Ethnopharmacology,* 15(3), 279–288 (March 1986).

6. Huang, Y.X., "Treatment of osteomyelitis of the fingers by steeping in a coptis decoction," *Chung-Kuo Chung Hsi I Chieh Ho Tsa Chih—Chinese Journal of Modern Developments in Traditional Medicine,* 5(10), 579 (October 1985).

7. Bensky, D., Gamble, A., Kaptchuk, T., Bensky, L.L., p. 79.

8. Shen, Z.F., Xie, M.Z., "Determination of berberine in biological specimen by high performance TLC and fluoro-densitometric method," *Yao Hsueh Hsueh Pao—Acta Pharmaceutica Sinica,* 28(7), 532–536 (1993).

9. Song, L.C., Chen, K.Z., Zhu, J.Y., "The effect of *Coptis chinensis* on lipid peroxidation and antioxidase activity in rats," *Chung-Kuo Chung Hsi I Chieh Ho Tsa Chih—Chinese Journal of Modern Developments in Traditional Medicine,* 12(7), 423–421, 390 (July 1992).

10. Namba, T., Sekiya, K., Toshinal, A., Kadota, S., Hatanaka, T., Katayama, K., Koizumi, T., "Study on baths with crude drug. II.: the effects of coptidis rhizoma extracts as skin permeation enhancer," *Yakugaku Zasshi—Journal of the Pharmaceutical Society of Japan,* 115(8), 618–625 (August 1995).

11. Chi, C.W., Chang, Y.F., Chao, T.W., Chiang, S.H., P'eng, F.K., Lui, W.Y., Liu, T.Y., "Flowcytometric analysis of the effect of berberine on the expression of glucocorticoid receptors in human hepatoma HepG2 cells," *Life Sciences,* 54(26), 2099–2107 (1994).

Cornelian Cherry

1. Huang, K.C. *The Pharmacology of Chinese Herbs* (Boca Raton, Florida: CRC Press, 1993), p. 244.

Corydalis

1. Bruneton, J. *Pharmacognosy, Phytochemistry, Medicinal Plants* (Paris: Lavoisier Publishing, 1995), p. 748.

2. Reimeier, C., Schneider, I., Schneider, W., Schafer, H.L., Elstner, E.F., "Effects of ethanolic extracts from *Eschscholtzia californica* and *Corydalis cava* on dimerization and oxidation of enkephalins," *Arzneimittel-Forschung,* 45(2), 132–136 (February 1995).

3. Bensky, D., Gamble, A., Kaptchuk, T., Bensky, L.L. *Chinese Herbal Medicine: Materia Medica,* Revised Edition (Seattle: Eastland Press, 1993), p. 270.

4. Dharmananda, S., personal communication with author, 17 April 1996.

5. Kubo, M., Matsuda, H., Tokuoka, K., Kobayashi, Y., Ma, S., Tanaka, T., "Studies of anti-cataract drugs from natural sources. I. Effects of a methanolic extract and the alkaloidal components from *Corydalis* tuber on in vitro aldose reductase activity," *Biological & Pharmaceutical Bulletin,* 17(3), 458–459 (March 1994).

6. Huang, K.C. *The Pharmacology of Chinese Herbs* (Boca Raton, Florida: CRC Press, 1993), p. 142.

Cuscuta

1. Huang, K.C. *The Pharmacology of Chinese Herbs* (Boca Raton, Florida: CRC Press, 1993), p. 210.

Dan Shen

1. Huang, K.C. *The Pharmacology of Chinese Herbs* (Boca Raton, Florida: CRC Press, 1993), pp. 83–84.

2. Huang, K.C., p. 82.

3. Ibid.

4. Shanghai Hospital Team, *Chinese Medical Journal,* 11, 68 (1976).

5. Ibid.

6. Liu, J., Hua, G., Liu W., Cui, Y., et al., "The effect of IH764-3 on fibroblast proliferation and function," *Chinese Medical Science Journal,* 7(3), 142–147 (September 1992).

7. Winston, D., "Eclectic specific condition review: uterine fibroids," *Protocol Journal of Botanical Medicine*, 1(4), 211 (Spring 1996).

8. Li, W., Zhou, C.H., Lu, Q.L., "Effects of Chinese materia medica in activating blood stimulating menstrual flow on the endocrine function of ovary-uterus and its mechanisms," *Chung Hsi I Chieh Ho Tsa Chih*, 12(30), 165–168 (1992).

Dandelion

1. Racz-Kotilla, E., Racz, G., Solomon, A., "The action of *Taraxacum officinale* extracts on the body weight and diuresis of laboratory animals," *Planta Medica*, 26(3), 212–217 (November 1974).

2. Faber, K., "The dandelion—*Taraxacum officinale* Weber," *Pharmazie*, 13, 423–435 (1958).

3. Chakurski, I., Matev, M., Koichev, A., Angelova, I., Stefanov, G., "Treatment of chronic colitis with an herbal combination of *Taraxacum officinale, Hypericum perforatum, Melissa officinalis, Calendula officinalis* and *Foeniculum vulgare*," *Vutreshni Bolesti*, 20(6), 51–54 (1981).

4. Swanston-Flatt, S.K., Day, C., Flatt, P.R., Gould, B.J., Bailey, C.J., "Glycaemic effects of traditional European plant treatments for diabetes. Studies in normal and streptozotocin diabetic mice," *Diabetes Research*, 10(2), 69–73 (February 1988).

5. Racz-Kotilla, E., Racz, G., Solomon, A., pp. 212–217.

6. Zheng, M., "Experimental study of 472 herbs with antiviral action against the herpes simplex virus," *Chung Hsi I Chieh Ho Tsa Chih—Chinese Journal of Modern Developments in Traditional Medicine*, 10(1), 39–41, 6 (January 1990).

Dendrobium

1. Fellows, L.E., Kite, G.C., Nash, R.J., Simmonds, M.J.S., Scofield, A.M., "Castanospermine, swainsonine and related polyhydroxyalkaloids: structure, distribution and biological activity," *Recent Advances in Phytochemistry*, 23, 395–427 (1989).

2. Dharmananda, S., "Traditional Chinese specific condition review," *Protocol Journal of Botanical Medicine*, 2(2), 43 (1997).

Dioscorea

1. Iwu, M.M., Okunji, C.O., Ohiaeri, G.O., Akah, P., Corley, D., Tempesta , M.S., "Hypoglycaemic activity of dioscoretine from tubers of *Dioscorea dumetorum* in normal and alloxan diabetic rabbits," *Planta Medica*, 56(3), 264–267 (June 1990).

2. Undie, A.S., Akubue, P.I., "Pharmacological evaluation of *Dioscorea dumetorum* tuber used in traditional antidiabetic therapy," *Journal of Ethnopharmacology*, 15(2), 133–144 (February 1986).

3. Huang, K.C. *The Pharmacology of Chinese Herbs* (Boca Raton, Florida: CRC Press, 1993), p. 162.

Inset: Beauty Served by Dioscorea

1. Accolla, D., Yates, P. *Back to Balance: A Holistic Self-Help Guide to Eastern Remedies* (New York: Kodansha International, 1996), pp. 55–56.

Dracaena Lily

1. Bensky, D., Gamble, A., Kaptchuk, T., Bensky, L.L. *Chinese Herbal Medicine: Materia Medica*, Revised Edition (Seattle: Eastland Press, 1993), p. 288.

Drynaria Rhizome

1. Bensky, D., Gamble, A., Kaptchuk, T., Bensky, L.L. *Chinese Herbal Medicine: Materia Medica*, Revised Edition (Seattle: Eastland Press, 1993), p. 350.

Ephedra

1. Toubro, S., Astrup, A.V., Breum, L., Quaade, F., "Safety and efficacy of long-term treatment with ephedrine, caffeine and an ephedrine/caffeine mixture," *International Journal of Obesity*, 17(Suppl 1), S69–S72 (1993).

2. Pasquali, R., Casimirri, F., "Clinical aspects of ephedrine in the treatment of obesity," unpublished paper.

3. Williamson, D.F., Madan, S.J., Anda, R.F., et al., "Smoking cessation and severity of weight gain in a national cohort," *New England Journal of Medicine*, 324, 739 (14 March 1991).

4. Dulloo, A.G., "Ephedrine, xanthines and prostaglandin-inhibitors: actions and interactions in the stimulation of thermogenesis," *International Journal of Obesity*, 17(Suppl 1), S35–S40 (1993).

5. White, L.M., Gardner, S.F., Gurley, B.J., Marx, M.A., Wang, P.L., Estes, M., "Pharmacokinetics and cardiovascular effects of ma-huang (*Ephedra sinica*) in normotensive adults," *Journal of Clinical Pharmacology*, 37(2), 116–122 (February 1997).

6. Huang, K.C. *The Pharmacology of Chinese Herbs* (Boca Raton, Florida: CRC Press, 1993), p. 231.

Epimedium

1. Huang, K.C. *The Pharmacology of Chinese Herbs* (Boca Raton, Florida: CRC Press, 1993), p. 91.

2. Bensky, D., Gamble, A., Kaptchuk, T., Bensky, L.L. *Chinese Herbal Medicine: Materia Medica*, Revised Edition (Seattle: Eastland Press, 1993), p. 342.

Eucommia

1. Huang, K.C. *The Pharmacology of Chinese Herbs* (Boca Raton, Florida: CRC Press, 1993), p. 75.

2. Oshima, Y., Takata, S., Hikino, H., Deyama, T., Kinoshita, G., "Anticomplementary activity of the constituents of *Eucommia ulmoides* bark," *Journal of Ethnopharmacology*, 23(2–3), 159–164 (July–August 1988).

3. Nakano, M., Nakashima, H., Itoh, Y., "Anti-human immunodeficiency virus activity of oligosaccharides from rooibos tea (*Aspalathus linearis*) extracts in vitro," *Leukemia*, 11(Suppl 3), 128–130 (April 1997).

4. Nakamura, T., Nakazawa, Y., Onizuka, S., Satoh, S., Chiba, A., Sekihashi, K., Miura, A., Yasugahira, N., Sasaki, Y.F., "Antimutagenicity of Tochu tea (an aqueous extract of *Eucommia ulmoides* leaves): 1. The clastogen-suppressing effects of Tochu tea in CHO cells and mice," *Mutation Research*, 388(1), 7–20 (January 1997).

5. Metori, K., Furutsu, M., Takahashi, S., "The preventive effective effect of ginseng with *du-zhong* leaf on protein metabolism in aging," *Biological and Pharmaceutical Bulletin*, 20(3), 237–242 (March 1997).

6. Sasaki, Y.F., Chiba, A., Murakami, M., Sekihashi, K., Tanaka, M., Takahoko, M., Moribayashi, S., Kudou, C., Hara, Y., Nakazawa, Y., Nakamura, T., Onizuka, S., "Antimutagenicity of Tochu tea (an aqueous extract of *Eucommia ulmoides* leaves): 2. Sup-

pressing effect of Tochu tea on urine mutagenicity after ingestion of raw fish and cooked beef," *Mutation Research,* 371(3–4), 203–214 (20 December 1996).

Eupatorium

1. Amman, M., Suter, K., *Deutsche Apotheke Zeitung,* 127, 853 (1987).

2. Wagner, H., Jurcic, K., "Immunologic studies of plant combination preparations. In-vitro and in-vivo studies on the stimulation of phagocytosis," *Arzneimittel-Forschung,* 41(10), 1072–1076 (October 1991).

3. Wagner, H., Proksch, A., Riess-Maurer, I., Vollmar, A., Odenthal, S., Stuppner, H., Jurcic, K., Le Turdu, M., Fang, J.N., "Immunostimulatory effects of polysaccharides (heteroglycans) of higher plants," *Arzneimittel-Forschung,* 35(7), 1069–1075 (1985).

Evodia

1. Bensky, D., Gamble, A., Kaptchuk, T., Bensky, L.L. *Chinese Herbal Medicine: Materia Medica,* Revised Edition (Seattle: Eastland Press, 1993), p. 304.

2. Huang, K.C. *The Pharmacology of Chinese Herbs* (Boca Raton, Florida: CRC Press, 1993), p. 197.

3. Bensky, D., Gamble, A., Kaptchuk, T., Bensky, L.L., p. 304.

4. Kong, Y.C., "*Evodia rutaecarpa,* from Pents'ao to action mechanism," *Advances in Pharmacological Therapeutics,* 6, 239–243 (1982).

Fennel Seed

1. Bensky, D., Gamble, A., Kaptchuk, T., Bensky, L.L. *Chinese Herbal Medicine: Materia Medica,* Revised Edition (Seattle: Eastland Press, 1993), p. 307.

2. Ibid.

Forsythia

1. Huang, K.C. *The Pharmacology of Chinese Herbs* (Boca Raton, Florida: CRC Press, 1993), 293.

2. Bruneton, J. *Pharmacognosy, Phytochemistry, Medicinal Plants* (Paris: Lavoisier Publishing, 1995), p. 215.

Fritillaria (Cirrhosa)

1. Bensky, D., Gamble, A., Kaptchuk, T., Bensky, L.L. *Chinese Herbal Medicine: Materia Medica,* Revised Edition (Seattle: Eastland Press, 1993), p. 177.

Fritillaria (Thunberg Fritillaria Bulb)

1. Lee, G.I., Ha, J.Y., Min, K.R., Nakagawa, H., Tsurufuji, S., Chang, I.M., Kim, Y., "Inhibitory effects of Oriental herbal medicines on IL-8 induction in lipopolysaccharide-activated rat macrophages," *Planta Medica,* 61(1), 26–30 (February 1995).

2. Huang, K.C. *The Pharmacology of Chinese Herbs* (Boca Raton, Florida: CRC Press, 1993), p. 217.

Galangal

1. Bensky, D., Gamble, A., Kaptchuk, T., Bensky, L.L. *Chinese Herbal Medicine: Materia Medica,* Revised Edition (Seattle: Eastland Press, 1993), p. 308.

2. Itokawa, H., Morita, M., Mihashi, S., *Chemical Pharmacy Bulletin,* 29, 2382 (1981). Also Kiuchi, F., Shibura, M., Sankawa, U., *Chemical Pharmacy Bulletin,* 30, 2279 (1982).

Gambir

1. Liu, J., Mori, A., "Antioxidant and free radical scavenging activities of *Gastrodia elata* Bl. and *Uncaria rhynchophylla* (Miq.) Jacks," *Neuropharmacology,* 31(12), 1287–1298 (December 1992).

Gardenia

1. Tseng, T.H., Chu, C.Y., Huang, J.M., Shiow, S.J., Wang, C.J., "Crocetin protects against oxidative damage in rat primary hepatocytes," *Cancer Letters,* 97(1), 61–67 (20 October 1995).

2. Kaji, T., Hayashi, T., Miezi, N., Kaga, K., Ejiri, N., Sakuragawa, N., "Gardenia fruit extract does not stimulate the proliferation of cultured vascular smooth muscle cells, A10," *Chemical & Pharmaceutical Bulletin,* 39(5), 1312–1314 (1991).

3. Jia, Y.J., Jiang, M.N., Pei, D.K., Ji, X.P., Wang, J.M., "Effect of *Gardenia jasminoides* Ellis (GJE) on the blood flow of internal organs at the early stage of acute necrotizing hemorrhagic pancreatitis in rats," *Chung-Kuo Chung Yao Tsa Chih—China Journal of Chinese Materia Medica,* 18(7), 431–433, 448 (July 1993).

4. Bensky, D., Gamble, A., Kaptchuk, T., Bensky, L.L. *Chinese Herbal Medicine: Materia Medica,* Revised Edition (Seattle: Eastland Press, 1993), p. 58.

5. Huang, K.C. *The Pharmacology of Chinese Herbs* (Boca Raton, Florida: CRC Press, 1993), p. 203.

6. Pei-Gen, X., Nai-Gong, W., "Can ethnopharmacology contribute to the development of anti-fertility drugs?" *Journal of Ethnopharmacology,* 32(1–3), 167–177 (April 1991).

Garlic

1. Phelps, S., Harris, W.S., "Garlic supplementation and lipoprotein oxidation susceptibility," *Lipids,* 28, 475–477 (1993).

2. Adler, A.J., Holub, B.J., "Effect of garlic and fish-oil supplementation on serum lipid and lipoprotein concentrations in hypercholesterolemic men," *American Journal of Clinical Nutrition,* 65(2), 445–450 (February 1997).

3. Chang, H.M., But, P.P.H. *Pharmacology and Applications of Chinese Materia Medica,* Volume 1 (Singapore: World Scientific Publishing, 1986), p. 90.

4. Villar, R., Alvarino, M.T., Flores, R., "Inhibition by ajoene of protein tyrosine phosphatase activity in human platelets," *Biochimica et Biophysica Acta,* 1337(2), 233–240 (8 February 1997).

5. Bordia, A., Verma, S.K., Srivastava, K.C., "Effect of garlic on platelet aggregation in humans: a study in healthy subjects and patients with coronary artery disease," *Prostaglandins Leukotrienes & Essential Fatty Acids,* 55(3), 201–205 (September 1996).

6. Batirel, H.F., Aktan, S., Aykut, C., Yegen, B.C., Coskun, T., "The effect of aqueous garlic extract on the levels of arachidonic acid metabolites (leukotriene C4 and prostaglandin E2) in rat forebrain after ischemia-reperfusion injury," *Prostaglandins Leukotrienes & Essential Fatty Acids,* 54(4), 289–292 (April 1996).

7. Numagami, Y., Sato, S., Ohnishi, S.T., "Attenuation of rat ischemic brain damage by aged garlic extracts: a possible protecting mechanism as antioxidants," *Neurochemistry International,* 29(2), 135–143 (August 1996).

8. Augusti, K.T., Benaim, M.E., "Effect of essential oil of onion (allyl propyl disulphide) on blood glucose, free fatty acid, and

insulin levels of normal subjects," *Chemical Abstracts*, 83(22), 593 (1975).

9. Brosche, T., Platt, N., "Garlic therapy and cellular immunocompetence in the elderly," *Zeitschrift für Phytotherapie*, 15, 23–24 (1994).

10. Abdullah, T.H., Kirkpatrick, D.V., Carter, J., "Enhancement of natural killer cell activity in AIDS with garlic," *Deutsche Zeitschrift für Onkologie*, 21, 52–53 (1989).

11. Koch, H.P., Lawson, L.D. *Garlic: The Science and Therapeutic Application of Allium sativum L. and Related Species*, Second Edition (Baltimore: Williams & Wilkins, 1996) p. 177.

12. Milner, J.A., "Garlic: its anticarcinogenic and antitumorigenic properties," *Nutrition Reviews*, 54(11 Pt 2), S82–S86 (November 1996).

13. Ishikawa, K., Naganawa, R., Yoshida, H., Iwata, N., Fukuda, H., Fujino, T., Suzuki, A., "Antimutagenic effects of ajoene, an organosulfur compound derived from garlic," *Bioscience, Biotechnology & Biochemistry*, 60(12), 2086–2088 (December 1996).

14. Polasa, K., Krishnaswamy, K., "Reduction of urinary mutagen excretion in rats fed garlic," *Cancer Letters*, 114(1–2), 185–186 (19 March 1997).

15. Sivam, G.P., Lampe, J.W., Ulness, B., Swanzy, S.R., Potter, J.D., "*Helicobacter pylori*—in vitro susceptibility to garlic (*Allium sativum*) extract," *Nutrition & Cancer*, 27(2), 118–121 (1997).

16. Sigounas, G., Hooker, J., Anagnostou, A., Steiner, M., "S-allylmercaptocysteine inhibits cell proliferation and reduces the viability of erythroleukemia, breast, and prostate cancer cell lines," *Nutrition & Cancer*, 27(2), 186–191 (1997).

17. Schaffer, E.M., Liu, J.Z., Milner, J.A., "Garlic powder and allyl sulfur compounds enhance the ability of dietary selenite to inhibit 7,12-dimethylbenz[a]anthracene-induced mammary DNA adducts," *Nutrition & Cancer*, 27(2), 162–168 (1997).

18. Jaiswal, S.K., Bordia, A., "Radio-protective effect of garlic *Allium sativum* Linn. in albino rats," *Indian Journal of Medical Sciences*, 50(7), 231–233 (July 1996).

19. Romano, E.L., Montano, R.F., Brito, B., Apitz, R., Alonso, J., Romano, M., Gebran, S., Soyano, A., "Effects of Ajoene on lymphocyte and macrophage membrane-dependent functions," *Immunopharmacology & Immunotoxicology*, 19(1), 15–36 (February 1997).

20. Feng, Z.H., Zhang, G.M., Hao, T.L., Zhou, B., Zhang, H., Jiang, Z.Y., "Effect of diallyl trisulfide on the activation of T-cell and macrophage-mediated cytotoxicity," *Journal of Tongji Medical University*, 14, 142–147 (1994).

21. Schinzel, W., Graf, T., "Hypertension and garlic," *Deutsche Ärtzeblatt*, 76, 1974–1975 (1979).

22. Chander, J., Maini, S., Subrahmanyan, S., Handa, A., "Otomycosis—a clinico-mycological study and efficacy of mercurochrome in its treatment," *Mycopathologia*, 135(1), 9–12 (1996).

23. Nok, A.J., Williams, S., Onyenekwe, P.C., "*Allium sativum*-induced death of African trypanosomes," *Parasitology Research*, 82(7), 634–637 (1996).

Gastrodia

1. Huang, J.H., "Comparison studies on pharmacological properties of Injectio Gastrodia Elata, gastrodin-free fraction and gastrodin," *Chung-Kuo i Hsueh Ko Hsueh Yuan Hsueh—Pao Acta Academiae Medicinae Sinicae*, 11(2), 147–150 (April 1989).

2. Liu, J., Mori, A., "Antioxidant and free radical scavenging activities of *Gastrodia elata* Bl. and *Uncaria rhynchophylla* (Miq.) Jacks," *Neuropharmacology*, 31(12), 1287–1298 (December 1992).

Gentian

1. Huang, K.C. *The Pharmacology of Chinese Herbs* (Boca Raton, Florida: CRC Press, 1993), p. 161.

2. Zhang, J.Q., Zhou, Y.P., "Inhibition of aldose reductase from rat lens by some Chinese herbs and their components," *Chung-Kuo Chung Yao Tsa Chih—China Journal Of Chinese Materia Medica*, 14(9), 557–559, 576 (September 1989).

3. Yuan, Z.Z., Feng, J.C., "Observation on the treatment of systemic lupus erythematosus with a *Gentiana macrophylla* complex tablet and a minimal dose of prednisone," *Chung Hsi I Chieh Ho Tsa Chih*, 9(3), 156–157 (March 1989).

Ginger

1. Tanabe, M., Chen, Y.D., Saito, K., Kano, Y., "Cholesterol biosynthesis inhibitory component from *Zingiber officinale* Roscoe," *Chemical & Pharmaceutical Bulletin*, 41(4), 710–713 (April 1993).

2. Meyer, K., Schwartz, J., Crater, D., Keyes, B., "*Zingiber officinale* (ginger) used to prevent 8-MOP associated nausea," *Dermatology Nursing*, 7(4), 242–244 (August 1995).

3. Srivastava, K.C., "Effects of aqueous extracts of onion, garlic and ginger on platelet aggregation and metabolism of arachidonic acid in the blood vascular system: in vitro study," *Prostaglandins in Medicine*, 13, 227–235 (1984).

4. Verma, S.K., Singh, J., Khamesra, R., Bordia, A., "Effect of ginger on platelet aggregation in man," *Indian Journal of Medical Research*, 98, 240–242 (October 1993).

5. Kawakishi, S., Morimitsu, Y., Osawa, T., "Chemistry of ginger components and inhibitory factors of the arachidonic acid cascade," in Ho, C.T., Osawa, T., Huang, M.T., Rosen, R. (eds). *Food Phytochemicals for Cancer Prevention II: Teas, Spices, and Herbs* (Washington: American Chemical Society, 1994), pp. 244–249.

6. Wu, H., Ye, D.J., Zhao, Y.Z., Wang, S.L., "Effect of different preparations of ginger on blood coagulation time in mice," *Chung-Kuo Chung Yao Tsa Chih—China Journal of Chinese Materia Medica*, 18(3), 147–149, 190 (March 1993).

7. Sharma, J.N., Srivastava, K.C., Gan, E.K., "Suppressive effects of eugenol and ginger oil on arthritic rats," *Pharmacology*, 49(5), 314–318 (November 1994).

8. Srivastava, K.C., Mustafa, T., "Ginger (*Zingiber officinale*) in rheumatism and musculoskeletal disorders," *Medical Hypotheses*, 39(4), 342–348 (December 1992).

9. Denyer, C.V., Jackson, P., Loakes, D.M., Ellis, M.R., Young, D.A., "Isolation of antirhinoviral sesquiterpenes from ginger (*Zingiber officinale*)," *Journal of Natural Products*, 57(5), 658–662 (May 1994).

10. Chang, C.P., Chang, J.Y., Wang, F.Y., Chang, J.G., "The effect of Chinese medicinal herb Zingiberis rhizoma extract on cytokine secretion by human peripheral blood mononuclear cells," *Journal of Ethnopharmacology*, 48(1), 13–19 (11 August 1995).

11. Yamahara, J., Hatakeyama, S., Taniguchi, K., Kawamura, M., "Stomachic principles in ginger. II. Pungent and anti-ulcer effects of low polar constituents isolated from ginger, dried rhizome of *Zingiber officinale* Roscoe cultivated in Taiwan. The absolute stereostructure of a new diarylheptanoid," *Yakugaku Zasshi—Journal of*

the Pharmaceutical Society of Japan, 112(9), 645–655 (September 1992).

12. Goso, Y., Ogata, Y., Ishihara, K., Hotta, K., "Effects of traditional herbal medicine on gastric mucin against ethanol-induced gastric injury in rats," *Comparative Biochemistry & Physiology. Part C Pharmacology, Toxicology, Endocrinology,* 113(1), 17–21 (January 1996).

13. Cai, R., Zhou, A., Gao, H., "Study on correction of abnormal fetal position by applying ginger paste at *zhiying* acupoint A. Report of 133 cases," *Chen Tzu Yen Chiu—Journal of Acupuncture Research,* 15(2), 89–91 (1990).

14. Mowrey, D., Clayson, D., "Motion sickness, ginger, and psychophysics," *Lancet,* 8, 655–657 (1982).

15. Grontbved, A., Braks, T., Kambskard, J., Hentzer, E., "Ginger root against seasickness: A controlled trial on the open sea," *Acta Otolaryngolica,* 105, 45–49 (1988).

16. Meyer, K., Schwartz, J., Crater, D., Keyes, B., pp. 242–244.

17. Cao, Z.F., Chen, Z.G., Guo, P., Zhang, S.M., Lian, L.X., Luo, L., Hu, W.M., "Scavenging effects of ginger on superoxide anion and hydroxyl radical," *Chung-Kuo Chung Yao Tsa Chih—China Journal of Chinese Materia Medica,* 18(12), 750–751, 764 (December 1993).

18. Kikuzaki, H., Kawasaki, Y., Nobuji, N., "Structure of antioxidative compounds in ginger," in Ho, C.T., Osawa, T., Huang, M.T., Rosen, R. (eds). *Food Phytochemicals for Cancer Prevention II: Teas, Spices, and Herbs* (Washington: American Chemical Society, 1994), pp. 237–243.

19. Minematsu, S., Taki, M., Watanabe, M., Takahashi, M., Wakui, Y., Ishihara, K., Takeda, S., Fujii, Y., "Effects of *Shosaiko-to-go-keishikashakuyaku-to* (TJ-960) on the valproic acid induced anomalies of rat fetuses," *Nippon Yakurigaku Zasshi—Folia Pharmacologica Japonica,* 96(5), 265–273 (November 1990).

20. Vogel, H. *The Nature Doctor* (New Canaan, Connecticut: Keats Publishing, 1991), p. 446.

21. Goto, C., Kasuya, S., Koga, K., Ohtomo, H., Kagei, N., "Lethal efficacy of extract of from *Zingiber officinale* (traditional Chinese medicine) or [6]-shogaol and [6]-gingerol in *Anisakis* larvae in vitro," *Parasitology Research,* 76(8), 653–656 (1990).

22. Adewunmi, C.O., Oguntimein, B.O., Furu, P., "Molluscicidal and antischistosomal activities of *Zingiber officinale," Planta Medica,* 56(4), 374–376 (August 1990).

23. Kiuchi, F., "Nematocidal activity of some anthelmintics, traditional medicines, and spices by new assay method using larvae of *Toxocara canis," Shoyakugaku Zasshi,* 43(4), 279–287 (1989).

24. Fulder, S., Tenne, M., "Ginger as an anti-nausea remedy in pregnancy: the issue of safety," *HerbalGram,* 38, 49 (Fall 1996).

25. Janssen, P.L., Meyboom, S., van Staveren, W.A., de Vegt, F., Katan, M.B., "Consumption of ginger (*Zingiber officinale* Roscoe) does not affect ex vivo platelet thromboxane production in humans," *European Journal of Clinical Nutrition,* 50(11), 772–774 (November 1996).

Ginkgo Nut

1. Guinot, P. et. al., "Tanakan inhibits platelet-activating aggregation in healthy male volunteers," *Haemostasis,* 19, 219–223 (1986).

2. Bensky, D., Gamble, A., Kaptchuk, T., Bensky, L.L. *Chinese Herbal Medicine: Materia Medica,* Revised Edition (Seattle: Eastland Press, 1993), p. 390.

Ginseng

1. Bensky, D., Barolet, R. *Chinese Herbal Medicine: Formulas and Strategies* (Seattle: Eastland Press, 1990), p. 236–237.

2. Chen, X., Lee, T.J., "Ginsenosides-induced nitric oxide-mediated relaxation of the rabbit corpus cavernosum," *British Journal of Pharmacology,* 115(1), 15–18 (May 1995).

3. Salvati, G., Genovesi, G., Marcellini, L., Paolini, P., De Nuccio, I., Pepe, M., Re, M., "Effects of *Panax ginseng* C.A. Meyer saponins on male fertility," *Panminerva Medica,* 38(4), 249–254 (December 1996).

4. Yun, T.K., Choi, S.Y., "Preventive effect of ginseng intake against various human cancers, a case-control study on 1987 pairs," *Cancer Epidemiology, Biomarkers & Prevention,* 4(4), 401–408 (June 1995).

5. Matsunaga, H., Katano, M., Saita, T., Yamamoto, H., Mori, M., "Potentiation of cytotoxicity of mitomycin C by a polyacetylenic alcohol, panaxytriol," *Cancer Chemotherapy & Pharmacology,* 33(4), 291–297 (1994).

6. Yi, R.L., Li, W., Hao, X.Z., "Differentiation effect of ginsenosides on human acute non-lymphocytic leukemic cells in 58 patients,"*Chung-Kuo Chung Hsi I Chieh Ho Tsa Chih—Chinese Journal of Modern Developments in Traditional Medicine,* 13(12), 722–724, 708 (December 1993).

7. Kim, S.H., Cho, C.K., Yoo, S.Y., Koh, K.H., Yun, H.G., Kim, T.H., "In vivo radioprotective activity of *Panax ginseng* and diethyldithiocarbamate," *In Vivo,* 7(5), 467–470 (September–October 1993).

8. Han, M.Q., Liu, J.X., Gao, H., "Effects of 24 Chinese medicinal herbs on nucleic acid, protein and cell cycle of human lung adenocarcinoma cell," *Chung-Kuo Chung Hsi I Chieh Ho Tsa Chih—Chinese Journal of Modern Developments in Traditional Medicine,* 15(3), 147–149 (1995).

9. Cha, R.J., Zeng, D.W., Chang, Q.S., "Non-surgical treatment of small cell lung cancer with chemo-radio-immunotherapy and traditional Chinese medicine," *Chung-Hua Nei Ko Tsa Chih—Chinese Journal of Internal Medicine,* 33(7), 462–466 (July 1994).

10. Sato, K., Mochizuki, M., Saiki, I., Yoo, Y.C., Samukawa, K., Azuma, I., "Inhibition of tumor angiogenesis and metastasis by asaponin of *Panax ginseng,* ginsenoside-Rb2," *Biological & Pharmaceutical Bulletin,* 17(5), 635–639 (May 1994).

11. Lee, Y.S., Chung, I.S., Lee, I.R., Kim, K.H., Hong, W.S., Yun, Y.S., "Activation of multiple effector pathways of immune system by the antineoplastic immunostimulator acidic polysaccharide ginsan isolated from *Panax ginseng," Anticancer Research,* 17(1A), 323–331 (January–February 1997).

12. Lin, J.H., Wu, L.S., Tsai, K.T., Leu, S.P., Jeang, Y.F., Hsieh, M.T., "Effects of ginseng on the blood chemistry profile of dexamethasone-treated male rats," *American Journal of Chinese Medicine,* 23(2), 167–172 (1995).

13. Park, H.J., Park, K.M., Rhee, M.H., Song, Y.B., Choi, K.J., Lee, J.H., Kim, S.C., Park, K.H., "Effect of ginsenoside Rb1 on rat liver phosphoproteins induced by carbon tetrachloride," *Biological & Pharmaceutical Bulletin,* 19(6), 834–838 (June 1996).

14. Huang, K.C. *The Pharmacology of Chinese Herbs* (Boca Raton, Florida: CRC Press, 1993), p. 43.

15. Ding, D.Z., Shen, T.K., Cui, Y.Z., "Effects of red ginseng on

the congestive heart failure and its mechanism," *Chung-Kuo Chung Hsi I Chieh Ho Tsa Chih—Chinese Journal of Modern Developments in Traditional Medicine,* 15(6), 325–327 (1995).

16. Toh, H.T., "Improved isolated heart contractility and mitochondrial oxidation after chronic treatment with *Panax ginseng* in rats," *American Journal of Chinese Medicine,* 22(3–4), 275–284 (1994).

17. Zhang, Y.G., Liu, T.P., "Influences of ginsenosides Rb1 and Rg1 on reversible focal brain ischemia in rats," *Chung-Kuo Yao Li Hsueh Pao—Acta Pharmacologica Sinica,* 17(1), 44–48 (January 1996).

18. Kim, Y.H., Park, K.H., Rho, H.M., "Transcriptional activation of the Cu,Zn-superoxide dismutase gene through the AP2 site by ginsenoside Rb2 extracted from a medicinal plant, *Panax ginseng,*" *Journal of Biological Chemistry,* 271(40), 24539–24543 (4 October 1996).

19. Kang, S.Y., Schini-Kerth, V.B., Kim, N.D., "Ginsenosides of the protopanaxatriol group cause endothelium-dependent relaxation in the rat aorta," *Life Sciences,* 56(19), 1577–1586 (1995).

20. Park, H.J., Lee, J.H., Song, Y.B., Park, K.H., "Effects of dietary supplementation of lipophilic fraction from *Panax ginseng* on cGMP and cAMP in rat platelets and on blood coagulation," *Biological & Pharmaceutical Bulletin,* 19(11), 1434–1439 (November 1996).

21. Huang, K.C., p. 43.

22. See, D.M., Broumand, N., Sahl, L., Tilles, J.G., "In vitro effects of echinacea and ginseng on natural killer and antibody-dependent cell cytotoxicity in healthy subjects and chronic fatigue syndrome or acquired immunodeficiency syndrome patients," *Immunopharmacology,* 35(3), 229–235 (January 1997).

23. Rosenfeld, M.S., "Evaluation of the efficacy of a standardized ginseng extract in patients with psychophysical asthenia and neurological disorders," *La Semana Médica,* 173, 148–154 (1989).

24. Hiai, S., Yokoyama, K., Oura, H., Yano, S., "Features of ginseng saponin-induced corticosterone secretion," *Endocronologica Japonica,* 26(6), 661 (1979).

25. Kiyohara, H., Hirano, M., Wen, X.G., Matsumoto, T., Sun, X.B., Yamada, H., "Characterisation of an anti-ulcer pectic polysaccharide from leaves of *Panax ginseng* C.A. Meyer," *Carbohydrate Research,* 263(1), 89–101 (3 October 1994).

26. Mitra, S.K., Chakraborti, A., Bhattacharya, S.K., "Neuropharmacological studies on *Panax ginseng,*" *Indian Journal of Experimental Biology,* 34(1), 41–47 (January 1996).

27. Nguyen, T.T., Matsumoto, K., Yamasaki, K., Nguyen, M.D., Nguyen, T.N., Watanabe, H., "Crude saponin extracted from Vietnamese ginseng and major constituent majonoside-R2 attenuate the psychological stress- and foot-shock stress-induced antinociception in mice," *Pharmacology, Biochemistry & Behavior,* 52(2), 427–432 (1995).

28. Nishiyama, N., Wang, Y.L., Saito, H., "Beneficial effects of S-113m, a novel herbal prescription, on learning impairment model in mice," *Biological & Pharmaceutical Bulletin,* 18(11), 1498–1503 (November 1995).

29. Okamura, N., Kobayashi, K., Akaike, A., Yagi, A., "Protective effect of ginseng saponins against impaired brain growth in neonatal rats exposed to ethanol," *Biological & Pharmaceutical Bulletin,* 17(2), 270–274 (1994).

30. Kim, H.S., Kang J.G., Oh, K.W., "Inhibition by ginseng total saponin of the development of morphine reverse tolerance and dopamine receptor supersensitivity in mice," *General Pharmacology,* 26(5), 1071–1076 (September 1995).

31. Kim, H.S., Kang, J.G., Rheu, H.M., Cho, D.H., Oh, K.W., "Blockade by ginseng total saponin of the development of methamphetamine reverse tolerance and dopamine receptor supersensitivity in mice," *Planta Medica,* 61(1), 22–25 (February 1995).

32. Kim, H.S., Kang, J.G., Seong, Y.H., Nam, K.Y., Oh, K.W., "Blockade by ginseng total saponin of the development of cocaine induced reverse tolerance and dopamine receptor supersensitivity in mice," *Pharmacology, Biochemistry & Behavior,* 50(1), 23–27 (January 1995).

33. "Chinese herbs and immunity," *Bulletin of the OHAI,* 9(8), 395 (1984).

Green Tea

1. Hara, Y., "Prophylactic functions of tea polyphenols," in Ho, C.T., Osawa, T., Huang, M.T., Rosen, R. (eds). *Food Phytochemicals for Cancer Prevention II: Teas, Spices, and Herbs* (Washington: American Chemical Society, 1994), p. 42.

2. Huang, K.C. *The Pharmacology of Chinese Herbs* (Boca Raton, Florida: CRC Press, 1993), p. 168.

3. Bruneton, J. *Pharmacognosy, Phytochemistry, Medicinal Plants* (Paris: Lavoisier Publishing, 1995), p. 886.

4. Hara, Y., pp. 36, 39, 43.

5. Iwata, S., Fukaya, Y., Nakazawa, K., Okuda, T.J., *Ocular Pharmacology,* 3, 227 (1987).

6. Hara, Y., p. 44.

7. Hara, Y., pp. 44–45.

8. Nanjo, F., Hara, Y., Kikuchi, Y., "Effects of tea polyphenols on blood rheology in rats fed a high-fat diet," in Ho, C.T., Osawa, T., Huang, M.T., Rosen, R. (eds). *Food Phytochemicals for Cancer Prevention II: Teas, Spices, and Herbs* (Washington: American Chemical Society, 1994), pp. 76–82.

9. Kinae, N., Shimoi, K., Masumoria, S., Harusawa, M., Furugori, M., "Suppression of the formation of advanced glycosylation products by tea extracts," in Ho, C.T., Osawa, T., Huang, M.T., Rosen, R. (eds), pp. 68–75.

10. Honda, M., Nanjo, F., Hara, Y., "Inhibition of saccharide digestive enzymes by tea polyphenols," in Ho, C.T., Osawa, T., Huang, M.T., Rosen, R. (eds), pp. 83–89.

11. Terada, A., Hara, H., Nakajyo, S., Ichikawa, H., Hara, Y., Fukai, K., Kabayashi, Y., Mitsuoka, T., *Microbial Ecology in Health and Disease,* 6, 3–9 (1993).

12. Kim, M., Hagiwara, N., Smith, S.J., Yamamoto, T., Yaamane, T., Takahashi, T., "Preventive effect of green tea polyphenols on colon carcinogenesis," in Ho, C.T., Osawa, T., Huang, M.T., Rosen, R. (eds), pp. 51–55.

13. Hara, Y., p. 47.

14. Shimamura, T., "Inhibition of influenza virus infection by tea polyphenols," in Ho, C.T., Osawa, T., Huang, M.T., Rosen, R. (eds), pp. 101–104.

Hawthorn

1. Petkov, V., "Plants and hypotensive, antiatheromatous and coronarodilatating action," *American Journal of Chinese Medicine,* 7(3), 197–236 (1979).

2. He, G., "Effect of the prevention and treatment of atherosclerosis of a mixture of hawthorn and motherwort," *Chung Hsi I Chieh Ho Tsa Chih—Chinese Journal of Modern Developments in Traditional Medicine,* 10(6), 361, 326 (June 1990).

3. Petkov, E., Nikolov, N., Uzunov, P., "Inhibitory effect of some flavonoids and flavonoid mixtures on cyclic AMP phosphodiesterease activity of rat heart," *Planta Medica,* 43, 183–186 (1981).

4. Schussler, M., Holzl, J., Fricke, U., "Myocardial effects of flavonoids from *Crataegus* species," *Arzneimittel-Forschung,* 45(8), 842–845 (August 1995).

5. Blumenthal, M., Busse, W.R., Goldberg, A., Gruenwald, J., Hall, T., Riggins, C.W., Rister, R.S., eds., Klein, S., Rister, R.S., trans. *The Complete German Commission E Monographs: Therapeutic Guide to Herbal Medicines* (Boston: Integrative Medicine Communications, 1998) p. 135.

6. Leuchtgens, H., "Crataegus Special Extract WS 1442 in NYHA II heart failure. A placebo-controlled randomized double-blind study," *Fortschritte der Medizin,* 111(20–21), 352–354 (20 July 1993).

7. Rajendran, S., Deepalakshmi, P.D., Parasakthy, K., Devaraj, H., Devaraj, S.N., "Effect of tincture of *Crataegus* on the LDL-receptor activity of hepatic plasma membrane of rats fed an atherogenic diet," *Atherosclerosis,* 123 (1–2), 235–241 (June 1996).

8. Shanthi, S., Parasakthy, K., Deepalakshmi, P.D., Devaraj, S.N., "Hypolipidemic activity of tincture of *Crataegus* in rats," *Indian Journal of Biochemistry & Biophysics,* 31(2), 143–146 (April 1994).

9. Rakotoarison, D.A., Gressier, B., Trotin, F., Brunet, C., Dine, T., Luyckx, M., Vasseru, J., Cazin, M., Cazin, J.C., Pinkas, M., "Antioxidant activities of polyphenolic extracts from flowers, in vitro callus and cell suspension cultures of *Crataegus monogyna,*" *Pharmazie,* 52(1), 60–64 (January 1997).

10. Bahorun, T., Gressier, B., Trotin, F., Brunet, C., Dine, T., Luyckx, M., Vasseru, J., Cazin, M., Cazin, J.C., Pinkas, M., "Oxygen species scavenging activity of phenolic extracts from hawthorn fresh plant organs and pharmaceutical preparations," *Arzneimittel-Forschung,* 46(110), 1086–1089 (November 1996).

11. Della Loggia, R., Tubaro, A., Redaelli, C., "Evaluation of the activity on the mouse CNS of several plant extracts and a combination of them," *Rivista di Neurologia,* 51(5), 297–310 (September–October 1981).

12. Shahat, A.A., Hammouda, F., Ismail, S.I., Azzam, S.A., De Bruyne, T., Lasure, A., Van Poel, B., Pieters, L., Vlietinck, A.J., "Anti-complementary activity of *Crataegus sinaica,*" *Planta Medica,* 62(1), 10–13 (February 1996).

13. Bensky, D., Gamble, A., Kaptchuk, T., Bensky, L.L. *Chinese Herbal Medicine: Materia Medica,* Revised Edition (Seattle: Eastland Press, 1993), p. 224.

14. Vibes, J., Lasserre, B., Gleye, J., Declume, C., "Inhibition of thromboxane A2 biosynthesis in vitro by the main components of *Crataegus oxycantha* (hawthorn) flower heads," *Prostaglandins Leukotrienes & Essential Fatty Acids,* 50(4), 175–176 (April 1994).

15. Havsteen, B., "Flavonoids, a class of natural products of high pharmacological potency," *Biochemical Pharmacology,* 32, 1141–1148 (1982).

16. Saenz, M.T., Ahumada, M.C., Garcia, M.D., "Extracts from *Viscum* and *Crataegus* are cytotoxic against larynx cancer cells," *Zeitschrift für Naturforschung,* 52(1–2), 42–44 (January–February 1997).

17. Ciplea, A.G., Richter, K.D., "The protective effect of *Allium sativum* and *Crataegus* on isoprenaline-induced tissue necroses in rats," *Arzneimittel-Forschung,* 38(110), 1583–1592 (November 1988).

18. Kuhnau, J., "The flavonoids. A class of semi-essential food components: their role in human nutrition," *World Review of Nutrition and Dietetics,* 24, 117–191 (1976).

19. Pourrat, H., "Anthocyanidin drugs in vascular disease," *Plant Medicinal Phytotherapy,* 11, 143–151 (1977).

Hoelen

1. Chen, J., "An experimental study on the anti-senility effects of *shou xing bu zhi,*" *Chung Hsi I Chieh Ho Tsa Chih—Chinese Journal of Modern Developments in Traditional Medicine,* 9(4), 226–227, 198 (April 1989).

2. Hattori, T., Hayashi, K., Nagao, T., Furuta, K., Ito, M., Suzuki, Y., "Studies on antinephritic effects of plant components (3): Effect of pachyman, a main component of *Poria cocos* Wolf. on original-type anti-GBM nephritis in rats and its mechanisms," *Japanese Journal of Pharmacology,* 59(1), 89–96 (May 1992).

3. Ding, X., "Effects of poriatin on mouse peritoneal macrophages," *Zhongguo Y'lxue Kexueyuan,* 9, 433–438 (1987).

4. Wang, G., "Effect of poriatin on mouse immune system," *South China Journal of Antibiotica,* 17, 42–47 (1992).

5. Yu, S.J., Tseng, J., "*Fu-ling,* a Chinese herbal drug, modulates cytokine secretion by human peripheral blood monocytes," *International Journal of Immunopharmacology,* 18(1), 37–44 (January 1996).

6. Narui, T., Takahashi, K., Kobayashi, M., Shibata, S., "Polysaccharide produced by laboratory cultivation of *Poria cocos* Wolf.," *Carbohydrate Research,* 87, 161–163 (1980).

7. Guo, D., "Preliminary observation on carboy-methyl *Poria cocos* polysaccharide (CMPLP) in treating chronic viral hepatitis," *Journal of Traditional Chinese Medicine,* 4, 282 (1984).

8. Ding, X., pp. 433–438.

9. Wang, G., "Effect of poriatin on mouse immune system," *South China Journal of Antibiotica,* 17, 42–47 (1992).

10. Narui, T., Takahashi, K., Kobayashi, M., Shibata, S., pp. 161–163.

Houttynia

1. Huang, K.C. *The Pharmacology of Chinese Herbs* (Boca Raton, Florida: CRC Press, 1993), p. 296.

2. Chang, H.M., But, P.P.H. *Pharmacology and Applications of Chinese Materia Medica,* Volume 1 (Singapore: World Scientific Publishing, 1986).

Japanese Mint

1. Ding, A.W., Wu, H., Kong, L.D., Wang, S.L., Gao, Z.Z., Zhao, M.X., Tan, M., "Research on hemostatic mechanism of extracts from carbonized *Schizonepeta tenuifolia* Brig.," *Chung-Kuo Chung Yao Tsa Chih—China Journal of Chinese Materia Medica,* 18(10), 598–600 (October 1993).

2. Huang, K.C. *The Pharmacology of Chinese Herbs* (Boca Raton, Florida: CRC Press, 1993), p. 153.

Japanese Watermelon

1. Bensky, D., Gamble, A., Kaptchuk, T., Bensky, L.L. *Chinese Herbal Medicine: Materia Medica,* Revised Edition (Seattle: Eastland Press, 1993), p. 109.

Jujube Fruit

1. Kurihara, Y., "Characteristics of antisweet substances, sweet proteins, and sweetness-inducing proteins," *Critical Reviews in Food Science and Nutrition,* 32(3), 231–252 (1992).

2. Bensky, D., Gamble, A., Kaptchuk, T., Bensky, L.L. *Chinese Herbal Medicine: Materia Medica,* Revised Edition (Seattle: Eastland Press, 1993), p. 323.

3. Wang, W., Chen, W.W., "Antioxidative activity studies on herbs also used as foods," *Chung Hsi I Chieh Ho Tsa Chih—Chinese Journal of Modern Developments in Traditional Medicine,* 11(30), 159–161 (March 1991).

4. Hsu, H.Y., Chen, Y.P., Hong, M. *The Chemical Constituents of Chinese Herbs* (Long Beach, California: Oriental Healing Arts Press, 1985), p. 752.

5. Yao, G.S., Li, Y.J., Chang, X.Q., Lu, J.H., "Vitamin C content in vegetables and fruits in the Shenyang (China) market during four season," *Acta Nutritica Sinica,* 5, 373–379 (1983).

Kelp

1. Long, A., "Vitamin B_{12} for vegans," *British Medical Journal,* 2(6080), 192 (16 July 1977).

2. Tyler, V.E. *The Honest Herbal: A Sensible Guide to the Use of Herbs and Related Remedies,* Third Edition (New York: Pharmaceutical Products Press, 1993), p. 190.

3. Teas, J., "The dietary intake of *Laminaria,* a brown seaweed, and breast cancer prevention," *Nutrition and Cancer,* 4(3), 217–222 (1983).

4. Becer, G., Osterloh, K., Schafer, S., Forth, W., Paskins-Hurburt, A.J., Tanaka, G., Skoryna, S.C., "Influence of fucoidan on the intestinal absorption of iron, cobalt, manganese and zinc in rats," *Digestion,* 21(1), 6–12 (1981).

5. Castelman, M. *The Healing Herbs* (Emmanus, Pennsylvania: Rodale Press, 1991), pp. 230–231.

6. Beress, A., Wassermann, O., Tahhan, S., Bruhn, T., Beress, L., Kraiselburd, E.N., Gonzalez, L.V., de Motta, G.E., Chavez, P.I., "A new procedure for the isolation of anti-HIV compounds (polysaccharides and polyphenols) from the marine alga *Fucus vesiculosus,*" *Journal of Natural Products,* 56(4), 478–488 (April 1993).

7. Grauffle, V., Kloareg, B., Mabeau, S., et al., "New natural polysaccharides with potent antithrombic activity, fucans from brown algae," *Biomaterials,* 10(6), 363–368 (1989).

8. Lamela, M., Anca, J., Villar, R., Otero, J., Callleja, J.M., "Hypoglycemic activity of several seaweed extracts," *Journal of Ethnopharmacology,* 27(1–2), 35–43 (November 1989).

9. Sakata, T., "A very-low-calorie conventional Japanese diet: its implications for prevention of obesity," *Obesity Research,* 3(suppl 2), 233S–239S (September 1995).

10. Konno, N., Makita, H., Yuri, K., Iizuka, N., Kawasaki, K., "Association between dietary iodine intake and prevalence of subclinical hypothyroidism in the coastal regions of Japan," *Journal of Clinical Endocrinology and Metabolism,* 78(2), 393–397 (February 1994).

Kudzu

1. Bruneton, J., *Pharmacognosy, Phytochemistry, Medicinal Plants* (Paris: Lavoisier Publishing, 1995), pp. 296–297.

2. Jing, Y., Nakaya, K., Han, R., "Differentiation of promyeloctic leukemia cells HL-60 induced by daidzen in vitro and in vivo," *Anticancer Research,* 13(4), 1049–1054 (1993).

3. Han, R., "Highlight on the studies of anticancer drugs derived from plants from China," *Stem Cells,* 12(1), 53–63 (1994).

4. Jing, Y., Han, R., "Differentiation of B16 melanoma cells induced by daidzein," *Chinese Journal of Pharmacology and Toxicology,* 6(4), 278–280 (1993).

5. Adlercreutz, H., "Diet, breast cancer and sex hormone metabolism," *Annals of the New York Academy of Sciences,* 595, 281 (1990).

6. Adlercreutz, H., Markkanen, H., Watanabe, S., "Plasma concentrations of phyto-estrogens in Japanese men," *Lancet,* 342 (8881), 1209–1210 (13 November 1993).

7. Bruneton, J., p. 298.

8. Lu, X.R., et al., *Acta Pharmacologica Sinica,* 7, 537–538 (1986).

9. Song, X.P., et al., *Acta Pharmacologica Sinica,* 9, 55–58 (1988).

10. Xie, C.I., Lin, R.C., Antony, V., Lumeng, L., Li, T.K., Mai, K., Liu, C., Wang, Q.D., Zhao, Z.H., Wang, G.F., "Daidzin, an antioxidant isoflavonoid, decreases blood alcohol levels and shortens sleep time induced by ethanol intoxication," *Alcoholism, Clinical & Experimental Research,* 18(6), 1443–1447 (December 1994).

Ledebouriella

1. Bensky, D., Gamble, A., Kaptchuk, T., Bensky, L.L. *Chinese Herbal Medicine: Materia Medica,* Revised Edition (Seattle: Eastland Press, 1993), p. 33.

Licorice

1. Shibata, S., "Antitumor-promoting and anti-inflammatory activities of licorice principles and their modified compounds," in Ho, C.T., Osawa, T., Huang, M.T., Rosen, R. (eds). *Food Phytochemicals for Cancer Prevention II: Teas, Spices, and Herbs* (Washington: American Chemical Society, 1994), p. 310.

2. Plyasunova, O.A., "Inhibition of HIV reproduction in cells cultures by glycyrrhizic acid," *International Conference on AIDS,* 8, 31 (1992).

3. Mori, K., "Effects of glycyrrhizin (SNMC: stronger neominophagen C) in hemophilia patients with HIV-1 infection," *Tohoku Journal of Experimental Medicine,* 162, 183–193 (1990).

4. Takahara, T., Watanabe, A., Shiraki, K., "Effects of glycyrrhizin on hepatitis B surface antigen, a biochemical and morphological study," *Journal of Hepatology,* 21(4), 601–609 (October 1994).

5. Tajiri, H., Kozaiwa, K., Ozaki, Y., Miki, K., Shimuzu, K., Okada, S., "Effect of *sho-saiko-to (xiao-chai-hu-tang)* on HBeAg clearance in children with chronic hepatitis B virus infection and with sustained liver disease," *American Journal of Chinese Medicine,* 19(2), 121–129 (1991).

6. Abe, Y., Ueda, T., Kato, T., Kohli, Y., "Effectiveness of interferon, glycyrrhizin combination therapy in patients with chronic hepatitis C," *Nippon Rinsho—Japanese Journal of Clinical Medicine,* 52(7), 1817–1822 (July 1994).

7. Nagai, T., Yamada, H., "In vivo anti-influenza virus activity of Kampo (Japanese herbal) medicine '*sho-seiryu-to*' and its mode

of action," *International Journal of Immunopharmacology,* 16(8), 605–613 (August 1994).

8. Baschetti, R., "Chronic fatigue syndrome and neurally mediated hypotension," *Journal of the American Medical Association,* 275, 359 (1996).

9. Demitrack, M.A., "Evidence for impaired activation of the hypothalamic-pituitary-adrenal axis in patients with chronic fatigue syndrome," *Journal of Clinical Endocrinology and Metabolism,* 73, 1224–1234 (1991).

10. Baschetti, R., "Chronic fatigue syndrome and liquorice," *New Zealand Medical Journal,* 108(1002), 259 (28 June 1995).

11. Tangi, K.K., et al., "Biochemical study of anti-inflammatory and anti-arthritic properties of glycyrrhetic acid," *Biochemical Pharmacology,* 14, 1277–1281 (1965).

12. Murray, M., Pizzorno, J. *Encyclopedia of Natural Medicine* (Rocklin, California: Prima Publishing, 1996), p. 522.

13. Wichtl, M., ed., Grainger-Bissett, N., trans. *Herbal Drugs and Phytopharmaceuticals: A Handbook for Practice on a Scientific Basis* (Boca Raton, Florida: CRC Press, 1995), p. 303.

14. Kassir, Z.A., "Endoscopic controlled trial of four drug regimens in the treatment of chronic duodenal ulceration," *Irish Medical Journal,* 78, 153–156 (1985).

15. Tewari, S.N., Wilson, A.K., "Deglycyrrhizinated liquorice in duodenal ulcer," *Practitioner,* 210, 820–825 (1972).

16. Chen, M.F., et al., "Effect of glycyrrhizin on the pharmacokinetics of prednisolone following low dosage of prednisolone hemisuccinate," *Endocronologica Japonica,* 37, 331–341 (1990).

17. Ibid.

18. Hiai, S., Yokoyama, H., Nagasawa, T., Oura, H., "Stimulation of the pituitary-adrenocortical axis by saikosaponin of Bupleuri Radix," *Chemical Pharmacology Bulletin,* 29, 495–499 (1981).

19. Wang, Z.Y., et al., "Inhibition of mutagencitiy in *Salmonella typhimurium* and skin tumor initiating and tumor promoting activities in sencar mice by glycyrrhetinic acid: comparison of the 18-α and 18-β steroisomers," *Carcinogenesis,* 12, 187–192 (1991).

20. Bensky, D., Gamble, A., Kaptchuk, T., Bensky, L.L. *Chinese Herbal Medicine: Materia Medica,* Revised Edition (Seattle: Eastland Press, 1993), p. 325.

21. Schambelan, M., "Licorice ingestion and blood pressure regulating hormones," *Steroids,* 59(2), 127–130 (February 1994).

22. Wichtl, M., p. 303.

23. Takeuchi, T., Nishii, O., Okamura, T., Yaginuma, T., "Effects of paeoniflorin, glycyrrhizin, and glycyrrhetic acid on ovarian androgen production," *American Journal of Chinese Medicine,* 19(1), 73–78 (1991).

24. Westman, E.C., "Does smokeless tobacco cause hypertension?" *Southern Medical Journal,* 88(7), 716–720 (July 1995).

Ligusticum

1. Beck, J.J., Stermitz, F.R., "Addition of methyl thioglycolate and benzylamine to (Z)-ligustilide, a bioactive unsaturated lactone constituent of several herbal medicines. An improved synthesis of (Z)-ligustilide," *Journal of Natural Products,* 58(7), 1047–1055 (July 1995).

2. Jin, R., Wan, L.L., Mitsuishi, T., "Effects of *shi-ka-ron* and Chinese herbs in mice treated with anti-tumor agent mitomycin C," *Chung-Kuo Chung Hsi I Chieh Ho Tsa Chih—Chinese Journal of Modern Developments in Traditional Medicine,* 15(2), 101–103 (February 1995).

Ligustrum

1. Lau, B.H., Ruckle, H.C., Botolazzo, T., Lui, P.D., "Chinese medicinal herbs inhibit growth of murine renal cell carcinoma," *Cancer Biotherapy,* 9(2), 153–161 (Summer 1994).

2. Wang, S.S., Chen, J.H., Liu, X.J., "Preliminary study on pharmacologic action of *Ligustrum japonicum," Chung-Kuo Chung Hsi I Chieh Ho Tsa Chih—Chinese Journal of Modern Developments in Traditional Medicine,* 14(11), 670–672 (November 1994).

Lily Bulb

1. Bensky, D., Gamble, A., Kaptchuk, T., Bensky, L.L., *Chinese Herbal Medicine: Materia Medica,* Revised Edition (Seattle: Eastland Press, 1993), pp. 363–364.

Lindera

1. Yu, S.M., Hsu, S.Y., Ko, F.N., Chen, C.C., Huang, Y.L., Huang T.F., Teng, C.M., "Haemodynamic effects of dicentrine, a novel alpha 1-adrenoceptor antagonist: comparison with prazosin in spontaneously hypertensive and normotensive Wistar-Kyoto rats," *British Journal of Pharmacology,* 106(4), 797–801 (August 1992).

2. Zheng, M., "Experimental study of 472 herbs with antiviral action against the herpes simplex virus," *Chung Hsi I Chieh Ho Tsa Chih,* 10(1), 39–41 (January 1990).

3. Mimaki, Y., Kameyama, A., Sashida, Y., Miyata, Y., Fujii, A., "A novel hexahydrodibenzofuran derivative with potent inhibitory activity on melanin biosynthesis of cultured B-16 melanoma cells from *Lindera ambulate* bark," *Chemical Pharmacy Bulletin* (Tokyo), 43(5), 893–895 (May 1995).

Lithospermum

1. Konoshima, T., Kozuka, M., Tokuda, H., Tanabe, M., "Antitumor promoting activities and inhibitory effects on Epstein-Barr virus activation of *Shi-un-kou* and its constituents," *Yakugaku Zasshi—Journal of the Pharmaceutical Society of Japan,* 109(11), 843–846 (November 1989).

2. Jin, R., Wan, L.L., Mitsuishi, T., "Effects of *shi-ka-ron* and Chinese herbs in mice treated with anti-tumor agent mitomycin C," *Chung-Kuo Chung Hsi I Chieh Ho Tsa Chih—Chinese Journal of Modern Developments in Traditional Medicine,* 15(2), 101–103 (February 1995).

3. Grases, F., Melero, G., Costa-Bauza, A., Prieto, R., March, J.G., "Urolithiasis and phytotherapy," *International Urology & Nephrology,* 26(5), 507–511 (1994).

Lobelia

1. Murray, M., Pizzorno, J. *Encyclopedia of Natural Medicine* (Rocklin, California: Prima Publishing, 1996), p. 154.

Longan

1. Bensky, D., Gamble, A., Kaptchuk, T., Bensky, L.L. *Chinese Herbal Medicine: Materia Medica,* Revised Edition (Seattle: Eastland Press, 1993), p. 335.

Lonicera

1. Taguchi, H., Iketani, Y., Niitsu, K., Mork, K., "Phar-

maceuticals for treatment of influenza virus infection," *Kokai Tokkyo Koho* JP, 40, 243, 016, cited in Tang, W., Eisenbrand, G. *Chinese Drugs of Plant Origin: Chemistry, Pharmacology, and Use in Traditional and Modern Medicine* (Berlin: Springer-Verlag, 1992), p. 624.

2. Huang, K.C. *The Pharmacology of Chinese Herbs* (Boca Raton, Florida: CRC Press, 1993), p. 292.

3. Yan, H.J., "Clinical and epxerimental study of the effect of *kang-er xin-i* on viral myocarditis," *Chung Hsi I Chieh Ho Tsa Chih,* 11(8), 468–470 (August 1991).

4. Li, Y.Q., Yuan, W., Zhang, S.L., "Clinical and experimental study of *xiao er ke cuan ling* oral liquid in the treatment of infantile bronchopneumonia," *Chung-Kuo Chung Hsi I Chieh Ho Tsa Chih—Chinese Journal of Modern Developments in Traditional Medicine,* 12(12), 719–721 (December 1992).

5. Chang, C.W., Lin, M.T., Lee, S.S., Liu, K.C., Hsu, F.L., Lin, J.Y., "Differential inhibition of reverse transcriptase and cellular DNA polymerase-alpha activities by lignans isolated from Chinese herbs, *Phyllanthus myrtifolius* Moon, and tannins from *Lonicera japonica* Thunb. and *Castanopsis hystrix,*" *Antiviral Research,* 27(4), 367–374 (August 1995).

Loranthus

1. Zhu, H.G., Zollner, T.M., Klein-Franke, A., Anderer, F.A., "Enhancement of MHC-unrestricted cytotoxic activity of human CD56+ CD3- natural killer (NK) cells and CD3+ T cells by rhamnogalacturonan: target cell specificity and activity against NK-insensitive targets," *Journal of Cancer Research and Clinical Oncology,* 120(7), 383–388 (1994).

2. Mueller, E.A., Anderer, F.A., "Chemical specificity of effector cell/tumor cell bridging by a *Viscum album* rhamnogalacturonan enhancing cytotoxicity of human NK cells," *Immunopharmacology,* 19(1), 69–77 (January 1991).

3. Nikolai, G., Friedl, P., Werner, M., Zanker, K.S., "Donor-dependent and dose-dependent variation in the induction of T lymphocyte locomotion in a three-dimensional collagen matrix system by a mistletoe preparation (Iscador)," *Anticancer Drugs,* 8(Supp 1), S61–S64 (April 1997).

4. Timoshenko, A.V., Kayser, K., Drings, P., Kolb, G., Havemann, K., Gabius, H.J., "Modulation of lectin-triggered superoxide release from neutrophils of tumor patients with and without chemotherapy," *Anticancer Research,* 13(5C), 1782–1792 (September 1993).

5. Kovacs, E., Hajto, T., Hostanska, K., "Improvement of DNA repair in lymphocytes of breast cancer patients treated with *Viscum album* extract (Iscador)," *European Journal of Cancer,* 27(12), 1672–1676 (1991).

6. Antony, S., Kuttan, R., Kuttan, G., "Effect of *Viscum album* in the inhibition of lung metastasis in mice induced by B16F10 melanoma cells," *Journal and Experimental and Clinical Cancer Research,* 16(2), 159–162 (June 1997).

7. Kuttan, G., Kuttan, R., "Reduction of leukopenia in mice by *Viscum album* administration during radiation and chemotherapy," *Tumori,* 79(1), 74–76 (28 February 1993).

Lotus

1. Shoji, N., Umeyama, A., Saito, N., Iuchi, A., Takemoto, T., Kajiwara, A., Ohizume, Y., "Asimilobine and lirinidine, serotonergic receptor antagonists, from *Nelumbo nucifera,*" *Journal of Natural Products,* 50(4), 773–774 (July 1987).

2. Mukherjee, P.K., Das, J., Saha, K., Giri, S.J.N., Pal, M., Saha, B.P., "Antipyretic activity of *Nelumbo nucifera* rhizome," *Indian Journal of Experimental Biology,* 34(3), 275–276 (March 1996).

3. Mukherjee, P.K., Saha, K., Das, J., Pal, M., Saha, B.P., "Studies on the anti-inflammatory activity of rhizomes of *Nelumbo nucifera,*" *Planta Medica,* 63(4), 367–369 (August 1997).

4. Mukherjee, P.K., Saha, K., Balasubramanian, R., Pal, M., Saha, B.P., "Studies on psychopharmacological effects of *Nelumbo nucifera* Gaertn. Rhizome extract," *Journal of Ethnopharmacology,* 54(2–3), 63–67 (November 1996).

5. Mukherjee, P.K., Saha, K., Pal, M., Saha, B.P., "Effect of *Nelumbo nucifera* rhizome extract on blood sugar level in rats," *Journal of Ethnopharmacology,* 58(3), 207–213 (November 1997).

Lycium

1. Huang, K.C. *The Pharmacology of Chinese Herbs* (Boca Raton, Florida: CRC Press, 1993), p. 279.

2. Kim, S.Y., Choi, Y.H., Huh, H., Kim, J., Kim, Y.C., Lee, H.S., "New antihepatotoxic cerebroside from *Lycium chinense* fruits," *Journal of Natural Products,* 60(3), 274–276 (March 1997).

3. Ren, B., Ma, Y., Shen, Y., Gao, B., "Protective action of *Lycium barbarum* L. (LbL) and betaine on lipid peroxidation of erythrocyte membrane induced by H_2O_2," *Chung-Kuo Chung Yao Tsa Chih—China Journal of Chinese Materia Medica,* 20(5), 303–304, inside cover (May 1995).

4. Cao, G.W., Yang, W.G., Du, P., "Observation of the effects of LAK/IL-2 therapy combining with *Lycium barbarum* polysaccharides in the treatment of 75 cancer patients," *Chung-Hua Chung Liu Tsa Chih—Chinese Journal of Oncology,* 16(6), 428–431 (November 1994).

5. Lu, C.X., Cheng, B.Q., "Radiosensitizing effects of *Lycium barbarum* polysaccharide for Lewis cell lung cancer," *Chung-Kuo Chung Hsi I Chieh Ho Tsa Chih—Chinese Journal of Modern Developments in Traditional Medicine,* 11(10), 611–612, 582 (October 1991).

6. Bensky, D., Gamble, A., Kaptchuk, T., Bensky, L.L. *Chinese Herbal Medicine: Materia Medica,* Revised Edition (Seattle: Eastland Press, 1993), p. 73.

Magnolia

1. Huang, K.C. *The Pharmacology of Chinese Herbs* (Boca Raton, Florida: CRC Press, 1993), p. 174.

2. Hong, C.Y., Huang, S.S., Tsai, S.K., "Magnolol reduces infarct size and suppresses ventricular arrhythmia in rats subjected to coronary ligation," *Clinical & Experimental Pharmacology & Physiology,* 23(8), 660–664 (August 1996).

3. Bensky, D., Gamble, A., Kaptchuk, T., Bensky, L.L. *Chinese Herbal Medicine: Materia Medica,* Revised Edition (Seattle: Eastland Press, 1993), p. 73.

Marijuana Seed

1. Huang, K.C. *The Pharmacology of Chinese Herbs* (Boca Raton, Florida: CRC Press, 1993), p. 187.

2. Bensky, D., Gamble, A., Kaptchuk, T., Bensky, L.L. *Chinese Herbal Medicine: Materia Medica,* Revised Edition (Seattle: Eastland Press, 1993), p. 120.

Morinda

1. Cui, C., Yang, M., Yao, Z., Cao, B., Luo, Z., Xu, Y., Chen, Y., "Antidepressant active constituents in the roots of *Morinda officinalis* How.," *Chung-Kuo Chung Yao Tsa Chih—China Journal of Chinese Materia Medica*, 20(1), 36–39 (January 1995).

2. Dharmananda, S. *Chinese Herbology: A Professional Training Program* (Portland: Institute for Preventative Medicine and Traditional Health Care, 1992), p. 256.

3. Huang, K.C. *The Pharmacology of Chinese Herbs* (Boca Raton, Florida: CRC Press, 1993), p. 211.

Motherwort

1. Blumenthal, M., Busse, W.R., Goldberg, A., Gruenwald, J., Hall, T., Riggins, C.W., Rister, R.S., eds., Klein, S., Rister, R.S., trans. *The Complete German Commission E Monographs: Therapeutic Guide to Herbal Medicines* (Boston: Integrative Medicine Communications, 1998), p. 172.

2. Ibid.

Moutan (Giant Peony)

1. Huang, K.C. *The Pharmacology of Chinese Herbs* (Boca Raton, Florida: CRC Press, 1993), p. 307.

2. Bensky, D., Gamble, A., Kaptchuk, T., Bensky, L.L. *Chinese Herbal Medicine: Materia Medica*, Revised Edition (Seattle: Eastland Press, 1993), p. 71.

3. Ishida, H., Takamatsu, M., Tsuji, K., Kosuge, T., "Studies on active substances in herbs used for *oketsu* ("stagnant blood") in Chinese medicine. V. On the anticoagulative principle in moutan cortex," *Chemical and Pharmaecutical Bulletin* (Tokyo), 35(2), 836–848 (February 1987).

4. Zhang, W.G., Zhang, Z.S., "Anti-ischemia reperfusion and damage and anti-lipid peroxidation effects of paeonol in rat heart," *Yao Hsueh Hsueh Pao—Acta Pharmaceutica Sinica*, 29(2), 145–148 (1994).

Mulberry Root

1. Yamatake, Y., Shibata, M., Nagai, M., "Pharmacological studies on root bark of mulberry tree (*Morus alba* L.)," *Japanese Journal of Pharmacology*, 26, 461–469 (1976).

2. Hikino, H., Mizuno, T., Oshima, Y., Konno, C., "Validity of the Oriental medicines. LXXX. Antidiabetes drugs. IV. Isolation and hypoglycemic activity of moran A, a glycoprotein of *Morus alba* root barks," *Planta Medica*, 51, 159–160 (1985).

3. Nomura, T., Fukai, T., Uno, J., Arai, T., "Mulberofuran A, a new isoprenoid 2-arylbenzo-furan from the root bark of the cultivated mulberry tree," *Heterocycles*, 16, 983–986 (1978).

4. Bensky, D., Gamble, A., Kaptchuk, T., Bensky, L.L. *Chinese Herbal Medicine: Materia Medica*, Revised Edition (Seattle: Eastland Press, 1993), pp. 203–204.

5. Takasugi, M., Munoz, L., Masamune, T., Shirata, A., Takahashi, K., "Stilbene phytoalexins from diseased mulberry, " *Chemical Letters*, 1241–1242 (1978).

Notopterygium

1. Okuyama, E., Nishimura, S., Ohmori, S., Ozaki, Y., Satake, M., Yamazaki, M., "Analgesic component of *Notopterygium incisum* Ting.," *Chemical & Pharmaceutical Bulletin*, 41(5), 926–929 (May 1993).

2. Yin, X.J., Liu, D.X., Wang, H.C., Zhou, Y., "A study on the mutagenicity of 102 raw pharmaceuticals used in Chinese traditional medicine," *Mutation Research*, 260(1), 73–82 (May 1991).

Nutmeg

1. Ozaki, Y., Soedigdo, S., Wattimena, Y.R., Suganda, A.G., "Antiinflammatory effect of mace, aril of *Myristica fragrans* Houtt., and its active principles," *Japanese Journal of Pharmacology*, 49(2), 155–163 (February 1989).

2. Rashid, A., Misra, D.S., "Antienterotoxic effect of *Myristica fragrans* (nutmeg) on enterotoxigenic *Escherichia coli*," *Indian Journal of Medical Research*, 79, 694–696 (May 1984).

3. Orabi, K.Y., Mossa, J.S., el-Feraly, F.S., "Isolation and characterization of two antimicrobial agents from mace (*Myristica fragrans*)," *Journal of Natural Products*, 54(3), 856–869 (May 1991).

4. Singh, A., Rao, A.R., "Modulatory effect of *Areca* nut on the action of mace (*Myristica fragrans*, Houtt.) on the hepatic detoxification system in mice," *Food Chemical Toxicology*, 31(7), 517–521 (July 1993).

5. Ram, A., Lauria, P., Gupta, R., Sharma, V.N., "Hypolipidaemic effect of *Myristica fragrans* fruit extract in rabbits," *Journal of Ethnopharmacology*, 55(1), 49–53 (December 1996).

6. A key scientific study was Forrest, J.E., Heacock, R.A., "Nutmeg and mace, the psychotropic spices from *Myristica fragrans*,"*Lloydia*, 35(4), 440–449 (December 1972).

Ophiopogon

1. Huang, K.C. *The Pharmacology of Chinese Herbs* (Boca Raton, Florida: CRC Press, 1993), p. 92.

Peach Seed

1. Shen, D., Shen, L., Wang, A.L., "Effect of *xiaoyu pian* on new platelet aggregation defect," *Chung-Kuo Chung Hsi I Chieh Ho Tsa Chih—Chinese Journal of Modern Developments in Traditional Medicine*, 14(10), 589–591 (October 1994).

Peony

1. Huang, K.C. *The Pharmacology of Chinese Herbs* (Boca Raton, Florida: CRC Press, 1993), p. 209.

2. Bruneton, J. *Pharmacognosy, Phytochemistry, Medicinal Plants* (Paris: Lavoisier Publishing, 1995), p. 401.

3. Sung, C.K., Kang, G.H., Yoon, S.S., Lee, I.K., Kim, D., Sankawa, U., Ebizuka, Y., "Glycosidases that converts natural glycosides to bioactive compounds," in Waller, G., Yamasaki, K., eds. *Saponins Used in Traditional and Modern Medicine*, Advances in Experimental Medicine and Biology Volume 404 (New York: Plenum Press, 1996), p. 24.

4. Ohta, H., Matsumoto, K., Shimizu, M., Watanabe, H., "Paeoniflorin attenuates learning impairment of aged rats in operant brightness discrimination task," *Pharmacology, Biochemistry & Behavior*, 49(1), 213–217 (September 1994).

5. Takeuchi, T., Nishii, O., Okamura, T., Yaginuma, T., "Effects of paeoniflorin, glycyrrhizin, and glycyrrhetic acid on ovarian androgen production," *American Journal of Chinese Medicine*, 19(1), 73–78 (1991).

Peppermint

1. Dew, M.J., "Peppermint oil for the irritable bowel syndrome:

a multicentre trial," *British Journal of Clinical Practice,* 38, 394–398 (1984).

2. Leicester, R., "Peppermint oil to reduce colonic spasm during endoscopy," *Lancet,* II, 989 (1982).

3. Tassou, C.C., Drosinos, E.H., Nychas, G.J., "Effects of essential oil from mint (*Mentha piperita*) on *Salmonella enteritidis* and *Listeria monocytogenes* in model food systems at 4 degrees and 10 degrees C," *Journal of Applied Bacteriology,* 78(6), 593–600 (January 1995).

4. Gobel, H., "Effectiveness of oleum menthae pipertae and paracetamol in therapy of headache of the tension type," *Nervenarzt,* 67(8), 672–681 (1996).

5. Kanjanapothi, D., Smitasiri, Y., Panthong, A., Taesotikul, T., Rattanapanone, V., "Postcoital antifertility effect of *Mentha arvensis,*" *Contraception,* 24(5), 559–567 (November 1981).

Perilla

1. Okuno, M., Kajiwara, K., Imai, S., Kobayashi, T., Honma, N., Maki, T., Suruga, K., Goda, T., Takase, S., Mujto, Y., Moriwaki, H., "Perilla oil prevents the excessive growth of visceral adipose tissue in rats by down-regulating adipocyte differentiation," *Journal of Nutrition,* 127(9), 1752–1757 (September 1997).

2. Ueda, H., Yamazaki, M., "Inhibition of tumor necrosis factor-alpha production by orally administering a perilla leaf extract," *Bioscience, Biotechnology, and Biochemistry,* 61(8), 1292–1295 (August 1997).

3. Reddy, B.S., Wang, C.X., Samaha, H., Lubet, R., Steele, V.E., Kelloff, G.J., Rao, C.V., "Chemoprevention of colon carcinogenesis by dietary perillyl alcohol," *Cancer Research,* 57(3), 420–425 (1 February 1997).

4. Crowell, P.L., Siar Ayoubi, A., Burke, Y.D., "Antitumorigenic effects of limonene and perillyl alcohol against pancreatic and breast cancer," *Advances in Experimental Medical Biology,* 401, 131–136 (1996).

Phellodenrdon

1. Mitscher, L.A., "Plant-derived antibiotics," in Weinstein, M.J., Wagman, G.H. (eds). *Antibiotics,* Volume 15 (New York: Plenum Press, 1978), pp. 363–477.

2. Uchiyama, T., Kamikawa H, et al., "Anti-ulcer effect of extract from phellodendri cortex," *Yakugaku Zasshi,* 109(9), 672–676 (September 1989).

3. Bensky, D., Gamble, A., Kaptchuk, T., Bensky, L.L. *Chinese Herbal Medicine: Materia Medica,* Revised Edition (Seattle: Eastland Press, 1993), p. 80–81.

Pinellia

1. Huang, K.C. *The Pharmacology of Chinese Herbs* (Boca Raton, Florida: CRC Press, 1993), p. 196.

2. Bensky, D., Gamble, A., Kaptchuk, T., Bensky, L.L. *Chinese Herbal Medicine: Materia Medica,* Revised Edition (Seattle: Eastland Press, 1993), p. 191.

Plantain

1. Bensky, D., Gamble, A., Kaptchuk, T., Bensky, L.L. *Chinese Herbal Medicine: Materia Medica,* Revised Edition (Seattle: Eastland Press, 1993), p. 143.

Platycodon

1. Huang, K.C. *The Pharmacology of Chinese Herbs* (Boca Raton, Florida: CRC Press, 1993), p. 223.

Polygonum

1. Mei, M.Z., Zhuang, Q.Q., Liu, G.Z., Xie, W.J., "Rapid screening method for hypocholesterolemic agents," *Acta Pharmaca Sinica,* 14, 8–11 (1979).

2. Kimura, Y., Ohminani, H., Okuda, H., Baba, K., Kozawa, M., Archi, S., "Effects of stilbene components of roots of *Polygonum* spp. on liver injury in peroxidized oil-fed rats," *Planta Medica,* 49, 51–54 (1983).

3. Boik, J. *Cancer and Natural Medicine: A Textbook of Basic Science and Clinical Research* (Princeton, Minnesota: Oregon Medical Press, 1995), pp. 112, 152, 196, 251.

Polyporus

1. Xiong, L.L., "Therapeutic effect of combined therapy of *Salvia miltiorrhizae* and *Polyporus umbellatus* polysaccharide in the treatment of chronic hepatitis B," *Chung-Kuo Chung Hsi I Chieh Ho Tsa Chih—Chinese Journal of Modern Developments in Traditional Medicine,* 13(9), 533–535, 516–517 (September 1993).

2. Sugiyama, K., Kawagishi, H., Tanaka, A., Saeki, S., Yoshida, S., Sakamoto, H., Ishiguro, Y., "Isolation of plasma cholesterol-lowering components from *ningyotake* (*Polyporus confluens*) mushroom," *Journal of Nutritional Science & Vitaminology,* 38(4), 335–342 (August 1992).

3. Rangelov, A., Toreva, D., Pisanets, M., "Cholagogic and choleretic activity of products from the high fungus *Polyporus squamosus* in test animals," *Folia Medica,* 32(1), 36–44 (1990).

4. You, J.S., Hau, D.M., Chen, K.T., Huang, H.F., "Combined effects of *chuling* (*Polyporus umbellatus*) extract and mitomycin C on experimental liver cancer," *American Journal of Chinese Medicine,* 22(1), 19–28 (1994).

5. Zhang, Y.H., Liu, Y.L., Yan, S.C., "Effect of *Polyporus umbellatus* polysaccharide on function of macrophages in the peritoneal cavities of mice with liver lesions," *Chung-Kuo Chung Hsi I Chieh Ho Tsa Chih—Chinese Journal of Modern Developments in Traditional Medicine,* 11(4), 225–226, 198 (April 1991).

6. Ohsawa, T., Yukawa, M., Takao, C., Murayama, M., Bando, H., "Studies on constituents of fruit body of *Polyporus umbellatus* and their cytotoxic activity," *Chemical & Pharmaceutical Bulletin,* 40(1), 143–147 (January 1992).

7. Inaoka, Y., Shakuya, A., Fukazawa, H., Ishida, H., Nukaya, H., Tsuji, K., Kuroda, H., Okada, M., Fukushima, M., Kosuge, T., "Studies on active substances in herbs used for hair treatment. I. Effects of herb extracts on hair growth and isolation of an active substance from *Polyporus umbellatus* F.," *Chemical Pharmaceutical Bulletin,* 42, 530–533 (1994).

Prunella

1. Zheng, M., "Experimental study of 472 herbs with antiviral action against the herpes simplex virus," *Chung Hsi I Chieh Ho Tsa Chih,* 10(1), 39–41 (January 1990).

2. Yamasaki, K., Otake, T., Mori, H., Morimoto, M., Ueba, N., Kurokawa, Y., Shiota, K., Yuge, T., "Screening test of crude drugs extract on anti-HIV activity," *Yakugaku Zasshi—Journal of the Pharmaceutical Society of Japan,* 113(11), 818–824 (November 1993).

3. Yao, X.J., Wainberg, M.A., Parniak, M.A., "Mechanism of inhibition of HIV-1 infection in vitro by purified extract of *Prunella vulgaris,*" *Virology,* 187(1), 56–62 (March 1992).

4. Tabba, H.D., Chang, R.S., Smith, K.M., "Isolation, purification, and partial characterization of prunellin, an anti-HIV component from aqueous extracts of *Prunella vulgaris,*" *Antiviral Research,* 11(5–6), 263–273 (June 1989).

Psoralea

1. Bensky, D., Gamble, A., Kaptchuk, T., Bensky, L.L. *Chinese Herbal Medicine: Materia Medica,* Revised Edition (Seattle: Eastland Press, 1993), p. 345.

2. Boik, J. *Cancer and Natural Medicine: A Textbook of Basic Science and Clinical Research* (Princeton, Minnesota: Oregon Medical Press, 1995), pp. 217–218.

Reed Root

1. Chang, H.M., But, P.P.H. *Pharmacology and Applications of Chinese Materia Medica,* Volume 2 (Teaneck, New Jersey: World Scientific Publishing, 1987), p. 822.

Rehmannia

1. Bensky, D., Gamble, A., Kaptchuk, T., Bensky, L.L. *Chinese Herbal Medicine: Materia Medica,* Revised Edition (Seattle: Eastland Press, 1993), p. 69.

2. Oshio, H., Inouye, H., "Iridoid glycosides of *Rehmannia glutinosa,*" *Phytochemistry,* 21, 133–138 (1981).

3. Naeser, M.A. *Outline Guide to Chinese Herbal Patent Medicines in Pill Form with Sample Pictures of the Boxes: An Introduction to Chinese Herbal Medicines,* Second Edition (Boston: Boston Chinese Medicine, 1996), p. 292.

Rhubarb Root

1. Castiglione, S., Paggi, M.G., Delpino, A., et al., "Inhibition of protein synthesis in neoplastic cells by rhein," *Biochemical Pharmacology,* 40(5), 967–973 (1990).

2. Chang, H.M., But, P.P.H. *Pharmacology and Applications of Chinese Materia Medica,* Volume 2 (Teaneck, New Jersey: World Scientific Publishing, 1987), p. 783.

3. Boik, J. *Cancer and Natural Medicine: A Textbook of Basic Science and Clinical Research* (Princeton, Minnesota: Oregon Medical Press, 1995), p. 196.

4. Miles, M.R., Olsen, L., Rogers, A., et al., "Recurrent vaginal candidiasis—importance of an intestinal reservoir," *Journal of the American Medical Association,* 238, 1863–1867 (1977).

5. Wang, H.H., "Antitrichomonal action of emodin in mice," *Journal of Ethnopharmacology,* 40(2), 111–116 (October 1993).

6. Huang, K.C. *The Pharmacology of Chinese Herbs* (Boca Raton, Florida: CRC Press, 1993), p. 185.

Saussurea

1. Chen, S.F., Li, Y.Q., He, F.Y., "Effect of *Saussurea lappa* on gastric functions," *Chung-Kuo Chung Hsi I Chieh Ho Tsa Chih—Chinese Journal of Modern Developments in Traditional Medicine,* 14(7), 406–408 (July 1994).

2. Yoshikawa, M., Hatakeyama, S., Inoue, Y., Yamahara, J., "Saussureamines A, B, C, D, and E, new anti-ulcer principles from Chinese Saussureae Radix," *Chemical & Pharmaceutical Bulletin,* 41(1), 214–216 (January 1993).

3. Bensky, D., Gamble, A., Kaptchuk, T., Bensky, L.L. *Chinese Herbal Medicine: Materia Medica,* Revised Edition (Seattle: Eastland Press, 1993), p. 238.

4. Chen, H.C., Chou, C.K., Lee, S.D., Wang, J.C., Yeh, S.F., "Active compounds from *Saussurea lappa* Clarks. that suppress hepatitis B virus surface antigen gene expression in human hepatoma cells," *Antiviral Research,* 27(1–2), 99–109 (May 1995).

Scallion

1. Goldman, I.L., Kopelberg, M., Debaene, J.E., Schwartz, B.S., "Antiplatelet activity in onion (*Allium cepa*) is sulfur dependent," *Thrombosis & Haemostasis,* 76(3), 450–452 (September 1996).

Schisandra

1. Ohkura, Y., Mizoguchi, Y., Sakagami, Y., Kobayashi, K., Yamamoto, S., Morisawa, S., Takeda, S., Aburada, M., "Inhibitory effect of TJN-101 ((+)-(6S,7S,R-biar)-5,6,7,8-tetrahydro-1,2,3,12-tetramethoxy-6,7-dimethyl-10,11-methylenedioxy-6-dibenzo[a,c]-cyclooctenol) on immunologically induced liver injuries," *Japanese Journal of Pharmacology,* 44(2), 179–185 (June 1987).

2. Ko, K.M., Ip, S.P., Poon, M.K., Wu, S.S., Che, C.T., Ng, K.H., Kong, Y.C., "Effect of a lignan-enriched Fructus Schisandrae extract on hepatic glutathione status in rats: protection against carbon tetrachloride toxicity," *Planta Medica,* 61(2), 134–137 (April 1995).

3. Chen, Y.Y., Yang, Y.Q., "Studies on the SGPT-lowering active component of the fruits of *Schisandra rubriflora* Rhed et Wils," *Yao Hsueh Hsueh Pao—Acta Pharmaceutica Sinica,* 17(4), 312–313 (April 1982).

4. Ohkura, Y., Mizoguchi, Y., Morisawa, S., Takeda, S., Aburada, M., Hosoya, E., "Effect of gomisin A (TJN-101) on the arachidonic acid cascade in macrophages," *Japanese Journal of Pharmacology,* 52(2), 331–336 (February 1990).

5. Ohkura, Y., Mizoguchi, Y., Sakagami, Y., Kobayashi, K., Yamamoto, S., Morisawa, S., Takeda, S., Aburada, M., pp. 179–185.

6. Kubo, S., Ohkura, Y., Mizoguchi, Y., Matsui-Yuasa, I., Otani, S., Morisawa, S., Kinoshita, H., Takeda, S., Aburada, M., Hosoya, E., "Effect of Gomisin A (TJN-101) on liver regeneration," *Planta Medica,* 58(6), 489–492 (December 1992).

7. Yasukawa, K., Ikeya, Y., Mitsuhashi, H., Iwasaki, M., Aburada, M., Nakagawa, S., Takeuchi, M., Takido, M., "Gomisin A inhibits tumor promotion by 12-O-tetradecanoylphorbol-13-acetate in two-stage carcinogenesis in mouse skin," *Oncology,* 49(1), 68–71 (1992).

8. Song, W., "Quality of *Schisandra incarnata* Stapf.," *Chung-Kuo Chung Yao Tsa Chih—China Journal of Chinese Materia Medica,* 16(4), 204–206, 253 (April 1991).

9. Bensky, D., Gamble, A., Kaptchuk, T., Bensky, L.L. *Chinese Herbal Medicine: Materia Medica,* Revised Edition (Seattle: Eastland Press, 1993), p. 378.

10. Nishiyama, N., Wang, Y.L., Saito H., "Beneficial effects of S-113m, a novel herbal prescription, on learning impairment model in mice," *Biological & Pharmaceutical Bulletin,* 18(11), 1498–1503 (November 1995).

11. Bensky, D., Gamble, A., Kaptchuk, T., Bensky, L.L., p. 378.

12. Takeda, S., Arai, I., Hasegawa, M., Tatsugi, A., Aburada, M., Hosoya, E., "Effect of gomisin A (TJN-101), a lignan compound isolated from schisandra fruits, on liver function in rats," *Nippon Yakurigaku Zasshi—Folia Pharmacologica Japonica,* 91(4), 237–244 (April 1988).

Scutellaria

1. Bensky, D., Gamble, A., Kaptchuk, T., Bensky, L.L. *Chinese Herbal Medicine: Materia Medica,* Revised Edition (Seattle: Eastland Press, 1993), p. 76.

2. Yang, D., Michel, D., Bevalot, F., Chaumont, J.P., Millet-Clerc, J., "Antifungal activity in vitro of *Scutellaria baicalensis* Georgi upon cutaneous and ungual pathogenic fungi," *Annales Pharmaceutiques Francaises,* 53(3), 138–141 (1995).

3. Li, B.Q., Fu, T., Yan, Y.D., Baylor, N.W., Ruscetti, F.W., Kung, H.F., "Inhibition of HIV infection by baicalin—a flavonoid compound purified from Chinese herbal medicine," *Cellular & Molecular Biology Research,* 39(2), 119–124 (1993).

4. Nagai, T., Suzuki, Y., Tomimori, T., Yamada, H., "Antiviral activity of plant flavonoid, 5,7,4'-trihydroxy-8-methoxyflavone, from the roots of *Scutellaria baicalensis* against influenza A (H3N2) and B viruses," *Biological & Pharmaceutical Bulletin,* 18(2), 295–299 (February 1995).

5. Nagai, T., Miyaichi, Y., Tomimori, T., Suzuki, Y., Yamada, H., "Inhibition of influenza virus sialidase and anti-influenza virus activity by plant flavonoids," *Chemical & Pharmaceutical Bulletin,* 38(5), 1329–1332 (May 1990).

6. Konoshima, T., Kokumai, M., Kozuka, M., Iinuma, M., Mizuno, M., Tanaka, T., Tokuda, H., Nishino, H., Iwashima, A., "Studies on inhibitors of skin tumor promotion. XI. Inhibitory effects of flavonoids from *Scutellaria baicalensis* on Epstein-Barr virus activation and their anti-tumor-promoting activities," *Chemical & Pharmaceutical Bulletin,* 40(2), 531–533 (February 1992).

7. Razina, T.G., Udintsev, S.N., Prishchep, T.P., Iaremenko, K.V., "Enhancement of the selectivity of the action of the cytostatics cyclophosphane and 5-fluorouracil by using an extract of the Baikal skullcap in an experiment," *Voprosy Onkologii,* 33(2), 80–84 (1987).

8. Bensky, D., Gamble, A., Kaptchuk, T., Bensky, L.L., p. 77.

9. Huang, H.C., Wang, H.R., Hsieh, L.M., "Antiproliferative effect of baicalein, a flavonoid from a Chinese herb, on vascular smooth muscle cell," *European Journal of Pharmacology,* 251(1), 91–93 (4 January 1994).

10. Bensky, D., Gamble, A., Kaptchuk, T., Bensky, L.L., p. 77.

11. Umeda, M., Amagaya, S., Ogihara, Y., "Effects of certain herbal medicines on the biotransformation of arachidonic acid, a new pharmacological testing method using serum," *Journal of Ethnopharmacology,* 23(1), 91–98 (May–June 1988).

12. Wong, B.Y., Lau, B.H., Yamasaki, T., Teel, R.W., "Inhibition of dexamethasone-induced cytochrome P450-mediated mutagenicity and metabolism of aflatoxin B1 by Chinese medicinal herbs," *European Journal of Cancer Prevention,* 2(4), 351–356 (July 1993).

13. Murray, M., Pizzorno, J. *Encyclopedia of Natural Medicine* (Rocklin, California: Prima Publishing, 1996), p. 153.

14. Zhang, H., Huang, J., "Preliminary study of traditional Chinese medicine treatment of minimal brain dysfunction: analysis of 100 cases," *Chung Hsi I Chieh Ho Tsa Chih—Chinese Journal of Modern Developments in Traditional Medicine,* 10(5), 278–279, 260 (May 1990).

15. Chung, C.P., Park, J.B., Bae, K.H., "Pharmacological effects of methanolic extract from the root of *Scutellaria baicalensis* and its flavonoids on human gingival fibroblast," *Planta Medica,* 61(2), 150–153 (April 1995).

16. Gao, D., Sakurai, K., Chen, J., Ogiso, T., "Protection by baicalein against ascorbic acid-induced lipid peroxidation of rat liver microsomes," *Research Communications in Molecular Pathology & Pharmacology,* 90(1), 103–114 (October 1995).

17. Zhang, J., Zhou, Y., "Research into the use of Chinese herbs which inhibit the mechanism responsible for diabetic opthamolopathy," *International Journal of Chinese Medicine,* 17(3), 160–164 (1992).

18. Yang, T., et al., "Inhibitory activity on aldose reductase and lipid peroxidation by components of four Chinese medicinal herbs," *Chinese Biochemical Journal,* 8(1), 169–173 (1992).

19. Costarella, L., "Naturopathic condition review: asthma," *Protocol Journal of Botanical Medicine,* 1(2), 103 (Autumn 1995).

Snake Gourd (Trichosanth) Fruit

1. Bensky, D., Gamble, A., Kaptchuk, T., Bensky, L.L. *Chinese Herbal Medicine: Materia Medica,* Revised Edition (Seattle: Eastland Press, 1993), p. 179.

Snake Gourd (Tricosanth) Root

1. Huang, K.C. *The Pharmacology of Chinese Herbs* (Boca Raton, Florida: CRC Press, 1993), p. 89.

2. Huang, Q., Liu, S., Tang, Y., Jin, S., Wang, Y., "Studies on crystal structures, active-centre geometry and depurinating mechanism of two ribosome-inactivating proteins," *Biochemical Journal,* 309(Pt 1), 285–298 (1 July 1995).

3. Yamashita, K., Fukushima, K., Sakiyama, T., Murata, F., Kuroki, M., Matsuoka, Y., "Expression of Sia alpha 2→6Gal beta 1→4GlcNAc residues on sugar chains of glycoproteins including carcinoembryonic antigens in human colon adenocarcinoma: applications of *Trichosanthes japonica* agglutinin I for early diagnosis," *Cancer Research,* 55(8), 1675–1679 (15 April 1995).

4. Zheng, Y.T., Zhang, W. F., Ben, K.L., Wang, J.H., "In vitro immunotoxicity and cytotoxicity of trichosanthin against human normal immunocytes and leukemia-lymphoma cells," *Immunopharmacology & Immunotoxicology,* 17(1), 69–79 (February 1995).

5. Huang, K.C., p. 252.

6. Bensky, D., Gamble, A., Kaptchuk, T., Bensky, L.L. *Chinese Herbal Medicine: Materia Medica,* Revised Edition (Seattle: Eastland Press, 1993), p. 181.

7. Chan, W.Y., Ng, T.B., Yeung, H.W., "Trichosanthin as an abortifacient for terminating early pregnancy," *International Journal of Fertility,* 38(2), 99–107 (March–April 1993).

Solomon's Seal

1. Bensky, D., Gamble, A., Kaptchuk, T., Bensky, L.L. *Chinese Herbal Medicine: Materia Medica,* Revised Edition (Seattle: Eastland Press, 1993), p. 363.

Stephania

1. Huang, K.C. *The Pharmacology of Chinese Herbs* (Boca Raton, Florida: CRC Press, 1993), pp. 121–122.

Tang-Kuei (Chinese Angelica)

1. Zheng, R.L., Zhang, H., "Effects of ferulic acid on fertile and asthenozoospermic infertile human sperm motility, viability, lipid peroxidation, and cyclic nucleotides," *Free Radical Biology & Medicine*, 22(4), 581–586 (1997).

2. Scott, B.C., Butler, J., Halliwell, B., Aruoma, O.I., "Evaluation of the antioxidant actions of ferulic acid and catechins," *Free Radical Research Communications*, 19(4), 241–253 (1993).

3. Huang, K.C. *The Pharmacology of Chinese Herbs* (Boca Raton, Florida: CRC Press, 1993), p. 248.

4. Ibid.

5. Raman, A., Lin, Z.X., Sviderskaya, E., Kowalska, D., "Investigation of the effect of *Angelica sinensis* root extract on the proliferation of melanocytes in culture," *Journal of Ethnopharmacology*, 54(2–3), 165–170 (November 1996).

6. Wang, S.R., Guo, Z.Q., Liao, J.Z., "Experimental study on effects of 18 kinds of Chinese herbal medicine for synthesis of thromboxane A2 and PGI2," *Chung-Kuo Chung Hsi I Chieh Ho Tsa Chih—Chinese Journal of Modern Developments in Traditional Medicine*, 13(3), 167–170, 134 (March 1993).

7. Chang, H.M., But, P.P.H. *Pharmacology and Applications of Chinese Materia Medica*, Volume 1 (Singapore: World Scientific Publishing, 1986), p. 446.

8. Ibid.

Turmeric

1. Oetari, S., Sudibyo, M., Commandeur, J.N., Samhoedi, R., Vermeulen, N.P., "Effects of curcumin on cytochrome P450 and glutathione S-transferase activities in rat liver," *Biochemical Pharmacology*, 51(1), 39–45 (12 January 1996).

2. Sreejayan, Rao, M.N., "Nitric oxide scavenging by curcuminoids," *Journal of Pharmacy & Pharmacology*, 49(1), 105–107 (January 1997).

3. Camoirano, A., Balansky, R.M., Bennicelli, C., Izzotti, A., D'Agostini, F., De Flora, S., "Experimental databases on inhibition of the bacterial mutagenicity of 4-nitroquinoline 1-oxide and cigarette smoke," *Mutation Research*, 317(2), 89–109 (April 1994).

4. Chan, T.A., Morin, P.J., Vogelstein, B., Kinzler, K.W., "Mechanisms underlying nonsteroidal antiinflammatory drug-mediated apoptosis," *Proceedings of the National Academy of Sciences of the USA*, 95(2), 681–686 (20 January 1998).

5. Chen, Y.C., Kuo, T.C., Lin-Shiau, S.Y., Lin, J.K., "Induction of HSP70 gene expression by modulation of Ca(+2) ion and cellular p53 protein by curcumin in colorectal carcinoma cells," *Molecular Carcinogenesis*, 17(4), 224–234 (December 1996).

6. Ibid.

7. Firozi, P.F., Aboobaker, V.S., Bhattacharya, R.K., "Action of curcumin on the cytochrome P450-system catalyzing the activation of aflatoxin B1," *Chemico-Biological Interactions*, 100(1), 41–51 (8 March 1996).

8. Jiang, M.C., Yang-Yen, H.F., Yen, J.J., Lin, J.K., "Curcumin induces apoptosis in immortalized NIH 3T3 and malignant cancer cell lines," *Nutrition & Cancer*, 26(1), 111–120 (1996).

9. Kuo, M.L., Huang, T.S., Lin, J.K., "Curcumin, an antioxidant and anti-tumor promoter, induces apoptosis in human leukemia cells," *Biochimica et Biophysica Acta*, 1317(2), 95–100 (15 November 1996).

10. Tanaka, T., Makita, H., Ohnishi, M., Hirose, Y., Wang, A., Mori, H., Satoh, K., Hara, A., Ogawa, H., "Chemoprevention of 4-nitroquinoline 1-oxide-induced oral carcinogenesis by dietary curcumin and hesperidin—comparison with the protective effect of beta-carotene," *Cancer Research*, 54(17), 4653–4659 (1 September 1994).

11. Ishizaki, C., Oguro, T., Yoshida, T., Wen, C.Q., Sueki, H., Iijima, M., "Enhancing effect of ultraviolet A on ornithine decarboxylase induction and dermatitis evoked by 12-o-tetradecanoylphorbol-13-acetate and its inhibition by curcumin in mouse skin," *Dermatology*, 193(4), 311–317 (1996).

12. Huang, M.T., Ma, W., Yen, P., Xie, J.G., Han, J., Frenkel, K., Grunberger, D., Conney, A.H., "Inhibitory effects of topical application of low doses of curcumin on 12-O-tetradecanoylphorbol-13-acetate-induced tumor promotion and oxidized DNA bases in mouse epidermis," *Carcinogenesis*, 18(1), 83–88 (January 1997).

13. Iersel, M.L., Ploemen, J.P., Struik, I., van Amersfoort, C., Keyzer, A.E., Schefferlie, J.G., van Bladeren, P.J., "Inhibition of glutathione S-transferase activity in human melanoma cells by alpha, beta-unsaturated carbonyl derivatives. Effects of acrolein, cinnamaldehyde, citral, crotonaldehyde, curcumin, ethacrynic acid, and trans-2-hexenal," *Chemico-Biological Interactions*, 102(2), 117–132 (21 October 1996).

14. Menon, L.G., Kuttan, R., Kuttan, G., "Inhibition of lung metastasis in mice induced by B16F10 melanoma cells by polyphenolic compounds," *Cancer Letters*, 95(1–2), 221–225 (16 August 1995).

15. Venkatesan, N., Chandrakasan, G., "Modulation of cyclophosphamide-induced early lung injury by curcumin, an anti-inflammatory antioxidant," *Molecular & Cellular Biochemistry*, 142(1), 79–87 (12 January 1995).

16. Thresiamma, K.C., George, J., Kuttan, R., "Protective effect of curcumin, ellagic acid and bixin on radiation induced toxicity," *Indian Journal of Experimental Biology*, 34(9), 845–847 (September 1996).

17. Kawashima, H., Akimoto, K., Shirasaka, N., Shimizu, S., "Inhibitory effects of alkyl gallate and its derivatives on fatty acid desaturation," *Biochimica et Biophysica Acta*, 1299(1), 34–38 (5 January 1996).

18. Nirmala, C., Puvanakrishnan, R., "Protective role of curcumin against isoproterenol induced myocardial infarction in rats," *Molecular & Cellular Biochemistry*, 159(2), 85–93 (21 June 1996).

19. Dikshit, M., Rastogi, L., Shukla, R., Srimal, R.C., "Prevention of ischaemia-induced biochemical changes by curcumin & quinidine in the cat heart," *Indian Journal of Medical Research*, 101, 31–35 (January 1995).

20. Sreejayan, Rao, M.N., "Curcuminoids as potent inhibitors of lipid peroxidation," *Journal of Pharmacy & Pharmacology*, 46(12), 1013–1016 (December 1994).

21. Babu, P.S., Srinivasan, K., "Influence of dietary curcumin and cholesterol on the progression of experimentally induced diabetes in albino rat," *Molecular & Cellular Biochemistry*, 152(1), 13–21 (8 November 1995).

22. Srivastava, K.C., Bordia, A., Verma, S.K., "Curcumin, a major component of food spice turmeric (*Curcuma longa*) inhibits aggregation and alters eicosanoid metabolism in human blood

platelets," *Prostaglandins Leukotrienes & Essential Fatty Acids,* 52(4), 223–227 (April 1995).

23. Yasni, S., Yoshiie, K., Oda, H., Sugano, M., Imaizumi, K., "Dietary *Curcuma xanthorrhiza* Roxb. increases mitogenic responses of splenic lymphocytes in rats, and alters populations of the lymphocytes in mice," *Journal of Nutritional Science & Vitaminology,* 39(4), 345–354 (August 1993).

24. Chandra, D., Gupta, S., "Anti-inflammatory and anti-arthritic activity of volatile oil of *Curcuma longa* (haldi)," *Indian Journal of Medical Research,* 60, 138–142 (1972).

25. Arora, R., Basu, N., Kapoor, V., Jain, A., "Anti-inflammatory studies on *Curcuma longa* (turmeric)," *Indian Journal of Medical Research,* 59, 1289–1295 (1971).

26. Sui, Z., Salto, R., Li, J., Craik, C., Ortiz de Montellano, P.R., "Inhibition of the HIV-1 and HIV-2 proteases by curcumin and curcumin boron complexes," *Bioorganic & Medicinal Chemistry,* 1(6), 415–422 (December 1993).

27. Mazumder, A., Wang, S., Neamati, N., Nicklaus, M., Sunder, S., Chen, J., Milne, G.W., Rice, W.G., Burke, T.R. Jr., Pommier, Y., "Antiretroviral agents as inhibitors of both human immunodeficiency virus type 1 integrase and protease," *Journal of Medicinal Chemistry,* 39(13), 2472–2481 (21 June 1996).

28. Chan, M.M., "Inhibition of tumor necrosis factor by curcumin, a phytochemical," *Biochemical Pharmacology,* 49(11), 1551–1556 (26 May 1995).

29. Patel, K., Srinivasan, K., "Influence of dietary spices or their active principles on digestive enzymes of small intestinal mucosa in rats," *International Journal of Food Sciences & Nutrition,* 47(1), 55–59 (January 1996).

30. Hussain, M.S., Chandrasekhara, N., "Biliary proteins from hepatic bile of rats fed curcumin or capsaicin inhibit cholesterol crystal nucleation in supersaturated model bile," *Indian Journal of Biochemistry & Biophysics,* 31(5), 407–412 (October 1994).

31. Unnikrishnan, M.K., Rao, M.N., "Inhibition of nitrite induced oxidation of hemoglobin by curcuminoids," *Pharmazie,* 50(7), 490–492 (July 1995).

32. South, E.H., Exon, J.H., Hendrix, K., "Dietary curcumin enhances antibody response in rats," *Immunopharmacology & Immunotoxicology,* 19(1),105–119 (February 1997).

33. Watanabe, A., Takeshita, A., Kitano, S., Hanazawa, S., "CD 14-mediated signal pathway of *Porphyromonas gingivalis* lipopolysaccharide in human gingival fibroblasts," *Infection & Immunity,* 64(11), 4488–4494 (November 1996).

34. Leri, A., Liu, Y., Malhotra, A., Li, Q., Stiegler, P., Claudio, P.P., Giordano, A., Kajstura, J., Hintze, T.H., Anversa, P., "Pacing-induced heart failure in dogs enhances the expression of p53 and p53-dependent genes in ventricular myocytes," *Circulation,* 97(2), 194–203 (20 January 1998).

Viola

1. Chang, R.S., Yeung, H.W., "Inhibition of growth of human immunodeficiency virus in vitro by crude extracts of Chinese medicinal herbs," *Antiviral Research,* 9(3), 163–175 (April 1998).

2. Ngan, F., Chang, R.S., Tabba, H.D., Smith, K.M., "Isolation, purification and partial characterization of an active anti-HIV compound from the Chinese medicinal herb *Viola yedoensis,*" *Antiviral Research,* 10(1–3), 107–116 (November 1988).

Vitex

1. Miliewicz, A., Gejdel, E., Sworen, H., Sienkiewicz, K., Jedrezjak, J., Teucher, T., Schmitz, H., "Vitex agnus castus extract in the treatment of luteal phase defects due to latent hyperprolactinemia. Results of a randomized placebo-controlled double-blind study," *Arzneimittel-Forschung,* 43(7), 752–756 (July 1993).

2. Sliutz, G., Speiser, P., Schultz, A.M., Spona, J., Zeillinger, R., "Agnus castus extracts inhibit prolactin secretion of rat pituitary," *Hormone and Metabolism Research,* 25(5), 253–255 (May 1993).

3. Hobbs, C., Amster, M., "Naturopathic specific condition review: premenstrual syndrome," *Protocol Journal of Botanical Medicine,* 1(4), 168–173 (Spring 1996).

4. Cahill, D.J., Fox, R., Wardel, P.G., Harlow, C.R., "Multiple follicular development associated with herbal medicine," *Human Reproduction,* 9(8), 1469–1470 (August 1994).

5. Bhargava, S.K., "Antiandrogenic effects of a flavonoid-rich fraction of *Vitex negundo* seeds: a histological and biochemical study in dogs," *Journal of Ethnopharmacology,* 27(3), 327–339 (December 1989).

Wheat

1. Paroli, E., "Opioid peptides from food (the exorphins)," *World Review of Nutrition and Dietetics,* 55, 58–97 (1988).

Zanthoxylum

1. Cichewicz, R.H., Thorpe, P.A., "The antimicrobial properties of chile peppers (*Capsicum* species) and their uses in Mayan medicine," *Journal of Ethnopharmacology,* 52(2), 61–70 (June 1996).

2. Bensky, D., Gamble, A., Kaptchuk, T., Bensky, L.L. *Chinese Herbal Medicine: Materia Medica,* Revised Edition (Seattle: Eastland Press, 1993), p. 305.

3. Adesany, S.A., Sofowora, A., "Phytochemical investigation of candidate plants for the management of sickle cell anaemia," in Hostettmann, K., Marston, A., Maillard, M., Hamburger, M. (eds). *Proceedings of the Phytochemical Society of Europe: 37, Phytochemistry of Plants Used in Traditional Medicine* (Oxford: Clarendon Press, 1995), pp. 189–204.

Zizyphus

1. Hans, B.H., Park, M.H. *Folk Medicine* (Washington: American Chemical Society, 1986), pp. 205–215.

Cordyceps

1. Hobbs, C. *Medicinal Mushrooms: An Exploration of Tradition, Healing, and Culture,* Second Edition (Santa Cruz, California: Botanica Press, 1995), p. 82.

2. Zhu, D., "Recent advances on the active components in Chinese medicines," *Abstracts of Chinese Medicines,* 1, 251–286 (1987).

3. Chen, J.R., Yen, J.H., Lin, C.C., Tsai, W.J., Liu, W.J., Tsai, J.J., Lin, S.F., Liu, H.W., "The effects of Chinese herbs on improving survival and inhibiting anti-ds DNA antibody production in lupus mice," *American Journal of Chinese Medicine,* 21(3–4), 257–262 (1993).

4. Yamaguchi, N., et al., "Augmentation of various immune reactivities of tumor-bearing hosts with an extract of *Cordyceps sinensis,*" *Biotherapy,* 2, 199–205 (1990).

5. Furuya, T., et al., "N6-(2-hydroxyethyl)adenosine, a biologi-

cally active compound from cultured mycelia of *Cordyceps* and *Isaria* species," *Phytochemistry*, 22, 2509–2511 (1983).

6. Naoki, T., et al., "Pharmacological studies on *Cordyceps sinensis* from China," *Fifth Mycological Congress Abstracts*, Vancouver, British Columbia: August 14–21, 1994.

7. Xu, N., Zhang, B., "Effect of Cordyceps on plasma lipids in normal, stressed, and hyperlipemic rats," *Abstracts of Chinese Medicines*, 2, 317 (1987).

8. Zhou, L., et al., "Short-term curative effect of cultured *Cordyceps sinensis* (Berk. Sacc.) Mycelia in chronic hepatitis B," *Chung-Kuo Chung-Yao Tsa Chi—China Journal of Chinese Materia Medica*, 15, 53–55, 65 (1990).

9. Chen, Y., et al., "Clinical effects of natural *Cordyceps* and cultured mycelia of *Cordyceps sinensis* in kidney failure," *Abstracts of Chinese Medicines*, 1, 547 (1986).

10. Zhuang, J., Chen, H., "Treatment of tinnitus with *Cordyceps* infusion: A report of 23 cases," *Abstracts of Chinese Medicines*, 1, 66 (1990).

11. Yang, Y., "Anticarcinogenic effect of the polysaccharide from *Laoshan polystictus versicolor*," *Abstracts of Chinese Medicines*, 1, 59 (1985).

12. Huang, Y., et al., "Toxicological studies on cultured *Cordyceps sinensis*, strain B414," *Abstracts of Chinese Medicines*, 2, 321 (1987).

Frankincense

1. Reddy, C.K., Chandrakasan, G., Dhar, S.C., "Studies on the metabolism of glycosaminoglycans under the influence of new herbal anti-inflammatory agents," *Biochemical Pharmacology*, 20, 3527–3534 (1989).

2. Kulkani, R.R., Patki, P.S., Jog, V.P., et al., "Treatment of osteoarthritis with a herbomineral formulation: a double-blind, placebo-controlled, cross-over study," *Journal of Ethnopharmacology*, 33, 91–95 (1991).

Gelatin

1. Bensky, D., Gamble, A., Kaptchuk, T., Bensky, L.L. *Chinese Herbal Medicine: Materia Medica*, Revised Edition (Seattle: Eastland Press, 1993), p. 333.

2. Huang, K.C. *The Pharmacology of Chinese Herbs* (Boca Raton, Florida: CRC Press, 1993), p. 261.

3. Fan, H.Z., Liu, Y.X., Xie, K.Q., Zhang, A., "Characterization and quantification of dermatan sulfate from donkey skin," *Chung-Kuo Chung Yao Tsa Chih—China Journal of Chinese Materia Medica*, 19(8), 477–480, 511 (August 1994).

Kaolin (Halloysite)

1. Huang, K.C. *The Pharmacology of Chinese Herbs* (Boca Raton, Florida: CRC Press, 1993), p. 194.

2. Bensky, D., Gamble, A., Kaptchuk, T., Bensky, L.L. *Chinese Herbal Medicine: Materia Medica*, Revised Edition (Seattle: Eastland Press, 1993), p. 380.

Malt Sugar

1. Shibamoto, T., Hagiwara, Y., Hagiwara, H., Osawa, T., "Flavonoid with strong antioxidative activity isolated from young green barley leaves," in , Ho, C.T., Osawa, T., Huang, M.T., Rosen, R., (eds). *Food Phytochemicals for Cancer Prevention II: Teas, Spices, and Herbs* (Washington: American Chemical Society, 1994), pp. 154–163.

Mirabilite (Epsom Salts)

1. Bensky, D., Gamble, A., Kaptchuk, T., Bensky, L.L. *Chinese Herbal Medicine: Materia Medica*, Revised Edition (Seattle: Eastland Press, 1993), p. 118.

Myrrh

1. Wichtl, M., ed., Grainger Bisset, N., trans. *Herbal Drugs and Phytopharmaceuticals: A handbook for practice on a scientific basis* (Boca Raton, Florida: CRC Press, 1995), p. 346.

Oyster Shell

1. Tsumura, A. *Kampo: How the Japanese Updated Traditional Herbal Medicine* (San Francisco: Kodansha, 1991), p. 168.

Talc

1. Bensky, D., Gamble, A., Kaptchuk, T., Bensky, L.L. *Chinese Herbal Medicine: Materia Medica*, Revised Edition (Seattle: Eastland Press, 1993), p. 134.

Ginkgo

1. Guinot, P., et al., "Tanakan inhibits platelet-activating aggregation in healthy male volunteers," *Haemostasis*, 19, 219–223 (1986).

2. Koltai, M., et al., "PAF: a review of its effects, antagonists, and possible future clinical implication. Part II," *Drugs*, 42, 174–204 (1991).

3. Yan, L.J., Droy-Lefaix, M.T., Packer, L., "*Ginkgo biloba* extract (EGb 761) protects human low density lipoproteins against oxidative modification mediated by copper," *Biochemical and Biophysical Research Communications*, 212(2), 360–366 (17 July 1995).

4. Rong, Y., Geng, Z., Lau, B.H., "*Ginkgo biloba* attenuates oxidative stress in macrophages and endothelial cells," *Free Radical Biology and Medicine*, 20(1), 121–127 (1996).

5. Seif-El-Nasr, M., El-Fattah, A.A., "Lipid peroxide, phospholipids, glutathione levels and superoxide dismutase activity in rat brain after ischaemia: effect of *Ginkgo biloba* extract," *Pharmacological Research*, 32(5), 273–278 (November 1995).

6. Ni, Y., Zhao, B., Hour, J., Xin, W., "Preventive effect of *Ginkgo biloba* extract on apoptosis in rat cerebellar neuronal cells induced by hydroxyl radicals," *Neuroscience Letters*, 214(2–3), 115–118 (23 August 1996).

7. Punkt, K., Unger, A., Welt, K., Hilbig, H., Schaffraniertz, L., "Hypoxia-dependent changes of enzyme activities in different fibre types of rat soleus and extensor digitorum longus muscles. A cytophotometrical study," *Acta Histochemica*, 98(3), 255–269 (July 1996).

8. Koc, R.K., Akdemir, H., Kurtsoy, A., Pasaoglu, H., Kavuncu, I., Pasaoglu, A., Krakucku, I., "Lipid peroxidation in experimental spinal cord injury. Comparision of treatment with *Ginkgo biloba*, TRH, and methylprednisolone," *Research in Experimental Medicine*, 195(2), 117–123 (1995).

9. Sohn, M., Sikora, R., "*Ginkgo biloba* extract in the therapy of erectile dysfunction," *Journal of Urology*, 141, 188A (1991).

10. Paick, J.S., Lee, J.H., "An experimental study of the effect of

Ginkgo biloba extract on human and rabbit corpus cavernosum tissue," *Journal of Urology,* 156(5), 1876–1880 (November 1996).

11. Haase, J., Halama, P., Horr, R., "Effectiveness of brief infusions with *Ginkgo biloba* Special Extract EGb 761 in dementia of the vascular and Alzheimer type," *Zeitschrift für Gerontologie und Geriatrie,* 29(4), 302–309 (July–August 1996).

12. Schubert, H., Halama, P., "Depressive episode primarily unresponsive to therapy in elderly patients: Efficacy of *Ginkgo biloba* extract (EGb 761) in combination with antidepressants," *Geriatrische Forschung,* 3, 45–53 (1993).

13. Hofferberth, B., "The efficacy of EGb 761 in patients with senile dementia of the Alzheimer type, a double blind, placebo-controlled study on different levels of investigation," *Human Psychopharmacology,* 9, 215–222 (1994).

14. Hasenorhl, R.U., Nichau, C.H., Frisch, C.H., De Sourza Silva, M.A., Huston, J.P., Mattern, C.M., Hacker, R., "Anxiolytic-like effect of combined extracts of *Zingiber officinale* and *Ginkgo biloba* in the elevated plus-maze," *Pharmacology, Biochemistry & Behavior,* 53(20), 271–275 (February 1996).

15. Barabasz, A., Barabasz, M., "Attention deficit hyperactivity disorder: neurological basis and treatment alternatives," *Journal of Neurotherapy,* 1, 1–10 (1985).

16. Itil, T., "Natural substances in psychiatry," *Psychopharmacology Bulletin,* 31, 147–158 (1995).

17. Knighton, D.R., Hunt, T.K., Scheuenstuhl, H., et al., "Oxygen tension regulates the expression of angiogenesis factor by macrophages," *Science,* 221, 1283–1285 (1983).

18. Wei, Y.Q., Zhao, X., Kariya, Y., Fukata, H., et al., "Induction of apoptosis by quercetin involvement of heat shock protein," *Cancer Research,* 54(18), 4952–4957 (1994).

19. Larocca, L.M., Teofili, L., Leone, G., Sica, S., et al., "Antiproliferative activity of quercetin on normal bone marrow and leukaemic progenitors," *British Journal of Haematology,* 79(4), 562–566 (1991).

20. Moongkarndi, P., Srivattana, A., Bunyaprprpphatsara, N., et al., "Cytotoxicity assay of hispidulin and quercetin using chlorimetric technique," *Warasan Phesetchasat,* 18(2), 25–31 (1991).

21. Ranelletti, F.O., Ricci, R., Larocca, L.M., Maggiano, N., et al., "Growth-inhibitory effect of quercetin and presence of type-II estrogen binding sites in human colon-cancer cell lines and primary colorectal tumors," *International Journal of Cancer,* 50(3), 486–492 (1992).

22. Larocca, L.M., Guistacchini, M., Maggiano, N., Ranelletti, F.O., et al., "Growth-inhibitory effect of quercetin and presence of type II estrogen binding sites in primary human transitional cell carcinomas," *Journal of Urology,* 1523(3), 1029–1033 (1994).

23. Scambia, G., Ranelletti, F.O., Benedetti, P.P., et al., "Quercetin potentiates the effect of adriamycin in a multidrug-resistant MCF-7 human breast-cancer cell line; P-glycoprotein as a possible target," *Cancer Chemotherapy and Pharmacology,* 28(4), 255–258 (1991).

24. Scambia, G., Ranelletti, F.O., Panici, P.B., et al., "Inhibitory effect of quercetin on OVCA 433 cells and presence of type II oestrogen binding sites in primary ovarian tumours and cultured cells," *British Journal of Cancer,* 62(6), 942–946 (1990).

25. Doly, M., Droy-Lefaix, M.T., Braquet, P., "Oxidative stress in diabetic retina," *EXS,* 62, 299–307 (1992).

26. Lanthony, P., Cosson, J.P., "The course of color vision in early diabetic retinopathy treated with *Ginkgo biloba* extract. A preliminary double-blind versus placebo study," *Journal Francais d'Ophthalmologie,* 11(10), 671–674 (February 1995).

27. Matsukawa, Y., Yoshida, M., Sakai, T., et al., "The effect of quercetin and other flavonoids on cell cycle progression growth of human gastric cancer cells," *Planta Medica,* 56, 677–678 (1990).

28. Winston, D., "Eclectic specific condition review: cataracts," *Protocol Journal of Botanical Medicine,* 2(2), 39 (1997).

29. Hoffmann, F., Beck, C., Schutz, A., Offermann, P., "Ginkgo extract EGb 761 (tenobin)/HAES versus naftidrofuryl (Dusodril)/HAES. A randomized study of therapy of sudden deafness," *Laryngo-Rhino-Otologie,* 73(3), 149–152 (March 1994).

30. Meyer, B., "Multi-center, randomized study of placebo vs. *Ginkgo biloba* extract in treatment of acute hearing loss," *Presse Med,* 15, 1562–1564 (1986).

31. Coles, R., "Trial of an extract of *Ginkgo biloba* (EGB) for tinnitus and hearing loss," *Clinical Otolaryngology,* 13, 501–504 (1988).

32. Howat, D.W., Chand, N., Braquet, P., Willoughby, D.A., "An investigation into the possible involvement of platelet activating factor in experimental allergic encephalomyelitis in rats," *Agents and Actions,* 27(3–4), 473–476 (June 1989).

33. Brochet, B., Orgogozo, J.M., Guinot, P., Dartigues, J.F., Henry, P., Loiseau, P., "Pilot study of Ginkgolide B, a PAF-acether specific inhibitor in the treatment of acute outbreaks of multiple sclerosis," *Revue Neurologique* (Paris), 148(4), 299–301 (1992).

34. Brochet, B., Guinot, P., Orgogozo, J.M., Confavreux, C., Rumbach, L., Lavergne, V., "Double blind placebo controlled multicentre study of ginkgolide B in treatment of acute exacerbations of multiple sclerosis," *Journal of Neurology, Neurosurgery, and Psychiatry,* 38(3), 360–362 (March 1995).

35. Amri, H., Ogwuegbu, S.O., Boujrad, N., Drieu, K., Papodopoulos, V., "In vivo regulation of peripheral-type benzodiazepine receptor and glucocorticoid synthesis by *Ginkgo biloba* extract EGb 761 and isolated ginkgolides," *Endocrinology,* 137(12), 5707–5718 (December 1996).

36. Emerit, I., Oganesian, N., Sarkisian, T., Arutyunyan, R., Pogosian, A., Asrian, K., Levy, A., Cernjavski, L., "Clastogenic factors in the plasma of Chernobyl accident recovery workers: anticlastogenic effect of *Ginkgo biloba* extract," *Radiation Research,* 144(20), 198–205 (November 1995).

37. Tosaki, A., Pali, T., Droy-Lefaix, M.T., "Effects of *Ginkgo biloba* extract and preconditioning on the diabetic rat myocardium," *Diabetologia,* 39(11), 1255–1262 (November 1996).

38. Tyler, V.E., "The honest herbalist: herbal medicine 101," *Prevention,* March 1997, p.150.

39. Hoffmann, F., Beck, C., Schutz, A., Offermann, P., pp. 149–152.

40. Rowin, J., Lewis, S.L., "Spontaneous bilateral subdural hematomas associated with chronic *Ginkgo biloba* ingestion," *Neurology,* 46(6), 1775–1776 (June 1996).

LEM

1. Breene, W., "Nutritional and medicinal value of specialty mushrooms," *Journal of Food Processing,* 53, 883–894 (1990).

2. Iizuka, C., et al., "Extract of *Basidomycetes,* especially *Lentinus edodes,* for treatment of human immnodeficiency virus (HIV)," Japanese Patent Application 88/287,316 (14 November 1988).

3. Tochikura, T.S., et al., "Inhibition (in vitro) of replication and of the cytopathic effect of human immunodeficiency virus by an extract of the culture medium of *Lentinus edodes* mycelia," *Medical Microbiology and Immunology* (Berlin), 177(5), 235–244 (1988).

4. Tochikura, T.S., et al., "Suppression of human immuno-deficiency virus replication by 3-azido-3-deoxythymidine in various human haematopoetic cells lines in vitro. Augmentation by the effect of lentinan," *Japanese Journal of Cancer Research,* 78, 583 (1987).

5. Chibata, I., et al., "Lentincin: a new hypocholseterolemic substance in *Lentinus edodes," Experientia,* 25, 1237–1238 (1969).

6. Rokujo, T., et al., "Lentysine: A new hypolipemic agent from a mushroom," *Life Sciences,* 9, 381–385 (1969).

7. Ying, J., et al. *Icones of Medicinal Fungi from China* (Beijing: Science Press, 1987).

8. Kimoto, M., et al., "Effects of 'shiitake' mushroom on plasma and liver lipid contents in rats," *Eiyo to Shokuryo,* 29, 275–281 (1976).

9. Amagase, H., "Treatment of hepatitis B patients with *Lentinus edodes* mycelium," *Proceedings of the XII International Congress of Gastroenterology* (Lisbon, 1987), p. 197.

10. Sugano, N., et al., "Anticarcinogenic actions of water-soluble and alcohol-insoluble fractions from culture medium of *Lentinus edodes* mycelia," *Cancer Letters,* 17, 109–114 (1982).

Lentinan

1. Aoki, T., "Lentinan," in Fenichel, R.I., Chirgis, M.A. (eds), "Immune modulation agents and their mechanisms," *Immunology Studies,* 25, 62–77 (1984).

2. Aoki, T., "Antibodies to HTLV I and HTLV II in sera from two Japanese patients, one with possible pre-AIDS," *Lancet,* 936–937 (20 October 1984).

3. Hobbs, C. *Medicinal Mushrooms: An Exploration of Tradition, Healing, and Culture,* Second Edition (Santa Cruz, California: Botanica Press, 1994), p. 134.

4. Ying, J., et al. *Icones of Medicinal Fungi From China* (Beijing: Science Press, 1987).

5. Moriyama, M., et al., "Anti-tumor effect of polysaccharide Lentinan on transplanted ascites hepatoma-134 in C3H/He mice," in Aoki, A., et al. (eds). *Manipulation of Host Defence Mechanisms* (Amsterdam: Excerpta Medica, 1981).

6. Maeda, Y.Y., et al., "Unique increase of serum protein components and action of antitumour polysaccharides," *Nature,* 252, 250 (1974).

7. Togami, M., et al., "Studies on *Basidiomycetes.* I. Antitumor polysaccharide from bagasse medium on which mycelia of *Lentinus edodes* (Berk.) Sing. had been grown," *Chemical Pharmacology Bulletin,* 30, 1134–1140 (1982).

8. Mashiko, H., et al., "A case of advanced gastric cancer with liver metastasis completely responding to a combined immunochemotherapy with UFT, mitomycin C and Lentinan," *Gan to Kagaku Ryoho—Japanese Journal of Cancer & Chemotherapy,* 19, 715–718 (1992).

9. Shimuzu, T., et al., "A combination of regional chemotherapy and systemic immunotherapy for the treatment of inoperable gastric cancer," in Aoki, A., et al.

10. Kosaka, A., et al., "Synergistic effect of Lentinan and surgical endocrine therapy on the growth of DMBA-induced mammary tumors of rats and of recurrent human breast cancer," *International Congress Series—Excerpta Medica,* 690, 138–150 (1985).

11. Taguchi, T., et al., "Phase I and II studies of lentinan," in Aoki, A., et al.

12. Yamasaki, K., et al., "Synergistic induction of lymphokine (IL-2)-activated killer activity by IL-2 and the polysaccharide lentinan, and therapy of spontaneous pulmonary metastases," *Cancer Immunology and Immunotherapy,* 29, 87–92 (1989).

13. Oka, M., et al., "Immunological analysis and clinical effects of intraabdominal and intrapleural injection of lentinan for malignant ascites and pleural effusion," *Biotherapy,* 5, 107–112 (1992).

14. Usuda, Y., et al., "Drug-resistant pulmonary tuberculosis treated with lentinan," in Aoki, A., et al., p. 50.

15. Kanai, K., Kondo, E., "Immunomodulating activity of lentinan as demonstrated by frequency limitation effect on post-chemotherapy relapse in experimental mouse tuberculosis," in Aoki, A., et al., p. 50.

Maitake

1. Mori, K., et al., "Antitumor activities of edible mushrooms by oral administration," in *Cultivating Edible Fungi* (Amsterdam: Elsevier, 1987), pp. 1–6.

2. Yang, D.A., Li, S.Q., Li, X.T., "Prophylactic effects of *zhuling* and BCG on postoperative recurrence of bladder cancer," *Chung-Hua Wai Ko Tsa Chih—Chinese Journal of Surgery,* 32(7), 433–434 (July 1994).

3. Nanba, H., "Activity of maitake D-fraction to prevent cancer growth and metastasis," *Journal of Naturopathic Medicine* (1994), cited in Hobbs, C. *Medicinal Mushrooms: An Exploration of Tradition, Healing, and Culture,* Second Edition (Santa Cruz, California: Botanica Press, 1994), p. 229.

4. Miller, D., Clinical protocol submitted to the NIH Scientific Director, Cancer Treatment Research Foundation, Arlington Heights, Illinois (1994).

5. Hobbs, C. *Medicinal Mushrooms: An Exploration of Tradition, Healing, and Culture,* Second Edition (Santa Cruz, California: Botanica Press, 1995), p. 114.

6. Ibid.

7. Wu, S., Zou, D., "Therapeutic effect of *Grifola* polysacharides in chronic hepatitis," unpublished paper (1994). Cited in Hobbs, C., p. 115.

8. Ooi, V.E.C., et al., "Protective effects of some edible mushrooms on paracetamol-induced liver injury," in *First International Conference on Mushroom Biology and Mushroom Products* (Hong Kong: Chinese University of Hong Kong, 1993), p. 139 (P-2-13).

9. Lee, J.W., et al., "Screening of hepatoprotective substances from higher fungi by primary cultured rat hepatocytes intoxicated with carbon tetrachloride," *Korean Journal of Mycology,* 10, 27–31 (1992).

10. Kabir, Y., Kimura, S., "Dietary mushrooms reduce blood pressure in spontaneously hypertensive rats (SHR)," *Journal of Nutritional Science and Vitaminology,* 34, 433–438 (1989).

11. Hobbs, C., pp. 114–115.

12. Kubo, M., "Anti-diabetic activity present in the fruit body of *Grifola frondosa* (Maitake). I.," *Biological Pharmaceutical Bulletin,* 17, 1106–1110 (1994).

13. Shimaoka, I., et al., "Preparation of therapeutic metal-bound

proteins from mushrooms," *Chemical Abstracts,* 114, 3250–3240 (1993).

14. Nouza, K., Krejcova, H., "Pathogenesis and therapy of multiple sclerosis," *Bratislavsky Lek Lísty,* 98(4), 199–203 (April 1997).

15. Squillacote, D., Martínez, M., Sheremata, W., "Natural alpha interferon for multiple sclerosis: results of three preliminary studies," *Journal of International Medical Research,* 24, 246–257 (1996).

16. Won, S.J., Lin, M.T., Wu, W.L., "*Ganoderma tsugae* mycelium enhances splenic natural killer cell activity and serum interferon production in mice," *Japanese Journal of Pharmacology,* 59(2), 171–176 (June 1992).

PSK

1. Fukushima, M., "The overuse of drugs in Japan," *Nature,* 342, 850–851 (1989).

2. Katsumatsu, T., "The radiation-sensitizing effect of PSK in treatment of cervical cancer patients," in Yamamura, Y., et al. (eds). *Immunomodulation by Microbial Products and Related Synthetic Compounds* (Amsterdam: Excerpta Medica, 1982), pp. 463–466.

3. Furuta, M., Niibe, H., "Effect of krestin (PSK) as adjuvant treatment on the prognosis after radical radiotherapy in patients with non-small cell lung cancer," *Anticancer Research,* 13(5C), 1815–1820 (September–October 1993).

4. Nishiwaki, Y., Furuse, K., Fukuoka, M., Ota, M., Niitani, H., Asakawa, M., Nakai, H., Sakai, S., Ogawa, N., "A randomized controlled study of PSK combined immuno-chemotherapy for adenocarcinoma of the lung," *Gan to Kagaku Ryoho—Japanese Journal of Cancer & Chemotherapy,* 17(1), 131–136 (January 1990).

5. Takashima, S., Kinami, Y., Miyazaki, I., "Clinical effect of postoperative adjuvant immunochemotherapy with the FT-207 suppository and PSK in colorectal cancer patients," *Gan to Kagaku Ryoho—Japanese Journal of Cancer & Chemotherapy,* 15(8), 2229–2236 (August 1988).

6. Ebina, T., Murata, K., "Antitumor effect of PSK at a distant site: tumor-specific immunity and combination with other chemotherapeutic agents," *Japanese Journal of Cancer Research,* 83(7), 775–782 (July 1992).

7. Harada, M., Matsunaga, K., Oguchi, Y., Iijima, H., Tamada, K., Abe, K., Takenoyama, M., Ito, O., Kimura, G., Nomoto, K., "Oral administration of PSK can improve the impaired antitumor CD4+ T-cell response in gut-associated lymphoid tissue (GALT) of specific-pathogen-free mice," *International Journal of Cancer,* 70(3), 362–372 (27 January 1997).

8. Sugiyama, Y., Saji, S., Miya, K., Fukada, D., Umemoto, T., Kunieda, K., Takao, H., Kato, M., Kawai, M., "Locoregional therapy for liver metastases of colorectal cancer," *Gan to Kagaku Ryoho—Japanese Journal of Cancer & Chemotherapy,* 23(11), 1433–1436 (September 1996).

9. Torisu, M., Uchiyama, A., Goya, T., Iwasaki, K., Katano, M., Yamamoto, H., Kimura, Y., "Eighteen-year experience of cancer immunotherapies—evaluation of their therapeutic benefits and future," *Nippon Geka Gakkai Zasshi—Journal of Japan Surgical Society,* 92(9), 1212–1216 (September 1991).

10. Yuan, C., Mei, Z., Liu, S., Yi, L., "PSK protects macrophages from lipoperoxide accumulation and foam cell formation caused by oxidatively modified low-density lipoprotein," *Atherosclerosis,* 124(2), 171–181 (1 August 1996).

11. Kawana, T., "Treatment of recurrent genital herpes with PSK," in *Proceedings of the International Symposium on Pharmacological and Clinical Approaches to Herpes Viruses and Virus Chemotherapy, Oiso, Japan, September 10–13, 1984,* reprinted in Kono, R., Nakajima, A. (eds). *Herpes Viruses and Chemotherapy: Pharmacological and Clinical Approaches* (Amsterdam: Excerpta Medica, 1985), pp. 271–272.

Reishi

1. Matsumoto, K. *The Mysterious Reishi Mushroom* (Santa Barbara, California: Woodbridge Press, 1979).

2. Huang, K.C. *The Pharmacology of Chinese Herbs* (Boca Raton, Florida: CRC Press, 1993).

3. Kohda, H., et al., "The biologically active constituents of *Ganoderma lucidum* (Fr.) Karst. Histamine release-inhibitory triterpenes," *Chemical Pharmacy Bulletin,* 33, 1367–1374 (1985).

4. Hobbs, C. *Medicinal Mushrooms: An Exploration of Tradition, Healing, and Culture,* Second Edition (Santa Cruz, California: Botanica Press, 1994), p. 104.

5. Lieu, C.W., Lee, S.S., Wang, S.Y., "The effect of *Ganoderma lucidum* on induction of differentiation in leukemic U937 cells," *Anticancer Research,* 12(4), 1211–1215 (July–August 1992).

6. Chang, H.M., But, P.P.H. *Pharmacology and Applications of Chinese Materia Medica,* Volume 1 (Singapore: World Scientific Publishing, 1986).

7. Ibid.

8. Ying, J., et al. *Icones of Medicinal Fungi from China* (Beijing: Science Press, 1987).

9. Kasahara, Y., Hikino, H., "Central actions of *Ganoderma lucidum,*" *Phytotherapy Research,* 1, 17–21 (1987).

10. Fu, H., Wang, Z., "The clinical effects of *Ganoderma lucidum* spore preparations in 10 cases of atrophic myotonia," *Journal of Traditional Chinese Medicine,* 2, 63–65 (1982).

11. Naeshiro, H., et al., "Skin-lightening cosmetics containing *Ganoderma lucidum* extract and vitamins," *Nihon Kokai Tokkyo Koho,* 4(9), 325 (1992).

Shiitake

1. Kimoto, M., et al., "Effects of shiitake mushroom on plasma and liver lipid contents in rats," *Eiyo to Shokuryo,* 29, 275–281 (1976).

2. Hobbs, C. *Medicinal Mushrooms: An Exploration of Tradition, Healing, and Culture,* Second Edition (Santa Cruz, California: Botanica Press, 1995), p. 104.

Siberian Ginseng (Eleuthero)

1. Barenboim, G.M., Koslova, N.B., "*Eleutherococcus* extract as an agent increasing the biological resistance of man exposed to unfavorable factors," in *Eleutherococcus: Strategy of the Use and New Fundamental Data* (Moscow: MedExport, not dated).

2. Wagner, H., "Immunostimulants from medicinal plants," in Chang, H.M., Yeung, W., Tso, W., Koo., A. (eds). *Advances in Chinese Medicinal Materials Research* (Singapore: World Scientific, 1985).

3. Ibid.

4. Murray, M. *Healing Power of Herbs* (Rocklin, California: Prima Publishing, 1991), p. 56.

5. Mar, S., "The 'adaptogens' (Part I): Can they really help your running?" *Running Research,* 11(5), 1–3 (June–July 1995).

6. Mar, S., personal communication with author, 5 June 1996.

Inset: Siberian Ginseng Goes to the Gym

1. Kalashnikov, B.N., "The effect of long-term prophylactic administration of *Eleutherococcus* on morbidity among coal miners in the far north," *Tesisi dokladov vsyesoyuznii konferenz po adaptatzii chegovyeka k razduchnii geografichyeskiim, klimatichyeskim i proizbochestbinim faktori* (Novosibirsk: USSR Academy of Medical Sciences, Far Eastern Division, 1977), pp. 43–44.

2. Mar, S., personal communication with author, 26 May 1996.

3. Dowling, E.A., Redondo, D.R., Branch, J.D., Jones, S., McNabb, G., Williams, M.H., "Effect of *Eleutherococcus senticosus* on maximal and submaximal exercise performance," *Medicine and Science in Sports and Medicine,* 28(4), 482–489 (April 1996).

4. Murano, S., Lo Russo, R.R., "Experiencia con ARM 229," *Prensa Medícinales de Argentina,* 71, 178–183 (1984).

5. Pieralisi, G., Ripari, P., Vecchiet, L., "Effects of s/a standardized ginseng extract combined with dimethylaminoethanol bitartrate, vitamins, minerals, and trace elements on physical performance during exercise," *Clinical Therapeutics,* 13, 373–382 (1991).

Snow Fungus

1. Yang, J., et al., "Stimulatory effect and kinetics of carboxymethylpachymaran on the induction of interferon by lymphoblastoid cell culture," *Chinese Journal of Microbiology and Immunology,* 6, 157–159 (1987).

2. Ma, L., Lin, Z., "Effect of *Tremella* polysaccharide on IL-2 production by mouse splenocytes," *Yaoxue Xuebao,* 27, 1–4 (1992).

3. Liu, S.H., et al., "Inhibition effect of *Tremella fuciformis* Berk. Preparation (TFB) on growth of transplanted mouse tumor cells," *Zhong Guo Zhong Liu Lin Chuang,* 21, 68–70 (1994).

4. Zheng, L., et al., "Effects of *ling zhi* on the production of interleukin-2. From Immunopharmacological Study (5)," *The Research on Ganoderma lucidum, Part One* (Shanghai: Shanghai Medical University Press, 1993), pp. 259–265.

5. Lin, Z., et al., "Studies on the pharmacology of *Tremella fuciformis,* preliminary research on the fermented solution and polysaccharides of *Tremella fuciformis* spores," *Journal of Traditional Chinese Medicine,* 2, 95–98 (1982).

6. Xiong, H.Z., "Clinical observation of 45 cases of chronic hepatitis by treatment with "*Tremella fuciformis* polysaccharide," *Chinese Journal of Antibiotics,* 10, 363–365 (1985).

7. Gao, Q., et al., "Polysaccharides and their antitumor activity of *Tremella fuciformis," Tianran Chanwu Yanjiu Yu Kaifa,* 3, 43–48 (1991).

8. Zican, W., et al., "Studies on the effects of *Tremella fuciformis* bark preparations on immunity and blood formation in rhesus monkeys," *Journal of Traditional Chinese Medicine,* 3, 13–16 (1983).

9. Hobbs, C. *Medicinal Mushrooms: An Exploration of Tradition, Healing, and Culture,* Second Edition (Santa Cruz, California: Botanica Press, 1994), p. 168.

Soy Isoflavones

1. Bruneton, J., *Pharmacognosy, Phytochemistry, Medicinal Plants* (Paris: Lavoisier Publishing, 1995), pp. 296–297.

2. Jing, Y., Nakaya, K., Han, R., "Differentiation of promyeloctic leukemia cells HL-60 induced by daidzein in vitro and in vivo," *Anticancer Research,* 13(4), 1049–1054 (1993).

3. Han, R., "Highlight on the studies of anticancer drugs derived from plants from China," *Stem Cells,* 12(1), 53–63 (1994).

4. Jing, Y., Han, R., "Differentiation of B16 melanoma cells induced by daidzein," *Chinese Journal of Pharmacology and Toxicology,* 6(4), 278–280 (1993).

5. Adlercreutz, H., Mousavia, Y., Höckerstedt, K., "Diet and breast cancer," *Acta Oncologica,* 31(2), 175–181 (1992).

6. Panno, M.L., Salerno, M., Pezzi, V., Sisci, D., Maggiolini, M., Mauro, L., Morrone, E.G., Ando, S., "Effect of oestradiol and insulin on the proliferative pattern and on oestrogen and progesterone receptor contents in MCF-7 cells," *Journal of Cancer Research & Clinical Oncology,* 122(12), 745–749 (1996).

7. Welshons, W.V., Murphy, C.S., Koch, R., Calaf, K.G., Jordan, V.C., "Stimulation of breast cancer cells in vitro by the environmental estrogen enterolactone and the phytoestrogen equol," *Breast Cancer Research and Treatment,* 10, 169–175 (1987).

8. Bowen, R., Barnes, S., Wei, H., "Antipromotional effect of the soybean isoflavone genistein," *Proceedings of the American Association for Cancer Research,* 34, 555 (1991).

9. Watanabe, T., Kondo, K., Oishi, M., "Induction of in vitro differentiation of mouse erytholeukemia cells by genistein, and inhibitor of tyrosine protein kinases," *Cancer Research,* 51, 764–768 (1991).

10. Fotsis, T., Pepper, M., Adlercreutz, H., Fleischmann, G., Hase, T., Montesano, R., Schweigerer, L., "Genistein, a dietary-derived inhibitor of in vitro angiogenesis," *Proceedings of the National Academy of Sciences of the USA,* 90, 2690–2694 (1993).

Chapter 4

The Formulas of Kampo

1. Kuwagi, T. *Ekisuzai ni Yoru Kampo Shinryo Handobukku (Handbook of Kampo Diagnosis and Treatment with Kampo Extracts)* (Tokyo: Sogensha, 1983), pp. 41–42.

2. Hosoya, E., Yamamura, Y., "Recent advances in the pharmacology of Kampo (Japanese herbal) medicines," *Excerpta Medica,* 1988, cited by Bakowky, H., personal communication with author, 20 October 1998.

3. Terasawa, K., "The significance of the combined preparations used in Kampo medicine," *Excerpta Medica,* 1988, cited by Bakowsky, H., personal communication with author, 20 October 1998.

4. Shibata, Y., Wu, J. *Kampo Treatment for Climacteric Disorders* (Brookline, Massachusetts: Paradigm Publications, 1997), p. 79.

Arrest Wheezing Decoction

1. Bensky, D., Gamble, A., Kaptchuk, T., Bensky, L.L. *Chinese Herbal Medicine: Materia Medica,* Revised Edition (Seattle: Eastland Press, 1993), p. 390.

Augmented Rambling Powder

1. Boik, J. *Cancer and Natural Medicine: A Textbook of Basic Science and Clinical Research* (Princeton, Minnesota: Oregon Medical Press, 1995), p. 253.

2. Sato, T., Yamaguchi, H., Fujii, T., Akiba, S., Tamura, A., Fujii, T., Tatsumi, Y., Miura, O., "Inhibitory effect of various traditional

Chinese medicines on rabbit platelet phospholipase A2 in vitro and suppressive effect of *toki-syakuyaku-san* on increased aggregability in hypercholesterolemic rabbit ex vivo," *Yakugaku Zasshi—Journal of the Pharmaceutical Society of Japan*, 109(11), 869–876 (November 1989).

Bupleurum Plus Dragon Bone and Oyster Shell Decoction

1. Tsumura, A. *Kampo: How the Japanese Updated Traditional Herbal Medicine* (San Francisco: Kodansha, 1991), pp. 67–68.

2. Fushitani, S., Tsuchiya, K., Minakuchi, K., Takasugi, M., Murakami, K.,"Studies on attenuation of post-ischemic brain injury by Kampo medicines—inhibitory effects of free radical production," *Yakugaku Zasshi—Journal of the Pharmaceutical Society of Japan*, 114(6), 388–394 (June 1994).

Cinnamon Twig and Poria Pill

1. Sakamoto, S., Kudo, H., Kawasaki, T., Kuwa, K., et al., "Effects of a Chinese herbal medicine, *keishi-bukuryo-gan*, on the gonadal system of rats," *Journal of Ethnopharmacology*, 23(2–3), 151–158 (July–August 1988).

2. Mori, T., Sakamoto, S., Singtripop, T., Park, M.K., Kato, T., Kawashima, S., Nagasawa, H., "Suppression of spontaneous development of uterine adenomyosis by a Chinese herbal medicine, *keishi-bukuryo-gan*, in mice," *Planta Medica*, 59(4), 308–311 (August 1993).

3. Ishikawa, H., et al., "Effects of *guizhi-fuling-wan* on male infertility with varicocele," *American Journal of Chinese Medicine*, 24, 327–331 (1996).

4. Sheng, F.Y., Ohta, A., Yamaguchi, M., "Inhibition of collagen production by traditional Chinese herbal medicine in scleroderma fibroblast cultures," *Internal Medicine*, 33(8), 466–471 (August 1994).

5. Fushitani, S., Tsuchiya, K., Minakuchi, K., Takasugi, M., Murakami, K., "Studies on attenuation of post-ischemic brain injury by Kampo medicines—inhibitory effects of free radical production. I.," *Yakugaku Zasshi—Journal of the Pharmaceutical Society of Japan*, 114(6), 388–394 (June 1994).

Coptis Decoction to Relieve Toxicity

1. Mori, M., Hojo, E., Takano, K., "Action of *oren-gedoku-to* on platelet aggregation in vitro," *American Journal of Chinese Medicine*, 19(2), 131–143 (1991).

2. Higaki, S., Nakamura, M., Morohashi, M., Hasegawa, Y., Yamagishi, T., "Activity of eleven Kampo formulations and eight Kampo crude drugs against *Propionibacterium acnes* isolated from acne patients: retrospective evaluation in 1990 and 1995," *Journal of Dermatology*, 23(12), 871–875 (December 1996).

3. Fushitani, S., Minakuchi, K., Tsuchiya, K., Takasugi, M., Murakami, K., "Studies on attenuation of post-ischemic brain injury by Kampo medicines—inhibitory effects of free radical production," *Yakugaku Zasshi—Journal of the Pharmaceutical Society of Japan*, 115(8), 611–617 (August 1995).

4. Takase, H., Inoue, O., Saito, Y., Yumioka, E., Suzuki, A., "Roles of sulfhydryl compounds in the gastric mucosal protection of the herb drugs composing *oren-gedoku-to* (a traditional herbal medicine)," *Japanese Journal of Pharmacology*, 56(4), 433–439 (August 1991).

5. Zhang, L., Yang, L.W., Yang, L.J., "Relation between *Helicobacter pylori* and pathogenesis of chronic atrophic gastritis and the research of its prevention and treatment," *Chung-Kuo Chung Hsi I Chieh Ho Tsa Chih—Chinese Journal of Modern Developments in Traditional Medicine*, 12(9), 521–523, 515–516 (September 1992).

6. Zhang, Q., Hsu, H.Y. *AIDS and Chinese Medicine: Applications of the Oldest Medicine to the Newest Disease* (Long Beach, California: Oriental Healing Arts Institute Press, 1990), p. 107.

7. Chang, K.S.S., Gao, C., Wang, L.C., "Berberine-induced morphologic differentiation and down-regulation of c-Ki-ras2 protooncogene expression in human teratocarcinoma cells," *Cancer Letters*, 55, 103–108 (1990).

8. Chang, K.S., "Down-regulation of c-Ki-ras2 gene expression associated with morphologic differentiation in human embryonal carcinoma cells treated with berberine," *Taiwan I Hsueh Hui Tsa Chih*, 90(1), 10–14 (1991).

Eight-Ingredient Pill With Rehmannia

1. Shoji, M., Sato, H., Hirai, Y., Oguni, Y., Sugimoto, C., "Pharmacological effects of *gosha-jinki-gan-ryo* extract, effects on experimental diabetes," *Nippon Yakurigaku Zasshi—Folia Pharmacologica Japonica*, 99(3), 143–152 (March 1992).

2. Kamei, A., Hisada, T., Iwata, S., "The evaluation of therapeutic efficacy of *hachimi-jio-gan* (traditional Chinese medicine) to rat galactosemic cataract," *Journal of Ocular Pharmacology*, 3(3), 239–248 (Fall 1987).

3. Kamei, A., Hisada, T., Iwata, S., "The evaluation of therapeutic efficacy of *hachimi-jio-gan* (traditional Chinese medicine) to mouse hereditary cataract," *Journal of Ocular Pharmacology*, 4(4), 311–319 (Winter 1988).

4. Ishikawa, H., Manabe, F., Zhongtao, H., Yoshii, S., Koiso, K., "The hormonal response to HCG stimulation in patients with male infertility before and after treatment with *hochuekkito*," *American Journal of Chinese Medicine*, 20(2), 157–165 (1992).

Ephedra Decoction

1. Ozaki, Y., "Studies on anti-inflammatory effect of Japanese Oriental medicines (Kampo medicines) used to treat inflammatory diseases," *Biological and Pharmaceutical Bulletin*, 18(4), 559–562 (April 1995).

2. Wang, C.M., Ohta, S., Shinoda, M., "Studies of chemical protectors against radiation. XXIX. Protective effects of methanol extracts of various Chinese traditional medicines on skin injury induced by X-irradiation," *Yakugaku Zasshi—Journal of the Pharmaceutical Society of Japan*, 110(3), 218–224 (March 1990).

3. Wang, C.M., Ohta, S., Shinota, M., "Studies on chemical protectors against radiation. XXVII. Survival effects of methanol extracts of various Chinese traditional medicines on radiation injury," *Yakugaku Zasshi—Journal of the Pharmaceutical Society of Japan*, 109(12), 949–953 (December 1989).

Ephedra, Asiasarum, and Prepared Aconite Decoction

1. Naito, K., Ishihara, M., Senoh, Y., Takeda, N., Yokoyama, N., Iwata, S., "Seasonal variations of nasal resistance in allergic rhinitis and environmental pollen counts. II. Efficacy of preseasonal therapy," *Auris, Nasus, Larynx*, 20(1), 31–38 (1993).

Five-Ingredient Powder With Poria

1. Bensky, D., Barolet, R. *Chinese Herbal Medicine: Formulas and Strategies* (Seattle: Eastland Press, 1990), p. 175.

2. Hattori, T., Shindo, S., "Effects of *sairei-to* (TJ-114) on the expression of adhesion molecule in anti-GBM nephritic rats," *Nippon Jinzo Gakkai Shi—Japanese Journal of Nephrology,* 37(7), 373–383 (July 1995).

3. Guandong Medical Journal Editorial Department, "Clinical observation of curative effects of *wu long san* for treatment of glaucoma," *Guandong Medical Journal,* 3(2), 40 (1982).

Four-Gentleman Decoction

1. Hidaka, S., Abe, K., Liu, S.Y., "In vitro and in vivo evaluations of Chinese traditional (Kampo) medicines as anticalculus agents in the rat," *Archives of Oral Biology,* 38(4), 327–335 (April 1993).

Ginseng Decoction to Nourish the Nutritive Qi

1. Zhou, N.N., Nakai, S., Kawakita, T., Oka, M., Nagasawa, H., Himeno, K., Nomoto, K., "Combined treatment of autoimmune MRL/MP-lpr/lpr mice with a herbal medicine, *ren-shen-yang-rong-tang* (Japanese name, *ninjin-youei-to*) plus suboptimal dosage of prednisolone," *International Journal of Immunopharmacology,* 16(10), 845–854 (October 1994).

Kudzu Decoction

1. Nagasaka, K., Kurokawa, M., Imakita, M., Terasawa, K., Shiraki, K., "Efficacy of *kakkon-to,* a traditional herbal medicine, in herpes simplex virus type 1 infection in mice," *Journal of Medical Virology,* 46(1), 28–34 (May 1995).

2. Ibid.

Ledebouriella Powder That Sagely Unblocks

1. Yoshida, T., Sakane, N., Wakabayashi, Y., Umekawa, T., Kondo, M., "Thermogenic, anti-obesity effects of *bofu-tsusho-san* in MSG-obese mice," *International Journal of Obesity & Related Metabolic Disorders,* 19(10), 717–722 (October 1995).

Licorice, Wheat, and Jujube Decoction

1. Paroli, E., "Opioid peptides from food (the exorphins)," *World Review of Nutrition and Dietetics,* 55, 58–97 (1988).

2. Winston, D., "Eclectic specific condition review: depression," *Protocol Journal of Botanical Medicine,* 2(1), 72 (Spring 1997).

Lonicera and Forsythia Powder

1. Chang, H.M., But, P.P.H. *Pharmacology and Applications of Chinese Materia Medica,* Volume 1 (Singapore: World Scientific Publishing, 1986), p. 822.

2. Chang, H.M., But, P.P.H., p. 935.

Major Bupleurum Decoction

1. Goto, M., Hayashi, M., Todoroki, T., Seyama, Y., Yamashita, S., "Effects of traditional Chinese medicines (*dai-saiko-to, sho-saiko-to* and *hachimi-zio*) on spontaneously diabetic rat (WBN/Kob) with experimentally induced lipid and mineral disorders," *Nippon Yakurigaku Zasshi—Folia Pharmacologica Japonica,* 100(4), 353–358 (October 1992).

2. Shoda, J., Matsuzaki, Y., Tanaka, N., Miyamoto, J., Osuga, T., "The inhibitory effects of *dai-chai-hu-tang* (*dai-saiko-to*) extract on supersaturated bile formation in cholesterol gallstone disease [letter]," *American Journal of Gastroenterology,* 91(4), 828–830 (April 1996).

3. Saku, K., Hirata, K., Zhang, B., Liu, R., Ying, H., Okura, Y., Yoshinaga, K., Arakawa, K., "Effects of Chinese herbal drugs on serum lipids, lipoproteins and apolipoproteins in mild to moderate essential hypertensive patients," *Journal of Human Hypertension,* 6(5), 393–395 (October 1992).

4. Fushitani, S., Minakuchi, K., Tsuchiya, K., Takasugi, M., Murakami, K., "Studies on attenuation of post-ischemic brain injury by Kampo medicines—inhibitory effects of free radical production," *Yakugaku Zasshi—Journal of the Pharmaceutical Society of Japan,* 115(8), 611–617 (August 1995).

Major Construct the Middle Decoction

1. Lin, D.Z., Fang, Y.S. *Modern Study and Application of Materia Medica* (Beijing, China Ocean Press, 1990).

Major Ledebouriella Decoction

1. Takamura, S., Yoshida, J., Suzuki, S., "Effect of an extract prepared from *dai-bofu-to* on morphine withdrawal responses," *Nippon Yakurigaku Zasshi—Folia Pharmacologica Japonica,* 105(2), 87–95 (February 1995).

Minor Bluegreen Dragon Decoction

1. Nagai, T. Yamada, H., "In vivo anti-influenza virus activity of Kampo (Japanese herbal) medicine '*sho-seiryu-to*' and its mode of action," *International Journal of Immunopharmacology,* 16(8), 605–613 (August 1994).

2. Ikeda, K., Wu, D.Z., Ishigaki, M., Sunose, H., Takasaka, T., "Inhibitory effects of *sho-seiryu-to* on acetylcholine-induced responses in nasal gland acinar cells," *American Journal of Chinese Medicine,* 22(2), 191–196 (1994).

3. "Japan's health ministry confirms efficacy of another of Tsumura's Kampo drugs," *Kampo Today,* 2(1), 3 (February 1997).

4. Sakaguchi, M., Iizuka, A., Yuzurihara, M., Ishige, A., Komatsu, Y., Matsumiya, T., Takeda, H., "Pharmacological characteristics of *sho-seiryu-to,* an antiallergic Kampo medicine without effects on histamine H1 receptors and muscarinic cholinergic system in the brain," *Methods & Findings in Experimental & Clinical Pharmacology,* 18(1), 41–47 (January–February 1996).

Minor Bupleurum Decoction

1. Yamaoka, Y., Kawakita, T., Kaneko, M., Nomoto, K., "A polysaccharide fraction of *shosaiko-to* active in augmentation of natural killer activity by oral administration," *Biological & Pharmaceutical Bulletin,* 18(6), 846–849 (1995).

2. Yamashiki, M., Kosaka, Y., Nishimura, A., Takase, K., Ichida, F., "Efficacy of an herbal medicine '*sho-saiko-to*' on the improvement of impaired cytokine production or peripheral blood mononuclear cells in patients with chronic viral hepatitis," *Journal of Clinical and Laboratory Immunology,* 37(3), 111–121 (1992).

3. Yamamoto, S., Oka, H., Kanno, T., Mizoguchi, Y., Kobayashi, K., "Controlled prospective trial to evaluate *Syosakiko-to* in preventing hepatocellular carcinoma in patients with cirrhosis of the liver," *Gan to Kagaku Ryoho—Japanese Journal of Cancer and Chemotherapy,* 16(4, Part 2–2), 1519–1524 (April 1989).

4. Sakamoto, S., Muroi, N., Matsuda, M., Tajima, M., Kudo, H., Kasahara, N., Suzuki, S., Sugiura, Y., Kuwa, K., Namiki H., "Suppression by Kampo medicines in preneoplastic mammary hyperplastic alveolar nodules of SHN virgin mice," *Planta Medica,* 59(5), 425–427 (October 1993).

5. Ono, K., Nakane, H., Fukushima, M., Chermann, J.C., Barre-Sinoussi, F., "Differential inhibition of the activities of reverse transcriptase and various cellular DNA polymerases by a traditional Kampo drug, *sho-saiko-to,*" *Biomedicine and Pharmacotherapy,* 44(1), 13–16 (1990).

6. Satomi, N., Sakurai, A., Iimura, F., Haranaka, R., Haranaka, K., "Japanese modified traditional Chinese medicines as preventive drugs of the side effects induced by tumor necrosis factor and lipopolysaccharide," *Molecular Biotherapy,* 1(3), 155–162 (1989).

7. Zhou, N.N., Nakai, S., Kawakita, T., Oka, M., Nagasawa, H., Himeno, K., Nomoto, K., "Combined treatment of autoimmune MRL/MP-lpr/lpr mice with a herbal medicine, *ren-shen-yang-rong-tang* (Japanese name, *ninjin-youei-to*) plus suboptimal dosage of prednisolone," *International Journal of Immunopharmacology,* 16(10), 845–854 (October 1994).

8. Inoue, M., Kikuta, Y., Nagatsu, Y., Ogihara, Y., "Response of liver to glucocorticoid is altered by administration of *shosaikoto* (Kampo medicine)," *Chemical & Pharmaceutical Bulletin,* 38(2), 418–421 (February 1990).

9. Yoshida, K., Mizukawa, H., Honmura, A., Uchiyama, Y., Nakajima, S., Haruki, E., "The effect of *sho-saiko-to* on concentration of vitamin E in serum and on granuloma formation in carrageenin cotton pellet-induced granuloma rats," *American Journal of Chinese Medicine,* 22(2), 183–189 (1994).

10. Nakagawa, A., Yamaguchi, T., Tako, T., Amano, H., "Five cases of drug-induced pneumonitis due to *sho-saiko-to* or interferon-alpha or both," *Nippon Kyobu Shikkan Gakkai Zasshi,* 33(12), 1361–1366 (December 1995).

Ophiopogonis Decoction

1. Tamaoki, J., Chiyotani, A., Takeyama, K., Kanemura, T., Sakai, N., Konno, K., "Potentiation of beta-adrenergic function by *saiboku-to* and *bakumondo-to* in canine bronchial smooth muscle," *Japanese Journal of Pharmacology,* 62(2), 155–159 (June 1993).

2. Miyata, T., Fuchikami, J., Kai, H., Takahama, K., "Antitussive effects of *Bakumondo-to* and codeine in bronchitic guinea-pigs," *Nippon Kyobu Shikkan Gakkai Zasshi—Japanese Journal of Thoracic Diseases,* 27(10), 1157–1162 (October 1989).

3. Ohno, S., Suzuki, T., Dohi, Y., "The effect of *bakumondo-to* on salivary secretion in Sjögren's syndrome," *Ryumachi,* 30(1), 10–16 (February 1990).

4. Huang, K.C. *The Pharmacology of Chinese Herbs* (Boca Raton, Florida: CRC Press, 1992), p. 92.

Peony and Licorice Decoction

1. Kato, T., Okamoto, R., "Effect of *shakuyaku-kanzo-to* on serum estrogen levels and adrenal gland cells in ovariectomized rats," *Nippon Sanka Fujinka Gakkai Zasshi,* 44(4), 433–439 (1992).

2. Takahashi, K., Kitao, M., "Effect of TJ-68 (*shakuyaku-kanzo-to*) on polycystic ovarian disease," *International Journal of Fertility and Menopausal Studies,* 39(2), 69–76 (March–April 1994).

3. Sakamoto, K., Wakabayashi, K., "Inhibitory effect of glycyrrhetinic acid on testosterone production in rat gonads," *Endocrinologia Japonica,* 35(2), 333–342 (April 1988).

Pinellia and Magnolia Bark Decoction

1. Bensky, D., Barolet, R. *Chinese Herbal Medicine: Formulas and Strategies* (Seattle: Eastland Press, 1990), p. 291.

Pinellia Decoction to Drain the Epigastrium

1. Wang, C.M., Ohta, S., Shinoda, M., "Studies of chemical protectors against radiation. XXIX. Protective effects of methanol extracts of various Chinese traditional medicines on skin injury induced by X-irradiation," *Yakugaku Zasshi—Journal of the Pharmaceutical Society of Japan,* 110(3), 218–224 (March 1990).

2. Kase, Y., Hayakawa, T., Takeda, S., Ishige, A., Aburada, M., Okada, M., "Pharmacological studies on antidiarrheal effects of *hange-shashin-to,*" *Biological & Pharmaceutical Bulletin,* 19(10), 1367–1370 (October 1996).

3. Suzuki, M., Nikaido, T., Ohmoto, T., "The study of Chinese herbal medicinal prescription with enzyme inhibitory activity. V. The study of *hange-shashin-to, kanzo-shashin-to, shokyo-shashin-to* with adenosine 3',5'-cyclic monophosphate phosphodiesterase," *Yakugaku Zasshi—Journal of the Pharmaceutical Society of Japan,* 111(11), 695–701 (November 1991).

Polyporus Decoction

1. Sugaya, K., Nishizawa, O., Noto, H., Sato, K., Sato, K., Shimoda, N., Otomo, R., Tsuchida, S., "Effects of Tsumura *chorei-to* and Tsumura *chorei-to-go-shimotsu-to* on patients with urethral syndrome," *Hinyokika Kiyo—Acta Urologica Japonica,* 38(6), 731–735 (June 1992).

2. Ibid.

Rhubarb and Moutan Decoction

1. Fushitani, S., Minakuchi, K., Tsuchiya, K., Takasugi, M., Murakami, K., "Studies on attenuation of post-ischemic brain injury by Kampo medicines—inhibitory effects of free radical production," *Yakugaku Zasshi—Journal of the Pharmaceutical Society of Japan,* 115(8), 611–617 (August 1995).

Six-Ingredient Pill With Rehmannia

1. Naeser, M.A. *Outline Guide to Chinese Herbal Patent Medicines in Pill Form with Sample Pictures of the Boxes: An Introduction to Chinese Herbal Medicines,* Second Edition (Boston: Boston Chinese Medicine, 1996), p. 292.

2. Zhang, J.P., Zhou, D.J., "Changes in leucocytic estrogen receptor levels in patients with climacteric syndrome and therapeutic effect of *luiwei dihuang* pills," *Chung Hsi I Chieh Ho Tsa Chih,* 11(9), 521–523, 515 (September 1991).

Tang-Kuei and Peony Powder

1. Usuki, S., "Effects of *hachimijiogan, tokishakuyakusan, keishibukuryogan, ninjinto* and *unkeito* on estrogen and progesterone secretion in preovulatory follicles incubated in vitro," *American Journal of Chinese Medicine,* 19(1), 65–71 (1991).

2. Ibid.

3. Takahashi, K., Kitao, M., "Effect of TJ-68 (*shakuyaku-kanzo-to*) on polycystic ovarian disease," *International Journal of Fertility & Menopausal Studies,* 39(2), 69–76 (March–April 1994).

4. Imai, A., Horibe, S., Fuseya, S., Iida, K., Takagi, H., Tamaya, T., "Possible evidence that the herbal medicine *shakuyaku-kanzo-to* decreases prostaglandin levels through suppressing arachidonate turnover in endometrium," *Journal of Medicine,* 26(3–4), 163–174 (1995).

5. Benesova, M., Benes, L., "Effect of Kampo preparations on peptidase activity after damage by free radicals," *Cekoslovenska Farmacie,* 41(7–8), 246–249 (1992).

Ten-Significant Tonic Decoction

1. Zhang, Q., Hsu, H.Y. *AIDS and Chinese Medicine: Applications of the Oldest Medicine to the Newest Disease* (Long Beach, California: Oriental Healing Arts Institute Press, 1990), p. 30.

2. Zee-Cheng, R.K., "*Shi-quan-da-bu-tang* (ten significant tonic decoction), SQT. A potent Chinese biological response modifier in cancer immunotherapy, potentiation and detoxification of anticancer drugs," *Methods & Findings in Experimental & Clinical Pharmacology,* 14(9), 725–736 (November 1992).

3. Ohnishi, Y., Yasumizu, R., Ikehara, S., "Preventative effect of TJ-48 on recovery from radiation injury," *Gan to Kagaku Ryoho—Japanese Journal of Cancer & Chemotherapy,* 16(4–Part 2-2), 1494–1499 (April 1989).

Tonify the Middle and Augment the Qi Decoction

1. Yoshida, H., Tanifuji, T., Sakurai, H., Tashiro, H., Ogawa, H., "Clinical effects of Chinese herbal medicine (*hochu-ekki-to*) on infertile men," *Hinyokika Kiyo—Acta Urologica Japonica,* 32(2), 297–302 (February 1986).

2. Sudo, K., Honda, K., Taki, M., Kanitani, M., Fujii, Y., Aburada, M., Hosoya, E., Kimura, M., Orikasa, S., "Effects of TJ-41 (Tsumura *hochu-ekki-to*) on spermatogenic disorders in mice under current treatment with adriamycin," *Nippon Yakurigaku Zasshi—Folia Pharmacologica Japonica,* 92(4), 251–261 (October 1988).

3. Li, X.Y., Takimoto, H., Miura, S., Yoshikai, Y., Matsuzaki, G., Momoto, K., "Effects of a traditional Chinese medicine, *bu-zhong-yi-qi-tang* (Japanese name: *hochu-ekki-to*) on the protection against *Listeria monocytogenes* infection in mice," *Immunopharmacology and Immunotoxicology,* 14(3), 383–402 (1992).

4. Cho, J.M., Sato, N., Kikuchi, K., "Prophylactic anti-tumor effect of *hochu-ekki-to* (TJ41) by enhancing natural killer cell activity," *In Vivo,* 5(4), 389–391 (July–August 1991).

5. Ikeda, S., Kaneko, M., Kumazawa, Y., Nishimura, C., "Protective activities of a Chinese medicine, *hochu-ekki-to,* to impairment of hematopoietic organs and to microbial infection," *Yakugaku Zasshi—Journal of the Pharmaceutical Society of Japan,* 110(9), 682–687 (September 1990).

6. Kaneko, M., Kishihara, K., Kawakita, T., Nakamura, T., Takimoto, H., Nomoto, K., "Suppression of IgE production in mice treated with a traditional Chinese medicine, *bu-zhong-yi-qi-tang* (Japanese name: *hochu-ekki-to*)," *Immunopharmacology,* 36(1), 79–85 (April 1997).

Two-Cured Decoction

1. Zhang, G.L., "Treatment of breast proliferation disease with modified *xiao yao san* and *er chen* decoction," *Chung Hsi I Chieh Ho Tsa Chih,* 11(7), 400–402 (1988).

2. Ibid.

White Tiger Plus Ginseng Decoction

1. Goto, M., Inoue, H., Seyama, Y., Yamashita, S., Inoue, O., Yumioka, E., "Comparative effects of traditional Chinese medicines (*dai-saiko-to, hatimi-zio-gan* and *byakko-ka-ninzin-to*) on experimental diabetes and hyperlipidemia," *Nippon Yakurigaku Zasshi—Folia Pharmacologica Japonica,* 93(3), 179–186 (March 1989).

Part Two

Disorders Treated With Kampo

Acne

1. Sansone, G., Reisner, R., "Differential rates of conversion of testosterone to dihydrotestosterone in acne and normal human skin—a possible pathogenic factor in acne," *Journal of Investigational Dermatology,* 56, 366–372 (1971).

2. Schavone, F., Rietschel, R., Squotas, D., Harris, R., "Elevated free testosterone levels in women with acne," *Archives of Dermatology,* 119, 799–802 (1982).

3. Higaki, S., Nakamura, M., Morohashi, M., Hasegawa, Y., Yamagishi, T., "Activity of eleven Kampo formulations and eight Kampo crude drugs against *Propionibacterium acnes* isolated from acne patients: retrospective evaluation in 1990 and 1995," *Journal of Dermatology,* 23(12), 871–875 (December 1996).

4. Usuki, S., "Effects of *hachimijiogan, tokishakuyakusan, keishibukuryogan, ninjinto* and *unkeito* on estrogen and progesterone secretion in preovulatory follicles incubated in vitro," *American Journal of Chinese Medicine,* 19(1), 65–71 (1991).

AIDS

1. Zhang, B.Z., Ding, F., Tan, L.W., "Clinical and experimental study on *yi-gan-ning* granule in treating chronic hepatitis B," *Chung-Kuo Chung Hsi I Chieh Ho Tsa Chih—Chinese Journal of Modern Developments in Traditional Medicine,* 13(10), 597–599, 580 (October 1993).

2. Zhao, T.H., "Positive modulating action of *shenmaisan* with *Astralagus membranaceus* on anti-tumor activity of LAK cells," *Chung Hsi I Chieh Ho Tsa Chih,* 13(8), 471–472 (1993).

3. Tochikura, T.S., et al., "Inhibition (in vitro) of replication and of the cytopathic effect of human immunodeficiency virus by an extract of the culture medium of *Lentinus edodes* mycelia," *Medical Microbiology and Immunology* (Berlin), 177(5), 235–244 (1988).

4. Aoki, T., "Antibodies to HTLV I and HTLV II in sera from two Japanese patients, one with possible pre-AIDS," *Lancet,* 936–937 (20 October 1984).

5. Nanba, H., "Immunostimulant activity in vivo and anti-HIV activity in vitro of 3 branched b-1-6 glucans extracted from maitake mushroom (*Grifola frondosa*)," Eighth International Conference on AIDS, 1992.

6. Yao, X.J., Wainberg, M.A., Parniak, M.A., "Mechanism of inhibition of HIV-1 infection in vitro by purified extract of *Prunella vulgaris,*" *Virology,* 187(1), 56–62 (March 1992).

7. Li, B.Q., Fu, T., Yan, Y.D., Baylor, N.W., Ruscetti, F.W., Kung, H.F., "Inhibition of HIV infection by baicalin—a flavonoid compound purified from Chinese herbal medicine," *Cellular & Molecular Biology Research,* 39(2),119–124 (1993).

8. Li, C.J., et al., "Three inhibitors of human type 1 immunodeficiency virus long terminal repeat directed gene expression and virus replication," *Proceedings of the National Academy of Sciences,* 90, 1839–1841 (1993).

9. Mazumder, A., et al., "Inhibition of human immunodeficiency virus type-1 integrase by curcumin," *Biochemical Pharmacology,* 49, 1165–1170 (1995).

10. Singh, S., Aggarwal, B.B., "Activation of transcription factor NF-Kappa B is suppressed by curcumin (diferulolylmethane),"

Journal of Biological Chemistry, 270(42), 24995–25000 (20 October 1995).

11. Chang, R.S., Yeung, H.W., "Inhibition of growth of human immunodeficiency virus in vitro by crude extracts of Chinese medicinal herbs," *Antiviral Research,* 9(3), 163–175 (April 1998).

12. Ngan, F., Chang, R.S., Tabba, H.D., Smith, K.M., "Isolation, purification and partial characterization of an active anti-HIV compound from the Chinese medicinal herb *Viola yedoensis," Antiviral Research,* 10(1–3), 107–116 (November 1988).

13. Buimovici-Klein, E., Mohan, V., Lange, M., Fenamore, E., Inada, Y., Cooper, L.Z., "Inhibition of HIV replication in lymphocyte cultures of virus-positive subjects in the presence of *sho-saiko-to,* an Oriental plant extract," *Antiviral Research,* 14(405), 279–286 (October 1990).

14. Ono, K., Nakane, H., Fukushima, M., Chermann, J.C., Barre-Sinoussi, F., "Differential inhibition of the activities of reverse transcriptase and various cellular DNA polymerases by a traditional Kampo drug, *sho-saiko-to," Biomedical Pharmacotherapy,* 44(1), 13–16 (1990).

15. Piras, G., Makino, M., Baba, M., "*Sho-saiko-to,* a traditional Kampo medicine, enhances the anti-HIV-1 activity of lamivudine (3TC) in vitro," *Microbiology and Immunology,* 41(10), 835–839 (1997).

16. Zhang, Q., Hsu, H.Y. *AIDS and Chinese Medicine: Applications of the Oldest Medicine to the Newest Disease* (Long Beach, California: Oriental Healing Arts Institute Press, 1990), pp. 82–83.

17. Ono, K., et al., "Inhibition of HIV-reverse transcriptase by a Kanpo medicine, *sho-saiko-to,*" in *Proceedings of the Fifth International Conference on AIDS,* Montreal, Quebec, 4–9 June 1989, p. 565.

18. Zhang, Q., Hsu, H.Y., p. 30.

Alcoholism

1. Rubenstein, E., Federman, D. *Scientific American Textbook of Medicine* (New York: Scientific American, 1985), pp. 13–14.

2. Cruz-Coke, R., "Genetics and alcoholism," *Neurobehavioral Toxicology and Teratology,* 5, 179–180 (1983).

3. Tipton, K.F., Heneman, G.T.M., McCrodden, J.M., "Metabolic and nutritional aspects of alcohol," *Biochemical Society Transactions,* 11, 59–61 (1983).

4. Xie, C.I., Lin, R.C., Antony, V., Lumeng, L., Li, T.K., Mai, K., Liu, C., Wang, Q.D., Zhao, Z.H., Wang, G.F., "Daidzin, an antioxidant isoflavonoid, decreases blood alcohol levels and shortens sleep time induced by ethanol intoxication," *Alcoholism, Clinical & Experimental Research,* 18(6), 1443–1447 (December 1994).

5. Chang, H.M., But, P.P.H. *Pharmacology and Applications of Chinese Materia Medica,* Volume 1 (Singapore: World Scientific Company, 1987), pp. 144–146.

Allergies, Food

1. McGovern, J.J., "Correlation of clinical food allergy symptoms with serial pharmacological and immunological changes in the patient's plasma," *Annals of Allergy,* 44, 57 (1980).

2. Trevino, R.J., "Immunological mechanisms in the production of food sensitivities," *Laryngoscope,* 91, 1913 (1981).

Allergies, Respiratory

1. Nesse, R.M., Williams, G.C. *Why We Get Sick: The New Science of Darwinian Medicine* (New York: Random House, 1994), p. 169.

2. Tang, W., Eisenbrand, G. *Chinese Drugs of Plant Origin: Chemistry, Pharmacology, and Use in Traditional and Modern Medicine* (Berlin: Springer-Verlag, 1992), p. 44.

3. Huang, K.C. *The Pharmacology of Chinese Herbs* (Boca Raton, Florida: CRC Press, 1993), p. 152.

4. Lin, D.Z., Fang, Y.S. *Modern Study and Application of Materia Medica* (Beijing: China Ocean Press, 1990).

5. Mitchell, W., "Allergies: immediate-type hypersensitivity," *Protocol Journal of Botanical Medicine,* 1(2), 66 (Spring 1996).

6. Lu, H.C. *The Chinese System of Food Cures* (New York: Sterling Publishing Company, 1992).

7. Yi, R., "Treatment of 120 cases of allergic rhinitis with *Magnolia liliflora," Bulletin of Chinese Materia Medica,* 10(5), 237 (1985).

8. Khoda, H., et al., "The biologically active constituents of *Ganoderma lucidum* (Fr.) Karst. Histamine release-inhibitory triterpenes," *Chemical Pharmacology Bulletin,* 33, 2624–2627 (1985).

9. Shimuzu, A., et al., "Isolation of an inhibitor of platelet aggregation from a fungus, *Ganoderma lucidum," Chemical Pharmacology Bulletin,* 33, 3012–3015 (1985).

10. Naito, K., Ishihara, M., Senoh, Y., Takeda, N., Yokoyama, N., Iwata, S., "Seasonal variations of nasal resistance in allergic rhinitis and environmental pollen counts. II. Efficacy of preseasonal therapy," *Auris, Nasus, Larynx,* 20(1), 31–38 (1993).

11. Lin, D.Z., Fang, Y.S.

Alzheimer's Disease

1. Roberts, H.J., "Allopathic specific condition review: Alzheimer's disease," *Protocol Journal of Botanical Medicine,* 2(1), 94 (1997).

2. Gandy, S.E., Bhasin, R., Ramabhadran, V., et al., "Alzheimer B/A4-amyloid precursor protein: evidence for putative amyloidogenic fragment," *Journal of Neurochemistry,* 548, 383–386 (1992).

3. Ibid.

4. Frolich, L., Riederer, P., "Free radical mechanisms in dementia of the Alzheimer's type and the potential for antioxidative treatment," *Drug Research,* 45(1):3A, 443–446 (1995).

5. Le Bars P.L., et al., "A placebo-controlled, double-blind, randomized trial of an extract of *Ginkgo biloba* for dementia," *Journal of the American Medical Association,* 278, 1327–1332 (22 October 1997).

6. Mitchell, W.A., "Naturopathic specific condition review: Alzheimer's disease," *Protocol Journal of Botanical Medicine,* 2(1), 107–109 (Spring 1997).

7. Wu, S.X., Zhang, J.X., Xu, T., Li, L.F., Zhao, S.Y., Lan, M.Y., "Effects of seeds, leaves and fruits of *Ziziphus spinosa* and jujuboside A on central nervous system function," *Chung-Kuo Chung Yao Tsa Chih—China Journal of Chinese Materia Medica,* 18(11), 685–687, 703–704 (November 1993).

8. Nishiyama, N., Wang, Y.L., Saito, H., "Beneficial effects of S-113m, a novel herbal prescription, on learning impairment model in mice," *Biological & Pharmaceutical Bulletin,* 18(11), 1498–1503 (November 1995).

9. Liu, J., Mori, A., "Antioxidant and free radical scavenging

activities of *Gastrodia elata* Bl. and *Uncaria rhynchophylla* (Miq.) Jacks," *Neuropharmacology*, 31(12), 1287–1298 (December 1992).

Inset: Ginkgo—The Memory Herb and Alzheimer's Disease

1. DeFeudis, F.V. (ed). *Ginkgo biloba Extract (EGb 761): Pharmacological Activities and Clinical Activities* (Amsterdam: Elsevier, 1991).

2. Kanowski, S., et al., "Proof of the efficacy of the *Ginkgo biloba* special extract EGb 761 in patients suffering from mild to moderate primary degenerative dementia of the Alzheimer type of multi-infarct dementia," *Phytomedicine*, 4, 3–13 (1997).

3. Le Bars, P.L., et al., "A placebo-controlled, double-blind, randomized trial of an extract of *Ginkgo biloba* for dementia," *Journal of the American Medical Association*, 278, 1327–1332 (22 October 1997).

Anemia

1. Duke, J.A. *Handbook of Medicinal Herbs* (Boca Raton, Florida: CRC Press, 1985), p. 313.

Angina

1. Huang, K.C. *The Pharmacology of Chinese Herbs* (Boca Raton, Florida: CRC Press, 1993), p. 82.

2. Petkov, E., Nikolov, N., Uzunov, P., "Inhibitory effect of some flavonoids and flavonoid mixtures on cyclic AMP phosphodiesterease activity of rat heart," *Planta Medica*, 43, 183–186 (1981).

3. Schussler, M., Holzl, J., Fricke, U., "Myocardial effects of flavonoids from *Crataegus* species," *Arzneimittel-Forschung*, 45(8), 842–845 (August 1995).

4. Leuchtgens, H., "*Crataegus* Special Extract WS 1442 in NYHA II heart failure. A placebo-controlled randomized double-blind study," *Fortschritte der Medizin*, 111(20–21), 352–354 (20 July 1993).

5. Huang, J.H., "Comparison studies on pharmacological properties of Injectio Gastrodia Elata, gastrodin-free fraction and gastrodin," *Chung-Kuo I Hsueh Ko Hsueh Yuan Hsueh Pao Acta Academiae Medicinae Sinicae*, 11(2), 147–150 (April 1989).

6. Jones, T.W., Porter, P., Sherwin, R.S., Davis, E.A., O'Leary, P., Frazer, F., Byrne, G., Stick, S., Tamborlane, W.V., "Decreased epinephrine responses to hypoglycemia during sleep," *New England Journal of Medicine*, 338(23), 657–662 (4 June 1998).

7. Steinberg, D., et al., "Beyond cholesterol: modification of the low-density lipoprotein that increase its atherogenecity," *New England Journal of Medicine*, 320, 915–924 (1989).

Inset: Angina—Is Surgery Necessary?

1. Graboys, T.D., et al., "Results of a second-opinion program for coronary artery bypass surgery," *Journal of the American Medical Association*, 258, 1611–1614 (1987).

2. Graboys, T.D., et al., "Results of a second-opinion program for coronary artery bypass surgery," *Journal of the American Medical Association*, 268, 2537–2540 (1992).

3. CASS Principal Investigators and Their Associates, "Coronary Artery Surgery (CASS): A randomized trial of coronary artery bypass surgery," *Circulation*, 68, 939–950 (1983).

4. CASS Principal Investigators and Their Associates, "Myocardial infarction and mortality in the Coronary Artery Surgery Study (CASS) randomized trial," *New England Journal of Medicine*, 310, 750–758 (1984).

Anxiety

1. De Felipe, C., Herrero, J.F., O'Brien, J.A., Palmer, J.A., Doyle, C.A., Smith, A.J.H., Laird, J.M.A., Belmonte, C., Cerver, F., Hung, S.P., "Altered nociception, analgesia and aggression in mice lacking the receptor for substance P," *Nature*, 392, 394–397 (26 March 1998).

2. Reimeier, C., Schneider, I., Schneider, W., Schafer, H.L., Elstner, E.F., "Effects of ethanolic extracts from *Eschscholtzia californica* and *Corydalis cava* on dimerization and oxidation of enkephalins," *Arzneimittel-Forschung*, 45(2), 132–136 (February 1995).

3. Hasenohrl, R.U., Nichau, C.H., Frisch, C.H., De Souza Silva, M.A., Huston, J.P., Mattern, C.M., Hacker, R., "Anxiolytic-like effect of combined extracts of *Zingiber officinale* and *Ginkgo biloba* in the elevated plus-maze," *Pharmacology, Biochemistry & Behavior*, 53(2), 271–275 (February 1996).

4. Kim, H.S., Kang, J.G., Rheu, H.M., Cho, D.H., Oh, K.W., "Blockade by ginseng total saponin of the development of methamphetamine reverse tolerance and dopamine receptor supersensitivity in mice," *Planta Medica*, 61(1), 22–25 (February 1995).

5. Kim, H.S., Kang, J.G., Seong, Y.H., Nam, K.Y., Oh, K.W., "Blockade by ginseng total saponin of the development of cocaine induced reverse tolerance and dopamine receptor supersensitivity in mice," *Pharmacology, Biochemistry & Behavior*, 50(1), 23–27 (January 1995).

6. Kin, H.S., Kang, J.G., Oh, K.W., "Inhibition by ginseng total saponin of the development of morphine reverse tolerance and dopamine receptor supersensitivity in mice," *General Pharmacology*, 26(5), 1071–1076 (September 1995).

7. Nguyen, T.T., Matsumoto, K., Yamasaki, K., Nguyen, M.D., Nguyen, T.N., Watanabe, H., "Crude saponin extracted from Vietnamese ginseng and major constituent majonoside-R2 attenuate the psychological stress- and foot-shock stress-induced antinociception in mice," *Pharmacology, Biochemistry & Behavior*, 52(2), 427–432 (1995).

8. Murray, M., Pizzorno, J. *Encyclopedia of Natural Medicine*, Second Edition (Rocklin, California: Prima Publishing, 1998), p. 252.

Asthma

1. Vanderhoek, J.Y., Ekborg, S.L, Bailey, J.M., "Nonsteroidal anti-inflammatory drugs stimulate 15-lipoxygenase/leukotriene pathway in human polymorphonuclear leukocytes," *Journal of Allergy and Clinical Immunology*, 74, 412–417 (1984).

2. Tan, Y., Collins-Williams, C., "Aspirin-induced asthma in children," *Annals of Allergy*, 48, 1–5 (1982).

3. Kaliner, M., Lemanske, R., "Rhinitis and asthma," *Journal of the American Medical Association*, 268, 2807–2829 (1992).

4. Odent, M.R., Culpin, E.E., Kimmel, T., "Pertussis vaccination and asthma: Is there a link?" *Journal of the American Medical Association*, 272, 592–593 (1994).

5. Tang, W., Eisenbrand, G. *Chinese Drugs of Plant Origin: Chemistry, Pharmacology, and Use in Traditional and Modern Medicine* (Berlin: Springer-Verlag, 1992), p. 44.

6. Chang, H.M., But, P.P.H. *Pharmacology and Applications of Chi-*

nese Materia Medica, Volume 2 (Teaneck, New Jersey: World Scientific Publishing, 1987), p. 975.

7. Kawakishi, S., Morimitsu, Y., Osawa, T., "Chemistry of ginger components and inhibitory factors of the arachidonic acid cascade," in Ho, C.T., Osawa, T., Huang, M.T., Rosen, R. (eds). *Food Phytochemicals for Cancer Prevention II: Teas, Spices, and Herbs* (Washington: American Chemical Society, 1994), pp. 244–249.

8. Guinot, P., et al., "Tanakan inhibits platelet-activating aggregation in healthy male volunteers," *Haemostasis,* 19, 219–223 (1986).

9. Ciplea, A.G., Richter, K.D., "The protective effect of *Allium sativum* and *Crataegus* on isoprenaline-induced tissue necroses in rats," *Arzneimittel-Forschung,* 38(110), 1583–1592 (November 1988).

10. Chen, M.F., et al., "Effect of glycyrrhizin on the pharmacokinetics of prednisolone following low dosage of prednisolone hemisuccinate," *Endocronologica Japonica,* 37, 331–341 (1990).

11. Kohda, H., et al., "The biologically active constituents of *Ganoderma lucidum* (Fr.) Karst. Histamine release-inhibitory triterpenes," *Chemical Pharmacy Bulletin,* 33, 1367–1374 (1985).

12. Umeda, M., Amagaya, S., Ogihara, Y., "Effects of certain herbal medicines on the biotransformation of arachidonic acid, a new pharmacological testing method using serum," *Journal of Ethnopharmacology,* 23(1), 91–98 (May–June 1988).

13. Wong, B.Y., Lau, B.H., Yamasaki, T., Teel, R.W., "Inhibition of dexamethasone-induced cytochrome 450-mediated mutagenicity and metabolism of aflatoxin B1 by Chinese medicinal herbs," *European Journal of Cancer Prevention,* 2(4), 351–356 (July 1993).

14. Srivastava, K.C., Bordia, A., Verma, S.K., "Curcumin, a major component of food spice turmeric (*Curcuma longa*) inhibits aggregation and alters eicosanoid metabolism in human blood platelets," *Prostaglandins, Leukotrienes & Essential Fatty Acids,* 52(4), 223–227 (April 1995).

15. Homma, M., Oka, K., Ikeshima, K., Takahashi, N., Niitsuma, T., Fukuda, T., Itoh, H., "Different effects of traditional Chinese medicines containing similar herbal constituents on prednisolone pharmacokinetics," *Journal of Pharmacy & Pharmacology,* 47(8), 687–692 (August 1995).

16. Homma, M., Oka, K., Ikeshima, K., Takahashi, N., Niitsuma, T., Fukuda, T., Itoh, H., pp. 687–692.

17. Zhou, N.N., Nakai, S., Kawakita, T., Oka, M., Nagasawa, H., Himeno, K., Nomoto, K., "Combined treatment of autoimmune MRL/MP-lpr/lpr mice with a herbal medicine, *ren-shen-yang-rong-tang* (Japanese name, *ninjin-youei-to*) plus suboptimal dosage of prednisolone," *International Journal of Immunopharmacology,* 16(10), 845–854 (October 1994).

Inset: Managing Asthma With Nutrition

1. Ogle, K.A., Bullocks, J.D., "Children with allergic rhinitis and/or bronchial asthma treated with elimination diet: A five-year follow-up," *Annals of Allergy,* 44, 273–278 (1980).

2. Businco, L., et al., "Food allergy and asthma," *Pediatric Pulmonology,* 11 (Suppl), 59–60 (1995).

3. Bircher, A.J., et al., "IgE to food allergens are highly prevalent in patients allergic to pollens, with and without symptoms of food allergy," *Clinical and Experimental Allergy,* 24(4), 367–374 (1994).

4. Oehling, A., "Importance of food allergy in childhood asthma," *Allergology and Immunopathology Supplement,* 9, 71–73 (1981).

5. Bray, G.W., "The hypochlorhydria of asthma in childhood," *Quarterly Journal of Medicine,* 24, 181–197 (1931).

6. Benard, A., et al., "Increased intestinal permeability in bronchial asthma," *Journal of Allergy and Clinical Immunology,* 97, 1173–1178 (1996).

7. Bray, G.W., pp. 181–197.

8. Haury, V.G., "Blood serum magnesium in bronchial asthma and its treatment by the administration of magnesium sulfate," *Journal of Laboratory and Clinical Medicine,* 26, 340–344 (1944).

9. Tendelenburg, P., "Physiologische und pharmakologische Untersuchungen an der isolierten bronchial Muskulatur," *Archives of Experimental Pharmacology Therapy,* CI, 79 (1912).

10. Broughtonk, K.S., et al., "Reduced asthma symptoms with omega-3 fatty acid ingestion are related to 5-series leukotriene production," *American Journal of Clinical Nutrition,* 65, 1011–1017 (1997).

11. Hodge, L., et al., "Consumption of oily fish and childhood asthma risk," (*MJA*), 164, 137–140 (1989).

12. Unge, G., Grubbstrom, J., Olsson, P., et al., "Effect of dietary tryptophan restriction on clinical symptoms in patients with endogenous asthma," *Allergy,* 38, 211–212 (1983).

13. Reynolds, R.D., Natta, C.L., "Depressed plasma pyriodoxal phosphate concentrations in adult asthmatics," *American Journal of Clinical Nutrition,* 41, 684–688 (1985).

14. Hatch, G.E., "Asthma, inhaled oxidants, and dietary antioxidants," *American Journal of Clinical Nutrition,* 61(Suppl), 625S–630S (1995).

15. Olusi, S.O., Ojutiku, O.O., Jessop, W.J.E., Iboko, M.I., "Plasma and white blood cell ascorbic acid concentrations in patients with bronchial asthma," *Clinica Chimica Acta,* 92, 161–166 (1979).

16. Akiyama, K., et al., "Atopic asthma caused by *Candida albicans* acid protease: Case reports," *Allergy,* 49, 778–781 (1994).

Atherosclerosis

1. Guyton, A.C., Hall, J.E. *Medical Physiology,* Ninth Edition (Philadelphia: W.B. Saunders & Co., 1996), p. 873.

2. Liang, H., Wang, Z., Tian, F., Geng, B., "Effects of astragalus polysaccharides and ginsenosides of ginseng stems and leaves on lymphocytes membrane fluidity and lipid peroxidation in traumatized mice," *Chung-Kuo Chung Yao Tsa Chih—China Journal of Chinese Materia Medica,* 20(9), 558–560, inside backcover (September 1995).

3. Lu, D.C., Su, Z.J., Rui, T., "Effect of *jian yan ling* on serum lipids, apoprotein and lipoprotein-a," *Chung-Kuo Chung Hsi I Chieh Ho Tsa Chih—Chinese Journal of Modern Developments in Traditional Medicine,* 14(3), 142–144, 131–132 (March 1994).

4. Check, J.B., K'Ombut, F.O., "The effect on fibrinolytic system of blood plasma of Wistar rats after feeding them with coix mixed diet," *East African Medical Journal,* 72(1), 51–55 (January 1995).

5. Park, Y., Suzuki, H., Lee, Y.S., Hayakawa, S., Wada, S., "Effect of coix on plasma, liver, and fecal lipid components in the rat fed on lard- or soybean oil-cholesterol diet," *Biochemical Medicine & Metabolic Biology,* 39(1), 11–17 (February 1988).

6. Adler, A.J., Holub, B.J., "Effect of garlic and fish-oil supplementation on serum lipid and lipoprotein concentrations in hypercholesterolemic men," *American Journal of Clinical Nutrition,* 65(2), 445–450 (February 1997).

7. Villar, R., Alvarino, M.T., Flores, R., "Inhibition by ajoene of protein tyrosine phosphatase activity in human platelets," *Biochimica et Biophysica Acta*, 1337(2), 233–240 (8 February 1997).

8. Bordia, A., Verma, S.K., Srivastava, K.C., "Effect of garlic on platelet aggregation in humans: a study in healthy subjects and patients with coronary artery disease," *Prostaglandins, Leukotrienes & Essential Fatty Acids*, 55(3), 201–205 (September 1996).

9. Meyer, K., Schwartz, J., Crater, D., Keyes, B., "*Zingiber officinale* (ginger) used to prevent 8-MOP associated nausea," *Dermatology Nursing*, 7(4), 242–244 (August 1995).

10. Rong, Y., Geng, Z., Lau, B.H., "*Ginkgo biloba* attenuates oxidative stress in macrophages and endothelial cells," *Free Radical Biology and Medicine*, 20(1), 121–127 (1996).

11. Yan, L.J., Droy-Lefaix, M.T., Packer, L., "*Ginkgo biloba* extract (EGb 761) protects human low density lipoproteins against oxidative modification mediated by copper," *Biochemical and Biophysical Research Communications*, 212(2), 360–366 (17 July 1995).

12. Shanthi, S., Parasakthy, K., Deepalakshmi, P.D., Devaraj, S.N., "Hypolipidemic activity of tincture of *Crataegus* in rats," *Indian Journal of Biochemistry & Biophysics*, 31(2), 143–146 (April 1994).

13. Ren, B., Ma, Y., Shen, Y., Gao, B., "Protective action of *Lycium barbarum* L. (LbL) and betaine on lipid peroxidation of erythrocyte membrane induced by H_2O_2," *Chung-Kuo Chung Yao Tsa Chih—China Journal of Chinese Materia Medica*, 20(5), 303–304, inside cover (May 1995).

14. Yuan, C., Mei, Z., Liu, S., Yi, L., "PSK protects macrophages from lipoperoxide accumulation and foam cell formation caused by oxidatively modified low-density lipoprotein," *Atherosclerosis*, 124(2), 171–181 (1 August 1996).

15. Sreejayan, Rao, M.N., "Curcuminoids as potent inhibitors of lipid peroxidation," *Journal of Pharmacy & Pharmacology*, 46(12), 1013–1016 (December 1994).

16. Babu, P.S., Srinivasan, K., "Influence of dietary curcumin and cholesterol on the progression of experimentally induced diabetes in albino rat," *Molecular & Cellular Biochemistry*, 152(1), 13–21 (8 November 1995).

17. Song, L.C., Chen, K.Z., Zhu, J.Y., "The effect of *Coptis chinensis* on lipid peroxidation and antioxidase activity in rats," *Chung-Kuo Chung Hsi I Chieh Ho Tsa Chih—Chinese Journal of Modern Developments in Traditional Medicine*, 12(7), 421–423, 390 (July 1992).

18. Goldman, I.L., Kopelberg, M., Debaene, J.E., Schwartz, B.S., "Antiplatelet activity in onion (*Allium cepa*) is sulfur dependent," *Thrombosis & Haemostasis*, 76(3), 450–452 (September 1996).

Attention Deficit Disorder/Attention Deficit Hyperactivity Disorder (ADD/ADHD)

1. Lombard, J., Germano, C. *The Brain Wellness Plan: Breakthrough Medical, Nutritional and Immune-Boosting Therapies* (New York: Kensington Books, 1997), pp. 152–153.

2. Barabasz, A., Barabasz, M., "Attention deficit hyperactivity disorder: Neurological basis and treatment alternatives," *Journal of Neurotherapy*, 1, 1–10 (1985).

3. Mefford, I.N., et al., "A neuroanatomical and biochemical basis for attention deficit disorder with hyperactivity in children. A defect in tonic adrenal mediated inhibition of locus ceruleus stimulation," *Medical Hypotheses*, 29, 33–42 (1989).

4. Arnsten, A.F., Steer, J.C., Hunt, R.D., "The contribution of alpha 2-noradrenergic mechanisms of prefrontal corticol cognitive function. Potential significance for attention-deficit hyperactivity disorder," *Archives of General Psychiatry*, 53(5), 448–455 (May 1996).

5. Girardi, N.L., Shaywitz, F.S., Shaywitz, B.A., et al., "Blunted catecholamine responses after glucose ingestion in children with attention deficit disorder," *Pediatrics Research*, 4, 539–542 (October 1995).

6. Della Loggia, R., Tubaro, A., Redaelli, C., "Evaluation of the activity on the mouse CNS of several plant extracts and a combination of them," *Rivista di Neurologia*, 51(5), 297–310 (September–October 1981).

7. Murray, M. *Healing Power of Herbs* (Rocklin, California: Prima Publishing, 1991), p. 56.

8. Paroli, E., "Opioid peptides from food (the exorphins)," *World Review of Nutrition and Dietetics*, 55, 58–97 (1988).

9. Weiss, R.F. *Herbal Medicine* (Beaconsfield, England: Beaconsfield Publishers Ltd., 1988), p. 286.

10. Hirokawa, S., Nose, M., Ishige, A., Amagaya, S., Oyama, T., Ogihara, Y., "Effect of *hachimi-jio-gan* on scopolamine-induced memory impairment and on acetylcholine content in rat brain," *Journal of Ethnopharmacology*, 50(2), 77–84 (February 1996).

11. Naeser, M.A. *Outline Guide to Chinese Herbal Patent Medicines in Pill Form with Sample Pictures of the Boxes: An Introduction to Chinese Herbal Medicines*, Second Edition (Boston: Boston Chinese Medicine, 1996), p. 292.

Bedwetting, Children's

1. Rona, R.J., Li, L., Chinn, S., "Determinants of nocturnal enuresis in England and Scotland in the 90's," *Development and Medical Child Neurology*, 39(10), 677–681 (October 1997).

2. Hansen, A., Hansen, B., Dahm, T.L., "Urinary tract infection, day wetting and other voiding symptoms in seven- to eight-year-old Danish children," *Acta Paediatrica*, 86(12), 1345–1349 (December 1997).

3. Cleper, R., Davidovitz, M., Halevi, R., Eisenstein, B., "Renal functional reserve after acute poststreptococcal glomerulonephritis," *Pediatric Nephrology*, 11(40), 473–476 (August 1997).

4. Rona, R.J., Li, L., Chinn, S., pp. 677–681.

5. Wieting, J.M., Dykstra, D.D., Ruggiero, M.P., Robbins, G.B., Galusha, K., "Central nervous system ischemia after varicella infection and desmopressin therapy for enuresis," *Journal of the American Osteopathic Association*, 97(5), 293–295 (May 1997).

6. Paroli, E., "Opioid peptides from food (the exorphins)," *World Review of Nutrition and Dietetics*, 55, 58–97 (1988).

Bladder Cancer

1. Boik, J. *Cancer and Natural Medicine: A Textbook of Basic Science and Clinical Research* (Princeton, Minnesota: Oregon Medical Press, 1995), p. 237.

2. Isselbacher, K.J., Braunwald, E., Wilson, J., Martin, J.V., Fauci, A.S., Kasper, D.L., eds. *Harrison's Principles of Internal Medicine*, Thirteenth Edition (New York: McGraw-Hill, 1995), p. 1338.

3. Alvares, A.P., "Interactions between environmental chemicals and drug biotransformation in man," *Clinical Pharmacokinetics*, 3, 462 (1978).

4. Boik, J., p. 238.

5. Yeager, R.T., DeVries, S., Jarrard, D.F., Kao, C., Nakada, S.Y., Moon, T.D., Bruskewitz, R., Stadler, W.M., Meisner, L.F., Gilchrist, K.W., Newton, M.A., Waldman, F.M., Reznikoff, C.A., "Overcoming cellular senescence in human cancer pathogenesis," *Genes and Development,* 12(2), 163–174 (15 January 1998).

6. Baud, E., Catilina, P.P., Bignon, Y.J., "Tracking the gatekeeper gene in the stages of carcinogenesis in the bladder," *Bulletin d' Cancer,* 84(10), 971–975 (October 1997).

7. Larocca, L.M., Giustacchini, M., Maggiano, N., Ranelletti, F.O., et al., "Growth-inhibitory effect of quercetin and presence of type II estrogen binding sites in primary human transitional cell carcinomas," *Journal of Urology,* 152(3), 1029–1033 (1994).

8. Den Otter, W., Dobrowolski, Z., Bugajski, A., Papla, B., Van Der Meijden, A.P., Koten, J.W., Boon, T.A., Siedlar, M., Zembala, M., "Intravesical interleukin-2 in T1 papillary bladder carcinoma: regression of marker lesion in 8 of 10 patients," *Journal of Urology,* 159(4), 1183–1186 (April 1998).

9. Zhao, T.H., "Positive modulating action of *shenmaisan* with *Astralagus membranaceus* on anti-tumor activity of LAK cells," *Chung Hsi I Chieh Ho Tsa Chih,* 13(8), 471–472 (1993).

10. Larocca, L.M., Giustacchini, M., Maggiano, N., Ranelletti, F.O., et al., pp. 1029–1033.

11. Mori, K., et al., "Antitumor activities of edible mushrooms by oral administration," in *Cultivating Edible Fungi* (Amsterdam: Elsevier, 1987), pp. 1–6.

12. Yang, D.A., Li, S.Q., Li, X.T., "Prophylactic effects of *zhuling* and BCG on postoperative recurrence of bladder cancer," *Chung-Hua Wai Ko Tsa Chih—Chinese Journal of Surgery,* 32(7), 433–434 (July 1994).

13. Wagner, H., "Immunostimulants from medicinal plants," in Chang, H.M., Yeung, W., Tso, W., Koo, A. (eds). *Advances in Chinese Medicinal Materials Research* (Singapore: World Scientific, 1985).

14. Chen, Y.C., Kuo, T.C., Lin-Shiau, S.Y., Lin, J.K., "Induction of HSP70 gene expression by modulation of Ca(+2) ion and cellular p53 protein by curcumin in colorectal carcinoma cells," *Molecular Carcinogenesis,* 17(4), 224–234 (December 1996).

15. Venkatesan, N., Chandrakasan, G., "Modulation of cyclophosphamide-induced early lung injury by curcumin, an anti-inflammatory antioxidant," *Molecular & Cellular Biochemistry,* 142(1), 79–87 (12 January 1995).

16. Thresiamma, K.C., George, J., Kuttan, R., "Protective effect of curcumin, ellagic acid and bixin on radiation induced toxicity," *Indian Journal of Experimental Biology,* 34(9), 845–847 (September 1996).

Bladder Infection

1. Murray, M., Pizzorno, J. *Encyclopedia of Natural Medicine,* Second Edition (Rocklin, California: Prima Publishing, 1998), p. 285.

2. Lidefelt, K.J., Bollgren, I., Nord, C.E., "Changes in periurethral microflora after antimicrobial drugs," *Archives of Disease in Childhood,* 66, 683–685 (1991).

3. Reid, G., Bruce, A.W., Cook, R.L., "Effect on urogenital flora of antibiotic therapy of urinary tract infection," *Scandinavian Journal of Infectious Disease,* 22, 43–47 (1990).

4. "Differentiations to UTI protocol," *Protocol Journal of Botanical Medicine,* 1(1), 135 (Summer 1995).

5. Tang, W., Eisenbrand, G. *Chinese Drugs of Plant Origin: Chemistry, Pharmacology, and Use in Traditional and Modern Medicine* (Berlin: Springer-Verlag, 1992), p. 196.

6. "Differentiations to UTI protocol," p. 135.

7. Sabir, M., Bhide, N., "Study of some pharmacologic actions of berberine," *Indian Journal of Physiatrics and Pharmacy,* 15, 111–132 (1971).

8. Kumazawa, Y., Itagaki, A., Fukumoto, M., et al., "Activation of peritoneal macrophages by berberine-type alkaloids in terms of induction of cytostatic activity," *International Journal of Immunopharmacology,* 6, 587–592 (1984).

9. Amin, A.H., Subbaiah, T.V., Abbasi, K.M., "Berberine sulfate: antimicrobial activity, bioassay, and mode of action," *Canadian Journal of Microbiology,* 15, 1067–1076 (1969).

10. Johnson, C.C., Johnson, G., Poe, C.F., "Toxicity of alkaloids to certain bacteria," *Acta Pharmacologica et Toxicologica,* 8, 71–78 (1952).

11. Brosche, T., Platt, N., "Garlic therapy and cellular immunocompetence in the elderly," *Zeitschrift für Phytotherapie,* 15, 23–24 (1994).

12. "Differentiations to UTI protocol," p. 135.

13. Ergil, K., "Chinese specific condition review: urinary tract infections," *Protocol Journal of Botanical Medicine,* 1(1), 131 (Summer 1995).

14. Sugaya, K., Nishizawa, O., Noto, H., Sato, K., Sato, K., Shimoda, N., Otomo, R., Tsuchida, S.,"Effects of Tsumura *chorei-to* and Tsumura *chorei-to-go-shimotsu-to* on patients with urethral syndrome," *Hinyokika Kiyo—Acta Urologica Japonica,* 38(6), 731–745 (June 1992).

Inset: Cranberry Juice and Kampo

1. Sobota, A.E., "Inhibition of bacterial adherence by cranberry juice: potential use for the treatment of urinary tract infection," *Journal of Urology,* 131, 1013–1016 (1984).

2. Kahn, D.H., Panariello, V.A., Saeli, J., et al., "Effect of cranberry juice on urine," *Journal of the American Dietetic Association,* 51, 251 (1967).

3. Prodomos, P.N., Brusch, C.A., Cereisa, G.C., "Cranberry juice in the treatment of urinary tract infections," *Southwest Medical Journal,* 47, 17 (1968).

Bleeding Gums

1. Osawa, K., Matsumoto, T., Yasuda, H., Kato, T., Naito, Y., Okuda, K., "The inhibitory effect of plant extracts on the collagenolytic activity and cytotoxicity of human gingival fibroblasts by *Porphyromonas gingivalis* crude enzyme," *Bulletin of Tokyo Dental College,* 32(1), 1–7 (February 1991).

2. Bruneton, J. *Pharmacognosy, Phytochemistry, Medicinal Plants* (Paris: Lavoisier, 1995), p. 452.

3. Murray, M., Pizzorno, J. *Encyclopedia of Natural Medicine* (Rocklin, California: Prima Publishing, 1996), p. 87.

4. Lasure, A., Vanden Berghe, D.A., Vlietinck, A.J., "Anti-microbial activity and anti-complement activity of extracts obtained from selected Hawaiian medicinal plants," *Journal of Ethnopharmacology,* 49(1), 23–32 (17 November 1995).

5. Hara, Y., "Prophylactic functions of tea polyphenols," in Ho, C.T., Osawa, T., Huang, M.T., Rosen, R. (eds). *Food Phytochemicals for Cancer Prevention II: Teas, Spices, and Herbs* (Washington: American Chemical Society, 1994), p. 47.

6. Terada, A., Hara, H., Nakajyo, S., Ichikawa, H., Hara, Y., Fukai, K., Kabayashi, Y., Mitsuoka, T., *Microbial Ecology in Health and Disease,* 6, 3–9 (1993).

7. Wichtl, M., ed., Grainger-Bissett, N., trans. *Herbal Drugs and Phytopharmaceuticals: A Handbook for Practice on a Scientific Basis* (Boca Raton, Florida: CRC Press, 1995), p. 346.

8. Chung, C.P., Park, J.B., Bae, K.H., "Pharmacological effects of methanolic extract from the root of *Scutellaria baicalensis* and its flavonoids on human gingival fibroblast," *Planta Medica,* 61(2), 150–153 (April 1995).

9. Watanabe, A., Takeshita, A., Kitano, S., Hanazawa, S., "CD14-mediated signal pathway of *Porphyromonas gingivalis* lipopolysaccharide in human gingival fibroblasts," *Infection & Immunity,* 64(11), 4488–4494 (November 1996).

10. Hidaka, S., Abe, K., Liu, S.Y., "In vitro and in vivo evaluations of Chinese traditional (Kampo) medicines as anticalculus agents in the rat," *Archives of Oral Biology,* 38(4), 327–335 (April 1993).

11. Tamaoki, J., Chiyotani, A., Takeyama, K., Kanemura, T., Sakai, N., Konno, K., "Potentiation of beta-adrenergic function by *saiboku-to* and *bakumondo-to* in canine bronchial smooth muscle," *Japanese Journal of Pharmacology,* 62(2), 155–159 (June 1993).

12. Ohno, S., Suzuki, T., Dohi, Y., "The effect of *bakumondo-to* on salivary secretion in Sjögren's syndrome," *Ryumachi,* 30(1), 10–16 (February 1990).

Boils

1. Murray, M., Pizzorno, J. *Encyclopedia of Natural Medicine* (Rocklin, California: Prima Publishing, 1998), p. 292.

2. Hahn, F.F., Ciak, J., "Berberine," *Antibiotics,* 3, 577–588 (1976).

3. Sabir, M., Bhide, N., "Study of some pharmacologic actions of berberine," *Indian Journal of Physiatrics and Pharmacy,* 15, 111–132 (1971).

4. Higaki, S., Nakamura, M., Morohashi, M., Hasegawa, Y., Yamagishi, T., "Activity of eleven Kampo formulations and eight Kampo crude drugs against *Propionibacterium acnes* isolated from acne patients: retrospective evaluation in 1990 and 1995," *Journal of Dermatology,* 23(12), 871–875 (December 1996).

Bone Cancer

1. Salmon, S.E., Crowley, J.J., Balcerzak, S.P., Roach, R.W., Taylor, S.A., Rivkin, S.E., Samlowski, W., "Interferon versus interferon plus prednisone remission maintenance therapy for multiple myeloma: A Southwest Oncology Group study," *Journal of Clinical Oncology,* 16(3), 896–900 (March 1998).

2. Joshua, S.E., MacCallum, S., Gibson, J., "Role of alpha interferon in multiple myeloma," *Blood Review,* 11(4), 191–200 (December 1997).

3. Huang, K.C. *The Pharmacology of Chinese Herbs* (Boca Raton, Florida: CRC Press, 1993), p. 152.

4. Aoki, T., "Antibodies to HTLV I and HTLV II in sera from two Japanese patients, one with possible pre-AIDS," *Lancet,* 936–937 (20 October 1984).

5. Maeda, Y.Y., et al., "Unique increase of serum protein components and action of antitumour polysaccharides," *Nature,* 252, 250 (1974).

6. Togami, M., et al., "Studies on Basidiomycetes. I. Antitumor polysaccharide from bagasse medium on which mycelia of *Lentinus edodes* (Berk.) Sing. had been grown," *Chemical Pharmacology Bulletin,* 30, 1134–1140 (1982).

7. Yamasaki, K., et al., "Synergistic induction of lymphokine (IL-2)-activated killer activity by IL-2 and the polysaccharide lentinan, and therapy of spontaneous pulmonary metastases," *Cancer Immunology and Immunotherapy,* 29, 87–92 (1989).

8. Wagner, H., "Immunostimulants from medicinal plants," in Chang, H.M., Yeung, W., Tso, W., Koo, A. (eds). *Advances in Chinese Medicinal Materials Research* (Singapore: World Scientific, 1985).

9. Zhao, T.H., "Positive modulating action of *shenmaisan* with *Astralagus membranaceus* on anti-tumor activity of LAK cells," *Chung Hsi I Chieh Ho Tsa Chih,* 13(8), 471–472 (1993).

10. Mori, K., et al., "Antitumor activities of edible mushrooms by oral administration," in *Cultivating Edible Fungi* (Amsterdam: Elsevier, 1987), pp. 1–6.

11. Boik, J. *Cancer and Natural Medicine: A Textbook of Basic Science and Clinical Research* (Princeton, Minnesota: Oregon Medical Press, 1995), pp. 217–218.

12. Tamaoki, J., Chiyotani, A., Takeyama, K., Kanemura, T., Sakai, N., Konno, K., "Potentiation of beta-adrenergic function by *saiboku-to* and *bakumondo-to* in canine bronchial smooth muscle," *Japanese Journal of Pharmacology,* 62(2), 155–159 (June 1993).

13. Vacca, A., Ribatti, D., Iurlaro, M., Albini, A., Minischetti, M., Bussolino, F., Pellegrino, A., Ria, R., Rusnati, M., Presta, M., Vincenti, V., Persico, M.G., Dammacco, F., "Human lymphoblastoid cells produce extracellular matrix-degrading enzymes and induce endothelial cell proliferation, migration, morphogenesis, and angiogenesis," *International Journal of Clinical Laboratory Research,* 28(1), 55–68 (1998).

Breast Cancer

1. Morabia, A., Bernstein, M., Ruiz, J., Heritier, S., Diebold Berger, S., Borlach, B., "Relation of smoking to breast cancer by estrogen receptor status," *International Journal of Cancer,* 75(3), 339–342 (January 1998).

2. Hurd, C., Khattree, N., Dinda, S., Alban, P., Moudgil, V.K., "Regulation of tumor suppresser proteins, p53 and retinoblastoma, by estrogen and antiestrogens in breast cancer cells," *Oncogene,* 15(3), 991–995 (18 August 1997).

3. Ozer, E., Canda, T., Kuyucuodlu, F., "p53 mutations in bilateral breast carcinoma. Correlation with Ki-67 expression and the mean nuclear volume," *Cancer Letters,* 122(1–2), 100–106 (9 January 1998).

4. Kandioler, D., Dekan, G., End, A., Pasching, E., Buchmayer, H., Gnant, M., Langmann, F., Mannhalter, C., Eckersburger, F., Wolner, E., "Molecular genetic differentiation between primary lung cancers and lung metastases of other tumors," *Journal of Thoracic and Cardiovascular Surgery,* 111(4), 827–831 (April 1996).

5. Burke, H.B., Hoang, A., Iglehart, J.D., Marks, J.R., "Predicting response to adjuvant and radiation therapy in patients with early stage breast carcinoma," *Cancer,* 82(5), 874–877 (1 March 1998).

6. Loret de Mola, J.R., "Endometrial changes with chronic Tamoxifen use," *Current Opinion in Obstetrics and Gynecology,* 9(3), 160–164 (June 1997).

7. Zhao, T.H., "Positive modulating action of *shenmaisan* with *Astralagus membranaceus* on anti-tumor activity of LAK cells," *Chung Hsi I Chieh Ho Tsa Chih,* 13(8), 471–472 (1993).

8. Sigounas, G., Hooker, J., Anagnostou, A., Steiner, M., "S-

allylmercaptocysteine inhibits cell proliferation and reduces the viability of erythroleukemia, breast, and prostate cancer cell lines," *Nutrition & Cancer,* 27(2), 186–191 (1997).

9. Ishikawa, K., Naganawa, R., Yoshida, H., Iwata, N., Fukuda, H., Fujino, T., Suzuki, A., "Antimutagenic effects of ajoene, an organosulfur compound derived from garlic," *Bioscience, Biotechnology & Biochemistry,* 60(10), 1712–1713 (October 1996).

10. Schaffer, E.M., Liu, J.Z., Milner, J.A., "Garlic powder and allyl sulfur compounds enhance the ability of dietary selenite to inhibit 7,12-dimethylbenz[a]anthracene-induced mammary DNA adducts," *Nutrition & Cancer,* 27(2), 162–168 (1997).

11. Scambia, G., Ranelletti, F.O., Benedetti, P.P., et al., "Quercetin potentiates the effect of adriamycin in a multidrug-resistant MCF-7 human breast-cancer cell line; P-glycoprotein as a possible target," *Cancer Chemotherapy Pharmacology,* 28(4), 255–258 (1991).

12. Ibid.

13. Komori, A., Yatsunamni, J., Okabe, S., et al., "Anticarcinogenic activity of green tea polyphenols," *Japanese Journal of Clinical Oncology,* 23(30), 186–190 (1993).

14. Teas, J., "The dietary intake of *Laminaria,* a brown seaweed, and breast cancer prevention," *Nutrition and Cancer,* 4(3), 217–222 (1983).

15. Adlercreutz, H., Mousavi, Y., Clark, J., Hocerstedt, K., et al., "Dietary phytoestrogens and cancer: in vitro and in vivo studies," *Journal of Steroid Biochemistry and Molecular Biology,* 41(3–8), 331–337 (1992).

16. Adlercreutz, H., Markkanen, H., Watanabe, S., "Plasma concentrations of phyto-estrogens in Japanese men," *Lancet,* 342 (8881), 1209–1210 (13 November 1993).

17. Bruneton, J. *Pharmacognosy, Phytochemistry, Medicinal Plants* (Paris: Lavoisier Publishing, 1995), pp. 296–297.

18. Foptsis, T., Pepper, M., Adlercreutz, H., Fleischmann, G., et al., "Genistein, a dietary-derived inhibitor of in vitro angiogenesis," *Proceedings of the National Academies of Science of the US,* 90(7), 2690–2694 (1993).

19. Shao, Z.M., Alpaugh, M.L., Fontana, J.A., Barsky, S.H., "Genistein inhibits proliferation similarly in estrogen receptor-positive and negative human breast carcinoma cell lines characterized by P21WAF1/CIP1 induction, G2/M arrest, and apoptosis," *Journal of Cellular Biochemistry,* 69(1), 44–54 (1 April 1998).

20. Maeda, Y.Y., et al., "Unique increase of serum protein components and action of antitumour polysaccharides," *Nature,* 252, 250 (1974).

21. Togami, M., et al., "Studies on *Basidiomycetes.* I. Antitumor polysaccharide from bagasse medium on which mycelia of *Lentinus edodes* (Berk.) Sing. had been grown," *Chemical Pharmacology Bulletin,* 30, 1134–1140 (1982).

22. Yamasaki, K., et al., "Synergistic induction of lymphokine (IL-2)-activated killer activity by IL-2 and the polysaccharide lentinan, and therapy of spontaneous pulmonary metastases," *Cancer Immunology and Immunotherapy,* 29, 87–92 (1989).

23. Oka, M., et al., "Immunological analysis and clinical effects of intraabdominal and intrapleural injection of lentinan for malignant ascites and pleural effusion," *Biotherapy,* 5, 107–112 (1992).

24. Kovacs, E., Hajto, T., Hostanska, K., "Improvement of DNA repair in lymphocytes of breast cancer patients treated with *Viscum album* extract (Iscador)," *European Journal of Cancer,* 27(12), 1672–1676 (1991).

25. Mori, K., et al., "Antitumor activities of edible mushrooms by oral administration," In *Cultivating Edible Fungi* (Amsterdam: Elsevier, 1987), pp. 1–6.

26. Yang, D.A., Li, S.Q., Li, X.T., "Prophylactic effects of *zhuling* and BCG on postoperative recurrence of bladder cancer," *Chung-Hua Wai Ko Tsa Chih—Chinese Journal of Surgery,* 32(7), 433–434 (July 1994).

27. Miller, D. Clinical protocol submitted to the NIH Scientific Director, Cancer Treatment Research Foundation, Arlington Heights, Illinois (1994).

28. Castiglione, S., Paggi, M.G., Delpino, A., et al., "Inhibition of protein synthesis in neoplastic cells by rhein," *Biochemical Pharmacology,* 40(5), 967–973 (1990).

29. Chang, H.M., But, P.P.H. *Pharmacology and Applications of Chinese Materia Medica,* Volume 2 (Teaneck, New Jersey: World Scientific Publishing, 1987), p. 783.

30. Chen, Y.C., Kuo, T.C., Lin-Shiau, S.Y., Lin, J.K., "Induction of HSP70 gene expression by modulation of Ca(+2) ion and cellular p53 protein by curcumin in colorectal carcinoma cells," *Molecular Carcinogenesis,* 17(4), 224–234 (December 1996).

31. Venkatesan, N., Chandrakasan, G., "Modulation of cyclophosphamide-induced early lung injury by curcumin, an anti-inflammatory antioxidant," *Molecular & Cellular Biochemistry,* 142(1), 79–87 (12 January 1995).

32. Thresiamma, K.C., George, J., Kuttan, R., "Protective effect of curcumin, ellagic acid and bixin on radiation induced toxicity," *Indian Journal of Experimental Biology,* 34(9), 845–847 (September 1996).

33. Boik, J. *Cancer and Natural Medicine: A Textbook of Basic Science and Clinical Research* (Princeton, Minnesota: Oregon Medical Press, 1995), p. 253.

34. Sakamoto, S., Kudo, H., Kawasaki, T., Kuwa, K., et al., "Effects of a Chinese herbal medicine, *keishi-bukuryo-gan,* on the gonadal system of rats," *Journal of Ethnopharmacology,* 23(2–3), 151–158 (July–August 1988).

35. Usuki, S., "Effects of *hachimijiogan, tokishakuyakusan, keishibukuryogan, ninjinto* and *unkeito* on estrogen and progesterone secretion in preovulatory follicles incubated in vitro," *American Journal of Chinese Medicine,* 19(1), 65–71 (1991).

36. Ibid.

37. Takahashi, K., Kitao, M., "Effect of TJ-68 (*shakuyaku-kanzo-to*) on polycystic ovarian disease," *International Journal of Fertility & Menopausal Studies,* 39(2), 69–76 (March–April 1994).

38. Zhang, G.L., "Treatment of breast proliferation disease with modified *xiao yao san* and *er chen* decoction," *Chung Hsi I Chieh Ho Tsa Chih,* 11(7), 400–402 (1988).

39. Wilson, S.T., Blask, D.E., Lemus-Wilson, A.M., "Melatonin augments the sensitivity of MCF-7 human breast cancer cells to tamoxifen in vitro," *Journal of Endocrinology and Metabolism,* 75(2), 669–670 (August 1992).

Inset: Breast Cancer in Men

1. Wolf, D.A., Wang, S., Panzica, M.A., Bassily, N.H., Thompson, N.L., "Expression of a highly conserved oncofetal gene, TA1/E16, in human colon carcinoma and other primary cancers: homology to *Schistosoma mansoni* amino acid permease and

Caenorhabditis elegans gene products," *Cancer Research,* 56(21), 5012–5022 (1 November 1996).

2. Sloan, B.S., Rickman, L.S., Blau, E.M., Davis, C.E., "Schistosomiasis masquerading as carcinoma of the breast," *Southern Medical Journal,* 89(3), 345–347 (March 1996).

Bronchitis and Pneumonia

1. Orr, P.H., et al., "Randomized placebo-controlled trials of antibiotics for acute bronchitis: a critical review of the literature," *Journal of Family Practice,* 36, 507–512 (1993).

2. Murray, M., Pizzorno, J. *Encyclopedia of Natural Medicine,* Second Edition (Rocklin, California: Prima Publishing, 1998), p. 295.

3. Gonzales, R., Sande, M., "What will it take to stop physicians from prescribing antibiotics in acute bronchitis?" *Lancet,* 345, 665 (1995).

4. Bensky, D., Gamble, A., Kaptchuk, T., Bensky, L.L. *Chinese Herbal Medicine: Materia Medica,* Revised Edition (Seattle: Eastland Press, 1993), p. 201.

5. Yang, J., et al., "Stimulatory effect and kinetics of carboxymethylpachymaran on the induction of interferon by lymphoblastoid cell culture," *Chinese Journal of Microbiology and Immunology,* 6, 157–159 (1987).

6. Ma, L., Lin, Z., "Effect of *Tremella* polysaccharide on IL-2 production by mouse splenocytes," *Yaoxue Xuebao,* 27, 1–4 (1992).

7. Liu, S.H., et al., "Inhibition effect of *Tremella fuciformis* Berk. Preparation (TFB) on growth of transplanted mouse tumor cells," *Zhong Guo Zhong Liu Lin Chuang,* 21, 68–70 (1994).

8. Lin, Z., et al., "Studies on the pharmacology of *Tremella fuciformis,* preliminary research on the fermented solution and polysaccharides of *Tremella fuciformis* spores," *Journal of Traditional Chinese Medicine,* 2, 95–98 (1982).

9. Zheng, L., et al., "Effects of *ling zhi* on the production of interleukin-2. From Immunopharmacological Study (5)," in *The Research on Ganoderma lucidum, Part One* (Shanghai: Shanghai Medical University Press, 1993), pp. 259–265.

10. Ryan, H., "A double-blind clinical evaluation of bromelains in the treatment of acute sinusitis," *Headache,* 7, 13–17 (1967).

Burns

1. Zhang, L., Tizard, I.R., "Activation of a mouse macrophage cell line by acemannan, the majorcarbohydrate fraction from *Aloe vera* gel," *Immunopharmacology,* 35(2), 119–128 (November 1996).

2. Karaca, K., Sharma, J.M., Nordgren, R., "Nitric oxide production by chicken macrophages activated by Acemannan, a complex carbohydrate extracted from *Aloe vera," International Journal of Immunopharmacology,* 17(3), 183–188 (March 1995).

3. Chen, Y.C., "Experimental studies on the effects of *danggui buxue* decoction on IL-2 production of blood-deficient mice," *Chung-Kuo Chung Yao Tsa Chih—China Journal of Chinese Materia Medica,* 19(12), 739–741, 763 (December 1994).

4. Liang, H., Zhang, Y., Geng, B., "The effect of astragalus polysaccharides (APS) on cell mediated immunity (CMI) in burned mice," *Chung-Hua Cheng Hsing Shao Shang Wai Ko Tsa Chih—Chinese Journal of Plastic Surgery & Burns,* 10(2), 138–141 (March 1994).

5. Bensky, D., Gamble, A., Kaptchuk, T., Bensky, L.L. *Chinese Herbal Medicine: Materia Medica,* Revised Edition (Seattle: Eastland Press, 1993), p. 79.

Cancer

1. Sato, K., Mochizuki, M., Saiki, I., Yoo, Y.C., Samukawa, K,. Azuma, I., "Inhibition of tumor angiogenesis and metastasis by a saponin of *Panax ginseng,* ginsenoside-Rb2," *Biological & Pharmaceutical Bulletin,* 17(5), 635–639 (May 1994).

Cataracts

1. Varma, S.D., Schocket, S.S., Richards, R.D., "Implications of aldose reductase in cataracts in human diabetes," *Investigations in Ophthalmology and Vision Science,* 18(30), 237–241 (March 1979).

2. Srivastava, S.K., Petrash, J.M., Sadana, I.J., Ansari, N.H., Partridge, C.A., "Susceptibility of aldehyde and aldose reductases of human tissues to aldose reductase inhibitors," *Current Eye Research,* 2(6), 407–410 (1982).

3. McLauchlan, W.R., Sanderson, J., Williamson, G., "Quercetin protects against hydrogen peroxide-induced cataract," *Biochemical Society Transactions,* 25(4), S581 (November 1997).

4. Winston, D., "Eclectic specific condition review: cataracts," *Protocol Journal of Botanical Medicine,* 2(2), 39 (1997).

5. Awasthi, S., Srivatava, S.K., Piper, J.T., Singhal, S.S., Chaubey, M., Awasthi, Y.C., "Curcumin protects against 4-hydroxy-2-trans-noenal-induced cataract formation in rat lenses," *American Journal of Clinical Nutrition,* 64(5), 761–766 (November 1996).

6. Kamei, A., Hisada, T., Iwata, S., "The evaluation of therapeutic efficacy of *hachimi-jio-gan* (traditional Chinese medicine) to mouse hereditary cataract," *Journal of Ocular Pharmacology,* 4(4), 311–319 (Winter 1988).

7. Shoji, M., Sato, H., Hirai, Y., Oguni, Y., Sugimoto, C., "Pharmacological effects of *gosha-jinki-gan-ryo* extract, effects on experimental diabetes," *Nippon Yakurigaku Zasshi—Folia Pharmacologica Japonica,* 99(3), 143–152 (March 1992).

8. Kamei, A., Hisada, T., Iwata, S., "The evaluation of therapeutic efficacy of *hachimi-jio-gan* (traditional Chinese medicine) to rat galactosemic cataract," *Journal of Ocular Pharmacology,* 3(3), 239–248 (Fall 1987).

9. Taylor, A., "Cataract: relationship between nutrition and oxidation," *Journal of the American College of Nutritionists,* 12, 138–146 (1993).

10. Bouton, S., "Vitamin C and the aging eye," *Archives of Internal Medicine,* 63, 930–945 (1939).

11. Rathbun, W., Hanson, S., "Glutathione metabolic pathway as a scavenging system in the lens," *Ophthalmology Research,* 11, 172–176 (1979).

12. Murray, M., Pizzorno, J. *Encyclopedia of Natural Medicine,* Second Edition (Rocklin, California: Prima Publishing, 1998), p. 320.

13. Swanson, A., Truesdale, A., "Elemental analysis in normal and cataractous human lens tissue," *Biochemical and Biophysical Research Communications,* 45, 1488–1496 (1971).

Cervical Cancer

1. Boik, J. *Cancer and Natural Medicine: A Textbook of Basic Science and Clinical Research* (Princeton, Minnesota: Oregon Medical Press, 1995), p. 235.

2. Dillner, J., Lehtinene, M., Bjorge, T., Luostarinene, T., Youngman, L., Jellum, E., Lskela, P., Gislefoss, R.E., Hallmans, G., Paavonen, J., Sapp, M., Schiller, J.T., Hakulinen, T., Thoresen, S., Hakama, M., "Prospective seroepidemiologic study of human papillomavirus infection as a risk factor for invasive cervical can-

cer," *Journal of the National Cancer Institute,* 89(17), 1293–1299 (September 1997).

3. Sizemore, N., Mukhtar, H., Couch, L.H., Howard, P.C., Rorke, E.A., "Differential response of normal and HPV immortalized ectocervical epithelial cells to b[a]P," *Carcinogenesis,* 16(10), 2413–2416 (October 1995).

4. von Knebel Doeberitz, M., Spitkovsky, D., Ridder, R., "Interactions between steroid hormones and viral oncogenes in the pathogenesis of cervical cancer," *Verhandlungen der Deutscher Gesellschaft für Pathologie,* 81, 233–239 (1997).

5. Prabhu, N.S., Somasundaram, K., Satyamoorthy, K., Herlyn, M., El-Deiry, W.S., "p73, unlike p53, suppresses growth and induces apoptosis of human papillomavirus E6-expressing cancer cells," *International Journal of Oncology,* 13(1), 5–9 (July 1998).

6. Lu, X., Toki, T., Konishi, I., Nikaido, T., Fujii, S., "Expression of p21WAF1/C1P1 in adenocarcinoma of the uterine cervix: a possible immunohistochemical marker of a favorable prognosis," *Cancer,* 82(120), 2409–2417 (15 June 1993).

7. Hurd, C., Khattree, N., Dinda, S., Alban, P., Moudgil, V.K., "Regulation of tumor suppresser proteins, p53 and retinoblastoma, by estrogen and antiestrogens in breast cancer cells," *Oncogene,* 15(3), 991–995 (18 August 1997).

8. Colombo, A., Landoni, F., Cormio, G., Barni, S., Maneo, A., Nava, S., Pelegrino, A., Placa, F., Mangioni, C., "Concurrent carboplatin-5FU and radiotherapy compared to radiotherapy alone in locally advanced cervical carcinoma: a case-control study," *Tumori,* 83(6), 895–899 (November 1997).

9. Kim, H.S., Lee, B.M., "Inhibition of benzo[a]pyrene-DNA adduct formation by *Aloe barbadensis* Miller," *Carcinogenesis,* 18(4), 771–776 (April 1997).

10. Gribel, N.V., Pashinskii, V.G., "Antimetastatic properties of aloe juice," *Voprosii Onkologii,* 32(12), 38–40 (1986).

11. Zhao, T.H., "Positive modulating action of *shenmaisan* with *Astralagus membranaceus* on anti-tumor activity of LAK cells," *Chung Hsi I Chieh Ho Tsa Chih,* 13(8), 471–472 (1993).

12. Hara, Y., "Prophylactic functions of tea polyphenols," in Ho, C.T., Osawa, T., Huang, M.T., Rosen, R. (eds). *Food Phytochemicals for Cancer Prevention II: Teas, Spices, and Herbs* (Washington: American Chemical Society, 1994), pp. 36, 43.

13. Ying, J., et al. *Icones of Medicinal Fungi From China* (Beijing: Science Press, 1987).

14. Taguchi, T., et al., "Phase I and II studies of lentinan," in Aoki, A., et al. (eds). *Manipulation of Host Defence Mechanisms* (Amsterdam: Excerpta Medica, 1981), p. 138.

15. Katsumatsu, T., "The radiation-sensitizing effect of PSK in treatment of cervical cancer patients," in Yamamura, Y., et al. (eds). *Immunomodulation by Microbial Products and Related Synthetic Compounds* (Amsterdam: Excerpta Medica, 1982), pp. 463–466.

16. Satomi, N., Sakurai, A., Iimura, F., Haranaka, R., Haranaka, K., "Japanese modified traditional Chinese medicines as preventive drugs of the side effects induced by tumor necrosis factor and lipopolysaccharide," *Molecular Biotherapy,* 1(3), 155–162 (1989).

17. Razina, T.G., Udintsev, S.N., Prishchep, T.P., et al., "Enhancement of the selectivity of the action of the cytostatics cyclophosphamide and 5-fluoruracil by using an extract of the Baikal skullcap in an experiment," *Voprosii Onkologii,* 33(20), 80–84 (1987).

18. Razina, T.G., Udintsev, S.N., Tiutrin, I.I., et al., "The role of thrombocyte aggregation function in the mechanism of the antimetastatic action of an extract of Baikal skullcap," *Voprosii Onkologii,* 35(3), 331–335 (1989).

19. Chen, Y.C., Kuo, T.C., Lin-Shiau, S.Y., Lin, J.K., "Induction of HSP70 gene expression by modulation of Ca(+2) ion and cellular p53 protein by curcumin in colorectal carcinoma cells," *Molecular Carcinogenesis,* 17(4), 224–234 (December 1996).

20. Venkatesan, N., Chandrakasan, G., "Modulation of cyclophosphamide-induced early lung injury by curcumin, an anti-inflammatory antioxidant," *Molecular & Cellular Biochemistry,* 142(1), 79–87 (12 January 1995).

21. Thresiamma, K.C., George, J., Kuttan, R., "Protective effect of curcumin, ellagic acid and bixin on radiation induced toxicity," *Indian Journal of Experimental Biology,* 34(9), 845–847 (September 1996).

22. Zhang, G.L., "Treatment of breast proliferation disease with modified *xiao yao san* and *er chen* decoction," *Chung Hsi I Chieh Ho Tsa Chih,* 11(7), 400–402 (1988).

23. Xin, Y.L., "Direct current therapy for malignant tumors," *Chung-Hua Chung Liu Tsa Chih—Chinese Journal of Oncology,* 13(6), 467–469 (1992).

24. Xin, Y.L., "Traditional and Western medical treatment of 211 cases of late stage lung cancer," *Chung-Hua Chung Liu Tsa Chih—Chinese Journal of Oncology,* 13(6), 135–138 (1993).

Inset: Nutrition as a Weapon Against Cervical Cancer

1. Butterworth, E.E., et al., "Folate deficiency and cervical dysplasia," *Journal of the American Medical Association,* 267, 528–533 (1982).

2. Wassertheil-Smoller, S., Romney, S., Wylie-Rosett, J., et al., "Dietary vitamin C and uterine cervical dysplasia," *American Journal of Epidemiology,* 114, 714–724 (1981).

3. Creek, K.E., Geslani, G., Batova, A., Pirisi, L., "Progressive loss of sensitivity to growth control by retinoic acid and transforming growth factor-beta at late stages of human papillomavirus type 16-initiated transformation of human keratinocytes," *Advances in Experimental Medicine and Biology,* 375, 117–135 (1995).

4. Verreault, R., Chu, J., Mandelson, M., Shy, K., "A case-control study of diet and invasive cervical cancer," *International Journal of Cancer,* 43(6), 1050–1054 (15 June 1989).

5. Giuliano, A.R., Papenfuss, M., Nour, M., Canfield, L.M., Schneider, A., Hatch, K., "Antioxidant nutrients: associations with persistent human papillomavirus infection," *Cancer Epidemiology, Biomarkers, and Prevention,* 6(11), 917–923 (November 1997).

6. Martens, J.E., Smedts, F., ter Harmsel, B., Helmerhorst, T.J., Ramaekers, F.C., "Glutathione S-transferase pi is expressed in (pre) neoplastic lesions of the human uterine cervix irrespective of their degree of severity," *Anticancer Research,* 17(6D), 4305–4309 (November 1997).

Chemotherapy Side Effects

1. Lin, C., Lin, X., Yang, J., "An observation on combined use of chemotherapy and traditional Chinese medicine to relieve cancer pain," *Journal of Traditional Chinese Medicine,* 14(4), 267–269 (December 1996).

Chemotherapy Side Effects, Cisplatin

1. Zee-Cheng, R.K., "*Shi-quan-da-bu-tang* (ten significant tonic decoction), SQT. A potent Chinese biological response modifier in cancer immunotherapy, potentiation and detoxification of anticancer drugs," *Methods & Findings in Experimental & Clinical Pharmacology*, 14(9), 725–736 (November 1992).

Chemotherapy Side Effects, Cyclophosphamide

1. He, J., Li, Y., Wei, S., et al., "Effects of mixture of *Astragalus membranaceus, Fructus ligustri* and *Eclipta prostrata* on immune function in mice," *Hua Hsi I Ko Ta Hsueh Pao*, 23(4), 408–411 (1992).

2. Yamaguchi, N., et al., "Augmentation of various immune reactivities of tumor-bearing hosts with an extract of *Cordyceps sinensis*," *Biotherapy*, 2, 199–205 (1990).

3. Itokawa, H., Morita, M., Mihashi, S., *Chemical Pharmacy Bulletin*, 29, 2382 (1981). Also Kiuchi, F., Shibura, M., Sankawa, U., *Chemical Pharmacy Bulletin*, 30, 2279 (1982).

4. Lei, L., Lin, Z., "Effects of *Ganoderma* polysaccharides on the activity of DNA polymerase a in spleen cells stimulated by alloantigens in mice in vitro," *Beijing Yike Daxue Xuebao*, 23, 329–333 (1991).

5. Razina, T.G., Udintsev, S.N., Prishchep, T.P., et al., "Enhancement of the selectivity of the action of the cytostatics cyclophosphamide and 5-fluoruracil by using an extract of the Baikal skullcap in an experiment," *Voprosii Onkologii*, 33(20), 80–84 (1987).

6. Razina, T.G., Udintsev, S.N., Tiutrin, I.I., et al., "The role of thrombocyte aggregation function in the mechanism of the antimetastatic action of an extract of Baikal skullcap," *Voprosii Onkologii*, 35(3), 331–335 (1989).

7. Venkatesan, N., Chandrakasan, G., "Modulation of cyclophosphamide-induced early lung injury by curcumin, an anti-inflammatory antioxidant," *Molecular & Cellular Biochemistry*, 142(1), 79–87 (12 January 1995).

8. Zee-Cheng, R.K., "*Shi-quan-da-bu-tang* (ten significant tonic decoction), SQT. A potent Chinese biological response modifier in cancer immunotherapy, potentiation and detoxification of anticancer drugs," *Methods & Findings in Experimental & Clinical Pharmacology*, 14(9), 725–736 (November 1992).

9. Ohnishi, Y., Fujii, H., Hayakaway, Y., Sakukawa, R., Yamaura, T., Sakamoto, T., Tsudada, K., Fujimaki, M., Nunome, S., Komatsu, Y., Saiki, I., "Oral administration of a Kampo (Japanese herbal) medicine *juzen-taiho-to* inhibits liver metastasis of colon 26-L5 carcinoma cells," *Japanese Journal of Cancer Research*, 89(2), 206–213 (February 1998).

10. Jing, Y., Nakaya, K., Han, R., "Differentiation of promyeloctic leukemia cells HL-60 induced by daidzein in vitro and in vivo," *Anticancer Research*, 13(4), 1049–1054 (1993).

11. Jing, Y.K., Han, R., "Differentiation of B16 melanoma cells induced by daidzein," *Chinese Journal of Pharmacology and Toxicology*, 6(4), 278–280 (1992).

Chemotherapy Side Effects, Doxorubicin Hydrochloride (Adriamycin)

1. Wu, Y., Cao, Y., Shi, X., Shi, Y., "Inhibitory effect of Radix et Rhizoma Rhei on the production of lipid peroxides (LPO) in mice liver," *Chung Kuo Chung Yao Tsa Chih*, 21(4), 240–242, inside back cover (April 1996).

2. Lin, T.J., Liu, G.T., Pan, Y., Liu, Y., Xu, G.Z., "Protection by schisanhenol against adriamycin toxicity in rat heart mitochondria," *Biochemical Pharmacology*, 42(9), 1805–1810 (9 October 1991).

3. Lin, T.J., "Antioxidant mechanism of schizandrin and tanshinonatic acid A and their effects on the protection of cardiotoxic action of adriamycin," *Sheng Li Ko Hsueh Chin Chan*, 22(4), 342–345 (October 1991).

4. Lin, T.J., Liu, G.T., "Effect of schisanhenol on the antitumor activity of adriamycin," *Biochemistry and Biophysics Research Communications*, 178(1), 207–212 (15 July 1991).

5. Xu, J.P., "Research on *Liu Wei* Rehmannia oral liquid against side effect of drugs used in antitumor chemotherapy," *Chung Kuo Chung Hsi I Chieh Ho Tsa Chih*, 12(12), 709–710 (December 1992).

6. Sudo, K., Honda, K., Taki, M., Kanitani, M., Fujii, Y., Aburada, M., Hosoya, E., Kumura, M., Orikasa, S., "Effects of TJ-41 (Tsumura *hochu-ekki-to*) on spermatogenic disorders in mice under current treatment with adriamycin," *Nippon Yakurigaku Zasshi*, 92(4), 251–261 (October 1988).

Chemotherapy Side Effects, 5-fluorouracil

1. Taguchi, T., et al., "Phase I and II studies of Lentinan," in Aoki, A., et al. (eds). *Manipulation of Host Defence Mechanisms* (Amsterdam: Excerpta Medica, 1981).

Chemotherapy Side Effects, Mitomycin

1. Taguchi, T., et al., "Phase I and II studies of Lentinan," in Aoki, A., et al. (eds). *Manipulation of Host Defence Mechanisms* (Amsterdam: Excerpta Medica, 1981).

2. Nanba, H., "Activity of maitake D-fraction to prevent cancer growth and metastasis," *Journal of Naturopathic Medicine* (1994).

3. Yang, D.A., Li, S.Q., Li, X.T., "Prophylactic effects of *zhuling* and BCG on postoperative recurrence of bladder cancer," *Chung-Hua Wai Ko Tsa Chih—Chinese Journal of Surgery*, 32(7), 433–434 (July 1994).

4. Miller, D. Clinical protocol submitted to the NIH Scientific Director, Cancer Treatment Research Foundation, Arlington Heights, Illinois (1994).

Chemotherapy Side Effects, Steroid Drugs

1. Chen, M.F., et al., "Effect of glycyrrhizin on the pharmacokinetics of prednisolone following low dosage of prednisolone hemisuccinate," *Endocronologica Japonica*, 37, 331–341 (1990).

Chronic Fatigue Syndrome

1. Ablashi, D.V., Levine, P.H., De Vinci, C., Whitman, J.E Jr., Pizza, G., Viza, D., "Use of anti HHV-6 transfer factor for the treatment of two patients with chronic fatigue syndrome (CFS). Two case reports," *Biotherapy*, 9(1–3), 81–86 (1996).

2. Levine, P.H., "The use of transfer factors in chronic fatigue syndrome: prospects and problems," *Biotherapy*, 9(1–3), 77–79 (1996).

3. Lombard, J., Germano, C. *The Brain Wellness Plan* (New York: Kensington Press, 1998), p. 177.

4. Baschetti, R., "Chronic fatigue syndrome and neurally mediated hypotension," *Journal of the American Medical Association*, 275, 359 (1996).

5. Demitrack, M.A., "Evidence for impaired activation of the hypothalamic-pituitary-adrenal axis in patients with chronic

fatigue syndrome," *Journal of Clinical Endocrinology and Metabolism,* 73, 1224–1234 (1991).

6. Baschetti, R., "Chronic fatigue syndrome and liquorice," *New Zealand Medical Journal,* 108(1002), 259 (28 June 1995).

7. Isselbacher, K.J., Braunwald, E., Wilson, J., Martin, J.V., Fauci, A.S., Kasper, D.L. (eds). *Harrison's Principles of Internal Medicine,* Thirteenth Edition (New York: McGraw-Hill, 1995), pp. 2398–2400.

8. Kurokawa, M., Nagasaka, K., Hirabayashi, T., Uyama, S., Sato, H., Kageyama, T., Kadota, S., Ohyama, H., Hozumi, T., Namba, T., et al., "Efficacy of traditional herbal medicines in combination with acyclovir against herpes simplex virus type 1 infection in vitro and in vivo," *Antiviral Research,* 27(1–2), 19–37 (May 1995).

9. Huang, K.C. *The Pharmacology of Chinese Herbs* (Boca Raton, Florida: CRC Press, 1993), p. 82.

10. Rosenfeld, M.S., "Evaluation of the efficacy of a standardized ginseng extract in patients with psychophysical asthenia and neurological disorders," *La Semana Médica,* 173, 148–154 (1989).

11. Aoki, T., "Antibodies to HTLV I and HTLV II in sera from two Japanese patients, one with possible pre-AIDS," *Lancet,* 936–937 (20 October 1984).

12. Ostrom, N., "Another mushroom miracle?" *New York Native,* 29, 34–35 (1992).

13. Costarella, L., "Naturopathic condition review: asthma," *Protocol Journal of Botanical Medicine,* 1(2), 103 (Autumn 1995).

14. Zhang, Q., Hsu, H.Y. *AIDS and Chinese Medicine: Applications of the Oldest Medicine to the Newest Disease* (Long Beach, California: Oriental Healing Arts Institute Press, 1990), p. 30.

15. Morris, D.H., Stare, F.J., "Unproven diet therapies in the treatment of the chronic fatigue syndrome," *Archives of Family Medicine,* 2(2), 181–186 (February 1993).

16. Pollmer, U., personal communication with author, 6 January 1995.

17. Droge, W., Holm, E., "Role of cysteine and glutathione in HIV infection and other diseases associated with muscle wasting and immunological dysfunction," *FASEB Journal,* 11(13), 1077–1089 (November 1997).

18. See, D.M., Broumand, N., Sahl, L., Tilles, J.G., "In vitro effects of echinacea and ginseng on natural killer and antibody-dependent cell cytotoxicity in healthy subjects and chronic fatigue syndrome or acquired immunodeficiency syndrome patients," *Immunopharmacology,* 35(3), 229–235 (January 1997).

Cirrhosis, Alcoholic

1. Lieber, C.S., "Ethanol metabolism, cirrhosis and alcoholism," *Clinica Chimica Acta,* 257(1), 59–84 (January 1997).

2. Lieber, C.S., "Role of oxidative stress and antioxidant therapy in alcoholic and nonalcoholic liver disease," *Advances in Pharmacology,* 38, 601–628 (1997).

3. Scevola, D., et al., "Possible anti-endotoxin activity of (+)-Cyanidanaol-3 in experimental hepatitis in the rat," *Hepatogastroenterology,* 29, 178–182 (1982).

4. World, M., et al., "(+)-Cyanidanol-3 for alcoholic liver disease: results of a six-month clinical trial," *Alcohol and Alcoholism,* 19, 23–29 (1984).

5. Pizzorno, J. *Total Wellness* (Rocklin, California: Prima Publishing, 1996), p. 132.

6. Nagabhushan, M., Bhide, S.V., "Curcumin as an inhibitor of cancer," *Journal of the American College of Nutritionists,* 11, 192–198 (1992).

7. Cadranel, J.F., di Martino, V., Devergie, B., "Grapefruit juice for the pruritus of cholestatic liver disease," *Annals of Internal Medicine,* 126(11), 920–921 (1 June 1997).

8. He, K., Iyer, K.R., Hayes, R.N., Sinz, M.W., Woolf, T.F., Hollenberg, P.F., "Inactivation of cytochrome P450 3A4 by bergamottin, a component of grapefruit juice," *Chemical Research in Toxicology,* 11(40), 252–259 (April 1998).

9. Ferenci, P., Dragosics, B., Dittrich, H., Frank, H., Benda, L., Lochs, H., Meryn, S., Base, W., Schneider, B., "Randomized controlled trial of silymarin treatment in patients with cirrhosis of the liver," *Journal of Hepatology,* 9(1), 105–113 (July 1989).

10. Velussi, M., Cernigoi, A.M., De Monte, A., Dapas, F., Caffau, C., Zilli, M., "Long-term (12 months) treatment with an anti-oxidant drug (silymarin) is effective on hyperinsulinemia, exogenous insulin need and malondialdehyde levels in cirrhotic diabetic patients," *Journal of Hepatology,* 26(4), 871–879 (April 1997).

Colds

1. Murray, M., Pizzorno, J. *Encyclopedia of Natural Medicine* (Rocklin, California: Prima Publishing, 1996), p. 87.

2. Schinzel, W., Graf., T., "Hypertension and garlic," *Deutsche Ärtzeblatt,* 76, 1974–1975 (1979).

3. Feng, Z.H., Zhang, G.M., Hao, T.L., Zhou, B., Zhang, H., Jiang, Z.Y., "Effect of diallyl trisulfide on the activation of T-cell and macrophage-mediated cytotoxicity," *Journal of Tongji Medical University,* 14, 142–147 (1994).

4. Aoki, T., "Antibodies to HTLV I and HTLV II in sera from two Japanese patients, one with possible pre-AIDS," *Lancet,* 936–937 (20 October 1984).

5. Khoda, H., et al., "The biologically active constituents of *Ganoderma lucidum* (Fr.) Karst. Histamine release-inhibitory triterpenes," *Chemical Pharmacology Bulletin,* 33, 2624–2627 (1985).

6. Shimuzu, A., et al., "Isolation of an inhibitor of platelet aggregation from a fungus, *Ganoderma lucidum,*" *Chemical Pharmacology Bulletin,* 33, 3012–3015 (1985).

7. Nagai, T., Suzuki, Y., Tomimori, T., Yamada, H., "Antiviral activity of plant flavonoid, 5,7,4'-trihydroxy-8-methoxyflavone, from the roots of *Scutellaria baicalensis* against influenza A (H3N2) and B viruses," *Biological & Pharmaceutical Bulletin,* 18(2), 295–299 (February 1995).

Colorectal Cancer

1. Zhao, T.H., "Positive modulating action of *shenmaisan* with *Astralagus membranaceus* on anti-tumor activity of LAK cells," *Chung Hsi I Chieh Ho Tsa Chih,* 13(8), 471–472 (1993).

2. Li, N.Q., "Clinical and experimental study on *shen-qi* injection with chemotherapy in the treatment of malignant tumor of the digestive tract," *Chung Hsi I Chieh Ho Tsa Chih,* 12(10), 588–592, 579 (1992).

3. Chang, K.S.S., Gao, C., Wang, L.C., "Berberine-induced morphologic differentiation and down-regulation of c-Ki-ras2 protooncogene expression in human teratocarcinoma cells," *Cancer Letters,* 55, 103–108 (1990).

4. Chang, K.S., "Down-regulation of c-Ki-ras2 gene expression associated with morphologic differentiation in human embryon-

al carcinoma cells treated with berberine," *Taiwan I Hsueh Hui Tsa Chih*, 90(1), 10–14 (1991).

5. Koch, H.P., Lawson, L.D. *Garlic: The Science and Therapeutic Application of Allium sativum L. and Related Species*, Second Edition (Baltimore: Williams & Wilkins, 1996), p. 177.

6. Wargovich, M.J., Woods, C., Eng, V.W., Stephens, L.C., Gray, K., "Chemoprevention of N-nitrosomethylbenzylamine-induced esophageal cancer in rats by the naturally occurring thioether, diallyl sulfide," *Cancer Research*, 48(23), 6872–6875 (December 1988).

7. Milner, J.A., "Garlic: its anticarcinogenic and antitumorigenic properties," *Nutrition Reviews*, 54(11 Pt 2), S82–S86 (November 1996).

8. Polasa, K., Krishnaswamy, K., "Reduction of urinary mutagen excretion in rats fed garlic," *Cancer Letters*, 114(1–2), 185–186 (19 March 1997).

9. Weber, G., Shen, F., Prajda, N., Yeh, Y.A., Yang, H., Herenyiova, M., Look, K.Y., "Increased signal transduction activity and down-regulation in human cancer cells," *Anticancer Research*, 16(6A), 3271–3282 (November–December 1996).

10. Kuo, S.M., "Antiproliferative potency of structurally distinct dietary flavonoids on human colon cancer cells," *Cancer Letters*, 110(1–2), 41–48 (20 December 1996).

11. Kim, M., Hagiwara, N., Smith, S.J., Yamamoto, T., Yaamane, T., Takahashi, T., "Preventive effect of green tea polyphenols on colon carcinogenesis," in Ho, C.T., Osawa, T., Huang, M.T., Rosen, R. (eds). *Food Phytochemicals for Cancer Prevention II: Teas, Spices, and Herbs* (Washington: American Chemical Society, 1994), pp. 51–55.

12. Hara, Y., "Prophylactic functions of tea polyphenols," in Ho, C.T., Osawa, T., Huang, M.T., Rosen, R. (eds), pp. 36, 43.

13. Teas, J., "The dietary intake of *Laminaria*, a brown seaweed, and breast cancer prevention," *Nutrition and Cancer*, 4(3), 217–222 (1983).

14. Mori, K., et al., "Antitumor activities of edible mushrooms by oral administration." In *Cultivating Edible Fungi* (Amsterdam: Elsevier, 1987), pp. 1–6.

15. Miller, D. Clinical protocol submitted to the NIH Scientific Director, Cancer Treatment Research Foundation, Arlington Heights, Illinois (1994).

16. Torisu, M., Uchiyama, A., Goya, T., Iwasaki, K., Katano, M., Yamamoto, H., Kimura, Y., "Eighteen-year experience of cancer immunotherapies—evaluation of their therapeutic benefits and future," *Nippon Geka Gakkai Zasshi—Journal of Japan Surgical Society*, 92(9), 1212–1216 (September 1991).

17. Sugiyama, Y., Saji, S., Miya, K., Fukada, D., Umemoto, T., Kunieda, K., Takao, H., Kato, M., Kawai, M., "Locoregional therapy for liver metastases of colorectal cancer," *Gan to Kagaku Ryoho—Japanese Journal of Cancer & Chemotherapy*, 23(11), 1433–1436 (September 1996).

18. Takashima, S., Kinami, Y., Miyazaki, I., "Clinical effect of postoperative adjuvant immunochemotherapy with the FT-207 suppository and PSK in colorectal cancer patients," *Gan to Kagaku Ryoho—Japanese Journal of Cancer & Chemotherapy*, 15(8), 2229–2236 (August 1988).

19. Ebina, T., Murata, K., "Antitumor effect of PSK at a distant site: tumor-specific immunity and combination with other chemotherapeutic agents," *Japanese Journal of Cancer Research*, 83(7), 775–782 (July 1992).

20. Harada, M., Matsunaga, K., Oguchi, Y., Iijima, H., Tamada, K., Abe, K., Takenoyama, M., Ito, O., Kimura, G., Nomoto, K., "Oral administration of PSK can improve the impaired anti-tumor CD4+ T-cell response in gut-associated lymphoid tissue (GALT) of specific-pathogen-free mice," *International Journal of Cancer*, 70(3), 362–372 (27 January 1997).

21. Zhang, L.X., Mong, H., Zhou, X.B., "Effect of Japanese *Ganoderma lucidum* (GL) planted in Japan on the production of interleukin-2 from murine splenocytes," *Chung Hsi I Chieh Ho Tsa Chih*, 10(11), 672–674 (1993).

22. Haak-Frendscho, M., Kino, K., Sone, T., et al., "Ling Zhi-8: a novel T-cell mitogen induces cytokine production and upregulation of ICAM-1 expression," *Cellular Immunology*, 150(1), 101–113 (1993).

23. Adlercreutz, H., Markkanen, H., Watanabe, S., "Plasma concentrations of phyto-estrogens in Japanese men," *Lancet*, 342(8881), 1209–1210 (13 November 1993).

24. Adlercreutz, H., Mousavi, Y., Clark, J., Hocerstedt, K., et al., "Dietary phytoestrogens and cancer: in vitro and in vivo studies," *Journal of Steroid Biochemistry and Molecular Biology*, 41(3–8), 331–337 (1992).

25. Kuo, S.M., pp. 41–48.

26. Chen, Y.C., Kuo, T.C., Lin-Shiau, S.Y., Lin, J.K., "Induction of HSP70 gene expression by modulation of Ca(+2) ion and cellular p53 protein by curcumin in colorectal carcinoma cells," *Molecular Carcinogenesis*, 17(4), 224–234 (December 1996).

27. Jiang, M.C., Yang-Yen, H.F., Yen, J.J., Lin, J.K., "Curcumin induces apoptosis in immortalized NIH 3T3 and malignant cancer cell lines," *Nutrition & Cancer*, 26(1), 111–120 (1996).

28. Firozi, P.F., Aboobaker, V.S., Bhattacharya, R.K., "Action of curcumin on the cytochrome P450-system catalyzing the activation of aflatoxin B1," *Chemico-Biological Interactions*, 100(1), 41–51 (8 March 1996).

29. Thresiamma, K.C., George, J., Kuttan, R., "Protective effect of curcumin, ellagic acid and bixin on radiation induced toxicity," *Indian Journal of Experimental Biology*, 34(9), 845–847 (September 1996).

30. Sakamoto, S., Mori, T., Sawaki, K., Kawachi, Y., Kuwa, K., Kudo, H., Suzuki, S., Sugiura, Y., Kasahara, N., Nagasawa, H., "Effects of Kampo (Japanese herbal) medicine *'sho-saiko-to'* on DNA-synthesizing enzyme activity in 1,2-dimethylhydrazine-induced colonic carcinomas in rats," *Planta Medica*, 59(2), 152–154 (April 1993).

31. Das, U.N., Madhavi, N., Sravan Kumar, G., Padma, M., Sangeetha, P., "Can tumour cell drug resistance be reversed by essential fatty acids and their metabolites?" *Prostaglandins, Leukotrienes, Essential Fatty Acids*, 58(1), 39–54 (January 1998).

Inset: Using Kampo With Other Herbal Treatments for Colorectal and Liver Cancer

1. Lersch, C., Zeuner, M., Bauer, A., Siemens, M., Hart, R., Drescher, M., Fink, U., Dancygier, H., Classen, M., "Nonspecific immunostimulation with low doses of cyclophosphamide (LDCY), thymostimulin, and *Echinacea purpurea* extracts (echinacin) in patients with far advanced colorectal cancers: preliminary results," *Cancer Investigation*, 10(5), 343–388 (1992).

2. Lersch, C., Zeuner, M., Bauer, A., Siebenrock, K., Hart, R., Wagner, F., Fink, U., Dancygier, H., Classen, M., "Stimulation of the immune response in outpatients with hepatocellular carcino-

mas by low doses of cyclophosphamide (LDCY), *Echinacea purpurea* extracts (Echinacin) and thymostimulin," *Archiv für Geschwulstforschung,* 60(5), 379–383 (1990).

3. Woerdenbag, H.J., Merfort, I., Passreiter, C.M., Schmidt, T.J., Willuhn, G., van Uden, W., Pras, N., Kampinga, H.H., Konings, A.W., "Cytotoxicity of flavonoids and sesquiterpene lactones from *Arnica* species against the GLC4 and the COLO 320 cell lines," *Planta Medica,* 60(5), 434–437 (October 1994).

4. Puhlmann, J., Zenk, M.H., Wagner, H., "Immunologically active polysaccharides of *Arnica montana* cell cultures," *Phytochemistry,* 30(4), 1141–1145 (1991).

5. Wagner, H., Jurcic, K., "Immunologic studies of plant combination preparations. In-vitro and in-vivo studies on the stimulation of phagocytosis," *Arzneimittel-Forschung,* 41(10), 1072–1076 (October 1991).

Congestive Heart Failure

1. Hikino, H., Takahashi, M., Konno, C., Hashimoto, I., Namiki, T., "Pharmacological study of *Aconitum* roots. XV. Subacute and subchronic toxicity of *Aconitum* extracts and mesaconitine," *Sohyakugaku Zasshi,* 37, 1–9 (1983).

2. Petkov, E., Nikolov, N., Uzunov, P., "Inhibitory effect of some flavonoids and flavonoid mixtures on cyclic AMP phosphodiesterease activity of rat heart," *Planta Medica,* 43, 183–186 (1981).

3. Schussler, M., Holzl, J., Fricke, U., "Myocardial effects of flavonoids from *Crataegus* species," *Arzneimittel-Forschung,* 45(8), 842–845 (August 1995).

Inset: Nutritional Support for Congestive Heart Failure

1. Shimon, I., Almog, S., Vered, Z., Seligmann, H., Shefi, M., Peleg, E., Rosenthal, T., Motro, M., Halkin, H., Ezra, D., "Improved left ventricular function after thiamine supplementation in patients with congestive heart failure receiving long-term furosemide therapy," *American Journal of Medicine,* 98(5), 485–490 (May 1995).

2. Costello, R.B., Moser-Veillon, P.B., Bianco, R., "Magnesium supplementation in patients with congestive heart failure," *Journal of the American College of Nutritionists,* 16(1), 22–31 (February 1997).

3. Clinical Quality Improvement Network Investigators, "Mortality risk and patterns of practice in 4,606 acute care patients with congestive heart failure. The relative importance of age, sex, and medical therapy," *Archives of Internal Medicine,* 156(15), 1669–1673 (August 1996).

4. Struthers, A.D., "Aldosterone escape during angiotensin-converting enzyme inhibitor therapy in chronic heart failure," *Journal of Cardiac Failure,* 2(1), 47–54 (March 1996).

5. Douban, S., Brodsky, M.A., Whang, D.D., Whang, R., "Significance of magnesium in congestive heart failure," *American Heart Journal,* 132(3), 664–671 (September 1996).

6. Fernandes, J.S., et al., "Therapeutic effect of a magnesium salt in patients suffering from mitral valvular prolapse and latent tetany," *Magnesium,* 4, 283–289 (1985).

7. Galland, L.D., Baker, S.M., McLellan, R.K., "Magnesium deficiency in the pathogenesis of mitral valve prolapse," *Magnesium,* 5, 165–174 (1986).

8. Ferrari, R., De Giuli, F., "The propionyl-L-carnitine hypothesis: an alternative approach to treating heart failure," *Journal of Cardiac Failure,* 3(3), 217–224 (September 1997).

9. Kawasaki, N., Lee, J.D., Shimizu, H., Ueda, T., "Long-term 1-carnitine treatment prolongs the survival in rats with adriamycin-induced heart failure," *Journal of Cardiac Failure,* 2(4), 293–299 (December 1996).

10. CoQ10 Drug Surveillance Investigators, "Italian multicenter study on the safety and efficacy of coenzyme Q10 as adjunctive therapy in heart failure," *Molecular Aspects of Medicine,* 15(Suppl), S287–S294 (1994).

Constipation

1. Akao, T., Che, Q.M., Kobashi, K., Hattori, M., Namba, T., "A purgative action of barbaloin is induced by *Eubacterium* sp. strain BAR, a human intestinal anaerobe, capable of transforming barbaloin to aloe-emodin anthrone," *Biological & Pharmaceutical Bulletin,* 19(1), 136–138 (January 1996).

2. Yagi, T., Yamauchi, K., Kuwano, S., "The synergistic purgative action of aloe-emodin anthrone and rhein anthrone in mice, synergism in large intestinal propulsion and water secretion," *Journal of Pharmacy & Pharmacology,* 49(1), 22–25 (January 1997).

3. Tyler, V.E. *The Honest Herbal: A Sensible Guide to the Use of Herbs and Related Remedies,* Third Edition (New York: Pharmaceutical Products Press, 1993), p. 190.

4. Heckers, H., Zielinsky, D., "Fecal composition and colonic function due to dietary variables. Results of a long-term study in healthy young men consuming 10 different diets," *Motility* (Lisbon), 24–29 (1984).

5. Huang, K.C. *The Pharmacology of Chinese Herbs* (Boca Raton, Florida: CRC Press, 1993), p. 185.

Depression

1. American Psychiatric Association. *Diagnostic and Statistical Manual of Mental Disorders,* Fourth Edition (Washington, D.C.: American Psychiatric Association, 1994), p. 199.

2. Fuller, R.W., "The involvement of serotonin in regulation of pituitary adrenal cortical function," *Frontiers of Neuroendocrinology,* 13, 250–270 (1992).

3. Maes, M., et al., "The relationship between the viability of L-tryptophan to the brain. The spontaneous HPA axis activity and the HPA axis response to dexamethasone in depressed patients," *Amino Acids,* 1, 57–65 (1991).

4. Delgado, P.L., Charney, C.S., Price L.H., et al., "Neuroendocrine and behavioral effects of dietary tryptophan restriction in healthy subjects," *Life Science,* 45, 2323–2332 (1990).

5. Weiss, R.F. *Herbal Medicine* (Beaconsfield, England: Beaconsfield Publishers Ltd., 1988), p. 286.

6. Schubert, H., Halama, P., "Depressive episode primarily unresponsive to therapy in elderly patients: efficacy of *Ginkgo biloba* extract (EGb 761) in combination with antidepressants," *Geriatrische Forschung,* 3, 45–53 (1993).

7. Hofferberth, B., "The efficacy of EGb 761 in patients with senile dementia of the Alzheimer type, a double blind, placebo-controlled study on different levels of investigation," *Human Psychopharmacology,* 9, 215–222 (1994).

8. Baschetti, R., "Chronic fatigue syndrome and neurally mediated hypotension," *Journal of the American Medical Association,* 275, 359 (1996).

9. Dharmananda, S. *Chinese Herbology: A Professional Training Program* (Portland: Institute for Preventative Medicine and Traditional Health Care, 1992), p. 256.

10. Paroli, E., "Opioid peptides from food (the exorphins)," *World Review of Nutrition and Dietetics*, 55, 58–97 (1988).

11. Winston, D., "Eclectic specific condition review: depression," *Protocol Journal of Botanical Medicine*, 2(1), 72 (Spring 1997).

12. Bensky, D., Barolet, R. *Chinese Herbal Medicine: Formulas and Strategies* (Seattle: Eastland Press, 1990), p. 291.

13. Blair, J., Morar, C., Hamon, C., et al., "Tetrahydrobiopterin metabolism in depression," *Lancet*, 1, 163 (1984).

14. Abou-Saleh, M.T., Coppen, A., "The biology of folate in depression: implications for nutritional hypotheses of psychoses," *Journal of Psychiatric Research*, 20(2), 91–101 (1982).

15. Leeming, R., Harpey, J., Brown, S., Blair, J., "Tetrahydrofolate and hydroxycobolamin in the management of dihydropteridine reductase deficiency," *Journal of Mental Deficiency Research*, 26, 21–25 (1982).

16. Bell, I.R., Edman, J.S., Morrow, F.D., Marby, D.W., et al., "B complex vitamin patterns in geriatric and young adult in patients with major depression," *Journal of the American Geriatric Society*, 39(3), 252–257 (March 1991).

Inset: Kampo and St. John's Wort

1. Müller, W.E., Rossol, R., "Effects of hypericum extract on the expression of serotonin receptors," *Journal of Geriatric Psychiatry & Neurology*, 7(Suppl 1), S63–S64 (October 1994).

2. Suzuki, O., Katsumata, Y., Oya, M., Bladt, S., Wagner, H., "Inhibition of monoamine oxidase by hypericin," *Planta Medica*, 50, 272–274 (1984).

3. Thiele, B., Brink, I., Ploch, M., "Modulation of cytokine expression by Hypericum extract," *Journal of Geriatric Psychiatry and Neurology*, 7(Suppl 1), S60–S62 (October 1994).

4. Griffin, W.S., Yeralan, O., Sheng, J.G., Boop, F.A., Mrak, R.E., Rovnaghi, C.R., Burnett, B.A., Feoktistova, A., van Eldik, L.J., "Overexpression of the neurotrophic cytokine S100 beta in human temporal lobe epilepsy," *Journal of Neurochemistry*, 65(1), 228–233 (July 1995).

Diabetes

1. Agarwal, O.P., "Prevention of atheromatous heart disease," *Angiology*, 36, 485–492 (1985).

2. Ghannam, N., Kingston, M., Al-Meshall, I.A., Tariq, M., Parman, N.S., Woodhouse, N., "The antidiabetic activity of Aloes: Preliminary clinical and experimental observations," *Hormone Research*, 24, 288–294 (1986).

3. Kimura, Y., Ohminami, H., Arichi, H., Okuda, H., Baba, K., Kozawa, M., Arichi, S., "Effects of various courmarins from roots *Angelica dahurica* on actions of adrenaline, ACTH, and insulin in fat cells," *Planta Medica*, 45, 183–187 (1982).

4. Deng, C.Q., Ge, J.W., Wang, Q., "Comparison of effect of *Astragalus membranaceus* and *huoxuefang* on thromboxane, prostacyclin and adenosine cyclic monophosphate in cerebral reperfusion injury in rabbits," *Chung-Kuo Chung Hsi I Chieh Ho Tsa Chih—Chinese Journal of Modern Developments in Traditional Medicine*, 15(3), 165–167 (March 1995).

5. Lin, L., et al., "A clinical study on treatment of vascular complications of diabetes with the sugar-reducing and pulse-invigorating capsule," *Journal of Traditional Chinese Medicine* (English), 14(1), 3–9 (1994).

6. Bensky, D., Gamble, A., Kaptchuk, T., Bensky, L.L. *Chinese Herbal Medicine: Materia Medica*, Revised Edition (Seattle: Eastland Press, 1993), p. 217.

7. Chandrasekar, B., Mukherjee, B., Mukherjee, S.K., "Blood sugar lowering potentiality of selected *Cucurbitaceae* plants of Indian origin," *Indian Journal of Medical Research*, 90, 300–305 (August 1989).

8. Meir, P., Yaniv, Z., "An in vitro study on the effect of *Momordica charantia* on glucose uptake and glucose metabolism in rats," *Planta Medica*, 51, 12 (1985).

9. Huang, K.C. *The Pharmacology of Chinese Herbs* (Boca Raton, Florida: CRC Press, 1993), p. 140.

10. Kubo, M., Matsuda, H., Tokuoka, K., Kobayashi, Y., Ma, S., Tanaka, T., "Studies of anti-cataract drugs from natural sources. I. Effects of a methanolic extract and the alkaloidal components from *Corydalis* tuber on in vitro aldose reductase activity," *Biological & Pharmaceutical Bulletin*, 17(3), 458–459 (March 1994).

11. Dharmananda, S., "Traditional Chinese specific condition review," *Protocol Journal of Botanical Medicine*, 1(3), 147 (Winter 1996).

12. Undie, A.S., Akubue, P.I., "Pharmacological evaluation of *Dioscorea dumetorum* tuber used in traditional antidiabetic therapy," *Journal of Ethnopharmacology*, 15(2), 133–144 (February 1986).

13. Augusti, K.T., Benaim, M.E., "Effect of essential oil of onion (allyl propyl disulphide) on blood glucose, free fatty acid, and insulin levels of normal subjects," *Chemical Abstracts*, 83(22), 593 (1975).

14. Koch, H.P., Lawson, L.D. *Garlic: The Science and Therapeutic Application of Allium sativum L. and Related Species*, Second Edition (Baltimore: Williams & Wilkins, 1996), pp. 193–195.

15. Huang, K.C., p. 43.

16. Ibid.

17. Kinae, N., Shimoi, K., Masumoria, S., Harusawa, M., Furugori, M., "Suppression of the formation of advanced glycosylation products by tea extracts," in Ho, C.T., Osawa, T., Huang, M.T., Rosen, R. (eds). *Food Phytochemicals for Cancer Prevention II: Teas, Spices, and Herbs* (Washington: American Chemical Society, 1994), pp. 68–75.

18. Honda, M., Nanjo, F., Hara, Y., "Inhibition of saccharide digestive enzymes by tea polyphenols," in Ho, C.T., Osawa, T., Huang, M.T., Rosen, R., pp. 83–89.

19. Tobin, R.B., Friend, B., Berdaniet, C.D., Mehlman, M.A., De Vore, V., "Metabolic responses of rats to chronic theophylline ingestion," *Journal of Toxicology and Environmental Health*, 2, 361–369 (1976).

20. Aida, K., Tawata, M., Shindo, H., Onaya, T., Sasaki, H., Yamaguchi, T., Chin, M., Mitsuhashi, H., "Isoliquiritigenin, a new aldose reductase inhibitor from glycyrrhizae radix," *Planta Medica*, 56(3), 254–258 (June 1990).

21. Hobbs, C. *Medicinal Mushrooms: An Exploration of Tradition, Healing, and Culture*, Second Edition (Santa Cruz, California: Botanica Press, 1995), p. 104.

22. Hobbs, C., p. 104.

23. Costarella, L., "Naturopathic condition review: asthma," *Protocol Journal of Botanical Medicine*, 1(2), 103 (Autumn 1995).

24. Liang, X.C., Guo, S.S., Wang, X.D., "Study on relationship of

lipid peroxide in coronary heart disease with and without diabetes," *Chung-Kuo Chung Hsi I Chieh Ho Tsa Chih—Chinese Journal of Modern Developments in Traditional Medicine,* 16(1), 29–31 (January 1996).

25. Hobbs, C., p. 104.

26. Xia, P., Aiello, L.P., Ishii, H., Jiang, Z.Y., Park, D.J., Robinson, G.S., Takagi, H., Newsome, W.P., Jirousek, M.R., King, G.L., "Characterization of vascular endothelial growth factor's effect on the activation of protein kinase C, its isoforms, and endothelial cell growth," *Journal of Clinical Investigation,* 98(9), 2018–2026 (1 November 1996).

27. Zhang, Q., Hsu, H.Y. *AIDS and Chinese Medicine: Applications of the Oldest Medicine to the Newest Disease* (Long Beach, California: Oriental Healing Arts Institute Press, 1990), p. 107.

28. Shoji, M., Sato, H., Hirai, Y., Oguni, Y., Sugimoto, C., "Pharmacological effects of *gosha-jinki-gan-ryo* extract, effects on experimental diabetes," *Nippon Yakurigaku Zasshi—Folia Pharmacologica Japonica,* 99(3), 143–152 (March 1992).

29. Kamei, A., Hisada, T., Iwata, S., "The evaluation of therapeutic efficacy of *hachimi-jio-gan* (traditional Chinese medicine) to rat galactosemic cataract," *Journal of Ocular Pharmacology,* 3(3), 239–248 (Fall 1987).

30. Goto, M., Hayashi, M., Todoroki, T., Seyama, Y., Yamashita, S., "Effects of traditional Chinese medicines (*dai-saiko-to, sho-saiko-to* and *hachimi-zio-gan*) on spontaneously diabetic rat (WBN/Kob) with experimentally induced lipid and mineral disorders," *Nippon Yakurigaku Zasshi—Folia Pharmacologica Japonica,* 100(4), 353–358 (October 1992).

31. Goto, M., Hayashi, M., Todoroki, T., Seyama, Y., Yamashita, S., pp. 353–358.

32. Huang, K.C., p. 280.

33. Dharmananda, S., p. 143.

34. Huang, K.C., p. 280.

35. Dharmananda, S., p. 143.

36. Goto, M., Inoue, H., Seyama, Y., Yamashita, S., Inoue, O., Yumioka, E., "Comparative effects of traditional Chinese medicines (*dai-saiko-to, hatimi-zio-gan* and *byakko-ka-ninzin-to*) on experimental diabetes and hyperlipidemia," *Nippon Yakurigaku Zasshi—Folia Pharmacologica Japonica,* 93(3), 179–186 (March 1989).

37. Matsumoto, J., "Vanadate, molybdate and tungstate for orthomolecular medicine," *Medical Hypotheses,* 43(3), 177–182 (September 1994).

38. Suzuki, Y., Kadowaki, H., Taniyama, M., Kadowaki, T., Katagiri, H., Oka, Y., Atsumi, Y., Hosokawa, K., Tanaka, Y., Asahina, T., et al., "Insulin edema in diabetes mellitus associated with the 3243 mitochondrial tRNA(Leu(UUR)) mutation; case reports," *Diabetes Research & Clinical Practice,* 29(2), 137–142 (August 1995).

Diabetic Retinopathy

1. Wang, Q., Dills, D.G., Klein, R., Klein, B.E., Moss, S.E., "Does insulin-like growth factor I predict incidence and progression of diabetic retinopathy?" *Diabetes,* 44(2), 161–164 (February 1995).

2. Lin, L., et al., "A clinical study on treatment of vascular complications of diabetes with the sugar-reducing and pulse-invigorating capsule," *Journal of Traditional Chinese Medicine* (English), 14(1), 3–9 (1994).

Diarrhea

1. Huang, K.C. *The Pharmacology of Chinese Herbs* (Boca Raton, Florida: CRC Press, 1993), p. 158.

2. Bensky, D., Gamble, A., Bensky, L., Kaptchuk, T. *Chinese Herbal Medicine: Formulas and Strategies* (Seattle: Eastland Press, 1992), p. 35.

3. Bruneton, J. *Pharmacognosy, Phytochemistry, Medicinal Plants* (Paris: Lavoisier Publishing, 1995), pp. 280–281.

4. Huang, K.C., p. 177.

5. Choudry, V.P., Sabir, M., Bhide, V.N., "Berberine in giardiasis," *Indian Pediatrics Journal,* 9, 143–146 (1972).

6. Huang, K.C., p. 293.

7. Huang, K.C., p. 158.

8. Huang, K.C., p. 293.

9. Hattori, T., Shindo, S., "Effects of *sairei-to* (TJ-114) on the expression of adhesion molecule in anti-GBM nephritic rats," *Nippon Jinzo Gakkai Shi—Japanese Journal of Nephrology,* 37(7), 373–383 (July 1995).

10. Takamura, S., Yoshida, J., Suzuki, S., "Effect of an extract prepared from '*dai-bofu-to*' on morphine withdrawal responses," *Nippon Yakurigaku Zasshi—Folia Pharmacologica Japonica,* 105(2), 87–95 (February 1995).

11. Suzuki, M., Nikaido, T., Ohmoto, T., "The study of Chinese herbal medicinal prescription with enzyme inhibitory activity. V. The study of *hange-shashin-to, kanzo-shashin-to, shokyo-shashin-to* with adenosine 3',5'-cyclic monophosphate phosphodiesterase," *Yakugaku Zasshi—Journal of the Pharmaceutical Society of Japan,* 111(11), 695–701 (November 1991).

12. Kase, Y., Hayakawa, T., Takeda, S., Ishige, A., Aburada, M., Okada, M., "Pharmacological studies on antidiarrheal effects of *hange-shashin-to," Biological & Pharmaceutical Bulletin,* 19(10), 1367–1370 (October 1996).

13. Wang, C.M., Ohta, S., Shinoda, M., "Studies of chemical protectors against radiation. XXIX. Protective effects of methanol extracts of various Chinese traditional medicines on skin injury induced by X-irradiation," *Yakugaku Zasshi—Journal of the Pharmaceutical Society of Japan,* 110(3), 218–224 (March 1990).

14. Sakata, Y., Suzuki, H., Kamataki, T., "Preventive effect of TJ-14, a Kampo (Chinese herb) medicine, on diarrhea induced by irinotecan hydrochloride (CPT-11)," *Gan to Kagaku Ryoho—Japanese Journal of Cancer & Chemotherapy,* 21(8), 1241–1244 (July 1994).

15. Bensky, D., Gamble, A., Bensky., L, Kaptchuk, T., p. 57.

Ear Infections

1. Batchelder, H.J., "Allopathic specific condition review: otitis media," *Protocol Journal of Botanical Medicine,* 2(2), 95 (1997).

2. Saarinen, U.M., Savilahti, E., Arjomaa, P., "Increased IgM-type betalactoglobulin antibodies in children with recurrent otitis media," *Allergy,* 38(3), 571–576 (November 1983).

3. Cantekin, et al., "Antimicrobial therapy for otitis media with effusion," *Journal of the American Medical Association,* 266, 3309–3317 (1991).

4. Klein, J.O., "Role of nontypeable *Haemophilus influenzae* in pediatric respiratory tract infections," *Pediatric Infectious Disease Journal,* 16(2 Suppl), S5–S8 (February 1997).

5. Kleinman, L.C., Kosecoff, J., Dubois, R.W., Brook, R.H., "The medical appropriateness of tympanostomy tubes proposed for

children younger than 16 years in the United States," *Journal of the American Medical Association,* 271(16), 1250–1255 (27 April 1994).

6. Kabelik, J., Hejtmankova-Uhrova, N., "The antifungal and antibacterial effects of certain drugs and other substances," *Chemical Abstracts,* 70(36), 264 (1969).

7. Shimamura, T., "Inhibition of influenza virus infection by tea polyphenols," in Ho, C.T., Osawa, T., Huang, M.T., Rosen, R. (eds). *Food Phytochemicals for Cancer Prevention II: Teas, Spices, and Herbs* (Washington: American Chemical Society, 1994), pp. 101–104.

8. Nagai, T., Suzuki, Y., Tomimori, T., Yamada, H., "Antiviral activity of plant flavonoid, 5,7,4'-trihydroxy-8-methoxyflavone, from the roots of *Scutellaria baicalensis* against influenza A (H3N2) and B viruses," *Biological & Pharmaceutical Bulletin,* 18(2), 295–299 (February 1995).

9. Nagai, T., Miyaichi, Y., Tomimori, T., Suzuki, Y., Yamada, H., "Inhibition of influenza virus sialidase and anti-influenza virus activity by plant flavonoids," *Chemical & Pharmaceutical Bulletin,* 38(5), 1329–1332 (May 1990).

10. Ozaki, Y., "Studies on antiinflammatory effect of Japanese Oriental medicines (Kampo medicines) used to treat inflammatory diseases," *Biological & Pharmaceutical Bulletin,* 18(4), 559–562 (April 1995).

11. Bray, G.W., "The hypochlorhydria of asthma in childhood," *Quarterly Journal of Medicine,* 24, 181–197 (1931).

12. Bernard, A., et al., "Increased intestinal permeability in bronchial asthma," *Journal of Allergy and Clinical Immunology,* 97, 1173–1178 (1996).

Eczema

1. Gfesser, M., Abeck, D., Rugemer, J., Schreiner, V., Stabh, F., Disch, R., Ring, J., "The early phase of epidermal barrier regeneration is faster in patients with atopic eczema," *Dermatology,* 195(4), 332–336 (1997).

2. Hutter, J.A., Salman, M., Stavinoha, W.B., Satsangi, N., Williams, R.F., Streeper, R.T., Weintraub, S.T., "Antiinflammatory C-glucosyl chromone from *Aloe barbadensis,*" *Journal of Natural Products,* 59(5), 541–543 (May 1996).

3. Davis, R.H., Parker, W.L., Murdoch, D.P., "Aloe vera as a biologically active vehicle for hydrocortisone acetate," *Journal of the American Podiatric Medical Association,* 81(1), 1–9 (January 1991).

4. Pizzorno, J.E., Murray, M.T. *A Textbook of Natural Medicine* (Seattle: John Bastyr College Publications, 1985), p. IV: Food A1.

5. Bensky, D., Gamble, A., Kaptchuk, T., Bensky, L.L. *Chinese Herbal Medicine: Materia Medica,* Revised Edition (Seattle: Eastland Press, 1993), p. 42.

6. Huang, K.C. *The Pharmacology of Chinese Herbs* (Boca Raton, Florida: CRC Press, 1993), p. 293.

7. Evans, F.Q., "The rational use of glycyrrhetinic acid in dermatology," *British Journal of Clinical Practice,* 12, 269–279 (1958).

8. Kawana, T., "Treatment of recurrent genital herpes with PSK," *Proceedings of the International Symposium on Pharmacological and Clinical Approaches to Herpes Viruses and Virus Chemotherapy, Oiso, Japan, September 10–13, 1984,* reprinted in Kono, R., Nakajima, A. (eds). *Herpes Viruses and Chemotherapy: Pharmacological and Clinical Approaches* (Amsterdam: Excerpta Medica, 1985), pp. 271–272.

9. Huang, K. C., p. 248.

10. Chang, H.M., But, P.P.H. *Pharmacology and Applications of Chinese Materia Medica,* Volume 1 (Singapore: World Scientific Publishing, 1986), p. 446.

11. Wang, S.R., Guo, Z.Q., Liao, J.Z., "Experimental study on effects of 18 kinds of Chinese herbal medicine for synthesis of thromboxane A2 and PGI2," *Chung-Kuo Chung Hsi I Chieh Ho Tsa Chih—Chinese Journal of Modern Developments in Traditional Medicine,* 13(3), 167–170, 134 (March 1993).

12. Raman, A., Lin, Z.X., Sviderskaya, E., Kowalska, D., "Investigation of the effect of *Angelica sinensis* root extract on the proliferation of melanocytes in culture," *Journal of Ethnopharmacology,* 54(2–3), 165–170 (November 1996).

13. Chandra, D., Gupta, S., "Anti-inflammatory and anti-arthritic activity of volatile oil of *Curcuma longa* (haldi)," *Indian Journal of Medical Research,* 60, 138–142 (1972).

14. Arora, R., Basu, N., Kapoor, V., Jain, A., "Anti-inflammatory studies on *Curcuma longa* (turmeric)," *Indian Journal of Medical Research,* 59, 1289–1295 (1971).

15. Nagasaka, K., Kurokawa, M., Imakita, M., Terasawa, K., Shiraki, K., "Efficacy of *kakkon-to,* a traditional herbal medicine, in herpes simplex virus type 1 infection in mice," *Journal of Medical Virology,* 46(1), 28–34 (May 1995).

16. Latchman, Y., Bungy, G.A., Atherton, D.J., Rustin, M.H., Brostoff, J., "Efficacy of traditional Chinese herbal therapy in vitro. A model system for atopic eczema: inhibition of CD23 expression on blood monocytes," *British Journal of Dermatology,* 132(4), 592–598 (April 1995).

17. Sheehan, M.P., Atherton, D.J., "A controlled trial of traditional Chinese medicinal plants in widespread non-exudative atopic eczema," *British Journal of Dermatology,* 126(2), 179–184 (1992).

18. Saarinen, U.M., Kajosaari, M., "Breast feeding as prophylaxis against atopic disease: prospective follow-up study until 17 years old," *Lancet,* 346(8982), 1065–1069 (21 October 1995).

Inset: Managing Eczema Through Diet

1. Van Bever, H.P., Docx, M., Stevens, W.J., "Food and food additives in severe atopic dermatitis," *British Journal of Dermatology,* 117, 301–310 (1987).

2. Agata, H., et al., "Effect of elimination of food-specific IgE antibodies and lymphocyte proliferative responses to food antigens in atopic dermatitis patients exhibiting sensitivity to food allergens," *Journal of Allergy and Clinical Immunology,* 91, 668–679 (1993).

3. Sampson, H.A., Scanlon, S.M., "Natural history of food hypersensitivity in children with atopic dermatitis," *Journal of Pediatrics,* 115, 23–27 (1993).

4. Savolainen, J., et al., "*Candida albicans* and atopic dermatitis," *Clinical Experience in Allergy,* 23, 332–339 (1993).

5. Caffarelli, C., Cavagni, G., Menzie, I.S., Bertoline, P., Atherton, D.J., "Elimination diet and intestinal permeability in atopic eczema: a preliminary study," *Clinical Experience in Allergy,* 23(1), 28–31 (January 1993).

6. Bjorneboe, A., et al., "Effect of dietary supplementation of eicosapentanoic acid in the treatment of atopic dermatitis," *British Journal of Dermatology,* 117, 463–469 (1987).

Endometrial Cancer

1. Koch, H.P., Lawson, L.D. *Garlic: The Science and Therapeutic Application of Allium sativum L. and Related Species*, Second Edition (Baltimore: Williams & Wilkins, 1996), p. 177.

2. Komori, A., Yatsunamni, J., Okabe. S., et al., "Anticarcinogenic activity of green tea polyphenols," *Japanese Journal of Clinical Oncology*, 23(30), 186–190 (1993).

3. Hara, Y., "Prophylactic functions of tea polyphenols," in Ho, C.T., Osawa, T., Huang, M.T., Rosen, R. (eds). *Food Phytochemicals for Cancer Prevention II: Teas, Spices, and Herbs* (Washington: American Chemical Society, 1994), p. 36, 43.

4. Katsumatsu, T., "The radiation-sensitizing effect of PSK in treatment of cervical cancer patients," in Yamamura, Y., et al. (eds). *Immunomodulation by Microbial Products and Related Synthetic Compounds* (Amsterdam: Excerpta Medica, 1982), pp. 463–466.

5. Boik, J. *Cancer and Natural Medicine: A Textbook of Basic Science and Clinical Research* (Princeton, Minnesota: Oregon Medical Press, 1995), p. 253.

6. Sakamoto, S., Kudo, H., Kawasaki, T., Kuwa, K., et al., "Effects of a Chinese herbal medicine, *keishi-bukuryo-gan*, on the gonadal system of rats," *Journal of Ethnopharmacology*, 23(2–3), 151–158 (July–August 1988).

7. Usuki, S., "Effects of *hachimijiogan, tokishakuyakusan, keishibukuryogan, ninjinto* and *unkeito* on estrogen and progesterone secretion in preovulatory follicles incubated in vitro," *American Journal of Chinese Medicine*, 19(1), 65–71 (1991).

8. Zhang, G.L., "Treatment of breast proliferation disease with modified *xiao yao san* and *er chen* decoction," *Chung Hsi I Chieh Ho Tsa Chih*, 11(7), 400–402 (1988).

9. Adlercreutz, H., Markkanen, H., Watanabe, S., "Plasma concentrations of phyto-estrogens in Japanese men," *Lancet*, 342 (8881), 1209–1210 (13 November 1993).

10. Adlercreutz, H., Mousavi, Y., Clark, J., Hocerstedt, K., et al., "Dietary phytoestrogens and cancer: in vitro and in vivo studies," *Journal of Steroid Biochemistry and Molecular Biology*, 41(3–8), 331–337 (1992).

Inset: Lowering Estrogen Levels Through Diet

1. Tegelman, R., Lindeskog, P., Carlström, K., Pousette, A., Blomstrand, R., "Peripheral hormone levels in healthy subjects during fasting," *Acta Endocrinologica (Denmark)*, 133, 457 (1986).

2. Adlercreutz, H., "Diet, breast cancer and sex hormone metabolism," *Annals of the New York Academy of Sciences*, 595, 281 (1990).

3. Longcope, C., Gorbach, S., Goldin, B., Woods, M., Wyer, J., Morril, A., Warram, J., "The effect of a low fat diet on estrogen metabolism," *Journal of Clinical Endocrinology and Metabolism*, 46, 146 (1987).

4. de Waard, F., Poortman, J., de Pedro-Alvarez, M., Ferrero, M., Baandersvan Halewijn, E.A., "Weight reduction and oestrogen excretion in obese post-menopausal women," *Maturitas*, 4, 155 (1982).

Endometriosis

1. Misao, R., Fujimoto, J., Nakanishi, Y., Tamaya, T., "Expression of estrogen and progesterone receptors and their mRNAs in ovarian endometriosis," *Gynecological Endocrinology*, 10(5), 303–310 (October 1996).

2. Bulun, S.E., Noble, L.S., Takayama, K., Michael, M.D., Agarwal, V., Fisher, C., Zhao, Y., Hinshelwood, M.M., Ito, Y., Simpson, E.R., "Endocrine disorders associated with inappropriately high aromatase expression," *Journal of Steroid Biochemistry and Molecular Biology*, 61(3–6), 133–139 (April 1997).

3. Winston, D., "Eclectic specific condition review: endometriosis," *Protocol Journal of Botanical Medicine*, 1(4), 35 (Spring 1996).

4. Hudson, T., Lewin, A., "Naturopathic specific condition review: endometriosis," *Protocol Journal of Botanical Medicine*, 1(4), 32 (Spring 1996).

5. Hiai, S., "Chinese medicinal material and the secretion of ACTH and corticosteroid," in Chang, H.M., Yeung, W., Tso, W., Koo, A. (eds). *Advances in Chinese Medicinal Materials Research* (Singapore: World Scientific, 1985), pp. 49–60.

6. Awasthi, S., Srivatava, S.K., Piper, J.T., Singhal, S.S., Chaubey, M., Awasthi, Y.C., "Curcumin protects against 4-hydroxy-2-transnoenal-induced cataract formation in rat lenses," *American Journal of Clinical Nutrition*, 64(5), 761–766 (November 1996).

7. Miliewicz, A., Gejdel, E., Sworen, H., Sienkiewicz, K., Jedrezjak, J., Teucher, T., Schmitz, H., "Vitex agnus castus extract in the treatment of luteal phase defects due to latent hyperprolactinemia. Results of a randomized placebo-controlled double-blind study," *Arzneimittel-Forschung*, 43(7), 752–756 (July 1993).

8. Usuki, S., "Effects of *hachimijiogan, tokishakuyakusan, keishibukuryogan, ninjinto* and *unkeito* on estrogen and progesterone secretion in preovulatory follicles incubated in vitro," *American Journal of Chinese Medicine*, 19(1), 65–71 (1991).

9. Imai, A., Horibe, S., Fuseya, S., Iida, K., Takagi, H., Tamaya, T., "Possible evidence that the herbal medicine *shakuyaku-kanzo-to* decreases prostaglandin levels through suppressing arachidonate turnover in endometrium," *Journal of Medicine*, 26(3–4), 163–174 (1995).

10. Usuki, S., pp. 65–71.

11. Takahashi, K., Kitao, M., "Effect of TJ-68 (*shakuyaku-kanzo-to*) on polycystic ovarian disease," *International Journal of Fertility & Menopausal Studies*, 39(2), 69–76 (March–April 1994).

Eye Disorders, Bloodshot Eyes

1. Mitchell, W., "Allergies: immediate-type hypersensitivity," *Protocol Journal of Botanical Medicine*, 1(2), 66 (Spring 1996).

2. Boik, J. *Cancer and Natural Medicine: A Textbook of Basic Science and Clinical Research* (Princeton, Minnesota: Oregon Medical Press, 1995), p. 253.

Eye Disorders, Blurred Vision

1. Jarry, H., Harnischfeger, G., Düker, E., "Studies on the endocrine effects of the contents of *Cimicifuga racemosa*. 2. In vitro binding of compounds to estrogen receptors," *Planta Medica*, 51, 316–319 (1985).

Fibrocystic Breast Disease

1. Isselbacher, K.J., Braunwald, E., Wilson, J., Martin, J.V., Fauci, A.S., Kasper, D.L., eds. *Harrison's Principles of Internal Medicine*, Thirteenth Edition (New York: McGraw-Hill, 1995), p. 1841.

2. Noble, L.S., Takayama, K., Zeitoun, K.M., Putman, J.M., Johns, D.A., Hinshelwood, M.M., Agarwal, V.R., Zhao, Y., Carr, B.R., Bulun, S.E., "Prostaglandin E2 stimulates aromatase expression in endometriosis-derived stromal cells," *Journal of Clinical Endocrinology and Metabolism*, 82(2), 600–606 (February 1997).

3. Srivastava, K.C., Mustafa, T., "Ginger (*Zingiber officinale*) in rheumatism and musculoskeletal disorders," *Medical Hypotheses*, 39(4), 342–348 (December 1992).

4. Kuo, S.M., "Dietary flavonoid and cancer prevention: evidence and potential mechanism," *Critical Reviews in Oncogenesis*, 8(1), 47–69 (1997).

5. Schwitters, B., Masquelier, J. *OPC in Practice: Bioflavonoids and Their Application* (Rome: Alfa Omega Group, 1993), p. 43.

6. Miksicek, R.J., "Interaction of naturally occurring nonsteroidal estrogen with expressed recombinant human estrogen receptor," *Journal of Steroid Biochemistry and Molecular Biology*, 29(2–3), 153–160 (June 1994).

7. Foptsis, T., Pepper, M., Adlercreutz, H., Fleischmann, G., et al., "Genistein, a dietary-derived inhibitor of in vitro angiogenesis," *Proceedings of the National Academies of Science of the US*, 90(7), 2690–2694 (1993).

8. Boik, J. *Cancer and Natural Medicine: A Textbook of Basic Science and Clinical Research* (Princeton, Minnesota: Oregon Medical Press, 1995), p. 253.

9. Usuki, S., "Effects of *hachimijiogan, tokishakuyakusan, keishibukuryogan, ninjinto* and *unkeito* on estrogen and progesterone secretion in preovulatory follicles incubated in vitro," *American Journal of Chinese Medicine*, 19(1), 65–71 (1991).

10. Ibid.

11. Takahashi, K., Kitao, M., "Effect of TJ-68 (*shakuyaku-kanzo-to*) on polycystic ovarian disease," *International Journal of Fertility & Menopausal Studies*, 39(2), 69–76 (March–April 1994).

12. Zhang, G.L., "Treatment of breast proliferation disease with modified *xiao yao san* and *er chen* decoction," *Chung Hsi I Chieh Ho Tsa Chih*, 11(7), 400–402 (1988).

Inset: Diet Items to Avoid, Supplements to Take for Fibrocystic Breast Disease

1. Minto, J.P., Abou-Issa, H., Reiches, N., Roseman, J.M., "Clinical and biochemical studies on methylxanthine-related fibrocystic breast disease," *Surgery*, 90, 299–304 (1981).

2. Sasano, H., Frost, A.R., Saitoh, R., Matsunaga, G., Nagura, H., Krozowski, Z.S., Silverberg, S.G., "Localization of mineralocorticoid receptor and 11 beta-hydroxysteroid dehydrogenase type II in human breast and its disorders," *Anticancer Research*, 17(3C), 2001–2007 (May 1997).

3. Audisio, M., Mastroiacovo, P., Martinoli, L., Fidanza, A., Cappelli, L., Pasquali Lasagni, R., Tirelli, C., Jacobelli, G., "Serum values of vitamins A, E, C and carotenoids in healthy adult subjects and those with breast neoplasia," *Bolletina de Societe Italiana de Biologia*, 65(5), 473–480 (May 1989).

4. Pasquali, D., Bellastella, A., Valente, A., Botti, G., Capasso, I., del Vecchio, S., Salvatore, M., Colantuoni, V., Sinisi, A.A., "Retinoic acid receptors alpha, beta and gamma, and cellular retinol binding protein-I expression in breast fibrocystic disease and cancer," *European Journal of Endocrinology*, 137(4), 410–414 (October 1997).

5. Rock, C.L., Saxe, G.A., Ruffin, M.T. 4th, August, D.A, Schottenfeld, D., "Carotenoids, vitamin A, and estrogen receptor status in breast cancer," *Nutrition and Cancer*, 25(3), 281–296 (1996).

Fibroids (Uterine Myomas)

1. The Boston Women's Health Book Collective, *The New Our Bodies, Ourselves: A Book by and for Women* (New York: Simon & Schuster Touchstone Books, 1992), p. 597.

2. Govan, A. *Gynecology Illustrated*, Fourth Edition (New York: Churchhill-Livingstone, 1993), pp. 242–243.

3. Viville, B., Charnock-Jones, D.S., Sharkey, A.M., Wetzka, B., Smith, S.K., "Distribution of the A and B forms of the progesterone receptor messenger ribonucleic acid and protein in uterine leiomyomata and adjacent myometrium," *Human Reproduction*, 12(4), 815–822 (April 1997).

4. Anania, C.A., Stewart, E.A., Quade, B.J., Hill, J.A., Nowak, R.A., "Expression of the fibroblast growth factor receptor in women with leiomyomas and abnormal uterine bleeding," *Molecules in Human Reproduction*, 3(8), 685–691 (August 1997).

5. Felter, H.W., Lloyd, J.U. *King's American Dispensatory* (Cincinnati: The Ohio Valley Company, 1898), pp. 529–532.

6. Winston, D., "Eclectic specific condition review: uterine fibroids," *Protocol Journal of Botanical Medicine*, 1(4), 211 (Spring 1996).

7. Ibid.

8. Li, W., Zhou, C.H., Lu, Q.L., "Effects of Chinese materia medica in activating blood stimulating menstrual flow on the endocrine function of ovary-uterus and its mechanisms," *Chung Hsi I Chieh Ho Tsa Chih*, 12(30), 165–168 (1992).

9. Kohda, H., et al., "The biologically active constituents of *Ganoderma lucidum* (Fr.) Karst. Histamine release-inhibitory triterpenes," *Chemical Pharmacy Bulletin*, 33, 1367–1374 (1985).

10. Lin, J.M., Lin, C.C., Chen, M.F., Ujiie, T., Takada, A., "Radical scavenger and antihepatotoxic activity of *Ganoderma formosanum, Ganoderma lucidum* and *Ganoderma neo-japonicum*," *Journal of Ethnopharmacology*, 47(1), 33–41 (23 June 1995).

11. Boik, J. *Cancer and Natural Medicine: A Textbook of Basic Science and Clinical Research* (Princeton, Minnesota: Oregon Medical Press, 1995), p. 253.

12. Sakamoto, S., Kudo, H., Kawasaki, T., Kuwa, K., et al., "Effects of a Chinese herbal medicine, *keishi-bukuryo-gan*, on the gonadal system of rats," *Journal of Ethnopharmacology*, 23(2–3), 151–158 (July–August 1988).

13. Mori, T., Sakamoto, S., Singtripop, T., Park, M.K., Kato, T., Kawashima, S., Nagasawa, H., "Suppression of spontaneous development of uterine adenomyosis by a Chinese herbal medicine, *keishi-bukuryo-gan*, in mice," *Planta Medica*, 59(4), 308–311 (August 1993).

14. Usuki, S., "Effects of *hachimijiogan, tokishakuyakusan, keishibukuryogan, ninjinto* and *unkeito* on estrogen and progesterone secretion in preovulatory follicles incubated in vitro," *American Journal of Chinese Medicine*, 19(1), 65–71 (1991).

15. Takahashi, K., Kitao, M., "Effect of TJ-68 (*shakuyaku-kanzo-to*) on polycystic ovarian disease," *International Journal of Fertility & Menopausal Studies*, 39(2), 69–76 (March–April 1994).

16. Imai, A., Horibe, S., Fuseya, S., Iida, K., Takagi, H., Tamaya, T., "Possible evidence that the herbal medicine *shakuyaku-kanzo-to* decreases prostaglandin levels through suppressing arachidonate turnover in endometrium," *Journal of Medicine*, 26(3–4), 163–174 (1995).

Gallstones

1. Sasaki, T., Ohta, S., Kamogawa, A., Shinoda, M., "Choleretic effects of methanol extracts obtained from various Chinese tradi-

tional medicine," *Yakugaku Zasshi—Journal of the Pharmaceutical Society of Japan*, 109(7), 487–495 (July 1989).

2. Wichtl, M., ed., Grainger-Bissett, N., trans. *Herbal Drugs and Phytopharmaceuticals: A Handbook for Practice on a Scientific Basis* (Boca Raton, Florida: CRC Press, 1995), p. 234.

3. Wichtl, M., Grainger-Bisset, N., p. 337.

4. Shoda, J., Matsuzaki, Y., Tanaka, N., Miyamoto, J., Osuga, T., "The inhibitory effects of *dai-chai-hu-tang (dai-saiko-to)* extract on supersaturated bile formation in cholesterol gallstone disease [letter]," *American Journal of Gastroenterology*, 91(4), 828–830 (April 1996).

Gastritis

1. Long, S.D., Li, C.M., Yang, Q.G., "Clinical observation on verrucous gastritis with combined therapy of traditional Chinese and Western medicine," *Chung-Kuo Chung Hsi I Chieh Ho Tsa Chih—Chinese Journal of Modern Developments in Traditional Medicine*, 14(3), 150–151 (March 1994).

2. Zhang, L., Yang, L.W., Yang, L.J., "Relation between *Helicobacter pylori* and pathogenesis of chronic atrophic gastritis and the research of its prevention and treatment," *Chung-Kuo Chung Hsi I Chieh Ho Tsa Chih—Chinese Journal of Modern Developments in Traditional Medicine*, 12(9), 521–523, 515–516 (September 1992).

3. Matsuta, M., Kanita, R., Tsutsui, F., Yamashita, A., "Antiulcer properties of *shosaiko-to*," *Nippon Yakurigaku Zasshi*, 108(4), 217–225 (October 1996).

4. Yeoh, K.G., Kang, J.Y., Yap, I., Guan, R., Tan, C.C., Wee, A., Teng, C.H., "Chili protects against aspirin-induced gastroduodenal mucosal injury in humans," *Digestive Diseases and Sciences*, 40(3), 580–583 (March 1995).

Glaucoma

1. Mertge, H.J., Merkle, W., "Long-term treatment with *Ginkgo biloba* extract of circulatory disturbances of the retina and optic nerve," *Klinische Monatsblatt für Augenheilkunde*, 177(5), 577–583 (1980).

2. Hagerman, A., Butler, L., "The specificity of proanthocyanidin-protein interactions," *Journal of Biological Chemistry*, 256, 4494–4497 (1981).

3. Gabor, M., "Pharmacologic effects of flavonoids on blood vessels," *Angiologica*, 9, 355–374 (1972).

4. Monboisse, J., Braquet, P, Borel, J., "Oxygen-free radicals as mediators of collagen breakage," *Agents and Actions*, 15, 49–50 (1984).

5. Kadar, A., Robert, L., Miskulin, M., Tixier, J.M., Brechemier, D., Robert, A.M., "Influence of anthocyanoside treatment on the cholesterol-induced atherosclerosis in the rabbit," *Paroi Arterielle*, 5(4), 187–205 (December 1979).

6. Kang, R.X., "The intraocular pressure depressive effect of peurarin," *Chung Hua Yen Ko Tsa Chih*, 29(6), 336–339 (November 1993).

7. Hattori, T., Shindo, S., "Effects of *sairei-to* (TJ-114) on the expression of adhesion molecule in anti-GBM nephritic rats," *Nippon Jinzo Gakkai Shi—Japanese Journal of Nephrology*, 37(7), 373–383 (July 1995).

8. Guandong Medical Journal Editorial Department, "Clinical observation of curative effects of *wu long san* for treatment of glaucoma," *Guandong Medical Journal*, 3(2), 40 (1982).

9. Higginbotham, E.J., Kilimanjaro, H.A., Wilensky, J.T., Batenhorst, R.L., Hermann, D., "The effect of caffeine on intraocular pressure in glaucoma patients," *Ophthalmology*, 96(5), 624–626 (May 1989).

Hair Loss

1. Hoffmann, R., Wenzel, E., Huth, A., van der Steen, P., Schaufele, M., Konig, A., Happle, R., "Growth factor mRNA levels in alopecia areata before and after treatment with the contact allergen diphenylcyclopropenone," *Acta Dermato-Venereologica*, 76(1), 17–20 (January 1996).

2. Sharma, V.K., "Pulsed administration of corticosteroids in the treatment of alopecia areata," *International Journal of Dermatology*, 35(2), 133–136 (February 1996).

3. Bensky, D., Barolet, R. *Chinese Herbal Medicine: Formulas and Strategies* (Seattle: Eastland Press, 1990), p. 350.

Hangover

1. Tipton, K.F., Heneman, G.T.M., McCrodden, J.M., "Metabolic and nutritional aspects of alcohol," *Biochemical Society Transactions*, 11, 59–61 (1983).

2. Sakai, K., Saitoh, Y., Ikawa, C., Nishihata, T., "Effect of water extracts of aloe and some herbs in decreasing blood ethanol concentration in rats. II," *Chemical & Pharmaceutical Bulletin*, 37(1), 155–159 (January 1989).

3. Chung, J.H., Cheong, J.C., Lee, J.Y., Roh, H.K., Cha, Y.N., "Acceleration of the alcohol oxidation rate in rats with aloin, a quinone derivative of *Aloe*," *Biochemical Pharmacology*, 52(9), 1461–1468 (8 November 1996).

4. Hobbs, C. *Ginseng: The Energy Herb* (Santa Cruz, California: Botanica Press, 1996), p. 34.

5. Nishiyama, N., Wang, Y.L., Saito H., "Beneficial effects of S-113m, a novel herbal prescription, on learning impairment model in mice," *Biological & Pharmaceutical Bulletin*, 18(11), 1498–1503 (November 1995).

6. Wickramasinghe, S.N., Hasan, R., Khalpey, Z., "Differences in the serum levels of acetaldehyde and cytotoxic acetaldehyde-albumin complexes after the consumption of red and white wine: in vitro effects of flavonoids, vitamin E, and other dietary antioxidants on cytotoxic complexes," *Alcoholism, Clinical & Experimental Research*, 20(5), 799–803 (August 1996).

Hemorrhoids

1. Ikeuchi, T., Ueno, M., Yogi, S., Hasegawa, K., Sasaki, H., Hamashima., T., "Clinical studies on chronic prostatitis and prostatitis-like syndrome. (5) Evaluation of prostatitis complicated by anal disease," *Hinyokika Kiyo*, 37(120), 1677–1682 (December 1991).

2. Wadworth, A.N., Faulds, D., "Hydroxyethylrutosides: a reivew of its pharmacology and therapeutic efficacy to venous insufficiency and related disorders," *Drugs*, 44, 1013–1032 (1992).

3. Saggloro, A., et al., "Treatment of hemorrhoidal syndrome with mesoglycan," *Minerva Dietética é Gastroenterlogica*, 31, 311–315 (1985).

Hepatitis

1. Wang, X., "Treatment of 100 cases of viral hepatitis with Compound 370," *Shanghai Journal of Traditional Chinese Medicine*, 4,5, cited by C. Hobbs in *Medicinal Mushrooms: An Exploration of*

Tradition, Healing, and Culture, Second Edition (Botanica Press: Santa Cruz, California, 1995), p. 241.

2. Guo, D., "Preliminary observation on carboy-methyl *Poria cocos* polysaccharide (CMPLP) in treating chronic viral hepatitis," *Journal of Traditional Chinese Medicine,* 4, 282 (1984).

3. Sato, H., Goto, W., Yamamura, J., Kurokawa, M., Kageyama, S., Takahara, T., Watanabe, A., Shiraki, K., "Therapeutic basis of glycyrrhizin on chronic hepatitis B," *Antiviral Research,* 30(2–3), 171–177 (May 1996).

4. Takahara, T., Watanabe, A., Shiraki, K., "Effects of glycyrrhizin on hepatitis B surface antigen, a biochemical and morphological study," *Journal of Hepatology,* 21(4), 601–609 (October 1994).

5. Abe, Y., Ueda, T., Kato, T., Kohli, Y., "Effectiveness of interferon, glycyrrhizin combination therapy in patients with chronic hepatitis C," *Nippon Rinsho—Japanese Journal of Clinical Medicine,* 52(7), 1817–1822 (July 1994).

6. Crance, J.M., Leveque, F., Chousterman, S., Jouan, A., Terpo, C., Deloince, R., "Antiviral activity of recombinant interferon-alpha on hepatitis A virus replication in human liver cells," *Antiviral Research,* 28(1), 69–80 (September 1995).

7. Chen, Y.Y., Yang, Y.Q., "Studies on the SGPT-lowering active component of the fruits of *Schisandra rubriflora* Rhed et Wils," *Yao Hsueh Hsueh Pao—Acta Pharmaceutica Sinica,* 17(4), 312–313 (April 1982).

8. Ko, K.M., Ip, S.P., Poon, M.K., Wu, S.S., Che, C.T., Ng, K.H., Kong, Y.C., "Effect of a lignan-enriched Fructus Schisandrae extract on hepatic glutathione status in rats: protection against carbon tetrachloride toxicity," *Planta Medica,* 61(2), 134–137 (April 1995).

9. Kubo, S., Ohkura, Y., Mizoguchi, Y., Matsui-Yuasa, I., Otani, S., Morisawa, S., Kinoshita, H., Takeda, S., Aburada, M., Hosoya, E., "Effect of Gomisin A (TJN-101) on liver regeneration," *Planta Medica,* 58(6), 489–492 (December 1992).

10. Yamaoka, Y., Kawakita, T., Kaneko, M., Nomoto, K., "A polysaccharide fraction of *shosaiko-to* active in augmentation of natural killer activity by oral administration," *Biological & Pharmaceutical Bulletin,* 18(6), 846–849 (1995).

11. Yamamoto, S., Oka, H., Kanno, T., Mizoguchi, Y., Kobayashi, K., "Controlled prospective trial to evaluate *syosakiko-to* in preventing hepatocellular carcinoma in patients with cirrhosis of the liver," *Gan to Kagaku Ryoho—Japanese Journal of Cancer and Chemotherapy,* 1 (4, Pt 2–2), 1519–1524 (April 1989).

12. Yamashiki, M., Asakawa, M., Kayaba, Y., Kosaka, Y., Nishimura, A., "Herbal medicine '*sho-saiko-to*' induces in vitro granulocyte colony-stimulating factor production on peripheral blood mononuclear cells," *Journal of Clinical & Laboratory Immunology,* 37(2), 83–90 (1992).

13. Yamashiki, M., Nishimura, A., Suzuki, H., Sakaguchi, S., et al., "Effects of the Japanese herbal medicine '*sho-saiko-to*' (TJ-9) on in vitro interleukein-10 production by peripheral blood mononuclear cells of patients with chronic hepatitis C," *Hepatology,* 25(6), 1390–1397 (June 1987).

14. Bensky, D., Barolet, R. *Chinese Herbal Medicine: Formulas and Strategies* (Seattle, Washington: Eastland Press, 1990), p. 137.

15. Wang, X., "Treatment of 100 cases of viral hepatitis with Compound 370," *Shanghai Journal of Traditional Chinese Medicine,* 4:5, cited by C. Hobbs in *Medicinal Mushrooms: An Exploration of Tradition, Healing, and Culture,* Second Edition (Botanica Press: Santa Cruz, California, 1995), p. 241.

Inset: The ABCs of Hepatitis

1. Polish, L.B., Gallagher, M., Fields, H.A., Hadler, S.C., "Delta hepatitis: molecular biology and clinical and epidemiologic features," *Clinical Microbiology Review,* 6, 211–219 (1993).

2. Feinman, S.V., Kim, J.P., Blajchman, M.A., Harding, G., Herst, R., Minuk, G., et al., "Post-transfusion hepatitis G (PTH-G)," *Hepatology,* 24, 415A (1996).

3. Pilot-Matias, T.J., Carrick, R.J., Coleman, P.F., Leary, T.P., Surowy, T.K., Simons, J.N., et al., "Expression of the GB virus C E2 glycoprotein using the Semliki Forest virus vector system and its utility as a serologic marker," *Virology,* 225, 282–292 (1996).

Herpes

1. Akiba, M., Yoshida, I., Suzutani, T., Ogasawara, M., Azuma, M., "Relationship of the strain and the intraocular amount of herpes simplex virus types 1 and 2 in the induction of anterior-chamber-associated immune deviation," *Ophthalmic Research,* 28(5), 289–295 (1996).

2. Richards, C.M., Shimeld, C., Williams, N.A., Hill, T.J., "Induction of mucosal immunity against herpes simplex virus type 1 in the mouse protects against ocular infection and establishment of latency," *Journal of Infectious Disease,* 77(6), 451–457 (June 1998).

3. Nagasaka, K., Kurokawa, M., Imakita, M., Terasawa, K., Shiraki, K., "Efficacy of *kakkon-to,* a traditional herb medicine, in herpes simplex virus type 1 infection in mice," *Journal of Medical Virology,* 46(1), 28–34 (May 1995).

4. Kurokawa, M., Nagasaka, K., Hirabayashi, T., Uyama, S., Sato, H., Kageyama, T., Kadota, S., Ohyama, H., Hozumi, T., Namba, T., et al., "Efficacy of traditional herbal medicines in combination with acyclovir against herpes simplex virus type 1 infection in vitro and in vivo," *Antiviral Research,* 27(1–2), 19–37 (May 1995).

5. Tangi, K.K., et al., "Biochemical study of anti-inflammatory and anti-arthritic properties of glycyrrhetic acid," *Biochemical Pharmacology,* 14, 1277–1281 (1965).

6. Sydiskis, R.J., Owen, D.G., Lohr, J.L., Rosler, K.H., Blomster, R.N., "Inactivation of enveloped viruses by anthraquinones extracted from plants," *Antimicrobial Agents in Chemotherapy,* 35(12), 2463–2466 (December 1991).

7. Andersen, D.O., Weber, N.D., Wood, S.G., Hughes, B.G., Murray, B.K., North, J.A., "In vitro virucidal activity of selected anthraquinones and anthraquinone derivatives," *Antiviral Research,* 16(2), 185–196 (September 1991).

8. Bourinbaiar, A.S., Lee-Huang, S., "The activity of plant-derived antiretroviral proteins MAP30 and GAP31 against herpes simplex virus in vitro," *Biochemical & Biophysical Research Communications,* 219(3), 923–929 (February 1996).

9. Kurokawa, M., Nagasaka, K., Hirabayashi, T., Uyama, S., Sato, H., Kageyama, T., Kadota, S., Ohyama, H., Hozumi, T., Namba, T., et al., pp. 19–37.

10. Vonka, V., Petrovska, P., Borecky, L., Roth, Z., "Increased effects of topically applied interferon on herpes simplex virus-induced lesions by caffeine," *Acta Virologica,* 39(3), 125–130 (June 1995).

11. Nagasaka, K., Kurokawa, M., Imakita, M., Terasawa, K., Shiraki, K., pp. 28–34.

12. Saito, S., Nagase, S., Ichinose, K., "New steroidal saponins from the rhizomes of *Anemarrhena asphodeloides* Bunge. (Liliaceae)," *Chemical Pharmacology Bulletin* (Tokyo), 42(11), 2342–2345 (November 1994).

13. Zheng, M.S., Lu, Z.Y., "Antiviral effect of mangiferin and isomangiferin on herpes simplex virus," *Chinese Medical Journal*, 103(2), 160–165 (February 1990).

High Blood Pressure

1. Wong, N.D., Ming, S., Zhou, H.Y., Black, H.R., "A comparison of Chinese traditional and Western medical approaches for the treatment of mild hypertension," *Yale Journal of Biology and Medicine*, 64(1), 79–87 (January 1991).

2. Ogawa, S., Nishimoto, N., Matsuda, H., "Pharmacology of ecdysones in vertebrates," in Burdette, W.J. (ed). *Invertebrate Endocrinology and Hormonal Heterophylly* (Berlin: Springer-Verlag, 1974), pp. 341–344.

3. Huang, K.C. *The Pharmacology of Chinese Herbs* (Boca Raton, Florida: CRC Press, 1993), p. 140.

4. Kang, S.Y., Schini-Kerth, V.B., Kim, N.D., "Ginsenosides of the protopanaxatriol group cause endothelium-dependent relaxation in the rat aorta," *Life Sciences*, 56(19), 1577–1586 (1995).

5. Hara, Y., "Prophylactic functions of tea polyphenols," in Ho, C.T., Osawa, T., Huang, M.T., Rosen, R. (eds). *Food Phytochemicals for Cancer Prevention II: Teas, Spices, and Herbs* (Washington: American Chemical Society, 1994), p. 44–45.

6. Petkov, V., "Plants and hypotensive, antiatheromatous and coronarodilatating action," *American Journal of Chinese Medicine*, 7(3), 197–236 (1979).

7. Blumenthal, M., Busse, W.R., Goldberg, A., Gruenwald, J., Hall, T., Riggins, C.W., Rister, R.S., eds., Klein, S., Rister, R.S., trans. *The Complete German Commission E Monographs: Therapeutic Guide to Herbal Medicines* (Boston: Integrative Medicine Communications, 1998), p. 172.

8. Huang, K C., p. 279.

9. Bensky, D., Gamble, A., Kaptchuk, T., Bensky, L.L. *Chinese Herbal Medicine: Materia Medica*, Revised Edition (Seattle: Eastland Press, 1993), p. 77.

10. Wei, M.J., Shintania, F., Kanba, S., Yagi, G., Asai, M., Kato, R., Nakaki, T., "Endothelium-dependent and -independent vasoactive actions of a Japanese kampo medicine, *Saiko-ka-ryukotsu-borei-to*," *Biomedical Pharmacotherapy*, 51(1), 38–43 (1997).

11. Mori, M., Hojo, E., Takano, K., "Action of *oren-gedoku-to* on platelet aggregation in vitro," *American Journal of Chinese Medicine*, 19(2), 131–143 (1991).

12. Hirawa, N., Uehara, Y., Kawabata, Y., Numabe, A., Takad, S., Nagoshi, H., Gomi, T., Ikeda, T., Omata, M., "*Hachimi-jio-gan* extract protects the kidney from hypertensive injury in Dahl salt-sensitive rat," *American Journal of Chinese Medicine*, 24(3–4), 241–254 (1996).

13. Hiwara, N., Uehara, Y., Takada, S., Kawabata, Y., Ohshima, N., Nagata, T., Ishimitsu, T., Gomi, T., Goto, A., Ikeda, T., et al., "Antihypertensive property and renal protection by *shichimotsu-koka-to* extract in salt-induced hypertension in Dahl strain rats," *American Journal of Chinese Medicine*, 22(1), 51–62 (1994).

14. Murakami, Y., Kato, Y., "Sleep disorders in several pathologic states—endocrine diseases," *Nippon Rinsho*, 56(2), 457–460 (February 1998). American studies have reached similar conclusions.

15. Takashima, Y., Iwase, Y., Yoshida, M., Kokaze, A., Takagi, Y., Tsubono, Y., Tsugane, S., Takahashi, T., Iitoi, Y., Akabane, M., Watanabe, S., Akamatsu, T., "Relationship of food intake and dietary patterns with blood pressure levels among middle-aged Japanese men," *Journal of Epidemiology*, 8(2), 106–115 (June 1998).

High Cholesterol

1. Huang, Y., et al., "Toxicological studies on cultured *Cordyceps sinsensis*, strain B414," *Zhongchengyao Yanjiu*, 10, 24–25 (1987).

2. Harenberg, J., Giese, C., Zimmermann, R., "Effect of dried garlic on blood coagulation, fibrinolysis, platelet aggregation and serum cholesterol levels in patients with hyperlipoproteinemia," *Atherosclerosis*, 74, 247–249 (1988).

3. Augusti, K.T., Benaim, M.E., "Effect of essential oil of onion (allyl propyl disulphide) on blood glucose, free fatty acid, and insulin levels of normal subjects," *Chemical Abstracts*, 83(22), 593 (1975).

4. Kimoto, M., et al., "Effects of shiitake mushroom on plasma and liver lipid contents in rats," *Eiyo to Shokuryo*, 29, 275–281 (1976).

5. Tsumura, A. *Kampo: How the Japanese Updated Traditional Herbal Medicine* (San Francisco: Kodansha, 1991), pp. 67–68.

6. Yoshida, K., Mizukawa, H., Honmura, A., Uchiyama, Y., Nakajima, S., Haruki, E., "The effect of *sho-saiko-to* on concentration of vitamin E in serum and on granuloma formation in carrageenin cotton pellet-induced granuloma rats," *American Journal of Chinese Medicine*, 22(2), 183–189 (1994).

7. Muldoon, M.F., Kritchevsky, S.B., Evans, R.W., Kagan, V.E., "Serum total antioxidant activity in relative hypo- and hypercholesterolemia," *Free Radical Research*, 25(3), 239–245 (September 1996).

8. Glueck, C.J., Tieger, M., Kunkel, R., Hamer, T., Tracy, T., Speirs, J., "Hypocholesterolemia and affective disorders," *American Journal of the Medical Sciences*, 308(4), 218–225 (October 1994).

9. Kereveur, A., Cambillau, M., Kazatchkine, M., Moatti, N., "Lipoprotein anomalies in HIV infections," *Annales de Medicine Interne*, 147(5), 333–343 (1996).

Inset: Cholesterol and Diet—The Whole Picture

1. Cited in Bernstein, R. *Dr. Bernstein's Diabetes Solution* (New York: Little, Brown & Company, 1997), p. 314.

2. Ibid.

HIV Infection

1. Huss, R., "Inhibition of cyclophilin function in HIV-1 infection by cyclosporin A," *Immunology Today*, 17, 259–260 (1996).

2. Zinkernagel, R.M., "MHC-restricted T-cell recognition," *Journal of the American Medical Association*, 274, 1069–1071 (1995).

3. Andrieu, J.M., Lu, W., "Viro-immunopathogenesis of HIV disease: implications for therapy," *Immunology Today*, 16, 5–7, 1995.

4. Arora, P.K., Fride, E., Petitio, J., et al., "Morphine-induced immune alterations in vivo," *Cellular Immunology*, 126, 343–353 (1990).

5. Piras, G., Makino, M., Baba, M., "*Sho-saiko-to*, a traditional Kampo medicine, enhances the anti-HIV-1 activity of lamivudine

(3TC) in vitro," *Microbiology and Immunology,* 41(10), 835–839, (1997).

6. Zhang, B.Z., Ding, F., Tan, L.W., "Clinical and experimental study on *yi-gan-ning* granule in treating chronic hepatitis B," *Chung-Kuo Chung Hsi I Chieh Ho Tsa Chih—Chinese Journal of Modern Developments in Traditional Medicine,* 13(10), 597–599, 580 (October 1993).

7. Tochikura, T.S., et al., "Inhibition (in vitro) of replication and of the cytopathic effect of human immunodeficiency virus by an extract of the culture medium of *Lentinus edodes* mycelia," *Medical Microbiology and Immunology* (Berlin), 177(5), 235–244 (1988).

8. Nanba, H., "Immunostimulant activity in-vivo and anti-HIV activity in vitro of 3 branched b-1-6 glucans extracted from maitake mushroom (*Grifola frondosa*)," Eighth International Conference on AIDS, 1992.

9. Yao, X.J., Wainberg, M.A., Parniak, M.A., "Mechanism of inhibition of HIV-1 infection in vitro by purified extract of *Prunella vulgaris,*" *Virology,* 187(1), 56–62 (March 1992).

10. Li, B.Q., Fu, T., Yan, Y.D., Baylor, N.W., Ruscetti, F.W., Kung, H.F., "Inhibition of HIV infection by baicalin—a flavonoid compound purified from Chinese herbal medicine," *Cellular & Molecular Biology Research,* 39(2), 119–124 (1993).

11. Li, C.J., et al., "Three inhibitors of human type 1 immunodeficiency virus long terminal repeat directed gene expression and virus replication," *Proceedings of the National Academy of Sciences,* 90, 1839–1841 (1993).

12. Mazumder, A., et al., "Inhibition of human immunodeficiency virus type-1 integrase by curcumin," *Biochemical Pharmacology,* 49, 1165–1170 (1995).

13. Singh, S., Aggarwal, B.B., "Activation of transcription factor NF-Kappa B is suppressed by curcumin (diferulolylmethane)," *Journal of Biological Chemistry,* 270(42), 24995–25000 (20 October 1995).

14. Chang, R.S., Yeung, H.W., "Inhibition of growth of human immunodeficiency virus in vitro by crude extracts of Chinese medicinal herbs," *Antiviral Research,* 9(3), 163–175 (April 1998).

15. Ngan, F., Chang, R.S., Tabba, H.D., Smith, K.M., "Isolation, purification and partial characterization of an active anti-HIV compound from the Chinese medicinal herb *Viola yedoensis,*" *Antiviral Research,* 10(1–3), 107–116 (November 1988).

16. Buimovici-Klein, E., Mohan, V., Lange, M., Fenamore, E., Inada, Y., Cooper, L.Z., "Inhibition of HIV replication in lymphocyte cultures of virus-positive subjects in the presence of *sho-saiko-to,* an Oriental plant extract," *Antiviral Research,* 14(405), 279–286 (October 1990).

17. Ono, K., Nakane, H., Fukushima, M., Chermann, J.C., Barre-Sinoussi, F., "Differential inhibition of the activities of reverse transcriptase and various cellular DNA polymerases by a traditional Kampo drug, *sho-saiko-to,*" *Biomedical Pharmacotherapy,* 44(1), 13–16 (1990).

18. Zhang, Q., Hsu, H.Y. *AIDS and Chinese Medicine: Applications of the Oldest Medicine to the Newest Disease* (Long Beach, California: Oriental Healing Arts Institute Press, 1990), pp. 82–83.

19. Ono, K., et al., "Inhibition of HIV-reverse transcriptase by a Kampo medicine, *sho-saiko-to,*" *Proceedings of the Fifth International Conference on AIDS, Montreal, Quebec, Canada, June 4–9, 1989,* p. 565.

20. Zhang, Q., Hsu, H.Y., p. 30.

21. Stanley, S.K., et al., "Effective immunization with a common recall antigen on viral expression in patients infected with HIV1," *New England Journal of Medicine,* 334, 1222–1230 (1996).

22. Munro, S., Thomas, K.L., Abu-Shaar, M., "Molecular characterization of peripheral receptor for cannabinoids," *Nature,* 365, 61–65 (1993).

Hodgkin's Disease

1. Liang, H., Zhang, Y., Geng, B., "The effect of astragalus polysaccharides (APS) on cell mediated immunity (CMI) in burned mice," *Chung-Hua Cheng Hsing Shao Shang Wai Ko Tsa Chih—Chinese Journal of Plastic Surgery & Burns,* 10(2), 138–141 (March 1994).

2. Wagner, H., "Immunostimulants from medicinal plants," in Chang, H.M., Yeung, W., Tso, W., Koo, A. (eds). *Advances in Chinese Medicinal Materials Research* (Singapore: World Scientific, 1985).

Hyperthyroidism

1. Hidaka, Y., Masai, T., Sumizaki, H., Takeoka, K., Tada, H., Amino, N., "Onset of Graves' thyrotoxicosis after an attack of allergic rhinitis," *Thyroid,* 6(4), 349–351 (August 1996).

2. Yanagawa, T., Ito, K., Kaplan, E.L., Ishikawa, N., DeGroot, L.J., "Absence of association between human spumaretrovirus and Graves' disease," *Thyroid,* 5(5), 379–382 (October 1995).

3. Mizokami, T., Okamura, K., Kohno, T., Sato, K., Ikenoue, H., Kuroda, T., Inokuchi, K., Fujishima, M., "Human T-lymphotropic virus type I-associated uveitis in patients with Graves' disease treated with methylmercaptoimidazole," *Journal of Clinical Endocrinology & Metabolism,* 80(6), 1904–1907 (June 1995).

4. Nagai, T., Suzuki, Y., Tomimori, T., Yamada, H., "Antiviral activity of plant flavonoid, 5,7,4'-trihydroxy-8-methoxyflavone, from the roots of *Scutellaria baicalensis* against influenza A (H3N2) and B viruses," *Biological & Pharmaceutical Bulletin,* 18(2), 295–299 (February 1995).

5. Nagai, T., Miyaichi, Y., Tomimori, T., Suzuki, Y., Yamada, H., "Inhibition of influenza virus sialidase and anti-influenza virus activity by plant flavonoids," *Chemical & Pharmaceutical Bulletin,* 38(5), 1329–1332 (May 1990).

6. Isselbacher, K.J., Braunwald, E., Wilson, J., Martin, J.V., Fauci, A.S., Kasper, D.L., eds. *Harrison's Principles of Internal Medicine,* Thirteenth Edition (New York: McGraw-Hill, 1995), pp. 1952–1953.

Hypothyroidism

1. Chen, H.P., He, J.S., Hu, G.S., "Analysis on the traditional Chinese medicine syndromes of the patients with autoimmune thyroid diseases. Changes in the thyroid and immune functions in 109 cases," *Chung Hsi I Chieh Ho Tsa Chih,* 10(9), 538–539 (September 1990).

2. Nagai, T., Suzuki, Y., Tomimori, T., Yamada, H., "Antiviral activity of plant flavonoid, 5,7,4'-trihydroxy-8-methoxyflavone, from the roots of *Scutellaria baicalensis* against influenza A (H3N2) and B viruses," *Biological & Pharmaceutical Bulletin,* 18(2), 295–299 (February 1995).

3. Nagai, T., Miyaichi, Y., Tomimori, T., Suzuki, Y., Yamada, H., "Inhibition of influenza virus sialidase and anti-influenza virus activity by plant flavonoids," *Chemical & Pharmaceutical Bulletin,* 38(5), 1329–1332 (May 1990).

4. Isselbacher, K.J., Braunwald, E., Wilson, J., Martin, J.V., Fauci, A.S., Kasper, D.L., eds. *Harrison's Principles of Internal Medicine,* Thirteenth Edition (New York: McGraw-Hill, 1995), pp. 1952–1953.

Impotence

1. Huang, K.C. *The Pharmacology of Chinese Herbs* (Boca Raton, Florida: CRC Press, 1992), p. 35.

2. Kang, S.Y., Schini-Kerth, V.B., Kim, N.D., "Ginsenosides of the protopanaxatriol group cause endothelium-dependent relaxation in the rat aorta," *Life Sciences,* 56(19), 1577–1586 (1995).

3. Fujihira, K., Hays, N.K. *Common Health Complaints* (Long Beach, California: Oriental Healing Arts Press, 1981), p. 31.

4. Mar, S., personal communication with author, 5 June 1996.

Incontinence

1. "Differentiations to UTI protocol," *Protocol Journal of Botanical Medicine,* 1(1), 135 (Summer 1995).

Indigestion, Belching

1. Brandt, W., "Spasmolytische Wirkung ätherischer Öle," in *Phytotherapie* (Stuttgart, Germany: Hippokrates, 1988), pp. 77–89.

2. Sigmund, C.J., McNally, E.F., "The action of a carminative on the lower esophageal sphincter," *Gastroenterology,* 56, 13–18 (1969).

Indigestion, Bloating and Flatulence

1. Hebbard, G.S., Sun, W.M., Dent, J., Horowitz, M., "Hyperglycaemia affects proximal gastric motor and sensory function in normal subjects," *European Journal of Gastroenterology and Hepatology,* 8(3), 211–217 (March 1996).

2. Suarez, F.L., Furne, J.K., Springfield, J., Levitt, M.D., "Bismuth subsalicylate markedly decreases hydrogen sulfide release in the human colon," *Gastroenterology,* 114(5), 923–929 (May 1998).

Infertility, Female

1. Sakamoto, S., Kudo, H., Kawasaki, T., Kuwa, K., Kasahara, N., Sassa, S., Okamoto, R., "Effects of a Chinese herbal medicine, *keishi-bukuryo-gan,* on the gonadal system of rats," *Journal of Ethnopharmacology,* 23 (2–3), 151–158 (July–August 1988).

2. Takahashi, K., Kitao, M., "Effect of TJ-68 (*shakuyaku-kanzo-to*) on polycystic ovarian disease," *International Journal of Fertility and Menopausal Studies,* 39(2), 69–76 (March–April 1994).

Infertility, Male

1. Hong, C.Y., Ku, J., Wu, P., "*Astragalus membranaceus* stimulates human sperm motility in vitro," *American Journal of Chinese Medicine,* 20(3–4), 289–294 (1992).

2. Ishikawa, H., et al., "Effects of *guizhi-fuling-wan* on male infertility with varicocele," *American Journal of Chinese Medicine,* 24, 327–331 (1996).

3. Sudo, K., Honda, K., Taki, M., Kanitani, M., Fujii, Y., Aburada, M., Hosoya, E., Kimura, M., Orikasa, S., "Effects of TJ-41 (Tsumura *hochu-ekki-to*) on spermatogenic disorders in mice under current treatment with adriamycin," *Nippon Yakurigaku Zasshi—Folia Pharmacologica Japonica,* 92(4), 251–261 (October 1988).

Influenza

1. Shimamura, T., "Inhibition of influenza virus infection by tea polyphenols," in Ho, C.T., Osawa, T., Huang, M.T., Rosen, R. (eds). *Food Phytochemicals for Cancer Prevention II: Teas, Spices, and Herbs* (Washington: American Chemical Society, 1994), pp. 101–104.

2. Nagai, T., Suzuki, Y., Tomimori, T., Yamada, H., "Antiviral activity of plant flavonoid, 5,7,4'-trihydroxy-8-methoxyflavone, from the roots of *Scutellaria baicalensis* against influenza A (H3N2) and B viruses," *Biological & Pharmaceutical Bulletin,* 18(2), 295–299 (February 1995).

3. Nagai, T., Miyaichi, Y., Tomimori, T., Suzuki, Y., Yamada, H., "Inhibition of influenza virus sialidase and anti-influenza virus activity by plant flavonoids," *Chemical & Pharmaceutical Bulletin,* 38(5), 1329–1332 (May 1990).

Irritable Bowel Syndrome

1. Swiatkowski, M., Klopocka, M., Suppan, K., "Hypersensitivity reactions in patients with irritable colon syndrome," *Wiadomosci Lekarskie,* 46(13–14), 482–488 (July 1993).

2. Zhou, N.N., Nakai, S., Kawakita, T., Oka, M., Nagasawa, H., Himeno, K., Nomoto, K., "Combined treatment of autoimmune MRL/MP-lpr/lpr mice with a herbal medicine, *ren-shen-yang-rong-tang* (Japanese name, *ninjin-youei-to*) plus suboptimal dosage of prednisolone," *International Journal of Immunopharmacology,* 16(10), 845–854 (October 1994).

Kidney Cancer (Renal Cell Carcinoma)

1. Negrier, S., Escudier, B., Lasset, C., Douillard, J.Y., Savary, J., Chervreau, C., Ravaud, A., Mercatello, A., Peny, J., Mousseau, M., Philip, T., Tursz, T., "Recombinant human interleukin-2, recombinant human interferon alfa-2a, or both in metastatic renal-cell carcinoma. Groupe Francais d'Immunotherapie," *New England Journal of Medicine,* 338(18), 1271–1278 (April 1998).

2. California Kidney Cancer Center, personal communication with author, 31 August 1998.

3. Negrier, S., et al., pp. 1271–1278.

4. Kushi, M., Jack, A. *The Cancer Prevention Diet* (New York: St. Martin's Griffin, 1993), pp. 196–197.

5. Zhao, T.H., "Positive modulating action of *shenmaisan* with *Astralagus membranaceus* on anti-tumor activity of LAK cells," *Chung Hsi I Chieh Ho Tsa Chih,* 13(8), 471–472 (1993).

6. Chu, D., Sun, Y., Lin, J., Wong, W., Mavligit, G., "F3, a fractionated extract of *Astragalus membranaceus,* potentiates lymphokine-activated killer cell cytotoxicity generated by low-dose recombinant interleukin-2," *Chung Hsi I Chieh Ho Tsa Chih,* 10(1), 34–36 (January 1990).

7. Liu, C.X., Lu, S., Ji, M.R., "Effects of *Cordyceps sinensis* on in vitro natural killer cells," *Chung-Kuo Chung Hsi I Chieh Ho Tsa Chih—Chinese Journal of Modern Developments in Traditional Medicine,* 12 (5), 267–269, 259 (1992).

8. Ying, J., et al. *Icones of Medicinal Fungi From China* (Beijing: Science Press, 1987).

9. Suzuki, F., Schmitt, D.A., Utsunomiya, T., Pollard, R.B., "Stimulation of host resistance against tumors by glycyrrhizin, an active component of licorice roots," *In Vivo,* 6(6), 589–596 (November 1992).

10. Zhang, L.X., Mong, H., Zhou, X.B., "Effect of Japanese *Gano-*

derma lucidum (GL) planted in Japan on the production of interleukin-2 from murine splenocytes," *Chung Hsi I Chieh Ho Tsa Chih,* 10(11), 672–674 (1993).

11. Haak-Frendscho, M., Kino, K., Sone, T., et al., "Ling Zhi-8: a novel T-cell mitogen induces cytokine production and upregulation of ICAM-1 expression," *Cellular Immunology,* 150(1), 101–113 (1993).

12. Wagner, H., "Immunostimulants from medicinal plants," in Chang, H.M., Yeung, W., Tso, W., Koo, A. (eds). *Advances in Chinese Medicinal Materials Research* (Singapore: World Scientific, 1985).

13. Zee-Cheng, R.K., "*Shi-quan-da-bu-tang* (ten significant tonic decoction), SQT. A potent Chinese biological response modifier in cancer immunotherapy, potentiation and detoxification of anticancer drugs," *Methods & Findings in Experimental & Clinical Pharmacology,* 14(9), 725–736 (November 1992).

Kidney Disease

1. Hattori, T., Nagamatsu, T., Ito, M., Suzuki, Y., "Studies on the antinephritic effect of TJ-8014, a new Japanese herbal medicine, and its mechanisms (2): Effect on the release of corticosterone from adrenal glands," *Japanese Journal of Pharmacology,* 51(1), 117–124 (September 1989).

2. Li, P., Kawachi, H., Morioka, T., Orikasa, M., Oite, T., Shi, Z.S., Shimizu, F., "Suppressive effects of *sairei-to* on monoclonal antibody 1-22-3-induced glomerulonephritis: analysis of effective components," *Pathology International,* 47(7), 430–435 (July 1997).

3. Hattori, T., Fujitsuka, N., Kurogi, A., Shindo, S., "*Sairei-to* may inhibit the synthesis of endothelin-1 in nephritic glomeruli," *Nippon Jinzo Gakkai Shinbun,* 39(2), 121–128 (March 1997).

4. Yoshikawa, N., Ito, H., Sakai, T., Takekoshi, Y., Honda, M., Awazu, M., Ito, K., Iitaka, K., Koitabashi, Y., Yamaoka, K., Nakagawa, K., Nakamura, H., Matsuyama, S., Seino, Y., Takeda, N., Hattori, S., Ninomiya, M., "A prospective controlled study of *sairei-to* in childhood IgA nephropathy with focal/minimal mesangial proliferation (Japanese Pediatric IgA Nephropathy Treatment Study Group)," *Nippon Jinzo Gakkai Shinbun,* 39(5), 503–506 (July 1997).

5. Hattori, T., Shindo, S., "Effects of *sairei-to* (TJ-114) on the expression of adhesion molecule in anti-GBM nephritic rats," *Nippon Jinzo Gakkai Shinbun,* 37(7), 373–383 (July 1995).

6. Li, P., Kawachi, H., Morioka, T., Orikasa, M., Oite, T., Shi, Z.S., Shimizu, F., pp. 430–435.

7. Huang, Y., Marumo, K., Urai, M., "Antitumor effects and pharmacological interaction of *xiao-chai-hu-tang (sho-saiko-to)* and interleukin 2 in murine renal cell carcinoma," *Keio Medical Journal,* 46(3), 132–137 (September 1997).

8. Goto, M., Hayashi, M., Todoroki, T., Seyama, Y., Yamashita, S., "Effects of traditional Chinese medicines (*dai-saiko-to, sho-saiko-to,* and *hachimi-zio-gan*) on spontaneously diabetic rat (WBN/Kob) with experimentally induced lipid and mineral disorders," *Nippon Yakurigaku Zasshi,* 100(4), 353–358 (October 1992).

Kidney Stones

1. Berg, W., et al., "Influence of anthraquinones on the formation of urinary calculi in experimental animals," *Urologe A,* 15, 188–191 (1976).

2. Anton, R., Haag-Berrurier, M., "Therapeutic use of natural anthraquinone for other than laxative actions," *Pharmacology,* 20, 104–112 (1980).

3. Berg, W., et al., pp. 188–191.

4. Anton, R., Haag-Berrurier, M., pp. 104–112.

5. Sugaya, K., Nishizawa, O., Noto, H., Sato, K., Sato, K., Shimoda, N., Otomo, R., Tsuchida, S., "Effects of Tsumura *chorei-to* and Tsumura *chorei-to-go-shimotsu-to* on patients with urethral syndrome," *Hinyokika Kiyo—Acta Urologica Japonica,* 38(6), 731–745 (June 1992).

6. Huang, K.C. *The Pharmacology of Chinese Herbs* (Boca Raton, Florida: CRC Press, 1993), p. 293.

Inset: Using Diet to Prevent Kidney Stones

1. Zechner, O., et al., "Nutritional factors in urinary stone disease," *Journal of Urology,* 125, 51–55 (1981).

2. Robertson, W., et al., "Prevalence of urinary stone disease in vegetarians," *European Urology,* 8, 334–339 (1982).

3. Griffith, H., et al., "A control study of dietary factors in renal stone formation," *British Journal of Urology,* 53, 416–420 (1981).

4. Shaw, P., "Idiopathic hypercalciuria: its control with unprocessed bran," *British Journal of Urology,* 52, 426–249 (1980).

5. Robertson, W., et al., pp. 334–339.

6. Rose, G., Westbury, E., "The influence of calcium content of water, intake of vegetables and fruit and of other food factors upon the incidence of renal calculi," *Urology Research,* 3, 61–66 (1975).

Leukemia

1. "Smoking tied to leukemia risk," *New York Times,* 23 February 1993.

2. Kobayashi, I., Hamasaki, Y., Yamamoto, S., Hayasaki, R., Zaitsu, M., Muro, E., Matsumoto, S., Ichimaru, T., Miyazaki, S., "Inhibitory effects of *saiboku-to* and component herbs on the production of peptide leukotrienes LTs and LTB4," *Arerugi,* 45(6), 577–583 (June 1996).

3. Zheng, S., Yang, H., Zhang, S., Wang, X., Yu, L., Lu, J., Li, J., "Initial study on naturally occurring products from traditional Chinese herbs and vegetables for chemoprevention," *Journal of Cellular Biochemistry* (Suppl), 27, 106–112 (1997).

4. Lea, M.A., Xiao, Q., Sadhukhan, A.K., Cottle, S., Wang, Z.Y., Yang, C.S., "Inhibitory effects of tea extracts and (-)-epigallocatechin gallate on DNA synthesis and proliferation of hepatoma and erythroleukemia cells," *Cancer Letters,* 68(2–3), 231–236 (February 1993).

5. Fujie, K., Aoki, T., Ito, Y., Maeda, S., "Sister-chromatid exchanges induced by trihalomethanes in rat erythroblastic cells and their suppression by crude catechin extracted from green tea," *Mutation Research,* 300(3–4), 241–246 (August 1993).

6. Naasani, I., Seimiya, H., Tsuruo, T., "Telomerase inhibition, telomere shortening, and senescence of cancer cells by tea catechins," *Biochemistry and Biophysics Research Communications,* 249(2), 391–396 (August 1998).

7. Zhen, Y., Cao, S., Xue, Y., Wu, S., "Green tea extract inhibits nucleoside transport and potentiates the antitumor effect of antimetabolites," *Chinese Medical Science Journal,* 6(1), 1–5 (March 1991).

8. Asano, Y., Okamura, S., Ogo, T., Eto, T., Otsuka, T., Niho, Y., "Effect of (-)-epigallocatechine gallate on leukemic blast cells

from patients with acute myeloblastic leukemia," *Life Sciences,* 60(2), 135–142 (1997).

9. Jing, Y., Nakaya, K., Han, R., "Differentiation of promyeloctic leukemia cells HL-60 induced by daidzein in vitro and in vivo," *Anticancer Research,* 13(4), 1049–1054 (1993).

10. Satoh, K., Sakagami, H., Nakamura, K., "Enhancement of radical intensity and cytotoxic activity of ascorbate by PSK and lignins," *Anticancer Research,* 16(5A), 2981–2986 (September–October 1996).

11. Ebina, T., Murata, K., "Antitumor effect of intratumoral administration of a *Coriolus* preparation, PSK: inhibition of tumor invasion in vitro," *Gan to Kagaku Ryoho—Japanese Journal of Cancer & Chemotherapy,* 21(13), 2241–2243 (September 1994).

12. Kawa, K., Konishi, S., Tsujino, G., Mabuchi, S., "Effects of biological response modifiers on childhood ALL being in remission after chemotherapy," *Biomedicine & Pharmacotherapy,* 45(2–3), 113–116 (1991).

13. Conney, A.H., Lou, Y.R., Xie, J.G., Osawa, T., Newmark, H.L., Liu, Y., Chang, R.L., Huang, M.T., "Some perspectives on dietary inhibition of carcinogenesis: studies with curcumin and tea," *Proceedings of the Society for Experimental Biology and Medicine,* 216(2), 234–245 (November 1997).

14. Zhang, Q., Hsu, H.Y. *AIDS and Chinese Medicine: Applications of the Oldest Medicine to the Newest Disease* (Long Beach, California: Oriental Healing Arts Institute Press, 1990), pp. 82–83.

15. Ono, K., et al., "Inhibition of HIV-reverse transcriptase by a Kampo medicine, *Sho-Saiko-To,*" *Proceedings of the Fifth International Conference on AIDS, Montreal, Quebec, Canada, June 4–9, 1989,* p. 565.

16. Ohsawa, T., Yukawa, M., Takao, C., Murayama, M., Bando, H., "Studies on constituents of fruit body of *Polyporus umbellatus* and their cytotoxic activity," *Chemical & Pharmaceutical Bulletin,* 40(1), 143–147 (January 1992).

17. Yamada. H., "Chemical characterization and biological activity of the immunologically active substances in *Juzen-taiho-to,*" *Gan to Kagaku Ryoho—Japanese Journal of Cancer & Chemotherapy,* 16(4 Pt 2–2), 1500–1505 (April 1989).

Liver Cancer

1. Ishak, K.G., "Hepatic neoplasia associated with contraceptive and anabolic steroids," *Recent Results in Cancer Research,* 66, 73–128 (1979).

2. Zhao, T.H., "Positive modulating action of *shenmaisan* with *Astralagus membranaceus* on anti-tumor activity of LAK cells," *Chung Hsi I Chieh Ho Tsa Chih,* 13(8), 471–472 (1993).

3. Zhang, B.Z., Ding, F., Tan, L.W., "Clinical and experimental study on *yi-gan-ning* granule in treating chronic hepatitis B," *Chung-Kuo Chung Hsi I Chieh Ho Tsa Chih—Chinese Journal of Modern Developments in Traditional Medicine,* 13(10), 597–599, 580 (October 1993).

4. Ling, J., Liu, W.Y., "Cytotoxicity of two new ribosome-inactivating proteins, cinnamomin and camphorin, to carcinoma cells," *Cell Biochemistry & Function,* 14(3), 157–161 (September 1996).

5. Chi, C.W., Chang, Y.F., Chao, T.W., Chiang, S.H., P'eng, F.K., Lui, W.Y., Liu, T.Y., "Flowcytometric analysis of the effect of berberine on the expression of glucocorticoid receptors in human hepatoma HepG2 cells," *Life Sciences,* 54(26), 2099–2107 (1994).

6. Sugano, N., et al., "Anticarcinogenic actions of water-soluble and alcohol-insoluble fractions from culture medium of *Lentinus edodes* mycelia," *Cancer Letters,* 17, 109–114 (1982).

7. Amagase, H., "Treatment of hepatitis B patients with *Lentinus edodes* mycelium," *Proceedings of the XII International Congress of Gastroenterology* (Lisbon), 197 (1987).

8. Toth, J.O., et al., "Les acides ganoderques T à Z: Triterpenes cytotoxiques de *Ganoderma lucidum* (Polyporacée)," *Tetrahedron Letters,* 24, 1081–1084 (1983).

9. Castiglione, S., Paggi, M.G., Delpino, A., et al., "Inhibition of protein synthesis in neoplastic cells by rhein," *Biochemical Pharmacology,* 40(5), 967–973 (1990).

10. Chang, H.M., But, P.P.H. *Pharmacology and Applications of Chinese Materia Medica,* Volume 2 (Teaneck, New Jersey: World Scientific Publishing, 1987), p. 783.

11. Razina, T.G., Udintsev, S.N., Prishchep, T.P., et al., "Enhancement of the selectivity of the action of the cytostatics cyclophosphamide and 5-fluoruracil by using an extract of the Baikal skullcap in an experiment," *Voprosii Onkologii,* 33(20), 80–84 (1987).

12. Razina, T.G., Udintsev, S.N., Tiutrin, I.I., et al., "The role of thrombocyte aggregation function in the mechanism of the antimetastatic action of an extract of Baikal skullcap," *Voprosii Onkologii,* 35(3), 331–335 (1989).

13. Yano, H., Mizoguchi, A., Fukuda, K., Haramaki, M., Ogasawara, S., Momosaki, S., Kojiro, M., "The herbal medicine *sho-saiko-to* inhibits proliferation of cancer cell lines by inducing apoptosis and arrest at the B-/G1 phase," *Cancer Research,* 54(2), 448–454 (15 January 1994).

14. Shimoda, S., "The herbal medicine *sho-saiko-to* induces nitric oxide synthase in rat hepatocytes," *Life Sciences,* 56(7), PL143–148 (1995).

15. Yamamoto, S., Oka, H., Kanno, T., Mizoguchi, Y., Kobayashi, K., "Controlled prospective trial to evaluate *Syosakiko-to* in preventing hepatocellular carcinoma in patients with cirrhosis of the liver," *Gan to Kagaku Ryoho—Japanese Journal of Cancer and Chemotherapy,* 16(4, Part 2–2), 1519–1524 (April 1989).

16. Inoue, M., Kikuta, Y., Nagatsu, Y., Ogihara, Y., "Response of liver to glucocorticoid is altered by administration of *shosaikoto* (Kampo medicine)," *Chemical & Pharmaceutical Bulletin,* 38(2), 418–421 (February 1990).

17. Wang, Z.Y., et al., "Inhibition of mutagencitiy in *Salmonella typhimurium* and skin tumor initiating and tumor promoting activities in sencar mice by glycyrrhetinic acid: Comparison of the 18-α and 18-β steroisomers," *Carcinogenesis,* 12, 187–192 (1991).

18. Nakagawa, A., Yamaguchi, T., Tako, T., Amano, H., "Five cases of drug-induced pneumonitis due to *sho-saiko-to* or interferon-alpha or both," *Nippon Kyobu Shikkan Gakkai Zasshi—Japanese Journal of Thoracic Diseases,* 33(12), 1361–1366 (December 1995).

19. Dehmlow, C., Erhard, J., de Groot, H., "Inhibition of Kupffer cell functions as an explanation for the hepatoprotective properties of silibinin," *Hepatology,* 23(4), 749–754 (April 1996).

Inset: Schisandra—Kampo's Supreme Liver Herb

1. Ko, K.M., Ip, S.P., Poon, M.K., Wu, S.S., Che, C.T., Ng, K.H., Kong, Y.C., "Effect of a lignan-enriched Fructus Schisandrae extract on hepatic glutathione status in rats: protection against carbon tetrachloride toxicity," *Planta Medica,* 61(2), 134–137 (April 1995).

2. Hikino, H., "Oriental plant antihepatotoxins," in *Proceedings of the Alfred Benzon Symposium,* p. 384.

3. Ko, K.M., Ip, S.P., Poon, M.K., Wu, S.S., Che, C.T., Ng, K.H., Kong, Y.C., pp. 134–137.

4. Chen, Y.Y., Yang, Y.Q., "Studies on the SGPT-lowering active component of the fruits of *Schisandra rubriflora* Rhed et Wils," *Yao Hsueh Hsueh Pao—Acta Pharmaceutica Sinica,* 17(4), 312–313 (April 1982).

5. Ohkura, Y., Mizoguchi, Y., Morisawa, S., Takeda, S., Aburada, M., Hosoya, E., "Effect of gomisin A (TJN-101) on the arachidonic acid cascade in macrophages," *Japanese Journal of Pharmacology,* 52(2), 331–336 (February 1990).

6. Kubo, S., Ohkura, Y., Mizoguchi, Y., Matsui-Yuasa, I., Otani, S., Morisawa, S., Kinoshita, H., Takeda, S., Aburada, M., Hosoya, E., "Effect of Gomisin A (TJN-101) on liver regeneration," *Planta Medica,* 58(6), 489–492 (December 1992).

Lung Cancer

1. Isselbacher, K.J., Braunwald, E., Wilson, J., Martin, J.V., Fauci, A.S., Kasper, D.L., eds. *Harrison's Principles of Internal Medicine,* Thirteenth Edition (New York: McGraw-Hill, 1995), p. 1221.

2. Zhao, T.H., "Positive modulating action of *shenmaisan* with *Astralagus membranaceus* on anti-tumor activity of LAK cells," *Chung Hsi I Chieh Ho Tsa Chih,* 13(8), 471–472 (1993).

3. He, J., Li, Y., Wei, S., et al., "Effects of mixture of *Astragalus membranaceus, Fructus ligustri* and *Eclipta prostrata* on immune function in mice," *Hua Hsi I Ko Ta Hsueh Pao,* 23(4), 408–411 (1992).

4. Oka, M., et al., "Immunological analysis and clinical effects of intraabdominal and intrapleural injection of lentinan for malignant ascites and pleural effusion," *Biotherapy,* 5, 107–112 (1992).

5. Taguchi, T., et al., "Phase I and II studies of lentinan," in Aoki, A., et al. (eds). *Manipulation of Host Defence Mechanisms* (Amsterdam: Excerpta Medica, 1981).

6. Furuta, M., Niibe, H., "Effect of krestin (PSK) as adjuvant treatment on the prognosis after radical radiotherapy in patients with non-small cell lung cancer," *Anticancer Research,* 13(5C), 1815–1820 (September–October 1993).

7. Nishiwaki, Y., Furuse, K., Fukuoka, M., Ota, M., Niitani, H., Asakawa, M., Nakai, H., Sakai, S., Ogawa, N., "A randomized controlled study of PSK combined immuno-chemotherapy for adenocarcinoma of the lung," *Gan to Kagaku Ryoho—Japanese Journal of Cancer & Chemotherapy,* 17(1), 131–136 (January 1990).

8. Torisu, M., Uchiyama, A., Goya, T., Iwasaki, K., Katano, M., Yamamoto, H., Kimura, Y., "Eighteen-year experience of cancer immunotherapies—evaluation of their therapeutic benefits and future," *Nippon Geka Gakkai Zasshi—Journal of Japan Surgical Society,* 92(9), 1212–1216 (September 1991).

9. Boik, J. *Cancer and Natural Medicine: A Textbook of Basic Science and Clinical Research* (Princeton, Minnesota: Oregon Medical Press, 1995), pp. 217–218.

10. Tanno, Y., Kakuta, Y., Aikawa, T., Shindoh, Y., Ohno, I., Takishima, T., "Effects of *qing-fei-tang (seihai-to)* and baicalein, its main component flavonoid, on lucigenin-dependent chemiluminescence and leukotriene B4 synthesis of human alveolar macrophages," *American Journal of Chinese Medicine,* 16(3–4), 145–154 (1988).

11. Razina, T.G., Udintsev, S.N., Prishchep, T.P., et al., "Enhancement of the selectivity of the action of the cytostatics cyclophosphamide and 5-fluoruracil by using an extract of the Baikal skullcap in an experiment," *Voprosii Onkologii,* 33(20), 80–84 (1987).

12. Razina, T.G., Udintsev, S.N., Tiutrin, I.I., et al., "The role of thrombocyte aggregation function in the mechanism of the antimetastatic action of an extract of Baikal skullcap," *Voprosii Onkologii,* 35(3), 331–335 (1989).

13. Sakata, Y., Suzuki, H., Kamataki, T., "Preventive effect of TJ-14, a Kampo (Chinese herb) medicine, on diarrhea induced by irinotecan hydrochloride (CPT-11)," *Gan to Kagaku Ryoho—Japanese Journal of Cancer & Chemotherapy,* 21(8), 1241–1244 (July 1994).

14. Liu, X.Y., Ang, N.Q., "Effect of *liu we di huang* or *jin gui shen qi* decoction on adjuvant treatment in small cell lung cancer," *Chung Hsi I Chieh Ho Tsa Chih,* 10(12), 720–722, 708 (1990).

Lupus

1. Lappe, M. *Evolutionary Medicine: Rethinking the Origins of Disease* (San Francisco: Sierra Club Books, 1994), pp. 141–147.

2. Zhao, X.Z., "Effects of *Astragalus membranaceus* and *Tripterygium hypoglancum* on natural killer cell activity of peripheral blood mononuclear in systemic lupus erythematosus," *Chung-Kuo Chung Hsi I Chieh Ho Tsa Chih—Chinese Journal of Modern Developments in Traditional Medicine,* 12(11), 669–671, 645 (November 1992).

3. Chen, Y.R., Yen, J.H., Lin, C.C., Tsai, W.J., Liu, W.J., Tsai, J.J., Lin, S.F., Liu, H.W., "The effects of Chinese herbs on improving survival and inhibiting anti-ds DNA antibody production in lupus mice," *American Journal of Chinese Medicine,* 21(3–4), 257–262 (1993).

4. Yuan, Z.Z., Feng, J.C., "Observation on the treatment of systemic lupus erythematosus with a *Gentiana macrophylla* complex tablet and a minimal dose of prednisone," *Chung Hsi I Chieh Ho Tsa Chih,* 9(3), 156–157 (March 1989).

5. Nagai, T., Suzuki, Y., Tomimori, T., Yamada, H., "Antiviral activity of plant flavonoid, 5,7,4'-trihydroxy-8-methoxyflavone, from the roots of *Scutellaria baicalensis* against influenza A (H3N2) and B viruses," *Biological & Pharmaceutical Bulletin,* 18(2), 295–299 (February 1995).

6. Nagai, T., Miyaichi, Y., Tomimori, T., Suzuki, Y., Yamada, H., "Inhibition of influenza virus sialidase and anti-influenza virus activity by plant flavonoids," *Chemical & Pharmaceutical Bulletin,* 38(5), 1329–1332 (May 1990).

7. Zhou, N.N., Nakai, S., Kawakita, T., Oka, M., Nagasawa, H., Himeno, K., Nomoto, K., "Combined treatment of autoimmune MRL/Mp-lpr/lpr mice with a herbal medicine, *ren-shen-yang-rong-tang* (Japanese Name: *ninjin-youei-to*) plus suboptimal dosage of prednisolone," *International Journal of Immunopharmacology,* 16(10), 845–854 (October 1994).

8. Kanauchi, H., Imamura, S., Takigawa, M., Furukawa, F., "Evaluation of the Japanese-Chinese herbal medicine, Kampo, for the treatment of lupus dermatoses in autoimmune prone MRL/Mp-lpr/lpr mice," *Journal of Dermatology,* 21(12), 935–939 (December 1994).

9. "Japan's health ministry confirms efficacy of another of Tsumura's Kampo drugs," *Kampo Today,* 2(1), 3 (February 1997).

Macular Degeneration

1. Young, R.W., "Pathophysiology of age-related macular degeneration," *Survey of Ophthalmology,* 31, 291–306 (1987).

2. Yuzawa, M., Tamakoshi, A., Kawamura, T., Ohno, Y., Uyama, M., Honda, T., "Report on the nationwide epidemiological survey of exudative age-related macular degeneration in Japan," *International Ophthalmology,* 21(1), 1–3 (1997).

3. Tobe, T., Takahashi, K., Ohkuma, H., Uyama, M., "The effect of interferon-beta on experimental choroidal neovascularization," *Nippon Ganka Gakkai Zasshi,* 99(5), 571–581 (May 1995).

4. Kliffen, M., Sharma, H.S., Mooy, C.M., Kerkvliet, S., de Jong, P.T., "Increased expression of angiogenic growth factors in age-related maculopathy," *British Journal of Ophthalmology,* 81(2), 154–162 (February 1997).

5. Caprioli, J., Kitano, S., Morgan, J.E., "Hyperthermia and hypoxia increase tolerance of retinal ganglion cells to anoxia and excitotoxicity," *Investigative Ophthalmology & Visual Science,* 37(12), 2376–2381 (November 1996).

6. Morazzoni, P., Magistretti, M.J., "Activity of Myrtocian®, an anthocyanoside complex from *Vaccinium myrtillus* (vma), on platelet aggregation and adhesiveness," *Fitoterapia,* 61, 13–21 (1990).

7. Ishihara, N., Yuzawa, M., Tamakoshi, A., "Antioxidants and angiogenetic factor associated with age-related macular degeneration," *Nippon Ganka Gakkai Zasshi,* 101(3), 248–251 (March 1997).

8. Miyamoto, H., Ogura, Y., Honda, Y., "Hyperbaric oxygen treatment for macular edema after retinal vein occlusion—fluorescein angiographic findings and visual prognosis," *Nippon Ganka Gakkai Zasshi,* 99(2), 220–225 (February 1995).

Mastitis

1. Takeuchi, S., Ishiguro, K., Ikegami, M., Kaidoh, T., Hayakawa, Y., "Production of toxic shock syndrome toxin by *Staphylococcus aureus* isolated from mastitic cow's milk and farm bulk milk," *Veterinary Microbiology,* 59(4), 251–258 (January 1998).

2. Bodley, V., Powers, D., "Long-term treatment of a breastfeeding mother with fluconazole-resolved nipple pain caused by yeast: a case study," *Journal of Human Lactation,* 13(4), 307–311 (December 1997).

3. Franzblau, S.G., Cross C., "Comparative in vitro antimicrobial activity of Chinese medicinal herbs," *Journal of Ethnopharmacology,* 15(3), 279–288 (March 1986).

4. Mitscher, L.A., "Plant-derived antibiotics," in Weinstein, M.J., Wagman, G.H. (eds). *Antibiotics,* Volume 15 (New York: Plenum Press, 1978), pp. 363–477.

5. Hunfeld, K.P., Bassler, R., "Lymphocytic mastitis and fibrosis of the breast in long-standing insulin-dependent diabetics. A histopathologic study on diabetic mastopathy and report of ten cases," *General Diagnosis and Pathology,* 143(1), 49–58 (July 1997).

Measles

1. Burney, P.G.J., Chinn, S., Rona, R.J., "Has the prevalence of asthma increased in children? Evidence from the national study of health and growth, 1973–1986," *British Medical Journal,* 300, 1306–1310 (1990).

2. Shaheen, S.O., Aaby, P., Hall, A.J., et al., "Measles and atopy in Guinea-Bisseau," *Lancet,* 347, 1792–1796 (1996).

3. Christian, P., West, Jr., K.P., "Interactions between zinc and vitamin A: an update," *American Journal of Clinical Nutrition,* 68, 435S–441S (1998).

Melanoma

1. Boik, J. *Cancer and Natural Medicine: A Textbook of Basic Science and Clinical Research* (Princeton, Minnesota: Oregon Medical Press, 1995), p. 227.

2. Zhao, T.H., "Positive modulating action of *shenmaisan* with *Astralagus membranaceus* on anti-tumor activity of LAK cells," *Chung Hsi I Chieh Ho Tsa Chih,* 13(8), 471–472 (1993).

3, He, J., Li, Y., Wei, S., et al., "Effects of mixture of *Astragalus membranaceus, Fructus ligustri* and *Eclipta prostrata* on immune function in mice," *Hua Hsi I Ko Ta Hsueh Pao,* 23(4), 408–411 (1992).

4. Jing, Y.K., Han, R., "Differentiation of B16 melanoma cells induced by daidzein," *Chinese Journal of Pharmacology and Toxicology,* 6(4), 278–280 (1992).

5. Ebina, T., Murata, K.," Antitumor effect of intratumoral administration of BRM: inhibition of tumor cell invasion in vitro," *Gan to Kagaku Ryoho—Japanese Journal of Cancer & Chemotherapy,* 22(11), 1626–1628 (September 1995).

6. Matsunaga, K., Ohhara, M., Oguchi, Y., Iijima, H., Kobayashi, H., "Antimetastatic effect of PSK, a protein-bound polysaccharide, against the B16-BL6 mouse melanoma," *Invasion & Metastasis,* 16(1), 27–38 (1996).

7. Ueno, Y., Kohgo, Y., Sakamaki, S., Itoh, Y., Takahashi, M., Hirayama, Y., Niitsu, Y., "Immunochemotherapy in B-16-melanoma-cell-transplanted mice with combinations of interleukin-2, cyclophosphamide, and PSK," *Oncology,* 51(3), 296–302 (May–June 1994).

8. Zhang, L.X., Mong, H., Zhou, X.B., "Effect of Japanese *Ganoderma lucidum* (GL) planted in Japan on the production of interleukin-2 from murine splenocytes," *Chung Hsi I Chieh Ho Tsa Chih,* 10(11), 672–674 (1993).

9. Haak-Frendscho, M., Kino, K., Sone, T., et al., "Ling Zhi-8: a novel T-cell mitogen induces cytokine production and upregulation of ICAM-1 expression," *Cellular Immunology,* 150(1), 101–113 (1993).

10. Mar, S., "The 'adaptogens' (Part I): can they really help your running?" *Running Research,* 11(5), 1–3 (June–July 1995).

11. Boik, J., p. 253.

12. Sakamoto, S., Kudo, H., Kawasaki, T., Kuwa, K., et al., "Effects of a Chinese herbal medicine, *keishi-bukuryo-gan,* on the gonadal system of rats," *Journal of Ethnopharmacology,* 23(2–3), 151–158 (July–August 1988).

13. Usuki, S., "Effects of *hachimijiogan, tokishakuyakusan, keishibukuryogan, ninjinto* and *unkeito* on estrogen and progesterone secretion in preovulatory follicles incubated in vitro," *American Journal of Chinese Medicine,* 19(1), 65–71 (1991).

Memory Problems

1. Dharmananda, S. *Chinese Herbology: A Professional Training Program* (Portland, Oregon: Institute for Traditional Medicine and Preventative Health Care, 1992), p. 233.

2. Wu, S.X., Zhang, J.X., Xu, T., Li, L.F., Zhao, S.Y., Lan, M.Y., "Effects of seeds, leaves and fruits of *Ziziphus spinosa* and jujuboside A on central nervous system function," *Chung-Kuo Chung Yao Tsa Chih—China Journal of Chinese Materia Medica,* 18(11), 685–687, 703–704 (November 1993).

3. Fushitani, S., Minakuchi, K., Tsuchiya, K., Takasugi, M., Murakami, K., "Studies on attenuation of post-ischemic brain

injury by Kampo medicines—inhibitory effects of free radical production," *Yakugaku Zasshi—Journal of the Pharmaceutical Society of Japan,* 115(8), 611–617 (August 1995).

4. Liu, J., Mori, A., "Antioxidant and free radical scavenging activities of *Gastrodia elata* Bl. and *Uncaria rhynchophylla* (Miq.) Jacks," *Neuropharmacology,* 31(12), 1287–1298 (December 1992).

Ménière's Disease

1. Rosingh, H.J., Wit, H.P., Albers, F.W., "Perilymphatic pressure dynamics following posture change in patients with Ménière's disease and in normal hearing subjects," *Acta Otolaryngolica* (Stockholm), 118(1), 1–5 (January 1998).

2. López-Gónzales, M.A., Guerrero, J.M., Sánchez, B., Delgado, F., "Melatonin induces hyporeactivity caused by type II collagen in peripheral blood lymphocytes from patients with autoimmune hearing losses," *Neuroscience Letters,* 239(1), 1–4 (December 1997).

3. Silverstein, H., Isaacson, J.E., Olds, M.J., Rowan, P.T., Rosenberg, S., "Dexamethasone inner ear perfusion for the treatment of Ménière's disease: a prospective, randomized, double-blind, crossover trial," *American Journal of Otology,* 19(2), 196–201 (March 1998).

4. Wagner, H., "Immunostimulants from medicinal plants," in Chang, H.M., Yeung, W., Tso, W., Koo, A. (eds). *Advances in Chinese Medicinal Materials Research* (Singapore: World Scientific, 1985).

Menopause-Related Problems

1. Hudson, T., "Naturopathic specific condition review: menopause," *Protocol Journal of Botanical Medicine,* 1(4), 100 (Spring 1996).

2. Düker, E.M., et al., "Effects of extracts from *Cimicifuga racemosa* on gonadotropin release in menopausal women and ovariectomized rats," *Planta Medica,* 57(5), 420–424 (1992).

3. Hirata, J.D., Swiersz, L.M., Zell, B., Small, R., Ettinger, B., "Does dong quai have estrogenic effects in postmenopausal women? A double-blind, placebo-controlled trial," *Fertility and Sterility,* 68(6), 981–986 (December 1997).

Menstrual Problems

1. Sakamoto, S., Yoshino, H., Shirahata, Y., Shimodairo, K., Okamoto, R., "Pharmacotherapeutic effects of *kuei-chih-fu-ling-wan (keishi-bukuryo-gan)* on human uterine myomas," *American Journal of Chinese Medicine,* 20(3–4), 313–317 (1992).

Inset: Using Shepherd's Purse With Kampo to Stop Bleeding

1. Kuroda, K., Takagi, K., "Physiologically active substance in *Capsella bursus-pastoris,*" *Nature* (London), 220, 707 (1968).

Migraine

1. Srivastava, K.C., Mustafa, T., "Ginger (*Zingiber officinale*) in rheumatism and musculoskeletal disorders," *Medical Hypotheses,* 39(4), 342–348 (December 1992).

2. Fushitani, S., Tsuchiya, K., Minakuchi, K., Takasugi, M., Murakami, K., "Studies on attenuation of post-ischemic brain injury by Kampo medicines—inhibitory effects of free radical production," *Yakugaku Zasshi—Journal of the Pharmaceutical Society of Japan,* 114(6), 388–394 (June 1994).

3. MacGregor, E.A., Guillebaud, J., "Combined oral contraceptives, migraine and ischaemic stroke," *British Journal of Family Planning,* 24(2), 55–60 (July 1998).

4. Kupersmith, M.J., Frohman, L., Sanderson, M., Jacobs, J., Hirschfeld, J., Ku, C., Warren, F.A., "Aspirin reduces the incidence of second eye NAION: a retrospective study," *Journal of Neuroophthalmology,* 17(4), 250–253 (December 1997).

Multiple Sclerosis

1. Haeren, A.F., Tourtellotte, W.W., Richard, K.A., et al., "A study of the blood cerebrospinal fluid-brain barrier in multiple sclerosis," *Neurology,* 14, 345–351 (1964).

2. Cullen, C.F., Swank, R.L., "Intravascular aggregation and adhesiveness of the blood elements associated with alimentary lipemia and injection of large molecular substances: effect on blood-brain barrier," *Circulation,* 9, 335–346 (1954).

3. Howat, D.W., Chand, N., Braquet, P, Willoughby, D.A., "An investigation into the possible involvement of platelet activating factor in experimental allergic encephalomyelitis in rats," *Agents and Actions,* 27(3–4), 473–476 (June 1989).

4. Brochet, B., Orgogozo, J.M., Guinot, P., Dartigues, J.F., Henry, P., Loiseau, P., "Pilot study of Ginkgolide B, a PAF-acether specific inhibitor in the treatment of acute outbreaks of multiple sclerosis," *Revue Neurologique* (Paris), 148(4), 299–301 (1992).

5. Brochet, B., Guinot, P., Orgogozo, J.M., Confavreux, C., Rumbach, L., Lavergne, V., "Double blind placebo controlled multicentre study of ginkgolide B in treatment of acute exacerbations of multiple sclerosis," *Journal of Neurology, Neurosurgery, and Psychiatry,* 38(3), 360–362 (March 1995).

6. Tong, X.W., Xue, Q.M., "Alterations of serum phopholipids in patients with multiple sclerosis," *Chinese Medical Journal,* 106(9), 650–654 (September 1993).

7. "Japan's health ministry confirms efficacy of another of Tsumura's Kampo drugs," *Kampo Today,* 2(1), 3 (February 1997).

8. Bernsohn, J., Stephanides, L.M., "Aetiology of multiple sclerosis," *Nature,* 10, 523–530 (1963).

Mumps

1. Ruther, U., Stilz, S., Rohl, E., Nunnensiek, C., Rassweiler, J., Dorr, U., Jipp, P., "Successful interferon-alpha 2 a therapy for a patient with acute mumps orchitis," *European Urologist,* 27(2), 174–176 (1995).

2. Isselbacher, K.J., Braunwald, E., Wilson, J., Martin, J.V., Fauci, A.S., Kasper, D.L., eds. *Harrison's Principles of Internal Medicine,* Thirteenth Edition (New York: McGraw-Hill, 1995), p. 830.

3. Wagner, H., Proksch, A., Riess-Maurer, I., Vollmar, A., Odenthal, S., Stuppner, H., Jurcic, K., Le Turdu, M., Fang, J.N., "Immunostimulatory effects of polysaccharides (heteroglycans) of higher plants," *Arzneimittel-Forschung,* 35(7), 1069–1075 (1985).

Obesity

1. Kimura, Y., Ohminami, H., Arichi, H., Okuda, H., Baba, K., Kozawa, M., Arichi, S., "Effects of various courmarins from roots *Angelica dahurica* on actions of adrenaline, ACTH, and insulin in fat cells," *Planta Medica,* 45, 183–187 (1982).

2. Wichtl, M., ed., Grainger-Bissett, N., trans. *Herbal Drugs and Phytopharmaceuticals: A Handbook for Practice on a Scientific Basis* (Boca Raton, Florida: CRC Press, 1995), pp. 486–488.

3. Ozaki, Y., "Studies on anti-inflammatory effect of Japanese Oriental medicines (Kampo medicines) used to treat inflammatory diseases," *Biological and Pharmaceutical Bulletin,* 18(4), 559–562 (April 1995).

4. Wang, C.M., Ohta, S., Shinoda, M., "Studies of chemical protectors against radiation. XXIX. Protective effects of methanol extracts of various Chinese traditional medicines on skin injury induced by X-irradiation," *Yakugaku Zasshi—Journal of the Pharmaceutical Society of Japan,* 110(3), 218–224 (March 1990).

5. Hara, Y., "Prophylactic functions of tea polyphenols," in Ho, C.T., Osawa, T., Huang, M.T., Rosen, R. (eds). *Food Phytochemicals for Cancer Prevention II: Teas, Spices, and Herbs* (Washington: American Chemical Society, 1994), p. 42.

6. Yoshida, T., Sakane, N., Wakabayashi, Y., Umekawa, T., Kondo, M., "Thermogenic, anti-obesity effects of *bofu-tsusho-san* in MSG-obese mice," *International Journal of Obesity and Related Disorders,* 19(10), 717–722 (October 1995).

Osteoarthritis

1. Summers, M.M., et al., "Radiographic assessment and psychologic variables as predictors of pain and functional impairment in osteoarthritis of the knee or hip," *Arthritis and Rheumatology,* 31, 204–209 (1988).

2. Havsteen, B., "Flavonoids, a class of natural products of high pharmacological potency," *Biochemical Pharmacology,* 32, 1141–1148 (1982).

3. Ciplea, A.G., Richter, K.D., "The protective effect of *Allium sativum* and *Crataegus* on isoprenaline-induced tissue necroses in rats," *Arzneimittel-Forschung,* 38(110), 1583–1592 (November 1988).

Inset: Complementing Kampo With Other Therapies in Osteoarthritis

1. Duwiejua, M,, Zeitlin, I.J., Waterman, P.G., Chapman, J., Mhango, G.J., Provan, G.J., "Anti-inflammatory activity of resins from some species of the plant family Burseraceae," *Planta Medica,* 59(1), 12–16 (February 1993).

2. Morales, T.K., Wahl, L.M., Hascall, V.C., "The effect of lipopolysaccharides on the biosynthesis and release of proteoglycans from calf articular cartilage cultures," *Journal of Biological Chemistry,* 259, 6720–6729 (1984).

3. Moussard, C., Alber, D., Toubin, M.M., Thevenon, N., Henry, J.C., "A drug used in traditional medicine, *Harpagophytum procumbens*: no evidence for NSAID-like effect on whole blood eicosanoid production in humans," *Prostaglandins Leukotrienes & Essential Fatty Acids,* 46(4), 283–286 (August 1992).

Ovarian Cancer

1. Isselbacher, K.J., Braunwald, E., Wilson, J., Martin, J.V., Fauci, A.S., Kasper, D.L., eds. *Harrison's Principles of Internal Medicine,* Thirteenth Edition (New York: McGraw-Hill, 1995), pp. 1853–1854.

2. McGuire, W.P., Hoskins, W.J., Brady, M.F., et al., "Cyclophosphamide and cisplatin compared with paclitaxel and cisplatin in patients with stage II and stage IV ovarian cancer," *New England Journal of Medicine,* 334(1), 1–6 (1996).

3. Gersshenson, D.M., Mitchell, M.F., Atkinson, N., et al., "The effect of prolonged cisplatin-based chemotherapy on progression-free survival in patients with optimal epithelial ovarian cancer: 'maintenance' therapy reconsidered," *Gynecologic Oncology,* 47(1), 7–13 (1992).

4. Hara, Y., "Prophylactic functions of tea polyphenols," in Ho, C.T., Osawa, T., Huang, M.T., Rosen, R. (eds). *Food Phytochemicals for Cancer Prevention II: Teas, Spices, and Herbs* (Washington: American Chemical Society, 1994), pp. 36, 44.

5. Komori, A., Yatsunamni, J., Okabe. S., et al., "Anticarcinogenic activity of green tea polyphenols," *Japanese Journal of Clinical Oncology,* 23(30), 186–190 (1993).

6. Kikuchi, Y., Kizawa, I., Oomori, K., Iwano, I., Kita, T., Kato, K., "Effects of PSK on interleukin-2 production by peripheral lymphocytes of patients with advanced ovarian carcinoma during chemotherapy," *Japanese Journal of Cancer Research,* 79(1), 125–130 (January 1988).

7. Wagner, H., "Immunostimulants from medicinal plants," in Chang, H.M., Yeung, W., Tso, W., Koo, A. (eds). *Advances in Chinese Medicinal Materials Research* (Singapore: World Scientific, 1985).

8. Scalzo, R., "Therapeutic botanical protocol for ovarian cancer," *Protocol Journal of Botanical Medicine,* 2(3), 152.

9. Chang, K.S.S., Gao, C., Wang, L.C., "Berberine-induced morphologic differentiation and down-regulation of c-Ki-ras2 protooncogene expression in human teratocarcinoma cells," *Cancer Letters,* 55, 103–108 (1990).

10. Chang, K.S., "Down-regulation of c-Ki-ras2 gene expression associated with morphologic differentiation in human embryonal carcinoma cells treated with berberine," *Taiwan I Hsueh Hui Tsa Chih,* 90(1), 10–14 (1991).

Ovarian Cysts

1. Winston, D., "Eclectic specific condition review: endometriosis," *Protocol Journal of Botanical Medicine,* 1(4), 35 (Spring 1996).

2. Hudson, T., Lewin, A., "Naturopathic specific condition review: endometriosis," *Protocol Journal of Botanical Medicine,* 1(4), 32 (Spring 1996).

3. Milewicz, A., Gejdel, E., Sworen, H., Sienkeiwicz, K., Jedrzejak, J., Teucher, T., Schmitz, Z.H., "Vitex agnus-castus extract in the treatment of luteal phase defects due to latent hyperprolactinemia: results of a randomized placebo-controlled double-blind study," *Arzneimittel-Forschung,* 43, 752–756 (1993).

4. Boik, J. *Cancer and Natural Medicine: A Textbook of Basic Science and Clinical Research* (Princeton, Minnesota: Oregon Medical Press, 1995), p. 253.

5. Sakamoto, S., Kudo, H., Kawasaki, T., Kuwa, K., et al., "Effects of a Chinese herbal medicine, *keishi-bukuryo-gan,* on the gonadal system of rats," *Journal of Ethnopharmacology,* 23(2–3), 151–158 (July–August 1988).

6. Dharmananda, S., "Traditional Chinese specific condition review: ovarian cysts," *Protocol Journal of Botanical Medicine,* 1(4), 138 (Spring 1996).

7. Takeuchi, T., Nishii, O., Okamura, T., Yaginuma, T., "Effects of paeoniflorin, glycyrrhizin, and glycyrrhetic acid on ovarian androgen production," *American Journal of Chinese Medicine,* 19(1), 73–78 (1991).

8. Usuki, S., "Effects of *hachimijiogan, tokishakuyakusan, keishibukuryogan, ninjinto* and *unkeito* on estrogen and progesterone secretion in preovulatory follicles incubated in vitro," *American Journal of Chinese Medicine,* 19(1), 65–71 (1991).

9. Takahashi, K., Kitao, M., "Effect of TJ-68 (*shakuyaku-kanzo-to*) on polycystic ovarian disease," *International Journal of Fertility & Menopausal Studies*, 39(2), 69–76 (March–April 1994).

10. Imai, A., Horibe, S., Fuseya, S., Iida, K., Takagi, H., Tamaya, T., "Possible evidence that the herbal medicine *shakuyaku-kanzo-to* decreases prostaglandin levels through suppressing arachidonate turnover in endometrium," *Journal of Medicine*, 26(3–4), 163–174 (1995).

11. Zhang, G.L., "Treatment of breast proliferation disease with modified *xiao yao san* and *er chen* decoction," *Chung Hsi I Chieh Ho Tsa Chih*, 11(7), 400–402 (1988).

Pelvic Inflammatory Disease

1. Isselbacher, K.J., Braunwald, E., Wilson, J., Martin, J.V., Fauci, A.S., Kasper, D.L., eds. *Harrison's Principles of Internal Medicine*, Thirteenth Edition (New York: McGraw-Hill, 1995), p. 544.

2. Landers, D.V., et al., "Combination antimicrobial therapy in treatment of acute pelvic inflammatory disease," *American Journal of Obstetrics and Gynecology*, 164, 849 (1991).

3. Kaneda, Y., Tanaka, T., Saw, T., "Effects of berberine, a plant alkaloid, on the growth of anaerobic protozoa in axenic culture," *Tokai Journal of Experimental & Clinical Medicine*, 15(6), 417–423 (November 1990).

4. Suzuki, T., Higashi, H., Saitoh, K., Kurokawa, K., Ohma, C., Yamanaka, H., "Effects of *gosha-jinki-gan* on urinary bladder contract in dogs," *Hinyokika Kiyo*, 43(4), 271–274 (April 1997).

5. Takahashi, K., Kitao, M., "Effect of TJ-68 (*shakuyaku-kanzo-to*) on polycystic ovarian disease," *International Journal of Fertility and Menopausal Studies*, 39(2), 69–76 (March–April 1994).

6. Omura, Y., Beckman, S.L., "Role of mercury (Hg) in resistant infections and effective treatment of *Chlamydia trachomatis* and *Herpes* family viral infections (and potential treatment for cancer) by removing localized Hg deposits with Chinese parsley and delivering effective antibiotics using various drug uptake enhancement methods," *Acupuncture and Electrotherapy Research*, 20(3–4), 195–229 (August 1995).

Peptic Ulcer

1. Hikino, H., "Recent research on Oriental medicinal plants," in Wagner, H., Hikino, H., Farnsworth, N.R. (eds). *Economic and Medicinal Plant Research*, Volume 1 (London: Academic Press, 1985), pp. 53–85.

2. Takase, H., Imanishi, K., Miura, O., Yumioka, E., Watanabe, H., "Features of the anti-ulcer effects of *Oren-gedoku-to* (a traditional Chinese medicine) and its component herb drugs," *Japanese Journal of Pharmacology*, 49(3), 301–308 (March 1989).

Premenstrual Syndrome (PMS)

1. Winston, D., "Eclectic specific condition review: premenstrual syndrome," *Protocol Journal of Botanical Medicine*, 1(4), 179 (Spring 1996).

2. Jarry, H., Harnischfeger, G., Düker, E., "Studies on the endocrine effects of the contents of *Cimicifuga racemosa*. 2. In vitro binding of compounds to estrogen receptors," *Planta Medica*, 51, 316–319 (1985).

3. Winston, D., p. 179.

4. Blumenthal, M., Busse, W.R., Goldberg, A., Gruenwald, J., Hall, T., Riggins, C.W., Rister, R.S., eds., Klein, S., Rister, R.S., trans. *The Complete German Commission E Monographs: Therapeutic Guide to Herbal Medicines* (Boston: Integrative Medicine Communications, 1998).

5. Harada, M., Suzuki, M., Ozaki, Y., "Effect of Japanese angelica root and peony root on uterine contraction in the rabbit in situ," *Journal of Pharmacodynamics*, 7, 304–311 (1984).

6. Hobbs, C., Amster, M., "Naturopathic specific condition review: premenstrual syndrome," *Protocol Journal of Botanical Medicine*, 1(4), 168–173 (Spring 1996).

7. Cahill, D.J., Fox, R., Wardel, P.G., Harlow, C.R., "Multiple follicular development associated with herbal medicine," *Human Reproduction*, 9(8), 1469–1470 (August 1994).

8. Boik, J. *Cancer and Natural Medicine: A Textbook of Basic Science and Clinical Research* (Princeton, Minnesota: Oregon Medical Press, 1995), p. 253.

Prostate Cancer

1. Ergil, K.V., "Traditional Chinese medicine specific condition review: prostate cancer," *Protocol Journal of Botanical Medicine*, 2(3), 188–191.

2. Horhammer, L., Wagner, H., König, H. *Um die Bestandteil des* Lithospermum officinale *L. II Teil.* (Munich, Germany: Institut für Pharmazeutisches Arzneimittel, 1964), Chapter 14, pp. 34–40.

3. Mickey, D.D., Bencuya, P.S., Foulkes, K., "Effects of the immunomodulator PSK on growth of human prostate adenocarcinoma in immunodeficient mice," *International Journal of Immunopharmacology*, 11(7), 829–838 (1989).

4. Bergan, R., Kyle, E., Nguyen, P., Trepel, J., Ingui, C., Neckers, L., "Genistein-stimulated adherence of prostate cancer cells is associated with the binding of focal adhesion kinase to beta-1-integrin," *Clinical & Experimental Metastasis*, 14(4), 389–398 (September 1996).

5. Bhagarva, S.K., "Antiandrogenic effects of a flavonoid-rich fraction of *Vitex negundo* seeds: a histological and biochemical study in dogs," *Journal of Ethnopharmacology*, 27(3), 327–339 (December 1989).

6. Kato, T., Okamoto, R., "Effect of *shakuyaku-kanzo-to* on serum estrogen levels and adrenal gland cells in ovariectomized rats," *Nippon Sanka Fujinka Gakkai Zasshi*, 44(4), 433–439 (1992).

7. Sakamoto, K., Wakabayashi, K., "Inhibitory effect of glycyrrhetinic acid on testosterone production in rat gonads," *Endocrinologia Japonica*, 35(2), 333–342 (April 1988).

8. Matzkin, H., Eber, P., Todd, B., et al., "Prognostic significance of changes in prostate-specific markers after endocrine treatment of stage D2 prostatic cancer," *Cancer*, 70(9), 2302–2309 (1992).

9. Catalona, W.J., Smith, D.S., Ratliff., T.L., et al., "Measurement of prostate-specific antigen in serum as a screening test for prostate cancer," *New England Journal of Medicine*, 324(17), 1156–1161 (1991).

10. Zentner, P.G., Pao, L.K., Benson, M.C., et al., "Prostate-specific antigen density: a new prognostic indicator for prostate cancer," *International Journal of Radiation Oncology, Biology, Physics*, 27(1), 47–58 (1993).

11. Adlercreutz, H., Markkanen, H., Watanabe, S., "Plasma concentrations of phyto-estrogens in Japanese men," *Lancet*, 342(8881), 1209–1210 (13 November 1993).

12. Adlercreutz, H., Mousavi, Y., Clark, J., Hocerstedt, K., et al., "Dietary phytoestrogens and cancer: in vitro and in vivo stud-

ies," *Journal of Steroid Biochemistry and Molecular Biology,* 41(3–8), 331–337 (1992).

Inset: Saw Palmetto and the Prostate

1. Tolino, A., Petrone, A., Sarnacchiaro, F., Cirillo, D., Ronsini, S., Lombardi, G., Nappi, C., "Finasteride in the treatment of hirsutism: new therapeutic perspectives," *Fertility and Sterility,* 66(1), 61–65 (July 1996).

2. Shimada, H., Tyler, V.E., McLaughlin, J.L., "Biologically active acylglycerides from the berries of saw-palmetto (*Serenoa repens*)," *Journal of Natural Products,* 60(4), 417–418 (April 1997).

Prostate Enlargement, Benign

1. Roehrborn, C.G., Oesterling, J.E., Auerbach, S., Kaplan, S.A., Lloyd, L.K., Milam, D.E., Padley, R.J., "The Hytrin Community Assessment Trial study: a one-year study of terazosin versus placebo in the treatment of men with symptomatic benign prostatic hyperplasia," *Urology,* 47(2), 159–168 (February 1996).

2. Sakamoto, S., Kudo, H., Kawsasaki, T., Kasahara, N., Okamoto, R., "Effect of *ba-wei-di-huang-wan (hachimi-jio-gan)* on thymidine kinase and its isozyme activities in the prostate glands in rats," *American Journal of Chinese Medicine,* 16(1–2), 29–36 (1988).

3. Ibid.

4. Utsugi, T., Igarashi, M., Yazaki, C., Hasegawa, Y., Miyamoto, K., Taniguchi, Y., Nomura, S., Shinkawa, T., "Effects of *hachimijiogan* on the hypothalamo-pituitary-testicular system," *Nippon Sanka Fujinka Gakkai Zasshi,* 35(120), 2305–2310 (December 1983).

5. Yachiku, S., Kaneko, S., Matsuura, T., Akiyama, T., Kurita, T., "Conservative treatment of benign prostatic hypertrophy—clinical effects of increased administration of *hachimijiogan* and the relation between these effects and the 'sho' of Chinese medicine," *Hinyokika Kiyo,* 31(30), 545–551 (March 1985).

6. Tozawa, K., Akita, H., Yamamoto, H., Nakahira, Y., Kawai, T., Kohri, K., "Clinical efficacy of *sairei-to* in prevention of recurrence of urethral stenosis: report of two cases," *Hinyokika Kiyo,* 44(1), 49–51 (January 1998).

7. Rugendorff, E.W., Weidner, W., et al., "Results of treatment with pollen extract (Cernilton) in chronic prostatitis and prostaodynia," *British Journal of Urology,* 71, 433–438 (1993).

8. Yablonsky, F., Nicolas, V., Riffaud, J.P., Bellamy, F., "Antiproliferative effect of *Pygeum africanum* extract on rat prostatic fibroblasts," *Journal of Urology,* 157(6), 2381–2387 (June 1997).

9. Paubert-Braquet, M., Cave, A., Hocquemiller, R., Delacroix, D., Dupont, C., Hedef, N., Borgeat, P., "Effect of *Pygeum africanum* extract on A23187-stimulated production of lipoxygenase metabolites from human polymorphonuclear cells," *Journal of Lipid Mediators & Cell Signalling,* 9(3), 285–290 (May 1994).

Psoriasis

1. Proctor, M., et al., "Lowered cutaneous and urinary levels of polyamines with clinical improvement in treated psoriasis," *Archives of Dermatology,* 15, 945–949 (1979).

2. Scholzen, T., Armstrong, C.A., Bunnett, N.W., Luger, T.A., Olerud, J.E., Ansel, J.C., "Neuropeptides in the skin: interactions between the neuroendocrine and the skin immune systems," *Experimental Dermatology,* 7(2–3), 81–96 (April 1998).

3. Misery, L., "Skin, immunity and the nervous system," *British Journal of Dermatology,* 137(6), 843–850 (December 1997).

4. Seveille, R.H., "Psoriasis and stress," *British Journal of Dermatology,* 97, 297 (1977).

5. Liu, H.C., "Correlation between types of syndrome differentiation and erythrocyte deformability and membrane ATPase activity in psoriatic patients," *Chung-Kuo Chung Hsi I Chieh Ho Tsa Chih—Chinese Journal of Modern Developments in Traditional Medicine,* 14(4), 210–212 (April 1994).

6. Hikino., H., et al., "Antihepatotoxic actions of flavanolignans from *Silybum marianum* fruits," *Plant Medica,* 50, 248–250 (1984).

7. Evans, F.Q., "The rational use of glycyrrhetinic acid in dermatology," *British Journal of Clinical Practice,* 12, 269–279 (1958).

8. Komine, M., Freedberg, I.M., Blumenberg, M., "Regulation of epidermal expression of keratin K17 in inflammatory skin diseases," *Journal of Investigative Dermatology,* 107(4), 569–575 (October 1996).

9. Bensky, D., Barolet, R. *Chinese Herbal Medicine: Formulas and Strategies* (Seattle: Eastland Press, 1990), p. 35.

10. Iijima, S., Otsuka, F., Kikuchi, Y., "*Unsei-in* inhibits rheological activity of leukocytes, mechanism of action in neutrophil-related skin diseases," *American Journal of Chinese Medicine,* 23(1), 81–90, 1995.

11. Rosenberg, E., Belew, P., "Microbial factors in psoriasis," *Archives of Dermatology,* 118, 1434–1444 (1982).

12. Monk, B.E., Neill, S.M., "Alcohol consumption and psoriasis," *Dermatologica,* 173, 57–60 (1986).

13. van Ruissen, F., Le, M., Carroll, J.M., van der Valk, P.G., Schalkwijk, J., "Differential effects of detergents on keratinocyte gene expression," *Journal of Investigational Dermatology,* 110(4), 358–363 (April 1998).

14. Winchell, S.A., Watts, R.A., "Relaxation therapies in the treatment of psoriasis and possible pahtophysicologic mechanisms," *Journal of the American Academy of Dermatology,* 20, 601–608 (1981).

Radiation Therapy Side Effects

1. Hara, Y., "Prophylactic functions of tea polyphenols," in Ho, C.T., Osawa, T., Huang, M.T., Rosen, R. (eds). *Food Phytochemicals for Cancer Prevention II: Teas, Spices, and Herbs* (Washington: American Chemical Society, 1994), p. 36, 43.

2. Kuttan, G., Kuttan, R., "Reduction of leukopenia in mice by *Viscum album* administration during radiation and chemotherapy," *Tumori,* 79(1), 74–76 (28 February 1993).

3. Katsumatsu, T., "The radiation-sensitizing effect of PSK in treatment of cervical cancer patients," in Yamamura, Y., et al. (eds). *Immunomodulation by Microbial Products and Related Synthetic Compounds* (Amsterdam: Excerpta Medica, 1982), pp. 463–466.

4. Zican, W., et al., "Studies on the effects of *Tremella fuciformis* bark preparations on immunity and blood formation in rhesus monkeys," *Journal of Traditional Chinese Medicine,* 3, 13–16 (1983).

5. Suzuki, M., Nikaido, T., Ohmoto, T., "The study of Chinese herbal medicinal prescription with enzyme inhibitory activity. V. The study of *hange-shashin-to, kanzo-shashin-to, shokyo-shashin-to* with adenosine 3',5'-cyclic monophosphate phosphodiesterase," *Yakugaku Zasshi—Journal of the Pharmaceutical Society of Japan,* 111(11), 695–701 (November 1991).

6. Wang, C.M., Ohta, S., Shinoda, M., "Studies of chemical protectors against radiation. XXIX. Protective effects of methanol extracts of various Chinese traditional medicines on skin injury

induced by X-irradiation," *Yakugaku Zasshi—Journal of the Pharmaceutical Society of Japan,* 110(3), 218–224 (March 1990).

7. Ohnishi, Y., Yasumizu, R., Ikehara, S., "Preventative effect of TJ-48 on recovery from radiation injury," *Gan to Kagaku Ryoho—Japanese Journal of Cancer & Chemotherapy,* 16 (4, Part 2–2), 1494–1499 (April 1989).

8. Li, X.Y., Takimoto, H., Miura, S., Yoshikai, Y., Matsuzaki, G., Momoto, K., "Effects of a traditional Chinese medicine, *bu-zhong-yi-qi-tang* (Japanese name: *hochu-ekki-to*) on the protection against *Listeria monocytogenes* infection in mice," *Immunopharmacology and Immunotoxicology,* 14(3), 383–402 (1992).

9. Clemens, M.R., Müller-Ladner, C.I., Gey, K.F., "Vitamins during high dose chemo- and radiotherapy," *Zeitschrift für Ernährungswissenschaft,* 31(2), 110–120 (June 1992).

10. Hartmann, A., Vormstein, M., Schnabel, T., Kehren, H., Stein, T., Schmitt, G., Makropoulos, W., "An absent correlation between antioxidant blood concentrations and the remission response of preopreatively treated breast carcinomas," *Strahlentherapie und Onkologie,* 72(8), 434–438 (August 1996).

Rheumatoid Arthritis

1. Lappé, M. *Evolutionary Medicine: Rethinking the Origins of Disease* (San Francisco: Sierra Club Books, 1994), p. 137.

2. Fleischer, B., et al., "An evolutionary conserved mechanism to T cell activation by microbial toxins," *Journal of Immunology,* 146, 11–17 (1991).

3. Zaphiropoulos, G.C., "Rheumatoid arthritis and the gut," *British Journal of Rheumatology,* 25, 138–140 (1986).

4. Jenkins, R., Rooney, P., Jones, D., et al., "Increased intestinal permeability in patients with rheumatoid arthritis: a side effect of oral nonsteroidal anti-inflammatory drug use," *Gastroenterology,* 96, 647–655 (1989).

5. Tang, W., Eisenbrand, G. *Chinese Drugs of Plant Origin: Chemistry, Pharmacology, and Use in Traditional and Modern Medicine* (Berlin: Springer-Verlag, 1992), p. 351.

6. Bensky, D., Barolet, R. *Chinese Herbal Medicine: Formulas and Strategies* (Seattle: Eastland Press, 1990), p. 159.

7. Murray, M., Pizzorno, J. *Encyclopedia of Natural Medicine* (Rocklin, California: Prima Publishing, 1998), p. 784.

8. Srivastava, K.C., Mustafa, T., "Ginger (*Zingiber officinale*) in rheumatism and musculoskeletal disorders," *Medical Hypotheses,* 39(4), 342–348 (December 1992).

9. Sharma, J.N., Srivastava, K.C., Gan, E.K., "Suppressive effects of eugenol and ginger oil on arthritic rats," *Pharmacology,* 49(5), 314–318 (November 1994).

10. Srivastava, K.C., Mustafa, T., "Ginger (*Zingiber officinale*) and rheumatic disorders," *Medical Hypotheses,* 29, 25–28 (1989).

11. Ding, X., "Effects of poriatin on mouse peritoneal macrophages," *Y'lxue Kexueyuan,* 9, 433–438 (1987)

12. Wang, G., "Effect of poriatin on mouse immune system," *South China Journal of Antibiotica,* 17, 42–47 (1992).

13. Srivastava, R., "Inhibition of neutrophil response by curcumin," *Agents and Actions,* 28, 298–303 (1989).

14. Shankar, T.N.B., Shantha, N.V., Ramesh, H.P., et al., "Toxicity studies on turmeric (*Curcuma longa*): acute toxicity studies in rats, guinea pigs, and monkeys," *Indian Journal of Experimental Biology,* 18, 735–775 (1980).

15. Deodhar, S.D., Sethi, R., Srimal, R.C., "Preliminary studies on antirheumatic activity of curcumin (diferuloyl methane)," *Indian Journal of Medical Research,* 71, 632–634 (1980).

16. Ohno, S., Suzuki, T., Dohi, Y., "The effect of *bakumondo-to* on salivary secretion in Sjögren's syndrome," *Ryumachi,* 30(1), 10–16 (February 1990).

17. Wakabayashi, K., Inoue, M., Ogihara, Y., "The effect of *keishi-bushi-to* on collagen-induced arthritis," *Biological Pharmacology Bulletin,* 20(4), 376–380 (April 1997).

18. Kawakatsu, T., Nomura, S., Kido, H., Yamaguchi, K., Fukuroi, T., Suzuki, M., Yanabu, M., Kokawa, T., Yasunaga, K., "Effect of three Japanese Kampo medicines on platelet activation by monoclonal anti-platelet membrane glycoprotein antibodies," *American Journal of Chinese Medicine,* 22(1), 71–76 (1994).

19. Watanabe, M., Kanitani, M., Kobayashi, Y., Taki, M., Minematsu, S., Maemura, S., Fujii, Y., Oyama, T., Takeda, K., "Combined effect of glucocorticoid and TJ-114 (Tsumura *Sairei-to*)," *Nippon Yakurigaku Zasshi,* 101(1), 39–51 (January 1993).

20. Suzuki, J., Watanabe, K., Kobayashi, T., Yoshida, K., Watanabe, Y., Kumada, K., Suzuki, S., Kume, K., Suzuki, H., "Effect of *sairei-to* on prostaglandin #2-induced phosphatidylinositol breakdown in aminonucleoside nephrotic rat," *Nephron,* 75(2), 208–212 (1997).

Seizure Disorders

1. Hardman, J.G., Limbird, L.E., Molinoff, P.B., Ruddon, R.W., Gilman, A.G. *Goodman & Gilman's The Pharmacological Basis of Therapeutics* (New York: McGraw-Hill, 1996), p. 461.

2. Minematsu, S., Taki, M., Watanabe, M., Takahashi, M., Wakui, Y., Ishihara, K., Takeda, S., Fujii, Y., "Effects of *Shosaiko-to-go-keishikashakuyaku-to* (TJ-960) on the valproic acid induced anomalies of rat fetuses," *Nippon Yakurigaku Zasshi—Folia Pharmacologica Japonica,* 96(5), 265–273 (November 1990).

3. Liu, J., Mori, A., "Antioxidant and free radical scavenging activities of *Gastrodia elata* Bl. and *Uncaria rhynchophylla* (Miq.) Jacks," *Neuropharmacology,* 31(12), 1287–1298 (December 1992).

Skin Cancer (Basal Cell Carcinoma)

1. Desai, K.N., Wei, H., Lamartiniere, C.A., "The preventive and therapeutic potential of the squalene-containing compound, Roidex, on tumor promotion and regression," *Cancer Letters,* 101(1), 93–96 (19 March 1996).

2. Zhang, G.L., "Treatment of breast proliferation disease with modified *xiao yao san* and *er chen* decoction," *Chung Hsi I Chieh Ho Tsa Chih,* 11(7), 400–402 (1988).

3. Namba, T., Sekiya, K., Toshinal, A., Kadota, S., Hatanaka, T., Katayama, K., Koizumi, T., "Study on baths with crude drug. II.: the effects of coptidis rhizoma extracts as skin permeation enhancer," *Yakugaku Zasshi—Journal of the Pharmaceutical Society of Japan,* 115(8), 618–625 (August 1995).

4. Yasukawa, K., Ikeya, Y., Mitsuhashi, H., Iwasaki, M., Aburada, M., Nakagawa, S., Takeuchi, M., Takido, M., "Gomisin A inhibits tumor promotion by 12-O-tetradecanoylphorbol-13-acetate in two-stage carcinogenesis in mouse skin," *Oncology,* 49(1), 68–71 (1992).

5. Ishizaki, C., Oguro, T., Yoshida, T., Wen, C.Q., Sueki, H., Iijima, M., "Enhancing effect of ultraviolet A on ornithine decarboxylase induction and dermatitis evoked by 12-O-tetradecanoylphorbol-13-acetate and its inhibition by curcumin in mouse skin," *Dermatology,* 193(4), 311–317 (1996).

6. Huang, M.T., Ma, W., Yen, P., Xie, J.G., Han, J., Frenkel, K., Grunberger, D., Conney, A.H., "Inhibitory effects of topical application of low doses of curcumin on 12-O-tetradecanoylphorbol-13-acetate-induced tumor promotion and oxidized DNA bases in mouse epidermis," *Carcinogenesis,* 18(1), 83–88 (January 1997).

Stomach Cancer

1. Zhang, L., Yang, L.W., Yang, L.J., "Relation between *Helicobacter pylori* and pathogenesis of chronic atrophic gastritis and the research of its prevention and treatment," *Chung-Kuo Chung Hsi I Chieh Ho Tsa Chih—Chinese Journal of Modern Developments in Traditional Medicine,* 12(9), 521–523, 515–516 (September 1992).

2. Yin, G.Y., He, X.F., Yin, Y.F., "Study on mitochondrial ultrastructure, trace elements and correlative factors of gastric mucosa in patients with spleen deficiency syndrome," *Chung-Kuo Chung Hsi I Chieh Ho Tsa Chih—Chinese Journal of Modern Developments in Traditional Medicine,* 15(12), 719–723 (December 1995).

3. Linder, M.C., ed. *Nutritional Biochemistry and Metabolism,* Second Edition (New York: Elsevier Science Publishing Co., 1991), pp. 499, 512.

4. Fukushima, M., "Adjuvant therapy of gastric cancer: the Japanese experience," *Seminars in Oncology,* 23(3), 369–378 (June 1996).

5. Boik, J. *Cancer and Natural Medicine: A Textbook of Basic Science and Clinical Research* (Princeton, Minnesota: Oregon Medical Press, 1995), p. 231.

6. Koch, H.P., Lawson, L.D. *Garlic: The Science and Therapeutic Application of Allium sativum L. and Related Species,* Second Edition (Baltimore: Williams & Wilkins, 1996), p. 177.

7. Chang, H.M., But, P.P.H. *Pharmacology and Applications of Chinese Materia Medica,* Volume 1 (Singapore: World Scientific Publishing, 1986).

8. Mashiko, H. et al., "A case of advanced gastric cancer with liver metastasis completely responding to a combined immunochemotherapy with UFT, mitomycin C and lentinan," *Gan to Kagaku Ryoho—Japanese Journal of Cancer & Chemotherapy,* 19, 715–718 (1992).

9. Shimuzu, T., et al., "A combination of regional chemotherapy and systemic immunotherapy for the treatment of inoperable gastric cancer," in Aoki, A., et al. (eds). *Manipulation of Host Defence Mechanisms* (Amsterdam: Excerpta Medica, 1981).

10. Maeda, Y.Y., et al., "Unique increase of serum protein components and action of antitumour polysaccharides," *Nature,* 252, 250 (1974).

11. Togami, M., et al., "Studies on Basidiomycetes. I. Antitumor polysaccharide from bagasse medium on which mycelia of *Lentinus edodes* (Berk.) Sing. had been grown," *Chemical Pharmacology Bulletin,* 30, 1134–1140 (1982).

12. Moriyama, M., et al., "Anti-tumor effect of polysaccharide Lentinan on transplanted ascites hepatoma-134 in C3H/He mice," in Aoki, A., et al.

13. Ying, J., et al. *Icones of Medicinal Fungi From China* (Beijing: Science Press, 1987).

14. Osawa, S., Shiroto, H., Kondo, Y., Nakanishi, Y., Fujisawa, J., Miyakawa, K., Oku, T., Nishimura, A., Uchino, J., "Randomized controlled study on adjuvant immunochemotherapy with carmofur (HCFU) for noncuratively resected and unresected gastric cancer," *Gan to Kagaku Ryoho—Japanese Journal of Cancer & Chemotherapy,* 23(3), 327–331 (February 1996).

15. Chang, K.S.S., Gao, C., Wang, L.C., "Berberine-induced morphologic differentiation and down-regulation of c-Ki-ras2 protooncogene expression in human teratocarcinoma cells," *Cancer Letters,* 55, 103–108 (1990).

16. Chang, K.S., "Down-regulation of c-Ki-ras2 gene expression associated with morphologic differentiation in human embryonal carcinoma cells treated with berberine," *Taiwan I Hsueh Hui Tsa Chih,* 90(1), 10–14 (1991).

17. Takase, H., Inoue, O., Saito, Y., Yumioka, E., Suzuki, A., "Roles of sulfhydryl compounds in the gastric mucosal protection of the herb drugs composing *oren-gedoku-to* (a traditional herbal medicine)," *Japanese Journal of Pharmacology,* 56(4), 433–439 (August 1991).

Strep Throat

1. Badgett, J.T., Hersterberg, L.K., "Management of Group A streptococcus pharyngitis with a second-generation rapid strep screen: Strep A O1A," *Microbial Drug Resistance,* 2, 371–376 (1996).

2. McIsaac, W.J., et al., "Reconsidering sore throats, part 2: alternative approach and practical office tool," *Canadian Family Physician,* 43, 497–500 (1997).

3. McIsaac, W.J., et al., "Reconsidering sore throats, part 1: problems with current clinical practice," *Canadian Family Physician,* 43, 495–500 (1997).

4. Murray, M., Pizzorno, J. *Encyclopedia of Natural Medicine* (Rocklin, California: Prima Publishing, 1998), pp. 802–803.

5. Mitscher, L.A., "Plant-derived antibiotics," in Weinstein, M.J., Wagman, G.H. (eds). *Antibiotics,* Volume 15 (New York: Plenum Press, 1978), pp. 363–477.

6. Franzblau, S.G., Cross, C., "Comparative in vitro antimicrobial activity of Chinese medicinal herbs," *Journal of Ethnopharmacology,* 15(3), 279–288 (March 1986).

7. Chang, H.M., But, P.P.H. *Pharmacology and Applications of Chinese Materia Medica,* Volume 2 (Teaneck, New Jersey: World Scientific Publishing, 1987) p. 822.

8. Chang, H.M., But, P.P.H., p. 935.

Stress

1. Gillis, C.N., "*Panax ginseng* pharmacology: a nitric oxide link?" *Biochemical Pharmacology,* 54(1), 1–8 (July 1997).

2. Wang, S., Zhai, S., Wang, Y., Wang, L., "Effect of radix ginseng—faeces Trogopterori combination on pharmacodynamics and effective chemical composition of radix ginseng," *Chung Kuo Chung Yao Tsa Chih,* 20(10), 630–632 (October 1995).

3. Udintsev, S.N., Krylova, S.G., Konovalova, O.N., "Correction by natural adaptogens of hormonal-metabolic status disorders in rats during the development of adaptation syndrome using functional tests with dexamethasone and ACTH," *Builletin Eksperimentalnii Biologii I Medizina,* 112(12), 599–601 (December 1991).

4. Murray, M. *Healing Power of Herbs* (Rocklin, California: Prima Publishing, 1991), p. 56.

5. Wagner, H., "Immunostimulants from medicinal plants," in Chang, H.M., Yeung, W., Tso, W., Koo, A. (eds). *Advances in Chinese Medicinal Materials Research* (Singapore: World Scientific, 1985).

6. Sasaki, K., Suzuki, K., Yoshizaki, F., Ando, T., "Effect of *saiko-ka-ryukotsu-borei-to* on the stress-induced increase of serum corti-

costerone in mice," *Biological and Pharmaceutical Bulletin,* 18(4), 563–565 (April 1995).

7. Watanabe, S., "Psychotropic effects of Sino-Japanese traditional medicines," *Yakubutsu Seishin Kodo,* 13(2), 51–57 (April 1993).

8. Tozawa, F., Dobashi, I., Horiba, N., Sakai, Y., Sakai, K., Suda, T., "*Saireito* (a Chinese herbal drug) decreases inhibitory effect of prednisolone and accelerates the recovery of rat hypothalamic-pituitary-adrenal axis," *Endocrinology Journal,* 45(1), 69–74 (February 1998).

9. Amagaya, S., Ogihara, Y., "Effect of *shosaikoto,* an Oriental herbal medicinal mixture, on restraint-stressed mice," *Journal of Ethnopharmacology,* 28(3), 357–363 (March 1990).

10. Ueda, Y., Komatsu, M., Hiramatsu, M., "Free radical scavenging activity of the Japanese herbal medicine *toki-shakuyaku-san* (TJ-23) and its effect on superoxide dismutase activity, lipid peroxides, glutamate, and monoamine metabolites in aged rat brain," *Neurochemical Research,* 21(8), 909–914 (August 1996).

Stroke

1. McIntosh, T.K., Juhler, M., Wieloch, T., "Novel pharmacologic strategies in the treatment of experimental traumatic brain injury: 1998," *Journal of Neurotrauma,* 15(10), 731–769 (October 1998).

2. Hofferberth, B., "The efficacy of EGb 761 in patients with senile dementia of the Alzheimer type, a double blind, placebo-controlled study on different levels of investigation," *Human Psychopharmacology,* 9, 215–222 (1994).

3. Pourrat, H., "Anthocyanidin drugs in vascular disease," *Plant Medicinal Phytotherapy,* 11, 143–151 (1977).

4. Fushitani, S., Minakuchi, K., Tsuchiya, K., Takasugi, M., Murakami, K., "Studies on attenuation of post-ischemic brain injury by Kampo medicines—inhibitory effects of free radical production," *Yakugaku Zasshi—Journal of the Pharmaceutical Society of Japan,* 115(8), 611–617 (August 1995).

Tinnitus (Ringing in the Ears)

1. Zhuang, J., Chen, H., "Treatment of tinnitus with Cordyceps infusion: a report of 23 cases," *Fujian Medical Journal,* 7, 42, 53 (1985).

2. Meyer, B., "Multi-center, randomized study of placebo vs. *Ginkgo biloba* extract in treatment of acute hearing loss," *Presse Med,* 15, 1562–1564 (1986).

3. Coles, R., "Trial of an extract of *Ginkgo biloba* (EGB) for tinnitus and hearing loss," *Clinical Otolaryngology,* 13, 501–504 (1988).

Tuberculosis

1. Isselbacher, K.J., Braunwald, E., Wilson, J., Martin, J.V., Fauci, A.S., Kasper, D.L., eds. *Harrison's Principles of Internal Medicine,* Thirteenth Edition (New York: McGraw-Hill, 1995), p. 710.

2. Onodera, H., Kasamatsu, Y., Tsujimoto, S., Takemura, S., Okamoto, M., Seto, N., Nakanishi, S., Nakahara, R., Ichio, N., Doi, T., et al., "A case of pulmonary tuberculosis complicated with drug toxicosis—value of *shosaikoto* and *hochuekito* as anti-allergic agents," *Kekkaku,* 68(1), 23–29 (January 1993).

3. Bensky, D., Gamble, A., Kaptchuk, T., Bensky, L.L. *Chinese Herbal Medicine: Materia Medica,* Revised Edition (Seattle: Eastland Press, 1993), p. 254.

4. Bensky, D., Gamble, A., Kaptchuk, T., Bensky, L.L., p. 218.

5. Bensky, D., Gamble, A., Kaptchuk, T., Bensky, L.L., p. 307.

6. Piras, G., Makino, M., Baba, M., "*Sho-saiko-to,* a traditional Kampo medicine, enhances the anti-HIV-1 activity of lamivudine (3TC) in vitro," *Microbiology and Immunology,* 41(10), 835–839.

7. Galitskii, L.A., Barnaulov, O.D., Zaretskii, B.V., Malkov, M.I., Konenkov, S.I., Gol'm, N.P., Tomakov, V.S., Ogarkov, P.I., Batskov, S.S., "Effect of phytotherapy on the prevention and elimination of hepatotoxic responses in patients with pulmonary tuberculosis, carriers of hepatitis B virus markers," *Problemii Tuberkulosisa,* 4, 35–38 (1997).

Yeast Infections

1. Hobbs, C., "Naturopathic specific condition review: candidiasis," *Protocol Journal of Botanical Medicine,* 1(3), 56 (Winter 1996).

Index

Abalone shell, 96
Abdominal pain, corydalis and, 44
Abscesses, painful, viola and, 93
Acne, 143
  Cinnamon Twig and Poria Pill and, 115
  Coptis Decoction to Relieve Toxicity and, 117
Aconite, 19
Acorus, 19–20
Acquired immune deficiency syndrome (AIDS), 143–145
  astragalus and, 28
  burdock and, 36
  cinnamon and, 40
  garlic and, 54
  lentinan and, 102
  licorice and, 66
  Ten-Significant Tonic Decoction and, 136
  viola and, 93
  See also HIV infection; Kaposi's sarcoma.
Actinic keratosis, 43, 288
Acute cutaneous lupus erythematous (ACLE), 254
Acute lymphocytic (or lymphoblastic) leukemia (ALL), 249
Acute myelocytic leukemia (AML), 249
ADD; ADHD. *See* Attention Deficit Disorder / Attention Deficit Hyperactivity Disorder (ADD / ADHD).
Addison's disease, licorice and, 67
Adriamycin. *See* Doxorubicin hydrochloride.
Age-related memory loss. *See* Memory problems.
Agrimony, 20
AIDS. *See* Acquired immune deficiency syndrome.
Akebia, 20
Alcoholism, 145–146
  kudzu and, 65
  Kudzu Decoction and, 124
  See also Cirrhosis, alcoholic.
Alisma, 21
Allergies
  to cedar pollen, 119
  Cinnamon and Peony Decoction and, 115
  Ephedra, Asiasarum, and Prepared Aconite Decoction and, 119
  food, 146–147, 205
  forsythia and, 51
  ginger and, 56
  jujube fruit and, 63
  licorice and, 67
  Minor Bluegreen Dragon Decoction and, 127–128
  reishi and, 104
  respiratory, 147–148. *See also* Asthma.
All-Inclusive Great Tonifying Decoction. *See* Ten-Significant Tonic Decoction.
Aloe, 21
Alzheimer's disease, 149–150
  biota and, 31
  Bupleurum Plus Dragon Bone and Oyster Shell Decoction and, 114
  Coptis Decoction to Relieve Toxicity and, 117
  gastrodia and, 55
  ginkgo and, 101
  hawthorn and, 60
Amaranth, 22
American Association of Acupuncture and Oriental Medicine, 12
American ginseng, 23
Analgesics. *See* Pain relief.
Androgenetic alopecia (AGA), 219
Anemarrhena, 24
Anemia, 150–151
  dandelion and, 45
Angelica dahurica, 24
Angina, 151–152
  astragalus and, 28
  surgery and, 152
  See also Atherosclerosis; High cholesterol.
Anxiety, 152–154
  corydalis and, 44
Appetite loss, codonopsis and, 41
Apricot seed, 25
Arisaema, 25
Arnica, cancer and, 186
Arrest Wheezing Decoction, 111
Arrhythmia. *See* Congestive heart failure.
Artemisia, 26
Arteriosclerosis, decoction and, 114
Arthritis
  bupleurum and, 35
  clematis and, 40
  scutellaria and, 89
  turmeric and, 93

See also Osteoarthritis; Rheumatoid arthritis.
Asiasarum, 26
Asparagus root, 27
Asthma, 154–157
chrysanthemum and, 39
codonopsis and, 41
ginger and, 56
ginkgo and, 100
ginkgo nut and, 57
green tea and, 59
jujube fruit and, 63
licorice and, 67
lobelia and, 69–70
Minor Bupleurum Decoction and, 128
nutrition and, 156
reishi and, 104
scutellaria and, 89
trigger foods, 156
turmeric and, 93
See also Allergies, respiratory.
Astragalus, 27–28
Astragalus Decoction to Construct the Middle, 111
Atherosclerosis, 157–158
acorus and, 19
carthamus and, 37
garlic and, 54
ginger and, 56
ginkgo and, 100, 101
hawthorn and, 60
kelp and, 64
lycium and, 72
scutellaria and, 89
snow fungus and, 107
turmeric and, 92
See also High cholesterol.
Athlete's foot, cloves and, 41
Atopic dermatitis, 205
Atractylodis, red, 29
Atractylodis, white, 29
Attention Deficit Disorder / Attention Deficit Hyperactivity Disorder (ADD / ADHD), 158–160
gingko and, 101
hawthorn and, 60
rehmannia and, 84
scutellaria and, 89
Siberian ginseng and, 106
Six-Ingredient Pill With Rehmannia and, 135
Augmented Four-Substance Decoction, 111
Augmented Rambling Powder, 112

Bacterial infection, decoction and, 137
Bags beneath the eyes, 210
Balances of energy, blood, and fluids, 3
Bamboo and Hoelen Decoction. *See* Warm the Gallbladder Decoction.
Bamboo shavings, 29
Barley sprouts, 30
Basal cell carcinoma. *See* Skin cancer (basal cell carcinoma).
Bedwetting, children's, 160–161. *See also* Bladder infection.
Belching, 238–239
Benign prostatic hyperplasia (BPH). *See* Prostate enlargement, benign.
Benincasa, 30
Biota, 30–31
Biota Seed Pill to Nourish the Heart, 112
Bitter melon, 31–32
Bitter orange, 32
Bitter orange peel, 32–33
Black cardamom, 33
Black cohosh, 33
Bladder cancer, 161–162
Bladder infection, 163–164
artemisia and, 26
Bleeding
agrimony and, 20
kaolin and, 98
shepherd's purse and, 265
Bleeding gums, 164–165. *See also* Gingivitis.
Bletilla, 34
Bloating, 239
Blood, in Oriental medicine, 10
Blood pressure problems. *See* High blood pressure; Low blood pressure.
Bloodshot eyes, 210–211
Blue citrus, 34
Blurred vision, 211
Boils, 165–166
Bone cancer, 166–168
agrimony and, 20
asiasarum and, 27
psoralea and, 83
turmeric and, 92
See also Cancer.
Boneset. *See* Eupatorium.
Boswellia. *See* Frankincense.
Breast cancer
Augmented Rambling Powder and, 112
Cinnamon Twig and Poria Pill and, 115–116
garlic and, 54
ginkgo and, 101
green tea and, 59
kelp and, 64
kudzu and, 64–65
lentinan and, 102
loranthus and, 71
maitake and, 103
in men, 169
polygonum and, 82
rhubarb and, 85
soy isoflavones and, 108
Tang-Kuei and Peony Powder and, 135
Two-Cured Decoction and, 138
See also Cancer.
Breast pain
vitex and, 94
kaolin and, 98

Bronchitis, 171–172
green tea and, 59
snow fungus and, 107
white mustard seed and, 95
Broomrape. *See* Cistanche.
Brucea, 35
Buddhism and Kampo, 7
Bupleurum, 35–36
Bupleurum and Cinnamon Twig Decoction, 112
Bupleurum and Kudzu Decoction to Release the Muscle Layer From *Medical Revelations*, 113
Bupleurum, Cinnamon Twig, and Ginger Decoction, 113
Bupleurum Decoction to Clear the Liver, 113
Bupleurum Plus Dragon Bone and Oyster Shell Decoction, 114
Burdock, 36
Burns, 173–174
aloe and, 21
coptis and, 43
Bursitis, turmeric and, 93
Buying herbs, 13

Calm the Middle Powder, 114
Calm the Stomach Powder, 114
Caltrop, 36–37
Cancer, 174–175
aloe and, 21
asiasarum and, 27
astragalus and, 28
atractylodis, white, and, 29
burdock and, 36
cinnamon and, 40
codonopsis and, 41
epimedium and, 49
eupatorium and, 50
garlic and, 54
ginkgo and, 101
ginseng and, 58
green tea and, 59
hawthorn and, 60
kelp and, 64
kudzu and, 64
lentinan and, 102
licorice and, 66
ligustrum and, 68
lithospermum and, 69
loranthus and, 71
lycium and, 72
maitake and, 103
nutmeg and, 76
polygonum and, 82
polyporus and, 82
PSK and, 104
rhubarb and, 85
scutellaria and, 88
Siberian ginseng and, 106
snow fungus and, 107
soy isoflavones and, 108
Ten-Significant Tonic Decoction and, 136
Tonify the Middle and Augment the Qi Decoction and, 137
turmeric and, 88
See also Bladder cancer; Bone cancer; Breast cancer; Cervical cancer; Colorectal cancer; Endometrial cancer; Hodgkin's disease; Kidney cancer; Leukemia; Liver cancer; Lung cancer; Melanoma; Ovarian cancer; Prostate cancer; Skin cancer (basal cell carcinoma); Stomach cancer.
Candidiasis. *See* Yeast infections.
Capital Qi Pill, 114
Carboplatin, 178–179
Carbuncles. *See* Boils.
Cardamom, 37
Cardiomyopathy, 189
Carnitine, and congestive heart disease, 190
Carpal tunnel syndrome, turmeric and, 93
Carthamus, 37
Cassia. *See* Cinnamon.
Cataracts, 175–176
Eight-Ingredient Pill With Rehmannia, 118
scutellaria and, 89
Catechins. *See* Green tea.
Celiac sprue, 146, 147
Cervical cancer, 176–178
arisaema and, 25
brucea and, 35
nutrition and, 177
snow fungus and, 107
Cervical dysplasia, 176, 177
CFS. *See* Chronic fatigue syndrome.
Chebula, 38
Chelation therapy, angina and, 152
Chemotherapy side effects, 178–181
astragalus and, 28
Chen-pi. *See* Bitter orange peel.
Cheng Wu-Ji, 6
Chi Po, 5
Children
bedwetting and. *See* Bedwetting, children's.
constipation in, easing, 193
developmental disorders in. *See* Attention Deficit Disorder/Attention Deficit Hyperactivity Disorder (ADD/ADHD).
Kampo remedies and, 142
Chinese angelica. *See* Tang-kuei.
Chinese date. *See* Jujube fruit.
Chinese prickly ash. *See* Zanthoxylum.
Chinese rose. *See* Rose hips.
Chinese senega root, 38
Cholesterol problems. *See* High cholesterol.
Chondroitin, and osteoarthritis, 272
Chronic fatigue syndrome (CFS), 181–183
cloves and, 41
dan shen and, 45
ginseng and, 58
licorice and, 66

Chronic lymphocytic leukemia (CLL), 249
Chronic myelocytic (or granulocytic) leukemia (CML), 249
Chrysanthemum, 38–39
Cimicifuga and Kudzu Decoction, 115
Cinnamon, 39–40
Cinnamon and Peony Decoction, 115
Cinnamon Twig and Poria Pill, 115
Cinnamon Twig Decoction, 116
Cinnamon Twig Decoction Plus Dragon Bone and Oyster Shell, 116
Cinnamon Twig Decoction Plus Kudzu, 116
Cinnamon Twig, Licorice, Dragon Bone, and Oyster Shell Decoction, 117
Cirrhosis, alcoholic, 183–184. *See also* Alcoholism.
Cisplastin, 178–179
Cistanche, 40
Clear Summerheat and Augment the Qi Decoction, 117
Clematis, 40
Cloud fungus. *See* PSK.
Cloves, 41
Cocklebur. *See* Agrimony.
Codonopsis, 41
Coix, 41–42
Cold and heat, in Oriental medicine, 8–9
Colds, 184–186
  astragalus and, 28
  bupleurum and, 35
  Cinnamon and Peony Decoction and, 115
  Ephedra Decoction and, 119
  eupatorium and, 50
  garlic and, 54
  ginger and, 56
  kudzu and, 65
  Kudzu Decoction and, 124
  scallion and, 87
  Siberian ginseng and, 105–106
  Tang-Kuei and Peony Powder and, 135
  white mustard seed and, 95
  See also Allergies, respiratory; Influenza.
Colorectal cancer, 186–189
  astragalus and, 28
  ginkgo and, 101
  kelp and, 64
  maitake and, 103
  other herbal treatments and, 186
  PSK and, 104
  turmeric and, 92
Coltsfoot, 42
Congestive heart failure, 189–191
  aconite and, 18
  astragalus and, 28
  nutritional support for, 190
Conjunctivitis, 191–192. *See also* Allergies, respiratory.
Constipation, 192–194
  aloe and, 22
  in children, 193
  Cinnamon and Peony Decoction and, 115
  dandelion and, 45
  Hemp Seed Pill and, 123
  kelp and, 64
  marijuana seed and, 73
  mirabilite and, 99
  rhubarb and, 85
  See also Irritable bowel syndrome.
Contact dermatitis, 205
Coptis, 42–43
Coptis Decoction to Relieve Toxicity, 117
CoQ_{10}, and congestive heart disease, 190
Cordyceps, 96–97
Cornelian cherry, 43–44
Coronary artery disease, 189
Cortisone, 180–181
Corydalis, 44
Cranberry juice, bladder infection and, 163
Crohn's disease. *See* Irritable bowel syndrome.
Curcumin. *See* Turmeric.
Cuscuta, 44
Cushing's syndrome, 248
Cyclophosphamide, 179
Cystitis. *See* Bladder infection.
Cysts, ovarian. *See* Ovarian cysts.

Dan shen, 44–45
Dandelion, 45–46
Dendrobium, 46
Dental plaque, green tea and, 59
Depression, 194–196
  Drive Out Stasis From the Mansion of Blood Decoction and, 118
  ginkgo and, 101
  morinda and, 74
  Siberian ginseng and, 106
  St. John's wort and, 195
  See also Anxiety; Chronic fatigue syndrome; Insomnia; Memory problems.
Dermatitis, 205
Dexamethasone, 180–181
Diabetes, 196–200
  agrimony and, 20
  aloe and, 22
  anemarrhena and, 24
  angelica dahurica and, 24
  astragalus and, 28
  atractylodis, red, and, 29
  benincasa and, 30
  bitter melon and, 31
  burdock and, 36
  dioscorea and, 47
  Eight-Ingredient Pill With Rehmannia and, 118
  garlic and, 54
  ginkgo and, 101
  ginseng and, 58
  green tea and, 59
  kelp and, 64
  lotus and, 72
  lycium and, 72

maitake and, 103
Major Bupleurum Decoction and, 126
mulberry root and, 76
White Tiger Plus Atractylodis Decoction and, 140
White Tiger Plus Ginseng Decoction and, 140
Diabetic neuropathy, 197
Diabetic retinopathy, 197, 200–201
astragalus and, 28
dan shen and, 45
ginkgo and, 101
Diagnosis in Kampo, 8–10, 17
Diarrhea, 201–203
agrimony and, 20
anemarrhena and, 24
angelica dahurica and, 24
bamboo shavings and, 30
chebula and, 38
home care for, 202
kaolin and, 98
peppermint and, 79
phellodendron and, 80
Pinellia Decoction to Drain the Epigastrium and, 131
See also Allergies, food; Irritable bowel syndrome.
Diet
cholesterol and, 230
eczema and, 205
estrogen levels, lowering with, 207
fibrocystic breast disease and, 213
kidney stone prevention and, 248
Dioscorea, 46–47
Discoid lupus erythematous (DLE), 254
Diuretic. *See* Urination, stimulating.
Dong quai. *See* Tang-kuei.
Dopamine, 194
Doxorubicin hydrochloride (Adriamycin), 180
Dracaena lily, 47
Dragon bone, 97
Drive Out Stasis From the Mansion of Blood Decoction, 118
Drug addiction, acorus and, 19
Drynaria rhizome, 47
Duodenal ulcer. *See* Peptic ulcer.
Dysmenorrhea, 265
Dyspepsia. *See* Indigestion.

Ear infection, 203–205
coptis and, 43
echinacea and, 204
Earache, garlic and, 54
Ears, ringing in the. *See* Tinnitus.
Echinacea
and colorectal and liver cancer, 186
and ear infection, 204
Eczema, 205–207
aloe and, 21
burdock and, 36
diet and, 205
licorice and, 67
Ophiopogonis Decoction and, 129
PSK and, 104
psoralea and, 83
tang-kuei and, 91
turmeric and, 93
See also Psoriasis.
Eight-Ingredient Pill With Rehmannia, 118
Emperor of Heaven's Special Pill to Tonify the Heart, 118
Empress Suiko, 6
Endometrial cancer, 207–208. *See also* Cancer.
Augmented Rambling Powder and, 112
Cinnamon Twig and Poria Pill and, 115–116
kudzu and, 65
PSK and, 104
Endometriosis, 208–210
Cinnamon Twig and Poria Pill and, 116
Two-Cured Decoction and, 138
vitex and, 94
Energy meridians, 10
Ephedra, 47–49
Ephedra, Apricot Kernel, Gypsum, and Licorice Decoction, 119
Ephedra, Asiasarum, and Prepared Aconite Decoction, 119
Ephedra Decoction, 119
Epilepsy. *See* Seizure disorders.
Epimedium, 49
Epinephrine, 194
Epsom salts. *See* Mirabilite.
Epstein-Barr virus (EBV), 69, 88, 181, 233
Essential fatty acids (EFAs). *See* Omega-3 fatty acids; Omega-6 fatty acids.
Estrogen, 161, 169, 207, 209, 212, 214, 259, 263, 273, 274, 278
Augmented Rambling Powder and, 112
black cohosh and, 33
Cinnamon Twig and Poria Pill and, 115–116
kudzu and, 64
lowering levels of, 207
Estrogen replacement therapy, 263–264
Eucommia, 49–50
Eupatorium, 50
Evodia, 50–51
Evodia Decoction, 120
Excess and deficiency, in Oriental medicine, 9, 17
Eye disorders. *See* Bags beneath the eyes; Bloodshot eyes; Blurred vision; Cataracts; Conjunctivitis; Diabetic retinopathy; Floaters; Glaucoma; Macular degeneration.

Fennel seed, 51
Fever, reducing
bupleurum and, 35
kudzu and, 65
peony and, 78
Fibrocystic breast disease, 212–214
diet and, 213
Tang-Kuei and Peony Powder and, 135
Two-Cured Decoction and, 138
Fibroids (uterine myomas), 214–215
Five Elements theory, 1, 10
Five Paired Organs, theory of, 6

Five-Accumulation Powder, 120
5-fluorouracil (5-FU), 180
Five-Ingredient Powder With Poria, 120
Flatulence, 239
Floaters, 211–212
Flu. *See* Influenza.
Fluid extract, 13
Fluid imbalances, in Oriental medicine, 10
Fluid retention, dandelion and, 45
Folic acid and cervical cancer, 177
Food allergies. *See* Allergies, food.
Food intolerance, 146
Food poisoning. *See* Diarrhea.
Forgetfulness. *See* Memory problems.
Formula usage notes, 109–111. *See also* Medicines, Kampo.
Forsythia, 51
Four Emperors Combination. *See* Ephedra Decoction.
Four-Gentleman Decoction, 121
Four-Substance Decoction, 121
Foxglove. *See* Rehmannia.
Frankincense, 97
Frigid Extremities Decoction, 121
Frigid Extremities Powder, 122
Fritillaria (cirrhosa), 52
Fritillaria (Thunberg fritillaria bulb), 52
Fungal infection
 cloves and, 41
 longan and, 70
 scutellaria and, 88
Furuncles. *See* Boils.

Galangal, 52
Gallbladder problems
 dandelion and, 45
 gentian and, 55
Gallstones, 216–217
 Major Bupleurum Decoction and, 126
Gambir, 52–53
Gardenia, 53
Garlic, 53–55
Gastric ulcer. *See* Peptic ulcer.
Gastritis, 217–218.
 turmeric and, 93
 See also Peptic ulcer.
Gastrodia, 55
Gastrodia and Uncaria Decoction, 122
Ge Hong, 6
Gelatin, 97–98
Gene p53, 161, 169, 176, 187, 188
Geni Nagoya, 7, 8
Gentian, 14, 55–56
Gentiana Longdancao Decoction to Drain the Liver, 122
Giant peony. *See* Moutan.
Ginger, 56–57
Gingivitis, 164. *See also* Bleeding gums.
 cinnamon and, 39
 lycium and, 72
 scutellaria and, 89
 turmeric and, 93
Ginkgo, 100–101
 and Alzheimer's disease, 149
Ginkgo nut, 57
Ginseng, 57–59
Ginseng Decoction to Nourish the Nutritive Qi, 123
Glaucoma, 218–219
 Five-Ingredient Powder With Poria and, 121
Glomerulonephritis. *See* Kidney disease.
Glucosamine sulfate and osteoarthritis, 272
Glutathione and cervical cancer, 177
Good manufacturing practices, (GMP), 14
Grave's disease. *See* Hyperthyroidism.
Green tea, 59–60
Guide Out the Red Powder, 123
Gum problems. *See* Bleeding gums; Gingivitis.
Gypsum, 98

H. pylori. See Helicobacter pylori.
Hair darkener, Seven-Treasure Pill for Beautiful Whiskers as, 134
Hair loss, 219–220
 biota and, 31
 carthamus and, 37
 Cinnamon Twig Decoction Plus Dragon Bone and Oyster Shell and, 116
 psoralea and, 83
Hangover, 220–221
Hashimoto's thyroiditis, 235
Hawthorn, 60–61
Hay fever, 147
HDL. *See* High-density lipoprotein.
Headache, 221–223
 peppermint and, 79
 See also Migraine.
Hearing loss. *See also* Ménière's disease; Tinnitus.
 drynaria tinctures and, 47
 ginkgo and, 101
Heart attack aftercare. *See* Congestive heart failure.
Heartbeat regulation
 amaranth and, 22
 American ginseng and, 23
 astragalus and, 28
 bitter orange and, 32
 black cardamom and, 33
 cinnamon and, 39
 dan shen and, 45
 ephedra and, 48
 ginseng and, 58
 green tea and, 59
 kudzu and, 65
 pinellia and, 80
Heartburn, 239
Heavy metal poisoning
 garlic and, 54
 kelp and, 64
Helicobacter pylori, 217, 277, 289
Hemorrhoids, 222–223

Peach Blossom Decoction and, 129
Hemp. *See* Marijuana seed.
Hemp Seed Pill, 123
Hepatitis, 223–225
artemisia and, 26
bupleurum and, 35
Calm the Middle Powder and, 114
hoelen and, 62
jujube fruit and, 63
LEM and, 102
licorice and, 66
maitake and, 103
Minor Bupleurum Decoction and, 128
polyporus and, 82
reishi and, 105
saussurea and, 86
schisandra and, 87
snow fungus and, 107
soy lecithin and, 108
types of, 224
Herbal medicine, in Oriental medicine, 5, 7
Herbal products, forms of, 13
Herbs. *See* Medicines, Kampo.
Hernia, fennel seed and, 51
Herpes, 225–226
bitter melon and, 31
bupleurum and, 36
dandelion and, 46
Kudzu Decoction and, 124
lindera and, 69
prunella and, 83
Hiccups, 240
High blood pressure, 226–229
agrimony and, 20
alisma and, 21
amaranth and, 22
Coptis Decoction to Relieve Toxicity and, 117
epimedium and, 49
eucommia and, 50
green tea and, 59
hawthorn and, 60
lindera and, 69
lycium and, 72
magnolia and, 73
marijuana seed and, 73
morinda and, 74
moutan and, 75
mulberry root and, 75–76
scutellaria and, 89
tang-kuei and, 91
High cholesterol, 229–231
Bupleurum Plus Dragon Bone and Oyster Shell Decoction and, 114
coix and, 42
cordyceps and, 96
dan shen and, 45
garlic and, 54
ginger and, 56
ginseng and, 58
green tea and, 59
hawthorn and, 60
LEM and, 102
lonicera and, 70
Major Bupleurum Decoction and, 126
polygonum and, 82
polyporus and, 82
scutellaria and, 89
shiitake and, 105
soy lecithin and, 108
High-density lipoprotein (HDL), 157, 229, 263
HIV infection, 231–232
bitter melon and, 31
cinnamon and, 40
dendrobium and, 46
hoelen and, 62
kelp and, 64
LEM and, 102
licorice and, 66
Minor Bupleurum Decoction and, 128
prunella and, 83
scutellaria and, 88
snake gourd root and, 90
turmeric and, 93
viola and, 93
See also Acquired immune deficiency syndrome.
Hives, ginkgo nut and, 57
Hodgkin's disease, 233
Hoelen, 61–62
Honey-Fried Licorice Decoction, 123
Honeysuckle and Forsythia Powder. *See* Lonicera and Forsythia Powder.
Hong-Yen Hsu, 11
Houttynia, 62
Human immunodeficiency virus. *See* HIV infection.
Human papillomavirus (HPV), 176, 177
Hydrocortisone, 180–181
Hyperactivity. *See* Attention Deficit Disorder/Attention Deficit Hyperactivity Disorder (ADD/ADHD).
Hypertension. *See* High blood pressure.
Hyperthyroidism, 234–235
Hypothyroidism, 235–236

IBS. *See* Irritable bowel syndrome.
Idiopathic rapidly progressive glomerulonephritis (IRPG), 247
Immune system stimulation
agrimony and, 20
aloe and, 21
asiasarum and, 27
cordyceps and, 96
eupatorium and, 50
garlic and, 54
hawthorn and, 60
LEM and, 102
lentinan and, 102
lithospermum and, 69

loranthus and, 71
peony and, 78
perilla and, 79
shiitake and, 105
Siberian ginseng and, 106
snow fungus and, 107
turmeric and, 92
Impotence, 236–237
cistanche and, 40
ginkgo and, 101
Siberian ginseng and, 106
Incontinence, 237–238. *See also* Bladder infection; Diarrhea.
Indigestion, 238–240
Infection. *See types:* Bacterial, Bladder, Ear, Fungal, HIV, Respiratory tract, Skin, Staph, Strep, Viral, Yeast.
Infertility, female, 240–241
American ginseng and, 24
Peony and Licorice Decoction and, 130
Infertility, male, 241–242
astragalus and, 28
black cohosh and, 34
Cinnamon Twig and Poria Pill and, 116
cordyceps and, 97
epimedium and, 49
ginseng and, 58
tang-kuei and, 91
Tonify the Middle and Augment the Qi Decoction and, 137
Influenza, 242–243
bupleurum and, 35
green tea and, 59
kudzu and, 65
licorice and, 66
ligusticum and, 68
scutellaria and, 88
Siberian ginseng and, 105–106
See also Colds.
Injuries
aloe and, 21
Trauma Pill and, 137
Insomnia, 243–244
Cinnamon Twig Decoction Plus Dragon Bone and Oyster Shell and, 116
corydalis and, 44
schisandra and, 87
Interior and exterior, in Oriental medicine, 9, 17
Intermittent claudication, ginkgo and, 100
Intestinal ulcer. *See* Peptic ulcer.
Irritable bowel syndrome (IBS), 244–245
dandelion and, 45
peppermint and, 78–79

Jack-in-the-pulpit. *See* Arisaema.
Japanese hawthorn. *See* Hawthorn.
Japanese honeysuckle. *See* Lonicera.
Japanese lily. *See* Ophiopogon.
Japanese mint, 62–63
Japanese watermelon, 63
Job's tears. *See* Coix.
Jujube fruit, 63

Kampo
diagnosis in, 8–10, 17
differences between other healing traditions and, 3, 10, 11, 17, 109
formula usage notes, 109–111
history of, 5–7, 10–11
popularity of, recent, 11, 12
pregnancy and, 142
prescription drugs and, 142
scientific validity of, 11–12
side effects and, 1, 18
treating disorders with, 141–142
uses most suitable for, 11
See also Medicines, Kampo.
Kaolin, 98, 202
Kaposi's sarcoma, 62, 144
Keisetu Otsuka, 4, 11
Kelp, 63–64
Keratin, 143
Kidney cancer, 245–247
astragalus and, 28
See also Cancer.
Kidney disease, 247–248
hoelen and, 61
Kidney Qi Pill From *The Golden Cabinet,* 124
Kidney stones, 248–249
diet for the prevention of, 248
lithospermum and, 69
Polyporus Decoction and, 132
talc and, 100
Koho school of Kampo, 7
Kou Zong-Shi, 8
Kudzu, 64–65
Kudzu Decoction, 1, 2, 124
Kyushin Yumoto, 10

Lactobacillus acidophilus, 207, 294, 295
Lactose intolerance, 146, 147
Laxative. *See* Constipation.
LDL. *See* Low-density lipoprotein.
Leaky gut syndrome, food allergies and, 146
Ledebouriella, 65–66
Ledebouriella Powder That Sagely Unblocks, 125
Leg cramps
bitter orange peel and, 33
dandelion and, 45
LEM, 102
Lentinan, 102–103
Leukemia, 249–251
agrimony and, 20
asiasarum and, 27
ginkgo and, 101
hawthorn and, 60
kudzu and, 65
reishi and, 105

soy isoflavones and, 108
turmeric and, 92
See also Cancer.
Leukopenia
ligusticum and, 68
loranthus and, 71
snow fungus and, 107
Licorice, 66–67
Licorice, Wheat, and Jujube Decoction, 125
Ligusticum, 67–68
Ligusticum Chuanxiong Powder to Be Taken With Green Tea, 125
Ligustrum, 68
Lily bulb, 68
Lily Bulb Decoction to Preserve the Metal, 125
Lindera, 68–69
Lipoprotein. *See* High-density lipoprotein; Low-density lipoprotein.
Lithospermum, 69
Liver cancer, 251–253
LEM and, 102
Minor Bupleurum Decoction and, 128
other herbal treatments and, 186
rhubarb and, 85
schisandra and, 251
See also Cancer.
Liver. *See* Cirrhosis, alcoholic; Hepatitis; Liver cancer.
Lobelia, 69–70
Locoweed. *See* Astragalus.
Longan, 70
Lonicera, 70
Lonicera and Forsythia Powder, 126
Lophatherum, 70
Loranthus, 71
Lotus, 71–72
Low blood pressure
agrimony and, 20
bitter orange and, 32
Low-density lipoprotein (LDL), 157, 229, 263
Lung cancer, 253–254
aloe and, 21
astragalus and, 28
ginkgo and, 101
ginseng and, 58
lentinan and, 103
psoralea and, 83
rhubarb and, 85
turmeric and, 92
See also Cancer.
Lupus, 254–256
codonopsis and, 41
cordyceps and, 96
gentian and, 55
hoelen and, 61
Lycium, 72–73
Lymphoma
astragalus and, 28
cordyceps and, 96
snake gourd root and, 90

Ma huang. *See* Ephedra.
Macrocytic anemia, 151
Macular degeneration, 256–257
Augmented Rambling Powder and, 112
dan shen and, 45
ginkgo and, 101
Magnesium
and asthma, 156
and congestive heart failure, 190
Magnetite, 98
Magnolia, 73
Maitake, 103–104
Major Bupleurum Decoction, 126
Major Construct the Middle Decoction, 126
Major Ledebouriella Decoction, 127
Major Order the Qi Decoction, 127
Malaria, 26, 37, 72
Malt sugar, 98–99
Marijuana seed, 73–74
Mastitis, 257–258
Measles, 258–259
Medicines, Kampo
buying, 13–14
quality control, 14
tea-making instructions, basic, 14–15
usage notes, 17–19
Melanoma, 259–260
astragalus and, 28
Cinnamon Twig and Poria Pill and, 115–116
rhubarb and, 85
soy isoflavones and, 108
See also Skin cancer (basal cell carcinoma).
Memory problems, 260–262
acorus and, 19
American ginseng and, 23
biota and, 31
hawthorn and, 60
rose hips and, 86
schisandra and, 87
See also Alzheimer's disease; Stroke.
Ménière's disease, 262–263
Siberian ginseng and, 106
Menopause-related problems, 263–265
black cohosh and, 34
Peony and Licorice Decoction and, 130
vitex and, 94
Menorrhagia, 265
Menstrual problems, 265–266
Augmented Rambling Powder and, 112
dioscorea and, 47
morinda and, 74
moutan and, 75
vitex and, 94
See also Endometriosis; Fibroids (uterine myomas); Pelvic inflammatory disease; Premenstrual syndrome (PMS).
Methylprednisone, 180–181

Microcytic anemia, 151
Migraine, 267–268
 decoction and, 114
 See also Headache.
Milk production, stimulation of
 fennel seed and, 51
 vitex and, 94
Milk vetch. *See* Astragalus.
Minor Bluegreen Dragon Decoction, 127
Minor Bupleurum Decoction, 1, 6, 128
Minor Construct the Middle Decoction, 128
Mint. *See* Japanese mint.
Mirabilite, 99
Mistletoe, mulberry. *See* Loranthus.
Mitomycin (Mitocycin-C), 180
Monkshood, blue. *See* Aconite.
Monoamine oxidase inhibitors (MAOIs), 194
Mood elevation
 lotus and, 72
 opium poppy husk and, 77
 wheat and, 94
Morinda, 74
Morning sickness, ginger and, 56
Motherwort, 74–75
Motion sickness, ginger and, 56
Moutan, 75
Moxibustion, 3
MS. *See* Multiple sclerosis.
Mu tong. *See* Akebia.
Mulberry root, 75–76
Multiple myeloma. *See* Bone cancer.
Multiple sclerosis (MS), 268–269
 ginkgo and, 101
 Ophiopogonis Decoction and, 129
Mumps, 269–270
Muscle stiffness
 dioscorea and, 47
 gastrodia and, 55
 lindera and, 69
 magnolia and, 73
Musk, 99
Mustard seed. *See* White mustard seed.
Myasthenia gravis, astragalus and, 28
Myocardial infarction, 189
Myotonia dystrophica, reishi and, 105
Myrrh, 99

Nausea and vomiting
 codonopsis and, 41
 ginger and, 56
 phellodendron and, 80
 pinellia and, 80
Nephritis. *See* Kidney disease.
Nephrotic syndrome, 247
Nerve pain, gastrodia and, 55
Nonsteroidal anti-inflammatory drugs (NSAIDs), 154, 217, 277, 284
Nosebleed, 270
Notopterygium, 76
NSAIDs. *See* Nonsteroidal anti-inflammatory drugs.
Nutmeg, 76
Nutrition
 asthma and, 156
 cervical cancer and, 177
 congestive heart failure and, 189

Obesity, 270–272
 ephedra and, 48
 kelp and, 64
 Ledebouriella Powder That Sagely Unblocks and, 125
 Peach Pit Decoction to Order the Qi and, 130
 perilla and, 79
Omega-3 fatty acids, 156, 205
Omega-6 fatty acids, 205
Ophiopogon, 77
Ophiopogonis Decoction, 129
Opium poppy husk, 77
Oral contraceptives, cervical cancer and, 176, 177
Oriental Healing Arts Institute (OHAI), 11
Oriental medicine, principles of, 3
Osteoarthritis, 272–273
 frankincense and, 97
 hawthorn and, 60
 other therapies for, 272
 See also Rheumatoid arthritis.
Osteoporosis prevention, gelatin and, 97
Osteosarcoma. *See* Bone cancer.
Otitis media, 203
Ovarian cancer, 273–274
 agrimony and, 20
 asiasarum and, 27
 ginkgo and, 101
 turmeric and, 92
 See also Cancer.
Ovarian cysts, 274–275
 Augmented Rambling Powder and, 112
 Cinnamon Twig and Poria Pill and, 115–116
 Two-Cured Decoction and, 138
 vitex and, 94
Oyster shell, 99–100
Oyster Shell Powder, 129

Pain relief
 aconite and, 18
 gentian and, 55
 ginseng and, 58
 kudzu and, 65
 nutmeg and, 76
 opium poppy husk and, 77
 stephania and, 90
Pancreatitis, gardenia and, 53
Panic disorder, 153
Parasites
 agrimony and, 20
 ginger and, 56
 zanthoxylum and, 95

Peach Blossom Decoction, 129
Peach Pit Decoction to Order the Qi, 130
Peach seed, 77–78
Pelvic inflammatory disease (PID), 275–276
Peony, 78
Peony and Licorice Decoction, 130
Peppermint, 78–79
Peptic ulcer, 276–277
  aloe and, 22
  codonopsis and, 41
  Ophiopogonis Decoction and, 129
  saussurea and, 86
  See also Gastritis.
Perilla, 79
Periodontitis, 164
Pernicious anemia, tang-kuei and, 91
Phellodendron, 79–80
Phobias, 153
PID. *See* Pelvic inflammatory disease.
Pill for Deafness That Is Kind to the Left Kidney, 130
Pinellia, 80–81
Pinellia and Magnolia Bark Decoction, 130
Pinellia, Atractylodis Macrocephala, and Gastrodia Decoction, 131
Pinellia Decoction to Drain the Epigastrium, 131
Pinkeye. *See* Conjunctivitis.
Plantain, 81
Platycodon, 81
Plummer's disease, 234
PMS. *See* Premenstrual syndrome.
Pneumonia, 171–172
  houttynia and, 62
  ligusticum and, 68
  Pneumocystic carinii, 143–144
Poisoning, food. *See* Food poisoning.
Polygonum, 82
Polyporus, 82
Polyporus Decoction, 131
Poria. *See* Hoelen.
Prednisolone, 180–181
Prednisone, 180–181
Pregnancy, Kampo remedies and, 142
Premenstrual syndrome (PMS), 278–279
  asiasarum and, 27
  Augmented Rambling Powder and, 112
  black cohosh and, 34
  kudzu and, 65
  motherwort and, 75
  Two-Cured Decoction and, 138
  vitex and, 94
Prepared Aconite Decoction, 132
Prescription drugs, Kampo and, 142
Privet. *See* Ligustrum.
Progesterone, 143, 212, 214, 263
Prolong Life Decoction, 132
Prostate cancer, 279
  garlic and, 54
  Peony and Licorice Decoction and, 130
  saw palmetto and, 279
  vitex and, 94
Prostate enlargement, benign, 280–281
  Peony and Licorice Decoction and, 130
  saw palmetto and, 279
  vitex and, 94
Prostate-specific antigen (PSA) test, 279
Prunella, 82–83
PSK, 104
Psoralea, 83
Psoriasis, 281–282
  aloe and, 21
  tang-kuei and, 91
  turmeric and, 93
Psychosomatic complaints, Kampo and, 11
Psyllium seed. *See* Plantain.
Purpura, jujube fruit and, 63
Pyorrhea, 164

Qi, in Oriental medicine, 3, 10, 17
Qing pi. *See* Blue citrus.

RA. *See* Rheumatoid arthritis.
Radiation therapy side effects, 282–283
  aloe and, 21
  codonopsis and, 41
  Pinellia Decoction to Drain the Epigastrium and, 131
  Ten-Significant Tonic Decoction and, 136
Rambling Powder, 132
Red atractylodis. *See* Atractylodis, red.
Red peony. *See* Peony.
Red sage. *See* Dan shen.
Red tangerine peel. *See* Bitter orange peel.
Reed root, 84
Regulate the Stomach and Order the Qi Decoction, 132
Rehmannia, 84
Rehmannia-Eight Combination. *See* Eight-Ingredient Pill With Rehmannia.
Rehmannia-Six Combination. *See* Six-Ingredient Pill With Rehmannia.
Reishi, 104–105
Renal cell carcinoma. *See* Kidney cancer.
Residual ADD, 159
Respiratory allergies. *See* Allergies, respiratory.
Respiratory tract infection, cinnamon and, 39
Restore the Right Kidney Pill, 133
Restore the Spleen Decoction, 133
Rheumatoid arthritis (RA), 283–285
  bupleurum and, 35
  frankincense and, 97
  ginger and, 56
  hawthorn and, 60
  hoelen and, 61
  licorice and, 67
  See also Osteoarthritis.
Rhubarb and Licorice Decoction, 133
Rhubarb root, 85–86
Ringing in the ears. *See* Tinnitus.

Ringworm, gardenia and, 53
Rose hips, 86
Rubeola. *See* Measles.

Safflower. *See* Carthamus.
Sairei-to, 133
Salvia. *See* Dan shen.
Saussurea, 86
Saw palmetto, 279
Scallion, 86–87
Schisandra, 87–88
  liver problems and, 251
Schistosomiasis, 53, 56, 95, 169
Scrophularia, 88
Scutellaria, 88–89
Sedatives
  cinnamon and, 39
  zizyphus and, 96
Seizure disorders, 285–286
  acorus and, 19
  gastrodia and, 55
Selective serotonin reuptake inhibitors (SSRIs), 194
Serotonin, 72, 194, 278
Settle the Emotions Pill, 133
Seven-Treasure Pill for Beautiful Whiskers, 134
Shen Nung, 5
Shepherd's purse, and bleeding, 265
Shiitake, 105
Shingles. *See* Herpes.
Sho (symptom pattern), 1, 8, 10
Sho Kan Ron, 5, 6, 7, 14
Shut the Sluice Pill, 134
Siberian ginseng, 105–107
Sickle cell anemia, zanthoxylum and, 95
Side effects, safeguards against, 110
Sinusitis, 286–287
  coptis and, 43
Six-Gentleman Decoction, 134
Six-Ingredient Pill With Rehmannia, 134
Sjögren's syndrome, Ophiopogonis Decoction and, 129
Skin cancer (basal cell carcinoma), 287–288
  carthamus and, 37
  coptis and, 43
  schisandra and, 87
  turmeric and, 92
  See also Melanoma.
Skin infection
  asparagus root and, 27
  burdock and, 36
  dracaena lily and, 47
  Japanese mint and, 62
  lithospermum and, 69
  white mustard seed and, 95
Skin irritation. *See* Acne; Eczema; Psoriasis.
Skullcap. *See* Scutellaria.
Snake gourd fruit, 89
Snake gourd root, 89–90
Snake gourd seed. *See* Benincasa.
Snakeroot, black. *See* Black cohosh.
Snow fungus, 107
Solomon's seal, 90
Sore throat, agrimony and, 20
Soy isoflavones, 108
Soy lecithin, 108
St. John's wort and depression, 195
Staph infection, 166, 201, 257
  anemarrhena and, 24
  asparagus root and, 27
  bamboo shavings and, 30
  chrysanthemum and, 39
  cloves and, 41
  coptis and, 43
  epimedium and, 49
  forsythia and, 51
  galangal and, 52
  houttynia and, 62
  ledebouriella and, 66
  lonicera and, 70
  magnolia and, 73
  moutan and, 75
  psoralea and, 83
  scutellaria and, 88
Stephania, 90–91
Stephania and Astragalus Decoction, 135
Steroid drugs, 180–181
Sting, wasp, cinnamon and, 39
Stomach cancer, 288–289
  Coptis Decoction to Relieve Toxicity and, 117
  houttynia and, 62
  lentinan and, 102
  See also Cancer.
Stomach ulcer. *See* Peptic ulcer.
Strep infection
  asiasarum and, 27
  asparagus root and, 27
  cloves and, 41
  galangal and, 52
  magnolia and, 73
  moutan and, 75
  scutellaria and, 88
  zanthoxylum and, 95
  See also Strep throat.
Strep throat, 289–290
  coptis and, 43
  forsythia and, 51
  Lonicera and Forsythia Powder and, 126
Stress, 290–291
  American ginseng and, 23–24
  Siberian ginseng and, 106
Stroke, 291–292
  acorus and, 19
  dan shen and, 45
  garlic and, 54
  gastrodia and, 55
  ginkgo and, 100
  ginseng and, 58

Rhubarb and Moutan Decoction and, 133
Subacute cutaneous lupus erythematous (SCLE), 254
Sun Si-Miao, 6
Sun-damaged skin, aloe and, 21
Sweet flag. *See* Acorus.
Systemic lupus erythematous (SLE), 254
Szechuan pepper. *See* Zanthoxylum.

Talc, 100
Tang-kuei, 91
Tang-Kuei and Peony Powder, 135
Tang-Kuei, Gentiana Longdancao, and Aloe Pill, 136
TB. *See* Tuberculosis.
TCM. *See* Traditional Chinese Medicine.
Tea. *See* Green tea.
Tea-making, basic instructions, 14–15
Tea-making, directions for
abalone shell, 96
aconite, 19
agrimony, 20
amaranth, 22
American ginseng, 24
angelica dahurica, 24
apricot seed, 25
artemisia, 26
asparagus root, 27
astragalus, 28
atractylodis, red, 29
bamboo shaving, 30
barley sprouts, 30
benincasa, 30
biota, 31
bitter orange, 32
bitter orange peel, 33
blue citrus, 34
bupleurum, 36
burdock, 36
caltrop, 37
cardamom, 37
Chinese senega root, 38
cinnamon, 40
clematis, 40
codonopsis, 41
coltsfoot, 42
dan shen, 45
dandelion, 46
dragon bone, 97
ephedra, 48
eupatorium, 50
fennel seed, 51
forsythia, 51
galangal, 52
gardenia, 53
ginger, 56–57
ginseng, 58–59
green tea, 59–60
gypsum, 98
hawthorn, 61
hoelen, 62
Japanese mint, 63
kudzu, 65
licorice, 67
ligustrum, 68
lycium, 73
morinda, 74
motherwort, 75
peppermint, 79
plantain, 81
prunella, 83
oyster shell, 100
reishi, 105
rhubarb, 85
schisandra, 87
scrophularia, 88
scutellaria, 89
Siberian ginseng, 107
tang-kuei, 91
turmeric, 93
viola, 93
Tendonitis, turmeric and, 93
Ten-Significant Tonic Decoction, 136
Testosterone, 143, 212, 274, 279, 281
Thiamin, and congestive heart failure, 190
Thrush, 39, 294
Thyroid function, kelp and, 64
Thyroid storm, 234
Tinctures, 14
Tinnitus, 292–293
black cohosh and, 34
drynaria rhizome and, 47
cordyceps and, 96
ginkgo and, 101
See also Ménière's disease.
Todo Yoshimasu, 7
Tonify the Middle and Augment the Qi Decoction, 136
Toothache
asiasarum and, 27
cloves and, 41
Toyo Yamawaki, 7
Traditional Chinese Medicine (TCM)
concepts borrowed by Kampo, 1, 4, 10
development of, 5–6
differences between Kampo and, 10, 11, 109
simplification by Japanese herbalists, 6–7
Transient ischemic attacks (TIA), 291
acorus and, 19
Trauma Pill, 137
Tricyclic antidepressants, 194
True Man's Decoction to Nourish the Organs, 137
True Warrior Decoction, 137
Tryptophan, role in children's asthma, 156
Tuberculosis (TB), 293–294
bletilla and, 34
cardamom and, 37
coptis and, 43
Lily Bulb Decoction to Preserve the Metal and, 126

Tuckahoe. *See* Hoelen.
Turmeric, 92–93
Two-Cured Decoction, 138
Type 1 diabetes, 197
Type 2 diabetes, 197

Ubiquinone. *See* CoQ_{10}.
Ulcer. *See* Peptic ulcer.
Unblock the Orifices and Invigorate the Blood Decoction, 138
Upper respiratory infection. *See* Colds; Influenza; Sinusitis.
Upset stomach. *See* Indigestion.
Urinary tract infection. *See* Bladder infection.
Urination, stimulating
- akebia and, 20
- atractylodis, white, and, 29
- caltrop and, 37
- Cornelian cherry and, 43
- dandelion and, 45
- eucommia and, 50
- green tea and, 59
- houttynia and, 62
- Japanese watermelon and, 63
- mulberry root and, 75

Uterine bleeding, abnormal. *See* Endometrial cancer; Fibroids (uterine myomas); Menopause-related problems; Menstrual problems; Ovarian cancer; Ovarian cysts; Pelvic inflammatory disease.
Uterine cancer. *See* Endometrial cancer.
Uterine myomas. *See* Fibroids.

Varicocele, 241
Ventricular fibrillation, 28, 189
Viola, 93
Viral hepatitis. *See* Hepatitis.
Viral infection
- aloe and, 21
- astragalus and, 28
- coix and, 42
- Kampo and, 11
- prunella and, 83

Viral myocarditis, astragalus and, 28
Vision, blurred. *See* Blurred vision.
Vitamin A, and fibrocystic breast disease, 213
Vitamin C, 156, 177, 213
- herbal sources of, 63, 74, 86

Vitamin E, 177, 213
Vitex, 93–94
Vitiligo, psoralea and, 83
Vomiting. *See* Nausea and vomiting.
Vulvovaginitis, 294

Warm the Gallbladder Decoction, 138
Warm the Menses Decoction, 139
Warming and Clearing Decoction, 139
Warts, coix and, 42
Water plantain. *See* Alisma.
Watermelon. *See* Japanese watermelon.
Weight loss. *See* Obesity.
Wheat, 94
White atractylodis. *See* Atractylodis, white.
White blood cells, deficient. *See* Leukopenia.
White mustard seed, 94–95
White Tiger Decoction, 139
White Tiger Plus Atractylodis Decoction, 140
White Tiger Plus Ginseng Decoction, 140
Wild angelica. *See* Angelica dahurica.
Wild yam. *See* Dioscorea.
Wolfbane. *See* Aconite.
Wolfberry. *See* Lycium.
Wrinkles and/or age spots
- eucommia bark and, 50
- reishi and, 105

Wu Shu-He, 6

Xu Yin-Song, 6

Yang and yin, 3, 8, 9, 17
Yasuyori Tamba, 7
Yeast infection, 156, 294–295
- cinnamon and, 39
- reishi and, 105
- shiitake and, 105

Yellow Dragon Decoction, 140
Yellow Emperor, 5

Zanthoxylum, 95–96
Zhang Zhongjing, 5, 6, 205, 222
Zhu Dan-xi, 284
Zizyphus, 96